OTOLOGIC SURGERY

Editor

Derald E. Brackmann, MD, FACS
Clinical Professor of Otolaryngology/Head and Neck Surgery
Clinical Professor of Neurosurgery
University of Southern California
School of Medicine
President, House Ear Clinic; Board of Directors, House Ear Institute
Los Angeles, California

Associate Editor

Clough Shelton, MD, FACS
Associate Professor of Otolaryngology/Head and Neck Surgery
University of Utah School of Medicine
Salt Lake City, Utah

Associate Editor

Moises A. Arriaga, MD
Director of Otology and Neurotology
Wilford Hall Medical Center
Lackland Air Force Base;
Assistant Clinical Professor of Otolaryngology
University of Texas, San Antonio
San Antonio, Texas

Illustrated by
Anthony Pazos

W.B. SAUNDERS COMPANY
A Division of Harcourt Brace & Company
Philadelphia London Toronto Montreal Sydney Tokyo

W. B. SAUNDERS COMPANY
A Division of
Harcourt Brace & Company

The Curtis Center
Independence Square West
Philadelphia, Pennsylvania 19106

Library of Congress Cataloging-in-Publication Data

Otologic surgery / editor, Derald E. Brackmann ; associate editors, Clough Shelton, Moises A. Arriaga ; illustrated by Anthony Pazos.

    p.   cm.

ISBN 0–7216–6639–6

1. Ear—Surgery.   I. Brackmann, Derald E.   II. Shelton, Clough.
III. Arriaga, Moises A.

[DNLM: 1. Ear—surgery. WV 200 0878 1994]

RF126.O87 1994

617.8′059—dc20

DNLM/DLC   93-40738

OTOLOGIC SURGERY   ISBN 0–7216–6639–6

Printed in the United States of America.

Last digit is the print number: 9 8 7 6 5 4 3 2 1

Dedication

This book is dedicated to our mentors and teachers, Drs. Howard P. House, William F. House, and James L. Sheehy. Each of these outstanding physicians has special talents and characteristics that, when melded together, resulted in an outstanding clinical, research, and educational facility, The House Ear Clinic and Institute.

Howard House, the founder of our Institutions, was among the first to concentrate his activities in the field of otology. He has devoted his career to the treatment of otosclerosis. In addition to his surgical genius, Howard is recognized as an outstanding statesman and fundraiser. Without him the House Ear Institute, which has provided so many opportunities for all of us, would not exist.

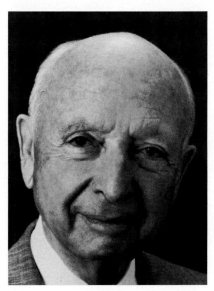

Howard P. House

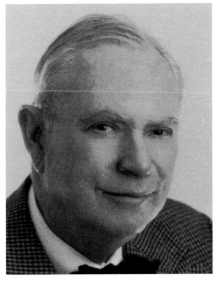

William F. House

William F. House joined his brother in practice after completing his residency. A creative genius, Bill recognized that the future of otology lay in the diagnosis and treatment of diseases of the inner ear. He introduced the operating microscope and microsurgical techniques to the field of neurosurgery and revolutionized the treatment of acoustic tumors and other neurotologic problems. Bill is also recognized as instrumental in bringing the cochlear implant to the state of a practical clinical device that is now widely applied.

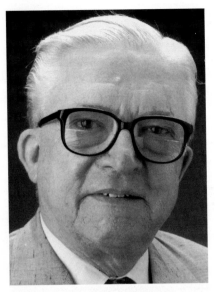

James L. Sheehy

The final link in the chain that resulted in the success of the House Ear Clinic and Institute is Dr. James L. Sheehy. His special interest is in the field of chronic otitis media. In addition to his outstanding surgical ability, Jim possesses exceptional talent in organizational ability and teaching. Jim was responsible for developing all the patient educational materials as well as serving as the editor for all of the many publications produced by members of the House Ear Clinic. His course development, panel discussions, and slide preparation techniques became standards for our specialty.

It was our great privilege to be under the personal tutelage of each of these outstanding men. In addition to all the attributes enumerated above, first and foremost each is an outstanding physician. They practice the art and science of surgery in the finest fashion, making it most appropriate that this book on surgical technique be dedicated to them.

DERALD E. BRACKMANN, M.D.
CLOUGH SHELTON, M.D.
MOISES A. ARRIAGA, M.D.

Contributors

SEAN R. ALTHAUS, M.D., F.A.C.S.

Associate Clinical Professor, Department of Otolaryngology/Head and Neck Surgery, University of California, San Francisco, School of Medicine; Active Staff, San Ramon Regional Medical Center, John Muir Medical Center, Summit Medical Center; Courtesy Staff, Children's Hospital, Oakland, California
TRAUMATIC PERFORATION—OFFICE TREATMENT OF THE CHRONICALLY DRAINING EAR

MOISES A. ARRIAGA, M.D.

Assistant Clinical Professor of Otolaryngology, University of Texas Medical School at San Antonio; Director of Otology and Neurotology, Wilford Hall Medical Center, Lackland Air Force Base, San Antonio, Texas
SURGERY FOR GLOMUS TUMORS

GREGORY A. ATOR, M.D.

Assistant Professor, Director of Otology, University of Kansas Medical Center; Staff, University of Kansas Medical Center, Kansas City, Kansas; Staff, Veterans Affairs Medical Center, Kansas City, Missouri
TRAUMATIC FACIAL PARALYSIS

R. STANLEY BAKER, M.D.

Clinical Assistant Professor, Department of Otorhinolaryngology–Head Neck Surgery, University of Oklahoma College of Medicine; Clinical Adjunct Professor, Department of Communication Disorders, University of Oklahoma; Baptist Medical Center of Oklahoma, University Hospital, Children's Memorial Hospital, Veterans Administration Hospital, Oklahoma City, Oklahoma
STAPEDECTOMY: USE OF NATURAL MATERIAL

GEORGE P. BAUER, M.D.

Private Practice, Ear Medical Center, Cincinnati, Ohio
MANAGEMENT OF COMPLICATIONS OF CHRONIC OTITIS MEDIA

JAMES E. BENECKE, JR., M.D., F.A.C.S.

Department of Clinical Neurosciences, St. John's Mercy Medical Center, Missouri Baptist Medical Center, St. Mary's Health Center, St. Joseph's Hospital, Cardinal Glennon Children's Hospital, St. Louis, Missouri
OTOLOGIC INSTRUMENTATION

CHARLES D. BLUESTONE, M.D.
Professor of Otolaryngology, University of Pittsburgh School of Medicine; Director, Department of Pediatric Otolaryngology, Children's Hospital of Pittsburgh, Pittsburgh, Pennsylvania
THE ABNORMALLY PATULOUS EUSTACHIAN TUBE

DERALD E. BRACKMANN, M.D., F.A.C.S.
Clinical Professor of Otolaryngology/Head and Neck Surgery, Clinical Professor of Neurosurgery, University of Southern California School of Medicine; President, House Ear Clinic; Board of Directors, House Ear Institute, Los Angeles, California
DRAINAGE PROCEDURES FOR PETROUS APEX LESIONS
SURGERY FOR GLOMUS TUMORS
MANAGEMENT OF POSTOPERATIVE CEREBROSPINAL FLUID LEAKS

GRAHAM BRYCE, M.D., F.R.C.S.(C)
Clinical Instructor, Division of Otolaryngology, University of British Columbia, Vancouver; Active Staff, University of British Columbia Representative, Saint Mary's Hospital, New Westminster, British Columbia
STAPEDECTOMY: USE OF NATURAL MATERIAL

ROBERT L. CAMPBELL, M.D.
Betsy Barton Professor of Neurosurgery, Indiana University School of Medicine, Indianapolis, Indiana
TREATMENT OF BILATERAL ACOUSTIC NEUROMAS

STEPHEN P. CASS, M.D.
Assistant Professor, Department of Otolaryngology, University of Pittsburgh School of Medicine; Presbyterian University Hospital, Pittsburgh, Pennsylvania
CHEMICAL LABYRINTHECTOMY: METHODS AND RESULTS

SUJANA S. CHANDRASEKHAR, M.D.
Former Clinical Fellow, House Ear Clinic, Los Angeles; Assistant Professor, Department of Surgery, Section of Otolaryngology; Assistant Professor of Otology and Neurotology, University of Medicine and Dentistry of New Jersey, Newark, New Jersey
CONGENITAL MALFORMATION OF THE TEMPORAL BONE
TRANSCOCHLEAR APPROACH TO CEREBELLOPONTINE ANGLE LESIONS

JOSEPH M. CHEN, M.D., F.R.C.S.C.
Assistant Professor, Department of Otolaryngology, University of Toronto; Staff Otolaryngologist, Sunnybrook Health Science Centre, Toronto, Ontario
MIDDLE CRANIAL FOSSA—VESTIBULAR NEURECTOMY
THE TRANSOTIC APPROACH

C. PHILLIP DASPIT, M.D.
Clinical Lecturer, Department of Surgery, Arizona Health Sciences Center, Tucson; Active Staff, St. Joseph's Hospital and Medical Center, Barrow Neurological Institute, Phoenix, Arizona
THE PETROSAL APPROACH

ANTONIO DE LA CRUZ, M.D.
Clinical Professor of Otolaryngology, University of Southern California; St. Vin-

cent Medical Center, LAC/USC Medical Center, USC University Hospital, Los Angeles, California
CONGENITAL MALFORMATION OF THE TEMPORAL BONE
TRANSCOCHLEAR APPROACH TO CEREBELLOPONTINE ANGLE LESIONS

UGO FISCH, M.D.

Professor of ENT, University of Zurich; Head of ENT Department, University Hospital, Zurich, Switzerland
MIDDLE CRANIAL FOSSA—VESTIBULAR NEURECTOMY
THE TRANSOTIC APPROACH

RICHARD R. GACEK, M.D.

Professor and Chairman, Department of Otolaryngology and Communication Sciences, SUNY Health Science Center at Syracuse; Chief of Otolaryngology, University Hospital, Syracuse, New York
POSTERIOR AMPULLARY NERVE SECTION
FOR BENIGN PAROXYSMAL POSITIONAL VERTIGO

BRUCE J. GANTZ, M.D.

Professor and Interim Head, Department of Otolaryngology–Head and Neck Surgery, University of Iowa College of Medicine, Iowa City, Iowa
MANAGEMENT OF BELL'S PALSY AND RAMSAY HUNT SYNDROME

GEORGE A. GATES, M.D.

Professor of Otolaryngology–Head and Neck Surgery; Director, Virginia Merrill Bloedel Hearing Research Center, University of Washington; University of Washington Medical Center; Children's Hospital of Seattle; Veteran's Administration Hospital, Seattle, Washington
SURGERY OF VENTILATION AND MUCOSAL DISEASE

NEIL A. GIDDINGS, M.D.

Sacred Heart and Deaconess Medical Centers, Spokane, Washington
DRAINAGE PROCEDURES FOR PETROUS APEX LESIONS

MICHAEL E. GLASSCOCK, III, M.D.

Clinical Professor of Surgery (Otology and Neurotology), Vanderbilt University School of Medicine; Clinical Associate Professor of Neurosurgery, Vanderbilt University School of Medicine, Nashville, Tennessee
TYMPANOPLASTY: THE UNDERSURFACE GRAFT TECHNIQUE—
POSTAURICULAR APPROACH

MALCOLM D. GRAHAM, M.D.

Georgia Ear Institute, Savannah, Georgia
MISCELLANEOUS EXTERNAL AUDITORY CANAL PROBLEMS
DURAL HERNIATION AND CEREBROSPINAL FLUID LEAKS

JAN J. GROTE, M.D., Ph.D.

Professor and Chairman, ENT Department, University of Leiden, Leiden, The Netherlands
BIOCOMPATIBLE MATERIALS IN CHRONIC EAR SURGERY

HAL HANKINSON, M.D.
Clinical Professor, University of New Mexico; Staff Neurosurgeon, St. Joseph Medical Center, Presbyterian Medical Center, Albuquerque, New Mexico
THE MIDDLE FOSSA TRANSPETROUS APPROACH FOR ACCESS TO THE PETROCLIVAL REGION (EXTENDED MIDDLE FOSSA APPROACH)

STEVEN A. HARVEY, M.D.
Assistant Professor, Department of Otolaryngology and Human Communication, Medical College of Wisconsin; Active Staff, Froedtert Memorial Lutheran, John L. Doyne Hospital, Veterans Affairs Hospital; Courtesy Staff, Children's Hospital of Wisconsin, Milwaukee, Wisconsin
MANAGEMENT OF COMPLICATIONS OF CHRONIC OTITIS MEDIA

WILLIAM E. HITSELBERGER, M.D.
St. Vincent's Hospital, Los Angeles, California
THE MIDDLE FOSSA TRANSPETROUS APPROACH FOR ACCESS TO THE PETROCLIVAL REGION (EXTENDED MIDDLE FOSSA APPROACH)
AUDITORY BRAINSTEM IMPLANT

DIETER F. HOFFMANN, M.D.
Assistant Clinical Professor, Department of Otolaryngology/Head and Neck Surgery, Oregon Health Sciences University; Staff Otolaryngologist, Kaiser Sunnyside Medical Center, Portland, Oregon
FACIAL REANIMATION TECHNIQUES

KARL L. HORN, M.D.
Medical Director, Presbyterian Ear Institute; Associate Clinical Professor, University of New Mexico Medical School; Presbyterian Hospital, St. Joseph's Hospital, University of New Mexico Hospital, Albuquerque, New Mexico
THE MIDDLE FOSSA TRANSPETROUS APPROACH FOR ACCESS TO THE PETROCLIVAL REGION (EXTENDED MIDDLE FOSSA APPROACH)

J. V. D. HOUGH, M.D.
Clinical Professor, University of Oklahoma Health Sciences Center; Baptist Medical Center, Oklahoma City, Oklahoma
STAPEDECTOMY: USE OF NATURAL MATERIAL
THE AUDIANT BONE CONDUCTOR DEVICE

HOWARD P. HOUSE, M.D., F.A.C.S
Clinical Professor of Otology, University of Southern California School of Medicine, St. Vincent Medical Center, California Medical Center, Hospital of the Good Samaritan, Children's Hospital of Los Angeles, Los Angeles County/USC Medical Center, Los Angeles, California
TOTAL STAPEDECTOMY

JAMES R. HOUSE, III, M.D.
Assistant Professor of Surgery (Otolaryngology), University of Mississippi School Medicine; Jackson, Mississippi
HYPOGLOSSAL FACIAL ANASTOMOSIS

JOHN W. HOUSE, M.D.
Clinical Associate Professor, Otolaryngology, University of Southern California; St. Vincent Medical Center, Huntington Memorial Hospital, Good Samaritan Hospital, Children's Hospital, LAC and USC Medical Center, USC University Hospital, Los Angeles, California
TRANSLABYRINTHINE APPROACH

WILLIAM F. HOUSE, M.D.

Hoog Hospital, Newport Beach, California
THE MIDDLE FOSSA APPROACH

ROBERT K. JACKLER, M.D.

Associate Professor of Otolaryngology and Neurological Surgery, University of California, San Francisco; Attending Staff, Medical Center at the University of California, San Francisco, California
RETROSIGMOID APPROACH TO TUMORS OF THE CEREBELLOPONTINE ANGLE

IVO P. JANECKA, M.D.

Professor of Otolaryngology and Neurological Surgery, University of Pittsburgh; Director, Center for Cranial Base Surgery, University of Pittsburgh Medical Center, Pittsburgh, Pennsylvania
MALIGNANCIES OF THE TEMPORAL BONE—RADICAL TEMPORAL BONE RESECTION

PETER JANNETTA, M.D., D.Sc.

Walter E. Dandy Professor of Neurological Surgery; Chairman, Department of Neurological Surgery, University of Pittsburgh School of Medicine, Pittsburgh, Pennsylvania
OPERATIONS FOR MICROVASCULAR COMPRESSION SYNDROMES

HERMAN A. JENKINS, M.D.

Professor and Vice Chairman, Baylor College of Medicine; Active Staff, The Methodist Hospital, Texas Children's Hospital, Ben Taub General Hospital; Attending, VA Medical Center; Courtesy Staff, St. Luke's Episcopal Hospital, Houston, Texas
TRAUMATIC FACIAL PARALYSIS

SAM E. KINNEY, M.D.

Associate Clinical Professor, Case Western Reserve University; Cleveland Clinic Foundation, Cleveland, Ohio
MALIGNANCIES OF THE TEMPORAL BONE—LIMITED TEMPORAL BONE RESECTION

JED A. KWARTLER, M.D.

Clinical Assistant Professor, Section of Otolaryngology, Department of Surgery, University of Medicine and Dentistry of New Jersey; Director of Neurotology, United Hospitals, Newark, New Jersey
TOTAL STAPEDECTOMY

MICHAEL LaROUERE, M.D.

Attending Staff Physician, Michigan Ear Institute, Providence Hospital, Southfield, Michigan
MISCELLANEOUS EXTERNAL AUDITORY CANAL PROBLEMS

ROBERT E. LEVINE, M.D.

Clinical Professor of Ophthalmology, University of Southern California School of Medicine; Active Staff, St. Vincent Medical Center, USC University Hospital; Consulting Staff, Kaiser Hospitals; Attending Staff, LA County General Hospital, Los Angeles, California
CARE OF THE EYE IN FACIAL PARALYSIS

WILLIAM H. LIPPY, M.D.

Trumbull Memorial Hospital, Saint Joseph's Hospital, Warren, Ohio
SPECIAL PROBLEMS OF OTOSCLEROSIS SURGERY

LARRY B. LUNDY, M.D.

Director, Otology and Neurotology Fellowship; Director, Cochlear Implant Program; Michigan Ear Institute; Providence Hospital, Southfield; William Beaumont Hospital, Royal Oak, Michigan
DURAL HERNIATION AND CEREBROSPINAL FLUID LEAKS
LASER REVISION STAPEDECTOMY

WILLIAM M. LUXFORD, M.D.

Associate, House Ear Clinic; Clinical Associate Professor of Otolaryngology, University of Southern California School of Medicine; St. Vincent Medical Center, Los Angeles, California
SURGERY FOR COCHLEAR IMPLANTATION
HYPOGLOSSAL FACIAL ANASTOMOSIS

ANTHONY E. MAGIT, M.D.

Assistant Professor, University of California at San Diego School of Medicine; Full-time Faculty, UCSD Medical Center, San Diego, California
THE ABNORMALLY PATULOUS EUSTACHIAN TUBE

DOUGLAS E. MATTOX, M.D.

Professor of Surgery and Director of Otolaryngology–Head and Neck Surgery, University of Maryland Medical System, Baltimore, Maryland
THE LATERAL INFRATEMPORAL FOSSA APPROACHES

MARK MAY, M.D.

Clinical Professor, Department of Otolaryngology/Head and Neck Surgery, University of Pittsburgh; Director, Facial Paralysis and Sinus Surgery Center, Shadyside Hospital, Pittsburgh, Pennsylvania
FACIAL REANIMATION TECHNIQUES

MICHAEL McGEE, M.D.

Associate Professor of Otolaryngology, University of Oklahoma Health Sciences Center; Chairman of the Department of Otolaryngology, Baptist Medical Center, Oklahoma City, Oklahoma
STAPEDECTOMY: USE OF NATURAL MATERIAL
THE AUDIANT BONE CONDUCTOR DEVICE

T. MANFORD McGEE, M.D.*

LASER REVISION STAPEDECTOMY
*Deceased

MICHAEL J. McKENNA, M.D.

Assistant Professor in Otology and Laryngology, Harvard Medical School; Assistant Surgeon in Otolaryngology, Massachusetts Eye and Ear Infirmary, Boston, Massachusetts
COCHLEOSACCULOTOMY
TRANSCANAL LABYRINTHECTOMY

RICHARD T. MIYAMOTO, M.D.
Arilla Spence DeVault Professor and Chairman, Department of Otolaryngology–Head and Neck Surgery, Indiana University School of Medicine; Medical Director of Audiology and Speech/Language Pathology, Indiana University Hospitals, Indianapolis, Indiana
TREATMENT OF BILATERAL ACOUSTIC NEUROMAS

AAGE R. MØLLER, Ph.D., D.M.Sc.
Professor of Neurological Surgery, University of Pittsburgh School of Medicine, Pittsburgh, Pennsylvania
INTRAOPERATIVE NEUROPHYSIOLOGIC MONITORING

MARGARETA B. MØLLER, M.D., D.M.Sc.
Associate Professor, Department of Neurological Surgery and Otolaryngology, University of Pittsburgh School of Medicine, Pittsburgh, Pennsylvania
OPERATIONS FOR MICROVASCULAR COMPRESSION SYNDROMES

EDWIN M. MONSELL, M.D., Ph.D.
Head, Division of Otology and Neurotology, Department of Otolaryngology–Head and Neck Surgery, Henry Ford Hospital, Detroit, Michigan
CHEMICAL LABYRINTHECTOMY: METHODS AND RESULTS

JOSEPH B. NADOL, Jr., M.D.
Walter Augustus Lecompte Professor and Chairman, Harvard Medical School; Professor, Massachusetts Institute of Technology; Professor and Chairman, Department of Otology and Laryngology, Harvard Medical School; Chief of Otology and Chief of Otolaryngology, Massachusetts Eye and Ear Infirmary, Boston, Massachusetts
TRANSCANAL LABYRINTHECTOMY

J. GAIL NEELY, M.D., F.A.C.S
Professor and Director, Otology, Neurotology, Base of Skull Surgery, Department of Otolaryngology–Head and Neck Surgery, Washington University School of Medicine, St. Louis, Missouri
SURGERY OF ACUTE INFECTIONS AND THEIR COMPLICATIONS

RALPH A. NELSON, M.D., M.S.
Associate Clinical Professor, University of Southern California; Active Staff, St. Vincent Medical Center; Los Angeles County Hospital; Courtesy Staff, Good Samaritan Hospital, Children's Hospital of Los Angeles; Provisional, University Hospital, Los Angeles, California
TRANSLABYRINTHINE VESTIBULAR NEURECTOMY

MICHAEL M. PAPARELLA, M.D.
Clinical Professor and Chairman Emeritus, Department of Otolaryngology, University of Minnesota; Fairview Riverside Medical Center, Minneapolis, Minnesota
ENDOLYMPHATIC SAC PROCEDURES

LORNE PARNES, M.D.
Associate Professor, Department of Otolaryngology, University of Western Ontario; Chief, Department of Otolaryngology, University Hospital, London, Ontario
POSTERIOR SEMICIRCULAR CANAL OCCLUSION FOR BENIGN PAROXYSMAL POSITIONAL VERTIGO

RODNEY PERKINS, M.D.

Professor of Surgery, Stanford University School of Medicine; Medical Staff, Stanford University Hospital, El Camino Hospital, Sequoia Hospital, Palo Alto, California

CANALPLASTY FOR EXOSTOSES OF THE EXTERNAL AUDITORY CANAL LASER STAPEDOTOMY

SANJAY PRASAD, M.D.

Clinical Assistant Professor, Georgetown University Medical Center; Clinical Assistant Professor, George Washington University Medical Center, Washington, D.C.

MALIGNANCIES OF THE TEMPORAL BONE—RADICAL TEMPORAL BONE RESECTION

MIRIAM I. REDLEAF, M.D.

Research Fellow—Temporal Bone Histopathology Laboratories, University of Chicago Medical Center, Chicago, Illinois

MANAGEMENT OF BELL'S PALSY AND RAMSAY HUNT SYNDROME

JOSEPH B. ROBERSON, Jr., M.D.

Assistant Professor, California Ear Institute at Stanford University, Palo Alto; Fellow, House Ear Clinic, Los Angeles, California

AVOIDANCE AND MANAGEMENT OF COMPLICATIONS

MENDELL ROBINSON, M.D., F.A.C.S.

Clinical Associate Professor of Surgery, Brown University Medical School; Director, Division of Otolaryngology, Miriam Hospital; Consultant in Otolaryngology, Rhode Island Hospital, Roger Williams Hospital, Women and Infants Hospital; Surgeon in Chief–Otology, Rhode Island Hospital, Providence, Rhode Island

PARTIAL STAPEDECTOMY

GRAYSON K. RODGERS, M.D.

Assistant Medical Director, Birmingham Ear Institute, Birmingham Otology Center, Birmingham, Alabama

MANAGEMENT OF POSTOPERATIVE CEREBROSPINAL FLUID LEAKS

KAREN L. ROOS, M.D.

Associate Professor of Neurology, Indiana University School of Medicine, Indianapolis, Indiana

TREATMENT OF BILATERAL ACOUSTIC NEUROMAS

SETH ROSENBERG, M.D.

Assistant Professor, Department of Otorhinolaryngology, University of Pennsylvania School of Medicine, Philadelphia, Pennsylvania; Sarasota Memorial Hospital, Doctors Hospital, Sarasota, Florida

RETROLABYRINTHINE/RETROSIGMOID VESTIBULAR NEURECTOMY

LEONARD P. RYBAK, M.D., Ph.D.

Professor, Departments of Surgery and Pharmacology, Southern Illinois University School of Medicine, Springfield, Illinois

CHEMICAL LABYRINTHECTOMY: METHODS AND RESULTS

HAROLD F. SCHUKNECHT, M.D.

Professor Emeritus in Otology and Laryngology, Harvard Medical School; Emeritus Chief of Otolaryngology, Massachusetts Eye and Ear Infirmary, Boston, Massachusetts
COCHLEOSACCULOTOMY

M. COYLE SHEA, M.D.

Associate Clinical Professor, Department of Otolaryngology–Head and Neck Surgery, University of Tennessee Center for the Health Sciences; Active Staff, Baptist Memorial Hospitals; Associate Staff, City of Memphis Hospitals; Courtesy Staff, Methodist Hospitals, St. Francis Hospital, Memphis, Tennessee
TYMPANOPLASTY: THE UNDERSURFACE GRAFT TECHNIQUE—TRANSCANAL APPROACH

JAMES L. SHEEHY, M.D.

Clinical Professor of Otolaryngology–Head and Neck Surgery, University of Southern California School of Medicine; St. Vincent Medical Center; Los Angeles, California
TYMPANOPLASTY: OUTER SURFACE GRAFTING TECHNIQUE
TYMPANOPLASTY: CARTILAGE AND POROUS POLYETHYLENE
MASTOIDECTOMY: THE INTACT CANAL WALL PROCEDURE
TYMPANOPLASTY: STAGING AND USE OF PLASTIC

CLOUGH SHELTON, M.D., F.A.C.S.

Associate Professor of Otolaryngology/Head and Neck Surgery, University of Utah School of Medicine, Salt Lake City, Utah
FACIAL NERVE TUMORS
THE MIDDLE FOSSA APPROACH

HERBERT SILVERSTEIN, M.D.

Clinical Professor, Department of Otorhinolaryngology and Head and Neck Surgery, University of Pennsylvania, Philadelphia, Pennsylvania; Clinical Professor of Surgery, Division of Otolaryngology, University of South Florida; Sarasota Memorial Hospital, Doctors Hospital, Sarasota, Florida
RETROLABYRINTHINE/RETROSIGMOID VESTIBULAR NEURECTOMY

DAVID W. SIM, F.R.C.S. Ed.(URL)

Clinical Tutor, University of Edinburgh, Edinburgh, Scotland
RETROSIGMOID APPROACH TO TUMORS OF THE CEREBELLOPONTINE ANGLE

GEORGE T. SINGLETON, M.D.

Professor of Otolaryngology, University of Florida College of Medicine; Attending Staff, Shands Hospital; Chief of Otolaryngology, VA Hospital, Gainesville, Florida
PERILYMPHATIC FISTULA

WILLIAM H. SLATTERY, III, M.D.

Associate, House Ear Clinic; Research Physician, House Ear Institute, Los Angeles, California
PERILYMPHATIC FISTULA

MANSFIELD F. W. SMITH, M.D., M.S.

Clinical Professor of Surgery (Otology), Stanford University, Palo Alto; O'Connor Hospital, Good Samaritan Hospital, San Jose; El Camino Hospital, Mountain View, California
AVOIDANCE AND MANAGEMENT OF COMPLICATIONS

GORDON D. L. SMYTH, M.D., F.R.C.S.*

Late Consultant Laryngologist, Royal Victoria Hospital, Belfast, Northern Ireland

MASTOIDECTOMY: CANAL WALL DOWN TECHNIQUES

*Deceased

ROBERT F. SPETZLER, M.D.

Barrow Neurological Institute, Phoenix, Arizona

THE PETROSAL APPROACH

BARBARA A. STAHL, R.N., B.S.N.

Self-employed Registered Nurse; Surgical Assistant, Dr. W. E. Hitselberger (Neurosurgeon); St. Vincent's Medical Center, Doheny Operating Room, Los Angeles, California

OTOLOGIC INSTRUMENTATION

BARRY STRASNICK, M.D.

Assistant Professor, Director of Otology/Neurotology, Eastern Virginia Medical School, Norfolk, Virginia

TYMPANOPLASTY: THE UNDERSURFACE GRAFT TECHNIQUE—POSTAURICULAR APPROACH

FRED F. TELISCHI, M.E.E., M.D.

Assistant Professor, University of Miami School of Medicine; Jackson Memorial Hospital; Chief of Otolaryngology, Veterans Administration Hospital, Miami, Florida

AUDITORY BRAINSTEM IMPLANT

ANDERS TJELLSTRÖM, M.D., Ph.D.

Associate Professor, Department of Otolaryngology, University of Göteborg; Associate Professor, Department of Otolaryngology, Sahlgrens Hospital, Göteborg, Sweden

THE BONE-ANCHORED HEARING AID

JOSEPH G. TONER, M.B., F.R.C.S.

Clinical Tutor, Queen's University; Consultant Otolaryngologist, Belfast City Hospital, Belfast, Northern Ireland

MASTOIDECTOMY: CANAL WALL DOWN TECHNIQUES

ROGER E. WEHRS, M.D.

Clinical Professor, University of Oklahoma College of Medicine; Active Staff, Saint Francis Hospital; Courtesy Staff, Saint John's Hospital, Hillcrest Medical Center, Tulsa, Oklahoma

TYMPANOPLASTY: HOMOGRAFT TYMPANIC MEMBRANE TECHNIQUE
TYMPANOPLASTY: OSSICULAR TISSUE AND HYDROXYAPATITE
CANAL WALL RECONSTRUCTION WITH HOMOGRAFT KNEE CARTILAGE

RICHARD J. WIET, M.D.

Professor of Clinical Otolaryngology; Associate Professor of Clinical Neurosurgery; Director of Otology, Neurotology, and Skull Base Surgery Fellowship, Northwestern University Medical School; Attending Staff, Northwestern Memorial Hospital, Chicago; Hinsdale Hospital, Hinsdale; Consulting Physician at Children's Memorial Hospital, Chicago, Illinois

MANAGEMENT OF COMPLICATIONS OF CHRONIC OTITIS MEDIA

Preface

Approximately two years ago, I was approached by one of the senior editors at the W. B. Saunders Company, who requested that I consider developing a book on otologic surgery techniques. It had been noted that a volume that described and illustrated various otologic surgical techniques would fill a deficiency in our field.

After a review of available textbooks, it became apparent that there was no single source where one could go to study varied surgical techniques. Many authors had described their particular techniques in papers or book chapters, but nowhere were these methods conveniently assembled. Recognizing this deficiency, I accepted the challenge and sought the help of two of my younger associates with the prodigious task.

Our first step was to define the varied otologic surgical techniques. We then sought authorship for each technique by the person best identified as an expert in that procedure. We were gratified by the overwhelming response of these noted clinicians.

What has resulted is a detailed description of the great majority of the surgical techniques used in our field. The publisher made a major commitment to ensure the excellence of the volume by employing Anthony Pazos to illustrate the entire volume. We are sure that you will agree that he has become the preeminent illustrator in our field.

Our intent was to produce a volume that will be a ready resource for residents wishing to learn the various techniques as well as a reference for clinicians in practice who may wish to renew and sharpen their skills. We hope that you agree that we accomplished our goal.

DERALD E. BRACKMANN, M.D.

Acknowledgments

Publication of a book of this scope requires a tremendous effort on the part of many, all of whom I wish to sincerely thank.

First, my thanks to my lovely wife, Charlotte, who supports all my efforts and forgave my absence for the time devoted to this project. No less supportive are our four sons, David, Douglas, Mark, and Steven, who provide diversion and pleasure by taking me hunting and fishing.

My associate editors, Dr. Shelton and Dr. Arriaga, worked tirelessly to bring this volume to fruition.

Anthony Pazos deserves special recognition. He spent countless hours in the temporal bone laboratory learning at first hand the various operations that he then illustrated. All the authors have appreciated his attention to detail and willingness to work with them until everything was "just right."

The publishers have been extremely supportive throughout the development of this book. From the beginning they made a major commitment to ensure that this volume was of the highest quality. I wish to thank particularly Lawrence McGrew and Faith Voit.

Finally, I wish to thank our office staff, who work tirelessly on behalf of both us and our patients. I would particularly like to thank Carol O'Reilly, my secretary, who maintains my focus and orientation on a daily basis, and Rita Koechowski, my surgery counselor, who not only schedules my surgery but also offers tremendous encouragement and support to all my patients.

DERALD E. BRACKMANN, M.D.

I would like to thank my wife, Kay, and my children, Jordan and Bill, for their support and encouragement during my career development as well as their understanding regarding the demands of my profession.

I would also like to take this opportunity to thank my teachers, friends, and associates at the House Ear Clinic, and my teachers at Stanford, all of whom gave me the skills necessary to practice otologic surgery.

Special gratitude goes to Jim Sheehy and Blair Simmons, both of whom spent much time and effort teaching me to write scientific papers.

CLOUGH SHELTON, M.D.

I am particularly grateful to Derald Brackmann for the opportunity to participate in this book; his rational approach to patient care, incomparable surgical skills, innovations, patience as a teacher, and genuine personal warmth make him a role model to all young otologists.

Rosie, Becca, Moi-Moi, and Toby are continuing sources of encouragement and support. Thanks to Moises Agusto and Leticia for their personal sacrifices and conviction that education is the only permanent gift from a parent to a child.

MOISES A. ARRIAGA, M.D.

Contents

xxi

1

Otologic Instrumentation

JAMES E. BENECKE, JR., M.D., F.A.C.S.

BARBARA A. STAHL, R.N.

Sophisticated micro-otosurgical techniques mandate that the otologic surgeon have an in-depth understanding of the operating room layout and surgical instrumentation. This chapter provides a detailed description of different surgical procedures. The operating room setup and the instruments necessary for the various types of otologic procedures are described. The Appendix provides a comprehensive list of instruments and equipment.

THE OPERATING ROOM

The operating theater for otologic surgery requires features that differ from those of operating rooms used for nonotologic surgery. The following sections elaborate on the general environment of the operating room (OR) designed for ear surgery. A word about the sterile field is in order before proceeding. Respecting the sterile field is vital during routine otologic surgery and takes on special significance during neurotologic procedures. Maintaining the proper environment means limiting traffic through the OR and keeping the number of observers to a minimum. It is preferable for observers to be in a remote room watching the procedure on video. Those individuals allowed in the OR should be experienced in sterile technique and should be wearing jackets over their scrubs so that all skin surfaces are covered. Some surgeons prefer that observers be mummified (Fig. 1–1).

The psychologic environment of the OR must be respected, as many otologic procedures are performed on alert patients under local anesthesia. Members of the surgical team and visitors must use discretion when making comments during surgery.

The first piece of OR equipment to be discussed is the operating table. The surgeon must be comfortable while performing microsurgery. Adequate legroom under the table can be achieved with older OR tables by placing the patient 180 degrees opposite the usual position; in other words, the patient's head is where the feet would normally go. This places the table controls near the anesthesiologist. Newer electrical tables easily accommodate the patient while allowing the surgeon ample legroom (Fig. 1–2). Once the patient is properly positioned, the table must be firmly locked in place.

All ORs are equipped with wall suction. The standard devices are acceptable for otologic surgery. However, when the suction from the operating field is connected to a multiple-canister suction system, few changes in suction bottles are necessary during the surgery (Fig. 1–3). Having a variable control device at the wall to adjust the amount of suction is helpful; this can be aided by placing a control clamp on the tubing in the sterile field (Fig. 1–4).

The tubing that is attached to the suction tips and suction irrigators should be of highly flexible, surgical rubber. The readily available disposable tubing is not flexible enough for microsurgery and places awkward torque on the surgeon's hand. Problems with the suction setup are frequent in every OR. Therefore, it is wise to troubleshoot the system in advance and have a backup system readily available.

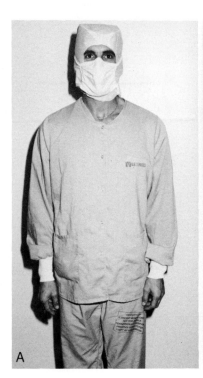
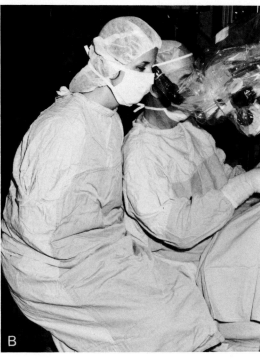

FIGURE 1–1. *A*, Observer in jacket. *B*, Observer mummified.

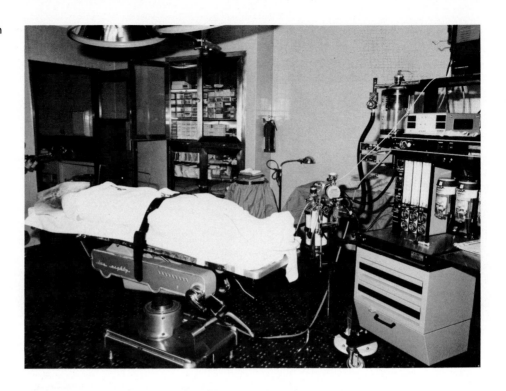

FIGURE 1-2. Operating table with patient's head at foot of bed.

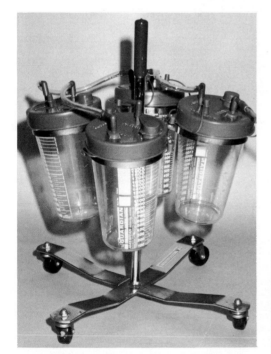

FIGURE 1-3. Multiple-suction canister setup.

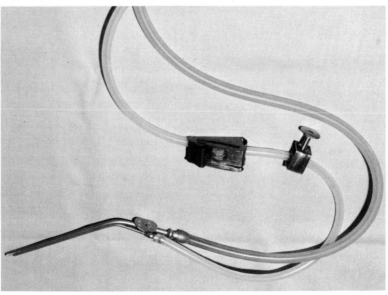

FIGURE 1-4. Suction tubing on sterile field with control clamp.

FIGURE 1–5. Skeeter microdrill for footplate work.

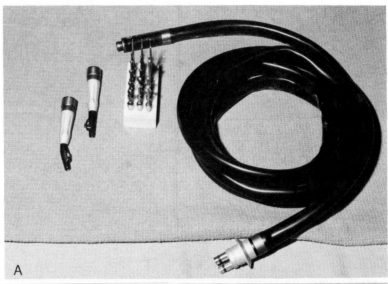

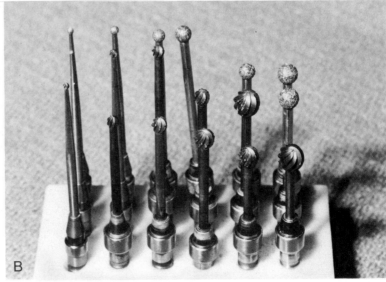

FIGURE 1–6. *A*, Osteon air-driven drill. *B*, Close-up of Osteon burrs.

Electrocautery equipment should be in a ready-to-use state on all procedures save, perhaps, stapes surgery. The patient should, of course, be properly grounded. It is advantageous to have both unipolar and bipolar cautery on the field for all chronic ear and neurotologic procedures. Surgeons are fortunate in having access to a wide variety of cautery devices. One should be thoroughly familiar with these electrical instruments prior to using them.

Another essential instrument for otologic surgery is the drill. The vast array of drills available makes it impossible to discuss every one. Basically, otologic drills fall into two categories: air-driven and electrical. There are advantages and disadvantages to each type, and most surgeons have a disinct preference based upon training and experience. For an air-driven drill, it is preferable to have a central supply of nitrogen as opposed to using tanks. Wall-delivered nitrogen removes the necessity for frequent changes of the nitrogen tanks.

High-speed drills capable of doing most of the bone work in the temporal bone include the ototome, Osteone, Fisch, and Midas Rex drill systems. These drills, in general, are not suitable for work in the middle ear, especially around the stapes footplate. For the latter purposes, a microdrill, such as the Skeeter drill, is suitable (Fig. 1–5). Whatever drill is used in the middle ear should have a variable speed and a wide array of drill bits.

The larger otologic drills must be equipped with both straight and angled handpieces. The straight handpiece is useful for the early gross removal of the mastoid cortex. For working deeper in the temporal bone, most surgeons prefer the angled handpiece. A full complement of both cutting and diamond burrs is mandatory. For example, cutting burrs should range

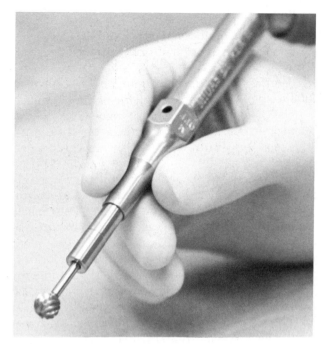

FIGURE 1–7. Midas Rex drill system.

from 1 to 6.5mm and have a length of 40 to 50mm in the smaller diameters in order to reach the deeper aspects of the temporal bone. Diamond burrs should be available in a similar array. Figures 1–6 and 1–7 show two of the available drill systems. Proper use of the drill should be emphasized. The otologic drill should be held like a pencil, with the hand resting comfortably on the sterile field. The side of the burr should be used to provide maximum contact between the bone and the flutes of the burr, affording safer and more efficient drilling (Fig. 1–8). Drill systems, like

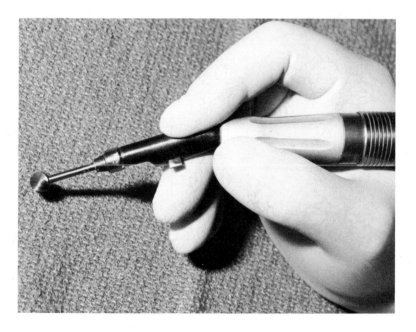

FIGURE 1–8. Proper holding of drill.

other OR equipment, are subject to malfunction. Careful inspection of the system should be performed prior to use, and a backup instrument should be available.

The introduction of the operating microscope revolutionized otologic surgery. The use of this instrument is well known to most otolaryngologists. Several brands of optically superior microscopes are available, most sufficiently similar to share the same general principles.

The otologic surgeon must be familiar with the adjustments on the microscope. For otologic surgery, the 200mm objective lens is preferred. If a laser micromanipulator is attached to the operating microscope, a 250mm or 300mm lens should be used. This, along with the other adjustments, should be done prior to draping out the microscope for surgery. The interpupillary distance is adjusted for maximal comfort. Par focal vision should be established so that the surgeon can change magnification without having to change focus. This is accomplished by first setting the diopter reading of both eyepieces to zero. The 40× magnification (or highest available setting) is selected. The locked microscope should be focused on a towel by using the focus knob. Without disturbing any of the settings, the magnification is now set at 6× (or the lowest available setting). The eyepieces are individually adjusted (with the opposite eye closed) to obtain the sharpest possible image. The diopter readings are recorded for future use. The surgeon should have par focal vision when these appropriate eyepiece settings are employed.

The microscope should be freely movable. All connections should be adjusted so that the microscope will not wander by itself, yet permit movement to any position with minimal effort. Needless to say, it is incumbent upon the surgeon to become intimately familiar with the peculiarities of his or her microscope.

Proper posture at the operating table is important so that the surgeon is comfortable. One should be seated in a comfortable chair with a back support adjusted to the proper height. The surgeon should have both feet comfortably on the floor. Fatigue is avoided by assuming a restful position in the chair rather than a military upright posture (Fig. 1–9).

The overall OR setup for routine otologic surgery is shown in Figure 1–10. For neurotologic surgery, more space must be available for additional necessary equipment. Middle cranial fossa procedures require modifications to the OR setup (Fig. 1–11). Basically, the surgeon and the microscope trade places such that the surgeon is at the head of the table. Cooperation and careful orchestration between surgeon, nursing personnel, and anesthesiologist are required for otologic surgery. The needs of the otologist are best served by having the anesthesiologist at the foot of the table and the scrub nurse opposite the surgeon.

STAPES SURGERY

The following description of the instrumentation and operative setup for stapes surgery will also prove use-

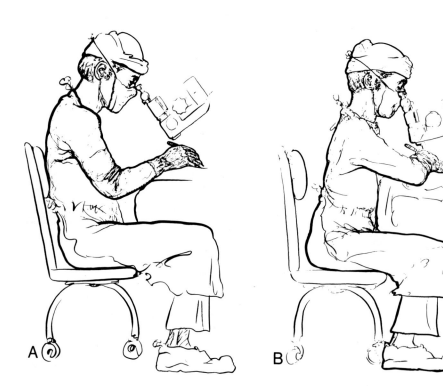

FIGURE 1–9. *A*, Proper surgeon's posture. *B*, Wrong posture for surgeon.

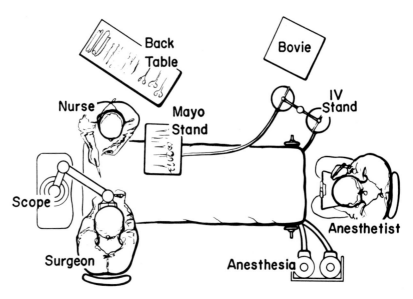

FIGURE 1-10. Usual otologic/neurotologic OR setup.

ful for other procedures involving the middle ear. In most settings, it is preferable to perform stapes surgery under local anesthesia; most surgeons provide some type of sedation for patients undergoing middle ear surgery under local anesthesia. Numerous regimens are available and are beyond the scope of this text. Sedation is safest when given in the form of a short-acting, and preferably reversible, substance. It is far safer for the patient to be psychologically prepared for the operation than to be oversedated. My choice for sedation during stapes surgery is very small increments (0.5mg) of intravenously administered Versed. I prefer that the patient be kept NPO, except for clear liquids, for at least 3 hours prior to surgery.

About 30 minutes before the operation, the patient is brought to the preoperative holding area. If the surgeon routinely harvests a postauricular graft, this area is now shaved. A plastic aperture drape is applied to the operative site and trimmed so as not to cover the patient's face (Fig. 1–12). An intravenous (IV) line is started, and the patient is now ready to go to the OR. Once the patient is positioned on the table, monitors are placed. These should include a blood pressure cuff (preferably automatic), electrocardiogram (EKG) electrodes, and a pulse oximeter. The ear and plastic drape are scrubbed with an iodine-containing solution, unless the patient is allergic to iodine. A head drape is applied, and the ear is draped with sterile towels so as not to cover the patient's face. This can be facilitated by supporting the drapes with a metal bar attached to the table or by fixing the drapes to the scrub nurse's Mayo stand (Fig. 1–13).

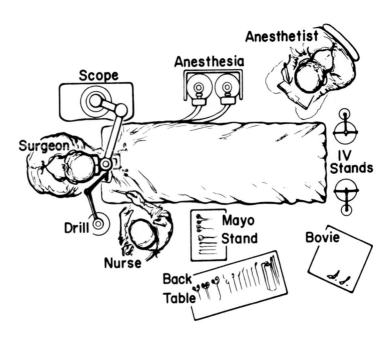

FIGURE 1-11. OR layout for middle fossa surgery.

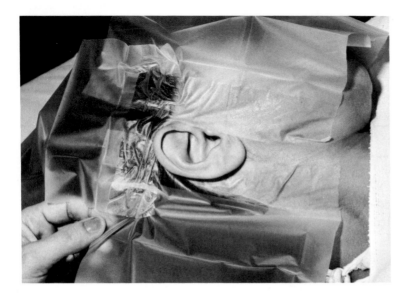

FIGURE 1-12. 3M plastic drape applied.

The patient's head is now gently rotated as far away from the ipsilateral shoulder as possible, and the table is placed in slight Trendelenburg position. These maneuvers increase the surgeon's working distance and help to straighten the external auditory canal (EAC). The EAC is gently irrigated with saline at body temperature. Vigorous cleaning of the canal is avoided until the ear is anesthetized. The local anesthesia is administered with a plastic Luer-Lok type syringe that has the finger and thumb control holes. A 27-gauge needle is firmly attached to the syringe. Surgeons differ in the concentrations of local solutions used. A solution of 1 per cent lidocaine with 1:100,000 epinephrine provides wonderful anesthesia and hemostasis if delivered slowly and strategically. Some surgeons prefer stronger concentrations of epinephrine, such as 1:40,000. The patient's blood pressure

and cardiac status must be considered when using stronger solutions, not to mention the possibility of error when mixing these substances.

The canal is injected slowly in four quadrants starting lateral to the bony-cartilaginous junction. The final injection is in the vascular strip. If one routinely harvests fascia or tragal perichondrium, these areas are now injected.

Before describing stapes surgery instruments, a few general comments are in order. All microsurgical instruments should be inspected periodically to ensure sharp points and cutting surfaces. The instruments for delicate work should have malleable shanks, enabling the surgeon to bend the instrument to meet the particular demands of the situation.

If the surgeon prefers a total stapedectomy to a small fenestra technique, an oval window seal must

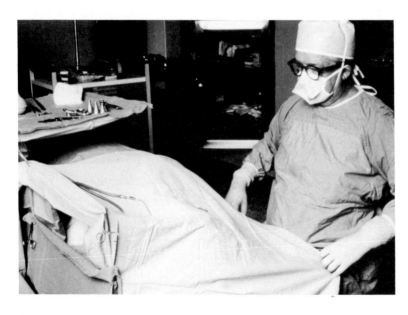

FIGURE 1-13. Patient draped in OR for stapes surgery.

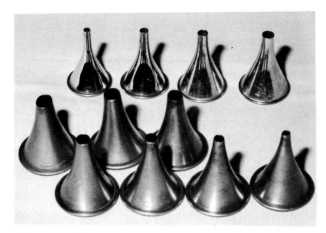

FIGURE 1-14. Speculum array.

from 4.5mm to 6.5mm (Fig. 1-14). The surgeon should always work through the largest speculum that the meatus will accommodate without lacerating the canal. Some surgeons use a speculum holder while performing transcanal surgery. The tympanomeatal flap is started with incisions made at the 6 and 12 o'clock positions with the No. 1, or "sickle," knife. These incisions are united with the No. 2, or lancet, knife. This instrument actually undermines the vascular strip, instead of cutting it. The strip is then cut with the Bellucci scissors. The defined flap is elevated to the tympanic annulus with the large round knife, known as the "weapon." The annulus, once properly identified, is elevated superiorly with the Rosen needle, and inferiorly with the annulus elevator, or "gimmick." Figure 1-15 shows the typical set of stapes instruments, including suction tips.

Adequate exposure usually requires removal of bone in the posterosuperior quadrant. This can be initiated with the Skeeter microdrill and completed with the stapes curette (Fig. 1-16).

From this point on, the steps differ depending upon the technique employed by the surgeon. The diagnosis of otosclerosis should be confirmed upon entering the middle ear and a measurement taken from incus to footplate with the measuring stick. The next step is to make a control hole in the footplate with a sharp needle (Barbara needle) or the laser. The incudostapedial joint is separated with the joint knife, the tendon

be selected. If fascia or vein is to be used, this tissue is harvested before the middle ear is exposed. The tissue is placed aside on the polytetrafluoroethylene (Teflon) block or fascia press to dry. If perichondrium is used, this may be harvested immediately prior to footplate removal. For the small fenestra technique, the patient's venous blood is obtained when the IV line is started. This is passed to the scrub nurse and placed in a vial on the sterile field.

A variety of ear specula should be available in both oval and round configurations. Sizes should range

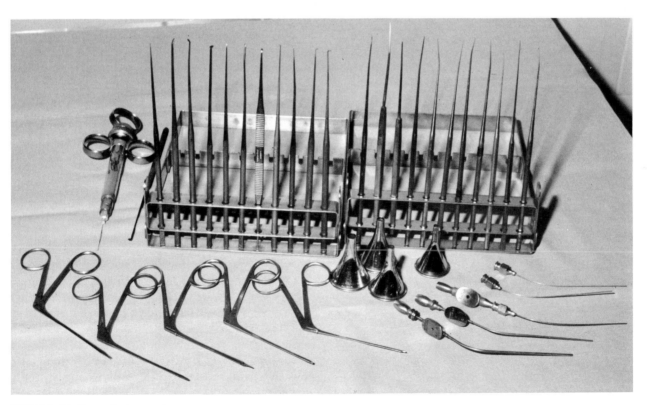

FIGURE 1-15. Stapes instruments.

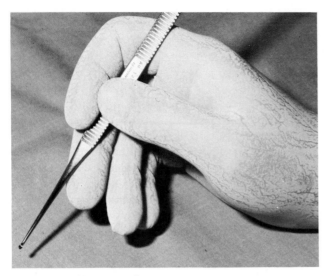

FIGURE 1-16. Stapes curette.

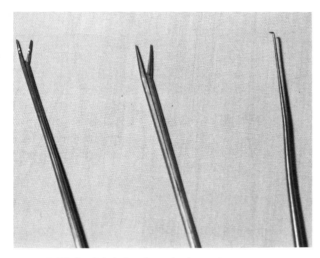

FIGURE 1-17. Footplate hook and crimpers.

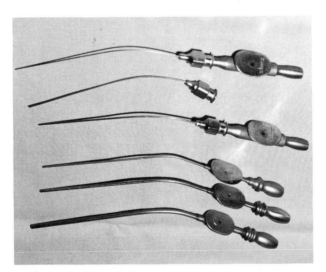

FIGURE 1-18. Rosen suction tubes with House adapter; Baron tubes.

cut with scissors or laser, and the superstructure fractured inferiorly and extracted.

For work on the footplate, the surgeon must have a variety of suitable instruments available. A stapedotomy can be created with a microdrill, a laser, or needles and hooks. The 0.3mm obtuse hook is useful for enlarging the fenestra.

For total footplate extraction, a right-angle hook or excavator (Hough hoe) is used. The harvested tissue graft is guided into place with a footplate chisel. The prosthesis is grasped with a smooth alligator or strut forceps and placed on the incus. It is positioned into the fenestra, or onto the graft, with a strut guide. The wire is secured onto the incus with a crimper. The McGee crimper is useful, especially if followed by a fine alligator forceps for the last gentle squeeze. A small right-angle hook may be necessary to fine-tune the position of the prosthesis (Fig. 1–17).

Suction tubes for stapes surgery include No. 3 to No. 7 Baron suctions plus Rosen needle suction tips (18- to 24-gauge) with the House adapter (Fig. 1–18). The Rosen tips are used when working near the oval window, and with the surgeon's thumb off the thumb port.

Ear canal packing following stapes surgery is accomplished with Kos-House cream or a suitable antibiotic ointment. A piece of cotton suffices as a dressing unless a postauricular incision has been made, in which case a mastoid dressing is applied.

For all middle ear procedures, the surgeon should hold the instruments properly. The instrument should rest, like a pencil, between the index finger and thumb, allowing easy rotation about the shank. The hands should always be resting on the patient and operating table. The middle and ring fingers should rest on the speculum, so that the hand moves as a unit with the patient. Proper hand position and holding of the instruments afford the surgeon an unimpeded view (Fig. 1–19).

TYMPANOPLASTY AND TYMPANOPLASTY WITH MASTOIDECTOMY SURGERY

The preparation and draping for tympanoplasty with or without mastoidectomy is very much the same as for stapes surgery. The major difference is the amount of hair shaved prior to draping. Usually about 3cm or 4cm of skin is exposed behind the postauricular sulcus. The plastic drape is applied to cover the remaining hair, as demonstrated in Figure 1–20.

The patient is taken to the OR and positioned on the table as described earlier. Whether the procedure is performed under local or general anesthesia depends on the extent of the surgery, the surgeon's pref-

FIGURE 1-19. Proper holding of instruments.

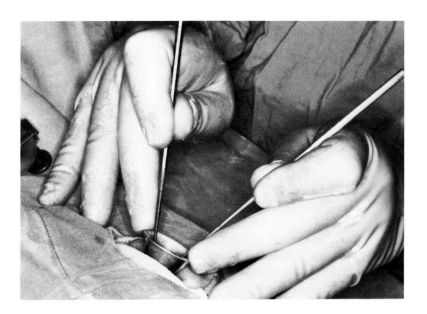

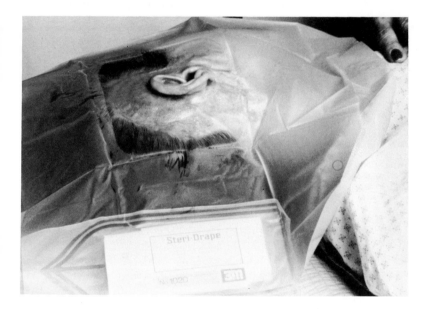

FIGURE 1-20. 3M 1020 Drape applied for chronic ear surgery.

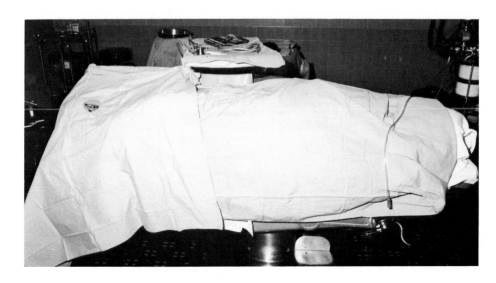

FIGURE 1-21. Chronic ear patient draped for local anesthesia.

erence, and, of course, the desire and concern of the patient. After appropriate sedation or induction of anesthesia, the ear and plastic drape are scrubbed with an iodine-containing prep solution. Many surgeons place cotton in the meatus when a perforation exists, preferring not to allow the prep solution to enter the middle ear. The field is draped as described earlier, the head is rotated toward the contralateral shoulder, and the table is placed in slight Trendelenburg position (Fig. 1–21). The postauricular area and canal are injected with 1 per cent lidocaine with 1:100,000 epinephrine for both local and general anesthesia.

Most chronic ear procedures begin in a similar fashion. Through an ear speculum, vascular strip incisions are made with the sickle or Robinson knife and united along the annulus with the lancet knife. The vascular strip incisions are completed with the No. 67 Beaver blade, which can also be used to transect the anterior canal skin just medial to the bony-cartilaginous junc-tion. The postauricular incision is then made with a No. 15 Bard-Parker blade behind the sulcus. The level of the temporalis fascia is identified, and a small self-retaining (Weitlaner) retractor is inserted. The fascia is cleared of areolar tissue and incised. A large area of fascia is undermined and removed with Metzenbaum scissors. This is thinned on the Teflon block and dehydrated by placing it under a 100-watt incandescent bulb. The fascia may also be dehydrated by placing it on a large piece of Gelfoam, and compressing the Gelfoam-fascia in a fascia press. Figure 1–22 shows the instruments used in the initial phases of chronic ear surgery.

Continued postauricular exposure is obtained by incising along the linea temporalis with a knife or with the electrocautery. A perpendicular incision is then made down to the mastoid tip. Soft tissues and periosteum are elevated with a Lempert elevator (Fig. 1–23), the vascular strip identified, and a large self-

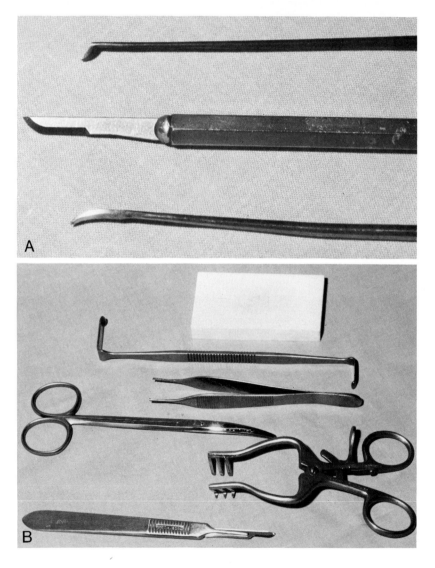

FIGURE 1–22. *A*, Instruments for canal incisions. *B*, Instruments for handling fascia.

FIGURE 1-23. Periosteal elevators.

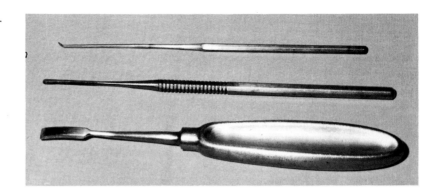

retaining retractor inserted. A very large retractor, such as an Adson cerebellar retractor with sharp prongs, is preferred. The self-retaining retractors can be modified as shown in Figure 1–24. Rings have been attached so that a small oxygen catheter can be threaded and attached to suction. This acts as a sump in the most dependent portion of the wound.

Next, under the microscope, the anterior canal skin is removed down to the level of the annulus with a weapon. The plane between the fibrous layer of the drum remnant and the epithelium is developed with a sickle knife, and the skin is removed with cup forceps. It is placed in a vial of saline to be used later as a free graft. The ear canal is enlarged with the drill and suction-irrigators. An angled handpiece and medium-size cutting burr are used. Irrigation is done with a physiologic solution such as Tis-U-Sol and is

delivered through flexible tubing to the House suction-irrigator. For convenience, two large bags of irrigant are connected by way of a three-way stopcock to the delivery system (Fig. 1–25).

For performing mastoidectomy, the surgeon must have a full array of cutting and diamond burrs as well as suction-irrigators in different sizes. In addition, bone wax and Surgicel should always be on the field. Middle ear instruments such as gimmick, weapon, and fine scissors are useful for removing cholesteatomas.

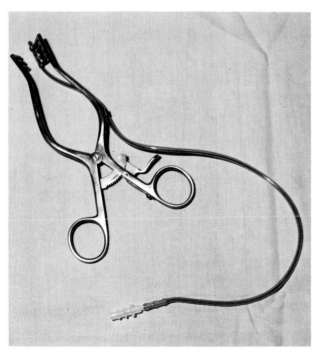

FIGURE 1–24. Modified Weitlaner retractor.

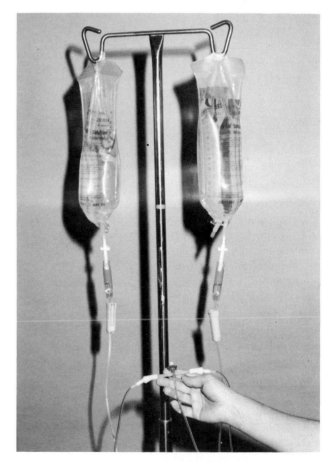

FIGURE 1–25. Irrigation setup with three-way stopcock.

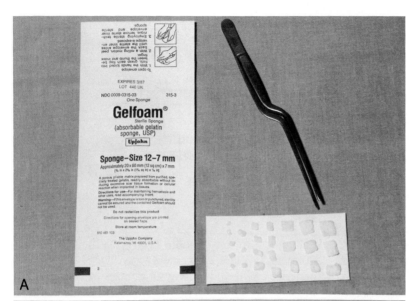

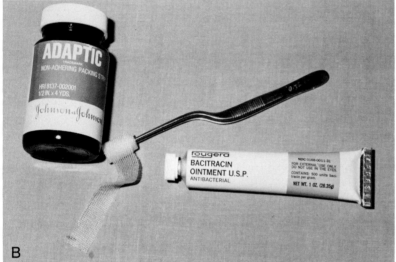

FIGURE 1–26. *A*, Gelfoam packing. *B*, Adaptic meatoplasty packing.

Although the setup for closing and packing following chronic ear surgery will vary with the specifics of the situation, a few generalities will cover most situations encountered by the otologist. To maintain the middle ear space, Silastic sheeting works well. This is available in a variety of thicknesses, ranging from 0.005 to 0.04 inches, with or without reinforcement. For middle ear packing, Gelfoam is the usual choice, soaked in saline or an antibiotic-containing suspension. This is also used to pack the EAC, though some surgeons prefer an ointment such as Kos-House or Aureomycin. For packing a meatoplasty, Adaptic gauze is saturated with an antibiotic ointment and rolled around the tips of a bayonet forceps. This creates a plug that conforms to the new meatus and is easily removed (Fig. 1–26).

Wound closure is done in two layers with absorbable sutures. The skin is closed with a running intradermal suture of 4.0 Vicryl or Dexon on a cutting needle. Steri-Strips are applied, and the wound is covered with a standard mastoid dressing.

There are some additional instruments that prove to be handy in many chronic ear cases. These include an ossicle holder, Crabtree dissectors, Zini mirrors, right-angle hooks, and the House-Dieter malleus nipper (Fig. 1–27). It is impossible to describe instruments for every conceivable situation, but the foregoing should cover most needs of the ear surgeon.

ENDOLYMPHATIC SAC SURGERY

There are many well-described procedures on the endolymphatic sac (ELS). It is not my purpose to outline the surgical options but rather to discuss the methodology for performing sac surgery. The preparation and draping of the patient for ELS surgery are essentially

FIGURE 1-27. Additional instruments.

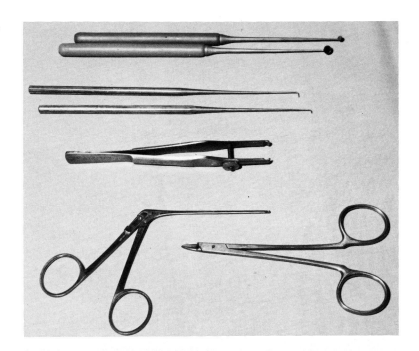

the same as for tympanoplasty with mastoidectomy surgery. In the preoperative holding area, the postauricular area is shaved so that at least 4cm of skin is available. Plastic adhesive drapes are applied, and the patient is transported to the OR. Endolymphatic sac surgery is performed under general anesthesia. The field is scrubbed and the patient positioned as described for chronic ear surgery.

The postauricular area is injected with 1 per cent lidocaine with 1:100,000 epinephrine. The incision is made 2cm to 3cm behind the sulcus. Periosteal incisions are made sharply or with the electrocautery as described earlier. Soft tissue and periosteum are elevated with the Lempert elevator up to the spine of Henle. A House narrow (canal) elevator is used to delineate the EAC, and a large self-retaining retractor is inserted. A complete mastoidectomy is performed with the drill and suction-irrigation. The antrum is not widely opened but is instead blocked with a large piece of Gelfoam to keep bone debris out of the middle ear.

Bone over the sigmoid sinus and posterior fossa dura is thinned with diamond burrs. The retrofacial air tract is widely opened to locate the ELS. The sac is decompressed with diamond burrs. Bone over the proximal sac can be removed with a stapes curette. There is some occasional bleeding from the surface of the sac or surrounding dura. This is best controlled with bipolar cautery. An alternative is to use the unipolar cautery turned to a low setting. The cautery tip is touched to an insulated Rosen or gimmick that is placed in contact with the offending vessel (Fig. 1–28).

Prior to opening of the sac, the wound is copiously irrigated with bacitracin solution or saline, and fresh towels are placed around the field. The sac is opened with a disposable Beaver ophthalmic blade (No. 59S, 5910, or 5920). The lumen can be probed with a blunt hook or a gimmick. The shunt tube preferred by the surgeon is inserted. One can fashion a shunt by using 0.005 inch Silastic sheeting. Figure 1–29 shows the materials used for the latter steps in ELS surgery. Like chronic ear procedures, the wound is closed in layers, usually beginning with 2.0 chromic suture and finishing with an intradermal 4.0 Vicryl or Dexon suture.

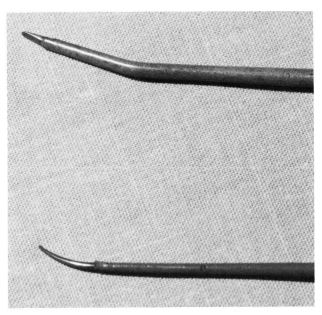

FIGURE 1-28. Insulated gimmick (top) and Rosen (bottom).

FIGURE 1-29. Endolymphatic sac instruments and materials.

NEUROTOLOGIC PROCEDURES

This section describes the layout for neurotologic procedures, the only exception being middle fossa surgery, which is discussed separately. For procedures involving exposure of intracranial structures, extraordinarily meticulous attention to detail is warranted. The preparation begins the evening prior to surgery by having the patient wash his or her hair with any of the widely available antiseptic shampoos. The day of surgery, the patient is seen by the surgeon in the preoperative holding area, at which time the ear to be operated is positively identified. The surgical site is shaved so that at least 6cm of scalp is exposed behind the postauricular sulcus. The area is sprayed with an adhesive and the plastic drapes applied so as to surround the field (Fig. 1–30). At the same time, the abdomen is shaved from below the umbilicus to the inguinal ligaments, in preparation for harvesting a fat graft. In the OR, the abdomen is surrounded by disposable adhesive drapes after the area is scrubbed (Fig. 1–31).

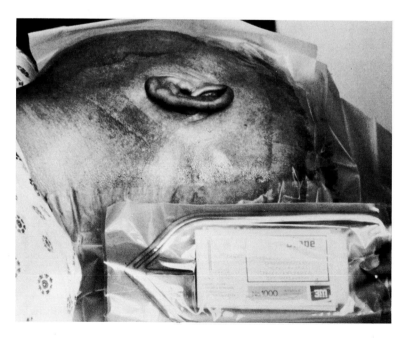

FIGURE 1-30. 3M 1000 drapes applied for neurotologic surgery.

FIGURE 1–31. Abdominal area prepared.

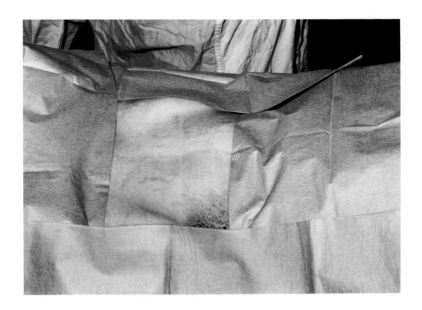

After anesthetic induction and intubation, there are a number of important matters to attend to. A catheter is aseptically inserted. When indicated, arterial and central venous catheters are placed. Electrodes for monitoring cranial nerves VII and VIII (and possibly other nerves) are positioned. The patient's head is supported on towels or blankets as needed and rotated toward the opposite shoulder. Preparation of the skin is performed, with the prepared area including the plastic drapes. The areas are blotted dry with towels. Plastic adhesive drapes (e.g., Steri-Drape, Ioban, cranial-incise) are positioned on the head and abdomen. Towels are used to block off the field, and a laparotomy aperture drape is placed over the abdominal area. The head is further draped with sheets and, finally, one additional layer of towels. This is important in preventing saturation of the drapes down to the level of the patient (Fig. 1–32).

Because the scrub nurse must handle a number of items attached to tubes and cords, it is helpful to have fastened to the field a plastic pouch into which the drill, suction, unipolar cautery, and bipolar cautery can be placed (Fig. 1–33). Two Mayo stands are kept close to the field. One holds the instruments for the neurotologic procedure, with the other containing the fat-harvesting instruments (Fig. 1–34).

The postauricular area is injected with 1 per cent lidocaine with 1:100,000 epinephrine. Suture scissors are used to cut away the plastic drape so as to expose the skin over the mastoid and lateral subocciput. As with other procedures, the skin incision is made; hemostasis is obtained; a Lempert elevator is used to elevate soft tissues and periosteum; and a large self-retaining retractor is inserted. Bone removal is accomplished with a drill and suction-irrigation. For neurotologic surgery, bone must be removed far posterior to the sigmoid sinus to expose posterior fossa dura. For this type of drilling, it is imperative that the surgeon have immediately available bipolar cautery, bone wax, and Surgicel. Some surgeons will completely decompress the sigmoid sinus, whereas others prefer to leave a thin shell of bone over the sinus (Bill's island). The essential equipment and material for controlling hemorrhage from large venous structures must always be on the sterile field.

The extent of bone removal will vary depending upon the nature of the neurotologic procedure. After appropriate bone removal, the field is irrigated prior to opening the dura. All retractors are removed from the wound and rinsed in bacitracin solution. The wound is also irrigated with bacitracin solution and fresh towels placed around the field. Bacitracin solution can be prepared by dissolving 50,000 U of bacitracin powder in 1 L of normal saline.

Dura may be opened with a No. 11 Bard-Parker scalpel blade or with the tips of the Jacobson scissors. The subdural space is entered, taking care not to violate the arachnoid. This avoids injury to vessels prior to gaining adequate exposure. The dural flap is carefully developed with the Jacobson scissors. Dural vessels are controlled with bipolar cautery. The arachnoid is carefully opened with a sharp hook, allowing for a brisk escape of cerebrospinal fluid (CSF). Figure 1–35 shows the instruments for opening dura and arachnoid. Once the subarachnoid space has been entered, all suction-irrigators should be of the fenestrated (Brackmann) variety (Fig. 1–36). A variety of moistened neurosurgical Cottonoids should be on the field. These are best positioned with bayonet forceps.

When the surgeon is performing a vestibular neurectomy, the plane between the cochlear and vestibular nerves is best developed with a blunt hook. The

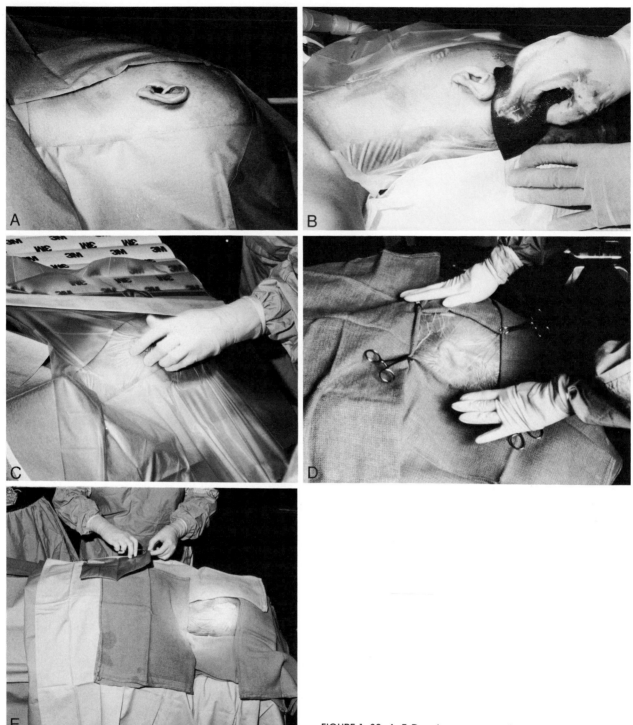

FIGURE 1-32. *A–E,* Draping sequence for neurotologic surgery.

FIGURE 1-33. SK-100 Surgi-kit for holding instruments.

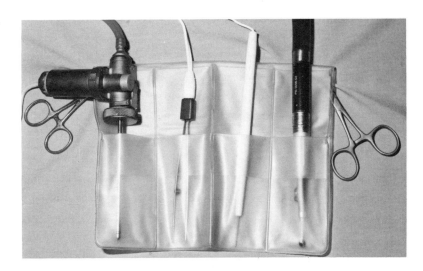

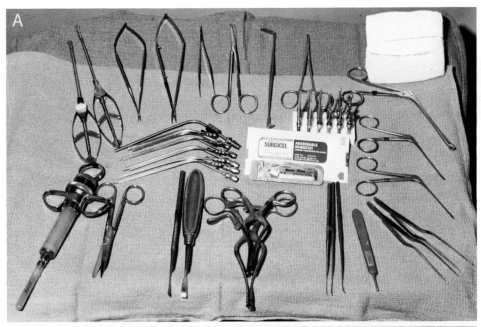

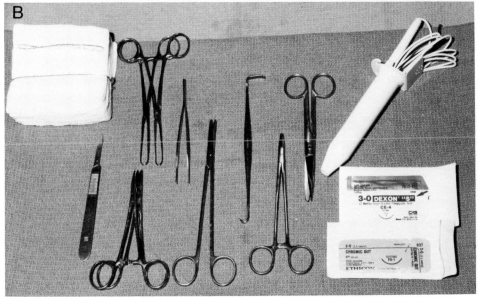

FIGURE 1-34. *A*, Mayo stand setup for tumor. *B*, Mayo stand setup for fat graft.

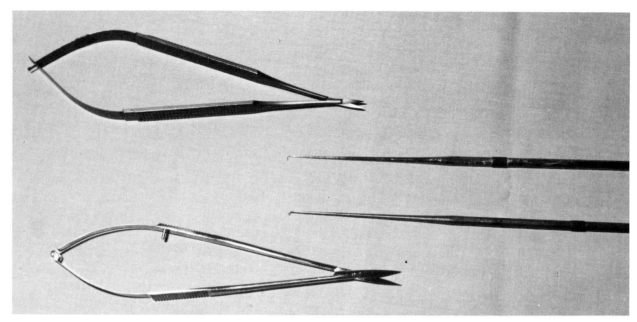

FIGURE 1–35. Hooks and scissors for opening dura and tumor dissection.

neurectomy can be completed with a sharp hook or microscissors (Fig. 1–37). A complete vestibular neurectomy is usually indicated by springing apart of the two cut ends. The same instrumentation is used to define the plane between an acoustic neuroma and the facial nerve. A right-angle sharp hook palpates Bill's bar and sections the superior vestibular nerve. The vestibulofacial fibers are cut with the hook. Once the proper plane between tumor and facial nerve has been identified, a blunt hook is used to separate tumor from facial nerve, taking care not to push or

stretch facial nerve fibers. Facial nerve monitoring has greatly facilitated this aspect of the dissection. For the small acoustic tumor, this technique might suffice to remove the entire lesion. Larger tumors are removed by gutting the tumor extensively, mobilizing the capsule, and then removing the capsule piecemeal. This is accomplished by morselizing the tumor with a large crushing forceps. The Urban rotary suction-dissector is used to extract the pieces (Fig. 1–38). The Urban dissector is held in the surgeon's right hand. Bayonet forceps direct the tumor into the suction port of the dissector. As the tumor is gutted the capsule collapses and can be removed from the brainstem.

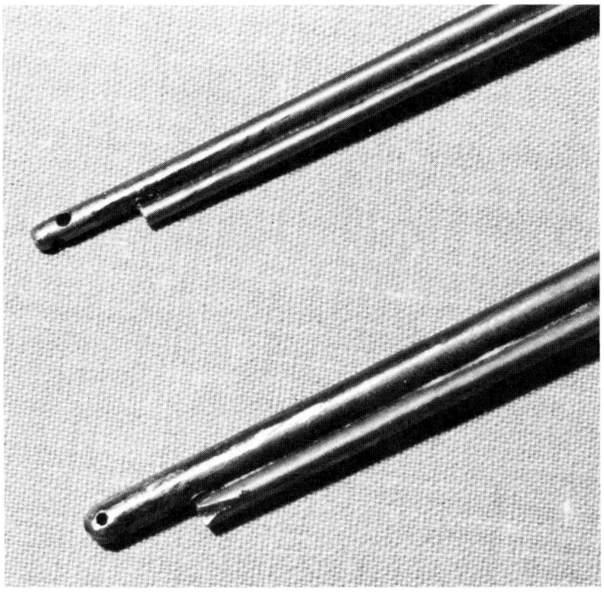

In addition to the Urban, the Cavitron ultrasonic suction aspirator is useful for gutting tumors. Proper use of these sophisticated devices should be learned from user manuals and appropriate in-service sessions.

Hemostasis during neurotologic surgery is accomplished by a number of different means. The surgeon should have immediate access to all possible items necessary to control bleeding from whatever the source. Unipolar and bipolar cautery have already been mentioned. Bone wax and Surgicel in varying sizes should be on the field. Microfibrillar collagen (Avitene) is a preferred means of achieving hemostasis in a tumor bed. Vascular clips and a reliable clip applicator should also be nearby. These clips are particularly useful for controlling bleeding from the petrosal vein and its tributaries (Fig. 1–39).

Infratemporal fossa and other approaches to the skull base are set up much like the above-mentioned neurotologic procedures. Incisions are generally

FIGURE 1–36. Brackmann fenestrated suction-irrigators.

FIGURE 1-37. Hooks for neurectomy and tumor dissection.

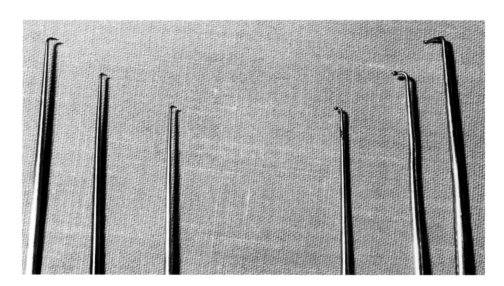

FIGURE 1-38. Urban dissector.

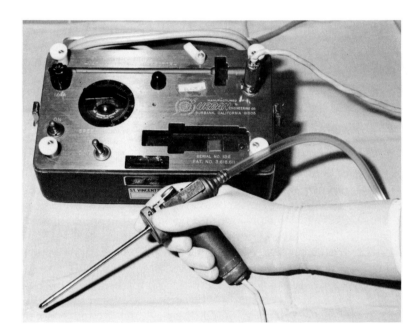

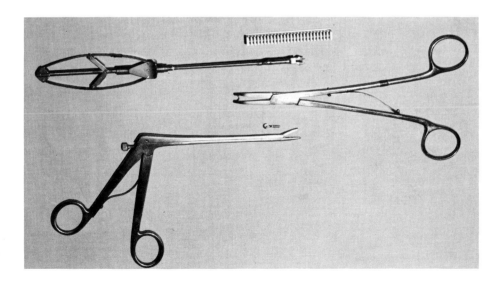

FIGURE 1-39. Clips and clip applicators.

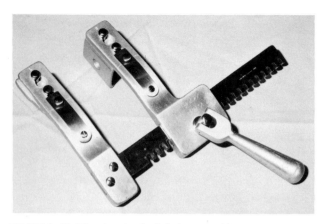

FIGURE 1-40. Rib retractor for infratemporal fossa surgery.

longer and extend into the neck to access major neurovascular structures. Silastic vessel loops should be placed around these structures for control and easy identification. Ligatures of 0 silk and transfixion sutures of 2.0 silk should be available for ligation of the jugular vein. Cardiovascular suture such as 5.0 and 6.0 Prolene should also be readily accessible.

The self-retaining retractors described earlier are usually insufficient for skull base surgery. The Fisch infratemporal fossa retractor or a pediatric rib retractor is better suited to these tasks, which include anteriorly displacing the mandible (Fig. 1-40). Oscillating saws may be necessary for mandibulotomy in these procedures.

There are some instruments that facilitate work on and near the facial nerve. For rerouting the facial nerve, bone is removed with a drill until an eggshell thickness remains. The rest of the bone is removed with a stapes curette. The nerve can be mobilized with a dental excavator or microraspatory. If a segment of the nerve is to be excised, as in a facial neuroma, this should be done sharply with a fresh knife blade. Likewise, prior to any neurorrhaphy, the ends of the nerve and graft should be freshened. A 9.0 monofilament suture is used for performing nerve anastomosis. Appropriate needle holder and forceps must be available (Fig. 1-41).

Prior to closing neurotologic and skull base wounds, abdominal fat is removed from the left lower quadrant, making use of the electrocautery to do most of the dissection. By this technique, hemostasis is usually excellent and a drain is rarely needed. The abdominal incision is closed in layers using 4.0 Vicryl or Dexon to run a continuous intradermal suture for skin approximation. The harvested fat is cut into strips and carefully insinuated into the dural defect. Continuous lumbar drainage is rarely necessary to prevent CSF leak, except in the extensive intracranial-extracranial resections. When the neck is opened, a suction drain is usually inserted into the depths of the wound prior to closure. Wounds are closed as in other otologic procedures and dressed with the standard mastoid dressing.

MIDDLE CRANIAL FOSSA SURGERY

Middle fossa procedures are discussed separately from other neurotologic procedures because they involve a different OR setup and some different instruments. The most obvious deviation from other procedures is the position from which the surgeon operates. The surgeon and the microscope trade locations, so that the surgeon operates from the head of the bed facing caudally (see Fig. 1-11).

As with other neurotologic procedures, middle

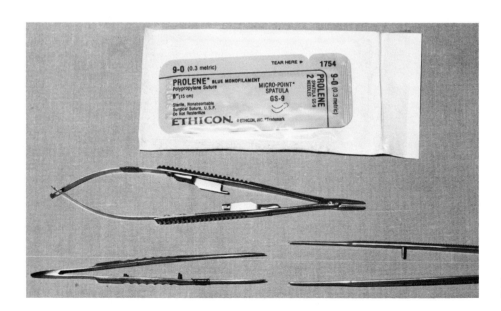

FIGURE 1-41. Nerve anastomosis equipment.

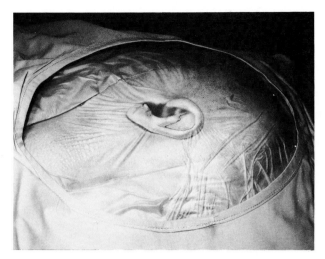

FIGURE 1-42. Patient draped for middle fossa surgery.

fossa surgery is performed under general anesthesia. Prior to surgery, the patient is transported to the preoperative holding area where the ipsilateral head is shaved to a distance of 6cm postauricularly and nearly to the midline above the ear in the temporal fossa. Plastic adhesive drapes are applied as with other procedures, and the patient is taken into the OR. After anesthesia, the surgical site and plastic drapes are scrubbed and then blotted dry with a sterile towel, and a plastic adhesive drape is placed over the area. Towels are positioned to block off the entire temporoparietal scalp, including the auricle and zygomatic arch. Sterile sheets complete the draping (Fig. 1–42). The abdomen is usually prepared for middle fossa surgery, as with other neurotologic procedures.

The incision is planned so that it begins in the preauricular incisura below the root of the zygoma, and extends cephalad to above the level of the superficial temporal line. A gentle curve facilitates exposure. Prior to the incision, the area is injected with 1 per cent lidocaine with 1:100,000 epinephrine. The plastic drape is cut away to expose the skin. After the skin incision is made, the superficial temporal vessels are identified and ligated. The dissection continues down to the level of the temporalis fascia. Instead of splitting the temporalis muscle, it is recommended that an inferiorly based flap be created, centered over the zy-

gomatic arch. This central portion of the temporalis muscle is elevated from the calvarium and reflected caudally by suturing the end of the flap to the drapes. Preserving the muscle with its neurovascular bundle does not compromise exposure and allows for the use of this muscle if facial reanimation surgery should ever be necessary. The rest of the temporalis muscle is elevated and reflected laterally. A large self-retaining retractor is inserted. A craniotomy is then performed with either a craniotome (e.g., Midas Rex) or cutting burrs and suction-irrigation. The size of the bone flap removed is dictated by the amount of exposure necessary. For tumor removal, it is wise to err on the large side.

The bone flap is carefully removed from the dura with an Adson periosteal elevator, otherwise known as a "joker" (Fig. 1–43). The bone flap is placed in saline. The edges of the craniotomy are smoothed with a rongeur and bleeding controlled with bone wax. Dural bleeding is stopped with bipolar cautery.

The joker is now used to begin dissecting the dura from the floor of the middle fossa. Adequate exposure mandates that the surgeon remove enough bone so as to be at the floor of the middle fossa. The surgeon is now ready to insert the House-Urban middle fossa retractor. The surgeon must be well acquainted with the mechanical workings of this retractor beforehand (Fig. 1–44). The retractor is used by first locking it onto the bony edges of the craniotomy site. The blade housing is positioned so that it allows good visualization of the field without placing excessive traction on the temporal lobe. This usually requires repositioning the apparatus several times during the early part of the dissection. Next, the blade of the retractor is inserted and the extradural dissection proceeds. The blade can be tilted with the hand and advanced with the thumb, leaving the other hand free for suctioning. Bleeding can be troublesome from the floor of the middle fossa, especially near the middle meningeal artery. Bipolar cautery should be on the field. Pieces of Surgicel and bayonet forceps must be within reach.

The surgeon elevates dura and temporal lobe until the arcuate eminence, superior petrosal sinus, and greater superficial petrosal nerve are visible. Bone over the internal auditory canal and geniculate ganglion is removed with a relatively large diamond burr.

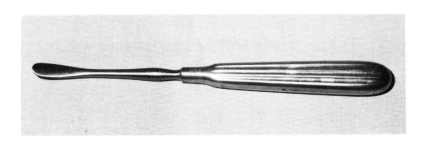

FIGURE 1-43. Adson periosteal elevator ("joker").

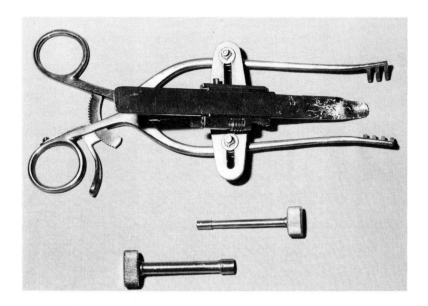

FIGURE 1-44. House-Urban middle fossa retractor.

When the dura over the internal auditory canal (IAC) has been completely skeletonized, the wound is irrigated with bacitracin solution and fresh towels applied to the edges of the sterile field. The dura of the IAC is opened posteriorly (away from the facial nerve) with a sharp hook. If a vestibular neurectomy is to be performed, the hook palpates Bill's bar and transects the superior vestibular nerve. Fine microscissors (e.g., Malis, Jacobson) are used to remove a segment of the nerve along with Scarpa's ganglion. Similarly, the inferior vestibular and singular nerves are cut. For acoustic tumor removal, significantly more bone removal is required for adequate exposure. The plane between the facial nerve and tumor is developed as in the translabyrinthine approach.

After the procedure is concluded, the defect over the IAC is reconstructed by filling it with small pieces of temporalis muscle or abdominal fat and covering it with a small piece of the bone flap that has been cut and trimmed to the appropriate size. The field is inspected for hemostasis and the middle fossa retractor slowly removed, allowing the brain to re-expand. The wound is irrigated with bacitracin solution. The bone flap is sutured in place with silk sutures and the wound closed in layers. The inferiorly based temporalis muscle flap should be sutured in its normal anatomic configuration. Some surgeons prefer to close the skin over a Penrose drain, which is removed the day after surgery. A mastoid-type dressing is placed at the completion of closing.

CONCLUSION

This chapter has provided a detailed description of the necessary instruments and the operating room setup for most situations that the otologist is likely to encounter. Although these descriptions by no means exhaust all the possibilities, they have proved to be satisfactory for many otologists. The Appendix lists the instruments and equipment that have been described.

Appendix

INSTRUMENTS AND EQUIPMENT FOR
OTOLOGIC SURGERY

General Operating Room Equipment
1. 3M 1000 plastic adhesive drapes
2. 3M 1020 aperture drapes
3. 3M Steri-Drape, Ioban drape, or cranial-incise drape
4. Pharmaseal preoperative skin preparation tray No. 4480
5. Dow-Corning flexible surgical tubing
6. Suction canisters
7. Electrocautery unit

Stapes Surgery
1. Assorted Farrior speculums
2. Finger-control Luer-Lok syringe
3. 1 1/2 inch 25-gauge needle
4. Small Weitlaner retractor
5. Sheehy fascia press
6. House cutting block
7. Scalpel, No. 15 Bard-Parker blade
8. Adson tissue forceps
9. Iris scissors
10. House-Baron suction tubes No. 3 Fr through No. 7 Fr
11. House suction tube adapter
12. Rosen suction tubes 18- through 24-gauge
13. Sickle knife (No. 1 knife)
14. Lancet knife (No. 2)
15. Robinson knife
16. Sheehy-House weapon (large and small)
17. Rosen needle
18. House elevator
19. Gimmick annulus elevator
20. House stapes curette
21. Incudostapedial joint knife
22. Bellucci scissors
23. Straight Barbara pick
24. Measuring struts, 4.0mm through 5.0mm
25. Measuring disk, 0.6mm
26. Hough hoe
27. Obtuse 30 degree, 0.25mm hook
28. Pick, 0.3mm, 90 degree
29. Strut guide
30. Footplate chisel
31. Skeeter drill; 1.0mm, 0.7mm, 0.6mm burrs
32. House strut forceps (nonserrated)
33. McGee wire closing forceps (crimper)
34. Kos-House ointment (or suitable antibiotic ointment)
35. Cotton balls, Band-Aids, mastoid dressing

Chronic Ear Surgery
1. Assorted Farrior speculums
2. Finger-control syringe
3. 1 1/2 inch 25-gauge needle
4. Small Weitlaner retractor
5. Large self-retaining retractor (Weitlaner, Adson cerebellar)
6. Scalpel, No. 15 Bard-Parker blade
7. No. 64 or 67 Beaver blade
8. House cutting block
9. Sheehy fascia press
10. House-Baron suction tubes No. 3 Fr through No. 7 Fr
11. Adson forceps
12. Iris scissors
13. Small Metzenbaum scissors
14. Sickle knife
15. Lancet knife
16. Robinson knife
17. Sheehy-House weapon (small and large)
18. Rosen needle
19. Gimmick
20. Crabtree dissector (large and small)
21. Lempert elevator
22. House narrow elevator
23. Pick, right angle, 0.6mm
24. Pick, right angle, 1.50mm
25. Pick, right angle, 3mm
26. Bellucci scissors
27. Hartmann forceps
28. House alligator forceps
29. House cup forceps
30. House-Dieter malleus nipper
31. Zini mirrors
32. Sheehy ossicle holder
33. Speculum, endaural (or nasal)
34. Drill with assortment of cutting and diamond burrs
35. House suction-irrigators, No. 2.5 Fr × No. 4 Fr through No. 8 Fr × No. 12 Fr
36. Needle holder, Webster
37. Suture scissors
38. Suture, 2.0 chromic and 4.0 Dexon (or Vicryl)
39. Gelfoam (saline- and Coly-Mycin-soaked)
40. Adaptic gauze
41. Silastic sheeting
42. Steri-Strips
43. Mastoid dressing
44. Bone wax
45. Surgicel
46. Sheehy bone paté collector

Endolymphatic Sac Surgery
1. Finger-control syringe
2. 1 1/2 inch 25-gauge needle
3. Scalpel, No. 15 Bard-Parker blade
4. Large self-retaining retractor
5. Lempert elevator
6. House narrow elevator
7. Drill and burrs
8. House suction-irrigators, No. 2.5 Fr × No. 4 Fr through No. 8 Fr × No. 12 Fr

9. Brackmann suction-irrigators, No. 4 Fr × No. 5 Fr, No. 5 Fr × No. 7 Fr
10. Stapes curette
11. Gimmick
12. Insulated gimmick
13. Bone wax
14. Surgicel
15. Malis bipolar cautery
16. Bacitracin irrigation solution
17. Beaver ophthalmic blade (No. 59S, 5910, or 5920)
18. Pick, right angle, 1.50mm
19. Hook, right angle, blunt
20. Rosen needle
21. House alligator forceps
22. Shunt tube or material
23. Suture, 2.0 chromic and 4.0 Dexon (or Vicryl)
24. Steri-Strips
25. Mastoid dressing

Neurotologic Surgery
1. Finger-control syringe
2. 1 1/2 inch 25-gauge needle
3. Scalpel, No. 15 Bard-Parker blade
4. Large self-retaining retractor
5. Lempert elevator
6. House narrow elevator
7. Drill and burrs
8. House suction-irrigators, No. 2.5 Fr × No. 4 Fr through No. 8 Fr × No. 12 Fr
9. Brackmann suction-irrigators, No. 4 Fr × No. 5 Fr, No. 5 Fr × No. 7 Fr
10. Stapes curette
11. Gimmick
12. Insulated gimmick
13. Bone wax
14. Surgicel
15. Malis bipolar cautery
16. Bacitracin irrigation solution
17. SK-100 Surgi-kit (Ethox Corp.)
18. Suture scissors
19. House-Urban dissector
20. Pick, right angle, 1mm
21. Pick, right angle, 1.5mm
22. Hook, right angle, blunt, 1.5mm
23. Bellucci scissors
24. House cup forceps
25. Blakesle nasal forceps (No. 1)
26. House alligator forceps
27. Myringoplasty knife
28. Jacobson scissors
29. Malis scissors
30. Allis forceps
31. Bayonet forceps
32. Adson tissue forceps
33. Microclip applicator
34. Assorted hemostats
35. Metzenbaum scissors
36. Senn retractor
37. US Army retractor
38. Pediatric rib retractor
39. Fisch infratemporal fossa retractor
40. Woodson elevator
41. Fisch microraspatory
42. Sagittal saw
43. Needle holder, Castroviejo
44. Needle holder, Crile-Wood
45. Needle holder, Webster
46. Avitene
47. Drains, Penrose and Jackson-Pratt
48. Vessel loops
49. Suture, 5.0 and 6.0 vascular Prolene
50. Suture, 0 and 2.0 chromic
51. Suture, 0 and 2.0 silk
52. Suture, 9.0 nylon or Prolene
53. Suture, 4.0 Dexon or Vicryl
54. Assorted neurosurgical Cottonoids
55. Steri-Strips
56. Mastoid dressing

Middle Fossa Surgery
1. Finger-control syringe
2. 1 1/2 inch 25-gauge needle
3. Scalpel, No. 15 Bard-Parker blade
4. Large self-retaining retractor
5. Lempert elevator
6. House narrow elevator
7. Drill and burrs
8. House suction-irrigators, No. 2.5 Fr × No. 4 Fr through No. 8 Fr × No. 12 Fr
9. Brackmann suction-irrigators, No. 4 Fr × No. 5 Fr, No. 5 Fr × No. 7 Fr
10. Stapes curette
11. Gimmick
12. Insulated gimmick
13. Bone wax
14. Surgicel
15. Malis bipolar cautery
16. Bacitracin irrigation solution
17. SK-100 Surgi-kit (Ethox Corp.)
18. Pick, right angle, 1mm
19. Pick, right angle, 1.5mm
20. Hook, right angle, blunt, 1.5mm
21. Bellucci scissors
22. House cup forceps
23. Metzenbaum scissors
24. House-Urban middle fossa retractor
25. Rongeur, Leksell
26. Adson tissue forceps
27. Microclip applicator
28. Assorted hemostats
29. Avitene
30. Cottonoids
31. Microclip applicator
32. Suture, 0 and 2.0 chromic
33. Suture, 4.0 Dexon or Vicryl
34. Steri-Strips and mastoid dressing

2

Canalplasty for Exostoses of the External Auditory Canal

RODNEY PERKINS, M.D.

Although the clinical disease caused by exostoses of the external auditory canal is not frequent, it occurs often enough to warrant that a method of surgical management be in the armamentarium of the otologic surgeon. Because it is not a high-incidence problem or one that is life-threatening, most otolaryngologists use a variety of independent approaches that, by and large, result in elimination of or damage to the canal skin. Unfortunately, these procedures frequently produce less than optimal results. A well-conceived approach addresses the problem of exostoses removal while maintaining the valuable residual skin of the external auditory canal. This chapter begins with clinical observations regarding this condition and then describes an operative procedure that has been very successful in its management.

The etiology of these benign growths is not completely understood. A widely held belief based on clinical information is that they occur primarily during the years of growth, their proliferation being enhanced or perhaps even caused by exposure to cold water during this period. This tends to be supported by historical information from patients with exostoses, who almost always indicate that they swam in cold water during their youth.[1-3] This is strongly corroborated by the high incidence of the problem in avid surfers who spend hours in the water almost daily. In my clinical experience, this problem occurs almost exclusively in males, who are more likely than females of the same age to have had frequent cold water exposure during their youth.

Most exostoses do not develop to a degree sufficient to cause clinical symptoms. Patients are frequently referred to otologists because the growths are observed, and not understood, by primary care physicians. This is particularly true with those that have a more pedunculated form than the more subtle sessile configuration. However, when exostoses become more marked, they obstruct the natural elimination of desquamated epithelium from the ear canal, and patients usually present with recurrent episodes of external otitis. In their most prolific expression, exostoses can lead to hearing impairment by causing the collection of epithelial debris that tamponades tympanic membrane movement, by impinging on and limiting the mobility of the malleus, or by markedly narrowing the aperture of the canal. These conditions may appear as a conductive hearing impairment on audiometric examination.

The external auditory canal is part of the hearing pathway. Essentially, it is a tube with resonant characteristics that amplify the incoming sound. The degree of amplification and the frequency at which it occurs is a function of the diameter and the length of the canal. When the diameter becomes small, it can interfere with the passage of sound and cause a hearing impairment. However, this effect does not become significant until the aperture becomes very small. With apertures under 3mm, high-frequency sounds begin to diminish, and further compromise of the channel diameter results in increased impairment and lower-frequency loss.

SURGICAL INDICATIONS

Surgery is indicated when chronic or recurrent external otitis exists or a conductive hearing impairment develops. The presence of chronic and recurrent infection over an extended period seems to debilitate the canal skin and can compromise the skin's ability to re-epithelialize in a robust and healthy manner in the postoperative period. For this reason, surgical therapy should be considered once a pattern of recurrent external otitis has been established in these patients. Patients who have significant external canal exostoses without recurrent infection or hearing impairment should be observed periodically, and surgery should be avoided until these symptoms occur.

PREOPERATIVE PREPARATION

Patient Preparation

There are two components of patient preparation for otologic surgery performed under local anesthesia: psychologic and pharmacologic.

Psychologic

To reduce anxiety and create rapport, the surgeon should provide the patient with a full explanation of the procedure, its objectives, benefits, and risks. In addition, a surgical nurse or medical assistant should explain what will happen to the patient in the operating room by describing such things as the operating room environment, use of an intravenous line for medication delivery, placement of monitor electrodes, and draping. By informing the patient of these things and making him or her part of the process, the clinician reduces the patient's anxiety, encourages cooperation, and reduces bleeding. Beyond the technical advantages achieved by such preparation, there is an ethical responsibility to inform the patient. In addition, the likelihood of the patient's becoming litigious because of a poor result is markedly reduced if he or she has been informed about the procedure and its risks and benefits and has had an opportunity to discuss them with the surgeon prior to the surgery.

Pharmacologic

The chemical preparation of the patient can be achieved in many ways. The chemical agents that I have employed in preparation have worked for me, but many premedication regimens achieve a similar result.

In the average adult, I give pentobarbital sodium (Nembutal), 150mg orally, 1 hour before surgery. One half hour prior to surgery meperidine (Demerol), 75mg, and diazepam (Valium), 10mg, are given by intramuscular injection. An intravenous catheter is started in the arm opposite the ear to be operated on before the patient arrives in the operating room, and five per cent dextrose in Ringer's solution is started with a Volutrol. Unless the patient appears very sedated, an additional 25mg dose of meperidine is placed in the Volutrol and infused slowly over 30 to 45 minutes. As the surgery proceeds, alternating supplements of intravenous diazepam and meperidine are infused as needed to maintain sedation. In addition, patients receive penicillin VK, 250mg, or another appropriate antibiotic 1 hour before surgery.

Site Preparation

The hair is shaved behind the ear to a distance of approximately 1.5 inches posterior to the postauricular fold. The auricle and the periauricular and postauricular areas are scrubbed with povidone-iodine (Betadine) solution. A plastic drape is placed over the area with the auricle and the postauricular area exteriorized through the opening in the drape. This drape is placed over an L-shaped bar that is fixed in the rail attachment of the operating table (Fig. 2–1). Attached to the bar is a small, low-volume office fan that provides a gentle cooling breeze to the patient's face during the procedure. The plastic drape forms a canopy, allowing the patient to see from under the drape and reducing the feeling of claustrophobia. In addition, a foam earpiece from an insert speaker is put into the opposite ear. The earpiece is connected to a compact disk player and input microphone that allows the patient to listen to relaxing music and provides a pathway to converse with the patient, if desired.

Analgesia

It is important not only to achieve analgesia but also to maximize canal hemostasis with injections into the external auditory meatus. Using two per cent lidocaine (Xylocaine) with 1:20,000 epinephrine solution in a ringed syringe with a 27-gauge needle, a classic quadratic injection is made such that each injection falls within the wheal of the previous injection. Another injection that I have found useful is an anterior canal injection, which is made with the bevel of the needle parallel to the bony wall of the external meatus (Fig. 2–2). In the patient with extensive exostoses, this injection is usually made into the lateral base of a large anterior sessile osteoma. After insinuation of the needle, it is advanced a few millimeters, and a few drops are injected extremely slowly. The solution infiltrates medially along the anterior canal wall and provides some analgesia to the auriculotemporal branch of cranial nerve V, which is usually unaffected by the quadratic injection and adds to the hemostasis anteriorly. The postauricular area is infiltrated with two per cent lidocaine with 1:100,000 epinephrine solution.

SURGICAL TECHNIQUE

Most surgical approaches for removal of external canal exostoses are done through the transmeatal route.[4–6] This approach has two distinct disadvantages. It usually results in significant loss of the remaining canal wall skin through damage by the drill, and it does not allow adequate visibility or instrument and drill access to safely remove the medial portion of the exostotic mass near the tympanic membrane. A large sessile anterior exostosis is almost uniformly present in these patients (Fig. 2–3). The approach described here is primarily postauricular and one that maximizes conservation of the canal wall skin and facilitates careful removal of the anterior exostosis, which is usually extremely close to the tympanic membrane.

A curvilinear postauricular incision is made approximately 1cm behind the postauricular fold (Fig. 2–4). The skin and subcutaneous tissues are elevated anteriorly to the area of the spine of Henle and the bony posterior canal, and a toothed, self-retaining retractor is placed (Fig. 2–5). Locating this area is facilitated by finding the plane of the lateral surface of the inferior border of the temporalis muscle and dissecting in this plane anteriorly to reach the meatus. Once this area is reached, the skin overlying the lateral slope of the posterior exostosis is elevated from its surface, and a Perkins bladed tympanoplasty retractor is inserted such that it holds elevated skin off the surface of the lateral portion of the bony mass (Fig. 2–6). Although there may be more than one posterior and anterior exostosis, predominant anterior and posterior exostoses are usually present along with others of lesser mass. These secondary masses may be handled similarly to the primary exostoses or may be removed directly. However, to simplify the description, this operation is divided into two major segments: removal of the posterior exostosis and removal of the anterior exostosis.

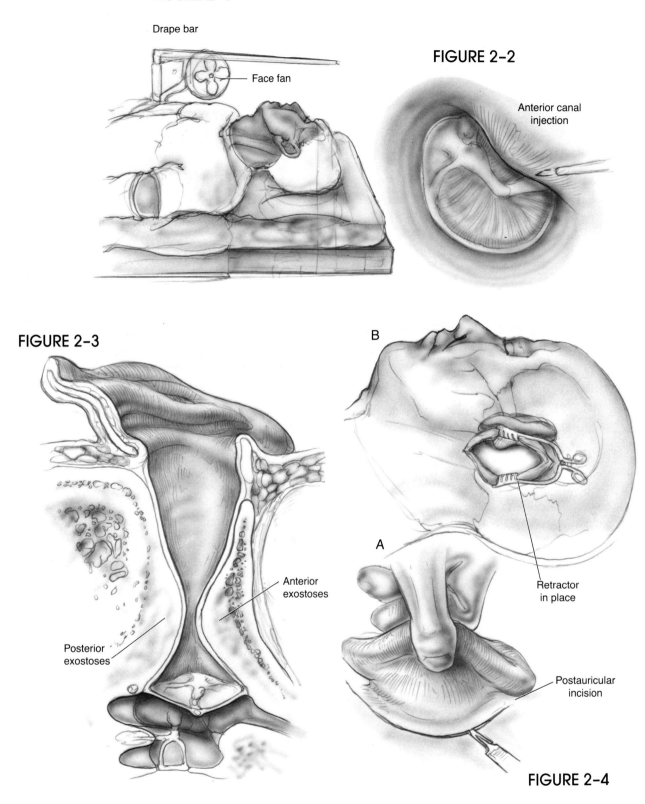

FIGURE 2-1

Drape bar

Face fan

FIGURE 2-2

Anterior canal
injection

FIGURE 2-3

Anterior
exostoses

Posterior
exostoses

B

A

Retractor
in place

Postauricular
incision

FIGURE 2-4

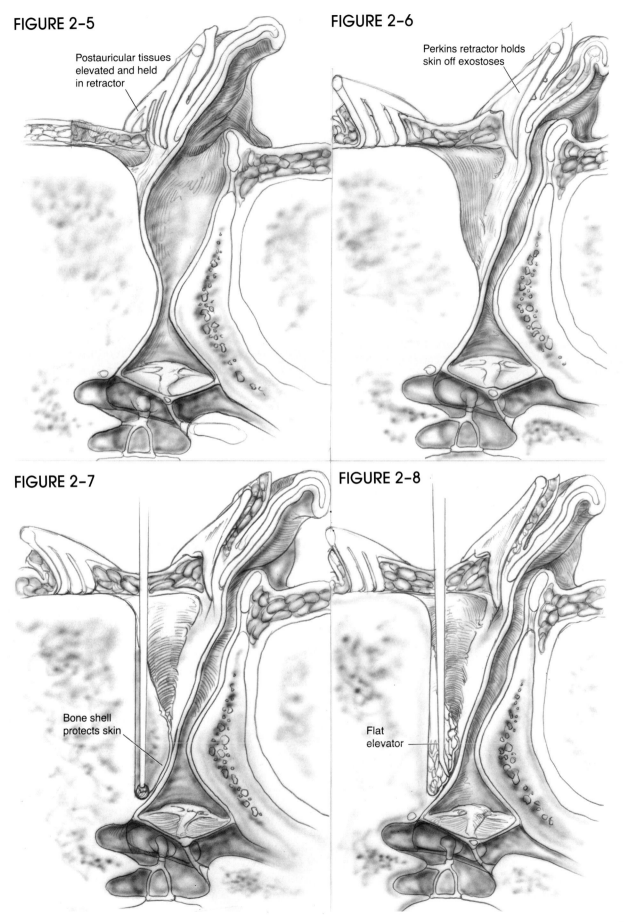

FIGURE 2–5

Postauricular tissues elevated and held in retractor

FIGURE 2–6

Perkins retractor holds skin off exostoses

FIGURE 2–7

Bone shell protects skin

FIGURE 2–8

Flat elevator

Removal of Posterior Exostoses

By use of a medium-sized cutting burr and an appropriately scaled suction-irrigator, the posterior exostosis is entered along its lateral sloping edge, and the bony removal is progressed medially, keeping a shell of bone over the area being burred anteriorly (Fig. 2–7). Thus, the remaining skin over the exostosis medial to that elevated earlier is protected from the burr. As this shell becomes thinner, it is advisable to switch to a diamond burr to prevent a sudden breakthrough to the skin that might occur if one continues with the cutting burr on the excessively thinned bone. The bone removal is continued medially and posteriorly until the estimated normal posterior canal contour and dimension is achieved. As one approaches a medial depth consistent with the posterior annulus of the tympanic membrane (which usually cannot be seen directly at this point), care must be taken to avoid damage to the chorda tympani nerve and the posterior aspect of the tympanic membrane. The thinned bony shell is collapsed, and a small elevator reveals the inside surface of the posterior canal skin that was over the exostosis (Fig. 2–8).

An incision is made midway along the posterior canal skin from the top of the canal to the bottom (Fig. 2–9). The posterior canal skin medial to this incision is then positioned onto the new contour of the posterior canal wall (Fig. 2–10). Then, the transmeatal approach is taken, and incisions are made with a sickle knife superiorly and inferiorly in the canal, extending from the ends of this previous incision laterally to the meatus and creating a laterally based posterior canal skin flap. This flap is then involuted back into the meatal portion of the canal and held there with the Perkins retractor (Fig. 2–11). Attention is then turned to the anterior exostosis, which has now been revealed.

Removal of Anterior Exostosis

By use of a round knife, an incision is made in the skin overlying the anterior exostosis from superior to inferior over the dome of the exostosis and as far medially as can be seen. This incision is connected to the incisions previously made superiorly and inferiorly in the canal that defined the posterior canal skin flap, and this anterior canal flap is elevated laterally (Fig. 2–12). By use of a back-angled Perkins tympanoplasty elevator, this laterally based anterior canal skin flap is elevated further to the cartilaginous portion of the anterior canal and is then smoothed so as to lie laterally near the posterior canal flap under the retractor (Fig. 2–13).

With a cutting burr and small suction irrigator, the anterior exostosis is removed in a manner similar to that of the posterior one, and a thin shell of bone that protects the canal skin is left over the anteromedial portion of the exostosis from the burr (Fig. 2–14). This bone removal is continued to the area of the anterior annulus of the tympanic membrane. The bony shell is then collapsed and removed, leaving the intact anterior canal skin (Fig. 2–15). Usually, it is necessary to finish up and smooth an edge of bone that remains at the anterior extent of this dissection to have a smooth contour near the annulus area. To protect the elevated anterior sulcus skin from the burr, a small tympanic membrane–size piece of silicone sheeting is placed on the inside surface of the anterior canal skin to hold it against the tympanic membrane during drilling. This prevents the skin flap from getting involved with the burr and also prevents damage to the tympanic membrane that might occur with the burr being used in such close proximity to the membrane. Subsequently, the Silastic is removed, the medial anterior canal skin is placed on the bone, and all skin flaps are folded back into position on the new contours of the bony canal (Fig. 2–16). The medial flaps are packed into place with chloramphenicol (Chloromycetin)–soaked absorbable gelatin sponge (Gelfoam) pledgets, and the postauricular incision is closed with interrupted subcuticular 4-0 Vicryl suture.

Through the transmeatal route the laterally based canal skin flaps are packed into place with gelatin sponge pledgets. A cotton ball is placed in the meatus, and a mastoid dressing is applied. The patient is returned to the outpatient recovery area and discharged 2 hours later.

POSTOPERATIVE CARE

The patient is placed on prophylactic antibiotics for 5 days and is instructed to remove the mastoid dressing the next morning. The gelatin sponge packing is removed using the stereo microscope and sterile instrumentation on the first office visit 1 week later. Antibiotic-steroid ear drops are prescribed for use twice daily for 1 week and once every 3 days for another 3 weeks. The second postoperative visit is at 1 month. If there is no evidence of infection, no additional drops are recommended. Because most of the cases in which this procedure is done have had recurrent external otitis, and because time is needed for epithelialization of uncovered bone, the ear canal may remain moist for a longer period of time than in a typical tympanoplasty. Until the ear canal is completely dry and healed, the patient should be seen every few weeks to inspect and clean debris from the canal as needed.

It should be remembered that the canal skin has usually been exposed to numerous infections and has been stretched over the exostoses; it therefore may not

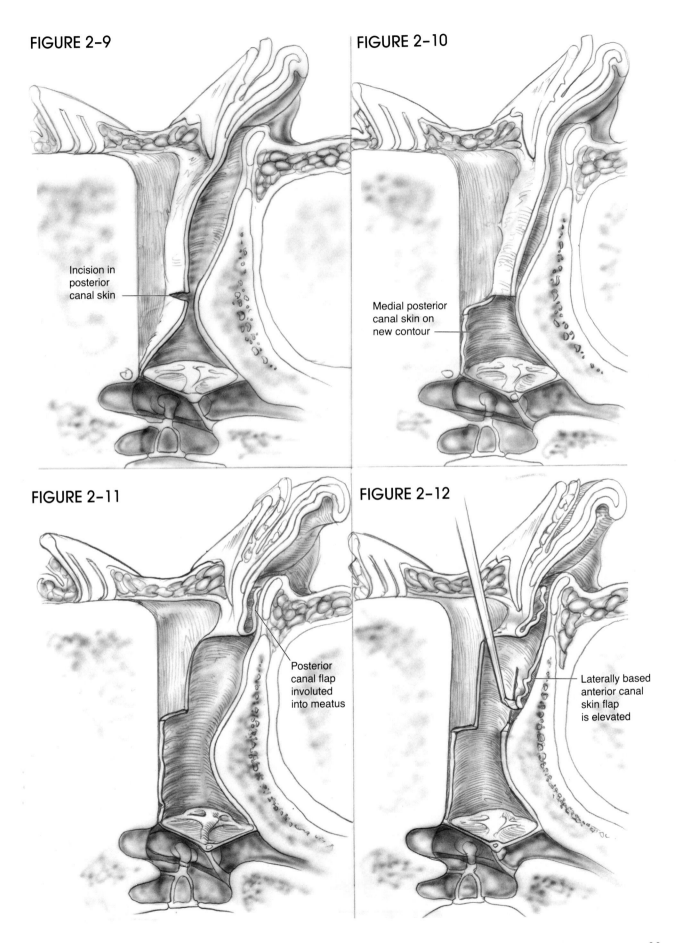

FIGURE 2-9

Incision in posterior canal skin

FIGURE 2-10

Medial posterior canal skin on new contour

FIGURE 2-11

Posterior canal flap involuted into meatus

FIGURE 2-12

Laterally based anterior canal skin flap is elevated

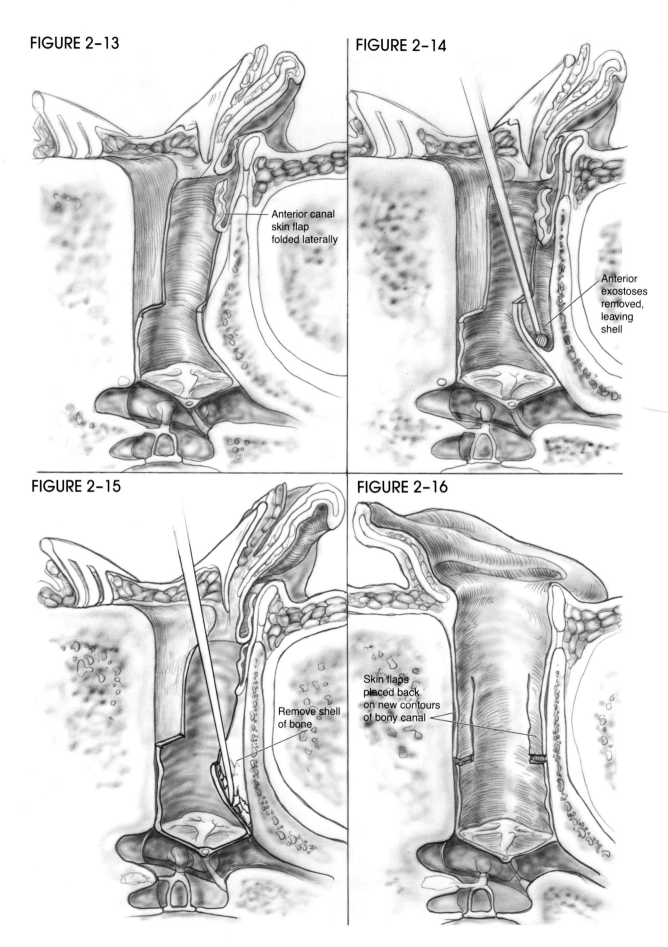

FIGURE 2–13

Anterior canal
skin flap
folded laterally

FIGURE 2–14

Anterior
exostoses
removed,
leaving
shell

FIGURE 2–15

Remove shell
of bone

FIGURE 2–16

Skin flaps
placed back
on new contours
of bony canal

be as resilient as normal canal skin. Return to water exposure should be avoided until 2 months after complete healing has occurred. If the patient is still in the growth years, further repeated exposure of the ear to cold water should be moderated. The bone may reproliferate under these conditions, and further surgery may become necessary. In patients who want to return to frequent surfing or similar water exposure, earplugs should be worn to prevent water entrance. This problem lessens in older surfers because they may be beyond their rapid growth phase, and the economic exigencies of life tend to decrease their frequency of exposure. It is advisable to see the patient annually for 2 years to assess the tendency for the problem to recur, although recurrence is infrequent.

PROBLEMS AND COMPLICATIONS

Although this procedure is not fraught with serious complications, complications can occur during several aspects of the operation. As the medial extent of the canal is approached in the removal of the posterior exostosis, the course of the chorda tympani nerve must be kept in mind. This portion of the bone removal is done largely without definite landmarks: the surgeon must rely on mental estimation of the distances in arriving at the posterior annulus. The chorda tympani nerve is beneath the bone near this field of dissection and could suffer damage. Also, it is important to remember the course of the facial nerve, which passes posterior and inferior to the canal, although this area is farther from the immediate area of dissection than is the chorda tympani nerve. When a burr is used very near the tympanic membrane and the malleus, a diamond burr should be used because it is less likely to run erratically than is the cutting burr.

Watch: ① FN/chorda
② TM
③ malleus
④ canal skin

SUMMARY

Exostoses of the external auditory canal usually present without attendant compromise in function or clinical disease. However, when recurrent external otitis or hearing impairment results, surgical removal is indicated. Canalplasty has significant advantages over commonly employed transmeatal approaches by maximizing conservation of canal skin and providing surgical access to the anterior medial zone of the canal. Complications are infrequent, but attention to the anatomy of the chorda tympani and facial nerve pathways and careful drill technique in the area of the tympanic membrane are important.

Although surgical techniques involving the external auditory canal have had little attention compared with other reconstructive procedures, they should be in the armamentarium of all otologic surgeons. This technique has proved to be effective for the management of exostoses of the external auditory canal.

References

1. Adams W: The aetiology of swimmer's exostoses of the external auditory canals and of associated changes in hearing. Part I. J Laryngol 65: 133–153, 1951.
2. Harrison D: Exostosis of the external auditory meatus. J Laryngol 65: 704–714, 1951.
3. Fowler EP, Jr, Osmun PM: New bone growth due to cold water in the ears. Arch Otolaryngol Head Neck Surg 36: 455–466, 1942.
4. Rauch SD: Management of soft tissue and osseous stenosis of the ear canal and canalplasty. *In* Nadol JB Jr, Schuknecht HF (eds): Surgery of the Ear and Temporal Bone. New York, Raven Press, 1993, pp 117–125.
5. Shambaugh GE Jr, Glasscock ME III: Operations on the auricle, external meatus, and tympanic membrane. *In* Shambaugh GE Jr, Glasscock ME III (eds): Surgery of the Ear. Philadelphia, WB Saunders, 1980, pp 194–215.
6. Dibartolomeo JR: Exostoses of the external auditory canal. Ann Otol Rhinol Laryngol 88(Suppl 61): 2–20, 1979.

3

Malignancies of the Temporal Bone— Limited Temporal Bone Resection

SAM E. KINNEY, M.D.

Malignant tumors involving the external auditory canal and temporal bone present a unique challenge to otologic and head and neck oncology surgeons. The most common primary lesion involving the temporal bone is squamous cell carcinoma originating in the skin of the external auditory canal. The lesion may remain confined to this anatomic area; however, it may extend medially through the tympanic membrane and into the various recesses of the middle ear and temporal bone and petrous apex. The origin of this tumor remains a mystery, for cutaneous squamous cell carcinoma most frequently results from the effect of ultraviolet radiation from the sun. The external canal does not receive direct radiation effect, and therefore the reason for the development of this particular cutaneous lesion remains unknown.

In addition to squamous cell carcinoma, there are lesions involving the auricle, such as basal cell carcinoma, which may extend to the bony portion of the external auditory canal and into the temporal bone. This tumor presents unique challenges that will be discussed further.

Primary neoplasms of the middle ear are quite rare. There is a question as to whether primary squamous cell carcinoma originates within the middle ear. There have been reported cases of adenocarcinomas beginning in the middle ear. There is also a series of adenomatous tumors of the middle ear that have been thought to be a form of adenocarcinoma of the middle ear. Primary connective tissue tumors of the ear, such as sarcomas, angiosarcomas, and rhabdomyosarcomas, are rare and carry a very poor prognosis.

Accurate assessment of therapeutic options for treating malignancy requires a staging system, the most commonly used being the tumor-node-metastasis (TNM) classification. To evaluate treatment modalities of squamous cell carcinoma of the ear canal and temporal bone an accurate TNM classification must be designed. Problems inherent in the system have been ameliorated with the advent of the newer imaging technologies. However, the accuracy of the staging system remains poor for patients with squamous cell carcinoma of the external auditory canal and temporal bone.

The first step in developing a TNM staging classification is careful physical examination. Most commonly a patient presents with pain in the ear associated with bloody drainage. The external auditory canal is examined under the microscope with attention to the extent of the lesion and involvement of the medial external auditory canal at the level of the tympanic membrane. The lesion is frequently granular in appearance, although it may present as an ulcer in the skin reaching to the periosteum of the bony portion of the canal. Because it is often confused with a form of external otitis, it may have undergone medical treatment. It is imperative that all physicians recognize that external otitis responds quickly to medical treatment with rapid resolution of pain. When pain persists, one should consider the possibility of a malignancy, particularly in an elderly patient. Biopsy should be done if there is doubt as to the nature of the lesion. If a patient referred with a negative biopsy still has evidence of an ulcer or granulation tissue as well as pain, biopsy should be repeated. The lesion is often circumferential when first identified, and its medial extent cannot be seen by physical examination.

A complete head and neck examination is performed, with particular care taken to evaluate the parotid gland. A firm lesion in the parotid gland can indicate direct extension of the tumor from the external auditory canal anteriorly. It may also represent a metastatic lesion into the superficial or deep lobe of the parotid gland. Careful examination is performed to evaluate the upper cervical jugular lymph nodes. The postauricular chain of lymph nodes off the mastoid tip must also be carefully examined. Direct spread or metastasis to this chain of lymph nodes may occur with a posterior lesion.

A complete cranial nerve examination of the head and neck should be performed. The most frequently involved cranial nerve from squamous cell carcinoma of the ear canal and temporal bone is the facial nerve. The nerves of the jugular foramen, including IX, X, and XI, may also be involved. Involvement of the third division of the fifth cranial nerve suggests extension of the tumor into the glenoid fossa along the floor of the middle fossa.

Imaging studies of the temporal bone are performed to evaluate soft tissue and bone involvement. The most consistently valuable imaging study is a high-resolution computed tomography (CT) scan with bone algorithm to identify changes within the bone of the external auditory canal or middle ear. Magnetic resonance imaging (MRI) scans enhanced with gadolinium may be of some benefit. Extension of tumor to the dura of the middle or posterior fossa may be seen on MRI scans. Digital subtraction angiography or interventional angiography may be of value in determining the extent of the lesion.

Upon completion of the entire head and neck examination and the imaging studies, an attempt is made to preoperatively stage the extent of the lesion. To date the accuracy of the imaging studies has not been confirmed by the intraoperative findings. Imaging studies do not show histologic involvement of the fissures of Santorini. Imaging studies may demonstrate soft tissue extension into the middle ear, which may represent neoplasm or the inflammatory response that so often accompanies the neoplasm. The preoperative evaluation and imaging studies may be a prognostic indicator based on an extensive tumor involvement of the temporal bone and skull base. If there is erosion to the dura of the middle or posterior fossa or involvement of the carotid jugular spine or glenoid fossa, the neoplasm would be staged as a T3 or T4 lesion. The prognosis for this patient's survival is very poor for all types of treatment modalities.

En bloc resection of the temporal bone is a sound principle of oncology. It is based on the ability to remove the entire tumor with clear, normal tissue margins around the tumor. Because of the inability to accurately define the extent of the tumor, attempts at en bloc resection result in one of the planes of resection transgressing the tumor mass. This necessitates further removal of tumor and normal tissue in a piecemeal fashion; therefore, the principle of en bloc resection becomes invalid. En bloc resection of the temporal bone involves significant morbidity and potential intraoperative mortality. This is because of the direct involvement of cranial nerves by the surgical resection and potential for major vascular catastrophes in the intraoperative period as well as the major difficulty of potential cerebrospinal fluid (CSF) leaks. The latter, combined with infection, may result in a terminal intracranial event.

The limitation of imaging studies in providing an accurate diagnosis of the extent of tumor will, in a significant number of cases, result in violation of the tumor with en bloc resection. Intraoperative morbidity and mortality of en bloc resection of the temporal bone mandate a more conservative approach to surgery, followed by postoperative radiation therapy. The agressive total removal of the tumor followed by irradiation provides effective control of tumor and significantly improved quality of life for the patient with a squamous cell carcinoma of the external auditory canal or middle ear.

PATIENT SELECTION

The average age of patients who develop squamous cell carcinoma of the external auditory canal is 62 years. These individuals may also have other medical conditions that may make a major surgical procedure more complicated; these need to be evaluated in the process of patient selection. The patients most frequently are experiencing severe pain that is not well controlled with medical treatment. Therefore, surgery becomes necessary both to control the lesion and to improve the patient's quality of life. Radiation therapy as the primary method of treatment may be effective temporarily in controlling pain; however, its long-term control of the primary neoplasm has not been found to be satisfactory.

There are specific lesions for which an attempt at formal temporal bone resection may be the only sur-gical option. Patients with such lesions include those who have residual disease following full radiation therapy as well as some in whom the disease has developed in a previous modified or radical mastoid-ectomy cavity. The attempt to remove these lesions without formal temporal bone resection would be unsatisfactory. If the lesion is identified early and confined to the external auditory canal without involvement of the tympanic membrane and middle ear or without extensive bone involvement of the external auditory canal, a lateral temporal bone resection or external auditory canal resection may be curative.

The limited temporal bone resection of squamous cell carcinoma of the external auditory and middle ear involves removal of the lesion as well as extensive removal of all gross tumor that is identified intraoperatively. This may include complete resection of the glenoid fossa, condyle of the mandible, base of the skull, and under the floor of the middle fossa, including the middle meningeal artery and the third division of the fifth cranial nerve. It may involve removal of the entire jugular bulb, carotid jugular spine, and, in some instances, the carotid artery itself preceded by balloon occlusion by interventional radiography. Resection of the entire skull base of the occiput to the foramen magnum may be necessary in an attempt to control spread of the tumor. Following total gross tumor resection the operative field is covered with a vascularized tissue flap, either muscle or free flap; afterward, full therapy radiation is administered to the involved field.

The lateral temporal bone or external auditory canal resection can be used as an important adjunct in managing other lesions that may not have their primary origin in the external auditory canal but that may originate either on the auricle or in the parotid gland and extend to the external canal. The external canal resection becomes a margin of normal tissue resection in order to control the lesion. Primary tumors of the parotid gland that extend posteriorly may require resection of the external auditory canal and the condyle of the mandible as a normal margin to control the extent of the lesion.

Basal cells carcinomas that have extended into the external auditory canal may best be controlled by resection of the bony portion of the canal with the tympanic membrane, malleus, and incus in order to provide a medial margin for these often difficult lesions. In all instances the extent of the resection is controlled by intraoperative frozen-section margin control.

Adenomatous tumors of the middle ear are quite rare. The patient presents with a blocked feeling in the ear and a conductive hearing loss; upon examination a mass is identified behind the eardrum. A mass that does not have the appearance of a cholesteatoma or the pulsatile character of a typical glomus tumor should be considered in the differential diagnosis to be an adenomatous tumor of the middle ear. A search of the literature suggests that opinions regarding the nature of this tumor have varied over time. Most pathologists propose that it is a benign tumor that can have aggressive local invasion. There have been suggestions that it is a low-grade adenocarcinoma. Most often, adenomatous tumors of the middle ear can be controlled with conservative therapy. This includes an intact canal wall tympanoplasty with mastoidectomy performed in such a way that all reaches of the middle ear mastoid epitympanum and eustachian tube can be examined; this may require resection of the malleus and incus. In most instances the tumor can be carefully dissected away from the stapes. This tumor has a high incidence of residual disease; therefore, the surgeon, both in the operative planning and in the preoperative counseling of the patient, should indicate the need for a planned second-stage evaluation of the middle ear and mastoid to make sure that there is no residual disease. The planned second-stage procedure can be performed approximately 1 year following the initial procedure. If there is no evidence of residual disease, a reconstruction of the middle ear transformer mechanism can be performed at that time.

PREOPERATIVE EVALUATION AND PATIENT COUNSELING

As noted earlier, following the complete head and neck examination, imaging studies are performed. The high-resolution CT scan with bone algorithm is the most important study, for it gives an evaluation of the bony structures of the temporal bone as well as soft tissue extension of the neoplasm within the structures of the temporal bone. When examining the scans, the first area of concern is the integrity of the bony portion of the external auditory canal. Invasion into the bone would place the tumor in a T2 or T3 classification.

An extensive lytic lesion involving the bony portion of the external auditory canal may carry a poor prognosis. If the lytic lesion has extended inferiorly, tumor may have reached into the space between the inner and outer tables of the skull base. The small likelihood of resecting this entire lesion makes the prognosis quite poor. A lytic lesion extending inferiorly in the external auditory canal may also go directly to the carotid jugular spine, suggesting tumor involvement of both the jugular vein and the carotid artery. Extension of tumor superiorly into the epitympanic space may suggest involvement of the middle fossa dura; extension posteriorly may suggest involvement of the

posterior fossa dura. In most instances, dura is a strong barrier against direct extension of squamous cell carcinoma. The tumor may spread along the surface of the dura, making resection of dura with a normal dural margin less likely, in either a lateral or a formal temporal bone resection.

The MRI scan may be of value in patients with extensive lesions. Involvement of the dura of the middle fossa seen on MRI scan may indicate direct extension of the tumor into the temporal lobe. This finding may be misleading, for there can be brain reaction around the tumor without direct extension of the tumor into the brain substance; this can be determined only during the operative procedure.

If the CT scans suggest involvement of the skull base in the area of the carotid jugular spine, or anteriorly in the middle ear to involve the carotid artery in its petrous portion, it may be advisable to attempt resection of the carotid artery. In this instance an interventional radiology procedure to temporarily occlude the carotid artery proximal to the ophthalmic artery may demonstrate the adequacy of collateral cross circulation and identify risk factors in the resection. This procedure is more likely to be considered in a younger patient. To date, however, there is minimal evidence to suggest that carotid artery resection, either as a part of an extended lateral temporal bone resection or as a part of a formal temporal resection, will improve control of the primary tumor.

Preoperative staging of the lesion, based on imaging studies, has been outlined previously. It is important to note that findings at surgery will often change the preoperative staging into a different level of intraoperative staging, with significant change of prognosis based on these findings.

It is important to counsel the patient as to the nature of the lesion and the necessity for surgical resection followed by planned postoperative radiation therapy. The emphasis is placed on planned postoperative radiation therapy, for experience has shown that if the radiation therapy is not given in a planned postoperative course or is delayed until there is evidence of residual or recurrent disease, its effectiveness in the patient with recurrent disease is very slight. In stage I disease, with the tumor limited to the external auditory canal without extensive bone invasion, an external auditory resection with skin grafting of the resultant cavity produces a 5-year survival rate of better than 90 per cent.

Stage II disease with limited extension into the bone of the external auditory canal and limited extension into the middle ear, treated with a lateral temporal bone resection followed by a full course of radiation therapy, results in a survival rate at 5 years of approximately 90 per cent. Stage III and stage IV disease with involvement of the medial wall of the middle ear, middle fossa dura, jugular bulb, and carotid artery, have a 5-year survival of less than 50 per cent. Experience has shown that if a stage III or stage IV squamous cell carcinoma of the external auditory canal and middle ear is not controlled by surgery combined with radiation therapy, the patient's survival will be less than 6 months.

SURGICAL TECHNIQUE

Although the surgical team may have only a head and neck surgeon with otologic surgical experience, it may include an otologist-neurotologist, head and neck surgeon, and, in some instances, a neurosurgeon. The team approach to dealing with these extensive lesions has proved most effective. Particular expertise can be brought to bear on the patient's problem by individual members. The operative procedure is performed under general anesthesia. The anesthesiologist will most often choose to place monitoring lines, including central venous catheters as well as arterial catheters, in order to observe the patient carefully throughout the procedure. This is particularly important in older patients and in those in whom major vascular structures are thought to be at risk as the result of the operative procedure.

The patient is placed on the operating table in the supine position as for otologic surgery, with foot-to-head reversed so that circulating nurses can have access to the controls of the table without disturbing the operative field. This position also allows the otologic portion of the procedure to be performed with the surgeon seated while having access to equipment under the end of the table. An indwelling bladder catheter is used to allow anesthesia personnel to monitor fluid balance. This also allows the intraoperative use of urea or mannitol to give greater intracranial access, should this become necessary as part of the surgery.

Facial nerve monitoring may be performed during the procedure. This procedure requires careful anatomic identification of the facial nerve, in both the temporal bone and the parotid gland. The potential risk to the facial nerve will have been described previously to the patient during preoperative counseling. In some instances, facial nerve alteration is to be expected as a result of the surgery. Perioperative antibiotics are not used unless it is anticipated that CSF will be encountered in the course of the procedure. In that case, antibiotics can be instituted at that time and continued for approximately 48 hours postoperatively. The use of steroids and diuretics would depend on the need to perform extensive intracranial surgery in order to resect the limits of the lesion.

The patient's head is rotated away from the involved ear toward the anesthesia personnel, who are positioned at the side of the table approximately two thirds of the way down from the head. The otologic nurse can sit directly in front of the patient's face. The patient's head is not placed in point fixation, for in these cases prolonged use of fixed brain retraction is not necessary. The patient's head is extended, possibly with a roll under the shoulders in order to expose the superior portion of the jugular digastric lymph nodes. The patient's head is prepared to include potential extension of the incision into the middle and posterior fossa as well as extension of the incision across the mastoid tip along the anterior border of the sternocleidomastoid muscle in order to expose the superior cervical lymph nodes. If a preoperative physical examination has suggested positive lymph nodes, the entire neck is exposed for the possibility of a formal radical neck dissection. The draping is also carried forward to the lateral canthus of the eye so that the flap elevation can include the entire parotid gland.

If it is anticipated that a regional flap, such as a pectoralis myocutaneous flap, will be necessary to cover the surgical site, this area is also included in the preoperative preparation. An area of the lower abdomen to obtain fat to obliterate dead space may also be prepared as may a site for a free microvascular flap positioned to obliterate a large surgical defect.

Instrumentation for this procedure is similar to that for otologic surgery, in addition to the instruments for radical neck dissection and possible free flap transfer. An oval burr approximately 4mm in diameter may be useful in expediting the epitympanic dissection over the ossicles into the temporal mandibular joint and eustachian tube. The operative plan is determined by the surgical team. The head and neck surgeon begins the procedure so that the operative field is clean and not involved with the bone dust.

A wide postauricular incision is performed as shown in Figure 3–1. This incision is carried approximately three fingerbreadths posterior to the auricle and approximately three to four fingerbreadths superior to the auricle, giving a wide base to the anterior portion of the flap. Care is taken not to limit the vascular pedicles anteriorly because there will be a hole in the center of the flap as the result of the tragal-conchal incisions on the lateral aspect of the external auditory canal. The incision is carried to the mastoid tip inferiorly so that it may be extended down along the anterior border of the sternocleidomastoid muscle in order to identify the structures in the superior neck.

The incision is carried down through the skin and subcutaneous tissues. If violation of CSF is anticipated, the incision should be made in two separate layers to include the deep layer of fascia and periosteum; a watertight seal can be accomplished when the wound is closed. The temporalis muscle is left in place with its blood supply originating underneath the zygomatic arch so that it may be used as a rotational flap at the conclusion of the procedure. A separate incision is made to outline the resection of the tragus and a portion of the conchal cartilage (see Fig. 3–1). This incision is carried down to the bone of the external auditory canal. Upon completion of this incision the external canal can be oversewn so that there is no spillage of cancer cells. If the entire auricle is involved and a complete auriculectomy is anticipated, the incisions may be modified to a pre- and postauricular Y-type incision or a circumferential incision, which must be closed with regional or distant vascularized flaps.

The postauricular flap is then elevated across the mastoid. Upon reaching the external auditory canal, it is elevated away from the tragal-conchal incision. The flap is elevated forward across the surface of the superficial lobe of the parotid gland. Approaching the mastoid tip from inferiorly, the facial nerve may be identified as it exits the temporal bone and may be traced out into the substance of the parotid gland for later removal of the superficial lobe of the parotid gland.

The ear canal resection portion of the procedure is performed next by the otologic surgeon. A complete mastoidectomy is performed as shown in Figure 3–2. The lateral dural sinus and middle fossa tegmen are identified. All the air cells in the mastoid down to the labyrinth are removed. The retrofacial air cells are opened primarily to examine this area for gross tumor. The external auditory canal is thinned, and the facial nerve is identified just inferior to the horizontal semicircular canal and traced to the stylomastoid foramen.

Figure 3–3 is a close-up view of the major portion of the bony resection of the external auditory canal. The facial recess is opened widely, identifying the annulus of the tympanic membrane as well as the chorda tympani nerve. Facial recess dissection is carried inferiorly and anteriorly to the facial nerve, sacrificing the chorda tympani nerve. Care is taken to recognize that the narrowest space in the facial recess is between the facial nerve and the annulus at the most posterior portion of the annular ring. From that point inferiorly the annulus will be moving medially at a rapid pace, and dissection must be carried significantly more medially in order to stay posterior to the tympanic annulus.

Using larger cutting burrs, the entire tympanic bone lateral to the facial nerve and inferior to the residual external auditory canal is removed. This dissection is carried forward into the temporal mandibular joint. The hypotympanic dissection is then performed by continuing to follow the annulus around inferiorly, remaining medial to the annulus and removing all bone of the inferior portion of the tympanic bone. As the surgeon proceeds medially the jugular bulb may

become apparent; as the surgeon moves forward the carotid artery will be identified. The dissection is carried forward along the external auditory canal until it completely joins the soft tissues of the temporal mandibular joint. The dissection is carried medially through the hypotympanum to the anterior wall of the mesotympanum medial to the bony annulus and the carotid artery. This portion of the dissection is important in order to obtain complete removal of the bony annulus at the time that it is fractured across the anterior wall of the middle ear.

The epitympanic resection is then performed by removing the bone between the dura of the middle fossa and the retained external auditory canal. Dissection is carried lateral to the body of the incus and the head of the malleus. As the dissection is carried forward the dura tends to dip inferiorly; therefore, the dissection must stay close to the curvature of the external auditory canal. The dissection is carried forward inferiorly until it again joins the soft tissues of the temporal mandibular joint. Anterior to the head of the malleus the dissection is carried medially into the anterior epitympanum and forward from the anterior epitympanum until it joins the eustachian tube medial to the tympanic annulus. In this dissection, care must be taken not to drop too medial, for the geniculate ganglion lies in the floor of the anterior epitympanum and can be inadvertently injured at that point.

With completion of both the hypotympanic and the epitympanic dissections, the final bar of bone separating the facial recess from the fossa incudis is carefully removed. The incudostapedial joint is separated, the tensor tympani tendon is cut, and the superior ligamentous attachments of the body of the incus and the head of the malleus and the anterior mallear ligament are cut. Gentle pressure is then placed with the thumb against the bony external auditory canal. If the hypotympanic and epitympanic dissections have been completed accurately and with minimal pressure, the anterior wall of the middle ear will fracture across the carotid artery, thus releasing the entire external auditory canal, tympanic membrane, malleus, and incus. The bony portion of the external auditory canal is then carefully separated from the soft tissues of the temporal mandibular joint using heavy Mayo scissors. There is often brisk bleeding from the parotid gland that can be controlled using bipolar coagulation. The external canal resection is then left attached to the superficial lobe of the parotid gland.

The entire bony tip of the mastoid has been removed in this procedure. The facial nerve can be traced out of the stylomastoid foramen to its anatomic direction into the parotid gland. The external canal and superficial lobe of the parotid gland can then be elevated off the facial nerve (see Fig. 3–3). The speci-

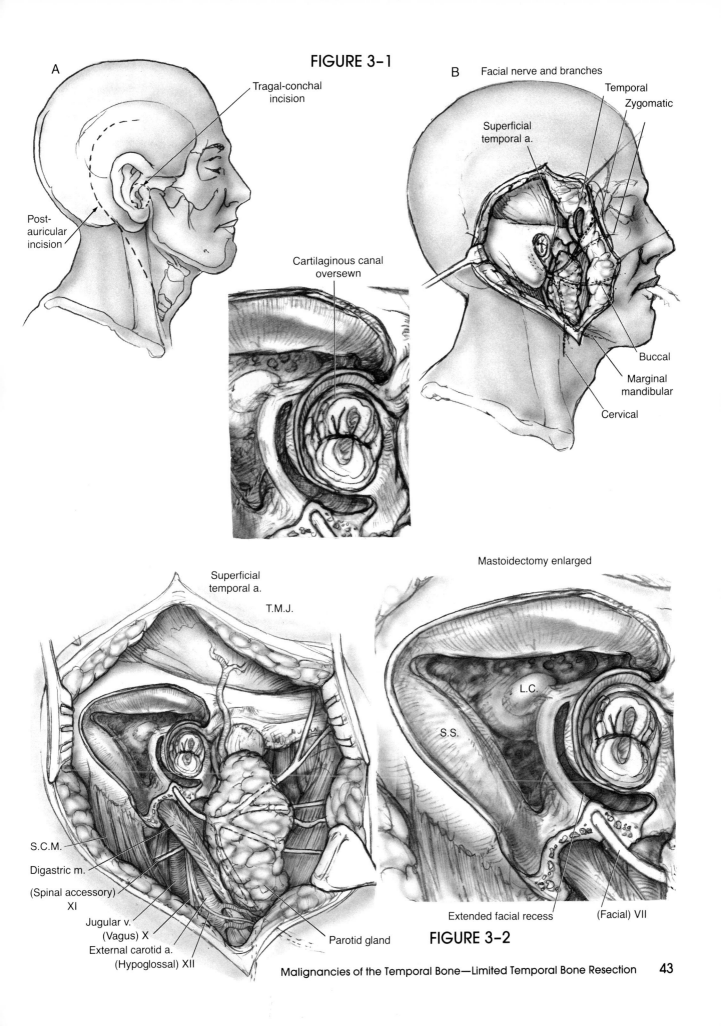

FIGURE 3-1

A

Tragal-conchal incision

Post-auricular incision

Cartilaginous canal oversewn

B Facial nerve and branches

Superficial temporal a.

Temporal

Zygomatic

Buccal

Marginal mandibular

Cervical

Superficial temporal a.

T.M.J.

Mastoidectomy enlarged

L.C.

S.S.

S.C.M.

Digastric m.

(Spinal accessory) XI

Jugular v. (Vagus) X

External carotid a. (Hypoglossal) XII

Parotid gland

Extended facial recess

(Facial) VII

FIGURE 3-2

Malignancies of the Temporal Bone—Limited Temporal Bone Resection   **43** men is removed with the external canal attached to the superficial lobe of the parotid gland.

Throughout the external canal resection the surgeon observes carefully for potential extension of the tumor outside the external canal. Particular notice is taken as the fissures of Santorini are approached anteriorly, for this may be a route of growth of the tumor. If there is direct extension of the tumor anteriorly, the soft tissues of the temporal mandibular joint, including the articular cartilage disk, are removed. The condyle of the mandible may be removed as an anterior margin of the tumor. If the tumor extends into the glenoid fossa, the middle fossa dura is followed forward, removing the bone of the glenoid fossa and sacrificing the middle meningeal artery and the third division of the fifth cranial nerve as necessary. If the tumor has extended to the middle fossa dura, the neurosurgeon can perform a bone flap craniectomy of the middle fossa using the Midas Rex drill. The dura of the middle fossa is then elevated until the tumor is encountered. The dura is further elevated in an attempt to identify a free margin of uninvolved dura medially. It may be necessary to resect the superior petrosal sinus in order to obtain a free tumor margin.

On occasion, the tumor will extend along the middle fossa dura deep to the petrous apex toward the clivus. In this case, the chances of completely removing the tumor begin to diminish significantly. If the tumor has extended to the posterior fossa dura, the entire lateral sinus can be uncovered of bone and the posterior fossa dura resected away from the tumor, again searching for a medial free margin of dura with which to attach a dural graft. If there is direct invasion of the cochlea or semicircular canals, these can be removed using the otologic drills until normal bone has been identified. If the facial nerve has been involved by the tumor, it can be resected segmentally, and a nerve graft from the great auricular or sural nerve may be placed from the tympanic bone segment to the parotid gland. If the tumor involves the stylomastoid foramen, the surgeon must have a high suspicion that this tumor will extend along the periosteum of the skull base. The tumor may extend into the plane between the outer and inner tables of the calvarium over the occiput. The tumor resection continues until the surgeon believes that no gross tumor remains. If the tumor extends into the carotid jugular spine, a decision may be made to sacrifice the jugular vein and jugular bulb. This would imply involvement of the carotid artery and a decision to occlude it; resection of the carotid artery may be made in specific cases. The principle remains constant: total removal of all gross tumor.

If the tumor appears to be confined to the external auditory canal, but the lesion was tightly packed into the anterior sulcus against the tympanic membrane, a decision may be made to perform a deep lobe parotidectomy as shown in Figure 3–4. The facial nerve may be completely mobilized off the deep lobe and the deep lobe dissected free off the masseter muscles as a second specimen.

Following the total removal of tumor the incision can be extended along the anterior border of the sternocleidomastoid muscle to expose the high jugular digastric chain of lymph nodes. If nodes are identified, they may be sent for frozen-section sampling (Fig. 3–5). The head and neck surgeon decides whether microscopic involvement of lymph nodes needs to be controlled with a radical neck dissection or by full therapy irradiation. If the lesion in the external auditory canal was located on the posterior and inferior canal wall, the surgeon must examine the area posterior to the mastoid tip and attempt to identify microscopic involvement of lymph nodes so that this area can be included in the radiation therapy field. If there are grossly positive lymph nodes in the neck, the incisions may be extended further inferiorly and a modified or formal radical neck dissection performed.

When total gross tumor removal, removal of the superficial and/or deep parotid lobes, and sampling of the superior cervical nodes have been completed, the plan for closure and postoperative irradiation therapy is determined. If the preoperative CT scan suggested a stage I lesion and the intraoperative findings did not suggest extension beyond the bony external canal, with an intact tympanic membrane, a decision may be made not to give postoperative irradiation with the potential of a 95 per cent chance of control of the primary lesion. A split-thickness skin graft is placed over the opening created by resection of the tragus and a portion of the conchal cartilage. It is depressed in its center until it completely fills the mastoid cavity and represents a graft over the middle ear, and it may come in contact with the capitulum of the stapes. The graft is then sutured to the resection line of the tragal-conchal incisions and gently held in place with gauze strip packing. Under these circumstances a split-thickness skin graft heals very effectively in the mastoid cavity. This is thought to be the result of removal of the cerumen gland system by the soft tissue canal resection. If the graft heals well and the lesion appears to be under control, a secondary procedure can be performed to install the middle ear transformer to improve hearing.

If a decision has been made either by the preoperative staging or by intraoperative findings to give the patient full therapy postoperative irradiation, it is most appropriate to sacrifice the attempt at reconstruction of hearing in order to cover the temporal bone with a vascularized flap of tissue. The long-term effects of osteoradionecrosis of the temporal bone and petrous apex in cases in which there is no covering of

FIGURE 3-3

Ear canal and superficial parotid gland removed

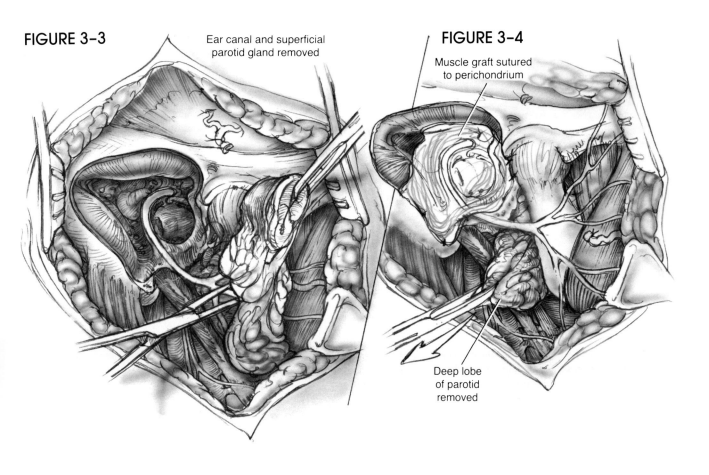

FIGURE 3-4

Muscle graft sutured to perichondrium

Deep lobe of parotid removed

FIGURE 3-5

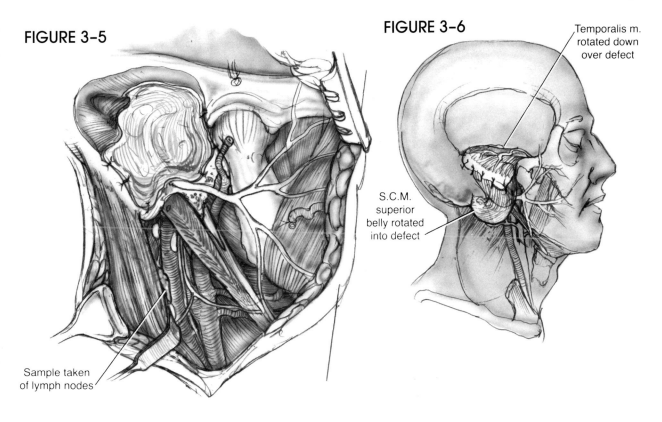

Sample taken of lymph nodes

FIGURE 3-6

Temporalis m. rotated down over defect

S.C.M. superior belly rotated into defect

vascularized free tissue can create complications that may become life-threatening. This includes loss of dura and resultant CSF leaks.

As shown in Figure 3–6 the temporalis muscle may be mobilized from its attachments along the linea temporalis and the superior temporal line and left attached at its insertion under the root of the zygoma with its associated blood supply. This flap can be rotated down to obliterate the mastoid cavity in the area of the tragal-conchal incision. The incision can then be covered with a split-thickness skin graft. It is also possible to mobilize the superior aspect of the sternocleidomastoid muscle. The sternocleidomastoid muscle receives its blood supply in three segments; if one attempts to detach the muscle at the clavicle and rotate the entire muscle superiorly, the blood supply to the more inferior portion of the muscle will be poor and the flap may not survive. A pectoralis myocutaneous flap may reach the area of the temporal bone as well as a trapezius flap rotated from posteriorly. If the soft tissue loss in the dead space obliteration seems to be extensive, a microvascular free flap from the rectus abdominis may be used to obliterate this space. It is important that viable tissue be used to cover the temporal bone in patients in whom postoperative irradiation therapy is to be delivered. If there has been no entrance into the CSF space, positive suction drain catheters are placed dependently in the wound in order to remove accumulated tissue fluids.

Once the wounds are closed and flaps placed into position, a formal mastoid ear dressing (or possibly other forms of dressings that would allow inspection and protection of a flap) may be chosen based on the recommendations of the head and neck surgeon. If there has been entrance into the CSF space, it is important that the eustachian tube be completely obliterated by removing the mucosa and tightly packing the eustachian tube with a free muscle graft. In these circumstances it is often important to use tissue to obliterate an opening into the dura. This may be abdominal fat or muscle or a free flap. Gentle pressure over the wound for a minimum of 3 days using a mastoid dressing may help prevent CSF from forming a pseudomeningocele under the flap.

The decision to use antibiotics postoperatively is based primarily on the entrance into the CSF space. Postoperative care of patients with lateral temporal bone resection is quite simple. If there has been involvement of the facial nerve, immediate eye care must be instituted. This may include patching of the eye and use of artificial tears and ointments. If the facial nerve has been resected and not regrafted, a decision to provide eye care (such as the implantation of a gold weight in the upper eyelid and a tensing of the lower eyelid by shortening at the lateral canthus) may be carried out, most often by an ophthalmologist.

The combination of the gold weight implant and tensing of the lower eyelid provides better protection as well as better appearance than the standard lateral tarsorrhaphy. If there was extensive involvement of the tumor in the jugular foramen, there may be paresis or paralysis of the ninth or tenth cranial nerve. Care must be taken to protect the airway and also provide nutrition, most often temporarily, through a nasogastric tube or possibly a longer term nutritional line through a percutaneous endoscopic gastrostomy, as determined in the postoperative period.

The greatest problem in surgery for squamous cell carcinoma of the external auditory canal and middle ear is removal of all gross tumor. In difficult cases with involvement of the deep petrous apex, the skills of the otologic surgeon, head and neck surgeon, and neurosurgeon must be brought to bear for complete removal of gross tumor. If the surgical team cannot remove all the gross tumor at the time of surgery, the patient's prognosis for salvage with radiation therapy is almost nonexistent.

The results of lateral temporal bone resection followed by total gross removal of all tumor and full therapy irradiation have been encouraging; however, they are not always successful. Great inconsistencies have been noted when the preoperative staging has been compared with the postoperative staging based on the intraoperative and histopathologic findings. Approximately 50 per cent of cases staged as a T1 or T2 tumor based on imaging studies were staged as T3 or T4 tumors at the time of surgery and histopathologic examination. This fact has led many surgeons to choose the lateral temporal bone resection approach as opposed to the formal temporal bone resection even though this is recognized as a violation of standard oncologic surgical procedures.

T1 lesions of the external auditory canal treated with a canal resection without postoperative radiation therapy have approximately a 95 per cent 5-year survival rate. The T2 lesions and some T3 lesions, in which total tumor removal has been obtained and the patient is given full therapy irradiation, have approximately an 85 per cent 5-year survival. For more extensive T3 and T4 lesions the 5-year survival drops below 50 per cent to approximately 43 per cent. Survival may also be altered by the histology of the tumor. Rare examples of verrucous carcinoma and carcinoma in situ may be staged as T3 or T4 lesions preoperatively. With total tumor removal followed by postoperative irradiation therapy, however, the prognosis may be quite good. Nevertheless, undifferentiated squamous cell carcinoma that has reached the dura, the carotid jugular spine, or the periosteum of the skull base will have limited potential for cure and survivability.

It is to be noted that patients with a T4 lesion by

imaging studies preoperatively have a very poor prognosis. However, palliative surgery using the lateral temporal bone resection approach, without the associated morbidity and mortality of a formal temporal bone resection, may be indicated. This may offer the patient a significant period of pain relief. Survival in these cases is often less than 6 months.

Postoperative irradiation is planned in conjunction with the radiotherapist. As noted earlier, the operative plan should include covering of the temporal bone by viable vascularized tissue in order to avoid potential for osteoradionecrosis in long-term survival cases. Radiation therapy portals are determined by the findings at the time of surgery and include not only the temporal bone but also the area of the parotid gland and neck region. Radiation is usually given in divided doses with portals to avoid injury to the central nervous system (CNS) structures. The dosage ranges from 5000 to 6500 rads, based on the recommendation of the radiotherapist. It is important that the decision to give radiation therapy be part of the planned treatment program and not reserved for an attempt to salvage a recurrence following the surgical procedure. The ability of radiation therapy to control the primary tumor or a recurrence has been demonstrated to be quite poor. On occasion, in a younger person with an aggressive undifferentiated squamous cell carcinoma, the treatment plan may include consultation with an oncologic physician for the purpose of giving chemotherapy. The role of chemotherapy in controlling squamous cell carcinoma of the temporal bone has not been determined. The incidence of the lesion is sufficiently small that entering these patients into a protocol that might help determine the effectiveness of chemotherapy has not been possible.

The lateral temporal bone resection associated with total gross tumor removal followed by irradiation therapy as a treatment for squamous cell carcinoma has been chosen for the following reasons. The imaging studies available have not yet been able to accurately diagnose the extent of tumor. Nor are they able to differentiate the presence of neoplasm and an inflammatory reaction resulting from the infection associated with the neoplasm. The lateral temporal bone resection with total gross tumor removal violates standard oncologic principles of en bloc resection. However, attempts at total temporal bone resection with en bloc tumor resection have a high incidence of transgression of the tumor, a situation that is based on the inability to accurately determine the extent of tumor with preoperative evaluations. Total temporal bone resection may once again become the procedure of choice if advances in imaging technology make possible the differentiation of tissue types. The surgical techniques for performing temporal bone resection are improving at a rapid pace. The time may come when total temporal bone resection can be performed with a level of morbidity and mortality that is acceptable and comparable to lateral temporal bone resection followed by gross tumor removal and postoperative irradiation therapy.

Bibliography

Arena S, Keen M: Carcinoma of the middle ear and temporal bone. Am J Otol 9(5): 351–356, 1988.

Arriaga M, Curtin H, Takahashi H, et al.: Staging proposal for external auditory meatus carcinoma based on preoperative clinical examination and computed tomography findings. Ann Otol Rhinol Laryngol 99(9.1): 714–721, 1990.

Benecke JE Jr, Noel FL, Carberry JN, et al.: Adenomatous tumors of the middle ear and mastoid. Am J Otol 11(1): 20–26, 1990.

Crabtree JA, Britton BH, Pierce MK: Carcinoma of the external auditory canal. Laryngoscope 86: 405–415, 1976.

Eby TL, Makek MS, Fisch U: Adenomas of the temporal bone. Ann Otol Rhinol Laryngol 97(6.1): 605–612, 1988.

Howard JD, Elster AD, May JS: Temporal bone: Three-dimensional CT. Part II, Pathologic alterations. Radiology 177(2): 427–430, 1990.

Kinney SE, Wood BG: Malignancies of the external ear canal and temporal bone: Surgical techniques and results. Laryngoscope 97: 158–164, 1987.

Lewis JS: Temporal bone resection. Arch Otolaryngol 101: 23–25, 1975.

Mafee MF, Valvassori GE, Kumar A, et al.: Tumors and tumor-like conditions of the middle ear and mastoid: Role of CT and MRI. An analysis of 100 cases. Otolaryngol Clin North Am 21(2): 349–375, 1988.

Meyerhoff WL, Mickey BE, Roland PS, Drummond JE: Magnetic resonance imaging in the diagnosis of temporal bone and skull base lesions. Am J Otol 10(2): 121–137, 1989.

Sataloff RT, Roberts BR, Myers DL, Spiegel JR: Total temporal bone resection—A radical but life-saving procedure. AORN J 48(5): 932–948, 1988.

Wiatrak BJ, Pensak ML: Rhabdomyosarcoma of the ear and temporal bone. Laryngoscope 99(11): 1188–1192, 1989.

4

Malignancies of the Temporal Bone— Radical Temporal Bone Resection

SANJAY PRASAD, M.D.
IVO P. JANECKA, M.D.

Primary malignancies of the temporal bone were first recognized in the late eighteenth century and histologically confirmed in the 1850s. By 1974, 250 cases had been reported in the English literature,[1] and the reported prevalence of the disease was six cases per million population.[2] The median age of presentation is 55 years, and there is a tendency for the disease to involve females,[1] although the reason for the latter remains unclear.

Based on the primary site of involvement, these lesions are divided into two types: those that involve the external ear, thought to be secondary to actinic exposure, such as basal cell carcinoma, and those that involve the external auditory canal, middle ear, and petrous apex, such as squamous cell carcinoma. Unlike squamous cell carcinoma of the upper aerodigestive tract, squamous cell carcinoma of the temporal bone does not appear to be related to tobacco or alcohol abuse. Temporal bone cancer also rarely metastasizes to regional and distant sites.

Multimodality treatment employing surgery and radiation therapy appears to be the best treatment. The efficacy of chemotherapy has not been clearly established, and it may play a role only in recalcitrant disease.

Lateral temporal bone resection (LTBR) involves the resection of the external auditory canal, tympanic membrane, malleus, and incus. Subtotal temporal bone resection (STBR) involves the additional removal of the otic capsule, whereas a total temporal bone resection (TTBR) involves the removal of the petrous apex in addition to the otic capsule.

LTBR is well accepted for T1 or T2 lesions; however, controversy arises in defining the optimal management of more extensive neoplasms. Some authors advocate LTBR with gross removal of middle ear disease followed by radiation therapy, whereas others prefer more radical surgery, namely STBR or TTBR, followed by radiation therapy. Cancerous invasion of the dura mater, brain parenchyma, and internal carotid artery (ICA) portend a poor prognosis, and the value of resection of these structures is unclear.

This chapter focuses on preoperative diagnostic evaluation, the surgical techniques of STBR and TTBR, postoperative management, and potential complications. Rehabilitation and adjuvant treatment for recalcitrant disease are briefly discussed. At the conclusion, we present a literature review of squamous cell carcinoma of the temporal bone in an effort to define the optimal management for middle ear disease and the prognostic significance of dural, brain, and ICA involvement.

DIAGNOSTIC EVALUATION

A thorough history and physical examination are imperative, with emphasis on the chronology of developing cranioneuropathies. The pathway of tumor spread can be deduced from a careful history. Facial nerve function and hearing should be carefully documented. The examination includes palpation of the parotid gland and cervical lymph glands for the presence of local spread and regional metastases, respectively. Patients should be questioned and tested for temporal lobe signs (e.g., memory loss, dysphasia, left-sided neglect, hemiparesis, and olfactory hallucinations) and cerebellar signs (e.g., dysmetria, truncal ataxia, nystagmus, and dysdiadochokinesia).

Imaging allows determination of the extent of tumor involvement. High-resolution axial and coronal computed tomographic imaging at 1.5mm intervals delineates the areas of bony involvement, and enhanced and unenhanced magnetic resonance imaging further delineates intracranial involvement.

Histologic confirmation of the lesion is essential in further treatment planning. The most accessible and expedient route for biopsy should be sought in every case. Malignant lesions, such as squamous cell carcinoma, adenoid cystic carcinoma, basal cell carcinoma, and ceruminous adenocarcinoma, should be treated in accordance with the extent of disease. The goal should be surgical extirpation of all visible tumor. Benign lesions, such as pleomorphic adenoma and ceruminous adenoma, require more conservative measures.

Angiography is used when involvement of the major vessels is suspected on preoperative imaging, or when surgical exposure of the petrous carotid artery is anticipated. Embolization of feeding vessels may reduce intraoperative blood loss, and the venous phase of the study can provide important information regarding blood flow through the dural venous sinuses.

Cerebral blood flow evaluation is indicated when involvement of the ICA is present. The patency of the anterior and posterior communicating arteries can be seen on angiography, but the sole use of this evaluation has proved inadequate. Our method of preoperative carotid artery testing is briefly described.[3]

A combination of temporary balloon occlusion (TBO) of the ICA and xenon computed tomographic cerebral blood flow measurements has allowed identification of patients who will most likely tolerate carotid artery sacrifice. Transfemoral introduction of a nondetachable intravascular balloon, inflated in the ICA, is performed in the awake patient while assessment of sensory, motor, and higher cortical function is made. Five per cent of the patients have a reversible neurologic deficit during the 15-minute period of oc-

clusion. These patients are at high risk for stroke following carotid sacrifice unless preoperative or intraoperative extracranial-to-intracranial arterial bypass is considered. These patients are thought to have a cerebral blood flow of less than 15ml per 100g per minute on the occluded side. Ninety-five per cent of the patients pass this portion of the test and are then studied using xenon computed tomography. The balloon is deflated, and the patient is transported to the computed tomographic scanner, where she or he inhales a mixture of 32 per cent stable xenon to 68 per cent oxygen for 4 minutes 20 seconds. A cerebral blood flow study is then obtained, first with temporary ICA occlusion and again 15 minutes later after the vessel is reopened. Several mirror-image zones of the brain are evaluated for changes in cerebral blood flow. In each hemisphere, three sections that are 1cm thick and separated by the same distance are evaluated. These are considered to represent the anterior, middle, and posterior arterial circulation.

Twenty-five per cent of the patients have a cerebral blood flow of 15 to 30ml per 100g per minute on the occluded side. These patients are at mild-to-moderate risk for stroke following permanent ICA occlusion. These patients tolerate temporary ICA occlusion, and a saphenous vein graft should be used to reconstruct the carotid artery at the time of sacrifice.

Seventy per cent of the patients have a cerebral blood flow over 35ml per 100g per minute on the occluded side, and these patients are at low risk for stroke following permanent ICA occlusion, provided a long "distal" stump is avoided. Hypotension and hypovolemia in the perioperative period should be avoided if permanent ICA occlusion is performed.

PREOPERATIVE PREPARATION

Preoperative preparation sets the stage for the operative and postoperative course. The evening before surgery, the operative site is shampooed and scrubbed with hexachlorophene. Intravenous phenytoin or phenobarbital, along with cefuroxime, is begun as prophylactic anticonvulsant and antibiotic measures. Communication between the surgeon and anesthesiologist is of vital importance in regard to airway management (intubation or tracheostomy) and the potential need for barbiturate or etomidate coma for cerebral protection in patients with a dominant carotid system or in those at mild-to-moderate risk for stroke. Barbiturates decrease cerebral metabolic demand, cause shunting of blood toward ischemic areas, and decrease intracranial pressure. The level of coma is titrated to cause burst suppression on the electroencephalogram when temporary occlusion of the carotid artery is performed. To facilitate intraoperative cranial nerve monitoring, short-acting neuromuscular blocking agents are used only for the induction of anesthesia and are not used during the operation.

On the morning of the operation, sequential compression stockings are placed on both legs to lessen chances of development of thromboembolic disease from venostasis. Following insertion of a central venous catheter and arterial line, the patient is intubated, and the endotracheal tube is secured by a circumdental or circummandibular wire. The operating table is then turned 90° from the anesthesiologist, giving him or her access to the contralateral arm. Somatosensory evoked potentials and electroencephalographic recording electrodes are placed in the scalp and secured. The head is positioned on a horseshoe (Mayfield) head holder to allow repositioning during the course of the operation. Temporary bilateral tarsorrhaphies are placed to prevent corneal abrasions. The operative site, which includes the temporal fossa, lateral half of the face, postauricular area, and neck as well as the ipsilateral thigh and lower leg (for the potential use of the tensor fascia lata, greater saphenous vein, and sural nerve), is shaved and scrubbed with an iodine-based solution. Bipolar facial electromyographic electrodes are placed in areas where facial function exists.

SURGICAL PROCEDURE

Incisions vary according to the extent of the tumor (Fig. 4–1). For lesions contained within the temporal bone, a C-shaped incision extending from the temporal fossa, postauricularly into the neck, and a blind-sac closure of the external auditory canal are employed. When the tumor is suspected to be in the vicinity of the conchal cartilage or periauricular skin, an appropriate skin island is incorporated into the overall design. The external auditory canal skin is then sutured shut to avoid tumor spillage. The outline of the incisions must preserve the blood supply to the remaining auricle.

The anterior and posterior skin flaps are elevated (Fig. 4–2A). The superficial temporal fat pad is elevated with the anterior skin flap in a subperiosteal plane over the zygomatic arch. The superficial temporal and middle temporal arteries are ligated. Management of the facial nerve varies according to the involvement of the parotid gland. When the gland may be involved, peripheral branches of the facial nerve are identified, with the help of the facial nerve monitor, and divided. The stumps of the anterior segments are secured to the anterior skin flap. The entire parotid gland is then dissected off the masseteric fascia, provided that the latter is free of disease and is mobilized posteriorly while the attachment to the ex-

ternal auditory canal is maintained. When the parotid is suspected to be free of tumor, the facial nerve trunk is located in the usual manner at the tympanomastoid suture and divided. The parotid gland along with the distal stump of the facial nerve is dissected free of the external auditory canal and mobilized anteriorly off the masseteric fascia.

The jugulodigastric region is then explored, and cervical lymph nodes are sent for frozen section pathologic analysis. The presence of regional metastases determines the need for a formal cervical lymphadenectomy. The uninvolved portion of cranial nerve XI, the greater auricular nerve, or cervical cutaneous nerves are harvested for use as cable grafts for facial nerve reconstruction. Cranial nerves IX, X, XI, and XII, the internal jugular vein, and the external and internal carotid arteries are dissected in a superior direction toward the temporal bone. The sternocleidomastoid and digastric muscles are detached from their attachment to the mastoid.

From this point, release of the masseter from its attachment to the zygomatic arch allows exposure for zygomatic and mandibular osteotomies (Fig. 4–2A). The meniscus of the temporomandibular joint is separated from the glenoid fossa, and the chorda tympani nerve emerging from the petrotympanic fissure is divided. The stylomandibular and sphenomandibular ligaments are divided and allow removal of the mandibular segment (Fig. 4–2B). The temporalis muscle is then elevated in a subperiosteal fashion and reflected inferiorly. The temporalis muscle must be separated from the lateral pterygoid muscle, and care should be taken not to injure the deep temporal arterial blood supply to the temporalis muscle. The lateral and medial pterygoid muscles are then resected either en bloc with the specimen or separately, depending on carcinomatous invasion. In a subperiosteal fashion, the contents of the infratemporal fossa are elevated off the floor of the middle fossa to expose the middle meningeal artery and vein in the foramen spinosum and the mandibular division of the trigeminal nerve in the foramen ovale. The contents of the foramen spinosum are bipolarly coagulated and divided. Frequently, the venous plexus of the foramen ovale requires bipolar coagulation and packing with oxidized cellulose. Infrequently, the lesser petrosal nerve may be seen emerging from a separate foramen, known as the innominate canal, on its way to the otic ganglion.

The stylohyoid, stylopharyngeus, and styloglossus muscles (Riolan's bouquet) are detached from the styloid process, which is then rongeured away. The branches of the external carotid artery are then dissected in the infratemporal fossa. The anterior tympanic and deep auricular branches of the internal maxillary artery are often divided before identification and may require bipolar coagulation. Unless it is diseased, the internal maxillary artery is preserved up to the branches of the deep temporal artery. When the internal maxillary artery must be sacrificed, brisk backflow from the anterior stump indicates that the temporalis muscle may derive its blood supply from reversed flow via the pterygoid system. If brisk backflow is not observed, the temporalis muscle cannot be relied on to reconstruct the surgical defect, and microvascular free flap options must be explored. The cartilaginous eustachian tube is divided and the anterior end sutured closed to prevent postoperative cerebrospinal fluid rhinorrhea (Fig. 4–3A).

The ICA is then dissected toward the carotid canal, and care is taken not to injure cranial nerve IX, which crosses its anterior surface. With Kerrison rongeurs, the vertical and horizontal petrous segments of the carotid artery are exposed to the precavernous segment (Fig. 4–3B). Occasionally, bleeding from the pericarotid venous plexus requires bipolar coagulation. The caroticotympanic artery is also divided when the petrous carotid artery is separated from the specimen. The extent of petrous carotid mobilization depends on whether an STBR or a TTBR is performed. When an STBR is performed, the vertical petrous carotid artery is mobilized from the carotid foramen and canal. When a TTBR is performed, the vertical and horizontal petrous carotid artery is mobilized to the foramen ovale.

A temporal craniectomy is then performed, and the intracranial portion of the middle meningeal vessels is coagulated (Fig. 4–3B). The patient is hyperventilated to keep the P_{CO_2} at 25mm Hg for adequate brain relaxation. Mannitol, furosemide, and dexamethasone can impart greater brain relaxation, if needed. Subtemporal dural elevation proceeds in a posterior to anterior direction. The greater superficial petrosal

---

FIGURE 4–1. Incisions vary according to whether or not the tumor is contained in the temporal bone.

FIGURE 4–2. *A*, The facial nerve can be divided peripherally at the distal branches or centrally at the facial nerve trunk, depending on involvement of the parotid gland. *B*, Following osteotomies and removal of the zygomatic arch and mandibular segments, dissection in the infratemporal fossa continues.

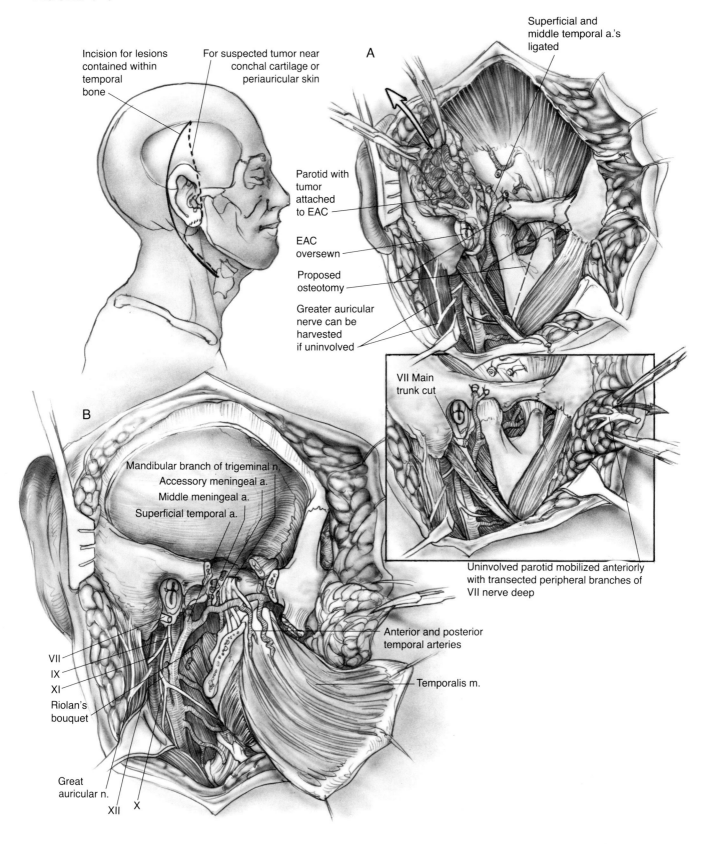

FIGURE 4-1

FIGURE 4-2

Incision for lesions contained within temporal bone

For suspected tumor near conchal cartilage or periauricular skin

Superficial and middle temporal a.'s ligated

A

Parotid with tumor attached to EAC

EAC oversewn

Proposed osteotomy

Greater auricular nerve can be harvested if uninvolved

VII Main trunk cut

Uninvolved parotid mobilized anteriorly with transected peripheral branches of VII nerve deep

B

Mandibular branch of trigeminal n.
Accessory meningeal a.
Middle meningeal a.
Superficial temporal a.

Anterior and posterior temporal arteries

Temporalis m.

VII
IX
XI
Riolan's bouquet

Great auricular n.

XII   X

FIGURE 4-3

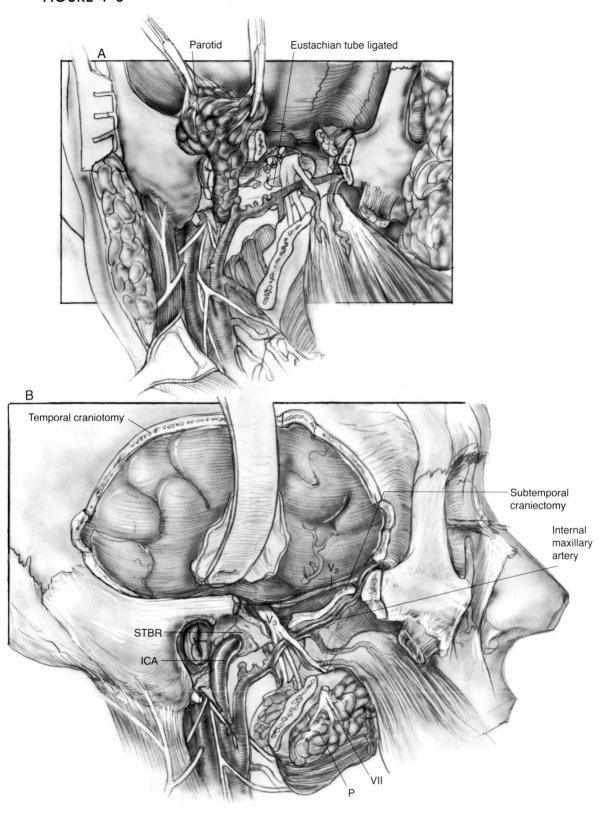

Parotid

Eustachian tube ligated

A

B

Temporal craniotomy

Subtemporal craniectomy

Internal maxillary artery

V₂

V₃

STBR

ICA

VII

P

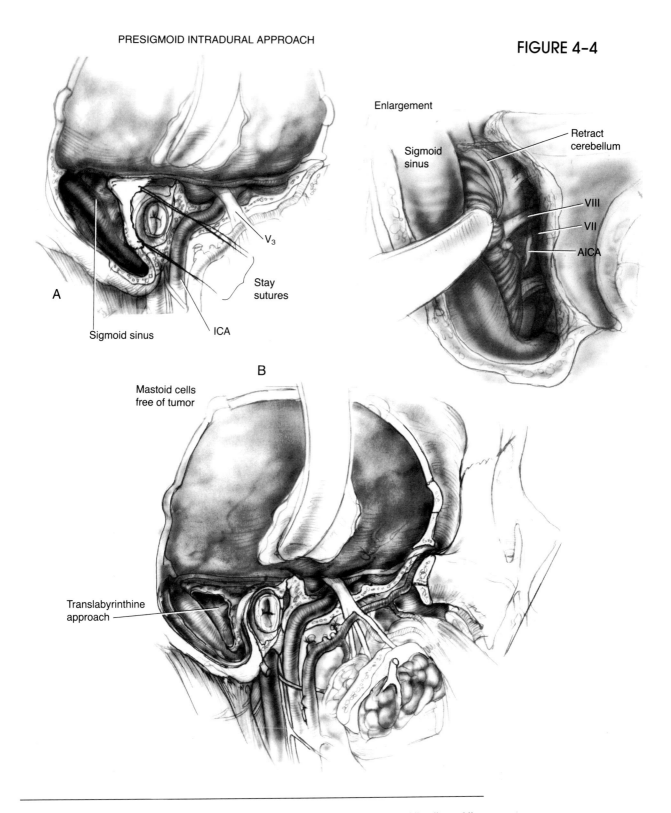

FIGURE 4-3. *A*, Further dissection in the infratemporal fossa allows division and ligation of the eustachian tube and exposure of the petrous carotid artery. *B*, The petrous carotid artery is further dissected according to whether a subtotal or total temporal bone resection is performed.

FIGURE 4-4. *A*, When tumor is thought to be present in the mastoid, a presigmoid intradural approach to the porus acusticus is used. *B*, When the mastoid is thought to be free of tumor, a translabyrinthine approach allows exposure of the internal auditory canal.

Malignancies of the Temporal Bone—Radical Temporal Bone Resection   55 nerve and accompanying petrosal artery to the geniculate ganglion are coagulated and divided to lessen traction on the geniculate ganglion. Similarly, the lesser petrosal nerve and superior tympanic artery are also divided. Subtemporal dural elevation then proceeds as far medially as possible to expose the superior petrosal sinus. When carcinomatous involvement of the middle fossa dura is suspected, an intradural approach keeps the involved dura attached to the specimen.

The extent of the mastoidectomy depends on whether tumor is present in the mastoid air cells. Care is taken to avoid exposure of tumor in the mastoid. In this case, the Midas Rex drill with the M-3 and M-8 dissecting tool is used to thin the bone over the confluence of the transverse, sigmoid, and superior petrosal sinuses. The bone over the sigmoid sinus and jugular bulb is also thinned. With a Freer or Cottle elevator, these sinuses are further decorticated to expose posterior fossa dura on either side of the sigmoid sinus. When posterior fossa dural involvement is suspected, a presigmoid intradural approach with retraction of the cerebellum (Fig. 4–4A) allows exposure to the vessels and nerves of the porus acusticus and internal auditory canal (IAC) while the involved dura is kept attached to the specimen. When the mastoid air cells are thought to be free of tumor, a translabyrinthine approach to the IAC is used (Fig. 4–4B). The anterior inferior cerebellar artery is retracted after the labyrinthine artery is bipolarly coagulated and divided. The superior and inferior vestibular nerves, cochlear nerve, facial nerve, and nervus intermedius (nerve of Wrisberg) are divided. A segment of the proximal facial nerve stump can be sent for frozen section pathologic examination if it is suggestive of carcinoma. The dome of the jugular bulb must be separated from the specimen when the dural venous sinuses are spared.

The surgical technique from here varies according to whether the internal jugular vein/dural venous sinuses or the ICA is preserved. When both are preserved and an STBR is being performed, an osteotome is inserted at the bony canal of the carotid artery at the junction of the vertical and horizontal segments (Fig. 4–5A). The osteotome is then aimed toward the fundus of the IAC. The petro-occipital synchondrosis

will sometimes require insertion of an osteotome just above the jugular bulb. This step releases the specimen en bloc from the attachment to the clivus. Bleeding from the inferior petrosal sinus can be controlled by intraluminal packing with oxidized cellulose. When both vascular structures are preserved and a TTBR is being performed, the osteotome is inserted at the posterior edge of the foramen ovale and aimed slightly posteriorly to avoid entry into the foramen lacerum (Fig. 4–5B). The petro-occipital synchondrosis may require an additional osteotomy before the specimen will be released.

When the dural venous sinuses are sacrificed, the internal jugular vein is double-ligated in the upper cervical area and mobilized toward the jugular bulb (Fig. 4–6). The superior petrosal sinus and sigmoid sinus are divided and intraluminally packed with oxidized cellulose. Care is taken not to overpack the sigmoid sinus proximally to avoid obstruction of the vein of Labbé, which can cause a hemorrhagic necrosis of the temporal lobe. Similarly, excessive packing of the inferior petrosal sinus can lead to cavernous sinus thrombosis. The sigmoid sinus is then opened toward the jugular bulb, which is then resected. Intraluminal rather than extraluminal packing of the inferior petrosal sinus is preferred to avoid injury to cranial nerves of the jugular foramen.

The results of the temporary balloon occlusion and xenon test determine whether the involved ICA can be safely resected. When the patient is at high risk for stroke following sacrifice of the ICA, the patient will require revascularization to ensure adequate cerebral blood flow. An extracranial-to-intracranial arterial bypass, such as a superficial temporal artery to middle cerebral artery bypass, must be considered. When the patient is at mild-to-moderate risk for stroke following ICA sacrifice, the carotid artery must be reconstructed with a saphenous vein bypass graft. The graft can run from the carotid bifurcation in the neck to the precavernous segment or to the supraclinoid segment, if the cavernous sinus appears involved with tumor. Hypothermia to 32° to 35°F and barbiturate or etomidate coma can decrease the cerebral metabolic rate during the period of occlusion. Pharmacologically, the systolic blood pressure is also kept at 20mm Hg to 30mm Hg above the normotensive state to ensure ad-

FIGURE 4-5. *A,* An osteotome, inserted at the junction of the vertical and horizontal petrous carotid canal, is aimed toward the fundus of the internal auditory canal to allow removal of the subtotal temporal bone specimen. *B,* An osteotome, inserted at the horizontal petrous carotid canal just posterior to the foramen ovale, is directed slightly posteriorly to avoid entry into the foramen lacerum. This releases the total temporal bone specimen.

FIGURE 4-6. When the dural venous sinus is sacrificed, the internal jugular vein is mobilized toward the cranial base as the sigmoid sinus is intraluminally packed.

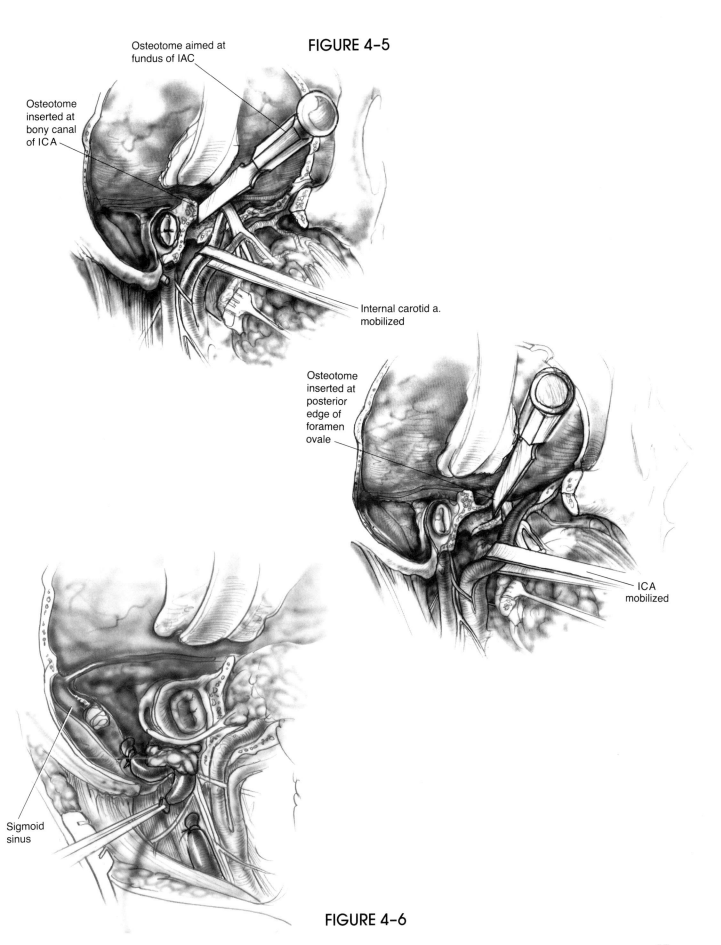

FIGURE 4-5

Osteotome aimed at
fundus of IAC

Osteotome
inserted at
bony canal
of ICA

Internal carotid a.
mobilized

Osteotome
inserted at
posterior
edge of
foramen
ovale

ICA
mobilized

Sigmoid
sinus

FIGURE 4-6

Malignancies of the Temporal Bone—Radical Temporal Bone Resection   57 equate cerebral blood flow through the contralateral carotid artery during the period of occlusion. When the patient is at low risk for stroke following ICA testing, the ICA is sacrificed either preoperatively, by permanent balloon occlusion of the ICA, or intraoperatively, by clipping of the supraclinoid ICA prior to the ophthalmic artery branch. The latter procedure requires a frontotemporal craniotomy with a transsylvian and subfrontal approach for exposure of the supraclinoid segment.

The middle and posterior fossa dura is then inspected for carcinomatous involvement, any involved areas are resected, and margins are sent for frozen-section pathologic examination. The temporal lobe and cerebellum are also examined, and limited involvement of the inferior temporal gyrus and cerebellum is resected. Once intradural hemostasis is achieved, the dura is then closed in a watertight fashion using pericranium, fascia lata, or cadaveric dura, depending on the size of the defect.

Reconstruction includes restoration of facial nerve continuity and filling of the surgical defect. The greater auricular, cervical cutaneous, or eleventh cranial nerve can be used as a cable graft from the facial nerve in the IAC to the peripheral branches. When greater length is required, the sural nerve can be harvested from the lower leg. Use of vascularized tissue, rather than autogenous fat grafts, is preferred to fill in the surgical defect. The temporalis muscle is rotated into the defect, and a split-thickness skin graft can be used over this for cutaneous defects. A small bolus dressing is placed to ensure adequate adhesion. When the temporalis is not available, microvascular free flaps are placed by the plastic surgery team. Jackson-Pratt drains are installed under the neck and scalp skin flaps to ensure tissue coaptation.

POSTOPERATIVE CARE

At extubation in the operating room, the patient is examined for unanticipated neurologic deficits, which are further studied by computed tomographic imaging to determine the presence of intracranial edema or bleeding. Intravenous contrast can help assess the patency of the saphenous vein graft or repaired ICA.

Antibiotics are continued postoperatively until the drains are removed or if an infectious process dictates otherwise. Anticonvulsant levels are carefully monitored and kept in the therapeutic range for 3 to 6 months. Dexamethasone is continued for 48 hours and then tapered over 5 days.

When the ICA has been sacrificed, great care is taken to avoid even minor hypotensive and hypovolemic periods. These events can reduce the cerebral blood flow through the remaining contralateral carotid artery and lead to cerebral ischemia.

Intermittent spinal drainage, through a lumbar drain installed at the end of the procedure, reduces the pressure in the subarachnoid space and accelerates healing of dural defects. Continuous spinal drainage can cause overdrainage and pneumocephalus and is not used. Fifty milliliters of spinal fluid is drained every 8 hours for 48 hours. The drain is then clamped for 24 hours and removed, provided that no evidence of cerebrospinal fluid leakage is noted.

POTENTIAL COMPLICATIONS

Inadvertent carotid artery injury is managed by local pressure to the site of entry with placement of temporary clips on either side. After systemic heparinization, the tear is examined, irrigated with heparinized saline, and repaired using 8-0 Novofil sutures. Prior to placement of the last suture, the lumen is irrigated with heparinized saline to clear any clots. The hemoclips are then released, and any minor leaks are managed with oxidized cellulose. If the tear is beyond repair, then the results of the preoperative temporary balloon occlusion and xenon test dictate further management.

Transient loss of somatosensory evoked potential waveforms during the course of the operation may indicate excessive temporal lobe retraction. Persistent loss of waveforms usually results from either detached recording electrodes or a high concentration of inhalation anesthetic. Blood pressure and carotid pulsations must also be checked. When all these factors are ruled out, sustained loss of somatosensory evoked potentials can be an ominous sign.

ADJUVANT TREATMENT

The treatment of temporal bone malignancies extending into the middle ear should consist of surgical resection of all visible disease followed by external-beam radiotherapy. Occasionally, large, aggressive tumors invading brain parenchyma, the dominant carotid artery, or dural venous sinus are encountered, and total tumor removal is not possible without serious neurologic deficits. In these instances, brachytherapy catheters have been inserted and localized radiotherapy used.

REHABILITATION

Facial palsy following temporal bone resection requires careful assessment and treatment. A temporary tarsorrhaphy at the conclusion of the operation af-

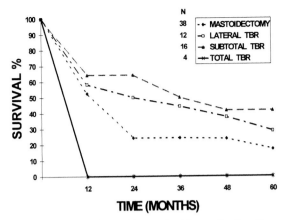

FIGURE 4-7. Treatment-specific survival for patients with carcinoma extending to involve the middle ear. (From Prasad S, Janecka IP: Efficacy of surgical treatments for squamous cell carcinoma of the temporal bone. Otol Head Neck Surg 110:270–280, 1994.)

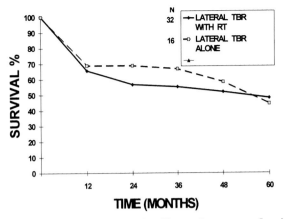

FIGURE 4-8. Survival of patients with carcinoma confined to the external auditory canal treated with LTBR with or without preoperative or postoperative radiation therapy. (From Prasad S, Janecka IP: Efficacy of surgical treatments for squamous cell carcinoma of the temporal bone. Otol Head Neck Surg 110:270–280, 1994.)

fords early corneal protection. Once the periorbital edema subsides, a gold-weight implant in the upper eyelid can offer long-term corneal protection. Elderly patients may also require lower-eyelid tightening procedures. Facial nerve recovery can be expected at 12 to 18 months. The best facial function a patient can expect with a cable graft, in our hands, is a House-Brackmann grade III.

Excessive packing of the inferior petrosal sinus can lead to lower cranial nerve dysfunction (IX, X, XI), which can be a debilitating handicap. Some patients require temporary tracheostomy and gastrostomy, and others will suffice with polytetrafluoroethylene (Teflon) injection of the vocal fold or an Isshiki thyroplasty.[4]

FOLLOW-UP

Patients are seen every month for the first year, and repeat imaging (computed tomography and magnetic resonance imaging) is obtained at 6 months and yearly thereafter. Enhancing tumors are best visualized by contrast-enhanced fat-suppression magnetic resonance imaging, which helps differentiate transposed flaps from tumor recurrence. Any suspicious areas have repeat biopsies directly or are needle-aspirated under computed tomographic guidance.

RESULTS

Temporal bone neoplasms occur infrequently, and the small experience, even at large institutions, makes analysis of treatment difficult. Because of this difficulty, we undertook a literature review of squamous cell carcinoma of the temporal bone[5] and present our findings.

All publications in the English language from 1915 to 1992 dealing with the treatment of squamous cell carcinoma of the temporal bone were reviewed. Ninety-six publications[1, 6–100] were encountered, of which twenty-six articles,[75–100] which contained information on 144 patients, were chosen for further analysis. The major reason for exclusion of a study was the lack of a descriptive table in which the extent of disease, type of treatment, and follow-up for each patient was carefully documented.

Several conclusions about overall survival can be made. When disease was confined to the external auditory canal, no statistically significant difference in 5-year survival was found between patients treated with LTBR (48.6 per cent) those treated with STBR (50 per cent). When disease extended into the middle ear, patients who had STBR had better 5-year survival (41.7 per cent) than those who had LTBR (28.6 per cent) (Fig. 4–7). The experience with carcinoma that invades the petrous apex was limited. Four patients treated with TTBR had a 50 per cent 1-year survival and zero per cent 2-year survival. One patient treated with STBR was dead of disease at 1 year.

The value of preoperative or postoperative radiation therapy was also analyzed. When disease was confined to the external auditory canal, the addition of either preoperative or postoperative radiation therapy to LTBR did not significantly improve 5-year survival (48.0 per cent with radiation therapy, 44.4 per cent without radiation therapy) (Fig 4–8). This was the only group in which a conclusion could be made.

The prognostic value of dural involvement was also studied. Resection of involved dura mater, surprisingly, did not improve overall 5-year survival (11.1 per cent with or without resection). The status of the margins of resection were not reported.

Four patients had extension of disease to involve the ICA. Of the two patients treated with TTBR and

ICA sacrifice, one died from postoperative cerebral ischemia and the other was dead of disease at 14 months of regional and distant failure. The other two patients who were treated in a method that spared the ICA were dead of disease shortly after resection.

Two patients with carcinomatous invasion of the temporal lobe who were treated with limited resection were also dead of disease shortly after resection. No patient was encountered who had resection of involved cerebral or cerebellar tissue.

Site of failure was also studied. Of 54 patients who died of their disease, 45 had local failure, five had locoregional failure, three had regional failure alone, and one had regional-distant failure.

Several other aspects of this disease could not be studied because of the lack of information provided by the authors. First the histologic differentiation of the tumor and its relationship to overall survival could not be analyzed. Second, the method of temporal bone removal, whether by en bloc resection, piecemeal resection or a drillout, and its relationship to survival remains unclear. The status of the margins of resection, in this disease, and overall survival has yet to be studied.

SUMMARY

Radical resection of the temporal bone requires thorough knowledge of the intricate anatomy of the temporal bone and surrounding structures. There is no substitute for laboratory dissection prior to embarking on such an endeavor. It also requires thorough preoperative imaging, delineation of the extent of tumor involvement, and preoperative carotid artery testing, when indicated.

The indications for the operation are slowly evolving as we gain experience and collate data for analysis. From our literature review,[5] it appears that cancerous involvement of the middle ear is best treated by STBR rather than LTBR with gross removal of middle ear disease. Once the tumor involves the petrous apex, we believe that TTBR can allow total tumor extirpation and possibly prolonged survival, although the latter remains to be proved. Prospective, randomized studies will be needed to define the value of margin-free dural, carotid artery, and brain parenchymal resection. The value of adjunctive radiation therapy for extensive lesions will also require further study.

References

1. Johns ME, Headington JT: Squamous cell carcinoma of the external auditory canal: A clinicopathologic study of 20 cases. Arch Otolaryngol Head Neck Surg 100: 45–49, 1974.
2. Kinney SE: Tumors of the external auditory canal, middle ear, mastoid and temporal bone. In Thawley SE, Panje WR, Batsakis JG, Lindberg RD (eds): Comprehensive Management of Head and Neck Tumors. Philadelphia, WB Saunders, 1987, p 182.
3. Janecka IP, Sekhar LN, Horton JA, Yonas H: Cerebral blood flow evaluation. In Cummings CW, Frederickson JM, Harlor LA, et al. (eds): Otolaryngology Head and Neck Surgery Update II. St. Louis, Mosby Year Book, 1990, pp 54–63.
4. Sasaki CT, Leder SB, Petcu L, Freidman CD: Longitudinal voice quality changes following Isshiki thyroplasty Type I: The Yale experience. Laryngoscope 100: 849–852, 1990.
5. Prasad S, Janecka IP: Efficacy of surgical treatments for squamous cell carcinoma of the temporal bone. Otol Head Neck Surg 110:270–280, 1994.
6. Campbell E, Volk BM, Burkland CW: Total resection of the temporal bone for malignancy of the middle ear. Ann Surg 134: 397–404, 1951.
7. Coleman CC, Khuri A: A rational treatment for advanced cancer of the external ear and temporal bone. VA Med Monthly 86: 21–24, 1959.
8. Hutcheon JR: Experiences with aural carcinoma over the past six years. Med J Aust 2:406–407, 1966.
9. Figi FA, Weisman PA: Cancer and chemodectoma in the middle ear and mastoid. JAMA 156: 1157–1162, 1954.
10. Wang CC: Radiation therapy in the management of carcinoma of the external auditory canal, middle ear or mastoid. Ther Rad 116: 713–715, 1975.
11. Sinha PP, Aziz HI: Treatment of carcinoma of the middle ear. Ther Rad 126: 485–487, 1978.
12. Boland J: The management of carcinomas of the middle ear. Radiology 80: 285, 1963.
13. Holmes KS: The treatment of carcinoma of the middle ear by the 4MV linear accelerator. Proc R Soc Med 53: 242–244, 1960.
14. Yamada S, Schuh FD, Marvin JS, Perot PL: En bloc subtotal temporal bone resection for cancer of the external ear. J Neurosurg 39: 370–379, 1973.
15. Hahn SS, Kim JA, Goodchild N, Constable WC: Carcinoma of the middle ear and external auditory canal. Int J Rad Oncol Biol Phys 9: 1003–1007, 1983.
16. Sorenson H: Cancer of the middle ear and mastoid. Acta Radiol 54: 460–468, 1960.
17. Frazer JS: Malignant disease of the external acoustic meatus and middle ear. Proc R Soc Med 23: 1235–1244, 1930.
18. Barnes EB: Carcinoma of the ear. Proc R Soc Med 23: 1231–1234, 1930.
19. Conley JS: Cancer of the middle ear and temporal bone. NY State J Med 1575–1579, 1974.
20. Kinney SE, Wood BG: Malignancies of the external ear canal and temporal bone: Surgical techniques and results. Laryngoscope 97: 158–164, 1987.
21. Kinney SE: Squamous cell carcinoma of the external auditory canal. Am J Otol 10: 111–116, 1989.
22. Graham MD, Sataloff RT, Kemink J, McGillicuddy JF: En bloc resection of the temporal bone and carotid artery for malignant tumors of the ear and temporal bone. Laryngoscope 94: 528–533, 1984.
23. Clark LJ, Narola AA, Morgan DAL, Bradley PJ: Squamous carcinoma of the temporal bone: A revised staging. J Laryngol Otol 105: 346–348, 1991.
24. Corey JP, Nelson E, Crawford M, et al.: Metastatic vaginal carcinoma to the temporal bone. Am J Otol 12: 128–131, 1991.
25. Hiraide F, Inouye T, Ishii T: Primary squamous cell carcinoma of the middle ear invading the cochlea: A histopathologic case report. Ann Otol Rhinol Laryngol 92: 290–294, 1983.
26. Schusterman MA, Kroll SS: Reconstruction strategy for temporal bone and lateral facial defects. Ann Plastic Surg 26: 233–294, 1983.
27. Haughey BH, Gates GA, Skerhut HE, Brown WE: Cerebral shift after lateral craniofacial resection and flap reconstruction. Otolaryngol Head Neck Surg 101: 79–86, 1989.
28. Bergetedt HF, Lind MG: Temporal bone scintigraphy. Acta Otolaryngol (Stockh) 89: 465–473, 1980.
29. Jahn AF, Farkashidy J, Berman JM: Metastatic tumors in the temporal bone—A pathophysiologic study. J Otolaryngol 8: 85–95, 1979.
30. Ruben RJ, Thaler SU, Holzer N: Radiation induced carcinoma of the temporal bone. Laryngoscope 87: 1613–1621, 1977.

31. Katsarkas A, Seemayer TA: Bilateral temporal bone metastases of a uterine cervix carcinoma. J Otolaryngol 5: 315–318, 1976.
32. Ramsden RT, Bulman CH, Lorigan BP: Osteoradionecrosis of the temporal bone. J Laryngol Otol 89: 941–955, 1975.
33. Vize G: Laryngeal metastasis to the temporal bone causing facial paralysis. J Laryngol Otol 88: 175–177, 1974.
34. Schuknecht HF, Allam AF, Murakami Y: Pathology of secondary malignant tumors of the temporal bone. Ann Otol Rhinol Laryngol 77: 5–22, 1968.
35. Lewis JS: Temporal bone resection: Review of 100 cases. Arch Otolaryngol Head Neck Surg 101: 23–25, 1975.
36. Arriaga M, Curtin H, Takahashi H, et al.: Staging proposal for external auditory meatus carcinoma based on preoperative clinical examination and computed tomography findings. Ann Otol Rhinol Laryngol 99: 714–721, 1990.
37. Adams WS, Morrison R: On primary carcinoma of the middle ear and mastoid. J Laryngol Otol 69: 115–131, 1955.
38. Gacek RR: Management of temporal bone carcinoma. Trans Penn Acad Otolaryngol Ophthalmol 32: 67–71, 1978.
39. Conley J, Schuller DE: Malignancies of the ear. Laryngoscope 86: 1147–1163, 1976.
40. Greer JA, Body DTR, Weiland LH: Neoplasms of the temporal bone. J Otolaryngol 5: 391–398, 1978.
41. Goodman ML: Middle ear and mastoid neoplasms. Ann Otol Rhinol Laryngol 80: 419–424, 1971.
42. Arena S, Keen M: Carcinoma of the middle ear and temporal bone. Am J Otol 9: 351–356, 1988.
43. Hilding DA, Selker R: Total resection of the temporal bone for carcinoma. Arch Otolaryngol Head Neck Surg 89: 98–107, 1969.
44. Cundy RL, Sando I, Hemenway WG: Middle ear extension of nasopharyngeal carcinoma via the eustachian tube. Arch Otolaryngol Head Neck Surg 98: 131–133, 1973.
45. Lewis JS: Squamous carcinoma of the ear. Arch Otolaryngol Head Neck Surg 97: 41–42, 1973.
46. Sekhar LN, Pomeranz S, Janecka IP, et al.: Temporal bone neoplasms: A report on 20 surgically treated cases. J Neurosurg 76:578–587, 1992.
47. Lessor RW, Spector GJ, Divinens VR: Malignant tumors of the middle ear and external auditory canal: A 20 year review. Otolaryngol Head Neck Surg 96: 43–47, 1987.
48. Kenyon GS, Marks PV, Scholtz CL, Dhillon R: Squamous cell carcinoma of the middle ear: A 25 year retrospective study. Ann Otol Rhinol Laryngol 94: 273–277, 1985.
49. Arthur K: Radiotherapy in carcinoma of the middle ear and auditory canal. J Laryngol Otol 90: 753–762, 1976.
50. Tucker WN: Cancer of the middle ear. Cancer 16: 642–650, 1965.
51. Conley JJ, Novack AJ: The surgical treatment of malignant tumors of the ear and temporal bone. Arch Otolaryngol Head Neck Surg 71: 635–652, 1960.
52. Conley JJ, Novack AJ: Surgical treatment of cancer of the ear and temporal bone. Trans Am Acad Ophthalmol Otolaryngol 64: 83–92, 1960.
53. Wagenfield DJH, Keane T, Norstrand AWP, Bryce DP: Primary carcinoma involving the temporal bone: Analysis of 25 cases. Laryngoscope 90: 912–919, 1980.
54. Lewis JS, Parsons H: Surgery for advanced ear cancer. Ann Otol Rhinol Laryngol 67: 364–399, 1958.
55. Lewis JS, Page R: Radical surgery for malignant tumors of the ear. Arch Otolaryngol Head Neck Surg 83: 56–61, 1966.
56. Lewis JS: Surgical management of tumors of the middle ear and mastoid. J Laryngol Otol 97: 299–311, 1983.
57. Lederman M: Malignant tumors of the ear. J Laryngol Otol 79: 85–119, 1965.
58. Frew I, Finney R: Neoplasms of the middle ear. J Laryngol Otol 77: 415–421, 1963.
59. Goodwin WJ, Jesse RH: Malignant neoplasms of the external auditory canal and temporal bone. Arch Otolaryngol Head Neck Surg 106: 675–679, 1980.
60. Lindahl JWS: Carcinoma of the middle ear and meatus. J Laryngol Otol 69: 457–467, 1955.
61. Bradley WH, Maxwell JH: Neoplasms of the middle ear and mastoid: Report of 54 cases. Laryngoscope 54: 533–556, 1954.
62. Miller D: Cancer of the external auditory meatus. Laryngoscope 65: 448–461, 1955.
63. Colledge L: Two cases of malignant disease of the temporal bone. J Laryngol Otol 58: 251–254, 1943.
64. Peele JC, Hauser GH: Primary carcinoma of the external auditory canal and middle ear. Arch Otolaryngol Head Neck Surg 34: 254–266, 1941.
65. Garnett-Passe ER: Primary carcinoma of the eustachian tube. J Laryngol Otol 62: 314–315, 1948.
66. Spencer FR: Malignant disease of the ear. Arch Otolaryngol Head Neck Surg 28: 916–940, 1938.
67. Means RG, Gersten J: Primary carcinoma of the mastoid process. Ann Otol Rhinol Laryngol 62: 93–100, 1953.
68. Spector JG: Management of temporal bone carcinomas: A therapeutic analysis of two groups of patients and long-term follow-up. Otolaryngol Head Neck Surg 104: 58–66, 1991.
69. Ariyan S, Sasaki CT, Spencer D: Radical en-bloc resection of the temporal bone. Am J Surg 142: 443–447, 1981.
70. Arena S: Tumor surgery of the temporal bone. Laryngoscope 84: 645–670, 1974.
71. Brooker GB: Bilateral middle ear carcinomas associated with Waldenström's macroglobulinemia. Ann Otol Rhinol Laryngol 91: 299–303, 1982.
72. Towson CE, Shofstall WH: Carcinoma of the ear. Arch Otolaryngol Head Neck Surg 51: 724–738, 1950.
73. Robinson GA: Malignant tumors of the ear. Laryngoscope 41: 467–473, 1931.
74. Kinney SE, Wood BG: Malignancies of the external ear canal and temporal bone: Surgical techniques and results. Laryngoscope 97: 158–164, 1987.
75. Buckmann LT, Barre W: Carcinoma of the middle ear and mastoid. Ann Otol Rhinol Laryngol 52: 194–201, 1943.
76. Liebeskind MM: Primary carcinoma of the external auditory canal, middle ear, and mastoid. Laryngoscope 61: 1173–1187, 1951.
77. Stokes HB: Primary malignant tumors of the temporal bone. Arch Otolaryngol Head Neck Surg 32: 1023–1030, 1990.
78. Rosenwasser H: Neoplasms involving the middle ear. Arch Otolaryngol Head Neck Surg 32: 38–53, 1940.
79. Grossman AA, Donnelly WA, Smithman MF: Carcinoma of the middle ear and mastoid process. Ann Otol Rhinol Laryngol 56: 709–721, 1947.
80. Mattick WL, Mattick JW: Some experience in management of cancer of the middle ear and mastoid. Arch Otolaryngol Head Neck Surg 53: 610–621, 1951.
81. Wahl JW, Gromet MT: Carcinoma of the middle ear and mastoid. Arch Otolaryngol Head Neck Surg 58: 121–126, 1953.
82. Crabtree JA, Britton BH, Pierce MK: Carcinoma of the external auditory canal. Laryngoscope 86: 405–415, 1976.
83. Hanna DC, Richardson GS, Gaisford JC: A suggested technique for resection of the temporal bone. Am J Surg 114: 553–558, 1967.
84. Adams GL, Paparella MM, Fiky FM: Primary and metastatic tumors of the temporal bone. Laryngoscope 81: 1273–1285, 1971.
85. Sataloff RT, Myers DL, Lowry LD, Spiegel JR: Total temporal bone resection for squamous cell carcinoma. Otolaryngol Head Neck Surg 96: 4–14, 1987.
86. Nadol JB, Schuknecht HF: Obliteration of the mastoid in the treatment of tumors of the temporal bone. Ann Otol Rhinol Laryngol 93: 6–12, 1984.
87. Arriaga M, Hirsch BE, Kamerer DB, Myers EN: Squamous cell carcinoma of the external auditory meatus (canal). Otolaryngol Head Neck Surg 101: 330–337, 1989.
88. Michaels L, Wells M: Squamous cell carcinomas of the middle ear. Clin Otolaryngol 5: 235–248, 1980.
89. McCrea RS: Radical surgery for carcinoma of the middle ear. Laryngoscope 82: 1514–1523, 1972.
90. Gacek RR, Goodman M: Management of malignancy of the temporal bone. Laryngoscope 87: 1622–1634, 1977.
91. Scholl LA: Neoplasms involving the middle ear. Arch Otolaryngol Head Neck Surg 22: 548–553, 1935.
92. Clairmont AA, Conley JJ: Primary carcinoma of the mastoid bone. Ann Otol Rhinol Laryngol 86: 306–309, 1977.

93. Beal DD, Lindsay JR, Ward PH: Radiation-induced carcinoma of the mastoid. Arch Otolaryngol Head Neck Surg 81: 9–16, 1965.
94. Coleman CC: Removal of the temporal bone for cancer. Am J Surg 112: 583–590, 1966.
95. Parsons H, Lewis JS: Subtotal resection of the temporal bone for cancer of the ear. Cancer 7: 995–1001, 1954.
96. Miller D, Silverstein H, Gacek RR: Cryosurgical treatment of carcinoma of the ear. Trans Am Acad Ophthalmol Otolaryngol 76: 1363–1367, 1972.
97. Tabb HG, Komet H, McLaurin JW: Cancer of the external auditory canal: Treatment with radical mastoidectomy and irradiation. Laryngoscope 74: 634–643, 1964.
98. Lodge WO, Jones HM, Smith MEN: Malignant tumors of the temporal bone. Arch Otolaryngol Head Neck Surg 61: 535–541, 1955.
99. Ward GE, Loch WE, Lawrence W: Radical operation for carcinoma of the external auditory canal and middle ear. Am J Surg 82: 169–178, 1951.
100. Newhart H: Primary carcinoma of the middle ear: Report of a case. Laryngoscope 27: 543–555, 1917.

5

Miscellaneous External Auditory Canal Problems

MALCOLM D. GRAHAM, M.D.

MICHAEL J. LAROUERE, M.D.

External auditory canal lesions are encountered uncommonly; their recognition may be difficult; and an early and specific diagnosis is essential. The surgical management, postoperative care, and potential complications are similar for each of the following conditions.

ACQUIRED STENOSIS OF THE EXTERNAL AUDITORY CANAL

Narrowing (stenosis) or closure (atresia) of the lumen of the external auditory canal may occur after acute, subacute, or chronic external otitis owing to thickened external auditory canal skin and the resulting organization of granulation tissue within the canal. Stenosis can also ensue following burns or after chemical injury and may occur spontaneously in individuals with chronic eczematoid external otitis. In these same individuals, the prolonged use of a hearing aid mold or repeated scratching of the external auditory canal with a foreign body is a factor that can predispose to canal stenosis.

Post-traumatic stenosis or atresia[1] may occur following temporal bone or tympanic bone fractures. A temporal bone fracture may lacerate the skin of the external auditory canal and tympanic membrane; a blow to the mandibular symphysis produces a posterior movement of the condyloid process, thereby fracturing the tympanic bone, which forms the anterior wall of the osseous canal. Laceration of the skin of the external auditory canal can thus predispose the patient to the development of an external canal stenosis.

Chronic ear surgery, such as tympanoplasty with or without mastoidectomy, may result in a blunting, or thickening, of the tympanic membrane graft or a stenosis of the external auditory canal. Stenosis of the external canal meatus can occur following lateral canal incisions such as those used to perform a meatoplasty.

KERATOSIS OBTURANS

Keratosis obturans is characterized by the abnormal accumulation of epithelial debris within an expanded bony external auditory canal.[1] It frequently presents with hearing loss and pain and occasionally otorrhea. This condition is often present bilaterally and may be associated with extensive erosion of the tympanic bone inferiorly, anteriorly into the glenoid fossa, or posteriorly into the mastoid segment. The inferior fibrous annulus, facial nerve, carotid artery, and jugular bulb may be skeletonized by the bone absorption or erosion. Faulty migration of the epithelial layer of the external auditory canal has been implicated as the underlying cause of keratosis obturans.

EXTERNAL AUDITORY CANAL CHOLESTEATOMA

It is essential to distinguish this entity from keratosis obturans and to appreciate that it may occur not only spontaneously[2] but also following trauma and chronic ear surgery.[3] In its spontaneous form, skin of the external auditory canal, usually located over the medial inferior bony canal, is ulcerated, thereby exposing underlying bone. The tympanic membrane is not affected, and hearing loss is uncommon; pain and discharge, however, are frequent. The condition is usually unilateral and frequently affects the elderly.

Post-traumatic cholesteatoma of the external auditory canal unrelated to previous otologic surgery is found uncommonly. Fracture of the tympanic or temporal bone may result in stenosis or atresia of the external auditory canal with secondary accumulation of squamous epithelial and keratin debris and associated erosion of adjacent bone.[3] Following otologic surgery, ear canal cholesteatoma may be encountered as a small epithelial pearl or as a large occluding mass. This entity results from the entrapment of squamous epithelial debris during the healing process.

HERNIATION OF TEMPOROMANDIBULAR JOINT SOFT TISSUE INTO THE EXTERNAL AUDITORY CANAL

Herniation of the temporomandibular joint (TMJ) soft tissue (usually fat) into the external auditory canal may occur spontaneously[4] or following trauma such as a mandibular condyle fracture with or without dislocation. Postoperatively herniation of TMJ contents can be seen following chronic ear surgery or TMJ arthroscopy. Rarely, it is present owing to low-grade inflammation following TMJ prosthetic surgery.

Temporomandibular joint tissue herniation is usually based anteriorly and medially in the external auditory canal. It is frequently invisible when the mouth is closed and protrudes impressively when the mouth is opened. Patients are most frequently disturbed by the loud sound present in the involved ear, particularly when chewing, at which time the mass comes in contact with the tympanic membrane.

OSTEONECROSIS OF THE TYMPANIC BONE

Tympanic bone osteonecrosis may occur spontaneously in individuals with uncontrolled chronic eczematoid external otitis and particularly in one using a hearing aid mold who suffers from diabetes mellitus. This entity may also occur in those patients who have received irradiation treatment for malignant lesions of the head and neck. Those receiving radiation to the brain, temporal bone, parotid gland, and nasopharynx seem to be particularly at risk. When necrosis of the tympanic bone occurs secondary to irradiation treatment, it is termed osteoradionecrosis, and inevitably the bone involvement is extensive.

Osteonecrosis of the tympanic bone is frequently painless. The ear canal is dry; generally, some crusting is present; and a nonhealing skin ulceration is evident. If the lesion results from irradiation treatment, debris accumulation may be present with secondary infection, drainage, and pain.

SPONTANEOUS ATTICOTOMY-MASTOIDECTOMY (AUTOMASTOIDECTOMY)

A variant of attic and middle ear cholesteatoma, "spontaneous atticotomy-mastoidectomy" is encountered infrequently. Although the disease process is primarily in the tympanomastoid cleft, the clinical manifestation mimics that of external canal cholesteatoma or keratosis obturans.

This entity generally presents in an individual with no prior history of ear surgery. Deep in the ear canal, a massive accumulation of squamous debris is usually found. Usually the ear is dry and pain is infrequent. Upon removal of the debris it is apparent that there is massive erosion of the scutum and posterior external auditory canal wall, with a mastoid cavity present.

MEDICAL MANAGEMENT AND INDICATIONS FOR SURGERY

Accurate diagnosis and treatment strategies for external auditory canal problems depend on a complete and thorough examination of the canal. Appropriate instrumentation for examination includes a head mirror or headlight, otoscope, operating microscope, several sizes of ear speculums, ear curettes, microhooks, metal applicators, bayonet forceps, alligator forceps, and several sizes of suction tips.

Once cleansing has been accomplished, the diagnosis is usually readily apparent. Repeated office visits may be required for cleansing and reevaluation in the acute and subacute conditions. As long as the condition continues to improve, as manifested by lessening of debris and secretions, resorption of granulation tissue, and elimination of pain and discharge, medical management should be conservative. It must be decided whether best to treat with moist agents, such as drops or solutions, or dry materials, such as powders, creams, or ointments. Occasionally if cellulitis is present in the external auditory canal, particularly in the lateral cartilaginous portion, oral or intravenously administered antibiotics may be of value.

Stenting with expanding cellulose wicks may be very useful to dilate immature stenosis of soft tissues in the ear canal and external meatus and to deliver creams, ointments, or drops to the skin of the external auditory canal. Once the acute and subacute stages have been eliminated, the chronic status of the particular disease should be considered.

Chronic external auditory canal problems can usually be treated medically on an indefinite basis. Office visits for a period of 3 to 6 months can allow for cleansing of the ear canal. The long-term use of 50/50 white household vinegar/water irrigations and steroid cream or drops on a daily to weekly basis is helpful. If osteoradionecrosis is present secondary to previous radiation therapy directed at or around the temporal bone, it may be prudent to continue long-term conservative management rather than embark upon surgical intervention. If a large accumulation of debris or crusting continues to present a problem, surgical intervention should be considered. This is especially true in the cases of keratosis obturans and external auditory canal cholesteatoma and when a sequestrum of bone is present.

SURGICAL PRINCIPLES AND TECHNIQUE

Surgical principles may be considered collectively for these various lesions. They include the following steps:

1. Postauricular approach
2. Identification of landmarks
3. Exposure of the bony external auditory canal
4. Preservation of structures and function
5. Removal of diseased tissue or exteriorization where required
6. Tissue coverage of exposed bone
   A. Skin
      a. Graft
      b. Flap
   B. Fascia
   C. Muscle obliteration
      a. Free muscle or flap
      b. Fat
7. Stenting
   A. Dry/wet
   B. Prevention of infection
   C. Stenting short/long
   D. Meatoplasty

The postauricular surgical approach (Fig. 5–1) is recommended in order to gain adequate exposure. Identification of major lateral landmarks includes the

FIGURE 5-2

Elevate vascular strip

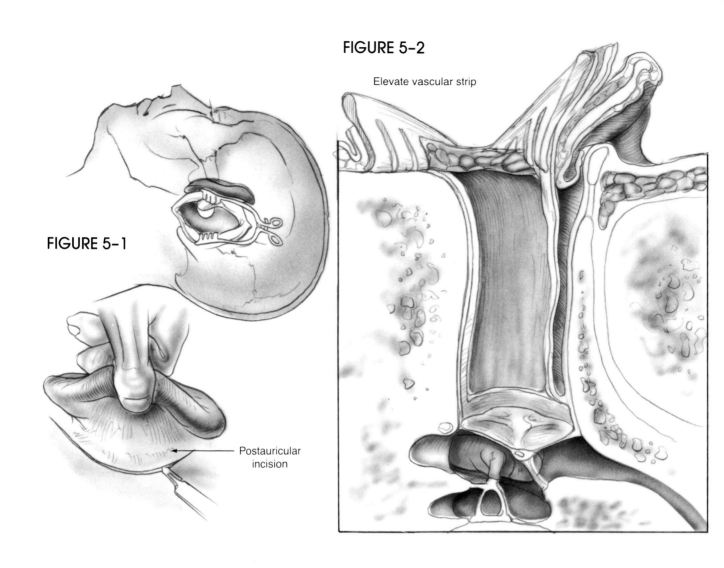

FIGURE 5-1

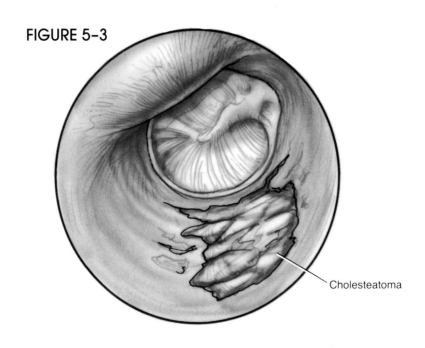

Postauricular
incision

FIGURE 5-3

Cholesteatoma

FIGURE 5-4

Mastoid tip cholesteatoma

Tympanic membrane
preserved

Cross section

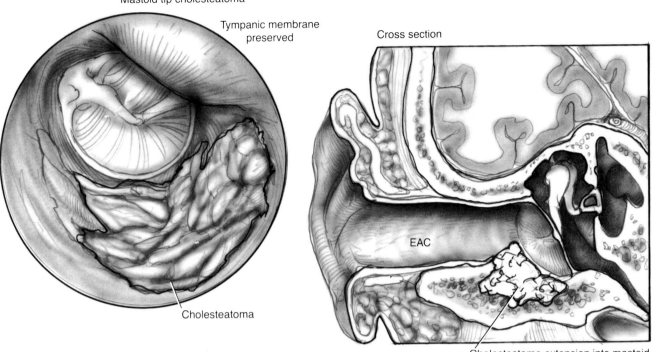

EAC

Cholesteatoma

Cholesteatoma extension into mastoid

Surgically enlarged bony canal

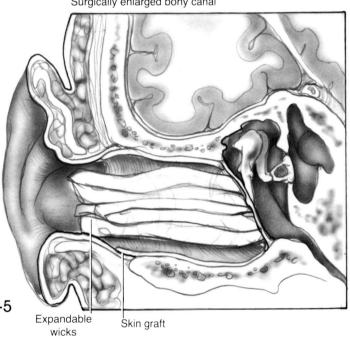

FIGURE 5-5

Expandable
wicks

Skin graft

mastoid tip, the spine of Henle, the inferior limb of the zygomatic arch, the anterior external auditory canal wall, the posterior external auditory canal wall, and the tympanic bone. Identification of these landmarks is particularly important in instances in which there has been significant bony erosion, such as in keratosis obturans, automastoidectomy, or tympanic bone fracture. Identification and preservation of deeper structures is an essential secondary step (Fig. 5–2). The tympanic membrane, ossicles, facial nerve, carotid artery, jugular bulb, and TMJ are usually normal both anatomically and functionally. The middle and posterior cranial fossa plates, digastric ridge, and horizontal semicircular canal may or may not be clearly apparent, depending upon the nature and extent of bone erosion. Having identified all major lateral and deep landmarks, one must then decide whether to remove diseased soft tissue and bone, such as in external auditory canal cholesteatoma, tympanic bone fractures, and osteonecrosis of the tympanic bone (Fig. 5–3), or to proceed with exteriorization of the epitympanum and mastoid segment, as in cases of keratosis obturans or automastoidectomy.

With removal of all diseased soft tissue and bone (Fig. 5–4), coverage of the exposed bone surfaces is now required.[2] This coverage may be accomplished by split-thickness skin grafts, skin flaps, or fascia (Fig. 5–5). In instances in which healing is predicted to be impaired, such as in osteoradionecrosis of the tympanic or temporal bone, free muscle or muscle flaps may be utilized under appropriate fascia or skin coverage. In certain conditions, fat may be used to obliterate major bony defects; the fat is then covered superficially with skin flaps.

Once the tissue coverage of bone is completed, it is necessary to determine whether or not a meatoplasty is indicated. Generally, if the bony external auditory canal has been enlarged or if an attic or mastoid defect has been found, a meatoplasty is essential in order to promote healing and subsequent cleansing of the external auditory canal.

Stenting (see Fig. 5–5) may be accomplished with expanding methocellulose wicks. It is almost always necessary in order to keep soft tissues approximated to bone and to splint a meatoplasty open. Topical antibiotic drops may be used in the immediate postoperative period, with the drops being placed upon the absorbing stenting material. It should be appreciated that the stenting material acts as an occlusive dressing and should be removed in approximately 1 week. In order to reduce pain it is advisable to soften the stenting material with hydrogen peroxide or antibiotic drops prior to extraction from the external auditory canal. The decision at this juncture is whether to continue further stenting of the external auditory canal. This is usually required if soft tissue, as opposed to bone, is still in the healing stages. Examples include TMJ soft tissue extrusion into the external auditory canal, cartilaginous canal stenosis, and the presence of a meatoplasty. Over a period of several weeks, while epithelialization is occurring, weekly changing of the stents in the physician's office is appropriate. Thereafter, the patient may change the stenting material. Finally, after 3 or 4 months, the stenting material may be left out during the daytime and used overnight. The recent availability of this stenting material has improved significantly the ability to prevent restenosis following surgery.

Long-term supervision and cleansing may be required in many of these lesions to prevent reaccumulation of cerumen, crusting, and the subsequent development of otorrhea. Agents such as 50/50 white household vinegar/water solution and a steroid cream may be very useful.

POSTOPERATIVE COMPLICATIONS AND THEIR MANAGEMENT

Intraoperative complications usually result in injury to the tympanic membrane, facial nerve, or jugular bulb and are generally the result of disorientation in patients in whom there has been significant bony erosion. Complications postoperatively are usually the result of nonhealing of the covering material, which may result in the formation of granulation tissue, otorrhea, crusting, and odor. The continuation of the steps in medical management, described earlier, often results in eventual healing. Occasionally, revision surgery may be required.

SUMMARY

Lesions of the external auditory canal are uncommon conditions, recognition of which may be difficult. Early and specific diagnosis is essential, as many conditions can be treated with effective medical management. Those that do not respond to medical therapy may be effectively stabilized by surgical intervention.

References

1. Piepergerdes JC, Kramer BM, Behnke EE: Keratosis obturans and external auditory canal cholesteatoma. Laryngoscope 90: 383–390, 1980.
2. Holt JJ: Ear canal cholesteatoma. Laryngoscope 102: 608–613, 1992.
3. Brookes GB: Post-traumatic cholesteatoma. Clin Otolaryngol 8: 31–38, 1983.
4. Hawke M, Kwok P, Shankar L, Wang RG: Spontaneous temporomandibular joint fistula into the external auditory canal. J Otolaryngol 17: 29–31, 1988.

6

Congenital Malformation of the Temporal Bone

ANTONIO DE LA CRUZ, M.D.

SUJANA S. CHANDRASEKHAR, M.D.

Congenital malformation of the temporal bone is characterized by aplasia or hypoplasia of the external auditory canal (EAC), often associated with absence or deformity of the auricle (microtia) and the middle ear, with occasional inner ear abnormalities. Aural atresia occurs in one in 10,000 to one in 20,000 live births,[1-5] with unilateral atresia being three times more common than bilateral atresia.[1] This disorder occurs more commonly in males and on the right side.[1] EAC atresia is more often bony rather than membranous, and bony atresia is regularly accompanied by malformation of the middle ear cavity and structures of the middle ear.[6-9] More severe forms of congenital microtia are usually associated with EAC atresia; in rare instances, canal atresia may be seen in patients with a normal pinna.[10] In general, a more severe external deformity implies a more severe middle ear abnormality.[11, 12]

In 1883, Kiesselbach performed the first deep operation attempting to correct this malformation.[8] Unfortunately, the procedure resulted in facial paralysis. Because of the lack of middle ear manipulation and the high complication rate, congenital aural atresia surgery was considered cosmetic at best, and dangerous and to be avoided in most cases. In 1914, Page[13] reported hearing improvement in five of eight cases after surgery. In 1917, Dean and Gittens[14] reported on an excellent hearing result in a patient and reviewed the various types of operations that had been tried by other surgeons. The prevailing attitude toward surgical correction in these cases remained generally pessimistic, despite these and other occasional reports of successful operations, until 1947. That year, Ombredanne, in France,[15] and Pattee, in the United States,[16] each reported on a series of patients successfully operated on to improve the hearing. Pattee's technique included removal of the incus to mobilize the stapes; Ombredanne added fenestration of the lateral semicircular canal (LSCC).

With the advent of tympanoplasty techniques in the 1950s, interest in atresiaplasty rose as the teachings of Wullstein and Zollner carried over into surgery of the congenital ear.[8] Larger series with greater success rates were reported as surgeons attempted to improve their results, using LSCC fenestration, ossiculoplasty, differing degrees of bone removal, and different types and techniques of graft placement.[2, 4, 15, 17-24] Ombredanne went on to report on over 600 "aplasia" cases by 1971,[24a] and 1600 cases with major and minor malformations by 1976.[8] Gill's series[2] of 83 cases is a landmark paper. In the past two decades, Crabtree,[25, 26] Jahrsdoerfer,[8, 27] Marquet[28, 29] and De La Cruz[6, 30] have reported on large surgical series, with modifications of classification and operative techniques.

Although the techniques of canalplasty, meatoplasty, tympanoplasty, and ossiculoplasty have improved considerably, surgical correction of congenital aural atresia remains one of the most challenging operations performed by otologists. This is a complicated surgical problem, requiring application of all modern tympanoplasty techniques and a thorough knowledge of the surgical anatomy of the facial nerve, oval window, and inner ear, as well as their congenital variants.[1, 6, 8, 15, 19, 24, 25, 27, 28, 30-33, 33a-33d] The temporomandibular joint is displaced posteriorly by the lack of development of the EAC, narrowing the distance between the glenoid fossa and the anterior wall of the mastoid tip.[17, 34] Fusion of the incus and malleus is common but because of its dual origin, the stapes footplate is usually normal.[4, 35]

The timing of repair must take into account any planned auricular reconstruction procedures, as well as the degree of pneumatization of the temporal bone.[6] Criteria for patient selection must be stringent when closure of the air-bone gap to within 20 to 30 dB is attempted. Preoperative counseling and several postoperative visits are essential for optimal results. In this chapter, we discuss these issues and provide guidelines for patient evaluation and selection, surgical techniques, and postoperative management.

EMBRYOLOGY

Understanding the normal embryologic development of the ear aids in the understanding of the myriad of possible combinations of malformations encountered in congenital aural atresia. The inner ear, middle ear, and external ear develop independently and in such a way that deformity of one does not necessarily presuppose deformity of another.[9, 36] Most frequently, abnormalities of the outer and middle ear are encountered in combination with a normal inner ear structure.[37, 38]

Microtia is a result of first branchial cleft and pouch anomalies. Growth of mesenchymal tissue from the first and second branchial arches forms six hillocks around the primitive meatus that fuse to form the auricle (Table 6–1). By the end of the third month, the primitive auricle has been completed. The external auditory meatus develops from the first branchial groove. During the second month, a solid core of epithelium migrates inward from the rudimentary pinna

TABLE 6–1. Development of the Auricle

FIRST BRANCHIAL ARCH	SECOND BRANCHIAL ARCH
First hillock—tragus	Fourth hillock—antihelix
Second hillock—helical crus	Fifth hillock—antitragus
Third hillock—helix	Sixth hillock—lobule and lower helix

toward the first branchial pouch. This core is the precursor of the EAC and starts to hollow out and take shape in the sixth month. It canalizes in the seventh month, causing the developing mastoid to become separated from the mandible. Its subsequent posterior and inferior development carries the middle ear and facial nerve to their normal positions.[1, 36, 39–41]

The first branchial pouch grows outward to form the middle ear cleft. The plaque of tissue where this cleft meets the epithelium of the EAC forms the tympanic membrane. While the pouch is forming the eustachian tube, tympanic cavity, and mastoid air cells, Meckel's cartilage (first branchial arch) is forming the neck and head of the malleus and incus. Reichert's cartilage (second branchial arch) forms the remainder of the first two ossicles and the stapes superstructure. The footplate has a dual origin from the second arch and the otic capsule. The ossicles attain their final shape by the fourth month. By the end of the seventh or eighth month, the expanding middle ear cleft surrounds the ossicles and covers them with a mucous membrane.[1, 38, 42]

The facial nerve is the nerve of the second branchial arch. At 4.5 weeks, this developing nerve divides the blastema, which is the condensation of the second arch mesenchymal cells, into the stapes, the interhyale (stapedius muscle precursor) and the laterohyale (precursor of the posterior wall of the middle ear). The nerve's intraosseous course is dependent on this bony expansion.[38, 40] The membranous portion of the inner ear develops during the third to the sixth week from an auditory placode on the lateral surface of the hindbrain. The surrounding mesenchyme transforms into the bony otic capsule.[43]

Congenital aural atresia can therefore range in severity from a thin membranous canal atresia to complete lack of tympanic bone, depending on the time of arrest of intrauterine development.[1, 44, 45] The usual finding of a normal inner ear is explained by the fact that the inner ear is already formed by the time of external/middle ear developmental arrest. Facial nerve course abnormalities are often seen. Only very severe congenital malformations of the external and middle ear are associated with inner ear deformities.[39, 43]

CLASSIFICATION SYSTEMS

A widely used classification system in congenital aural atresia was developed in 1955 by Altmann.[44] In this system, atresias are categorized into three groups. In group 1 (mild), some part of the EAC, although hypoplastic, is present. The tympanic bone is hypoplastic, and the ear drum is small. The tympanic cavity is either normal in size or hypoplastic. In group 2 (moderate), the EAC is completely absent, the tympanic cavity is small and its content deformed, and the "atresia plate" is partially or completely osseous. In group 3 (severe), the EAC is absent, and the tympanic cavity is markedly hypoplastic or missing.

Altmann's classification system is purely descriptive, and most surgical candidates fall into groups 2 and 3. De La Cruz has modified this system with more practical surgical guidelines.[6] The De La Cruz modification involves only advanced Altmann groups 2 and 3 and divides abnormalities into "minor" and "major" categories. Minor malformations consist of 1) normal mastoid pneumatization, 2) normal oval window, 3) reasonable facial nerve–oval window relationship, and 4) normal inner ear. Major malformations are 1) poor pneumatization, 2) abnormal or absent oval window, 3) abnormal course of the horizontal portion of the facial nerve, and 4) abnormalities of the inner ear. The clinical importance of this classification is that surgery in cases of minor malformations has a good possibility of yielding serviceable hearing, whereas cases of major malformations are frequently inoperable.

A point-grading system to guide surgeons in their preoperative assessment of the best candidates for hearing improvement has been developed by Jahrsdoerfer (Table 6–2).[46] This system takes into account the parameters of mastoid pneumatization, presence of the oval and round windows, facial nerve course, status of the ossicles, and external appearance. Point allocation is based primarily on the findings on high-resolution computed tomography (HRCT). Jahrsdoer-

TABLE 6–2. Grading System of Candidacy for Surgery of Congenital Aural Atresia

PARAMETER	POINTS
Stapes present	2
Oval window open	1
Middle ear space	1
Facial nerve normal	1
Malleus-incus complex present	1
Mastoid well pneumatized	1
Incus-stapes connection	1
Round window normal	1
Appearance of external ear	1
Total available points	10

RATING	TYPE OF CANDIDATE
10	Excellent
9	Very good
8	Good
7	Fair
6	Marginal
≤5	Poor

From Jahrsdoerfer RA, Yeakley JW, Aguilar EA, et al.: Grading system for the selection of patients with congenital aural atresia. Am J Otol 13(1): 6–12, 1992.

fer proposes that when the preoperative evaluation of the patient is incorporated into this grading system, the best results (>80 per cent success) will be achieved with a score of eight or better. A score of seven implies a fair chance, six is marginal, and below this the patient becomes a poor candidate.

Of note, Jahrsdoerfer credits presence of the stapes with two points. In our experience, this item is less important than the presence of an oval window and a well-pneumatized mastoid because 1) with current ossiculoplastic techniques, a good hearing result can be achieved with a footplate-to-drum prosthesis, and 2) the new EAC is fashioned at the expense of the mastoid. A large, well-pneumatized mastoid allows for greater ease of dissection with less risk to the facial nerve and inner ear structures, and also allows for the creation of a good-sized EAC.

Schuknecht's[47] system of classification of congenital aural atresia is based on a combination of clinical and primarily surgical observations. Type A (meatal) atresia is limited to the fibrocartilaginous part of the EAC. Meatoplasty is the surgical procedure of choice and, when performed in a timely fashion, prevents formation of canal cholesteatoma and conductive hearing loss. In type B (partial) atresia, narrowing of both the fibrocartilaginous and bony EAC occurs, but a patent dermal tract allows partial inspection of the tympanic membrane. The tympanic membrane is small and partly replaced by a bony septum. Minor ossicular malformations exist, and hearing loss may be mild to severe. Type C (total) atresia includes all cases with a totally atretic ear canal but a well-pneumatized tympanic cavity. There is a partial or total bony atretic plate, the tympanic membrane is absent, the heads of the ossicles are fused, there may be no connection to a possibly malformed stapes, and the facial nerve is more likely to have an aberrant course over the oval window. Type D (hypopneumatic total) atresia is a total atresia with poor pneumatization, common in dysplasias such as Treacher Collins syndrome. These patients with abnormalities of the facial nerve canal and the bony labyrinth are poor candidates for hearing improvement surgery.

In 1983, Chiossone presented a classification scheme based primarily on the location of the glenoid fossa.[48] In type I, the fossa is in the normal position; in type II, it is moderately displaced; in type III, the fossa overlaps the middle ear; and in type IV, in addition to the fossa overlapping the middle ear, there is lack of mastoid pneumatization. Cases with types I and II are ideal surgical candidates. Type III cases have a tendency toward graft lateralization. Type IV cases are not surgical candidates. In elective atresiaplasty surgery, a classification scheme is useful for surgical planning, patient counseling, and comparison of outcomes.

INITIAL EVALUATION AND PATIENT SELECTION

When aural atresia is noted in a newborn, several issues must be addressed. Where one congenital abnormality is found, others must be sought; a high-risk register for deafness is helpful in this regard.[49] After the degree of aural deformity is assessed by physical examination, evaluation of auditory function in both unilateral and bilateral atresia should be performed using auditory brainstem response audiometry within the first few days of life. The incidence of inner ear abnormality associated with congenital aural atresia is 11 per cent to 47 per cent.[12] In unilateral cases, a total sensorineural hearing loss may occur on the normal-appearing ear.[6, 30]

In bilateral cases, a bone-conduction hearing aid should be applied as soon as possible, ideally in the third or fourth week of life. In unilateral cases in which the opposite ear hears normally, a hearing aid is not necessary. We do not recommend implantable hearing aids in children because the surgical scars preclude future microtia repair. The syndromic child with aural atresia and associated cephalic abnormalities (e.g., Treacher Collins, Crouzon's, Klippel-Feil, Pierre Robin, and Goldenhar's syndromes, VATER, CHARGE, drug teratogenicity, and hemifacial microsomia) should be recognized.[49–53] In this subset, surgical correction yields poor results,[47] and long-term bone-conduction aiding is indicated.

Prompt and careful counseling of the parents of a child with sporadic (nonsyndromal) congenital aural atresia is necessary to alleviate concerns regarding possible occurrence in their subsequent children (no more than the general population), to answer questions regarding future auricular reconstruction, and, most importantly, to ensure that proper hearing amplification is instituted in a timely fashion. The child should be enrolled in special education at an early age to maximize speech and language acquisition, in preparation for mainstreaming at the preschool age. Radiologic and surgical evaluations are deferred until the child reaches age 6 and are discussed later in this chapter.

In the initial evaluation of an older individual with congenital aural atresia, the most crucial elements remain the functional and anatomic integrity of the inner ear. Audiometry and HRCT evaluation are necessary. Prognosis for hearing improvement is dependent on the presence and degree of malformations. Auricular reconstruction must be addressed prior to hearing restorative surgery to avoid alterations in the blood supply to the surrounding soft tissue that may compromise microtia repair.

A patient with congenital aural atresia may present with an infected or draining ear or acute facial palsy;

14% have congenital cholesteatoma.[6] The priority in these cases is removal of the cholesteatoma and resolution of the infection; however, preoperative audiometry and HRCT scanning are necessary.[6, 47, 54]

There are two indisputable requirements for surgery in congenital aural atresia: 1) radiographic evidence of an inner ear and 2) audiometric evidence of cochlear function.[8, 55] Other indications mandating prompt surgical intervention are congenital cholesteatoma, a draining postoperative atretic ear, or acute facial palsy. The computed tomographic scan should always be reviewed for cholesteatoma, which necessitates surgery at any age.[47, 54, 56] Cholesteatoma is not included in any of the grading systems because these systems are used only for predicting hearing results in elective atresiaplasty surgery.

TIMING OF AURICULAR RECONSTRUCTION AND ATRESIAPLASTY

In binaural atresia, auricular reconstruction and atresiaplasty are recommended when the patient is 6 years of age. By this time, the costal cartilage has developed sufficiently to allow for harvesting and transplantation to the auricle, and the mastoid has become as pneumatized as possible. The microtia repair should be done first because the complex flaps and use of autologous rib graft demand excellent blood supply.[57, 58] (Of note, many surgeons will not perform atresiaplasty on an ear reconstructed with silicone sheeting stent.[56]) The hearing restoration surgery is then performed 2 months after the microtia repair. Rehabilitation of severe auricular defects using tissue-integrated percutaneous mastoid implant prostheses with and without bone conduction aids has also been described in the literature.[3, 41, 59–61]

In unilateral atresia cases, atresiaplasty surgery is delayed until the patient is old enough to understand the significant risks to the cochlea, vestibular system, and facial nerve. The exception to this is the individual who has a very thin unilateral atresia plate with excellent pneumatization and normal middle ear, ossicles, and facial nerve. This deformity is a minor atresia. In these cases, surgery can be safely performed in childhood with the parents' consent.[30] We often see older adults with unilateral atresia who request surgery when their normal ear begins having high-frequency hearing loss (presbycusis).

PREOPERATIVE EVALUATION AND PATIENT COUNSELING

Early diagnosis with auditory brainstem response audiometry and auditory enhancement with bone-conduction hearing aids in bilateral cases should be done in the first weeks of life.[62] Imaging is deferred until the child reaches age 6 years. The only imaging acceptable today for preoperative evaluation is HRCT scanning in both the axial and coronal planes (Fig. 6–1).[5, 12, 55, 63] Three-dimensional reconstruction computed tomography is in its early stages of use for preoperative evaluation,[34, 64] but this new modality's utility is as yet unproven (Fig. 6–2). The computed tomographic scan must be examined carefully by the otologic surgeon and the otoradiologist because one interpretation often does not provide all of the information necessary for operative planning.

The four important imaging elements that are most helpful to the surgeon planning reconstruction of a congenitally malformed ear are 1) the degree of pneumatization of the temporal bone; 2) the course of the facial nerve, both the relationship of the horizontal portion to the oval window and the location of the mastoid segment; 3) the existence of the oval window and stapes footplate; and 4) the status of the inner ear.[5, 6, 55] Computed tomography also provides information on thickness and form of the bony atretic plate, size and status of the middle ear cavity, existence of congenital cholesteatoma, and soft tissue contribution to the atresia,[6] but this information is less critical for the repair.

Lack of pneumatization is the major cause of inoperability in congenital aural atresia.[6, 30] Fortunately, normal pneumatization is present in most cases. Prolapse of the facial nerve over the oval window may prevent ossiculoplasty and hearing improvement. If the oval window is absent, surgery with fenestration of the lateral semicircular canal or placement of a hearing aid is indicated. There is potential for facial nerve injury in atresia surgery.[65] The nerve may describe a more acute angle rather than its usual 120 degrees at the second genu and often lies more lateral than usual (Fig. 6–3).[66] On HRCT, it is important not to mistakenly identify the vertical lie of the facial nerve to the marrow bone of the styloid process (Fig. 6–4).[67] Even in atretic ears in which the facial nerve does not have an abnormal course, a significantly reduced distance is found between the facial canal and the temporomandibular joint,[34] and the facial canal and the posterior wall of the cavum tympani.[40]

An estimate of the size of the mastoid can be determined by palpation of the mastoid tip, suprameatal spine of Henle (if present), condyle, and zygomatic arch. This measure is useful because the new ear canal will be constructed at the expense of the mastoid air cell system.[6] To be considered a surgical candidate, the patient must have sufficient cochlear function by auditory brainstem response audiometry or on routine audiometry, a normal-appearing inner ear on computed tomographic scan, and, preferably, a well-

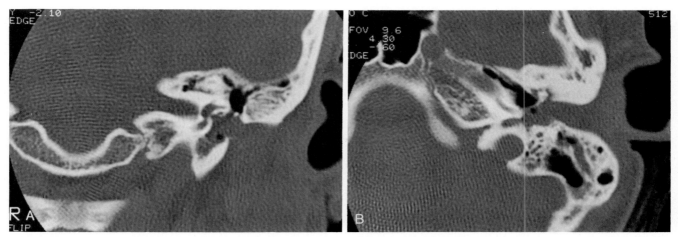

FIGURE 6-1

FIGURE 6-1. Congenital aural atresia, left ear. *A*, Coronal HRCT demonstrates atretic external auditory canal and underdeveloped mastoid system, with normal inner ear. *B*, Axial HRCT of the same case.

FIGURE 6-2. *A*, Three-dimensional CT imaging of normal ear demonstrating complete tympanic ring, normal mastoid development, and normal location of glenoid fossa. *B*, Three-dimensional CT image of opposite atretic ear shows only partial development of the tympanic ring and mastoid, with poor pneumatization, and posterior positioning of the glenoid fossa.

FIGURE 6-3. The facial nerve in congenital aural atresia. *A*, Normal intratemporal facial nerve anatomy. *B*, Intratemporal facial nerve anatomy in CAA.

FIGURE 6-4. Pitfalls in CAA surgery: facial nerve on coronal HRCT. *A*, Arrows point to marrow of the styloid process in an atretic ear. *B*, Arrows point to vertical segment of facial nerve in the same ear.

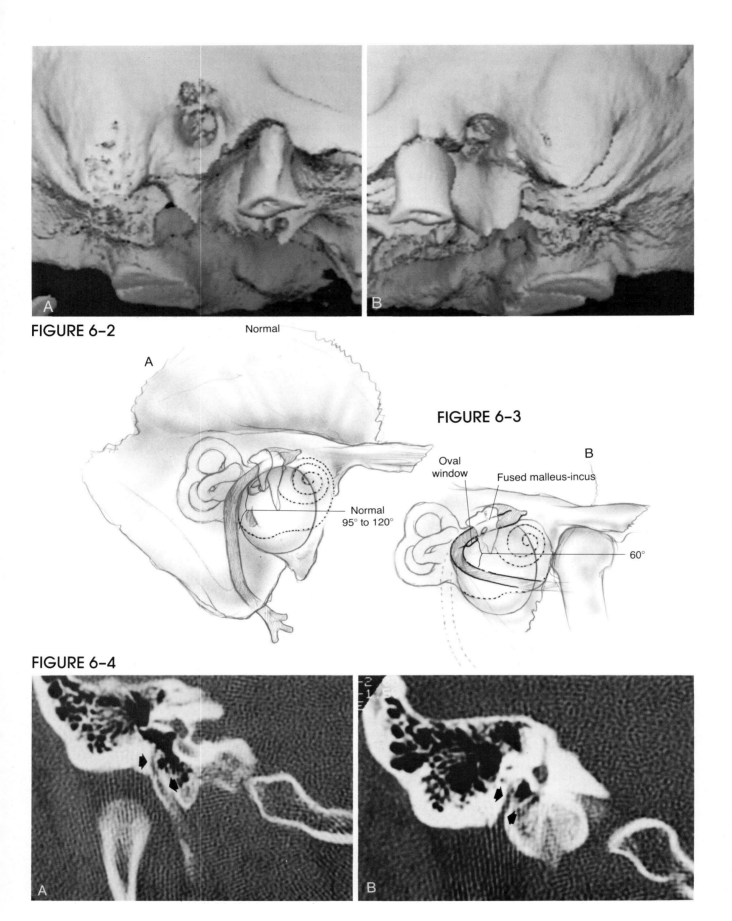

FIGURE 6-2

FIGURE 6-3

A

Normal

Normal
95° to 120°

B

Oval
window

Fused malleus-incus

60°

FIGURE 6-4

developed mastoid and a good oval window–facial nerve relationship.

Patient counseling integrates all of these issues. Patients with a degree of malformation equivalent to a seven or better on the Jahrsdoerfer grading scale are given a greater than 75 per cent chance of hearing improvement. The risk to the facial nerve is small and is made smaller by the use of the facial nerve monitor intraoperatively.[30, 66] Patients are informed that a split-thickness skin graft from the hypogastrium will be used to line the new EAC. Initially, frequent postoperative visits are necessary. The risk of graft lateralization is 26 to 28 per cent, the risk of sensorineural hearing loss is 2 per cent, and the risk of facial nerve palsy is 1 per cent. Otherwise, the risks and complications are similar to those for other mastoidectomy procedures.

SURGICAL TECHNIQUE

The first atresiaplasty operations failed because of poor tympanoplasty technique[16]; as this was improved, hearing restoration was added through lateral semicircular canal fenestration.[17, 24, 44] Simultaneously, advances in meatoplasty added to the success rate of atresiaplasty surgery.[17, 68] Although fenestration remains an option in congenital absence of the oval window, modern methods of ossiculoplasty are used preferentially and yield superior results. There has been debate in the literature over techniques of tympanoplasty and ossiculoplasty in atresia repair. Many materials have been used, including acrylic stents, full-thickness skin grafts, fascia and homografts, the intact (deformed) ossicular mass, stapes (with and without stapedectomy or mobilization), and ossicular replacement prostheses.[6, 8, 17, 21, 24, 28, 29, 31–33, 69, 70, 70a]

We use general endotracheal anesthesia and avoid using muscle relaxants. Facial nerve monitoring is used in all cases. The patient is in the otologic position, and the head is turned away. A large shave of the postauricular area is done, and the auricle and postauricular area are prepared with povidone-iodine (Betadine) and draped. Additionally, the lower abdomen is shaved, prepared, and draped for the skin graft donor site. Perioperative antibiotics are used routinely.

A postauricular temporo-occipital incision is made. In cases in which microtia repair has been done, care is taken not to expose the grafted costal cartilage. Subcutaneous tissue is elevated anteriorly to the temporomandibular joint. A T-shaped incision is made in the periosteum, which is elevated, exposing the mastoid cortex and, anteriorly, the temporomandibular joint space (Fig. 6–5). Care is taken to avoid injury to an anomalous facial nerve exiting the temporal bone in this area. A large piece of temporalis fascia is harvested, trimmed of excess soft tissue if needed, and placed aside to dry. The temporomandibular joint space is explored to verify that the facial nerve or tympanic bone is not lying within it.

The literature has fostered the belief that there are separate and distinct approaches to the bony work necessary in atresiaplasty: the anterior approach, the transmastoid approach, and modification of the anterior approach.[6, 8, 22, 30, 32, 49, 56] We feel that this strict distinction between these surgical approaches is unnecessary, as each can be used alone or in combination to facilitate the atresiaplasty. For purposes of discussion, however, each technique will be elucidated in detail.

Anterior Approach

If a remnant of tympanic bone is present, the new ear canal is begun either through it, or at the level of the middle fossa dura. If no such remnant is present, drilling begins at the level of the linea temporalis, just posterior to the glenoid fossa. The surgeon must always keep in mind that there are few landmarks through atretic bone. By use of cutting and diamond burrs, the dissection is carried anteriorly and medially. The middle fossa plate is identified and followed to the epitympanum, where the fused malleus head–incus body mass is identified (Fig. 6–6). Care is taken not to drill on the ossicular mass because the incudo-

---

FIGURE 6–5. Incision, harvesting temporalis fascia, T-incision, and elevation of periosteum.

FIGURE 6–6. Anterior approach: mastoidectomy completed, demonstrating LSCC, fallopian canal, atresia plate, and ossicles.

FIGURE 6–7. A–B, Anterior approach: removal of atretic plate and adhesions, exposing the ossicles.

FIGURE 6–8. Split-thickness skin graft used to line new EAC.

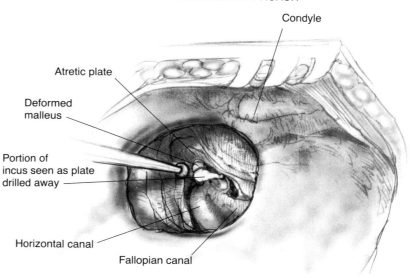

FIGURE 6-6

ANTERIOR APPROACH

Condyle

Atretic plate

Deformed malleus

Portion of incus seen as plate drilled away

Horizontal canal

Fallopian canal

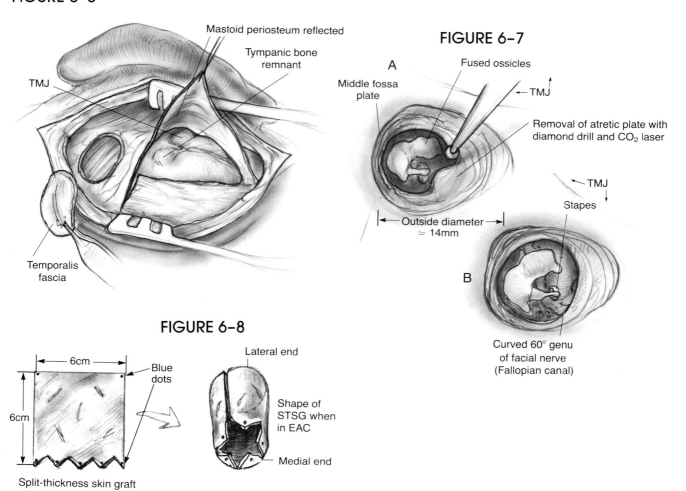

FIGURE 6-5

Mastoid periosteum reflected

Tympanic bone remnant

TMJ

Temporalis fascia

FIGURE 6-7

A

Middle fossa plate

Fused ossicles

TMJ

Removal of atretic plate with diamond drill and CO_2 laser

Outside diameter ≃ 14mm

TMJ

Stapes

B

Curved 60° genu of facial nerve (Fallopian canal)

FIGURE 6-8

Lateral end

6cm

6cm

Blue dots

Shape of STSG when in EAC

Medial end

Split-thickness skin graft

stapedial joint is presumed intact, and transmission of high-speed drill energy to the inner ear can result in sensorineural hearing loss. The epitympanic ossicular mass in the epitympanum is meticulously dissected free of the atresia plate and is left intact. This action helps protect the horizontal facial nerve, which lies medial to these structures.

The atresia plate is removed with diamond microdrills and curettes to completely expose the ossicles (Fig. 6–7A). While the inferior and posterior aspects are dissected, an aberrant facial nerve may be encountered as it passes laterally through the atresia plate in this area. Although deformed, if the ossicular chain is felt to be complete, it is left in place. The ever-present fibrous ligaments and adhesions are better vaporized with a carbon dioxide laser in the final phases of ossicular dissection, to avoid delayed refixation of the ossicles (Fig. 6–7B). Ossicular reconstruction with the patient's intact ossicular chain is preferred to the use of prostheses. When the ossicular chain is not complete, ossiculoplasty is performed by use of a total or partial ossicular reconstruction prosthesis to either a mobile footplate or to the stapes head. Infrequently, it is necessary to drill out an obliterated oval window.[35] The prosthesis is covered with cartilage prior to the grafting of the new drum. On occasion, the stapes footplate may not be seen well because of anomalous facial nerve anatomy, making placement of an ossicular prosthesis difficult or dangerous. In these instances, hearing restoration can be accomplished with LSCC fenestration, or the patient can be counseled to use a hearing aid.[4, 8, 15, 24, 29, 33, 35]

Drilling is continued to create a new ear canal measuring about 1.5 times the normal size, with the surgeon being careful not to violate the temporomandibular joint space or to expose an excessive number of mastoid air cells.

The previously prepared skin graft donor site is exposed. A 0.012-inch thick, 6cm × 6cm split-thickness graft is obtained by use of a Brown dermatome. Hemostasis of the donor site is accomplished by pressure with a gauze sponge wet with 1 per cent lidocaine with epinephrine 1:100,000U and thrombin solution. When the donor site is dry, a sterile Op-Site dressing is applied.[71] One edge of the skin graft is cut in a zigzag fashion such that four or five triangular points are created (Fig. 6–8). The points of the zigzag are colored with a skin marker, as are the two points on the other edge. This marking allows for easy inspection in the final stages of the procedure. The skin graft is kept moist and set aside.

The now-dry temporalis fascia is inspected and trimmed to size, ideally a 20mm × 15mm oval. Small 3mm × 6mm tabs are cut into the anterior and superior aspects of the fascia to prevent lateralization of this tympanic membrane graft.[72] Lateralization is the most common delayed cause of a poor hearing outcome, occurring in 22 per cent of patients.[6, 30] Nitrous oxide, if used by the anesthesiologist, must be discontinued 30 minutes before grafting begins.

The fascia is placed over the ossicular chain, medial to the malleus (Fig. 6–9A) or, when ossicular reconstruction is needed, over the cartilage covering the prosthesis (Fig. 6–9B). The tabs are placed medially into the protympanum and epitympanum in an attempt to prevent lateralization of the new tympanic membrane. The new ear canal is circumferentially lined with the split-thickness skin, and the zigzags are placed medially and partially overlap the fascia. All bone of the EAC is covered.[8, 27] The colored points allow the surgeon to be sure that no skin lies folded on itself, and that the entire width of the graft is being used (the number of points seen matches the number of points created). Two centimeters to 3cm of (apparent) excess skin remains laterally, to be tacked down later (Fig. 6–10). A single layer of antibiotic-soaked absorbable gelatin sponge (Gelfoam) is used to hold the fascia and skin of the new ear drum in place. A disk of 0.020-inch reinforced silicone sheeting is placed over the tympanic membrane to reproduce the anterior tympanomeatal angle (Fig. 6–11). A large Merocel wick is placed over this medial canal wall packing, and attention is then turned to meatoplasty.

A 14mm meatus is created, as 30 per cent of the diameter will eventually reduce as a result of the normal healing process. We avoid denuding or otherwise damaging the cartilage of the microtia repair. Skin, subcutaneous tissue, and cartilage are removed in a

---

FIGURE 6–9. A–B, Temporalis fascia graft with tabs used over ossicular mass or partial ossicular replacement prosthesis and cartilage.

FIGURE 6–10. STSG in place over fascia, lining new EAC (two views).

FIGURE 6–11. STSG with ear wicks to maintain contact with bony EAC, and wide meatus.

FIGURE 6–12. Skin graft sutured into place at meatus.

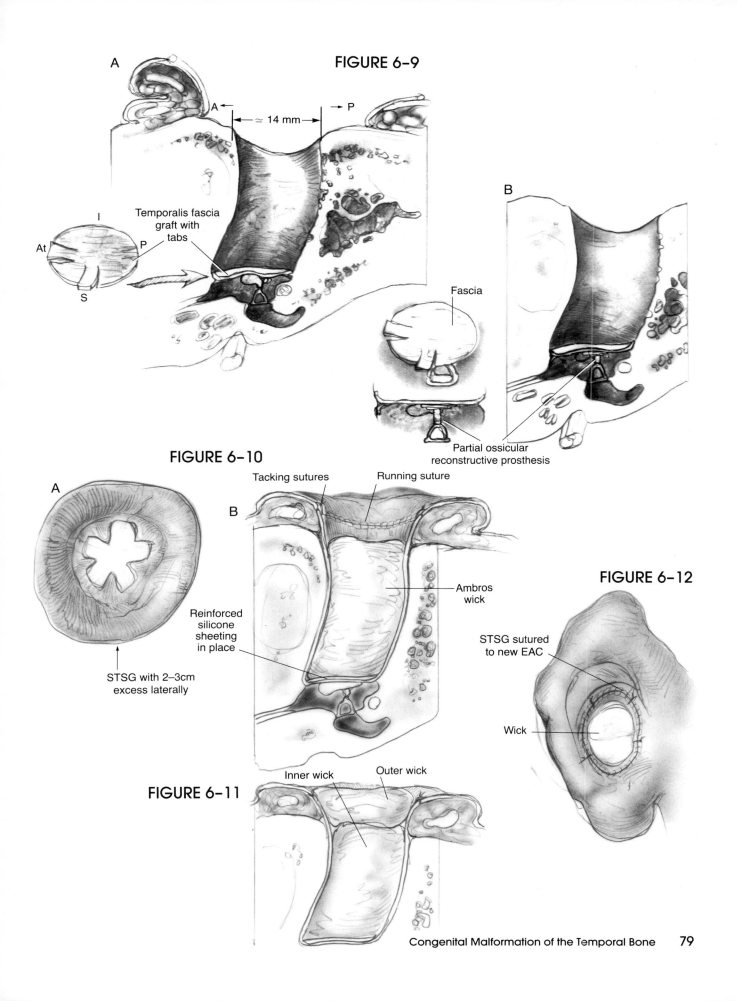

FIGURE 6-9

A

≈ 14 mm

A   P

Temporalis fascia
graft with
tabs

I

At   P

S

B

Fascia

Partial ossicular
reconstructive prosthesis

FIGURE 6-10

A

B   Tacking sutures   Running suture

Ambros
wick

Reinforced
silicone
sheeting
in place

STSG with 2–3cm
excess laterally

FIGURE 6-12

STSG sutured
to new EAC

Wick

Inner wick   Outer wick

FIGURE 6-11

1.4cm diameter core over the new meatus. The ear is turned, and the excess canal skin graft is brought through the meatoplasty. With one or two absorbable sutures bringing the periosteum back in place over the mastoid cortex, the pinna and meatus are stabilized. Six or seven tacking sutures of 5-0 Ti-Cron attach the lateral edge of the skin graft circumferentially to the meatal skin. Next, absorbable suture (6-0 fast-absorbing plain gut) is used in a running fashion between each Ti-Cron suture. The lateral portion of the EAC and the meatus are packed. We prefer to use the large Ambros Merocel ear wick, divided longitudinally as necessary, for diffuse pressure over the entire lateral skin graft and for wide packing of the meatus (Fig. 6–12).

The periosteum is sutured back into position. This action allows additional insurance that the meatus will heal wide open. The postauricular incision is closed with absorbable sutures (3-0 Dexon). Steri-Strips cover the incision, a mastoid dressing is applied, anesthesia is reversed, monitoring equipment is removed, and the patient leaves the operating room.

Transmastoid Approach

The authors have not used the transmastoid approach in over 10 years. Exposure of the mastoid cortex and glenoid fossa is obtained as for the anterior approach. Dissection is then begun at the level of the linea temporalis, well posterior to the temporomandibular joint. The sinodural angle is identified and followed medially to the antrum. Bone pate is obtained during drilling. The lateral semicircular canal, the malleus-incus complex, and the atresia plate are identified, and the atresia plate is removed carefully with microdrills to avoid inner ear acoustic trauma. Mastoid air cell exenteration and lowering of the facial ridge to the facial nerve allow access and creation of an EAC with a canal wall down technique (Fig. 6–13). The remainder of the operation (ossiculoplasty, tympanoplasty) proceeds as outlined earlier. The only additional step is bone pate or soft tissue obliteration of the large mastoid cells before meatoplasty and canal skin grafting are performed.

Modified Anterior Approach

In patients with thick, bony atresia plates, orientation may be difficult during the medial dissection. These patients typically have few air cells, making this approach particularly challenging. Dissection too far in either the inferior or the posterior direction risks inadvertent carotid, lateral canal, or facial nerve injury. Orientation is achieved in these cases with initial posterior dissection and limited posterior antrotomy at the sinodural angle only, enabling identification of the

levels of the lateral semicircular canal and the ossicular mass. A new ear canal is then created in a method similar to that used for the anterior approach by drilling just posterior to the glenoid fossa and following an intact canal wall mastoidectomy approach. The lateral canal can be used repeatedly as a landmark to indicate depth and anteroposterior and superoinferior directionality, thus making the dissection safer. An intact canal wall–like procedure is then carried out. The remainder of the surgery proceeds as described earlier.

POSTOPERATIVE CARE

The mastoid dressing is removed on the first postoperative day, and the Steri-Strips are left in place over the postauricular incision for 7 days. The patient is counseled to keep the operative site dry and to change the cotton ball over the canal-meatus packing once or twice daily. The Op-Site over the skin graft donor site is left on for at least 3 weeks and requires no special attention. Epithelization occurs under the plastic, and the typical pain associated with older methods of donor site dressing is absent.[71] The patient is given a 5-day course of oral antistaphylococcal antibiotics.

The patient is seen 1 week after surgery, at which time the postauricular strips are removed, the tacking Ti-Cron sutures at the meatus are removed, and the dried and crusted lateral end of the meatus pack is trimmed off. The donor site is inspected. The postauricular site can now be washed, but water precautions continue to apply to the canal. We see the patient again in 2 weeks, and at this time the dried portion of the Merocel pack is removed. The meatus is repacked with antibiotic-soaked gelatin sponge. At this point, the patient is instructed to begin applying antibiotic suspension to the packing in the EAC twice a day. By this time, also, the Op-Site has peeled off, and the donor site has completed the initial healing phase. At the third postoperative week, the gelatin sponge and silicone sheeting disk are removed. The patient continues to use the drops for 8 to 12 weeks.

The first postoperative audiogram is obtained at 6 to 8 weeks, when nearly all of the gelatin sponge is gone and the canal is healing well. Audiograms are then obtained at 6 months, 1 year, and yearly thereafter.

PITFALLS

In all cases, we prefer and often begin with an anterior approach; however, in atretic bone often no clearly identifiable landmarks exist. The only "knowns" are the middle fossa plate or the sinodural angle, and the

FIGURE 6-13. Transmastoid approach.

TRANSMASTOID APPROACH

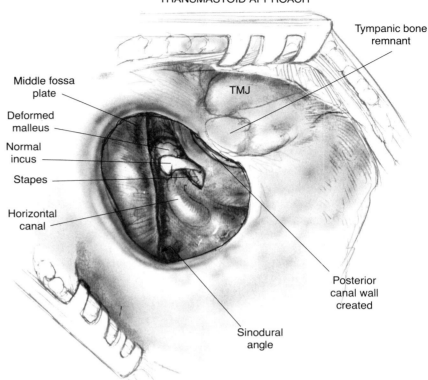

Labels on figure:
Tympanic bone remnant
Middle fossa plate
TMJ
Deformed malleus
Normal incus
Stapes
Horizontal canal
Posterior canal wall created
Sinodural angle

occasional atresiaplasty surgeon can follow these forward to reach the epitympanum. Complete communication between the surgeon and the anesthesiologist will ensure that the patient is not paralyzed during the procedure because facial nerve monitoring is essential in these cases. When the monitor is off transiently because of the use of electrocautery, we monitor the facial nerve manually with a hand on the patient's face. In poorly pneumatized mastoids, the otic capsule may be difficult to distinguish, resulting in blue lining, or worse, of the semicircular canals. In these cases, we recommend the modified anterior approach. We do not use the transmastoid approach.

Postoperative office care is important. Patients should know beforehand that they must precisely follow the instructions given and that they must keep all scheduled postoperative office visits. An infected graft in a patient who has missed appointments for a month is a serious and difficult problem. We recommend checking the circumference of the pack each week to ensure that there is no ingrowth of grafted skin into the pack, although we have not seen this problem with the Ambros packs. If the meatus appears to be narrowing, usually at the third month, it can be dilated every 2 weeks and restented effectively with the large Merocel wick and gelatin sponge for 12 to 24 months.

RESULTS

At the House Ear Clinic, a review of 302 atretic ears in 239 patients was done by De La Cruz et al. in 1985.[6] All of the cases were classified under "major" or "minor" malformation categories using the De La Cruz modification of the Altmann system. One hundred forty-one (59 per cent) of the patients were male, and the right ear was involved in 108 of 169 unilateral cases (64 per cent). There were 70 bilateral cases. Thirty patients had associated anomalies: cleft palate ($n=5$), Treacher Collins ($n=6$), Mondini's inner ear deformity ($n=7$), stenotic internal auditory canal ($n=1$), and congenital ipsilateral facial anomaly—either microtia or paralysis—($n=11$). There were two nonhearing ears before surgery. Of the unilateral patients, five had either nonhearing ears or cholesteatoma in the normal-appearing ear. Nine atretic ears had cholesteatoma, usually lateral to the atretic plate.

Sixty-five ears underwent a primary atresiaplasty. Hearing results were excellent: 16 per cent had a conductive deficit of less than 10dB; 53 per cent, under 20dB; and 73 per cent, under 30dB. Of the patients with poorer auditory outcomes, one developed a high-frequency sensorineural hearing loss but preserved the low tones, and one developed a nonhearing ear following an LSCC fenestration procedure. In six bilaterally atretic patients, the operated ear was so poorly pneumatized and the deformity so severe that the surgeon attempting the repair elected to close the ear without hearing restoration. No patient had post-operative facial palsy. Two cases of transient facial palsy were seen in 18 ears operated on elsewhere. Fourteen per cent had cholesteatoma.

Twenty patients needed revision surgery. The most common reason for failure was lateralization of the tympanic membrane, which occurred in 14 cases (22 per cent). This problem usually occurs within 12 months after surgery. Five other patients had canal stenoses and required reoperation. The other reason for revision surgery was persistent drainage. Eighteen of the 20 revision cases, including all five stenosis cases, had had full-thickness skin graft used to line the EAC initially. The change to split-thickness skin grafting has reduced the incidence of stenosis and the need for revision surgery. Hearing results following revision surgery have been very good: 10 per cent closed the air-bone gap to within 10dB, and 60 per cent did so to within 20dB. One patient had a profound sensorineural hearing loss following a drill-out for an absent oval window. There were no facial nerve injuries. Our revisions of two cases initially operated on elsewhere resulted in hearing within 20dB.

Molony and De La Cruz's review of 24 atresiaplasties from the House Ear Clinic between 1984 and 1988[30] revealed similar rates of air-bone gap closure, no sensorineural hearing losses, and 79 per cent and 60 per cent success rates for the anterior and transmastoid approaches, respectively. Four of the seven failures in this series were from the transmastoid approach, which also had the only instances of recurrent drainage. This approach has therefore gone into disuse.

COMPLICATIONS AND THEIR MANAGEMENT

Complications of atresiaplasty include lateralization of the tympanic membrane in up to 26 per cent, stenosis of the external auditory meatus in 8 per cent, sensorineural hearing loss in 2 per cent, and facial nerve palsy in 1 per cent.

Care taken at the time of surgery can help minimize the incidence of lateralization. The anesthesiologist should be alerted to shut off any nitrous oxide 30 minutes before grafting is begun. The graft should be anchored medially to the malleus, and the tabs placed into the hypotympanum and epitympanum. Use of an accurately sized silicone sheeting disk will help reform an anterior tympanomeatal angle and keep the graft in position. The patient must be followed up carefully for at least 12 to 16 months because laterali-

zation has been known to occur up to 12 months postoperatively.

The incidence of stenosis has been reduced with the use of large, split-thickness skin grafts. Careful inspection of the meatus at frequent intervals and early stenting with Merocel wicks can obviate reoperation. The importance of early identification and treatment of infection to prevent graft failure and stenosis cannot be overemphasized.

With better imaging techniques, oval window problems can be identified preoperatively, and problems of sensorineural hearing loss due to oval window drill-out can be avoided. Likewise, patients with computed tomographic evidence of severe malformations in whom surgery would be fraught with problems can be counseled against surgical intervention and fitted with hearing aids instead. The facial nerve can be imaged preoperatively. Along with intraoperative facial nerve electromyographic monitoring, this preoperative imaging will serve to reduce even further the incidence of facial nerve injury.

ALTERNATIVE TECHNIQUES

Patients with bilateral atresia must have auditory amplification. Initially, as we have discussed, newborns receive bone-conduction aids. At age 6, if evaluation reveals a high surgical risk or poor predicted outcome, a bone conduction aid is a good option. In patients with unilateral atresia and contralateral normal auditory function, no intervention is mandatory, but implantation of a bone-conduction hearing aid can be considered. These aids can also anchor synthetic auricular prostheses.[3, 41, 59–61] They are osseointegrated titanium devices that are implanted into the mastoid. Experience in the United States with these devices is limited. We do not recommend implantable bone-conduction hearing aids in children, because surgical scarring and disruption of vascular planes preclude future auricular reconstruction.

The two types of implantable bone aids available for clinical use are the bone-anchored hearing aid (BAHA), introduced in 1977 in Sweden, and the Audiant, introduced in 1984 and manufactured in the United States.[3, 41] Surgery for the BAHA is a two-stage procedure with an interval of 3 to 4 months between operations, allowing for osseointegration to start before a load is applied. The first stage is implantation of the fixture into the mastoid cortex. Following implantation, the skin flap is replaced, and healing is allowed to take place. At the second stage, a skin-penetrating abutment is secured to the fixture, reducing the amount of subcutaneous tissue and eliminating hair follicles in the site. Often, this step necessitates a hairless skin transplant. The aid is first useable 3 to 5 weeks following the second stage. Clinical trials are at present underway to convert the insertion of the BAHA into a one-stage procedure. The Audiant has two parts: an internal magnet housed in a titanium disk and coated with medical-grade silicone attached to the skull through an orthopedic screw, and an external device, which is the sound processor, which includes a second rare earth magnet and an induction coil. Transmission is transcutaneous through a thickness of 4mm to 6mm of skin and subcutaneous tissue.

For use of the Audiant, a bone conduction hearing threshold of better than 25dB for the speech frequencies is recommended. For the BAHA, 45dB or better bone thresholds result in subjective improvement in 90 per cent of patients. Further comparisons between the two types of devices are available in the literature.[59, 60]

SUMMARY

The treatment of congenital aural atresia poses a challenging problem. Early identification, amplification, and speech and language therapy are crucial in bilateral cases. Cooperation with the auricular reconstruction surgeon allows for both esthetic and functional success, and the use of strict radiologic and clinical criteria for operative candidates is necessary. Patients whose disorders are classified into categories of "minor" and "major" malformations should understand the prognosis for hearing improvement and the risks and results of surgery. A thorough understanding of embryologic maldevelopment and rigorous adherence to the surgical principles of mastoidectomy, facial nerve dissection, and tympanoplasty enable us to offer our patients optimal hearing restoration. Diligent postoperative office care is vital to maintaining the good results obtained at surgery.

References

1. Federspil P, Delb W: Treatment of congenital malformations of the external and middle ear. In Ars B (ed): Congenital External and Middle Ear Malformations: Management. Amsterdam, Kugler Publications, 1992, pp 47–70.
2. Gill NW: Congenital atresia of the ear—a review of the surgical findings in 83 cases. J Laryngol Otol 83: 551–587, 1969.
3. Granstrom G, Bergstrom K, Tjellstrom A: The bone-anchored hearing aid and bone-anchored epithesis for congenital ear malformations. Otolaryngol Head Neck Surg 109: 46–53, 1993.
4. House HP: Management of congenital ear canal atresia. Laryngoscope 63(10): 916–946, 1953.
5. Mehra YN, Dubey SP, Mann SBS, Suri S: Correlation between high-resolution computed tomography and surgical findings in congenital aural atresia. Arch Otolaryngol Head Neck Surg 114: 137–141, 1988.
6. De La Cruz A, Linthicum FH Jr, Luxford WM: Congenital atresia of the external auditory canal. Laryngoscope 95: 421–427, 1985.
7. Hiraide F, Nomura Y, Nakamura K: Histopathology of atresia auris congenita. J Laryngol Otol 88: 1249–1256, 1974.
8. Jahrsdoerfer RA: Congenital atresia of the ear. Laryngoscope 88(9 Suppl) 13: 1–48, 1978.
9. Kelemen G: Aural participation in congenital malformations of the organism. Acta Otolaryngol Suppl (Stockh) 321: 1–35, 1974.
10. Grundfast KM, Camilon F: External auditory canal stenosis and partial atresia without associated anomalies. Ann Otol Rhinol Laryngol 95: 505–509, 1986.
11. Harada O, Ishii H: The condition of the auditory ossicles in microtia: findings in 57 middle ear operations. Plast Reconstr Surg 50(1): 48–53, 1972.
12. Hasso AN, Broadwell RA: Congenital anomalies. In Som PM, Bergeron RT (eds): Head and Neck Imaging. St. Louis, CV Mosby, 1991, pp 960–966.
13. Page JR: Congenital bilateral microtia with total osseous atresia of the external auditory canals, operation and report of cases. Trans Am Otol Soc 13: 376–390, 1914.
14. Dean LW, Gittens TR: Report of a case of bilateral, congenital osseous atresia of the external auditory canal with an exceptionally good functional result following operation. Trans Am Laryngol Rhinol Otol Soc 296–309, 1917.
15. Ombredanne M: Chirurgie de la surdité: fenestration dans les aplasies de l'oreille avec imperforation du conduit. Resultats. Otorhinolaryngol Int 31: 229–236, 1947.
16. Pattee GL: An operation to improve hearing in cases of congenital atresia of the external auditory meatus. Arch Otolaryngol Head Neck Surg 45(5): 568–580, 1947.
17. Bellucci RJ: The problem of congenital auricular malformation. I. Construction of the external auditory canal. Trans Am Acad Ophthalmol Otolaryngol 64: 840–852, 1960.
18. Meurman Y: Congenital microtia and meatal atresia. Arch Otolaryngol Head Neck Surg 66(4): 443–463, 1957.
19. Nager GT: Aural atresia: anatomy and surgery. Postgrad Med 29(5): 529–541, 1961.
20. Ombredanne M: Malformations des osselets dans les embryopathies de l'oreille. Acta Otorhinolaryngol Belg 20(6): 623–652, 1965.
21. Ruedi L: The surgical treatment of the atresia auris congenita: a clinical and histological report. Laryngoscope 64: 666–684, 1954.
22. Scheer AA: Correction of congenital middle ear deformities. Arch Otolaryngol Head Neck Surg 85(3): 269–277, 1967.
23. Shambaugh Jr GE: Developmental anomalies of the sound conducting apparatus and their surgical correction. Ann Otol 74: 873–887, 1952.
24. Woodman DG: Congenital atresia of the auditory canal. Arch Otolaryngol Head Neck Surg 55: 172–181, 1952.
24a. Ombredanne M: Chirurgie des surdités congenitales par malformations ossiculaires. Acta Otolaryngol Belg 25: 837–869, 1971.
26. Crabtree JA: Congenital atresia: case selection, complications, and prevention. Otolaryngol Clin North Am 15(4): 755–762, 1982.
27. Jahrsdoerfer RA, Cole RR, Gray LE: Advances in congenital aural atresia. Adv Otolaryngol Head Neck Surg 5: 1–15, 1991.
27a. Jahrsdoerfer RA: Clinical aspects of temporal bone anomalies. AJNR 13: 821–825, 1992.
28. Marquet J: Homogreffes tympano-ossiculaires dans le traitement chirurgical de l'agenesie de l'oreille; rapport preliminaire. Acta Otorhinolaryngol Belg 25(6): 885–897, 1971.
29. Marquet J, Declau F, De Cock M, et al.: Congenital middle ear malformations. Acta Otorhinolaryngol Belg 42: 117–302, 1988.
30. Molony TB, De La Cruz A: Surgical approaches to congenital atresia of the external auditory canal. Otolaryngol Head Neck Surg 103: 991–1001, 1990.
31. Crabtree JA: Tympanoplastic techniques in congenital atresia. Arch Otolaryngol Head Neck Surg 88: 89–96, 1968.
32. Minatogawa T, Nishimura Y, Inamori T, Kumoi T: Results of tympanoplasty for congenital aural atresia and stenosis, with special reference to fascia and homograft as the graft material of the tympanic membrane. Laryngoscope 99: 632–638, 1989.
33. Schuknecht HF: Reconstructive procedures for congenital aural atresia. Arch Otolaryngol Head Neck Surg 101: 170–172, 1975.
33a. Bellucci RJ: Congenital auricular malformation: indications, contraindications, and timing of middle ear surgery: an otolo-

gist's viewpoint. *In* Converse JM (ed): Reconstructive Plastic Surgery, Vol 3. Philadelphia, WB Saunders, 1977, pp 1719–1724.

33b. Linthicum FH Jr: Surgery of congenital deafness. Otolaryngol Clin North Am 4(2): 401–409, 1971.

33c. Patterson ME, Linthicum FH Jr: Congenital hearing impairment. Otolaryngol Clin North Am 201–219, 1970.

33d. Ruben RJ: Management and therapy of congenital malformations of the external and middle ears. *In* Ruben RJ, Alberti PW (eds): Otologic Medicine and Surgery. New York, Churchill Livingstone, 1988, pp 1135–1154.

34. Jahrsdoerfer RA, Garcia ET, Yeakley JW, Jacobson JT: Surface contour three-dimensional imaging in congenital aural atresia. Arch Otolaryngol Head Neck Surg 119: 95–99, 1993.

35. Ombredanne M: Absence congenitale de fenetre ronde dans certaines aplasies mineures. Ann Otolaryngol (Paris) 85(5): 369–378, 1968.

36. Aase, JM: Microtia-clinica observations. Birth Defects 16(4): 289–297, 1980.

37. Sando I, Shibahara Y, Takagi A, et al.: Congenital middle and inner ear anomalies. Acta Otolaryngol Suppl (Stockh) 458: 76–78, 1988.

38. Van De Water TR, Maderson PFA, Jaskoll TF: The morphogenesis of the middle and external ear. Birth Defects 16(4): 147–180, 1980.

39. Barrios-Montes JM: Malformaciones auriculares. Acta Otorrinolaringol Esp 27(1): 17–46, 1976.

40. Savic D, Jasovic A, Djeric D: The relations of the mastoid segment of the facial canal to surrounding structures in congenital middle ear malformations. Int J Pediatr Otorhinolaryngol 18: 13–19, 1989.

41. Tjellstrom A, Bergstom K: Bone-anchored hearing aids and prostheses. *In* Ars B (ed): Congenital External and Middle Ear Malformations: Management. Amsterdam, Kugler Publications, 1992, pp 1–9.

42. Gill NW: Congenital atresia of the ear. J Laryngol Otol 85: 1251–1254, 1971.

43. Melnick M: The etiology of external ear malformations and its relation to abnormalities of the middle ear, inner ear, and other organ systems. Birth Defects 16(4): 303–331, 1980.

44. Altmann F: Congenital atresia of the ear in man and animals. Ann Otol Rhinol Laryngol 64: 824–858, 1955.

45. Bellucci RJ: Congenital aural malformations: diagnosis and treatment. Otolaryngol Clin North Am 14(1): 95–124, 1981.

46. Jahrsdoerfer RA, Yeakley JW, Aguilar EA, et al.: Grading system for the selection of patients with congenital aural atresia. Am J Otol 13(1): 6–12, 1992.

47. Schuknecht HF: Congenital aural atresia and congenital middle ear cholesteatoma. *In* Nadol JB Jr, Schuknecht HF (eds): Surgery of the Ear and Temporal Bone. New York, Raven Press, 1993, pp 263–274.

48. Chiossone E: Surgical management of major congenital malformations of the ear. Read at the Politzer Society International Conference. Montreux, Switzerland, September 1983.

49. Sando I, Suehiro S, Wood RP II: *In* Bluestone CD, Stool SE (eds): Congenital anomalies of the external and middle ear. Pediatric Otolaryngology. Philadelphia, WB Saunders, 1983, pp 309–326.

50. Fernandez AO, Ronis ML: The Treacher Collins syndrome. Arch Otolaryngol Head Neck Surg 80: 505–520, 1964.

51. Rapin I, Ruben RJ: Patterns of anomalies in children with malformed ears. Laryngoscope 86: 1469–1502, 1976.

52. Ruben RJ, Toriyama M, Dische MR, et al.: External and middle ear malformations associated with mandibulo-facial dysostosis and renal abnormalities: a case report. Ann Otol Rhinol Laryngol 78: 605–624, 1969.

53. Sanchez-Corona J, Garcia-Cruz D, Ruenes R, Cantu JM: A distinct dominant form of microtia and conductive hearing loss. Birth Defects 18(3B): 211–216, 1982.

54. Miyamoto RT, Fairchild TH, Daugherty HS: Primary cholesteatoma in the congenitally atretic ear. Am J Otol 5(4): 283–285, 1984.

55. Jahrsdoerfer RA, Yeakley JW, Hall III JW, et al.: High-resolution CT scanning and auditory brain stem response in congenital aural atresia: patient selection and surgical correlation. Otolaryngol Head Neck Surg 93: 292–298, 1985.

56. Jahrsdoerfer RA, Hall JW: Congenital malformations of the ear. Am J Otol 7(4): 267–269, 1986.

57. Brent B: The correction of microtia with autogenous cartilage grafts: I. The classic deformity. Plast Reconstr Surg 66(1): 1–12, 1980.

58. Brent B: Auricular repair with autogenous rib cartilage grafts: two decades of experience with 600 cases. Plast Reconstr Surg 90: 355–374, 1992.

59. Gates GA, Hough JV, Gatti WM, Bradley WH: The safety and effectiveness of an implanted electromagnetic hearing device. Arch Otolaryngol Head Neck Surg 115: 924–930, 1989.

60. Hakansson B, Liden G, Tjellstrom A, et al.: Ten years of experience with the Swedish bone-anchored hearing system. Ann Otol Rhinol Laryngol (Suppl) 151: 1–16, 1990.

61. Niparko JK, Langman AW, Cutler DS, Carroll WR: Tissue-integrated prostheses in the rehabilitation of auricular defects: results with percutaneous mastoid implants. Am J Otol 14(4): 343–348, 1993.

62. Sortini AJ: Hearing aids for children with bilateral congenital ear canal atresia. Hear Instrum 6: 20–23, 1981.

63. Zalzal GH, Shott SR, Towbin R, Cotton RT: Value of CT scan in the diagnosis of temporal bone diseases in children. Laryngoscope 96: 27–32, 1986.

64. Andrews JC, Anzai Y, Mankovich NJ, et al.: Three-dimensional CT scan reconstruction for the assessment of congenital aural atresia. Am J Otol 13(3): 236–240, 1992.

65. Crabtree JA: The facial nerve in congenital ear surgery. Otolaryngol Clin North Am 7(2): 505–510, 1974.

66. Linstrom CJ, Meiteles LZ: Facial nerve monitoring in surgery for congenital auricular atresia. Laryngoscope 103: 406–415, 1993.

67. Chandrasekhar SS, De La Cruz A, Lo WWM, Telischi FJ: Imaging of the facial nerve. *In* Jackler RA, Brackmann DE (eds): Neurotology. St. Louis, Mosby-Year Book, [In press].

68. Chole RA: Meatoplasty using inferiorly based island pedicle flap for congenital aural atresia. Laryngoscope 93(7): 954–955, 1983.

69. Colman BH: Congenital malformations of the ear—aspects of management. J Otolaryngol Soc Aust 4(3): 197–200, 1978.

70. Wigand ME: Tympano-meatoplastie enduarale pour les atresies congenitales severes de l'oreille. Rev Laryngol 99(1–2): 14–28, 1978.

70a. Ombredanne M: Transposition d'osselets dans certaines "aplasies mineures." Ann Otolaryngol (Paris) 83(45): 273–280, 1966.

71. Weymuller EA Jr: Dressings for split thickness skin graft donor sites. Laryngoscope 91:652–653, 1981.

72. Sheehy JL: Surgery of chronic otitis media. *In* English GE (ed): Otolaryngology, Vol 1. Harper & Row, 1977.

7

Surgery of Ventilation and Mucosal Disease

GEORGE A. GATES, M.D.

Otitis media with effusion (OME) is the most common indication for a surgical procedure in children. Given that at least a million tympanostomy tube (T-tube) insertion procedures are done annually in the United States, with charges for an outpatient surgical procedure now averaging over $7500, the aggregate cost may fall between 1.5 to 2 billion dollars.[1] In the current societal milieux of cost-containment and cost-effectiveness, there is increasing scrutiny of the treatment of common conditions such as OME. Over the past decade, several prospective, randomized clinical trials[2-5] have validated the efficacy of surgical therapy of OME. It would seem prudent to apply this knowledge to develop a cost-conscious treatment protocol to provide rational and effective care.

TERMINOLOGY

OME refers to an accumulation of inflammatory liquid in the middle ear cleft. Effusions due to barotrauma, head trauma, or cerebrospinal fluid otorrhea are specifically excluded. OME is a convenient term to use for inflammatory effusions of unknown duration. Because it is not possible to distinguish the etiology of such an effusion on the basis of its physical characteristics (i.e., serous, mucoid, purulent), OME is meant to include all types of inflammatory effusions.

OME may be acute or chronic. Acute OME is a middle ear effusion accompanied by signs of inflammation, such as redness of the tympanic membrane, fever, irritability, or pain. Acute OME in the older child has a substantially different clinical presentation: the older child may have no fever and little pain, but tympanic membrane redness and middle ear effusion will be present.

Chronic OME refers to an inflammatory middle ear effusion present for 30 days or more. Although the effusion may vary from serous to purulent to mucoid in character across patients or from the same patient at different times, the underlying pathologic disorder is the same. *Secretory otitis media* is a term used to describe a hyperplastic condition of the middle ear mucosa that produces continuing middle ear effusion, and this term has had a specific implication of a noninfectious etiology to some authors. More recently, however, secretory otitis media is being used interchangeably with chronic OME to indicate an asymptomatic (i.e., painless) middle ear effusion of any etiology. These terms will be used as synonyms in this chapter. To complicate terminology even more, the *International Coding of Diseases, 9th edition* coding manual separates suppurative otitis media, which would include acute OME (382), from nonsuppurative otitis media (381), which has subcategories of chronic serous otitis media (or chronic tubotympanic catarrh,

381.1), chronic mucoid otitis media (or glue ear, 381.2), and other (or otitis media, chronic: allergic, exudative, secretory, seromucinous, transudative, or with effusion, 381.3). It is no small wonder that these terms, which many use interchangeably, cause confusion.

Idiopathic hemotympanum describes the clinical syndrome of a patient with a dark blue–appearing tympanic membrane in whom there is no history of trauma. In reality, however, hemorrhage is not an etiologic factor in the development of this condition. Rather, it develops in cases of long-standing chronic OME for reasons that are not clear. Nonetheless, the term persists. The histopathologic correlate of idiopathic hemotympanum is cholesterol granuloma (see later).

RISK FACTORS

Susceptibility to OME is a genetic trait. Whether this is mediated through the immune system or by the anatomy of the family members, or both, is not easy to determine. Certain ethnic groups, notably Native Americans, have a high prevalence of OME, presumably because of differences in the anatomy of the eustachian tube and skull base.[6] Boys have more episodes of OME than girls, and whites have a higher incidence than blacks. Breast-fed babies have less OME than bottle-fed babies. Position of feeding appears to play a role: children held or placed supine are at greater risk for OME than those held upright. Cigarette smoking in the home appears to be a risk factor for OME. Children in day care have more OME than those reared at home because of endemic upper respiratory infections in groups. Similarly, children in the early school grades have an increased frequency of OME.

EFFECT OF OTITIS MEDIA WITH EFFUSION ON THE CHILD

Recurrent acute illness is often associated with fever, malaise, pain, anorexia, and inadequate sleep. These associated symptoms often produce behavioral changes in children that include inattentiveness, irritability, and social isolation. These may lead to impaired learning and poor socialization. In addition to the disruptive effects on the child's behavior, OME produces a mild-to-moderate conductive hearing loss secondary to the collection of liquid in the middle ear. Such hearing losses may impair communication and create additional difficulties in interpersonal relations, affect the development of speech and language skills, and, perhaps, retard intellectual achievement.[7, 8] A further problem is the effect of a sick child on the family dynamics. Time lost from work or social activities due to illness of a child may impose additional hardships on the status of the child in the family.

PATHOPHYSIOLOGY

Otitis Media With Effusion

Acute OME is an inflammatory disorder induced by microorganisms in the middle ear. The principal route of bacterial entry is retrogradely by reflux of material from the nasopharynx via the eustachian tube. Three factors appear to enhance bacterial reflux into the middle ear: bacterial colonization of the nasopharynx, incompetence of the protective function of the eustachian tube, and a pressure differential between the middle ear and the nasopharynx.

REFLUX. It is well documented clinically[9] and experimentally[10] that acute OME is a sequel to an upper respiratory infection (URI). Viral rhinitis breaks down mucosal barriers that prevent bacterial adherence and growth in both the nose and nasopharynx. In addition, swelling of the adenoid and nasal mucosa alters the aerodynamics of the upper airway. Pathogenic bacteria appear in the nasopharynx following a URI and are the same as those cultured from middle ear effusions, namely *Streptococcus pneumoniae* and *Hemophilus influenzae*.[11] Pillsbury et al.[12] demonstrated higher bacterial colony counts in the adenoids of children with recurrent otitis media than in those undergoing adenoidectomy for adenoid hypertrophy without otitis media. Thus, it appears that the adenoid is the source of the microorganisms that infect the middle ear.

EUSTACHIAN TUBE DYSFUNCTION. Eustachian tube dysfunction is generally held to be the underlying cause of OME. However, controversy remains about the nature of the dysfunction and whether it may be the cause or the result of OME. The eustachian tube has three functions: protection of the middle ear, clearance of middle ear secretions, and equalization of pressure between the nose and middle ear.

In children, in whom the tube is short, horizontal, and composed of relatively flaccid cartilage, the protective function of the tube is less effective, and retrograde reflux of nasopharyngeal secretions may occur.[13] Clearance results mainly from ciliary action. It is presumed that ciliary function of the middle ear and eustachian tube mucosa is impaired during acute OME to the same extent as the nasal mucosa during an acute URI. Thus, fluid that forms during acute OME accumulates in the middle ear primarily because

of ciliary paralysis, and clearance of fluid normally follows recovery of ciliary function. However, thick viscous fluid may occlude the tube secondarily because of its rheologic properties. Pressure equalization is the third function of the eustachian tube and is normally mediated by opening of the tube from contraction of the tensor veli palatini muscle in response to stimuli mediated by the tympanic plexus.[14] Altered pressure regulation is discussed in more detail next.

PRESSURE DIFFERENTIAL. The third factor in the genesis of acute OME—pressure differential—may result from either a negative pressure in the middle ear or positive pressure in the nasopharynx. Obstruction of the nose secondary to viral rhinitis may result in the equivalent of the Toynbee maneuver during swallowing. Because most URIs result in nasal obstruction, swallowing during a URI may increase the nasopharyngeal pressure, which will open the tube and tend to push secretions earward. Nose blowing also increases nasopharyngeal pressures. Sniffing is a common symptom of URI, and it is known to produce negative middle ear pressure,[15] which may facilitate reflux process by pulling any material in the eustachian tube into the middle ear.

Chronic Otitis Media With Effusion

Current concepts of the pathogenesis of chronic OME fall into two broad categories: 1) it is a common sequela of acute otitis media, or 2) it represents a chronically altered state of the middle ear due to multiple causes, of which eustachian tube dysfunction is the chief. There is evidence to support both concepts.

The Greater Boston Collaborative Otitis Media Study[16] demonstrated that persistent effusion is a sequela of acute OME and that effusion persists for 1 month in 40 per cent, for 2 months in 20 per cent, and for 3 or more months in 10 per cent of cases. Further support comes from the work of many investigators who, like Liu et al.,[17] demonstrated pathogenic bacteria in the fluid obtained from the middle ears of children with chronic OME. Stangerup and Tos[18] found a significantly higher incidence of abnormal tympanograms (suggesting OME) in those of a group of 360 children who had had an acute episode of infection in the preceding 3 months. It is likely that eustachian tube obstruction and retained secretion in these cases are the result of the acute infection rather than the cause of it. Thus, there is good evidence that chronic OME is a sequela of acute OME and should be classified as a stage in the pathologic spectrum of that disorder. However, whether this concept applies to all cases of asymptomatic OME in children is not known. The marked variation in prevalence of OME in young children with season[19] also supports an infectious etiology.

The theory that chronic OME is a primary disorder that predisposes to acute OME is supported by Sade[20] and Tos[21] who demonstrated a hypersecretory state of the middle ear mucosa in patients with OME. This state is attributed to multiple causes, infection included, but the primary pathogenic mechanism is classically ascribed to eustachian tube dysfunction. Such dysfunction is held to result sequentially in underaeration of the middle ear, negative middle ear pressure, and hypoxia and hypercapnia of the mucosa. These, in turn, are thought to lead to goblet cell hyperplasia and hypersecretion. Allergy and immune complex formation are also thought to play a role in the genesis of OME. However, more recent work has indicated that the normal middle ear gas is hypoxic and hypercapnic in relation to inspired air[22] and that eustachian tube obstruction per se does not result in severe negative middle ear pressure.[23] The available evidence lends support to the theory that the secretory changes in the middle ear that exist in cases of chronic OME are the histologic sequelae of chronic infection, rather than a separate pathologic disorder.

The therapeutic implications of these differing concepts is substantial. In the first case, antimicrobial therapy and removal of any source of infection is the logical primary treatment strategy; in the second, surgical drainage, ventilation, and pressure equalization would be indicated. There is growing acceptance of the theory that the majority of cases of chronic OME begin as acute infection of the middle ear, that post-inflammatory alterations in the middle ear mucosa and eustachian tube lead to persistence of effusion, and that obstruction of the eustachian tube is secondary to the infection, rather than the cause of it. This theory appears to satisfactorily explain the clinical phenomena of OME.

Idiopathic Hemotympanum

Patients with idiopathic hemotympanum usually experience symptoms similar to those of chronic OME, that is, hearing loss and a plugged or pressure sensation in the middle ear. Generally, these patients are older and often are adults, but this disorder is also seen in children with long-standing OME. The tympanic membrane appears dark and bluish in color. The fluid removed at myringotomy is dark brown and often syrupy in consistency, resembling thin molasses. Microscopic examination of the fluid reveals cholesterol-like crystals, hence the term *cholesterol granuloma*, which is the histopathologic correlate of the clinical term *idiopathic hemotympanum*. The term *hemotympanum* is probably a misnomer because hemorrhage is not a factor in its pathogenesis; its use

undoubtedly began because the bluish color of the tympanic membrane in this condition is reminiscent of the color occurring with frank hemorrhage, such as in temporal bone fracture.

The etiology of idiopathic hemotympanum is obscured by the relative infrequency of the disorder. Paparella and Lim,[24] Sheehy et al.[25] and Sade[26] indicate that idiopathic hemotympanum arises in long-standing cases of chronic OME that develop granulomatous deposits in the middle ear and mastoid. Clinically, there is a strong relation of cholesterol granuloma to hemorrhage because of the frequent finding of hemosiderin pigment in the granuloma. It has been produced experimentally by obstructing the eustachian tube of squirrel monkeys by Thomas et al.[27] who examined the relation of hemorrhage and negative middle ear pressure to cholesterol granuloma. Cholesterol granuloma contains cholesterol crystals and elemental iron deposited in the submucosa surrounded by phagocytes and giant cells. Sade[26] suggests that microorganisms' need for elemental iron is countered by lactoferrin production in the host, leading to chelation of iron and its subsequent deposition in tissue. He found immunohistochemical evidence of lactoferrin in the middle ear mucosa of patients with chronic otitis media and cholesterol granuloma.

TREATMENT

Recurrent Acute Otitis Media With Effusion

Treatment of an acute episode of OME relies on antimicrobial agents directed against the infecting organism. The majority of cases are due to aerobic organisms, with *S. pneumoniae*, *H. influenzae*, and *Moraxella catarrhalis* being the most frequent offenders in order. Patients with acute OME are usually referred for surgical therapy for one of two clinical syndromes: recurrent acute OME and status OME. In the first instance, the goal of treatment is to prevent new episodes of OME (surgical prophylaxis) and in the second, surgical drainage of the middle ear is meant to stop an episode of symptomatic acute OME that has resisted medical therapy.

For children with recurrent acute OME, prevention of additional episodes is the therapeutic goal. Gebhart[28] was the first to demonstrate a reduction in the number of new episodes of acute OME following the insertion of T-tubes. Subsequently, T-tube placement has become the primary surgical prophylaxis against recurrent acute OME as well as the principal method for prolonged drainage of the middle ear.

Although adenoidectomy has been found to be of

value in the treatment of chronic OME, Paradise et al.[5] also found a significant reduction in the incidence of acute OME in the first year following adenoidectomy (but not in the second). However, a formal study of adenoidectomy in the management of recurrent acute OME has not been done and extrapolation of the results of studies done for chronic OME may or may not be appropriate. Nonetheless, adenoidectomy is a logical surgical treatment for surgical prophylaxis against recurrent acute otitis media, particularly those with persistent effusion as well as recurrent infection. Adenoidectomy has been shown to be a safe procedure for children over 18 months.[29]

Chronic Otitis Media With Effusion

ANTIMICROBIAL THERAPY. Mandel et al.[30] demonstrated the efficacy of antimicrobial therapy in chronic OME. However, the effectiveness of antimicrobial therapy is reduced as the number of treatments increases. In the San Antonio study,[3] in which the majority of cases of OME had no prior therapy, the control rate at 2 months was nearly 50 per cent. In contrast, the Pittsburgh subjects[30] had more prior treatment and a correspondingly lower control rate. Thus, an argument can be made to treat new cases of OME with an antimicrobial agent and proceed with surgical therapy for cases failing adequate antimicrobial therapy. Children with persistent chronic OME have commonly received four or more courses of antimicrobials in a 3-month period. For these children, additional antimicrobial therapy is futile.

CORTICOSTEROID THERAPY. Short-term corticosteroid therapy has been studied, and with conflicting results. Schwartz et al.[31] found otoscopic improvement in the treated subjects, whereas Lambert[32] found no difference in outcomes between the corticosteroid group and the control group. Rosenfeld et al.[33] performed a meta-analysis of the published studies and found that the odds ratio for clearance was 3.6 in steroid-treated children. However, the long-term benefit of corticosteroid therapy has yet to be determined, and in balancing the long-term risks of corticosteroid therapy against the short-term control of effusion, most physicians are reluctant to recommend this treatment for any but the exceptional case.

SURGICAL THERAPY. The goal of surgical therapy is correction of the underlying pathophysiologic condition, if possible, to prevent recurrent OME and remediation of symptoms, primarily hearing loss. When inadequate ventilation of the middle ear is the principal problem, insertion of T-tubes is the treatment of choice. When infection of the middle ear from reflux of nasopharyngeal organisms is the chief problem, adenoidectomy is the treatment of choice. In most cases of chronic OME, both conditions exist concurrently and, thus, the combined operation would be indicated.

T-tubes were introduced in 1954 by Armstrong,[34] and insertion of the tubes is the most common operation performed in children. Adenoidectomy has been used more frequently since the publication of three randomized clinical trials[2, 3, 5] that validated the efficacy of this procedure.

Tympanostomy Tube Insertion. The T-tube serves as an artificial eustachian tube to ventilate the middle ear and equalize the middle ear pressure to atmospheric pressure. Ciliary clearance is also aided because negative pressure cannot build up as the fluid is transported down the eustachian tube.

The finding that the time to recurrence of OME after myringotomy is the same as after extrusion of T-tubes[3] suggests that ventilation of the middle ear provides palliation of the symptoms of OME rather than correction of the underlying problem. Therefore, using T-tubes that remain in place for long durations is a logical choice.[35, 36]

The major differences among the multitude of tubes that are available relate to lumen size, length, and retention time. In general, the short grommet tubes extrude sooner than the long, T-shaped tubes. The larger the bore of the tube and the longer it stays in place, the more likely is a persistent perforation of the tympanic membrane.[36]

Adenoidectomy. Adenoidectomy has been shown to significantly reduce morbidity from chronic OME in three separate, prospective, randomized clinical trials.[2, 3, 5] Given that 1) children in the San Antonio study receiving adenoidectomy had a significant reduction in morbidity as compared with those who did not have their adenoids removed, 2) if adenoidectomy was done, the outcome was similar whether a T-tube was used or not, and 3) the very low rate of complications from adenoidectomy and the modest additional cost when doing T-tube insertion, an argument can be made to perform adenoidectomy and myringotomy—with or without T-tube insertion—as the primary procedure for chronic OME.[37] Paradise et al.[38] argued that adenoidectomy, being slightly riskier and more expensive than T-tube insertion, should be reserved for recurrent cases.

Certainly, the reader will have to decide this matter in his or her own practice according to local costs and practices. However, a rather high rate of T-tube failure exists, leading to repeat surgery, whereas repeat adenoidectomy is seldom necessary and has never been necessary in the practice of this author.

Mastoidectomy. Mastoidectomy is seldom indicated for the treatment of chronic OME and only for recalcitrant cases of chronic OME with mastoid involvement (serous mastoiditis). Because of the relative rarity of these cases, the indications and results of mastoidectomy for chronic OME have not received systematic study, and, therefore, its value remains undocumented. Nonetheless, there are stubborn cases of chronic effusion in which mastoidectomy may be considered, and anecdotal experience indicates a satisfactory outcome. The rationale for the procedure is to remove secretory tissue from the mastoid and to improve ventilation by opening the middle ear to the mastoid via the aditus and the facial recess. However, given that ventilation of the middle ear via the eustachian tube is often inadequate and that the secretory epithelium is largely confined to the middle ear, mastoidectomy should clearly be restricted to only those cases with abnormal mucosa in the mastoid, that is, secretory (or serous) mastoiditis or cholesterol granuloma. Clouding of the entire mastoid air cell system is commonly found in cases of OME; therefore, clouding is not per se an indication. The decision to use mastoidectomy is therefore made based on experience and professional judgment. The few cases this author has treated in this way have been older children with unrelenting effusion and otorrhea through an existing T-tube for which conventional therapy has failed.

PATIENT SELECTION

Cure of OME depends on growth of the skull and eustachian tube and maturation of the immune system. The goals of treatment are reduction in the number of episodes of OME and relief of the conductive hearing loss. Specific objectives are removal of effusion, prolonged drainage of the middle ear, and removal of a septic focus in the nasopharynx.

Therapy for OME differs by the age of the patient and whether the process is acute or chronic. Because antimicrobial therapy is the standard of treatment for acute OME in the United States (this is a controversial issue in Europe), patients with occasional, isolated episodes of acute OME do not generally come to the attention of the otolaryngologist. Therefore, only recurrent or chronic cases are considered here.

Recurrent Acute Otitis Media With Effusion

Children with recurrent acute OME may exhibit normal middle ear examinations between episodes, and some retain effusion and could therefore also be categorized as having chronic OME. The chief goal for those whose effusion clears between episodes is prophylaxis, that is, to prevent new episodes of infection. Several studies have demonstrated efficacy of medical prophylaxis.[39–41] It is becoming generally accepted that children with multiple episodes of acute OME should be treated with long-term, low-dose antimicrobial therapy before surgical therapy is considered. Once a child has developed a new episode of acute OME when receiving prophylaxis, surgery should be considered. Depending on the child's age, T-tubes, adenoidectomy, or both, may be recommended.

T-tube insertion is recommended for infants and children under the age of 18 months who fail medical therapy whether there is residual fluid in the middle ear or not. In children 18 months and older, this author recommends adenoidectomy in addition to T-tube insertion. If the child is in the older range of the acute OME group (i.e., 3 years or older) and the middle ears are air-containing, adenoidectomy and myringotomy without T-tubes are done in selected cases. This treatment cannot be recommended for all children with recurrent acute OME, because the efficacy of adenoidectomy for prevention of acute OME has not been rigorously studied. The reduction in new episodes noted by Paradise et al.[5] in the first year after adenoidectomy and the beneficial effect of adenoidectomy in treatment of children with chronic OME justify study of this indication for adenoidectomy in children with recurrent acute OME.

Chronic Otitis Media With Effusion

Earlier theories of treatment for chronic OME were based on the theory that secretory otitis media was primarily due to eustachian tube obstruction and that ventilation of the middle ear was both necessary and sufficient treatment. It now appears that ventilation of the middle ear via T-tube bypasses the problem but does not correct the underlying disorder, whereas adenoidectomy appears to modify the underlying pathophysiology. Gates et al.[3] compared adenoidectomy with and without T-tube and found no significant difference in the outcome variables, including hearing. Further, outcome after adenoidectomy did not vary with the size of the adenoid. Previous theories held that adenoidectomy was indicated only for an enlarged adenoid. However, this newer evidence, which shows that the effect of adenoidectomy is independent of adenoid size, suggests that basing the indication for adenoidectomy on size is no longer valid. In fact, the small adenoid is apparently more likely to be chronically infected than the large adenoid, which is physiologically healthier.

Idiopathic Hemotympanum

Surgical treatment of patients with idiopathic hemotympanum follows the principles elaborated earlier for the treatment of patients with chronic OME, with the exception that mastoidectomy is necessary more often.

PREOPERATIVE EVALUATION AND PATIENT COUNSELING

Otitis Media With Effusion

The indication for surgery for recurrent acute OME is failure of medical therapy either to clear the middle ear or to prevent recurrences. However, the criteria for failure vary among specialists. Many authorities accept, as a minimum, four episodes of acute OME in 6 months. A more recent addition to this criterion is failure of medical prophylaxis, that is, a breakthrough episode of OME during prolonged antimicrobial therapy. Many children with recurrent episodes of acute OME also retain middle ear effusion between episodes and thus carry a diagnosis of chronic OME as well. In these situations, the prudent physician will act according to the diagnosis with the more serious implications.

The indication for surgery for chronic OME is failure of medical therapy to clear the middle ear effusion and restore hearing to normal levels within a reasonable time. Although controversy remains as to what constitutes a reasonable time, most clinicians and parents agree that if an effusion has not cleared in 3 months in spite of adequate antimicrobial therapy (three courses), the effusion is truly persistent and should be removed and additional steps taken (T-tube insertion and adenoidectomy) to prevent recurrence. In children with documented learning difficulties and bilateral conductive hearing loss, a case can be made to proceed with surgery after 60 days. It is helpful to note that the time criterion is used as an index of the likelihood of spontaneous resolution: many effusions will clear within 30 to 60 days, and surgery should not be performed in such self-limited cases. Once an effusion has persisted for 90 days, it is likely to persist for months or even years. In such a circumstance, there is little doubt that correction of the hearing loss should be done to avoid developmental delays. Although the evidence that mild-to-moderate conductive hearing loss causes developmental delays is inconsistent, these delays clearly occur in many cases, and it seems prudent, therefore, to prevent the problem rather than to seek remedial education after the fact.

Documentation

Current cost-containment strategies by third-party payers have led to increasing scrutiny of the indications for surgical treatment of OME. Various schemes have been developed to verify the history, physical findings, and prior treatment of the condition. The criteria for precertification vary among the payers, in spite of widely circulated indications used by otolar-yngologists. As a result, an increasing burden is placed on the staff of the surgeon's office to collect additional information over and above that needed for patient care. A written summary from the referring pediatrician will fulfill the documentation requirements of most payers.

Demonstration of an enlarged adenoid has been classically required to justify adenoidectomy. Now that it is known that the size of the adenoid is not related to outcome, basing the decision on adenoid size is no longer justified. Children being considered for adenoidectomy should be free of defects of the soft palate. The most insidious problem is that of submucous cleft of the soft palate, which can be suspected by a bifid uvula, a bluish-white band in the midline of the palate (where the muscles are absent), absence of a spine on the posterior edge of the hard palate, and a groove in the posterior surface of the soft palate seen on fiberoptic nasopharyngoscopy.

Counseling

Three aspects of surgical therapy for OME should be stressed: 1) benefits, 2) limitations, and 3) complications.

BENEFITS. The chief benefits of surgery are improved hearing and a reduction in the number of subsequent episodes of OME. Additional benefits are a reduction in the secondary problems of illness (e.g., behavior and time lost from work).

LIMITATIONS. Parents are advised that surgical therapy for OME is generally not curative, but it does correct the hearing loss and generally reduces the number and severity of subsequent episodes. T-tubes will correct the conductive hearing loss as long as the tubes remain open and in place. However, when the tube extrudes, many children experience recurrent OME. Adenoidectomy removes a source of infection from the nasopharynx and is associated with a reduction in the number of new episodes. Removal of the enlarged adenoid often improves sleep and decreases mouth breathing. However, if mouth breathing is an established pattern, the child may still breathe through the mouth, even with a patent nasal airway.

COMPLICATIONS. Purulent otorrhea is a frequent problem with T-tubes, requiring oral and topical antimicrobial agents for control and water precautions (keeping the ears dry) for prevention. Perforation of the tympanic membrane occurs in 1 to 15 per cent of cases, depending on the size of the tube, the number of intercurrent infections, and the duration of intubation. Adenoidectomy requires treatment for hemorrhage in about 1 case in 250 (0.4 per cent); transfusion has not been necessary in my practice, although it remains a theoretic risk. Temporary incompetence of velopharyngeal closure occurs in fewer than 5 per cent of patients and principally in those with a very large adenoid. Permanent velopharyngeal insufficiency is rare and seldom occurs in the absence of a submucous cleft palate.

Idiopathic Hemotympanum

Patients are counseled about the recalcitrant nature of idiopathic hemotympanum and its obscure etiology. Treatment is directed toward relief of symptoms, which in most case is aeration of the middle ear. Although T-tubes are usually ineffective in these cases, it is prudent to use them first and proceed with mastoid surgery if the effusion fails to resolve. The T-tubes often become plugged because of the thick nature of the effusion.

Preoperative thin-section, axial computed tomographic scan of the temporal bone will display the pneumatization pattern of the air cell system and indicate the extent of the hemotympanum. This information is useful for surgical planning and counseling about the extent of the surgery: removal of all affected mucosa via an intact canal wall, facial recess tympanomastoidectomy is the surgical goal. If the aeration pattern and extent of the disease are considerable, a long anesthetic can be anticipated.

The greatest problem with surgery for idiopathic hemotympanum is recurrent effusion. Insufficient data exist on which to base a risk estimate for recurrence; a conservative estimate is no more than a 50 per cent chance of cure. The patient and family are advised about the rare risk of facial nerve injury. The risk of transient paralysis is cited as being less than 1 per cent and permanent paralysis as less than 0.5 per cent.

SURGICAL TECHNIQUE

Preoperative Preparation

The child is kept without food or water for 4 to 6 hours prior to administration of the general anesthetic, depending on the child's age and the policies of the anesthesiologist and hospital. For T-tube insertion, a perioperative antibiotic is not used routinely, because the majority of cases have already received ample antimicrobial therapy. If the effusion is blatantly purulent and pulsatile, suggesting acute inflammation, another agent—one that is not inactivated by β-lactamase—is used for 10 days postoperatively.

For mastoid surgery, a general health assessment and anesthetic risk evaluation are done according to the needs of the patient and the policies of the hospital and anesthesia department. A broad-spectrum antimicrobial agent is administered as soon as the intravenous line is established.

Surgical Site Preparation and Draping

Tympanostomy Tubes

Sterilization of the external auditory canal is not routinely done, because of the low rate of infection and the lack of efficacy.[42, 43] Thorough cleaning of the canal is important for visualization of the tympanic membrane and for postoperative care.

Postoperative use of topical antimicrobial drops is controversial because of conflicting studies showing efficacy[44] and lack of efficacy.[45] They are generally deemed useful in younger children and in cases of purulent or mucoid effusion. However, the magnitude of the effect of these agents is small because infection in the control group is low. The ototoxicity of these preparations precludes their use in situations where absorption through the round window membrane is a possibility, such as in ears with uninflamed middle ear mucosa. In cases of thickened mucosa, the risk of absorption appears to be low, and there have been no documented episodes of sensorineural loss in humans attendant to their use in this instance. Unfortunately, no nonototoxic agents are available for topical prophylaxis, and, further, the manufacturer's recommendations of available agents specifically exclude patients with a perforated tympanic membrane.

Mastoidectomy

The supine position is used for mastoidectomy, with the patient's head at the foot of the table. Long tubing lines are used by the anesthesiologist, who is positioned at the patient's feet. The head is turned away from the affected side. Straps across the chest and pelvis are used to avoid sliding of the patient as the table is rotated from side to side to maximize operative exposure.

The postauricular area is shaved, and clear plastic drapes with sticky edges are applied to the skin edges after the skin is dried and coated with tincture of benzoin. These drapes keep unwanted hair out of the wound. An antibacterial soap is used to scrub the ear and postauricular area and the sticky drapes.

Towels are placed around the incision area, and a clear plastic sticky drape is applied to the entire operative field. This is later incised to expose the incision line. A neurosurgical drape with irrigation catchment will avoid water spillage on the field and floor when drilling with suction irrigation is used.

Instruments

Tympanostomy Tubes

Choice of T-tube is dictated by the surgeon's experience and the treatment goals. The choice of tubes available is staggering in number and variety, and many articles and presentations have discussed the advantages of each type of tube. However, direct comparison of tubes using a prospective randomized study design with stratification by important risk factors needs to be done. The discussions may be reduced to three considerations: duration of intubation, risk of water contamination, and ease of removal. For short-term intubation (as with placement for a severe acute otitis media), a short grommet is a logical choice. For long-term intubation (e.g., for an 11-month boy in day care with eight documented episodes of acute OME, persistent effusion, a strong family history of otitis media, and smoking in the family), a long-stemmed T-tube is a better choice. The short, wide-bore tubes offer little resistance to water entry into the middle ear, compared to the long-shafted T-tubes. Finally, the long tubes can be easily removed in the office, whereas removal of the short grommet tubes with rigid flanges may require a general anesthetic. The risk of otorrhea and permanent perforation increases with the duration of the intubation. However, the risk of recurrent effusion appears to lessen as the duration of intubation increases.

A set of metal speculums, cerumen curettes, and suction cannulas of several sizes are necessary. The operating microscope is vital for illumination and magnification. Myringotomy knives are manufactured in various shapes and configurations. It is useful to choose a knife with a blade width the size of the tube to aid in making the correct dimensions of the incision. Placement of long-stemmed T-tubes is facilitated by the use of an inserter in which the tube is positioned with the short arms of the tube folded forward (Fig. 7–1B). The purpose of the inserter is to avoid damage to the tympanic membrane (bleeding between the epithelial and fibrous layers, which is probably a factor in the genesis of tympanosclerosis. A small pistol-grip forceps may also be used to insert the tube. A fine-tipped otologic dissector is used to manipulate the tube to assure that it is in proper position with the arms fully unfolded. Failure to position the tube so that the lumen can be inspected may create problems if the tube becomes occluded and cleaning is necessary.

Adenoidectomy

Adenoid curettes are available in several sizes and configurations. Those with an angulated handle are easier to use than those with a straight handle. A No. 10 Fr catheter is used to retract the soft palate. Laryngeal mirrors of several sizes permit inspection of the nasopharynx with the use of a headlight or a binocular microscope as a light source. A malleable suction cautery is occasionally used to control bleeding.

Mastoidectomy

The ideal operating room table has motorized controls for adjustment of height and side-to-side rotation. The surgeon's stool has castors, easy height adjustment, and a flexible back that permits the surgeon to lean backwards as necessary while still receiving full support for his or her back. The operating microscope should be adjusted for the surgeon's refraction and interpupillary distance. A bright halogen light source connected to the microscope by a fiberoptic cable is vital for adequate illumination and ease of changing burned-out light bulbs without having to change the microscope drape. Several types of facial nerve monitors are available. The device manufactured by XOMED-Treace provides continuous monitoring of facial motion and also permits stimulation of the nerve for localization during the case.

Technical Details

Tympanostomy Tube Insertion

The ear canal is gently cleaned of all wax and debris. Contact with the anterior bony canal wall is avoided because of the risk of bleeding. The tympanic membrane is inspected and the short process of the malleus identified. This is a constant landmark that may be the only one available in cases of acute infection. The tympanic membrane is incised anteroinferiorly by using an incision that parallels the annulus fibrosus (see Fig. 7–1). This site is generally at right angles to the surgeon's line of vision. Use of a radial incision is satisfactory but may be limited by the overhanging bulge of the anterior ear canal. A posterior incision must be avoided, as it is difficult to make and places the ossicles at risk of injury. The incision is spread open with the side of the knife to accommodate the insertion of the tube. Beginning residents will find that comparing the width of the knife blade with the tube facilitates correct incision dimensions. Care is taken to avoid any major vessel in the tympanic membrane to prevent hemorrhage into the layers of the tympanic membrane, which predisposes to tympanosclerosis.

The middle ear should be evacuated by using a small diameter suction cannula. Usually a No. 5 Fr cannula suffices; occasionally, the gluey material in the middle ear is too viscous to pass through the cannula, and a larger one is necessary. It is not always possible, nor is it desirable, to attempt to remove all the effusion. As long as the middle ear has a near-normal air space into which to place the tube, the remainder of the effusion will be carried into the eustachian tube or will drain out the tube. Culture of the effusion is not done clinically, because in many cases there will be no growth because of prior antimicrobial therapy or technical reasons related to the need to break up the immunoglobulin matrix of the effusion.

It is important to position the tube such that the lumen is in line with the surgeon's line of sight, thereby facilitating postoperative examination of the middle ear mucosa in the office and, also, cleaning of the tube should it become plugged later on. When using T-tubes, the surgeon should assure that the short arms of the tube are completely unfolded. If one arm is not fully open, manipulating the tube from side to side or even twisting it will usually release it. If the tube has a removal wire, it can be used to make sure that the tube is positioned properly.

In patients with mucoid or purulent middle ear effusion, a topical polymicrobial-corticosteroid solution is placed on the tube and the tympanic membrane to reduce the likelihood of postoperative otorrhea and clotting within the tubal lumen. Where the middle ear is air-containing and the mucosa looks normal, these drops may be omitted to avoid the risk of cochlear toxicity that is known to follow absorption of the material through the round window membrane.

Adenoidectomy

The patient is given a general anesthetic and the airway is ensured by endotracheal intubation. The patient is placed in the Rose position with the neck extended over a rolled sheet. A mouth gag is inserted, and the soft palate is retracted with a catheter. The adenoid is excised with curved curettes of various sizes and shapes and the use of a large mirror and either a headlight or the operating microscope to inspect the nasopharynx to assure completeness of removal (Fig. 7–2A). Care must be taken to avoid injury to the prevertebral fascia and muscles, which may cause excessive bleeding. Curved biting forceps are useful to remove tissue not accessible by the curette.

The basket adenotome is seldom used because its curved shape may promote incomplete removal.

Bleeding usually stops promptly; pressure applied for a few minutes via sponges in the nasopharynx appears to assist the process, as does irrigation with saline at room temperature. Suction electrocautery permits precise coagulation of bleeding vessels and avoids the risk of stenosis from indiscriminate field cauterization (Fig. 7–2B).

The goal of the surgery is complete removal of the midline adenoid pad to achieve smooth re-epithelialization of the nasopharynx. Curettage of the tissue in the fossa of Rosenmüller is not done for fear of scar tissue formation and contracture that might contribute to eustachian tube reflux. Care must be taken to avoid direct injury to the eustachian tube that might result in stenosis.

Mastoidectomy

Incision of the external auditory canal skin is done first, if necessary, and the tympanic membrane is elevated forward to permit a look into the posterior mesotympanum. The incision is placed about 2mm behind the annulus and parallel to it. Longitudinal incisions are made at 6 and 12 o'clock, and a long posterior flap is elevated laterally. A small piece of absorbable gelatin sponge (Gelfoam) soaked in epinephrine 1:1000 is placed into the middle ear for hemostasis.

A postauricular incision is used in all cases, and it is based about one fingerbreadth behind the postauricular crease, roughly paralleling the free margin on the helix (Fig. 7–3). The further posterior the incision, the greater the ease of inspecting the middle ear and eustachian tube through the facial recess. The incision is made into the subcutaneous layer, and the postauricular muscles are cut and the pinna rotated forward and held with dural hooks. A second, more rectangular, incision is made through the deep tissues and periosteum down to the mastoid cortex. This flap, popularized by Tauno Palva of Helsinki, is based anteriorly and extends behind the skin incision. This flap is sutured back into place at the end of the case to provide support for the pinna and keep the ear from falling into the mastoid cavity. If needed, fascia from the temporalis muscle may be harvested for later use.

FIGURE 7–1. *A*, The incision in tympanic membrane. *B*, The placement of the T-tube within the inserter. *C*, The proper position of the tube.

FIGURE 7–2. *A*, The technique of adenoidectomy using the curette. It is important to keep the handle in the sagittal or parasagittal plane to prevent injury to the torus tubarius. *B*, The use of the suction cautery with mirror for hemostasis.

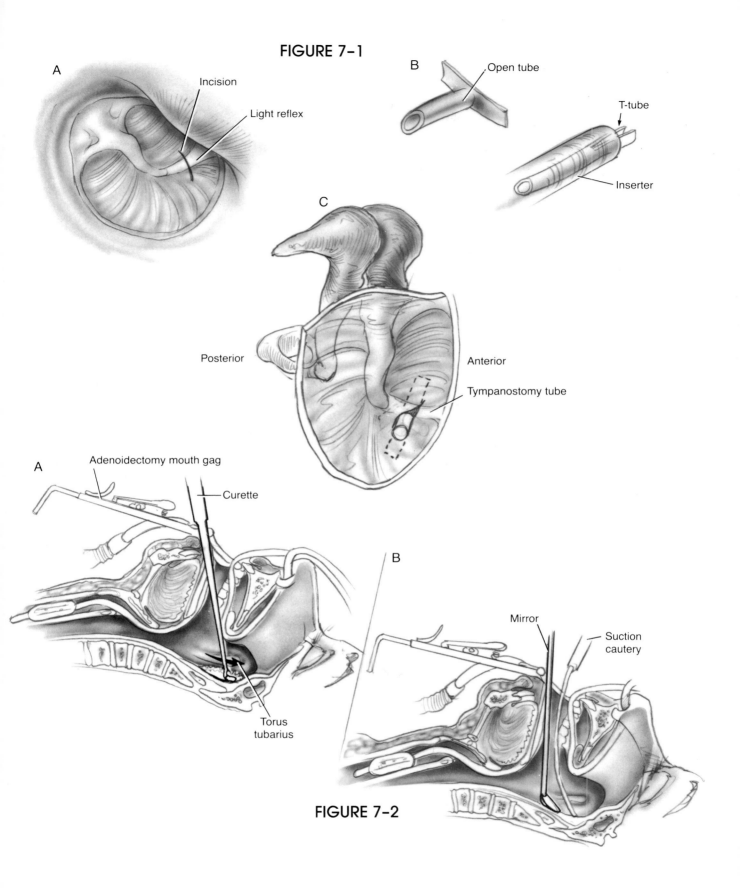

FIGURE 7-1

A — Incision, Light reflex

B — Open tube, T-tube, Inserter

C — Posterior, Anterior, Tympanostomy tube

A — Adenoidectomy mouth gag, Curette, Torus tubarius

B — Mirror, Suction cautery

FIGURE 7-2

The skin of the posterior wall of the external auditory canal, which was elevated earlier, is rotated posteriorly and held in place by the self-retaining retractor. A full view of the bony external auditory canal and middle ear is gained.

A large cutting burr on a straight handpiece is used to remove the lateral mastoid cortex. This procedure is done using a headlight or overhead light for illumination. After identification of the sigmoid sinus, posterior wall of the external auditory canal, tegmen, and mastoid antrum, the operating microscope is brought into the field, and the aditus and attic are opened laterally. The fossa incudis and the short process of the incus are uncovered. The extent of the mastoidectomy varies with the surgical pathology and extent of pneumatization. Generally, the temporal bone is well pneumatized in these cases, and it is desirable to take down all the cells in the mastoid portion of the temporal bone to reduce the surface area of the system. In this way, as the epithelium regenerates, there will be a single, large cavity rather than an extensive, honeycombed, spongiform mastoid, and correspondingly, less secretory epithelium. The mastoid tip is opened to the level of the digastric ridge, the retrofacial cell tract is opened to determine its contents (these are usually normal), and the bony plates over the posterior and middle fossa dura are skeletonized to form a smooth surface (Fig. 7–4). Care is taken to avoid exposing dura, especially in the middle cranial fossa, for fear of later brain herniation. Any osteitic bone is removed until healthy bleeding bone is encountered.

The facial recess is opened into the middle ear by the use of progressively smaller cutting burrs. The plane of the short process of the incus leads to the facial recess (Fig. 7–5). With experience, one learns the character of the bone of the recess and can identify the dense bone of the fallopian canal, the thin bone of the air cells, and the dull yellow, variegated-appearing supporting bone filling the recess. Once the fallopian canal and chorda tympani nerve are identified, the recess is opened between them into the middle ear. The internal opening of the facial recess, which is anteromedial to the facial nerve, may be flared to permit inspection of nearly all parts of the mesotympanum. Coupled with the tympanotomy, the ossicular chain is inspected, and any hyperplastic mucosa and secreting membranes are removed from the middle ear. If bone is exposed, a piece of absorbable gelatin film (Gelfilm) is placed through the facial recess and across the promontory toward the eustachian tube at the end of the case to prevent adhesions and to keep the recess open.

The tympanic membrane is returned to its position, and the canal wall flap is rotated forward to close the defect in the external auditory canal. The Palva flap is sutured tightly back into place. A drain may be placed into the subcutaneous space and brought out through the wound inferiorly. The subcutaneous layer is closed with interrupted 3-0 chromic sutures placed in an inverted manner so that the knots are down and the skin edges are tightly approximated. Skin sutures are generally not necessary if the subcutaneous layer is expertly closed. Steri-Strips may be applied as necessary, thereby avoiding the need for removal of skin sutures for patients who may have to travel long distances. They are particularly appropriate for children, for whom suture removal may be arduous.

A small drain is placed in the incision, and a form-fitting mastoid dressing is applied using gauze fluffs and a conforming gauze roll. An ear cup with head band is commercially available to substitute for the gauze wrap. This preparation has the advantage of allowing the patient to dress the ear at home. However, a pressure dressing is unnecessary in most cases after the second day at home, and a well-wrapped dressing will stay in place for several days. If a tympanoplasty was performed, the external auditory canal is dressed with an absorbable gelatin sponge and polymyxin B ointment.

Postoperative Care

A cotton ball is inserted into the ear canal to absorb any drainage and may be changed by the parents as often as necessary. A topical solution of polymicrobial and corticosteroid is used twice daily for 5 days, or until the drainage ceases. A postoperative office visit

FIGURE 7–3. The skin incision and the second incision for the Palva flap.

FIGURE 7–4. The mastoidectomy in progress. The sigmoid plate is skeletonized, and the bulge of the lateral semicircular canal in the antrum is visible. Note the positioning of the large retractor and dural hooks to keep the Palva flap rotated forward.

FIGURE 7–5. The completed mastoidectomy in the right ear with the facial recess opened. The dimensions of the facial recess are exaggerated by the artist to display the middle ear structures that may be seen by the surgeon after multiple repositionings of the viewing angle of the microscope.

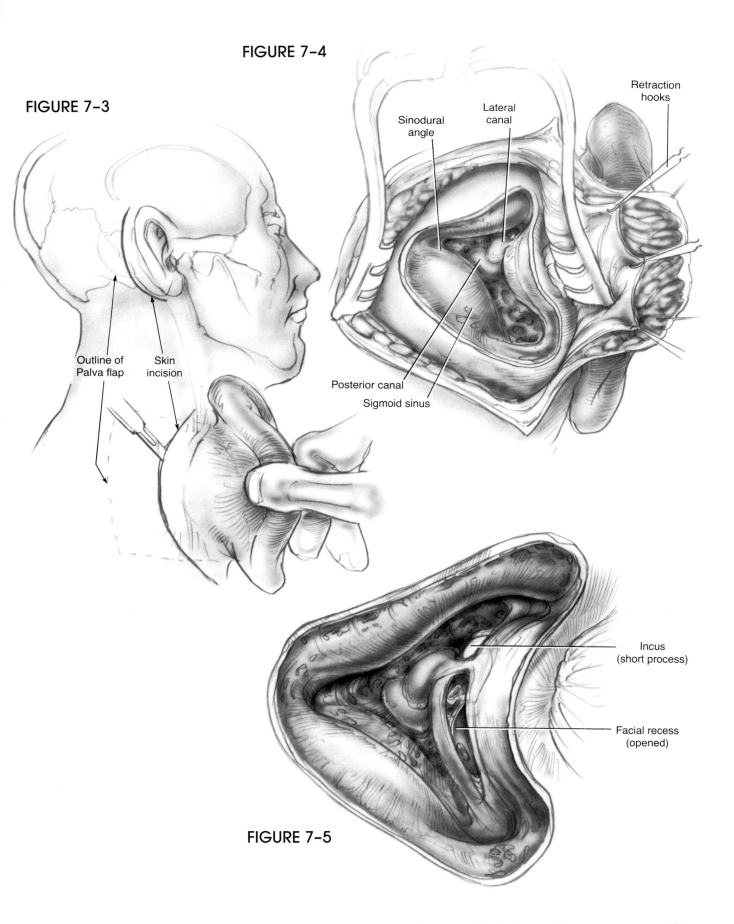

FIGURE 7–4

FIGURE 7–3

Retraction hooks

Sinodural angle

Lateral canal

Outline of Palva flap

Skin incision

Posterior canal

Sigmoid sinus

Incus (short process)

Facial recess (opened)

FIGURE 7–5

is made between the tenth and fourteenth days to assure that the tube is properly positioned and that the infection is under control. This visit provides an additional opportunity for counseling regarding water protection.

Following adenoidectomy, mild ear pain is common. Acetaminophen is prescribed for pain control. The child is able to eat normally as soon as nausea from the anesthetic has subsided. Transient nasal speech may occur in a small percentage of cases, but frank regurgitation of liquids through the nose is uncommon. These transient sequelae may occur after removal of a large adenoid mass. Palatal and pharyngeal wall compensation occurs quickly, and permanent voice change is rare.

After mastoidectomy, the patient receives pain medication and other supportive agents for the postoperative recovery period. The drain is removed on the morning of the first postoperative day, and the mastoid dressing is reapplied. The vast majority of patients undergoing mastoid surgery are discharged on the day after surgery, the so-called 23-hour admission. Home care is minimal. The postauricular wound and hair may be washed as soon as the patient is comfortable. Care is taken not to disturb or wet the ear canal packing. An office visit at 2 weeks permits cleaning of the canal and inspection of the wound. A second visit a month later is made for a final canal cleaning and audiogram.

Periodic Follow-up Visits

The modified T-tubes, which are slightly shorter than the original Goode T-tubes, are favored because these will remain in situ for 2 to 5 years. The child is examined at 6-month intervals to assure tubal patency, freedom from infection, and proper position of the tube. These tubes are well tolerated. Occasionally, granulation tissue will form around the base of the tube, and this usually responds well to the same topical solution used postoperatively.

Parents are instructed to treat any episode of otorrhea with the same topical drops, and if the episode continues for more than 48 hours, to obtain an oral antimicrobial agent effective against β-lactamase from the primary care physician. If the discharge fails to resolve promptly with this regimen, the child is seen in the office for cleaning of the canal, softening any debris in the tube (if necessary) with hydrogen peroxide, and opening by gentle suctioning, as well as for culturing for identification and antimicrobial sensitivity. Repeated office cleaning and continued use of topical drops usually suffices. If not, the tube is removed in the operating room, and the middle ear is inspected and cultured. If the middle ear looks healthy, the tube is replaced; if there is significant

inflammation, the tube is removed, and medical treatment is continued. Rarely, a resistant organism will be present that may require intravenous antimicrobial therapy, either at home (with visiting nurse support) or in the hospital. The choice of agent depends on the sensitivity of the organism. In most cases, a resistant *Pseudomonas* sp. is found. With home intravenous therapy becoming available in many cities, the prolonged used of intravenous antipseudomonal agents is increasingly more practical.

Surgical Pitfalls

TYMPANOSTOMY TUBE INSERTION. Trauma of the external auditory canal during cleaning or instrumentation is a common problem for the beginning resident. Great care should be taken to avoid trauma because the resultant bleeding, although minor in amount, obscures vision and often results in a clot that is difficult to remove later in the office. Irrigation with saline and application of a topical vasoconstrictive agent, such as phenylephrine (Neosynephrine) 1/8%, will usually bring this under control.

Bleeding within the tympanic membrane is commonly seen when a vessel is included in the incision. Such bleeding will dissect between the layers of the tympanic membrane and may result in the formation of a tympanosclerotic plaque. Various measures have been employed to prevent this: topical heat cautery, application of phenol, and laser myringotomy. Often, careful placement of the incision will avoid the problem.

Dislodgement of tube into the middle ear may be a problem with a large myringotomy and small tubes without wires or tabs but is not a problem with T-tubes. Early extrusion of the tube usually occurs because the incision is too large or the tube is only partially inserted.

ADENOIDECTOMY. The chief surgical pitfalls to avoid during adenoidectomy are trauma to the torus tubarius, which protects the opening of the eustachian tube, and deep removal of the posterior wall of the nasopharynx, which leads to excessive bleeding. Inadequate removal of adenoid tissue may be avoided by careful inspection of the nasopharynx with a mirror.

MASTOIDECTOMY. The chief pitfall of mastoidectomy is injury to the facial nerve in opening the facial recess. This trauma is rare in experienced hands, especially with continuous monitoring of the nerve during the procedure. Dural exposure in the tegmen should be avoided because of the risk of later encephalocele. Contact of the drill with the incus may result in mild-to-moderate high-frequency sensorineural loss due to vibratory energy transmitted to the cochlea.

Wound infection is uncommon. Copious irrigation during and after the procedure aids in removal of unwanted debris that might serve as a nidus for infection.

Results

The principal effect of surgery is to reduce the number of recurrences of OME and to restore hearing. The following discussion is based on data from 491 patients randomly assigned to one of four surgical treatment groups as presented in Gates et al.[3] Recurrent effusions were measured by how long they lasted, and the total duration of effusion was used as the chief outcome measure. Over the 2-year period after surgical treatment, the children treated with myringotomy had mean time with effusion of any type in either ear of 51 weeks, whereas those receiving T-tubes had effusions of 36 weeks, those with adenoidectomy and myringotomy had effusions of 31 weeks, and those receiving the combination of adenoidectomy and T-tubes had effusions of 27 weeks. Thus, using myringotomy only as the baseline, T-tubes reduced time with effusion by 29 per cent after T-tubes; by 38 per cent after adenoidectomy and myringotomy; and by 47 per cent after adenoidectomy and T-tubes. Statistically, the outcomes for the myringotomy-only group were significantly worse than each of the other three groups; effusion time was significantly less in the adenoidectomy plus T-tubes group than in the T-tubes–only group, but not in comparison with adenoidectomy-myringotomy; effusion time was not significantly different between the T-tube group and the adenoidectomy-myringotomy group.

Time with abnormal hearing was comparable among the patients in the three treatment groups, all of whom had significantly better hearing than the patients in the surgical control group, that is, myringotomy only. In addition, the patterns of recurrence and morbidity were altered: most recurrent effusions were unilateral and cleared faster than in the surgical control group.

Surgical retreatment was performed for 109 (22 per cent) of the 491 patients: once for 85, twice for 21, and three times for 3. Surgical retreatments were necessary more often in children initially treated with myringotomy (66 retreatments in 34 of 107 children [32 per cent]) or T-tubes (36 reoperations in 26 of 129 children [20 per cent]) than in those treated by adenoidectomy and myringotomy (17 operations in 13 of 130 children [10 per cent]) or adenoidectomy plus T-tubes (17 reoperations in 12 of 125 children [10 per cent]). The number of repeat operations in the two adenoidectomy groups was significantly less than in the two nonadenoidectomy groups ($P < 0.001$). None of the children needed a repeat adenoidectomy.

The most frequent sequela, purulent otorrhea, occurred one or more times in 22 per cent of the surgical control group, 29 per cent of the T-tube group, 11 per cent of the adenoidectomy-myringotomy group, and 24 per cent of the adenoidectomy–T-tube group. This difference was highly significant ($P < 0.001$).

Although most cases of idiopathic hemotympanum resolve satisfactorily, surgical management is generally successful. Often, it takes months for the ear to aerate and for satisfactory hearing to return. Nonetheless, persistence and patience are often rewarded.

Complications and Management

Tympanostomy Tubes

OTORRHEA. The most prevalent sequela of T-tubes is purulent otorrhea, from which *Pseudomonas* spp. are usually grown. Some cases are due to water contamination of the ear; others are the result of acute OME. Treatment is the same: a topical polymicrobial-steroid solution, an oral antibiotic agent, and, if the otorrhea continues, suction cleaning of the ear in the otologist's office. Fortunately, most episodes clear promptly. On rare occasions, an unusual organism may the cause. Therefore, in recalcitrant cases, the tube is removed, a culture the middle ear is done, a new tube is inserted, and topical therapy is continued. For those that fail to clear, tube removal is the next step. If the otorrhea continues, mastoidectomy with tympanoplasty is done. Fortunately, this problem is uncommon.

PERSISTENT PERFORATION. In from 1 to 15 per cent of cases, the tympanic membrane fails to heal following tube removal or extrusion. If the child is older, it may be possible to close the perforation with cautery to the edges with trichloroacetic acid and patching with a Steri-Strip. More often, however, the standard treatment—once the ear is dry—is to perform a fat graft myringoplasty.[46] This approach offers an uncomplicated and effective remedy that can be performed on an outpatient basis.

Adenoidectomy

BLEEDING. The most common complication of adenoidectomy is postoperative bleeding. However, the incidence is low: of 250 cases done by 13 surgeons, only one child required operative treatment for bleeding, and none needed or received blood transfusion.[3] Helmus et al.[47] noted that only four patients in 1000 (0.4 per cent) bled after outpatient adenoidectomy and that all instances occurred in the first 6 postoperative hours and were managed without transfusion.

VELOPHARYNGEAL INCOMPETENCE. Other less common complications include nasopharyngeal stenosis and velopharyngeal incompetence. Stenosis results from excessive tissue destruction, such as might occur from excessive use of the electrocautery, excessive curettage of the fossa of Rosenmüller, and removal of the lateral pharyngeal bands. Transient velopharyngeal insufficiency may occur after removal of a large adenoid but resolves quickly in the majority of cases. Persistent velopharyngeal incompetence is the most feared complication because it requires either a prosthesis or a secondary procedure (pharyngeal flap) for correction. The majority of such cases are due to an undetected submucous cleft palate. Preoperative evaluation with fiberoptic nasopharyngoscopy is useful in detecting an occult posterior submucous cleft.

Mastoidectomy

FACIAL PARALYSIS. Complications following mastoidectomy are rare. Wound infection is the most common, and recurrence of effusion is next. Facial paresis (weakness) occurs rarely in surgeries performed by experienced hands. Intraoperative nerve monitoring is a welcome and useful adjunct that frees the surgical team members from having to look at the face with a flashlight under the drapes when the surgeon is drilling close to the nerve. Heat injury to the nerve should not occur if continuous irrigation is used. Physical damage to the nerve should be rare.

RECURRENT HEMOTYMPANUM. Recurrent idiopathic hemotympanum is common. A second mastoid operation is not indicated in this event; instead, insertion or reinsertion of a large-bore T-tube should be done. Amplification may be necessary for hearing.

ALTERNATIVE TECHNIQUES

HEARING AIDS. Older children with persistent effusion for whom both medical and surgical treatment have failed should be evaluated in regard to hearing aid use, particularly when the child is in school.

ALLERGY TREATMENT

Children with symptomatic food or inhalant allergy deserve therapy whether they have OME or not. Given that the majority of cases of OME have had prior nasal infection and that children with nasal allergy have a higher prevalence of infection, allergy evaluation is appropriate for children with OME who also have nasal symptoms. However, we found a lower incidence of allergy in our subjects with OME

than in the general population.[3] Although a cause-and-effect relation between nasal allergy and OME has not been shown, the surgeon should inquire about allergic symptoms to provide proper therapy for those with dual problems.

References

1. Gates GA: Socioeconomic impact of otitis media. Pediatrics 71: 648–649, 1983.
2. Maw AR: Chronic otitis media with effusion (glue ear) and adenotonsillectomy: A prospective randomized controlled study. BMJ 287: 1586–1588, 1983.
3. Gates GA, Avery CA, Prihoda TJ, Cooper JC: Effectiveness of adenoidectomy and tympanostomy tubes in the treatment of chronic otitis media with effusion. N Engl J Med 317: 1444–1451, 1987.
4. Mandel EM, Bluestone CD, Paradise JL: Myringotomy with and without tympanostomy tube insertion in the treatment of chronic otitis media with effusion. Arch Otolaryngol Head Neck Surg 115: 1217–1224, 1989.
5. Paradise JL, Bluestone CD, Rogers KD, et al.: Efficacy of adenoidectomy for recurrent otitis media in children previously treated with tympanostomy-tube placement. JAMA 263: 2066–2073, 1990.
6. Doyle WJ: A functiono-anatomic description of eustachian tube vector relations in four ethnic populations: an osteology study. Ph.D. dissertation. University of Pittsburgh, 1977.
7. Klein JO, Teele DW, Mannos R, et al.: Otitis media with effusion during the first three years of life and development of speech and language. In Lim DJ, Bluestone CD, Klein JO, Nelson JD (eds): Recent Advances in Otitis Media with Effusion. Philadelphia, BC Decker, 1984, pp 332–335.
8. Hubbard TW, Paradise JL, McWilliams BJ, et al.: Consequences of unremitting middle-ear disease in early life: Otologic, audiologic, and developmental findings in children with cleft palate. N Engl J Med 312: 1529–1534, 1985.
9. Henderson FW, Collier AM, Sanyal MA, et al.: A longitudinal study of respiratory viruses and bacteria in the etiology of acute otitis media with effusion. N Engl J Med 306: 1377–1383, 1982.
10. Giebink GS, Payne EE, Mills EL, et al.: Experimental otitis media due to Streptococcus pneumoniae: Immunopathogenic response in the chinchilla. J Infect Dis 134: 595–604, 1976.
11. Howie VM, Ploussard JH: Simultaneous nasopharyngeal and middle ear exudate cultures in otitis media. Pediatr Digest 13: 31–35, 1971.
12. Pillsbury HC III, Kveton JF, Sasaki CT, Frazier W: Quantitative bacteriology in adenoid tissue. Otolaryngol Head Neck Surg 89: 355–363, 1981.
13. Bluestone CD, Paradise JL, Beery QC: Physiology of the eustachian tube in the pathogenesis and management of middle ear effusions. Laryngoscope 82: 1654–1670, 1972.
14. Eden AR, Laitman JT, Gannon PJ: Mechanisms of middle ear aeration: Anatomic and physiologic evidence in primates. Laryngoscope 100: 67–75, 1990.
15. Aschan G, Ekvall L, Magnusson B: Reverse aspiratory middle ear disease: A neglected pathogenic principle. In Munker G, Arnold W (eds): Physiology and Pathophysiology of Eustachian Tube and Middle Ear. New York, Thieme-Stratton, 1980, pp 90–96.
16. Teele DW, Klein JO, Rosner BA: Epidemiology of acute otitis media in children. Ann Otol Rhinol Laryngol 89(Suppl 68): 5–6, 1980.
17. Liu YS, Lang RW, Lim DJ: Microorganisms in chronic otitis media with effusion. Ann Otol Rhinol Laryngol 85: 245–249, 1976.
18. Stangerup SE, Tos M: The etiologic role of acute suppurative otitis media in chronic secretory otitis media. Am J Otolaryngol 6: 126–131, 1985.
19. Tos M, Holm-Jensen S, Sorensen CH, et al.: Spontaneous course and frequency of secretory otitis in four-year-old children. Arch Otolaryngol 108: 4–10, 1982.

20. Sade J: The natural history of the secretory otitis media syndrome. *In* Sade J (ed): Secretory Otitis Media and Its Sequelae. New York, Churchill Livingstone, 1979, pp 89–101.
21. Tos M: Production of mucus in the middle ear and eustachian tube: Embryology, anatomy, and pathology of the mucous glands and goblet cells in the eustachian tube and middle ear. Ann Otol Rhinol Laryngol 83(Suppl 11): 44–58, 1974.
22. Segal J, Ostfeld E, Yinon J, et al.: Mass spectrometric analysis of composition in the guinea pig middle ear–mastoid system. *In* Lim D, Bluestone C, Klein J, Nelson J (eds): Recent Advances in Otitis Media with Effusion. Philadelphia, BC Decker, 1983, pp 68–70.
23. Cantekin EI, Doyle WJ, Phillips DC, Bluestone CB: Gas absorption in the middle ear. Ann Otol Rhinol Laryngol 69(Suppl 68): 71–75, 1980.
24. Paparella MM, Lim DJ: Pathogenesis and pathology of the "idiopathic" blue drum. Arch Otolaryngol 85: 249–258, 1967.
25. Sheehy JL, Linthicum FH, Greenfield EC: Chronic serous mastoiditis, idiopathic hemotympanum and cholesterol granuloma of the mastoid. Laryngoscope 79: 1189–1217, 1969.
26. Sade J: The blue drum (idiopathic hemotympanum) and cholesterol granulomas. *In* Sade J (ed): Secretory Otitis Media and Its Sequelae. New York, Churchill Livingstone, 1979, p 12.
27. Thomas SM, Shimada T, Lim DJ: Experimental cholesterol granuloma. Arch Otolaryngol 91: 356–358, 1970.
28. Gebhart DE: Tympanostomy tubes in the otitis media prone child. Laryngoscope 91: 849–866, 1981.
29. Gates GA, Muntz H, Gaylis B: Adenoidectomy and otitis media. Ann Otol Rhinol Laryngol 101(Suppl 155): 24–32, 1992.
30. Mandel EM, Rockette HE, Bluestone CD, et al.: Efficacy of amoxicillin with and without decongestant-antihistamine for otitis media with effusion in children. N Engl J Med 316: 432–437, 1987.
31. Schwartz RH, Puglese J, Schwartz DM: Use of a short course of prednisone for treating middle ear effusion: A double-blind crossover study. Ann Otol Rhinol Laryngol 89(Suppl 68): 296–300, 1980.
32. Lambert PR: Oral steroid therapy for chronic middle ear effusion: A double-blind crossover study. Otolaryngol Head Neck Surg 95: 193–199, 1986.
33. Rosenfeld RM, Mandel EM, Bluestone CD: Systemic steroids for otitis media with effusion in children. Arch Otolaryngol Head Neck Surg 117: 984–989, 1991.
34. Armstrong BW: A new treatment for chronic secretory otitis media. Arch Otolaryngol 69: 653–654, 1954.
35. Goode RL: T tube for middle ear ventilation. Arch Otolaryngol 97: 402–403, 1973.
36. Per-Lee JH: Long-term middle ear ventilation. Laryngoscope 91: 1063–1072, 1981.
37. Gates GA, Avery CA, Prihoda TJ, Cooper JC Jr: Adenoidectomy and chronic otitis media. (Letter) N Engl J Med 318: 1470–1471, 1988.
38. Paradise JL, Bluestone CD: Adenoidectomy and chronic otitis media. (Letter) N Engl J Med 318: 1470, 1988.
39. Maynard JE, Fleshman JK, Tschopp CR: Otitis media in Alaskan Eskimo children: Prospective evaluation of chemoprophylaxis. JAMA 219: 597–599, 1972.
40. Perrin JM, Charney E, MacWhinney JB Jr, et al.: Sulfisoxazole as chemoprophylaxis for recurrent otitis media. N Engl J Med 291: 664–667, 1974.
41. Principi N, Marchisio P, Massironi E, et al.: Prophylaxis of recurrent acute otitis media and middle-ear effusion. Comparison of amoxicillin with sulfamethoxazole and trimethoprim. Am J Dis Child 143: 1414–1418, 1989.
42. Baldwin RL, Aland J: The effects of povidone-iodine preparation on the incidence of post-tympanostomy otorrhea. Otolaryngol Head Neck Surg 102: 631–634, 1990.
43. Giebink GS, Daly K, Buran DJ, et al.: Predictors for postoperative otorrhea following tympanostomy tube insertion. Arch Otolaryngol Head Neck Surg 118: 491–494, 1992.
44. Gates GA, Avery C, Prihoda TJ, Holt GR: Post-tympanostomy otorrhea. Laryngoscope 96: 630–634, 1986.
45. Scott BA, Strunk CJ: Post-tympanostomy otorrhea: A randomized clinical trial of topical prophylaxis. Otolaryngol Head Neck Surg 106: 34–41, 1992.
46. Gross C, Bessila M, Lazar RH, et al.: Adipose plug myringoplasty: An alternative to formal myringoplasty techniques in children. Otolaryngol Head Neck Surg 101: 617–620, 1989.
47. Helmus C, Grin M, Westfall R: Same-day stay adenotonsillectomy. Laryngoscope 100: 593–596, 1990.

8

The Abnormally Patulous Eustachian Tube

CHARLES D. BLUESTONE, M.D.
ANTHONY E. MAGIT, M.D.

The abnormally patulous eustachian tube presents as a spectrum of clinical signs and symptoms. Patient presentations range from subclinical disturbances to debilitating symptoms leading to significant psychologic impairment. The eustachian tube is closed in the normal physiologic state, with brief open periods primarily resulting from activity of the tensor veli palatini muscle. The abnormally patulous eustachian tube is permanently open. Patients with a patulous tube have abnormal gas flow from the nasopharynx to the middle ear throughout all phases of respiration and swallowing.

Schwartze was the first to describe the patulous eustachian tube with the report of a scarred atrophic eardrum moving synchronously with respiration.[1] In 1867, Jago reported having this affliction himself.[2] Zollner and Shambaugh noted that patients with abnormally patulous eustachian tubes complain of autophony.[3, 4] The abnormally patulous eustachian tube is not a rare condition. However, as noted by Rumbolt in 1873 and Bull in 1976,[5, 6] the diagnosis requires constant awareness and clinical vigilance. Heightened awareness is an important component to the increased frequency of the diagnosis. From 1940 to 1959, the diagnosis of a patulous eustachian tube was made 41 times at the Mayo Clinic. This diagnosis was made 95 times at the Mayo Clinic in the 7-year period from 1960 to 1966.[7] Zollner cited an incidence of 0.3 per cent in the general population.[3] Munker diagnosed an abnormally patulous eustachian tube in 6.6 per cent of 100 woman who had normal results on otoscopic examination.[8]

The diagnosis of an abnormally patulous eustachian tube necessitates an intensive search for an etiology in each patient because of the possibility of a serious underlying disease. Weight loss is the most common etiology and the one most easily treated. As little as 6 pounds of weight loss may lead to sufficient atrophy of soft tissue in the peritubal area to result in a patulous tube.[7, 9] Atrophy and scarring of the nasopharyngeal muscles secondary to a cerebral vascular accident, poliomyelitis, multiple sclerosis, radiotherapy, and iatrogenic and traumatic injuries to the fifth cranial nerve may result in a functionally patulous eustachian tube.[4, 10–12] Muscular dysfunction secondary to direct damage to the tensor veli palatini muscle during cleft palate surgery, combined with postoperative nasopharyngeal adhesions and fibrosis, may cause a patulous tube.[13] Shambaugh[4] and Pulec and Simonton[14] proposed that repeated tonsillar and pharyngeal infections can alter pharyngeal function to the point of causing a patulous eustachian tube. Palatal myoclonus has also been associated with this disorder.

Pregnancy and supplemental estrogen are implicated in the etiology of a patulous eustachian tube.[11, 14–16] High levels of estrogen may lead to thinning of intraluminal eustachian tube secretions or an increase in relaxin, a hormone known to increase ligamentous relaxation in the pelvis.[17] Estrogen also affects prostaglandin E levels, with a subsequent effect on surfactant levels.[18] Elevated surfactant levels may decrease the intraluminal surface tension, with the development of a more patulous eustachian tube. Less common conditions associated with a patulous eustachian tube are chronic gum chewing, dental malocclusion, continued voluntary or involuntary subluxation of the temporomandibular joint, and skull dysmorphology, such as brachycephaly.

PATIENT SELECTION

The most frequent symptom associated with an abnormally patulous eustachian tube is autophony, the awareness of hearing one's own voice.[13] Autophony may also be described as a roaring sound in the ear synchronous with respiration, fluctuating fullness and "blockage" in the ear, a feeling of talking into a barrel, or such loud perception of one's voice that normal conversation is impossible.[19, 20] Autophony is usually fluctuant and does not become apparent until the patient has been erect for several minutes. Relief comes from assuming a supine position, sniffing, or by placing one's head between the knees.[21] These maneuvers effectively increase venous congestion in the peritubal area. Acute rhinitis or any increase in edema of the nasal mucosa and postnasal space is usually associated with an improvement in symptoms.[13] Symptoms may be exacerbated by topical or systemic decongestants, exercise, fatigue, or nervousness.[19]

Patients with an abnormally patulous eustachian tube may present with an apparent psychoneurotic condition.[20, 22] Manipulation of the mandible as a means of closing off the eustachian tube may give the appearance of a tick or manifestation of neurotic behavior. Hyponasality and hyporhinolalia secondary to the attempt to close the eustachian tube is a less common presentation of a patulous eustachian tube.[13, 23] Ringing tinnitus, conductive hearing loss, and vestibular symptoms are uncommon characteristics of a patulous eustachian tube. Robinson and Hazell reported an association between patulous eustachian tubes and sensorineural hearing loss.[24]

The diagnostic evaluation of the patient suspected of having a patulous eustachian tube starts with a comprehensive history. Symptoms of autophony as previously described are the hallmark of the patulous eustachian tube. Autophony improves when the patient is supine or when the head is in a dependent position, and the onset of symptoms develop within minutes or hours of assuming an upright position.[21]

Otoscopic results may be normal; however, tympanic membrane findings may include atrophic changes. Synchronous movement of the tympanic membrane with respiration has been documented by Schwartze, Hartman, and Voltolini.[1, 25, 26] Otoscopy should be performed using a microscope with the patient in the upright position.[24] Movement of the tympanic membrane is enhanced by occlusion of one naris and closure of the mouth during forced inspiration and expiration, or by using the Toynbee or Valsalva maneuver. Gentle pneumatic pressure in the external auditory canal may give the appearance of a flail tympanic membrane. Rarely, respiration and speech may be heard by using a microphone placed in the external auditory canal.

In addition to video documentation of a flail tympanic membrane, objective evidence of a patulous eustachian tube is possible with tympanometry.[27] Two tympanograms are obtained while the patient is in the upright position. The first is done with the patient breathing normally, and the second, during breath holding. Fluctuations in the tympanometry tracing coincide with respiration. Fluctuations are enhanced by occluding one nostril and closing the mouth, or by the Toynbee maneuver. More detailed characterization of a patulous eustachian tube is possible after determination of the passive eustachian tube opening pressure when the tympanic membrane has a tube or hole present; the middle ear eustachian tube (which is patulous) will not maintain positive middle-ear pressure.[27] An intact tympanic membrane can be evaluated by performing the "nine-step" test.[27, 28] Virtanen is a proponent of sonotubometry for diagnosing the abnormally patulous eustachian tube.[29]

An audiogram should be obtained as part of the evaluation, as hearing loss is often a part of the constellation of complaints associated with a patulous eustachian tube. Although some reports describe a unilateral sensorineural hearing loss of unknown etiology on the same side as a patulous eustachian tube, no clear association has been established between a patulous eustachian tube and sensorineural hearing loss.[24]

TREATMENT

Once the diagnosis of a patulous eustachian tube has been established, an underlying cause should be sought. Initial therapy involves addressing the underlying cause, if found. When a clear etiology is not apparent, medical and surgical therapy are instituted and are aimed at ultimately decreasing patency of the eustachian tube lumen. The severity of symptoms will dictate the urgency with which treatment is implemented.

Children and adolescents rarely present with a patulous eustachian tube. In this population, therapy is usually not indicated, as the symptoms are self-limited. Minimal symptoms of a patulous tube may initially be treated with reassurance and an explanation of the benign nature of the affliction.[7] Weight loss is the most obvious etiology of a patulous eustachian tube, and the most responsive to nonsurgical therapy. Weight gain usually results in resolution of symptoms.

Elevated estrogen levels may lead to a patulous condition as previously described. Pregnant women can be assured that completion of the pregnancy will lead to stabilization of estrogen fluxes and a return to normal eustachian tube function.[11, 14-16] Prior to the introduction of low-dose estrogen birth control pills, patients complained more frequently of patulous symptoms. Nontheless, birth control pills may still be responsible for abnormal eustachian tube function.

When an etiology for the patulous eustachian tube condition is not found, or the contributing condition cannot be effectively treated, for example, emaciation due to terminal cancer, medical or surgical therapy is indicated.

Medical therapy intended to decrease eustachian tube patency may be started as an initial course of therapy for patients with moderate symptoms. The oral administration of a saturated solution of potassium iodide (SSKI, 10 drops in a glass of juice three times a day) has been reported to be efficacious in some patients. This may be combined with the use of conjugated estrogens (Premarin) nasal spray (25mg in 30ml of normal saline solution, three drops three times per day).[30] Medical therapy may be tried for 1 month in patients with moderate symptoms before surgery is recommended. Experimentally, atropine has been shown to reduce the inflation pressure and initial opening pressure of a patulous eustachian tube.[31] Medical therapy may not be a plausible first-line management for patients with grossly abnormal results on otoscopic examinations and debilitating symptoms and is rarely successful in the long term when the condition is chronic.

Procedures intended to cause irritation and inflammation of the eustachian tube orifice provide transient relief from patulous symptoms. Although not widely used in contemporary practice, several means of creating eustachian inflammation are available: eustachian tube catheterization and insufflation with a salicylic acid–boric acid solution in a 1:4 ratio,[32] eustachian tube diathermy,[24, 33] silver nitrate cautery,[13, 34] and the application of nitric acid and phenol.[35] In the authors' experience, these procedures have limited efficacy.

Surgical therapy is an alternative when less invasive methods of treatment have failed. Although the abnormally patulous eustachian tube allows abnormal air flow to the middle ear cleft, some physicians report success with myringotomy and tympanostomy tube placement.[14, 36, 37] Despite the lack of theoretical basis for the success of this procedure, myringotomy with tube placement continues to be used for the treatment of this condition.

Surgical reconstruction of the eustachian tube orifice is one treatment option for a patulous eustachian tube. Closure of the eustachian tube orifice involving the removal of cartilage is one method.[38] This procedure either has been unsuccessful in alleviating the symptoms, or has led to complete stenosis of the eustachian tube and refractory middle ear effusion. Transposition of the tendon of the tensor veli palatini muscle with and without hamulotomy has been reported in several small series.[21, 39] With limited follow-up, this procedure has been successful in approximately 70 per cent of cases; long-term follow-up of patients treated with this method has not been reported.

Various methods of blocking the pharyngeal opening of the eustachian tube have been reported. Zollner infiltrated paraffin around the eustachian tube orifice and saw transient improvement in patulous symptoms.[3] Ogawara et al. infused an absorbable gelatin sponge–glycerin mixture into the eustachian tube and found a high recurrence rate within 1 month of the procedure.[40] O'Connor and Shea introduced polytetrafluoroethylene (Teflon) paste into the eustachian tube orifice and saw transient relief.[13] Pulec succeeded in resolving patulous symptoms in 19 of 26 patients after an injection of polytetrafluoroethylene at the anteroinferior margin of the pharyngeal eustachian tube orifice.[7] Polytetrafluoroethylene injection is now contraindicated because of complications that include cerebral thrombosis and death.[13]

Because the authors have had limited success with either the nonsurgical or the surgical methods reported in the past, we prefer treating surgically the chronically abnormal patulous eustachian tube by inserting an indwelling catheter into the protympanic portion of the eustachian tube.[41] This procedure is combined with myringotomy and tympanostomy tube placement in anticipation of a middle ear effusion forming after the eustachian tube is obstructed. Patients are told that following surgery, water must be kept out of the ear because of the tympanostomy tube. No other limitation of activity is necessary. A tympanostomy tube placed in the anteroinferior portion of the tympanic membrane will not cause hearing loss. The patients should be followed up at least twice a year to assess the status of their symptoms and that of the tympanostomy tubes. Some patients will spontaneously extrude the tympanostomy tube and not develop middle ear effusion. Presumably, there is

enough gas exchange from the nasopharynx into the middle ear to effectively ventilate the middle ear. However, if middle ear negative pressure or effusion develops, then a tympanostomy tube must be reinserted. With this procedure, eustachian tube obstruction can be reversed by removing the indwelling catheter if, on a rare occasion, the patient desires it to be removed, or if there are postoperative complications or sequelae.

Surgical Technique

The surgical procedure may be performed with local anesthesia supplemented with systemic analgesia or under general anesthesia. The type of anesthetic is based on patient preference. Advantages of local anesthesia include the safety of the anesthetic and a reduced recovery time. Local anesthetic infiltration is used whether the procedure is performed under mild intravenous sedation or general anesthesia. A standard four-quadrant injection is made at the bony-cartilaginous junction of the external auditory canal by using a solution of 1 per cent lidocaine and 1:100,000 epinephrine injected from a 25-gauge needle. A significant blanching of the anterior canal wall may not be possible because of the thinness of the skin in this area.

Following injection of the ear canal, the ear is prepared with a povidone-iodine solution. If a tympanostomy tube is present, a piece of cotton is placed in the external auditory canal to prevent flow of the solution through the tube. The ear canal is irrigated with a sterile saline solution prior to beginning the surgical procedure.

Perioperative antibiotics are not used. Any sign or symptom of infection in the external auditory canal or middle ear is a contraindication to surgery until the condition is resolved.

The surgical procedure is performed with the aid of an operating microscope. Using a Rosen knife, or "round knife," an *anterior* circumferential incision is made 8mm from the annulus extending from 12 o'clock to 6 o'clock (Fig. 8–1). The initial elevation of the anterior tympanomeatal flap is done with a Moon elevator (Fig. 8–2). A No. 3 Fr suction is positioned behind the elevator to prevent trauma to the flap. If the patient has a large anterior bony overhang, it may require drilling with a Skeeter drill to provide adequate exposure. Caution must be exercised during any drilling of the anterior canal wall to avoid entrance into the temporomandibular joint. Once the level of the anterior annulus is reached, a cotton pledget soaked with 1:1000 adrenaline may be placed between the flap and anterior canal wall to prevent bleeding prior to entering the middle ear. The anterior annulus is drawn out of the sulcus with a Rosen

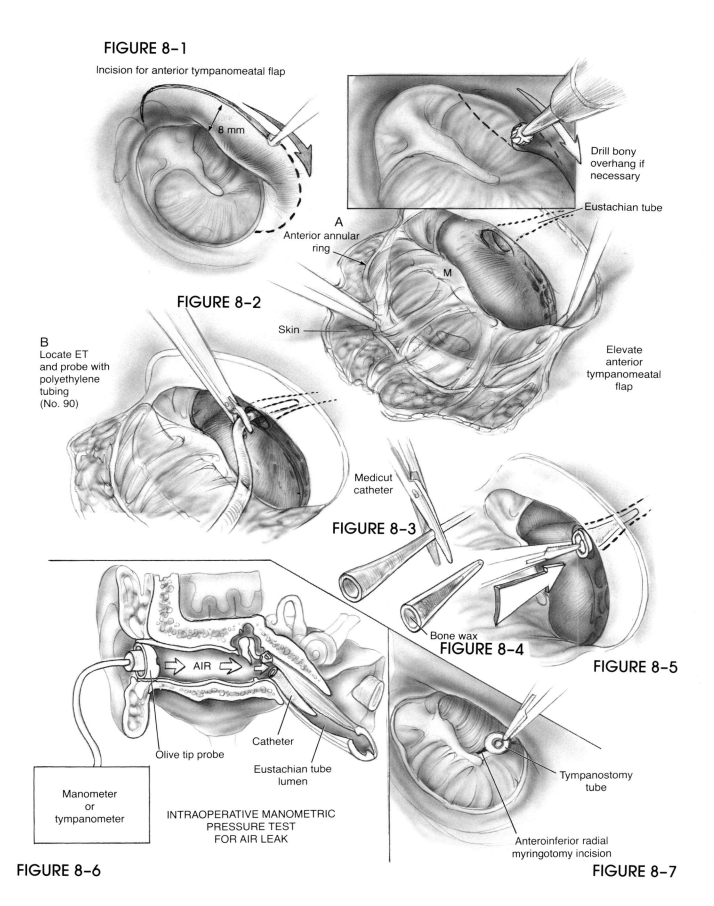

FIGURE 8-1

Incision for anterior tympanomeatal flap

8 mm

Drill bony overhang if necessary

Eustachian tube

A
Anterior annular ring

M

Skin

Elevate anterior tympanomeatal flap

FIGURE 8-2

B
Locate ET and probe with polyethylene tubing (No. 90)

Medicut catheter

FIGURE 8-3

Bone wax

FIGURE 8-4

FIGURE 8-5

AIR

Olive tip probe

Catheter

Eustachian tube lumen

Manometer or tympanometer

INTRAOPERATIVE MANOMETRIC PRESSURE TEST FOR AIR LEAK

FIGURE 8-6

Tympanostomy tube

Anteroinferior radial myringotomy incision

FIGURE 8-7

needle or a gently curved instrument. Once the middle ear is entered, the flap is further elevated with an annulus elevator, or "gimmick." The flap is elevated to the malleus. Care must be taken not to traumatize the ossicles; however, this does not usually pose a problem.

A modification of the anterior tympanomeatal flap approach to the middle ear involves using a large anterior myringotomy for access to the middle ear.[30] This method has been reported to be successful in a small series of patients but is not the method preferred by the authors.

The eustachian tube orifice is identified with direct vision or with a piece of No. 90 polyethylene tubing. The polyethylene tubing is helpful in assessing the orientation of the eustachian tube lumen. The eustachian tube catheter is fashioned using an 18-gauge Medicut angiocath (Argyle Medicut, Sherwood Medical Industries, St. Louis, MO). The narrowed end of the catheter is cut to leave a total catheter length of approximately 2cm (Fig. 8–3). The flared end of the catheter is occluded with bone wax (Fig. 8–4). The narrowed end of the catheter is introduced into the eustachian tube orifice using a forceps or large alligator (Fig. 8–5). Sufficient pressure is used to obtain a tight fit.

Once the catheter is secured, a manometer or tympanometer is used to assess the degree of occlusion of the eustachian tube. With the tympanomeatal flap still elevated, a sterile olive tip probe is inserted into the external auditory canal (Fig. 8–6). Using either the manometer or tympanometer, the pressure is slowly raised to 400mm to 600mm of water. Obtaining an opening pressure prior to inserting the Medicut catheter is helpful in assessing if the opening pressure is significantly higher after the catheter has been inserted; ideally, there will be no opening pressure and the middle ear and the obstructed eustachian tube will hold air pressure to the limit of the manometer or tympanometer. It should be noted that when the patient is in the supine position, there will be an opening pressure, albeit lower than normal, prior to inserting the Medicut catheter, because the eustachian tube is engorged in this position. Any leak of air below this level is considered an inadequate seal, and catheter placement is reassessed. If the Medicut catheter appears to be in place and there is still a leak of air, bone pate (taken from the anterior auditory canal) can be used around the edges of the catheter. After the pressure test is completed, the tympanomeatal flap is placed back into its anatomic position. At this point, an anterior radial myringotomy is performed, and a tympanostomy tube is placed (Fig. 8–7). The ear canal is filled with an antibiotic ointment to secure the flap. A cotton ball is then placed in the external meatus and serves as the only necessary dressing.

POSTOPERATIVE CARE

The patient is instructed to limit physical activity for 4 weeks to allow for healing of the tympanomeatal flap. Postoperative antibiotics are not routinely used. Patients are instructed to keep water out of their ears by using an ear plug and by avoiding submerging their heads. Ear plugs are not used until the patient is seen at the postoperative visit to assure that the canal incisions are well healed.

RESULTS *Success ~60%.*

Of nine patients with follow-up of between 2 and 15 years, five have had marked improvement in symptoms. These patients had failed previous medical and surgical interventions. Patients have not had complications related to the tympanostomy tubes. Two patients have extruded their eustachian tube catheters and tympanostomy tubes, with continued relief from their patulous tube symptoms. It is felt that these patients developed adequate scarring of the eustachian tube lumen to effectively eliminate the patulous condition. Two patients with catheters in place and extruded tympanostomy tubes with intact tympanic membranes have not experienced any episodes of middle ear effusion. This finding supports the concepts that in some patients there is gas exchange around the Medicut catheter. Because of the tympanostomy tube, patients have not complained of aural fullness following catheter placement. One patient who complained of postoperative tinnitus wanted the catheter removed, which was done without any complication. However, that patient still has symptoms of a patulous tube bilaterally and has persistent tinnitus in both the ear that was previously operated on and the one that was not.

References

1. Schwartze H: As cited by Ogawara S, et al. Arch Otolaryngol 102: 276–280, 1976.
2. Jago J: Functions of the tympanum. Br For Med Chir Rev 39: 496–520, 1867.
3. Zollner F: As cited by Ogawara S, et al. Arch Otolaryngol 102: 276–280, 1976.
4. Shambaugh GE Jr: Continuously open eustachian tube. Arch Otolaryngol 27: 420–425, 1938.
5. Rumbolt TF: The Functions of the Eustachian Tube. St. Louis, South Western Book and Publishing Company, 1873, p 98.
6. Bull TR: Abnormal patency of the eustachian tube. [Letter] Br Med J 283: 1390, 1976.
7. Pulec JL: Abnormally patent eustachian tubes: Treatment with injection of polytetrafluoroethylene (Teflon) paste. Laryngoscope 77: 1543–1554, 1967.
8. Munker G: Physiology and pathophysiology of eustachian tube and middle ear. In Munker G, Arnold W (eds): New York, Thieme-Stratton.
9. Perlman HB: The eustachian tube. Arch Otolaryngol 73: 310–321, 1961.
10. Virtanen H: Patulous eustachian tube. Arch Otolaryngol 86: 401–407, 1978.

11. Pulec JL, Horowitz MJ: Diseases of the eustachian tube. *In* Paparella MM, Shumrick PA (eds): Otolaryngology, Vol 2. Philadelphia, WB Saunders, 1973, pp 275–290.
12. Bluestone CD, Cantekin EI, Beery Q: Certain effects of adenoidectomy on eustachian tube ventilatory function. Laryngoscope 85: 113–127, 1975.
13. O'Connor AF, Shea JJ: Autophony and the patulous eustachian tube. Laryngoscope 91: 1427–1435, 1981.
14. Pulec JL, Simonton KM: Abnormal patency of the eustachian tube. Laryngoscope 74: 267–271, 1964.
15. Suehs GW: The abnormally open eustachian tube. Laryngoscope 70: 1418–1426, 1960.
16. Allen GW: Abnormal patency of the eustachian tube. JAMA 200: 412–413, 1967.
17. Flisberg K, Inglestet S: Middle-ear mechanics in patulous eustachian tube cases. Acta Otolaryngol 263: 18–22, 1969.
18. Davis LJ, Sheffield PA, Jackson RT: Drug induced patency changes in the eustachian tube. Arch Otolaryngol 92: 325–328, 1970.
19. Miller JB: Patulous eustachian tube: Report of 30 cases. Arch Otolaryngol 73: 310–321, 1961.
20. Moore PM, Miller JB: Patulous eustachian tube. Arch Otolaryngol 54: 643–650, 1951.
21. Stroud MH, Spector GT, Maisel RH: Patulous eustachian tube syndrome. Arch Otolaryngol 99: 419–421, 1974.
22. Perlman HB: The eustachian tube: Abnormal patency and normal physiologic state. Arch Otolaryngol 30: 212–238, 1939.
23. Landes BA: Hyporhinolalia associated with eustachian tube dysfunction. Laryngoscope 77: 244–246, 1967.
24. Robinson PJ, Hazell JWP: Patulous eustachian tube syndrome: The relationship with sensorineural hearing loss. Treatment with eustachian tube diathermy. J Laryngol Otol 103: 739–742, 1989.
25. Hartman A: Experimentelle Studien über die Function der Eustachischen Röhre. Veit Comp, 1879.
26. Voltolini R: Zwei eigenthümliche Ohrenkrenkheiten Monatsschr Ohrenheilkd 1883, 17: 1–6.
27. Bluestone CD: Otitis media, atelectasis, and eustachian tube dysfunction. *In* Bluestone CD, Stool SE (eds): Pediatric Otolaryngology. Philadelphia, WB Saunders, 1990, pp 350–356; 360–362; 416–418.
28. Bluestone CD: Assessment of eustachian tube function. *In* Jerger J, Northern J (eds): Clinical Impedance Audiometry. Acton, MA, American Electromedics Corporation, 1980, pp 83–108.
29. Virtanen H: Patulous eustachian tube: Diagnostic evaluation by sonotubometry. Acta Otolaryngol 86: 401–407, 1978.
30. Dyer RK, McElveen JT: The patulous eustachian tube: Management options. Otolaryngol Head Neck Surg 105: 832–835, 1991.
31. Morita M, Matsunaga T: Effects of an anti-cholinergic on the function of the patulous eustachian tube. Acta Otolaryngol (Stockh) 458: 63–66, 1988.
32. Bezold F, Siebenman F: Textbook of Otology for Physicians and Students (Translated by J. Holinger). Chicago, EH Colgrove Company, 1908, pp 154–155.
33. Halstead TH: Pathology and surgery of the eustachian tube. Arch Otolaryngol 4: 189–195, 1926.
34. Eisner MF, Alexander MH: Silver nitrate cautery. *In* Coates GM, Schenck MF (eds): Otolaryngology, Vol 1. Hagerstown, MD, Prior & Company, 1957, pp 17–19.
35. McAliffe GB: Dilatation and stenosis of the eustachian tube. N Y Eye Ear Infirm Rep 6: 116–118, 1898.
36. Thaler S, Yamagisawa E: The abnormally patent eustachian tube. Arch Otolaryngol 84: 418–421, 1966.
37. Chen DA, Luxford WM: Myringotomy and tube for relief of patulous eustachian tube symptoms. Am J Otol 11: 272–273, 1990.
38. Simonton KM: Abnormal patency of the eustachian tube—Surgical treatment. Laryngoscope 67: 342–359, 1957.
39. Virtanen H, Palva T: Surgical treatment for patulous eustachian tube. Arch Otolaryngol 108: 735–739, 1982.
40. Ogawara S, Satoh I, Tanaka H: Patulous eustachian tube. Arch Otolaryngol 102: 276–280, 1980.
41. Bluestone CD, Cantekin EI: Management of the patulous eustachian tube. Laryngoscope 91: 149–152, 1981.

9

Traumatic Perforation— Office Treatment of the Chronically Draining Ear

SEAN R. ALTHAUS, M.D., F.A.C.S.

TYMPANIC MEMBRANE PERFORATIONS, CHRONIC OTITIS MEDIA, AND CHOLESTEATOMA

Tympanic membrane perforations result from various pathologic conditions. Trauma, inflammatory disease within the middle ear and temporal bone, cholesteatoma, and, rarely, neoplastic disease can interrupt the interface between the external auditory canal and the middle ear cleft. These perforations are generally described as central, marginal, or epitympanic (attic retraction pocket) (Fig. 9–1).

The most common cause of persistent tympanic membrane perforations is suppurative or nonsuppurative chronic otitis media. Additionally, cholesteatoma, although less common now than in the past, continues to represent a significant problem in otologic practice.

A cholesteatoma, or keratoma, is defined as "an accumulation of exfoliated keratin in the middle ear or other pneumatized areas of the temporal bone arising from keratinizing squamous epithelium."[1] Generally, these lesions have a sac-like structure, occur in conjunction with a tympanic membrane perforation, and contain whitish debris composed of cholesterol crystals, hence the term *cholesteatoma*.[2] Cholesteatomas typically expand over time, resulting from the continuing process of desquamation and entrapment of epithelial debris within the sac, or from epithelial migration.[3, 4] The expansion process is thought to be due to a combination of erosive pressure on surrounding structures as the lesion grows in bulk, and a localized destruction of bone from pyogenic osteitis, enzymatic collagenolysis, and osteoclastic bone resorption.[5, 6] In addition to causing both conductive and sensorineural hearing loss, bone erosion from the expanding cholesteatoma may invade the bony covering of the facial nerve, semicircular canals, cochlea, dura, or sigmoid sinus, leading to the feared complications of facial paralysis, labyrinthitis, sensorineural hearing loss, brain abscess, meningitis, or thrombophlebitis of the sigmoid sinus.[7]

Generally, three types of cholesteatoma are recognized: attic retraction cholesteatoma, secondary acquired cholesteatoma, and congenital cholesteatoma. Attic retraction cholesteatoma represents the most common form of cholesteatoma and is generally felt to result from an invagination of the pars flaccida portion of the tympanic membrane, usually caused by chronic eustachian tubal dysfunction and negative middle ear pressures.[8, 9] Attic retraction cholesteatomas may be indolent and hidden beneath a small crust of epithelial debris or cerumen. Meticulous cleaning of the ear, preferably under the otomicroscope, will detect such a lesion. Typically, one will encounter a fairly small erosion of the superior osseous canal wall, just above the malleus short process, that yields moist epithelial debris on cleaning. On the other hand, the patient may present with a chronically discharging ear and the diagnosis, after the ear is cleaned, should be relatively easy.

Secondary acquired cholesteatoma typically arises through an existing posterior marginal tympanic membrane perforation, as squamous epithelium from the external auditory canal and lateral tympanic membrane surface migrates over the edges of the perforation, entering the middle ear cleft. In these cases, the posterior annular ligament of the tympanic membrane is usually attenuated or missing, favoring epithelial migration over the edge of the perforation. Skin ingrowth can involve the middle ear extensively and enter the epitympanic space and mastoid antrum.[10] Eventually, the epithelial contents of most cholesteatomas become contaminated by microbial organisms, leading to otorrhea, which may be foul smelling. The clinical diagnosis of secondary acquired cholesteatoma usually poses little difficulty for the otologist, as layers or accumulations of moist, whitish epithelial debris are found to occupy the involved portions of the middle ear on physical examination.

Congenital cholesteatomas of the temporal bone were first described in 1938.[11] They are thought to be caused by epithelial rests of embryonal origin or through basal cell papillary proliferation and ingrowth and may occur anywhere within the temporal bone.[12, 13] They are relatively rare and develop behind an intact ear drum, frequently in patients with no history of ear disease. Typically, a whitish globular mass is seen behind the anterior portion of the drum on otoscopy, adjacent to the malleus handle. Often, an alert pediatrician will spot the problem and request clarification from the otologist. On the other hand, congenital cholesteatomas deep within the temporal bone may remain silent for years, until progressive hearing loss, facial paresis, or disequilibrium alert the clinician to the possibility of such a lesion.

The diagnosis of cholesteatoma is generally made on clinical grounds. Imaging studies, such as computed tomographic scans or mastoid X-rays, are not obtained routinely in the preoperative assessment unless an unusual situation or threatening complication is suspected. The treatment of cholesteatoma is surgical and is detailed in the chapters following.

OFFICE TREATMENT OF THE CHRONICALLY DRAINING EAR

Obtaining a dry ear prior to surgery is an important and desirable goal in the surgical treatment of chronic otitis media. This objective can be achieved in the majority of "wet" ears, through thorough evaluation and meticulous medical management in the preoperative period. Careful and repeated cleaning of the middle ear and ear canal, the topical use of antimicrobial medications, and the creation of an unfavorable environment for bacterial and fungal growth are essential for achieving the goal of a dry ear preoperatively. On the other hand, in ears not selected for surgery, gaining a dry ear may improve the quality of life for the elderly or poor-risk surgical patient. In some ears, and in particular, some cholesteatoma cases, no amount of preoperative effort will lead to a dry ear, and the surgery itself must be relied on to achieve this goal.

Access to an otomicroscope is a basic requirement for proper cleaning of a wet ear, as is adequate suction equipment. A head mirror or hand-held otoscope simply does not provide the otologist with the necessary technical help to properly clean an ear.

Most chronic ear drainage results from mixed infections of aerobic and anaerobic pathogens, typically *Pseudomonas aeruginosa, Staphylococcus aureus, Proteus* species, *Escherichia coli*, and anaerobic streptococcal organisms.[14, 15] Rarely, uncommon pathogens, such as *Mycobacterium* species, are responsible for chronic resistant otorrhea.

Although there is a growing concern regarding the potential ototoxicity of otic drops, and while the majority of these products are theoretically ototoxic, they have been used in the medical management of chronic suppurative otitis media for years and appear to have a wide margin of safety. The more commonly used preparations contain neomycin or polymyxin, individually or in combination. These agents are active against the majority of middle ear bacterial pathogens. Research into the development of effective non-ototoxic topical medications continues, and the experimental use of topical fluoroquinolones has been reported.[16] Corticosteroids are a common component of otic drops, and they reduce itching and inflammation, while decreasing mucosal and ear canal edema. Antimicrobial dusting powders offer an effective alternative to otic drops in many instances, particularly in the presence of neomycin sensitivity or pain associated with the application of drops. Although some draining ears respond nicely to a regimen of boric acid, 95 per cent salicylic acid 5 per cent, three times a day, the majority of wet ears are truly suppurating, and antibacterial or antifungal preparations are necessary. With a combination of chloramphenicol (Chloromycetin), *p*-aminobenzene sulfonamide (Sulfanilamide), and amphotericin B–timerosal–titanium dioxide (Fungizone) powder delivered through an inexpensive insufflator twice a day, it is not unusual to see a chronically wet, noncholesteatomatous ear that is unresponsive to topical otic drops dry up quickly. The pharmacist is asked to compound chloramphenicol, 50mg, *p*-aminobenzene sulfonamide, 50mg, and amphotericin B (Fungizone), 5mg, in a number 4 gel capsule, and dispense a suitable starter supply with an Oto-Med Power Insufflator and instructions for use. Hydrocortisone, 1 mg, can be added to this preparation if desired, and the *p*-aminobenzene sulfonamide can be removed for patients allergic to it.

Measures aimed at promoting an undesirable environment for antimicrobial proliferation are very important in the effective medical management of the chronically draining middle ear. Avoiding water contact is mandatory. The patient is instructed in dry ear precautions and is advised to use a silicone ear plug or cotton–petroleum jelly dam when showering or shampooing. Swimming is discouraged. The careful use of a hand-held hair dryer after showering can facilitate drying of the ear and ear canal. Microbial growth is inhibited in an acidic medium, and steps are taken to lower the pH of the ear canal and middle ear. Irrigation of the canal with a diluted white vinegar solution can accomplish this goal while it cleans the canal of debris, which is also a desirable component of effective medical management. Many topical otic preparations contain acetic acid to acidify the pH.

The following approach in the office treatment of the chronically draining ear, in the author's experience, works well. At the first office visit, a history is obtained, and the ear is carefully examined under the otomicroscope and cleaned. A culture and sensitivity specimen of the drainage is not obtained routinely, unless the patient has been on prolonged systemic antibiotic therapy, or an unusual problem is suspected. Plans are made to obtain an audiogram at some point during the preoperative evaluation period. Instructions are given for cleaning the ear twice daily with a diluted acetic acid and water solution (half-strength white vinegar) using a medicine dropper or small bulb syringe. The patient is seen 7 to 10 days later, and the ear is re-examined. At this point, the ear usually looks less inflamed, with a minimal amount of debris in the canal. If the ear is not better, a culture and sensitivity specimen is obtained, and culture-specific oral antibiotic therapy is initiated. Ciprofloxacin and fluoroquinolones are not used in children under age 18 because of the potential to produce erosion of cartilage in weight-bearing joints and arthropathy in immature animals of various species.[17]

At this point, if the patient is a child, the parent is instructed to continue the vinegar rinses and to begin using an antibiotic-steroid–containing ear drop twice daily following vinegar cleaning of the ear. This regimen is continued for 10 days and is then discontinued. The ear is examined 3 to 4 days later and, if dry, surgery can be scheduled. If not, an antibiotic-antifungal powder insufflation regimen is initiated twice daily, following the vinegar rinse. This "dry program" will dry up a significant number of these wet ears. If the ear fails to clear on this regimen, a culture and sensitivity specimen is obtained, surgery is scheduled, and the parent is advised that mastoid disease is contributing to the problem, and that mastoid surgery will be required.

In adults, dry treatment is usually initiated at the second office visit, and the patient is instructed to clean the ear twice a day, before insufflating the powder, with a cotton-tipped wire applicator, which is supplied by the doctor's office. This regimen is continued until maximum improvement has been obtained, and surgery is then scheduled. Once again, not all discharging ears will dry on this regimen, and if the ear remains wet, the patient is advised that mastoid surgery will be required.

OFFICE TREATMENT OF THE DRAINING MASTOID CAVITY

The most common causes for a draining mastoid cavity are 1) inadequate or poorly performed surgery, 2) failure to seal the middle ear from the mastoid cavity at surgery, 3) suboptimal postoperative care, 4) neglect of the cavity, and 5) persistent suppurative disease in the temporal bone.

The principles of well-done canal wall down tympanomastoid surgery include beveling the edges of the mastoid cavity and removing all bone overhang, sealing off the middle ear space, obliterating mucosa-containing cell tracts, lowering the facial ridge and removing the anterior buttress, taking care of the large mastoid tip, and performing a generous meatoplasty. Details and surgical technique are thoroughly described in Chapter 19.

When the original surgery has been inadequate, leaving a high facial ridge, or when a small meatoplasty prevents adequate aeration and good access to the cavity for cleaning, cavity moisture may become a problem. With moisture due to a troublesome large mastoid tip, or failure to seal the middle ear space at surgery, a revision operation will generally prove necessary, with correction of these causative problems. Adequate and aggressive postoperative care is a requirement for obtaining a dry cavity. Following discharge from the surgical facility, the patient is seen weekly for cleaning and painting of granulation tissue with 1 per cent aqueous gentian violet or cauterization of granulations with silver nitrate. Subsequently, monthly visits are held until the mastoid cavity is dry and completely skin lined. The need for annual or semiannual inspection and cleaning of the mastoid cavity throughout life is emphasized.

The presence of a mucosal-skin interface in the mastoid cavity is a frequent reason for a chronically wet cavity. This abnormal relationship was never intended by nature and commonly results when the middle ear cleft is left open at canal wall down tympanomastoid surgery. On inspection under the otomicroscope, the nature of the problem becomes apparent, as the mastoid cavity is generally well lined with squamous epithelium, and the moisture comes from the middle ear space. Revisionary surgery, with placement of a fascia graft over the middle ear cleft, will usually lead to a dry ear and affords the possibility of ossicular reconstruction for hearing improvement. Occasionally, mucosalization of the cavity occurs, and this problem can be prevented by obliterating mucosa-containing cell tracts at the initial surgery with fibromuscular tissue.

Cavity neglect leads to the build-up of cerumen and epithelial debris, then secondary moisture and suppuration beneath the debris. A thorough cleaning under the otomicroscope, followed by a 5-day course of topical antibiotic drops or powder, will usually dry the cavity promptly. Persistent suppurative disease of the temporal bone will require further evaluation and, in most cases, secondary surgery.

From a practical standpoint, the author has found the following products useful in the office management of the chronic mastoid cavity:

NONSPECIFIC AGENTS
1. Vinegar swishes
2. Acetic acid, 2 per cent, and aluminum acetate otic solution
3. Silver nitrate
4. Povidone-iodine, 10 per cent
5. Five per cent boric acid–95 per cent isopropyl alcohol drops
6. Five per cent salicylic–95 per cent boric acid powder

ANTIBACTERIAL AGENTS
1. Neomycin-polymyxin–containing otic drops
2. Tobramycin (Tobrex) drops
3. Chloramphenicol otic drops (for patients allergic to neomycin or polymyxin).
4. Chloramphenicol, *p*-aminobenzene sulfonamide, and Fungizone powder (or chloramphenicol-Fungizone powder in *p*-aminobenzene sulfonamide–sensitive patients)

ANTIFUNGAL AGENTS
1. Gentian violet (aqueous)
2. One per cent Thymol–95 per cent isopropyl alcohol drops
3. Cresylate (a solution containing thimerosal [Merthiolate], *m*-cresyl-acetate, propylene glycol, and boric acid)
4. Castellani's paint (a nonspecific antifungal agent whose active ingredients are fuchsin, phenol, resor-

cinol [paraben], acetone, and 70 per cent isopropyl alcohol)
5. Merthiolate
6. Clotrimazole (Lotrimin)—the most effective antifungal agent in in vitro studies of common otomycotic pathogens.[18]

OTHER CONSIDERATIONS

1. EUSTACHIAN TUBE FUNCTION.

   The evaluation of eustachian tube function in the office management of the chronically wet ear is unnecessary, in the author's experience. Significant eustachian tubal dysfunction usually clears by age 6 and is rarely a persistent problem beyond childhood. Localized obstruction of the tubal orifice in the middle ear from inflammatory tissue or cholesteatoma does occur and can be corrected at the time of surgery.

2. ADENOTONSILLECTOMY.

   The child presenting with a chronically draining ear, with or without cholesteatoma, with persistent middle ear effusion in the contralateral ear, a history of previous myringotomies with tubes, and hypertrophic tonsils and adenoid is a candidate for adenotonsillectomy prior to definitive ear surgery. On the other hand, if the contralateral ear is normal, and the discharging ear clears on medical management, the tonsils and adenoid are probably not playing a major role in the chronic middle ear problem, and surgery can proceed.

3. NASAL PROBLEMS.

   Structural problems within the nose rarely contribute to chronic middle ear disease and generally need not be considered in the genesis of chronic middle ear drainage.

4. ALLERGY.

   The role of allergy in chronic middle ear disease remains controversial. The assistance of a competent allergist can optimize the preoperative status of the severely allergic individual, particularly in the presence of lower respiratory tract disease. Allergy management alone, however, rarely resolves long-standing otorrhea.

5. GENERAL HEALTH.

   On occasion, underlying systemic disease will confound the otologist's best efforts to obtain a dry ear preoperatively. Significant metabolic or vascular disease, autoimmune and other immune system disease, such as human immunodeficiency virus infection, can complicate the picture, and a general internist or infectious diseases consultant may be called on to assist in the evaluation and management strategy.

TRAUMATIC TYMPANIC MEMBRANE PERFORATIONS

Traumatic tympanic membrane perforations represent a fairly common problem for the otologist. Hand slaps, water skiing falls, cotton-tipped swab injuries, blast trauma, and penetrating injuries caused by high velocity missiles are some of the more common causative factors.

Typically, the patient presents acutely with a linear tear in the drum or a stellate opening of variable size, with some fresh blood at the margins. Complaints of aural fullness, tinnitus, altered hearing, and mild disequilibrium are common. After 72 hours, the perforation tends to become circular as the drum attempts to heal itself. A significant conductive hearing loss or mixed loss with persistent vertigo should alert the physician to the possibility of inner ear damage and the need for formal surgical exploration of the middle ear for possible perilymph fistula. Retained foreign body fragments in the middle ear must be considered if the ear begins to suppurate.

The initial evaluation of the patient consists of a complete ear, nose, and throat history, followed by a head and neck examination, which includes microotoscopic evaluation of the tympanic membranes. Debris and clots are carefully cleaned from the ear canal, and an initial assessment of the perforation is completed. If the injury is acute (within 48 to 72 hours), and the ear is uninfected, tympanic membrane patching is undertaken in the office in the following way: For a linear tear (Fig. 9–2) or a small circular defect, a piece of cigarette paper is trimmed to an appropriate shape, and antibiotic ointment is applied to its undersurface for adherence. The patch is applied to the surface of the tympanic membrane with alligator microforceps or suction tip and is gently tamped into place with a blunt hook (Fig. 9–3). No ear canal packing is used, and broad-spectrum oral antibiotic coverage is not started unless there has been water entry into the ear canal. On the other hand, if the ear is suppurating when the patient is first seen, gentle cleaning is carried out, and broad-spectrum antibiotic coverage is started. A culture specimen is not obtained routinely. The perforation is left to heal secondarily, and if it does not within 4 to 6 weeks, a formal myringoplasty is recommended.

With a stellate perforation (Fig. 9–4), when the patient is seen acutely without evidence of infection, local anesthesia is applied to the external auditory meatus in circumferential fashion, and the ear is carefully cleaned under the otomicroscope. A sterile piece of dry crushed absorbable gelatin sponge (Gelfoam) is moistened with normal saline and gently placed into the middle ear through the perforation (Fig. 9–5). The edges of the perforation are carefully everted with a

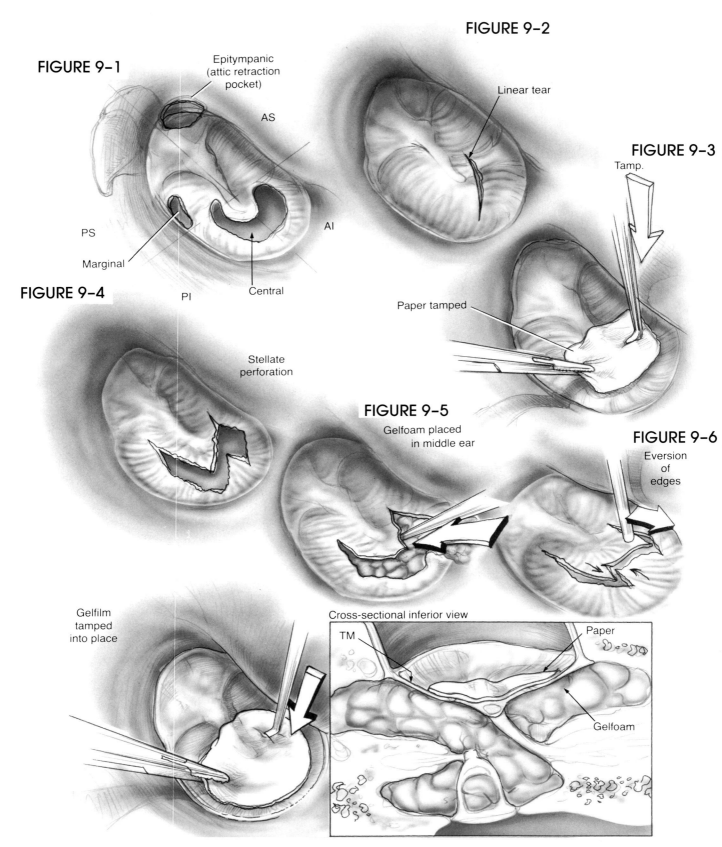

FIGURE 9-1

Epitympanic (attic retraction pocket)

AS

PS

Marginal

AI

PI

Central

FIGURE 9-2

Linear tear

FIGURE 9-3

Tamp.

Paper tamped

FIGURE 9-4

Stellate perforation

FIGURE 9-5

Gelfoam placed in middle ear

FIGURE 9-6

Eversion of edges

Gelfilm tamped into place

Cross-sectional inferior view

TM

Paper

Gelfoam

FIGURE 9-7

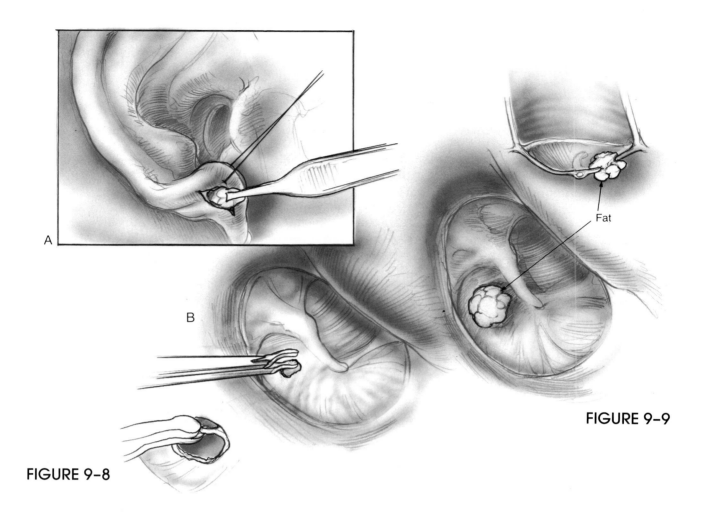

A

B

FIGURE 9-8

Fat

FIGURE 9-9

FIGURE 9-1. Tympanic membrane perforations: central, marginal, and epitympanic (attic retraction pocket).

FIGURE 9-2. Tympanic membrane showing linear perforation.

FIGURE 9-3. Paper patch applied to tympanic membrane perforation.

FIGURE 9-4. Tympanic membrane showing stellate perforation.

FIGURE 9-5. Placement of Gelfoam into middle ear.

FIGURE 9-6. Positioning of edges of stellate perforation over Gelfoam.

FIGURE 9-7. Paper patch applied to lateral surface of stellate perforation.

FIGURE 9-8. De-epithelization of margins of small perforation.

FIGURE 9-9. Placement of fat graft through perforation.

number 3 or 5 Baron suction tip and arranged in proper position (Fig. 9–6). Once this step has been completed, a piece of absorbable gelatin film (Gelfilm) or cigarette paper, trimmed to an appropriate shape with antibiotic ointment applied to its undersurface as an adhesive, is positioned over the lateral tympanic membrane surface and gently tamped into place (Fig. 9–7). No canal packing or dressing is used, and broad-spectrum antibiotic coverage is started if there has been water entry or other foreign material into the middle ear space. Antibiotic therapy is continued for 7 to 10 days.

The patient is advised to keep the ear dry and to not blow his or her nose or disturb the area in any other way and is seen in the office 1 week later. If the patch is in place and dry, it is not disturbed. At a secondary visit 4 to 6 weeks later, the patch is carefully removed and the drum inspected. If healing is complete, the patient is advised to keep the ear dry for another 2 weeks, and to then resume full activities. An audiogram is generally obtained at this point. If a persistent perforation is noted, however, formal repair is advised. In the author's experience, approximately 95 per cent of perforations handled in this fashion will heal, and the patient is so advised before treatment is undertaken. The option of no treatment is explained, as some authorities do not recommend patching traumatic tympanic membrane perforations.[19, 20]

When the patient is seen more than 72 hours following a traumatic tympanic membrane perforation, office patching is generally not recommended, and the drum is allowed to heal secondarily. In these subacute cases, antibiotics are not used unless the ear is suppurating. Patients with subacute perforations are told that the ear has an 85 to 90 per cent chance of healing within 4 to 6 weeks, and that formal repair will be recommended if healing has not occurred by then. Once again, water entry into the ear canal and vigorous nose blowing are avoided until healing is complete.

FAT GRAFT MYRINGOPLASTY

Fat graft myringoplasty is the procedure of choice for the repair of persistent small tympanic membrane perforations. This technique is well suited to the repair of small perforations due to chronic otitis media, myringoplasty failure, or following tympanostomy tube extrusion. The procedure represents a cost-effective alternative to standard tympanic membrane grafting techniques in such cases. In most cases, surgery is performed under local anesthesia in the office or outpatient surgery center and requires approximately 15 minutes of operating time. Within 12 to 16 weeks, the grafted tympanic membrane is fully healed and of normal thickness and appearance.

SURGICAL TECHNIQUE. Following premedication with agents of the surgeon's choice and the establishment of an intravenous line, the ear is prepared and draped in standard fashion. Local anesthesia is injected circumferentially at the external auditory meatus and into the posteromedial surface of the ear lobe. Through a 5mm to 8mm incision made on the posterior surface of the lobe, a small portion of adipose tissue is removed and placed in sterile normal saline. After hemostasis is achieved, the incision is closed with two or three 5.0 nylon sutures.

Under the otomicroscope, squamous epithelium is carefully removed from the margins of the tympanic membrane perforation with the microsurgical argon laser or a small cupped forceps (Fig. 9–8). A piece of adipose tissue approximately four times the diameter of the defect is inserted through the perforation, leaving one-half of its bulk medial and one-half lateral to the ear drum (Fig. 9–9). The ear canal is then packed with absorbable gelatin foam containing an antibiotic-steroid suspension, and a mastoid dressing is applied. Actually, the mastoid dressing is placed only to minimize postoperative earlobe swelling or seepage. The dressing is removed the following day, and the ear lobe sutures are removed on the fifth postoperative day. The patient then begins using otic drops to soften the packing, which is removed at 3 weeks after surgery. Instructions are given to avoid vigorous nose blowing for 3 weeks following the surgery, and to keep water out of the ear until healing is complete.

Over the years, numerous materials and techniques for myringoplasty have found favor among otologic surgeons. In experienced hands, both lateral and medial surface grafting procedures have been highly successful. Various graft materials have been used, including canal skin, temporalis fascia and prefascia, tragal perichondrium, and vein.[21] Adipose tissue has been used in other forms of otologic surgery, particularly stapedectomy, perilymph fistula repair,[22, 23] and mastoid obliteration following translabyrinthine operations.[24] Additionally, the use of fat tissue to repair small defects of the tympanic membrane has been previously reported by the author[25] and others.[26–29] When used to repair a tympanic membrane perforation, fat functions as both a lateral and a medial surface graft, and this flexibility may in part account for its high success rate.

In selecting cases suitable for this technique, the perforation should be less than 2mm in diameter, central, and dry and should present without signs of healing for at least 6 to 8 weeks. A wet ear would indicate the probability of more extensive middle ear or mastoid pathology requiring formal surgical intervention. The technique can be modified to permit repair of a posterior or anterior marginal perforation, provided that a tympanomeatal flap is turned before placement of the fat plug to ensure that there has been no growth of squamous epithelium into the middle ear. If such growth is found, it must obviously be removed.

When an ear with a small perforation and significant conductive hearing loss is encountered, the perforation can be repaired first, using the technique described, followed by the raising of a tympanomeatal flap to address the ossicular problem. Repairing the perforation first allows the surgeon to de-epithelialize the margins of the defect and place the graft while working on a stable and secure drum remnant, greatly facilitating the procedure.

The classic technique for repairing small tympanic membrane perforations has been fascia or perichondrial grafting. These more formal techniques are time consuming and carry a small potential for complications, such as graft lateralization. The success rate is certainly no higher. On the other hand, other limited procedures have been described, including paper graft patching of the drum,[30–33] absorbable gelatin film patch,[34] absorbable gelatin sponge plugs, and other materials.[35, 36]

The author has found adipose tissue an ideal material with which to repair small tympanic membrane perforations. This technique has yielded a success rate of 97 per cent in a series of 52 cases over the past 24 years. At 12 to 16 weeks after surgery, the graft site is of normal thickness and appearance and resembles the surrounding tympanic membrane. Postoperative hearing loss has not been encountered to date.

References

1. Shuknecht H: Pathology of the Ear. Cambridge, MA, Harvard University Press, 1974, p 228.
2. Glasscock ME, Shambaugh GE: Surgery of the Ear. Philadelphia, WB Saunders, 1990, p 187.
3. Abramson M, Gantz B, Asarch R, et al.: Cholesteatoma pathogenesis: Evidence for the migration theory. In McCabe B, Sade J, Abramson M (eds.): Cholesteatoma: First International Conference. Birmingham, AL, Aesculapius, 1977, pp 176–186.
4. Litton WB: Epidermal migration patterns in the ear and possible relationship to cholesteatoma genesis. In McCabe B, Sade J, Abramson M (eds): Cholesteatoma: First International Conference. Birmingham, AL, Aesculapius, 1977, pp 90–91.
5. Abramson M, Huang CC: Cholesteatoma and bone resorption. In McCabe B, Sade J, Abramson M (eds): Cholesteatoma: First International Conference. Birmingham, AL, Aesculapius, 1977, pp 162–166.
6. Gantz B, Clancy C, Abramson M: Decalcification factors in granulation tissue and ear canal skin. In McCabe B, Sade J, Abramson M (eds): Cholesteatoma: First International Conference. Birmingham, AL, Aesculapius, 1977, pp 167–169.
7. Glasscock ME, Shambaugh GE: Surgery of the Ear. Philadelphia, WB Saunders, 1990, p 187.
8. Bezold F: Cholesteatom, Perforation der membrana flaccida shrapnelli und tubenverschluss. Z Ohrenh 20: 5, 1890.
9. Wittmaack K: Wie entsteht ein genuines cholesteatom? Arch Ohren-Nasen-n. Kehlkopfh, 137: 306, 1933.
10. Jackler RK: The surgical anatomy of cholesteatoma. Otolaryngol Clin North Am 22: 883–896, 1989.
11. Jefferson G, Smalley AA: Progressive facial palsy produced by intratemporal epidermoids. J Laryngol Otol 53: 417–443, 1938.
12. Cawthorne T: Congenital cholesteatoma. Arch Otolaryngol 78: 248–252, 1963.
13. House JW, Sheehy JL: Cholesteatoma with intact tympanic membrane: A report of 41 cases. Laryngoscope 90: 70–75, 1980.
14. Glasscock ME, Shambaugh GE: Surgery of the Ear. Philadelphia, WB Saunders, 1990, p 187.
15. Hughes GB: Textbook of Clinical Otology. New York, Thieme-Stratton, 1985, p 306.
16. Brownlee RE, Hulka GF, Prazma J, et al.: Ciprofloxacin: Use as a topical otic preparation. Arch Otolaryngol Head Neck Surg 118: 392–396, 1992.
17. Physicians' Desk Reference. Montvale, NJ, Medical Economics Company, 1993, p 1634.
18. Stern JC, Shah MK, Lucente FE: In vitro effectiveness of 13 agents in otomycosis and review of the literature. Laryngoscope 98: 1173–1177, 1988.
19. Lindeman P, Edstrom S, Granstrom G, et al.: Acute traumatic tympanic membrane perforations. Cover or observe? Arch Otolaryngol Head Neck Surg 113: 1285–1287, 1987.
20. Kristensen S, Juul A, Gammelgaard NP, et al.: Traumatic tympanic membrane perforations: Complications and management. Ear Nose Throat J 68: 503–516, 1989.
21. Sheehy JL: Surgery of Chronic Otitis Media, vol 2. Hagerstown, MD, Harper & Row Publishers, 1972, p 15.
22. Althaus SR: Spontaneous and traumatic perilymph fistulas. Laryngoscope 87: 364–371, 1977.
23. Althaus SR: Perilymph fistulas. Laryngoscope 91: 538–562, 1981.
24. House JL, Hitselberger WE, House WF: Wound closure and cerebrospinal fluid leak after translabyrinthine surgery. Am J Otol 4: 126–128, 1982.
25. Althaus SR: "Fat plug" myringoplasty: A technique for repairing small tympanic membrane perforations. Same Day Surg 10: 88–89, 1986.
25. Althaus SR: "Fat plug" myringoplasty: A technique for repairing small tympanic membrane perforations. Same Day Surg 10: 88–89, 1986.
26. Ringenberg JC: Closure of tympanic membrane perforations by the use of fat. Laryngoscope 88: 982–993, 1978.
27. Terry RM, Bellini MJ, Clayton MI, et al: Fat graft myringoplasty—a prospective trial. Clin Otolaryngol 13: 227–229, 1988.
28. Gold SR, Chaffoo RAK: Fat myringoplasty in the guinea pig. Laryngoscope 101: 1–5, 1991.
29. Gross CW, Bassila M, Lazar RH, et al: Adipose plug myringoplasty: an alternative to formal myringoplasty techniques in children. Otolaryngol Head Neck Surg 101: 617–620, 1989.
30. Camnitz PS, Bost WS: Traumatic perforations of the tympanic membrane: early closure with paper patching. Otolaryngol Head Neck Surg 93: 220–223, 1985.
31. Kitchens GC: Theta myringoplasty. Laryngoscope 102: 588–589, 1992.
32. Laurent C, Soderberg O, Anniko M, et al: Repair of chronic tympanic membrane perforations using applications of hyaluronate or rice paper prostheses: ORL J Otorhinolaryngol Relat Spec 53: 37–40, 1991.
33. Merwin GE, Boies LR Jr: Paper patch repair of blast rupture of the tympanic membrane. Laryngoscope 90: 853–860, 1980.
34. Baldwin RL, Loftin L: Gelfilm myringoplasty: A technique for residual perforations. Laryngoscope 102: 340–342, 1992.
35. Saito H, Kazama Y, Yazawa Y: Simple maneuver for closing traumatic ear drum perforation by microscope strip tape patching. Am J Otol 11: 427–430, 1990.
36. Stenfors LE: Repair of tympanic membrane perforations using hyaluronic acid: an alternative to myringoplasty. J Laryngol Otol 103: 39–40, 1989.

10

Tympanoplasty: Outer Surface Grafting Technique

JAMES L. SHEEHY, M.D.

Elimination of disease and restoration of function are the aims of tympanoplasty. Restoration of function requires a tympanic membrane, an air-containing, mucosal-lined middle ear (so that the membrane will vibrate), and a secure connection between the tympanic membrane and the inner ear fluids.

Presented here is one of the three major techniques of tympanic membrane grafting: the outer surface, or onlay, procedure, the technique used with rare exceptions by doctors of the House Ear Clinic (HEC). Before describing the surgical procedure, comments will be made on the evolution of tympanic grafting techniques, patient selection, and evaluation and counseling prior to surgery.

HISTORICAL ASPECTS

Systematic reconstruction of the tympanic membrane, the sine qua non of the modern era of reconstructive ear surgery, had its beginning with reports of Wullstein[1] and Zollner.[2] Split-thickness or full-thickness skin was placed over the de-epithelized tympanic membrane remnant. The initial results were very encouraging, but unfortunately, graft eczema, inflammation, and finally, perforation were common.

As a result of these experiences, most surgeons had begun changing to undersurface (underlay) connective tissue grafts by the late 1950s (see Chapters 11 and 12). The HEC doctors continued using an onlay technique but changed to "canal skin", [3, 4] which actually was periosteum graft, covered by canal skin.

This change was made in 1958 and resulted in an immediate improvement in results. But draining ears and total perforations continued to have up to a 40 per cent failure rate.

In 1961, Storrs[5] published the results of a small series of cases in which temporalis fascia had been used as an outer surface graft. Changing to this technique resulted in a dramatic improvement in results over the next 3 years: over 90 per cent graft take.[6-8]

PATIENT SELECTION AND EVALUATION

The patient with chronic otitis media may consult a physician because of a hearing impairment or because of discharge from the ear. Occasionally, the patient may have symptoms of more advanced chronic ear pathology, such as pain, vertigo, or facial nerve paralysis.

Careful evaluation of the symptoms and findings allows the otologist to determine the need for surgery, its urgency, and the anticipated result. Only by so doing can the patient be advised properly. A good

surgical result should not be a disappointment to the patient if there is proper counseling.

Let us assume, for purposes of this chapter, that the patient has a dry central perforation. The ear may drain briefly with upper respiratory infections or if water is allowed to get into the ear. This discharge responds promptly to local medication. The preoperative treatment of the draining ear will be discussed in depth in Chapter 18.

When one is dealing with a dry central perforation, or inactive disease, surgery is elective, and the patient (or family) should be so informed. Assuming that the problem is unilateral, with only a mild hearing impairment, the only indication for surgery is to avoid further episodes of otorrhea.

In children, it is best (from the psychologic standpoint) to avoid elective surgery of any type between the ages of 4 and 7 years. Certainly, in ear surgery, it is wise to wait until after the age of 7 years so as not to lay the groundwork for serous otitis media. If the problem is bilateral, there is a hearing problem, and the ears do not drain often, fitting with hearing aids in each ear may be preferable for children under the age of 8; however, the parents have to make the decision. At age 8 years and thereafter, the patient (child) should be allowed to make the decision.

What about eustachian tube function? When contemplating tympanoplasty, the HEC doctors do not usually test to determine the status of the eustachian tube.[9] The philosophy has been that tubal malfunction per se is no contraindication to tympanoplasty but that the operation will not be successful unless tubal function is re-established.

Many persons showing no tubal function by various available tests used in the past have been operated on to eliminate a chronic drainage problem. Surprisingly, when the ear heals the drum is usually mobile. Re-exploration in some of these patients has demonstrated normal mucosa in the tubotympanum, where before surgery the mucosa was of a very poor quality. It would appear that surgery, in eliminating infection and sealing the ear, is in itself the best treatment for the obstructed tube.

PATIENT COUNSELING

What is the outlook with surgery, and what are the risks and complications? A surgeon must relate his or her own experience. HEC doctors explain that the likelihood of obtaining a permanently healed, dry ear, which may be treated normally, is better than 90 per cent. "The only complication that happens with any degree of regularity, and is serious, is a total loss of hearing in the operated ear. That likelihood is no more than 1 per cent. All of the other things listed here are either very remote or are temporary." ["Listed here" refers to the Risk and Complications section of a Patient Discussion Booklet. The actual Risk and Complications Sheet is given to the patient at the time the surgery is scheduled, which allows the patient to review the sheet leisurely. The Risk and Complications Sheet appears as Appendix 1.]

PREOPERATIVE PREPARATION

If the patient is a child, the preoperative visit occurs the day before surgery. Surgery is under general anesthesia the following morning, and the child is released to the parents' care in the afternoon.

For adults, the preoperative visit is often the morning of surgery. The patient goes to the hospital for afternoon surgery, which will occur under local anesthesia. The patient may be kept in the hospital overnight, depending on many circumstances.

PREPARATION IN SURGERY

The smoothness with which the operation proceeds depends not only on the ability of the surgeon but also on the organization of the team (anesthesiologist and surgical nurse) and arrangements in the operating room.

The patient's hair is shaved 3cm above and behind the ear. The skin is cleansed with an iodine-based soap, rinsed with water, and sprayed with tincture of benzoin. A sterile plastic adhesive drape is applied.

The mattress of the operating table is taped securely to the table to prevent it from slipping when the table is tipped from side to side or into the Trendelenburg position. The patient is placed on the table with his or her head at the *foot* of the table, which allows the circulating nurse or anesthesiologist free access to the table controls, which are then at the feet of the patient. The patient's head and shoulders should be as near to the surgeon's side of the table as possible. A pillow is placed under the patient's knees. The Bovie plate goes under the patient's buttocks.

Anesthesia

Ear surgery can be performed with the patient under local anesthesia in most cases. The decision on this depends on the age of the patient and other factors.

Lidocaine with 1:100,000 adrenalin is used for postauricular and meatal incisions. Some of the injection material should find its way under the skin of the posterior superior wall of the canal (the vascular strip) and into the middle ear.

General anesthesia is used in children, in most mastoid surgery, and in procedures that require more than 1 1/2 hours of operating time. The anesthetist should be at the feet of the patient (which is actually the head of the table) to allow the surgeon and scrub nurse complete freedom at the patient's head.

A few useful suggestions for the anesthesiologist are as follows:

1. Have extra long tubing for the gas machine to allow seating at the foot of the patient.
2. Start the intravenous infusion in the forearm and extend the tubing to the foot of the table.
3. The blood pressure cuff belongs on the arm *opposite* the ear to be operated on.
4. Be certain that the patient is secured to the table with wide adhesive tape. The eyes should be taped shut.

Arrangement and Instrumentation

Particular attention should be paid to operating room arrangement (Fig. 10–1). The anesthesiologist is at the patient's feet, far removed from the operating field, and the scrub nurse is directly across from the surgeon, where the nurse may be of the most assistance. The same arrangement, minus the anesthesiologist, is used for procedures occurring with the patient under local anesthesia.

It is important for the comfort of the surgeon that the patient be in a satisfactory position. The table is usually placed in a few degrees of Trendelenburg's position and rolled slightly toward the surgeon. The patient's head is adjusted as necessary, usually flexed slightly onto the opposite shoulder.

The surgeon should be comfortably seated on a chair with a back support. The surgeon should use the back support and be in a comfortable position so that all back and arm muscles will be relaxed.

SURGICAL TECHNIQUE

The lateral surface grafting technique involves eight steps: Transmeatal canal incisions and elevations of the vascular strip; postauricular exposure and removal and dehydration of the temporalis fascia; removal of canal skin; enlargement of the ear canal by removal of the anterior (and inferior) canal bulge; deepithelization of the tympanic membrane remnant; placement of the rehydrated fascia on the outer surface of the remnant, but under the manubrium; replacement of canal skin; and closure of the postauricular incision and replacement of the vascular strip transmeatally.[10]

Transmeatal Incisions

Incisions are made along the tympanomastoid and tympanosquamous suture lines, demarcating the vascular strip, with a No. 1 (sickle) knife (Fig. 10–2). The vascular strip is the area of the canal skin that covers the superior and posterior portions of the ear canal between these two suture lines. It is easily demarcated from the skin of the remainder of the ear canal because of its thickness and the fact that it balloons up when local anesthesia is injected into the area. The vascular strip is elevated from the bone, from within outward using a round knife (Fig. 10–3).

A semilunar incision is made in the outer third of the ear canal, using a Beaver knife with a No. 64 blade, connecting the two incisions already made along the border of the vascular strip (Fig. 10–4). The knife blade is angled toward the bone to thin the 1mm or 2mm section of the membranous canal included.

Postauricular Exposure and Removal of Fascia

The skin incision must provide adequate exposure for the operative field. It should extend far enough foreword, both superiorly and inferiorly, to allow adequate exposure of the bony meatus when the ear is retracted forward. Failure to do this may result in difficulty seeing structures in the posterior part of the middle ear.

The superior portion of the incision begins at the most anterior extent of, and 1cm above, the postauricular fold. It is then continued into the postauricular fold at the level of the lower border of the muscle and extends inferiorly under the lobule of the ear.

Exposure of the temporalis fascia is facilitated if ample local anesthetic has been injected to balloon the area. A retractor is inserted to retract the skin margins in this area and to obtain hemostasis. By lifting up on the retractor, one may pull the areolar tissue away from the fascia, facilitating the dissection and ensuring that all loose areolar tissue is lifted off the fascia prior to the fascia's removal.

Local anesthesia is injected under the fascia to elevate it slightly from the underlying muscle. A 2cm × 2cm piece of fascia is removed.

The fascia is spread on a polytetrafluoroethylene (Teflon) block, undersurface upward, and any adherent muscle is removed. The fascia is then placed on a fascia press, absorbable gelatin sponge (Gelfoam) is placed on the fascia, and the press is closed. The press is opened after 5 minutes, and the gelatin sponge is removed; the fascia, now smooth and partially dehydrated, is left attached to the press. The press, with the attached fascia, is placed under an electric lamp to complete the dehydration process.

An incision is made through the soft tissue above the meatus, from the root of the zygoma, horizontally, along the linea temporalis. This horizontal incision is extended posteriorly to the level of the skin incision. The incision is then extended inferiorly, below the linea temporalis, following the postauricular incision, incising the periosteum until the incision curves forward, down to the level of the floor of the ear canal.

The periosteum is elevated superiorly (under the temporalis muscle), posteriorly and anteriorly, using a Lempert elevator, to obtain adequate exposure of the mastoid cortex. A self-retaining retractor is inserted to retract the auricle and vascular strip forward, exposing the ear canal.

Removal of the Canal Skin

The periosteum and canal skin are elevated from the bone as far as the annular ligament (Fig. 10–5). Care should be taken not to elevate the ligament and the remnant of the middle fibrous layer. The dissection is superficial to the fibrous layer of the remnant in such a way that the remnant is de-epithelized in continuity with the canal skin, if possible. It is often easier to begin the final removal and de-epithelization by starting anterosuperiorly, using a cup forceps (Fig. 10–6). Removal of the canal skin and de-epithelization are continued inferiorly and posteriorly. The periosteum and canal skin are removed from the ear and kept moist in Tis-U-Sol irrigating solution.

In elevating the periosteum and the canal skin, one should remember to work perpendicular to the annular ligament and remnant, keeping the instrument on the bone at all times, until the dissection is completed to the level of the remnant. The dissection is then continued parallel to the annular ligament to avoid elevating it and the remnant (Fig. 10–7).

FIGURE 10–1. Operating room arrangement, right ear. Table controls and anesthesiologist are at the patient's feet. Scrub nurse is opposite the surgeon.

FIGURE 10–2. Tympanosquamous and tympanomastoid suture line incisions.

FIGURE 10–3. Vascular strip elevation.

FIGURE 10–4. Semilunar incision.

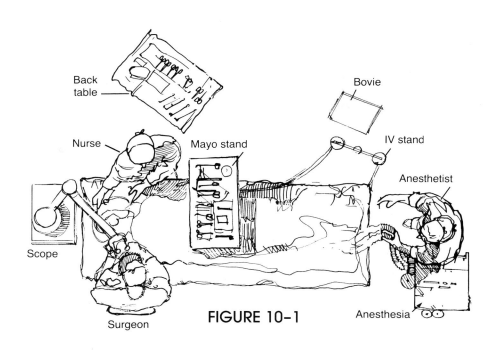

Back table

Nurse

Mayo stand

Bovie

IV stand

Anesthetist

Scope

Surgeon

Anesthesia

FIGURE 10-1

FIGURE 10-2

FIGURE 10-4

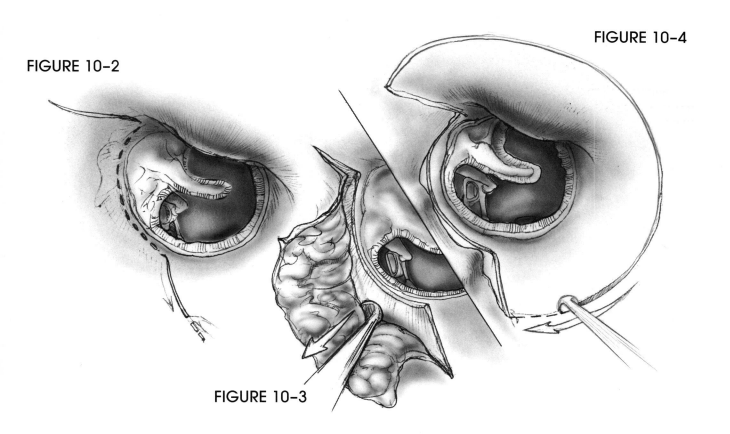

FIGURE 10-3

Enlarging the Ear Canal

Through the use of a drill and continuous suction-irrigation, the ear canal is enlarged by removal of the anterior and inferior canal bulges (Fig. 10–8).

The importance of this step in the lateral surface grafting technique must be emphasized. Removal of this bone enlarges the field of surgery. The anterior and inferior sulci are thoroughly exposed to allow de-epithelization and satisfactory graft placement. The acute angle that exists anteriorly is opened, helping to prevent postoperative blunting. There is no area hidden from postoperative observation. Enlarging the ear canal is routine in all lateral surface grafting procedures and is the main reason for removal of canal skin.

De-epithelization of the Tympanic Membrane Remnant

The lateral surface grafting technique demands a complete de-epithelization of the remnant. Although the graft may take without all the skin having been removed, postoperative epithelial cysts may develop.

Direct your attention first to the ear canal bone immediately adjacent to the bony annulus. Pay particular attention the anteroinferior bone 1mm lateral to the annulus, where a small vessel and nerve perforate the bone and where there is a particularly tight attachment to the skin.

Next, check the tympanic membrane remnant carefully for skin. If there is a question about whether de-epithelization has been thorough, remove a portion of the remnant to be certain. The size of the perforation is of no consequence in regard to graft take in the lateral surface technique.

Preparation of Packing

The surgical nurse should have begun preparing absorbable gelatin sponge packing prior to or shortly after the beginning of the operation. Uncompressed gelatin sponge is cut into an ample number of various-sized pieces and then soaked in antibiotic-cortisone solution. Pieces of gelatin sponge are then removed from the solution and compressed (on a tongue blade or a paper gelatin sponge packet) until most of the solution has been removed. The gelatin sponge is put aside and allowed to dry more until needed by the surgeon.

Placement of Fascia

When the perforation is large, or the fascia is unusually thin, it is helpful to fill the middle ear with gelatin sponge packing prior to placing the graft. The gelatin sponge serves as an artificial remnant and facilitates graft placement. The fascia will be placed under the malleus handle. When the manubrium is surrounded by remnant (small perforation), the remnant is separated from the malleus handle to allow proper placement of the fascia.

The dehydrated fascia is trimmed to an oval shape measuring approximately 1.3cm × 1.5cm. A slit is cut in the fascia to allow placement under the manubrium (Fig. 10–9); the two cut ends are grasped with the forceps, and then the fascia is immersed for a few seconds in Tis-U-Sol irrigating solution to dehydrate it.

The fascia is placed over the perforation and immediately slipped under the manubrium (Fig. 10–10). Be certain that the apex of the slit in the fascia comes into contact with the tensor tendon.

FIGURE 10–5. Elevation of canal skin and periosteum.

FIGURE 10–6. Cup forceps used, anterosuperiorly, to begin remnant de-epithelization in continuity with the periosteum and canal skin.

FIGURE 10–7. Direction of dissection: perpendicular to the remnant until reaching it, then parallel to the remnant.

FIGURE 10–8. Anterior canal bulge removed with cutting burrs and continuous suction-irrigation.

FIGURE 10–9. Slit in fascia for placement under malleus handle.

FIGURE 10–10. Placement of rehydrated fascia under malleus handle and on outer surface of remnant.

FIGURE 10–11. Covering the malleus handle with anterosuperior flap of fascia.

FIGURE 10–12. Fascia graft cut for tucking under bone of epitympanum for stability when malleus is absent.

FIGURE 10–13. Fascia in place; compare with Fig. 10–12.

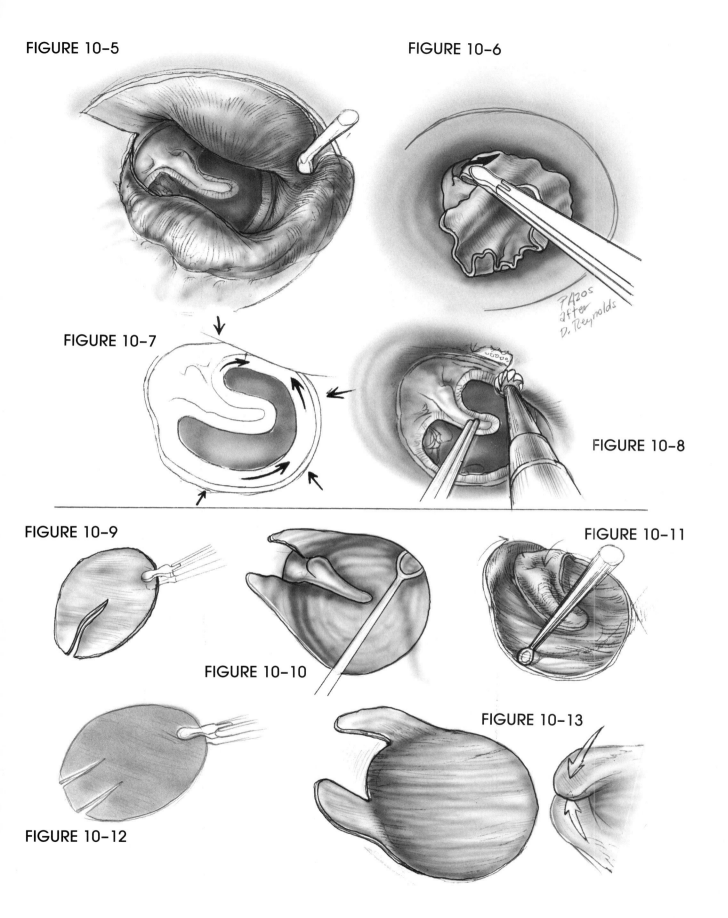

FIGURE 10-5

FIGURE 10-6

FIGURE 10-7

FIGURE 10-8

FIGURE 10-9

FIGURE 10-10

FIGURE 10-11

FIGURE 10-12

FIGURE 10-13

The fascia is then adjusted to the remnant anteriorly and inferiorly, with care being taken that it does not extend onto the bony wall anteriorly, unless there is no remnant at all, then only for a millimeter at the most. The anterior flap is turned back over the exposed manubrium, resulting in a better appearance of the membrane when healed (Fig. 10–11).

When the malleus is absent and there is only a small remnant present, it is necessary to insert the fascia in a different way to result in the stabilized graft (Fig. 10–12). The fascia is cut twice, creating a flap that can then be tucked under the lateral wall of the epitympanum. The anterosuperior edge of the fascia is then swung posteriorly to overlap the upper edge of the graft and secure the seal of the middle ear (Fig. 10–13).

Replacement of Canal Skin

The canal skin is replaced to cover the bone from which it was removed. It is positioned only slightly more medially, allowing it to overlap the fascia by a millimeter (Fig. 10–14), which helps promote rapid epithelization. Epithelization is particularly important in preventing blunting in the anterosuperior sulcus. There must be no edges of epithelium turned under, or small epithelial cysts may develop on the surface of the fascia during healing.

The first piece of packing is a small, dry, rolled up, (cigar-shaped) tightly compressed piece of absorbable gelatin sponge, placed in the sulcus anteriorly. The canal is packed tightly with pledgets of slightly moist gelatin sponge, leaving room posterosuperiorly for the vascular strip.

Closure and Replacement of the Vascular Strip

The retractors are released, and the vascular strip is pushed anteriorly to lie over the packing. One suture is placed subcutaneously postauricularly to stabilize the auricle.

Transmeatally, the vascular strip is lifted up, some packing is removed, and the vascular strip is then replaced in the ear canal in the exact position from which it came (Fig. 10–15). Gelatin sponge packing in the canal is then completed, and a plug of cotton is placed in the outer meatus. The postauricular incision is closed with subcutaneous sutures, and a mastoid dressing is applied.

POSTOPERATIVE CARE

The mastoid dressing is removed the day following surgery. The patient is given a postoperative instruc-tion card (Appendix 2) just before entering the hospital. It is important to review some aspects of this information with the patient. The patient should be reminded not to blow the nose and not to get water in the ear. An antibiotic has been prescribed and should be taken as directed on the bottle. There will be discomfort for a few days, and the patient should take aspirin or acetaminophen four times a day regularly for the first few days just to keep the pain under control. Nothing need be done with the cotton in the ear, but it may be changed if it becomes terribly soiled.

The patient should be asked to touch the edge of the auricle. Point out that the ear is numb and that it is going to take a few months for that numbness to go away. There is also tenderness on the incision behind the ear. This will diminish rapidly, but it may be 6 months before it is totally gone. Finally, the patient should be reminded of the first postoperative appointment, which should occur 7 to 10 days later in the doctor's office.

At the first postoperative visit, the cotton plug in the ear canal is removed and the ear inspected. The gelatin sponge should appear firm. Remove a piece of this to show to the patient so that the patient understands that it will eventually turn to a liquid and will run out of the ear. The patient is instructed to begin using ear drops (of one type or another) 3 weeks following the date of surgery, twice daily. The drops may be started sooner should the ear begin to drain, an indication of liquefaction of the gelatin sponge.

The second postoperative visit is scheduled for 6 to 8 weeks following the date of surgery. Eighty to 90 per cent of the ear will be totally healed at this point.

PROS AND CONS OF THE OUTER SURFACE TECHNIQUE

One of the problems faced by the novice is that there are many techniques and prostheses recommended as "the best—it always works well." Of course, how well a technique or prosthesis works for the individual depends on the technical ability of that individual—the person's judgment and manual dexterity.

The outer surface grafting technique has numerous advantages and disadvantages. The advantages are well known to all who have used the technique. The exposure is excellent—one can see everything necessary without moving the microscope. Secondly, one may remove as much remnant as necessary to eliminate the disease. There is no need to scrape in many different places. Certainly, the graft rate take is high. Finally, it is one technique that can be used in all cases.

However, there are disadvantages that may outweigh the advantages for some individuals. The tech-

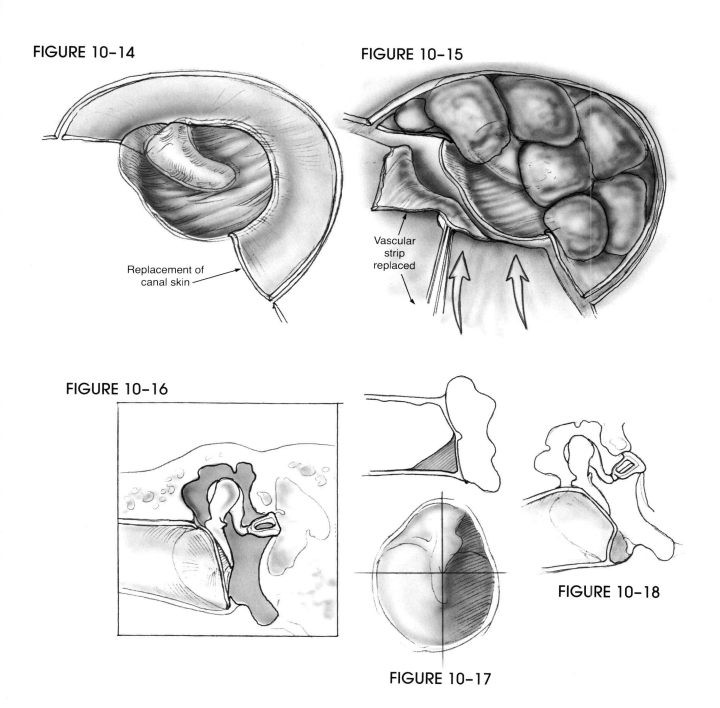

FIGURE 10-14

FIGURE 10-15

Replacement of canal skin

Vascular strip replaced

FIGURE 10-16

FIGURE 10-18

FIGURE 10-17

FIGURE 10-14. Canal skin is replaced.

FIGURE 10-15. Vascular strip is replaced.

FIGURE 10-16. Lateralization of the tympanic membrane.

FIGURE 10-17. Blunting in anterior sulcus may immobilize the malleus handle.

FIGURE 10-18. Epithelial cyst medial to fascia graft.

nique requires very precise surgery to avoid problems. The healing time is longer than with the undersurface technique. Finally, if the operation is not done extremely skillfully, one may develop either blunting in the anterior sulcus or lateral healing, both of which may result in a healed ear with worse hearing.

HEALING PROBLEMS

One of the disadvantages of the outer surface grafting technique, as already noted, is that although there is a very high graft take rate regardless of how the operation is performed, there are healing problems. These healing problems may outweigh the advantages for some individuals.[10]

These healing problems became evident soon after the technique was started in the early 1960s: lateralization of the graft, blunting in the anterior sulcus, excessive membrane thickness, epithelial cysts between the remnant and the fascia, and epithelial pearls on the drum surface and ear canal. Most of these have ceased to be major problems but they still occur in a small percentage of cases.

Lateralization of the Tympanic Membrane

The very first problem that was noticed with this technique was lateralization of the membrane (Fig. 10–16). This usually did not become apparent until 6 to 12 months following surgery and resulted from the fascia not being placed under the malleus handle when the technique was first introduced (see Fig. 10–10).

When lateralization has occurred, the patient's hearing will be reduced, but often not as much as anticipated. The appearance is of a smaller-than-normal-sized ear drum, mobile, and at a direct right angle to the line of vision. Treatment of this problem (if needed) requires reoperation and the placement of the new graft underneath the malleus handle.

Blunting in the Anterior Sulcus

Blunting in the anterior sulcus, particularly anterosuperiorly, occurs to a minor degree in most lateral surface cases but is of no consequence and results from the formation of excess fibrous tissue. Blunting is probably the most common healing problem encountered by the novice surgeon. It can interfere greatly with the hearing result if it is great enough to involve the malleus handle when the ossicular chain is intact (Fig. 10–17).

To prevent blunting, one should remove the anterior canal bulge so that the anterior angle is open. One should not place the fascia onto the anterior canal bone unless there is no alternative. Finally, one should make sure that the replaced canal skin overlaps the graft slightly anterosuperiorly. Finally, placing the

rolled-up piece of dried gelatin foam in the anterior sulcus as the first piece of packing also helps prevent blunting.

When severe blunting occurs, the manubrium becomes indistinguishable, and the anterior half of the tympanic membrane is immobile and takes on a concave appearance with no clear-cut distinction between the edge of the membrane and the bony wall. The posterior half of the membrane may show fair mobility. Should this appearance persist after 6 months, and should there be a hearing problem, reoperation would be required to correct it.

Other Problems

Two varieties of epithelial cysts may be noted. One of these is common and appears as a small "pearl" on the tympanic membrane or ear canal. It is the result of turning under the skin edges when replacing the canal skin. Spontaneous rupture and healing are common. The cyst might be marsupialized under the microscope in the office if desired.

An epithelial cyst may occur between the remnant and the fascia and enlarge slowly over 1 to 2 years (Fig. 10–18). This is an uncommon problem that results from inadequate de-epithelization of bone and the remnant adjacent to the bone. The only place where this is likely to occur is anteroinferiorly where the small vessel and nerve enter the ear canal a millimeter lateral to the drum. As opposed to blunting, where there is a concave appearance, the appearance here is convex, and it occurs anteroinferiorly. Once it is recognized, it can be corrected by merely incising the cyst and evacuating it.

Acknowledgment

Many of the illustrations are modified from *Otolaryngology*, Vol. 1, published by J. B. Lippincott Company.

References

1. Wullstein H: Theory and practice of tympanoplasty. Laryngoscope 66: 1076–1093, 1956.
2. Zollner F: Principles of plastic surgery of the sound conducting apparatus. J Laryngol Otol 69: 637–652, 1955.
3. House WF, Sheehy JL: Myringoplasty: Use of ear canal skin compared with other techniques. Arch Otolaryngol Head Neck Surg 73: 407–415, 1961.
4. Plester D: Skin and mucous membrane grafts in middle ear surgery. Arch Otolaryngol Head Neck Surg 72: 718–721, 1960.
5. Storrs LA: Myringoplasty with use of fascia graft. Arch Otolaryngol Head Neck Surg 74: 45–49, 1961.
6. Sheehy JL: Tympanic membrane grafting: Early and long term results. Laryngoscope 74: 985–988, 1964.
7. Sheehy JL, Glasscock ME: Tympanic membrane grafting with temporalis fascia: A report of four years' experience. Arch Otolaryngol Head Neck Surg 86: 391–402, 1967.
8. Sheehy JL, Anderson RG: Myringoplasty: A review of 472 cases. Ann Otol Rhinol Laryngol 89: 331–334, 1980.
9. Sheehy JL: Testing eustachian tube function. Ann Otol Rhinol Laryngol 90: 562–564, 1981.
10. Sheehy JL: Surgery of chronic otitis media. *In* English GM (ed): Otolaryngology. Philadelphia: Harper and Row, 1984.

Appendix 1

RISKS AND COMPLICATIONS OF MYRINGOPLASTY, TYMPANOPLASTY, MASTOID SURGERY, AND OTHER OPERATIONS FOR CORRECTION OF CHRONIC EAR INFECTIONS

(Operations to eliminate middle ear or mastoid infection, to repair the eardrum or the sound transmission mechanism)

Ear Infection

Ear infection with drainage, swelling, and pain may persist following surgery or, on rare occasions, may develop following surgery because of poor healing of the ear tissue. If this is the case, additional surgery may be necessary to control the infection.

Loss of Hearing

Further permanent impairment of hearing develops in 3 per cent of patients because of problems in the healing process. In 2 per cent this loss of hearing may be severe or total in the ear that was operated on. Nothing further can be done in these instances.

When a two-stage operation is necessary, the hearing is usually worse after the first operation.

Tinnitus

Should the hearing be worse following surgery, tinnitus (head noises) likewise may be more pronounced.

Dizziness

Dizziness may occur immediately following surgery because of irritation of the inner ear structures. Some unsteadiness may persist for a week postoperatively. Prolonged dizziness is rare unless there was dizziness prior to surgery.

Taste Disturbance and Mouth Dryness

Taste disturbance and mouth dryness are common for a few weeks following surgery. In some patients, this disturbance is prolonged.

Facial Paralysis

A rare postoperative complication of ear surgery is temporary paralysis of one side of the face. This may occur as a result of an abnormality or a swelling of the nerve and usually subsides spontaneously.

On very rare occasions, the nerve may be injured at the time of surgery or it may be necessary to excise it in order to eradicate infection. When this happens, a skin sensation nerve is removed from the upper part of the neck to replace the facial nerve. Paralysis of the face under these circumstances lasts 6 months to a year, and there would be a permanent residual weakness. Eye complications requiring treatment by a specialist could develop.

Hematoma

A hematoma (collection of blood) develops in a small percentage of cases, prolonging healing. Reoperation to remove the clot may be necessary if this complication occurs.

General Anesthesia Complications

Anesthetic complications are very rare but can be serious. You may discuss these with the anesthesiologist if you desire.

Complications Related to Mastoid Surgery

A cerebrospinal fluid leak (leak of fluid surrounding the brain) is a very rare complication. Reoperation may be necessary to stop the leak.

Intracranial (brain) complications, such as meningitis or brain abscess, or even paralysis, were common in cases of chronic otitis media prior to the antibiotic era. Fortunately, these now are extremely rare complications.

Appendix 2

POSTOPERATIVE INSTRUCTION FOLDER:
MYRINGOPLASTY, TYMPANOPLASTY, AND
MASTOIDECTOMY

Precautions

1. *Do not* blow your nose until your doctor has indicated that your ear is healed. Any accumulated secretions in the nose may be drawn back into the throat and expectorated if desired. This is particularly important if you develop a cold.
2. *Do not* "pop" your ears by holding your nose and blowing air through the eustachian tube into the ear. If it is necessary to sneeze, do so with your mouth open.
3. *Do not* allow water to enter the ear until advised by your doctor that the ear is healed. Until such time, when showering or washing your hair, lambswool or cotton may be placed in the outer ear opening and covered with vaseline. If an incision was made in the skin behind your ear, water should be kept away from this area for 1 week.
4. *Do not* take an unnecessary chance of catching cold. Avoid undue exposure or fatigue. Should you catch a cold, treat it in your usual way, reporting to us if you develop ear symptoms.
5. You may anticipate a certain amount of pulsation, popping, clicking, and other sounds in the ear, and also a feeling of fullness in the ear. Occasional sharp shooting pains are not unusual. At times, it may feel as if there is liquid in the ear.
6. *Do not* plan to drive a car home from the hospital. Air travel is permissible 2 days following surgery. When changing altitude, you should remain awake and chew gum to stimulate swallowing.

Dizziness

Minor degrees of dizziness may be present on head motion and need not concern you unless it increases.

Hearing

Rarely is a hearing improvement noted immediately following surgery. It may even be worse temporarily because of swelling of the ear tissues and packing in the ear canal. Six to 8 weeks after surgery, an improvement may be noted. Maximum improvement may require 4 to 6 months.

Discharge

A bloody or watery discharge may occur during the healing period. The outer ear cotton may be changed if necessary, but in general, the less done to the ear the better.

A yellow (infected) discharge at any time is an indication to call the appointment desk and arrange to see your doctor. Discharge with foul odor should also be reported.

Pain

Mild, intermittent ear pain is not unusual during the first 2 weeks. Pain above or in front of the ear is common when chewing. If you have persistent ear pain, not relieved by a few aspirins, call the appointment desk and arrange to see your doctor.

Eardrops

If you were given a prescription for ear drops, begin using these 3 weeks after surgery. Place a few drops in the ear twice daily to loosen the packing, which will run out of the ear as a liquid. Tip the head to the side, place two drops in the ear, and allow them to remain for 5 minutes. Then tip the head in the opposite direction to allow the ear drops to run out. Continue doing this twice daily until you have finished the drops or until advised otherwise by your doctor.

11

Tympanoplasty: The Undersurface Graft Technique— Transcanal Approach

M. COYLE SHEA, JR., M.D.

Many otologic surgeons prefer placing the connective tissue graft medial to the tympanic membrane remnant. This can be accomplished through either the transcanal or postauricular approach. In this chapter, the transcanal technique will be described in detail.

In transcanal tympanoplasty using the underlay technique, the grafting material may be any type of autogenous connective tissue, such as vein, fascia, or perichondrium. In 1957, Shea,[1] using vein, was the first to use the underlay grafting technique. Tabb,[2] Austin and Shea,[3] and others soon recognized the superiority of this method over onlay skin grafting and followed Shea's lead. The use of fascia as an underlay graft was first reported by Storrs.[4] Tragal perichondrium was first used in tympanoplasty by Goodhill et al.[5] as an onlay graft, and it is the material preferred by this writer. It is in the immediate surgical field, is extremely durable and, when pressed, is very easy to handle. Vein also is easy to position and if large enough (as from the antecubital fossa), can be used to repair perforations of any size. Our primary objection to the use of vein grafts is that in the event of a serious future illness, the large vein could be an important means of administering parenteral medications. Temporalis fascia, its overlying areolar tissue, or even scar tissue from the vicinity of a previous postauricular incision can be used with the transcanal undersurface technique, but it is not as easy to handle as vein or perichondrium. Pressing the fascia in a vein or fascia press makes it much more manageable by eliminating the tenacious loose strands and at the same time preventing the stiffness that occurs with drying. We do not recommend pressing vein for tympanoplasty (as done in stapedectomy) because it results in excessive thinning. Instead, we trim away the adventitia and stretch the vessel between the blades of a vein scissors before opening it.

PREOPERATIVE EVALUATION AND PATIENT SELECTION

If the canal is of adequate size, this technique is suitable for any tympanic membrane perforation in which tympanoplasty is indicated, regardless of size or location. If the canal is not large enough to accommodate a 5mm or larger ear speculum, this procedure may not be technically feasible.

The usual indications for closure of a tympanic membrane perforation are to reduce the incidence of middle ear infection and to improve hearing. Not every perforation needs to, or should be, closed. Each patient must be evaluated on what would be best for that patient. An elderly or debilitated patient with an asymptomatic perforation or a patient for which the ear under evaluation is the only hearing ear is not a good surgical candidate. In the case of a young child who developed a perforation from a ventilation tube that was initially inserted because the child could not ventilate the ear, it would be unwise to repair the tympanic membrane until it is apparent that eustachian tube function has significantly improved, lest the pathologic process repeat itself.

There is no infallible test of tubal function, but it is reasonable to assume that if the patient can autoinflate by the Valsalva maneuver preoperatively, he or she will be able to ventilate the ear postoperatively. Consequently, the patient is instructed in this procedure before surgery.

SURGICAL TECHNIQUE

Local anesthesia using 1 to 2 per cent lidocaine with 1:100,000 epinephrine is employed in combination with either a general endotracheal anesthetic or an intravenous sedation. The local anesthetic is administered at the time of the immediate preoperative preparation of the surgical area to ensure adequate vasoconstriction by the time the actual surgical procedure is begun. Perioperative antibiotics are rarely used. The hair and skin surrounding the ear are cleansed with 70 per cent alcohol. No hair is shaved unless fascia is to be taken, but it is combed away from the ear and sprayed with liquid spray bandage. The head is secured with tape in a standard foam headrest in the position most conducive to good vision for the surgeon. This usually involves tilting the head back and the chin up slightly (Fig. 11–1). For this reason, the surgeon rather than a nursing assistant should prepare and position the patient. The ear canal, auricle, and surrounding skin are cleansed with povidone-iodine scrub and then painted with povidone-iodine solution. The field is then draped in a sterile manner.

The sine qua non for successful transcanal surgery is adequate exposure. Inadequate visibility is probably the primary objection to this technique, but there are several moves that can significantly improve it. The external auditory meatus can be enlarged by making a small slit in the superior aspect of its lateral end with a No. 15 scalpel blade and stretching it with a nasal speculum. The largest-sized ear speculum that can be atraumatically inserted is used and secured with a speculum holder (Fig. 11–2). The speculum holder is essential because it allows the use of both hands and serves as a support for the surgeon's fingers. The holder is quite mobile and allows the speculum to be placed and secured in the optimal position. It should be repositioned as needed throughout the procedure. The microscope head should also be

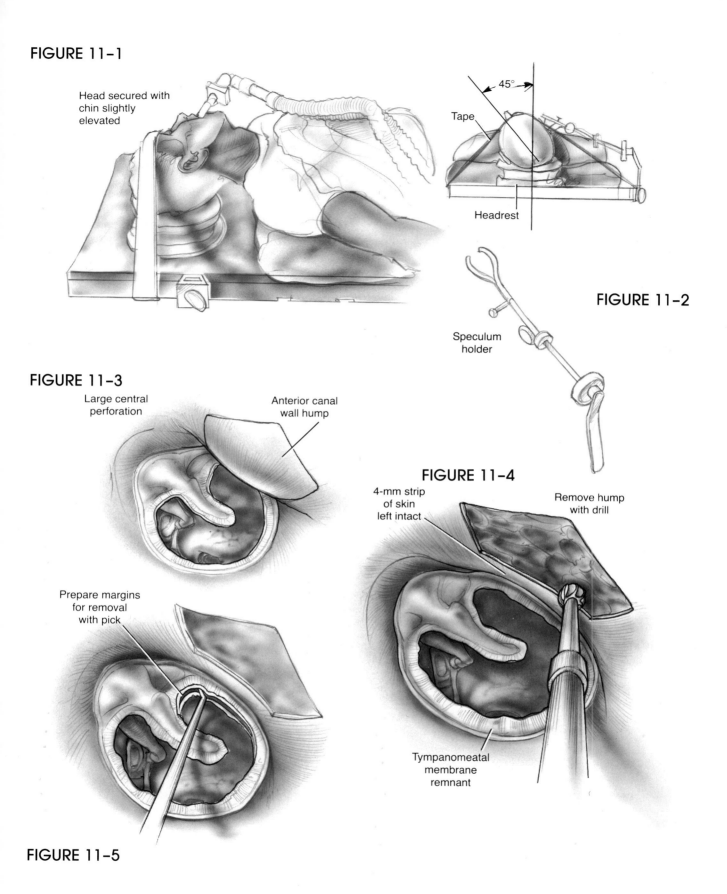

FIGURE 11-1

Head secured with chin slightly elevated

FIGURE 11-2

45°

Tape

Headrest

Speculum holder

FIGURE 11-3

Large central perforation

Anterior canal wall hump

FIGURE 11-4

4-mm strip of skin left intact

Remove hump with drill

Tympanomeatal membrane remnant

Prepare margins for removal with pick

FIGURE 11-5

moved about frequently to provide an unobstructed view of the operative field. In general, the less complex the microscope, the easier it is to use. Another item that is extremely helpful in improving visibility is the hydraulic chair. Because it can be lowered or raised in a matter of seconds, it rapidly allows the surgeon to change position in relation to the patient's ear without the need for a circulating nurse to tilt the operating table back and forth.

In anterior perforations and large central perforations, the anterior margin frequently cannot be seen because of a bulging anterior canal wall (Fig. 11–3). This problem can easily be remedied in 99 per cent of the cases by removing the hump. Sometimes the removal of a "dog-house" segment of anterior canal wall skin is all that is necessary. Frequently, the bony hump must also be removed, and this can be quickly done with a curette or small cutting burr (Fig. 11–4). It is important to leave a 2mm to 3mm strip of skin intact between the annulus and the medial end of the resected skin. The excised skin is preserved in physiologic solution until the end of the procedure, at which time it is replaced. Once the margins of the perforation can be adequately visualized, they are prepared by incising the edge with a sharp, slightly angulated pick (Fig. 11–5), removing the rim and about 1 or 2mm of the mucosa with a cup forceps (Fig. 11–6).

If the anterior perforation is marginal, the Austin "reverse elevator" (Fig. 11–7) is used to elevate the annulus and the 1mm to 2mm of the canal wall skin to provide a larger raw surface area for graft attachment. This elevated area gradually retracts back into its normal position spontaneously. It is an extremely important maneuver in the successful repair of the anterior perforation.

A posterior tympanomeatal incision is then made with the superior limb beginning 2mm to 3mm anterior to the malleus neck (Fig. 11–8). This makes it possible to completely elevate the drumhead remnant off of the malleus handle (Fig. 11–9). Removal of the drumhead remnant from the malleus handle is performed in most situations except those in which the perforation is in an inferior or extremely posterior position. The three most important things facilitated by this elevation are the removal of any squamous epithelial ingrowth along the medial aspect of the malleus handle, the ossicular chain reconstruction, and the placement of the graft along the lateral aspect of the malleus.

Some surgeons prefer to place the graft medial to the malleus handle.[6] If there is extreme medial retraction of the malleus handle so that the umbo is touching the promontory, the handle can be slowly elevated laterally with a right-angle pick to release the accom-

panying contracture of the tensor tympani tendon. When the mucosa is badly diseased or eroded, the medial wall of the middle ear can be lined with absorbable gelatin film (Gelfilm) cut to the desired size and shape. Because of the potential for delayed reaction, we do not use Silastic sheeting unless a second stage is planned, at which time the Silastic sheeting is removed.

Next, the tragal perichondrial graft is taken. If the perforation involves 60 per cent of the surface of the drumhead or less, the graft may be obtained from the posterior aspect of the tragus through an incision immediately posterior to the free border without removal of the cartilage itself (Fig. 11–10). If the perforation involves more than 60 per cent of the drumhead, the entire tragus with its perichondrium is removed through an incision along the free border. The excess soft tissue is removed from the perichondrium overlying the anterior surface of the tragus, and the entire perichondrium is removed from both sides of the cartilage and over the free border with a duckbill or Freer elevator and thumb forceps (Fig. 11–11). The cartilage is reinserted into the wound in its normal position to preserve the tragal contour, and the incision is closed with fine absorbable suture. The perichondrium is pressed with a vein or fascia press (Fig. 11–12). This process thins the graft for easier handling and enlarges it so that any size perforation can be closed.

The middle ear is then filled with gelatin sponge (Gelfoam) soaked in a physiologic solution, such as lactated Ringer's or Tis-U-Sol (Fig. 11–13). It is imperative that the tympanic cavity be filled with the gelatin sponge, especially in the anterior part at the eustachian tube orifice, to prevent medial displacement of the graft. The central part of the middle ear, however, should not be filled lateral to the umbo. If it is overfilled at this point, lateralization and loss of the conical contour of the drumhead may result.

For medium-sized or large perforations, the graft is then advanced under the tympanomeatal flap and over the malleus handle to the anterior-most extent of the perforation with the edges tucked under the margins of the drum remnant (Fig. 11–14). With smaller, inferior perforations, the graft may be inserted through the perforation and smoothed out posteriorly by elevating the tympanomeatal flap.

When using a perichondrial graft, the surface that was in contact with the cartilage should be positioned toward the middle ear. With a vein graft, the intimal surface should be medially placed. After the graft has been roughly positioned, the edges of the perforation are then carefully everted bimanually with a 20-gauge suction tip and a 90-degree pick to prevent the ingrowth of squamous epithelium. If the graft does not

FIGURE 11-6

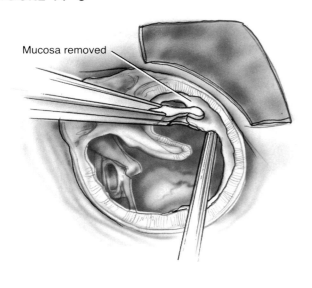

Mucosa removed

FIGURE 11-7

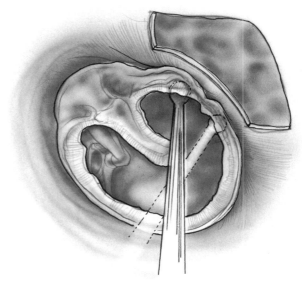

FIGURE 11-8

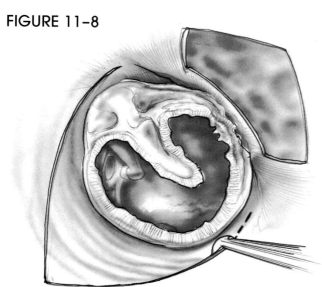

FIGURE 11-9

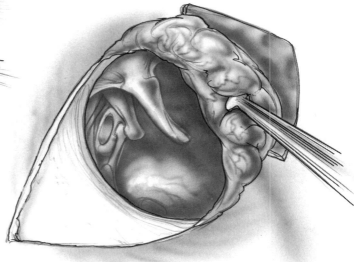

FIGURE 11-10

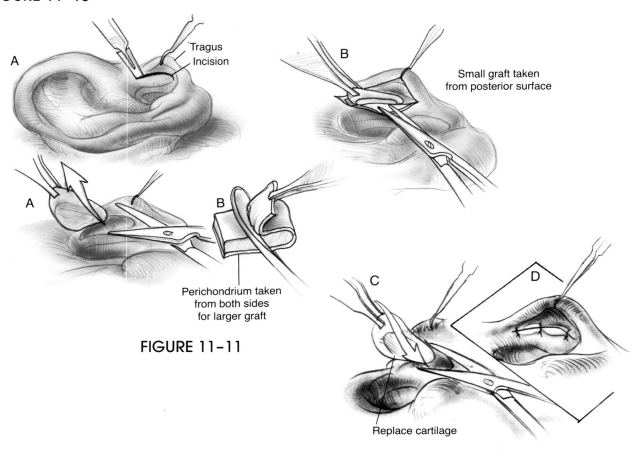

A   Tragus
     Incision

B   Small graft taken
     from posterior surface

A

B   Perichondrium taken
     from both sides
     for larger graft

FIGURE 11-11

C   Replace cartilage

D

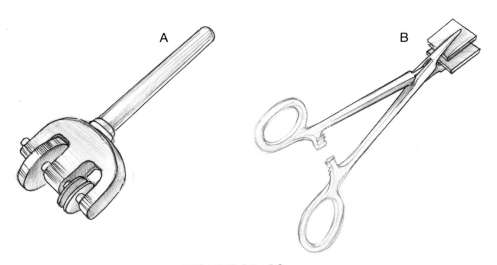

A   B

FIGURE 11-12

FIGURE 11-13

FIGURE 11-14

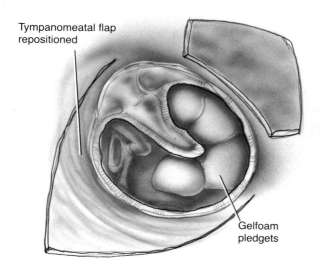

Tympanomeatal flap
repositioned

Gelfoam
pledgets

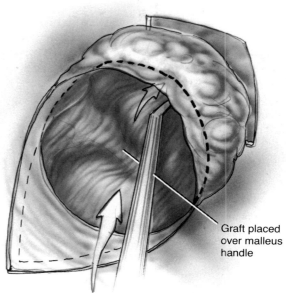

Graft placed
over malleus
handle

FIGURE 11-15

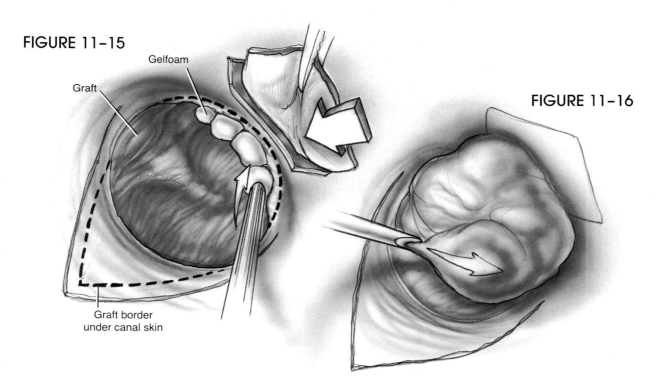

Graft

Gelfoam

Graft border
under canal skin

FIGURE 11-16

appear to be adequately supported by gelatin sponge, it can be reflected back and more gelatin sponge inserted.

If the anterior canal wall skin has been removed, it should now be replaced. Small pledgets of moist gelatin sponge are then used to overlap the junction of rim and graft circumferentially for further stabilization (Figs. 11–15 and 11–16).

Finally, the external canal is filled with an antibiotic ointment, such as polymyxin. In the event of antibiotic sensitivity, povidone-iodine ointment may be substituted.

POSTOPERATIVE CARE

The only dressing that is used is a small, sterile, cotton ball that is loosely placed in the conchal cavity to absorb drainage. Once the drainage stops, the cotton is discontinued, and the ear is allowed to ventilate. In the event that purulent discharge occurs, antibiotic otic drops are started and continued until the first postoperative visit. The patient is instructed to avoid getting water in the affected ear or blowing the nose until the first postoperative visit at 3 weeks. At that time, the ear is cleaned using the operating microscope, and the graft is inspected. Approximately 95 per cent of the time, the graft will have taken, and the drumhead will be intact. Autoinflation is now begun using the Valsalva maneuver. If the patient is unable to ventilate the middle ear within a week or 10 days, a small ventilation tube is inserted in the drumhead.

If the graft is intact but not completely epithelialized at the time of the first postoperative visit, antimicrobial drops or a vinegar-alcohol solution should be used for 1 to 3 weeks to promote healing.

Although frank graft failure is a rarity, a small area of residual perforation will occasionally be found. If this occurs, the edges can be cauterized with trichloroacetic acid and then covered with a cigarette paper patch impregnated with povidone-iodine solution. The area is re-examined in 2 to 3 weeks, at which time it is usually healed. If revision surgery is necessary, it should be delayed for at least 3 months to allow for resolution of postoperative inflammatory changes.

References

1. Shea JJ Jr: Vein graft closure of eardrum perforations. J Laryngol Otol 74: 358, 1960.
2. Tabb HG: Closure of perforations of the tympanic membrane by vein grafts: A preliminary report of twenty cases. Laryngoscope 70: 271, 1960.
3. Austin DF, Shea JJ Jr: A new system of tympanoplasty using vein graft. Laryngoscope 71: 596, 1961.
4. Storrs LA: Myringoplasty with the use of fascia grafts. Arch Otolaryngol Head Neck Surg 74: 45, 1961.
5. Goodhill V, Harris I, Brockman SJ: Tympanoplasty with perichondrial graft. Arch Otolaryngol Head Neck Surg 79: 131, 1964.
6. Hough JVD: Tympanoplasty with the interior fascial graft technique and ossicular reconstruction. Laryngoscope 80: 1385, 1970.

12

Tympanoplasty: The Undersurface Graft Technique — Postauricular Approach

MICHAEL E. GLASSCOCK, III, M.D., F.A.C.S.
BARRY STRASNICK, M.D.

Since the fundamental principles of tympanoplasty were first introduced by Wullstein and Zollner, there has been great diversity in the accepted surgical techniques used for repair of the tympanic membrane.[1, 2] The multitude of graft materials employed is a testimony to the difficulty of middle ear reconstruction. However, with advanced microsurgical techniques, the state of the art has now developed to the extent that graft success rates on the order of 90 to 97 per cent are to be expected.[3, 4, 5]

Over the years, two basic grafting techniques have evolved based on where the graft material is placed in relation to the drum remnant (overlay versus underlay techniques). In this chapter, a method of undersurface grafting is presented that combines the salient features of each approach. Detailed surgical techniques along with appropriate preoperative and postoperative care will be presented.

HISTORICAL ASPECTS

Modern middle ear reconstructive surgery represents the culmination of over a century of contributions by numerous dedicated and innovative otologic surgeons. The term *tympanoplasty* was originally defined in 1964 by what was then known as the American Academy of Ophthamology and Otolaryngology's Committee on Conservation of Hearing as "an operation to eradicate disease in the middle ear and to reconstruct the hearing mechanism without mastoid surgery, with or without tympanic membrane grafting."[6] Should a mastoid procedure be included, the term *tympanoplasty with mastoidectomy* is used.

The era of surgical repair of the tympanic membrane dates as far back as the nineteenth century. In 1853, Toynbee described closure of a perforation of the tympanic membrane using a small rubber disk attached to a silver wire.[7] Ten years later, Yearsley advocated placing a cotton ball over the perforation, whereas in 1887, Blake introduced the concept of placing a thin paper patch over the membrane.[8, 9] The use of cautery to promote spontaneous healing of tympanic membrane perforations was introduced by Roosa in 1876, who used silver nitrate.[10] Later, Joynt, Linn, and Derlacki would describe modifications of this technique using various forms of cautery and patches.[11, 12, 13] However, closure of tympanic membrane perforations was considered appropriate only for dry central perforations. That is, at this point, no one advocated the use of drum closure for the chronically draining ear.

It was not until 1952 that Wullstein and Zollner revolutionized middle ear surgery by advocating reconstructive grafting of the chronically diseased ear through the use of full- or split-thickness skin grafts.[1, 2]

House and Sheehy[14] and Plester[15] later used canal skin, believing that it more closely resembled the squamous layer of the tympanic membrane. However, the overall poor success rates of these grafts along with the development of iatrogenic cholesteatomas prompted the search for alternative grafting materials.

Shea and Tabb, working independently, described the use of autogenous vein to close the tympanic membrane.[16, 17] Goodhill advocated tragal perichondrium in the mid-1960s, and tympanic membrane homografts became popular a few years later.[18] The first sizable series of homograft tympanic membrane transplants was reported by Glasscock and House in 1968.[19] However, over the years, interest in homografts has waned largely because of the fear of transmission of infectious diseases.

Storrs is credited with performing the first fascia graft in the United States.[20] Although vein, perichondrium, and homografts still have their advocates, autogenous fascia has now become the standard by which all other grafting materials are measured.

The use of skin grafts required that the tympanic membrane perforation be repaired by laying the graft on top of the denuded drum remnant. This method of repair eventually became known as the overlay technique and was carried over to other forms of grafting material. With the use of connective tissue grafts, the graft material could be placed medial to the tympanic membrane remnant. The success of this approach eventually gave rise to the underlay technique of tympanic membrane grafting, of which a large series was reported by Austin and Shea.[3] Proponents of the underlay procedure submit that it eliminates many of the problems associated with overlay grafts, such as anterior blunting, epithelial pearl formation, and lateralization of the new drum.

In 1973, Glasscock described an underlay grafting technique that relied on a postauricular approach.[4] With minor modifications, this approach continues to be the preferred method of dealing with disorders of the tympanic membrane and middle ear.

PREOPERATIVE CONSIDERATIONS

Regardless of the grafting technique chosen, the preoperative evaluation and management of the patient with a tympanic membrane perforation remains the same. A complete clinical history along with a comprehensive head and neck examination is performed. Otoscopic examination is performed with the aid of an operating microscope, and all findings are diagrammed on the patient's chart. All patients receive a pure-tone air and bone conduction audiogram along with speech discrimination testing. Tuning fork tests should be done on all patients to confirm the audiologic findings. Depending on the clinical presentation, conventional mastoid X-rays, high-resolution computed tomographic scans, or magnetic resonance imaging studies may be obtained.

Every attempt is made to identify and treat coexistent inhalant allergies and sinus disease prior to surgery. The status of the upper respiratory tract directly influences eustachian tube function, and, therefore, the eventual outcome of surgery. Similarly, emphasis is placed on eradication or control of active infection in the involved ear. If the ear is draining at the initial visit, it is meticulously cleansed under microscopic vision through the use of otologic suction. The patient is instructed to irrigate the ear three times a day with a sterile 1.5 per cent acetic acid solution using a small rubber bulb ear syringe. This procedure allows purulent material to be removed from the middle ear and external canal and restores a more physiologic pH. It is important that the solution be used at body temperature to avoid caloric stimulation of the labyrinth. Following acetic acid irrigation, three drops of an antibiotic otic solution are instilled into the ear. Depending on the severity of the infection, systemic oral antibiotics may also be prescribed. The fluid from draining ears is not routinely cultured because the majority will respond to local care. If the ear continues to drain despite aggressive medical treatment, a culture and sensitivity test is performed, and the antibiotic regimen is adjusted appropriately. This regimen has been extremely successful in drying the majority

of ears prior to surgery. We have no reservations, however, in performing tympanoplasty on a "wet" ear and feel that no waiting period is necessary once the ear has become dry.

An assessment of eustachian tube function should be included as part of the preoperative evaluation. One of the most useful indications of proper eustachian tube function is a normal contralateral ear. Although a functioning eustachian tube is important to the success of the operation, a lack of eustachian tube function should not preclude surgical intervention. In fact, eustachian tube function may improve once the infection is removed and the middle ear space reconstructed.

The patient is counseled preoperatively as to the nature of the problem, proposed treatment as well as alternative therapies, and expected outcome. It is helpful to provide written explanations and instructions discussing preoperative and postoperative care of the ear. Videotaped discussions of the proposed procedure are also useful.

Surgical Technique

Surgical Preparation

A 2cm wide area of hair is shaved above and behind the auricle. Skin degreaser is applied to the shaved area, followed by tincture of benzoin. Nonsterile 3M (number 1010) plastic towel drapes are then placed on the skin to cover the hair. All procedures for chronic ear problems are performed using intraoperative facial nerve monitoring. Electrode insertion occurs prior to the surgical preparation. An iodine soap solution is used to wash the auricle and the skin around it, which is blotted dry with a sterile towel, and the ear itself is bathed in an iodine prep solution for 3 minutes. The solution is allowed to enter the external auditory canal. Finally, the area about the ear is prepared with an alcohol-based solution (DuraPrep).

The circulating nurse next injects the postauricular region and tragus with a 2 per cent lidocaine (Xylocaine) and 1:100,000 adrenalin solution. This procedure allows adequate time for the epinephrine to diffuse through the tissues, thereby reducing the amount of bleeding encountered at the time of incision.

Following injection, the scrub nurse drapes the auricle with three layers of sterile sheets. The first layer consists of four paper adhesive sheets placed in a squared-off fashion about the auricle. This is followed by a 3M plastic ear drape (number 1030). This waterproof sheet effectively isolates the patient and prevents contamination should the paper drapes become soaked with irrigation solution. Finally, a custom-designed paper otologic drape, along with a plastic drainage bag, is applied (Fig. 12–1).

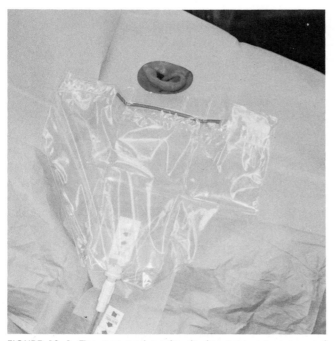

FIGURE 12–1. The ear and postauricular area are prepared and draped in a sterile fashion.

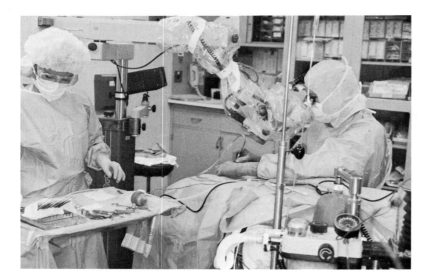

FIGURE 12-2. Operating room arrangement. The scrub nurse is located directly across from the surgeon, and the anesthesiologist is seated at the foot of the table.

Irrigation and suction tubing and cautery lines are secured to the field using Velcro adhesive pads. The scrub nurse attaches a compartmentalized plastic pouch to the Mayo stand to hold suction tips and Bovie's and bipolar cauteries.

Anesthesia

All patients receive general endotracheal anesthesia with an epinephrine-compatible anesthetic agent. Long circuits are used on the anesthesia machine to enable the anesthesiologist to be seated at the foot of the table, opposite the surgeon (Fig. 12-2).

The vascular strip and four quadrants of the ear canal are injected with a 2 per cent lidocaine and 1:50,000 adrenalin solution. The local anesthetic reduces pain and allows the patient to be kept relatively "light" during the procedure. No limitations on the use of nitrous oxide during graft placement are required. This is because the undersurface placement of the graft, along with packing of the eustachian tube orifice, precludes the graft being elevated off the drum remnant. Rather, the nitrous oxide bubbles will escape harmlessly up the posterior canal wall.

Every attempt is made to extubate the patient deeply to avoid straining and potentially detrimental Valsalva efforts. In addition, intravenous antiemetics, such as droperidol, are given in an attempt to reduce postsurgical nausea and vomiting.

Incisions

The vascular strip is outlined by making incisions at the tympanosquamous and tympanomastoid suture lines using a No. 67 Beaver knife blade. In addition, small inferiorly and superiorly based flaps are created by making right-angle incisions to the vascular strip incisions. The medial end of the vascular strip is formed by connecting the two primary incisions with a No. 72 Beaver blade approximately 2mm lateral to the annulus (Fig. 12-3).

Attention is now directed away from the ear canal and a Bard-Parker No. 15 blade is used to fashion a postauricular incision approximately 5mm behind the postauricular crease (Fig. 12-4). The surgeon firmly grasps the auricle in the left hand and forcefully pulls forward and outward. Constant tension allows identification of the loose areolar tissue overlying the temporalis fascia and creates a bloodless surgical plane. Bleeding is controlled with electrical cautery.

Harvesting Fascia

Once hemostasis is achieved, a small Weitlaner retractor is positioned to hold the auricle forward. The scrub nurse places a small Senn retractor under the upper part of the incision and pulls laterally, exposing the temporalis fascia. The loose areolar tissue overlaying the temporalis fascia is then ballooned up with a local anesthetic to facilitate its removal. An incision is made at the level of the linea temporalis, and the areolar tissue is dissected free from the temporalis fascia using Metzenbaum scissors (Fig. 12-5). This tissue is then pressed onto a polytetrafluoroethylene (Teflon) block and placed on the back table under a gooseneck lamp to dehydrate it.

Exposing the Middle Ear

The retractor is removed, and an incision is made along the linea temporalis, extending anteriorly over the external auditory canal. A T-shaped incision is then created by dropping a vertical limb from the midpoint of the linea temporalis to the mastoid tip (see Fig. 12–5). A Lempert elevator is used to mobilize the periosteum to the level of the ear canal. The vascular strip is then identified from posteriorly, grasped with an Adson forceps, and held forward in the blade of a Weitlaner retractor, along with the auricle (see Fig. 12–5). A second Weitlaner retractor is placed between the temporalis muscle and mastoid tip at right angles to the first retractor.

The ear canal is copiously irrigated with a physiologic saline solution to remove blood and debris. With a 20-gauge needle suction in the left hand and a House No. 2 lancet knife in the right, the skin of the inferior ear canal is elevated down to the fibrous annulus (Fig. 12–6), creating an inferiorly based flap. Next, a House No. 1 sickle knife is used to develop a superior flap just above the short process of the malleus. The fibrous annulus is mobilized out of its sulcus anterior to the malleus.

If the operating table is rotated away from the surgeon, the anterior drum remnant and annulus are easily seen. Should a bony overhang obscure complete vision, the canal skin may be reflected medially and the bone removed with a small diamond burr. Care must be taken to protect the anterior annulus and adjacent canal skin.

Eradication of Disease

With the middle ear now well exposed, the primary disease process can be addressed in a logical fashion. Cholesteatoma, granulation tissue, or polypoid disease can be removed through the middle ear itself, or in conjunction with a mastoidectomy if indicated. For better exposure of the middle ear, the facial recess is opened, leaving the posterior canal wall intact.

Preparation of the Tympanic Membrane Remnant

Once the disease in the middle ear and mastoid has been eradicated, the drum remnant is prepared for grafting. Small attic, marginal, or central perforations are prepared so as to preserve the normal drum remnant. In the case of an extensive perforation or a severely diseased membrane, the entire drum remnant is removed to the level of the annulus. The manubrium of the malleus is denuded, preserving the fibrous annulus. The mucosa of the undersurface of the drum remnant or annulus is then abraded through the use of a House No. 1 sickle knife and cup forceps to further ensure an adequate recipient surface for the graft (see Fig. 12–6).

A two-stage procedure is often planned in cases of massive cholesteatoma, extensive mucosal disease, or ossicular fixation. At the primary procedure, repair of the tympanic membrane along with removal of the middle ear disease is attempted, delaying ossicular reconstruction until approximately 6 to 8 months later. If, however, ossicular reconstruction is performed at the initial procedure, it is done prior to placement of the graft.

Placement of the Graft

It is imperative that excellent hemostasis be achieved prior to graft placement. Absorbable gelatin sponge (Gelfoam) saturated in 1:1000 adrenalin is packed into the middle ear space while the graft is being fashioned. The dried areolar tissue graft is then removed from the polytetrafluoroethylene block and trimmed to size (approximately 2 1/2cm by 1 1/2cm). A slit is made toward the superior aspect of the graft to accommodate placement medial to the malleus handle.

If mucosa has been removed from the middle ear, a sheet of absorbable gelatin film (Gelfilm) is trimmed and placed onto the promontory to prevent adhesions. The adrenalin-soaked gelatin sponge is removed, and the middle ear is packed with saline-moistened gelatin sponge starting from the eustachian tube and working posteriorly.

The graft is grasped with cup forceps, rehydrated in a physiologic saline solution (Tis-U-Sol), and placed in the middle ear. With a 22-gauge suction in the left hand and a right-angle hook in the other, the graft is slid under the manubrium of the malleus onto the lateral attic wall. A House annulus elevator is used to tuck the fascia under the drum remnant anteriorly and inferiorly (Fig. 12–7).

With this technique, there is a point in the inferior canal at approximately 6 o'clock where the graft makes a transition from lying medial to the annulus to being on top of it. The remaining graft is draped along the posterior canal wall, and the inferior canal flap with attached annulus is repositioned over the graft. Similarly, the superior flap is replaced, covering the fascia lying anterior to the malleus (see Fig. 12–7). A gimmick is used to even all edges of the annulus and smooth out the graft. Polymyxin B (Polysporin) ointment is then placed over the fascia graft, filling the anterior sulcus. The retractors are removed, and the vascular strip is carefully replaced in its original position. The mastoid periosteum incision is closed with 3.0 Dexon suture in interrupted fashion. A rubber-band drain is sutured in placed and left until the following morning. The postauricular incision is then closed with the same suture, using an interrupted subcuticular stitch. No skin sutures are used, obviating later removal. Proper position of the vascular strip is once again confirmed through an ear speculum, and the remainder of the ear canal is filled with the anti-

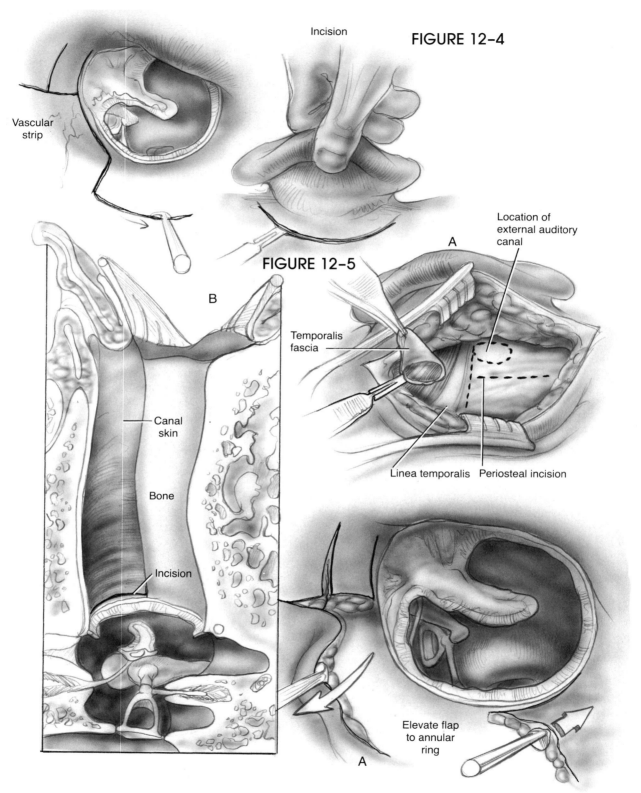

FIGURE 12-3

Vascular strip

Incision

FIGURE 12-4

FIGURE 12-5

B

Canal skin

Bone

Incision

A

Location of external auditory canal

Temporalis fascia

Linea temporalis   Periosteal incision

Elevate flap to annular ring

A

FIGURE 12-6

FIGURE 12-6

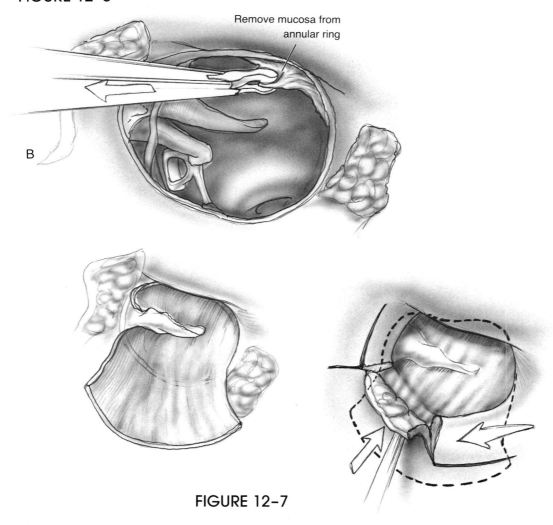

Remove mucosa from
annular ring

B

FIGURE 12-7

FIGURE 12-3. The vascular strip is outlined with a No. 67 and No. 72 Beaver blade.

FIGURE 12-4. A standard postauricular incision is fashioned approximately 5mm behind the postauricular crease.

FIGURE 12-5. *A*, The loose areolar tissue overlying the temporalis fascia is harvested as a free graft. Note the T incision through the mastoid periosteum used to expose the external auditory canal. *B*, The vascular strip is held forward along with the auricle.

FIGURE 12-6. *A*, The inferior canal flap is developed to the level of the fibrous annulus. *B*, The malleus is denuded and the undersurface of the drum remnant or annulus is abraded, while diseased mucosa is removed.

FIGURE 12-7. *A*, The fascia graft is directed under the fibrous annulus and malleus handle. *B*, The superior and inferior canal flaps are replaced over the fascia graft.

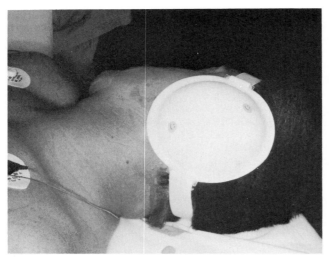

FIGURE 12–8. A sterile prepackaged mastoid dressing is applied.

biotic ointment. A cotton ball is placed in the meatus, and a sterile, prepackaged plastic bubble mastoid dressing is applied (Fig. 12–8).

Postoperative Care

On the first postoperative day the mastoid dressing along with the rubber-band drain is removed. A sterile, prepackaged postauricular dressing is applied behind the ear, and a fresh cotton ball is placed in the meatus of the ear canal to absorb the ointment as it liquifies. Patients are instructed to change the cotton ball at least three times per day and whenever it becomes soiled. The patient is instructed on dry ear precautions and advised to avoid blowing the nose. The patient is discharged to home with a 3-week follow-up appointment. Each individual is counseled as to the warning signs of infection and instructed to contact the office immediately should these occur. A prescription for analgesics is given; however, perioperative antibiotics are not employed on a routine basis in dry ears. Patients with ears that are infected at the time of surgery are placed on appropriate antibiotic coverage.

By the first postoperative visit, the postauricular wound should be well healed, the ear canal free of ointment, and the tympanic membrane epithelialized. All simple tympanoplasty patients undergo a pure-tone audiogram at this visit. If ossicular reconstruction was performed, then testing is delayed until 2 months following surgery. By 6 weeks, the grafted eardrum has thinned considerably and takes on the appearance of a normal tympanic membrane. Follow-up visits are arranged at 6 and 12 months, and thereafter the patient is seen at yearly intervals.

Results

In 1982, Glasscock et al. reported their experience in 1556 cases of tympanic membrane repair using the herein described postauricular undersurface grafting technique.[5] Of these cases, 663 were simple tympanoplasties, 687 involved a mastoidectomy, 54 were performed to repair a graft failure at a second stage, 38 involved a tympanoplasty with mastoid revision, and 114 were canal wall down mastoidectomies in which the tympanic membrane was grafted. Four hundred sixty-three ears (34 per cent) had undergone at least one previous surgery. All tympanic membranes were repaired using areolar tissue, temporalis fascia, or tragal perichondrium.

Of the 1556 ears, there were a total of 110 failures, for an overall graft success rate of 93 per cent. Of the failures, 19 occurred within 3 weeks of surgery, 31 at 3 months, 19 at 6 months, and 41 after 1 year. Successful grafting occurred in 91.5 per cent of patients under the age of 12, as compared with 93.3 per cent of patients over the age of 12. Similarly, the graft success rate was 92.7 per cent in draining ears, versus 93.1 per cent in dry. The presence of cholesteatoma had no apparent effect on success. Ears with cholesteatoma had a 92 per cent success rate, whereas those without averaged 93.2 per cent.

Complications were minimal in this series. Postoperative otorrhea occurred in 6 per cent, varying from a mild otitis externa to a severe middle ear infection promoting loss of the graft. True wound infections were seen is fewer than 0.5 per cent. Sensorineural hearing loss occurred in fewer than 1 per cent of cases. There were five cases of delayed facial paralysis, all of which recovered completely within 2 to 3 weeks. Serous otitis media occurred in 2 per cent, whereas perichondritis, stenosis of the external auditory canal, and epithelial pearls occurred in fewer than 0.5 per cent.

CARTILAGE GRAFT TYMPANOPLASTY

In cases of severe atelectasis of the tympanic membrane, a cartilage tympanoplasty is often indicated. Cartilage autografts have long been used in repair of canal wall defects as well as ossiculoplasty.[21–24] In 1982, the senior author first described the successful use of cartilage-perichondrial autografts for severe atelectasis attic cholesteatoma and posterior retraction pockets.[5] Since that time, others have reported their results with this technique.[25–27]

The goal of cartilage tympanoplasty is to prevent recurrent retractions along with their long-term sequelae, including cholesteatoma formation, ossicular erosion, and progressive hearing loss. Incorporation of cartilage in the repair of the eardrum provides sufficient structural integrity to resist recurrent retraction. This technique is ideally suited for patients who demonstrate persistent eustachian tube dysfunction, including cleft palate patients or those with recurrent atelectasis following standard fascia graft tympanoplasty.

Surgical Techniques

The components of the operation that have a general application are described in the preceding section. Once exposure of the middle ear is obtained, the next step is to excise all diseased and atelectic tympanic membrane. The posterior fibrous annulus is elevated from its bony sulcus with a House No. 2 lancet knife. Careful dissection is required to avoid tearing the atelectatic drum to ensure that no epithelium will be left in the middle ear. To verify complete removal of an attic retraction, it is often necessary to perform a tympanomastoidectomy. Posterosuperior retractions must be elevated in continuity with the remainder of the tympanic membrane. When elevating the drum off the lenticular process and stapes suprastructure, applying force in a posterior-to-anterior direction will allow the stapedius tendon to provide countertraction, thereby preventing inadvertent stapes mobilization. A House No. 1 sickle knife is used to elevate the diseased membrane off the manubrium and lateral process of the malleus. Fibrous adhesions are lysed and diseased middle ear mucus removed with a cup forceps (Fig. 12–9).

To harvest the cartilage-perichondrial graft, an incision is made on the medial aspect of the tragus (Fig. 12–10). A House No. 2 lancet elevator is used to elevate the perichondrium from one surface of the cartilage, leaving it hinged on the other side, like a book cover. The cartilage is trimmed to the proper dimensions, depending on the degree of disease present. A posterosuperior quadrant retraction often requires a cartilage graft of approximately 4mm in diameter. For cases of atelectasis of the entire tympanic membrane, the cartilage can be incorporated into the entire pars tensa. In this situation, a wedge-shaped area of cartilage is accessed to accommodate the manubrium, if present.

Once the middle ear has been packed with moistened absorbable gelatin sponge, the cartilage-perichondrial graft is placed with the perichondrium side facing laterally. The perichondrium is then tucked under the manubrium and draped over the ear canal posteriorly. The cartilage should not overlap the posterior canal wall. The areolar tissue graft is then trimmed to size and placed lateral to the cartilage-perichondrial graft and medial to the fibrous annulus and manubrium (Fig. 12–11). This areolar graft serves to cover any remaining defects in the tympanic membrane or exposed bone in the external canal. The superior- and inferior-based canal flaps are then returned to their original positions, covering the grafts as they extend onto the posterior canal wall. The external canal is then filled with polymyxin B ointment, and closure proceeds in the manner previously described. Ossicular reconstruction, if required, is typically performed at a second stage.

Results

Our results using cartilage tympanoplasty were recently reported.[28] During the period 1982 to 1990, cartilage tympanoplasty was performed on 100 ears. The retracted portion of the tympanic membrane was in the posterosuperior quadrant in 37 per cent, the entire drum in 34 per cent, the posterior half in 18 per cent, the pars flaccida alone in 16 per cent, the pars flaccida and pars tensa combined in 4 per cent, and the anterior half in 1 per cent. Thirty-three ears had cholesteatoma present. Fifty-two ears required ossicular reconstruction, of which 31 were performed simultaneously with the cartilage tympanoplasty, and 21 were staged.

Hearing results were reported in 79 ears by calculating the postoperative average air-bone gap for the speech frequencies (500, 1000, and 2000Hz) in 10dB increments. Of these 79 cases, 38 per cent achieved closure of the air-bone gap to within 10dB, whereas 39 per cent closed to within 20dB, and 18 per cent closed to within 30dB. Five per cent of patients failed to demonstrate closure to less than 30dB.

Of the 100 ears, there were four failures (4 per cent) in terms of the technique itself. There were two recurrent cholesteatomas, one perforation, and one recurrent retraction. Six patients (6 per cent) developed serous otitis media postoperatively. Of these six patients, three eventually required ventilation tubes. Fifteen patients had mild retractions that were easily controlled with modified Valsalva exercises. There were two wound infections and six cases of external auditory canal infections. Perichondritis and external canal stenosis did not occur in this series.

SUMMARY

The major objectives of tympanoplasty may be prioritized as follows: 1) control of infection, 2) creation of an air-containing middle ear space, and 3) hearing rehabilitation. To accomplish these goals, it is imperative that the otologic surgeon exercise sound clinical judgment in terms of selection of patients as well as surgical approach.

Over the years, two classical approaches to the repair of tympanic membrane perforations have evolved. In earlier years, the overlay method was extremely popular, owing to its high success rate and reproducibility.[29] With time, however, several bothersome complications with the overlay technique have become apparent. The most common of these complications is blunting of the anterior sulcus, which can be so excessive as to lead to fixation of the malleus handle and produce a conductive hearing loss. Another difficulty with this method of repair is the inability of the surgeon to completely denude the drum remnant of all squamous epithelium. Epithelial pearls as well as cholesteatoma can therefore arise anywhere in the new tympanic membrane. Lateral migration of the graft away from the malleus handle can also occur, producing a conductive hearing loss. One other problem associated with the operation is delayed healing because the canal skin is completely removed and replaced as a free graft.

The use of connective tissue as a grafting material has made it possible to place the graft under the drum remnant. The undersurface technique is generally perceived as being more technically difficult, leading to errors in graft placement and subsequent failure. In part, this problem occurs because the procedure is routinely performed through the ear canal, using a speculum and holder. Unless the surgeon is experienced with stapedectomies, the use of an ear speculum is typically a cumbersome procedure. The size and shape of the ear canal often impairs visualization of the entire drum remnant and anterior sulcus, making graft placement particularly difficult. Complete exposure of the middle ear and, particularly, the eustachian tube orifice is limited as well.

The postauricular approach using the vascular strip as a means to expose the ear canal has avoided many of the problems associated with the transcanal undersurface technique. Through the use of a postauricular incision, it is possible to work transmeatally without the need of a speculum. The inferior canal skin flap exposes the hypotympanum, whereas the posterior approach allows excellent visualization of the anterior

annulus and eustachian tube orifice. Overall exposure is improved, making graft placement more exact and leading to consistently higher graft success rates. Additionally, the aforementioned problems of blunting, lateralization, epithelial pearl formation, and delayed healing associated with the overlay technique are avoided.

For the average surgeon, the postauricular undersurface graft technique of myringoplasty will yield consistently superior functional results with fewer complications than those seen with classical transcanal undersurface procedures or overlay techniques. Rigid adherence to basic surgical principles along with the techniques described in this chapter should lead to a successful outcome in excess of 90 per cent of cases.

References

1. Wullstein H: Funktionelle Operations in Muttelokr met Hilfe des fresen Spalthappen-Tranplantes. Arch Ohr Nas Kehlhopfheilk, 161: 422, 1952.
2. Zollner F: The principles of plastic surgery of the sound-conducting apparatus. J Laryngol Otol 69: 637, 1955.
3. Austin DF, Shea JJ: A new system of tympanoplasty using vein graft. Laryngoscope 71: 596, 1961.
4. Glasscock ME: Tympanic membrane grafting with fascia: Overlay vs underlay technique. Laryngoscope 5: 754, 1973.
5. Glasscock ME, Jackson CJ, Nissen AJ, et al.: Postauricular undersurface tympanic membrane grafting: A follow-up report. Laryngoscope 92: 718, 1982.
6. Committee on Conservation of Hearing of the American Academy of Ophthamology and Otolaryngology: Standard Classification for Surgery of Chronic Ear Infection. Arch Otolaryngol Head Neck Surg 81: 204, 1964.
7. Toynbee J: On the Use of An Artificial Membrane Tympanic in Cases of Deafness Dependant Upon Perforations in Destruction of the Natural Organ. London, J. Churchill and Sons, 1853.
8. Yearsley J: Deafness, Practically Illustrated. Ecl. 6, London, J. Churchill and Sons, 1863.
9. Blake CJ: Transactions of the First Congress of the International Otological Society. New York, D. Appelton and Company, 1887, p 125.
10. Roosa DB, St. J: Disease of the Ear, 3rd ed. New York, William Wood and Company, 1876.
11. Joynt JA: Repair of the drum. J Iowa Med Soc 9: 51, 1919.
12. Linn EG: Closure of tympanic membrane perforations. Arch Otolaryngol Head Neck Surg 58: 405, 1953.

FIGURE 12-9. Standard vascular strip incisions are made. House sickle knife opens the middle ear and elevates the atelectic drum.

FIGURE 12-10. A, The tragal cartilage perichondrial graft is harvested by means of an incision on the posteromedial aspect of the tragus. B, The tragal perichondrium is elevated off the surface of the cartilage. C, The cartilage is trimmed to the desired size.

FIGURE 12-11. A, The cartilage perichondrial graft positioned medial to manubrium and fibrous annulus. The areolar tissue graft is then positioned lateral to the cartilage perichondrial graft but medial to the annulus and manubrium. B, Lateral view demonstrating cartilage-perichondrial graft in place. Ossiculoplasty is typically performed at a second stage.

FIGURE 12-9

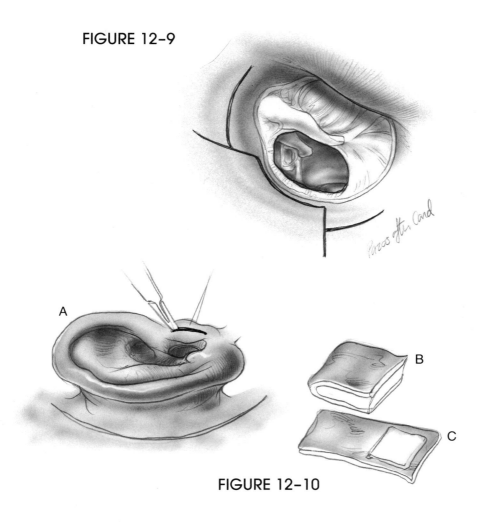

A

B

C

FIGURE 12-10

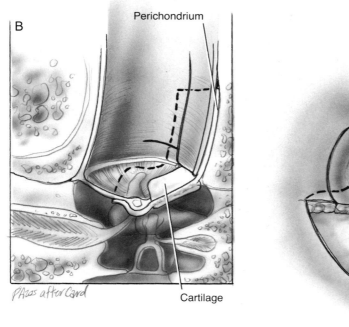

B

Perichondrium

Cartilage

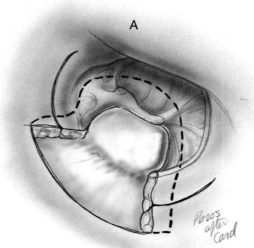

A

FIGURE 12-11

13. Derlacki EL: Repair of central perforations of the tympanic membrane. Arch Otolaryngol Head Neck Surg 58: 405, 1953.
14. House WF, Sheehy JL: Myringoplasty. Arch Otolaryngol 73: 407, 1961.
15. Plester D: Myringoplasty methods. Arch Otolaryngol 78: 310, 1963.
16. Shea JJ: Vein graft closure of eardrum perforations. J Otolaryngol 74: 358, 1960.
17. Tabb HG: Closure of perforations of the tympanic membrane by vein grafts: A preliminary report of 20 cases. Laryngoscope 70: 271, 1960.
18. Goodhill V: Tragal perichondrium and cartilage in tympanoplasty. Arch Otolaryngol 85: 480, 1967.
19. Glasscock ME, House WF: Homograft reconstruction of the middle ear. Laryngoscope 78: 1219, 1968.
20. Storrs LA: Myringoplasty with the use of fascia grafts. Arch Otolaryngol 74: 65, 1961.
21. Donald PJ, McCabe BF, Loevy SS, et al.: Atticotomy: A neglected otosurgical technique. Ann Otol Rhinol Laryngol 83: 652, 1974.
22. McCleve DE: Repair of boney canal wall defects in tympanomastoid surgery. Am J Otol 6: 76, 1985.
23. McCleve DE: Tragal reconstruction of the auditory canal. Arch Otolaryngol 90: 35, 1969.
24. Linda RE: The cartilage-perichondrium graft in the treatment of posterior tympanic membrane retraction packets. Laryngoscope 83: 747, 1973.
25. Schwaber MK: Postauricular undersurface tympanic membrane grafting: Some modifications of the "swinging door" technique. Arch Otolaryngol Head Neck Surg 95: 182, 1986.
26. Levenson RM: Cartilage-perichondrial composite graft tympanoplasty in the treatment of posterior marginal and attic retraction pockets. Laryngoscope 97: 1069, 1987.
27. Adkins W: Composite autograft for tympanoplasty and tympmastoid surgery. Laryngoscope 100: 244, 1990.
28. Glasscock ME, Hart MJ: Surgical treatment of the atelectic ear. Operative Tech Otolaryngol Head Neck Surg 3: 15, 1992.
29. Sheehy JL, Glasscock ME: Tympanic membrane grafting with temporalis fascia. Arch Otolaryngol 86: 391, 1967.

13

Tympanoplasty: Homograft Tympanic Membrane Technique

ROGER E. WEHRS, M.D.

In 1964, Chalet reported using homograft tympanic membranes in three patients with one success.[1] Over the next few years, several articles appeared in the literature describing the use of this new material.[2-6] The initial results were good; however, over the longer term, the breakdown and failure rate were high. Seventy per cent ethyl alcohol was the preservative most often employed in this country; however, in Europe, Cialit was used. In 1970, Perkins[7] introduced buffered formaldehyde as a preservative. This substance greatly enhanced the tensile strength of the homograft drum; however, the detoxification process was time consuming and technically demanding.

This author first used the homograft tympanic membrane in 1965.[8] Prior to this time, canal skin or fascia had been employed as the chief type of grafting material. An overlay type of technique was employed, and results were mixed in that if canal skin were used alone, the graft take rate was only 60 per cent, but the hearing results were good. If the canal skin was reinforced with the fascia, the graft take rate improved to 95 per cent, but this procedure produced a thick graft with blunting of the anterior angle and a poor hearing result. It was therefore decided to try the homograft tympanic membrane. These early tympanic membranes were preserved in alcohol and had the epithelial layer removed at the time of harvest. They were thin dead tissue. The homograft eardrum was used to give stiffness and a cone shape to the new drumhead. It was covered with the canal skin to produce early epithelization and a living graft. This technique increased the graft take rate to 96 per cent.[9] The hearing results were good: the cone shape and sharp anterior angle so important to obtaining good hearing were preserved. When the perforation was posterior or attic, an underlay technique was used, and the homograft tympanic membrane was covered with a fascial graft. Thus, the breakdown and recurrent perforation that had attended the early use of the homograft tympanic membrane alone was avoided, although the graft retained its cone shape and stiffness. In cases in which the patient's malleus was absent, another important function of the homograft tympanic membrane was to hold the malleus in anatomic position. This homograft and malleus became the main building block in ossicular reconstruction to restore hearing. This technique has been employed with only minor variations for 25 years. The survival and function of the homograft tympanic membrane in the middle ear point to it as a privileged site.[10]

Formaldehyde-preserved tympanic membranes were tried in a few cases with this technique; however, these healed poorly and suffered redness, thickening, granulations, and sloughing of the canal skin. Therefore, their use was discontinued.

Some authors reported good results with eardrums preserved in buffered formaldehyde.[11] Their technique is different than that described here, in that the homograft drum is the only grafting material used. Because it is dead tissue, it must be strong enough not to break down until epithelialization has taken place. It is therefore ideal to use in severely damaged ears that are wet and infected. In these ears, it is acceptable for the graft to granulate and heal slowly by secondary intention. Under these circumstances, this author has used the formaldehyde drum and has seen these findings and an eventual good result. Therefore, it is my opinion that both alcohol- and formaldehyde-preserved material should be available so that the technique used would fit the pathology of the ear undergoing surgery.

ANATOMY AND PHYSIOLOGY

The primary purpose of the tympanic membrane is to change air pressure waves to fluid pressure waves so that they may stimulate the hair cells of the cochlea. This process is accomplished primarily through the hydraulic principle of a small amount of pressure applied to a large surface area (tympanic membrane) and results in a large amount of pressure (fluid waves) being applied to a small surface area (stapedial footplate) (Fig. 13–1).

The ossicle's main task is mechanical. The ossicular chain exerts a lever action that increases the sound pressure transmitted. The hydraulic principle increases the hearing level by approximately 27dB, whereas the lever action of the ossicles contributes only 3dB (Fig. 13–2).

In applying these principles to the clinical situation, one finds that a small perforation of the tympanic membrane with an intact ossicular chain produces only minimal conductive hearing loss, whereas ossicular discontinuity with only a small perforation produces a substantial hearing loss.

FIGURE 13–1. Hydraulic principles as applied to hearing.

FIGURE 13–2. The lever action of the ossicles as applied to hearing.

FIGURE 13-1

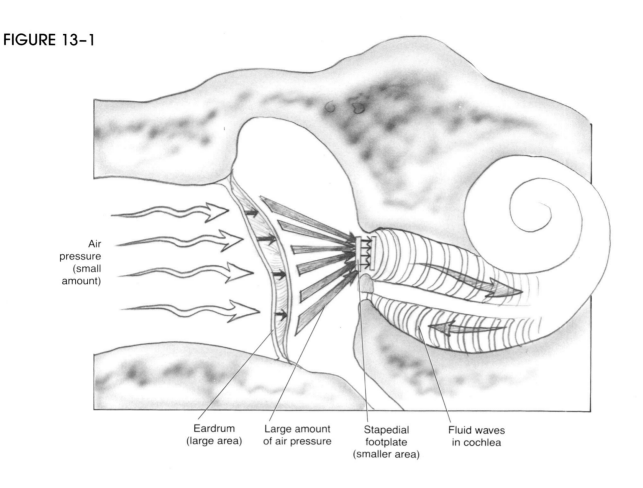

Air
pressure
(small
amount)

Eardrum
(large area)

Large amount
of air pressure

Stapedial
footplate
(smaller area)

Fluid waves
in cochlea

FIGURE 13-2

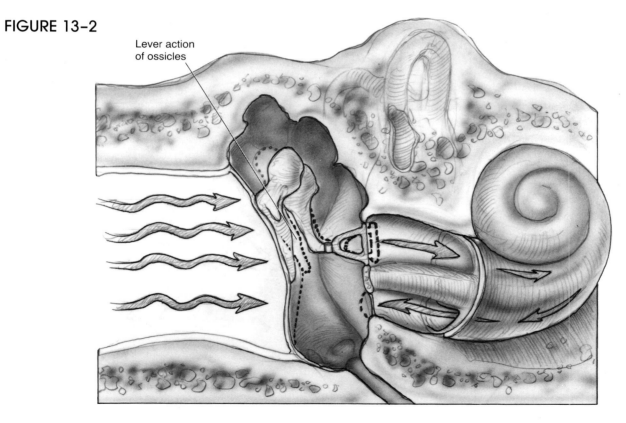

Lever action
of ossicles

In addition to its role in hydraulic force, the tympanic membrane also affords sound protection for the round window. This creates a phase differential so that the sound waves do not strike the oval and round windows at the same instant, thus, canceling each other and resulting in no movement of the inner ear fluids. In an ear with an intact tympanic membrane and discontinuity of the ossicular chain, the sound cannot reach either window, and a maximal conductive loss of approximately 60dB exists, whereas with a perforation, a phase differential is set up, and the hearing may improve by 20dB or 30dB.

The middle ear is an air-containing space that communicates with the outside through the eustachian tube. It also aerates the mastoid air cells through the mastoid antrum. The eustachian tube serves as a conduit for drainage of the middle ear and mastoid.

PATIENT SELECTION

The patients usually selected for homograft tympanoplasty with a transplant eardrum are those with a severely damaged drum. These include patients with a total perforation and an intact ossicular chain, those with squamous ingrowth beneath the remaining drum remnant even when the perforation is small, and those without a malleus or with a malleus that is so diseased that it must be removed. The homograft tympanic membrane then supports the homograft malleus in anatomic position so that the ossicular reconstruction can be accomplished. Patients selected for repair with homograft dura are those with small central perforations or revision cases.

In some cases of mastoid revision, in which a total perforation exists with absence of all ossicular tissue as well as the posterior bony wall, a total reconstruction is required. In these cases, one would use the homograft tympanic membrane with attached malleus as the main building block. Ossicular reconstruction would involve the use of the incus stapes prosthesis of hydroxyapatite. The posterior canal wall would be reconstructed with homograft knee cartilage. As these patients have often had several previous ear procedures, there is usually no remaining fascia. Homograft dura is an acceptable substitute in these cases.

Surgical Indications

All perforations of the eardrum pose a risk of infection and hearing loss and should be closed. However, mitigating circumstances, such as advanced age or poor physical condition, may exist that make surgery inadvisable. If the patient follows physiologic principles to prevent irritation or contamination of the middle ear, he or she can live with a perforation and suffer very little inconvenience. Any moisture in the middle ear or ear canal will lead to infection because of the fact that the external auditory meatus and tympanic membrane are skin and therefore dry. When they become moist, the ear canal, which is dark and warm, becomes an ideal incubator for bacterial as well as yeast and fungus infections.

This moisture often follows trauma of the ear canal, such as rubbing or scratching, which produces irritation and weeping of the thin canal skin. Another source of moisture is the middle ear itself, which is lined with mucous membrane. When this lining becomes irritated or infected, it produces considerable discharge, which is often caused by contamination with water in the ear canal or nasal secretions from violent nose blowing. Therefore, the patient must be instructed to blow the nose very gently, to never rub or scratch the ear or neck, and to sleep with affected ear toward the ceiling. The last precaution is to prevent the normal accumulation of moisture in the middle ear from exuding through the perforation to the ear canal. Therefore, the patient should not swim and should use special precautions when washing the hair. The patient is told to take a large piece of cotton, coat it with white petroleum jelly, and saturate it with the jelly by massaging it into the cotton with the fingers. The saturated cotton ball is then placed in the outer ear canal before the hair is washed. The patient should wash the hair over a lavatory or tub and not in a shower, as even this method of protection will not suffice if the patient stands upright in a shower. Avoidance of swimming would seem obvious, but unless the physician specifically mentions it, some patients will continue to participate in water sports and risk contamination. It is also my firm conviction that there is no ear plug with which the patient can safely swim. If the plug fits tight enough to keep water out it will irritate the ear and on its own produce infection, or the patient will loosen it to obtain relief and thus lose the supposed protection.

If the circumstances against surgery are valid and the patient has sufficient motivation to observe these precautions, he or she may coexist with the perforation for many years.

PREOPERATIVE EVALUATION AND MEDICAL TREATMENT

When a patient first presents with an infected perforation and hearing loss, the ear must be treated medically. The first priority is to carefully clean the ear under microscopic vision so that the pathology can be more accurately evaluated and the proper medications can reach the skin of the ear canal and mucous membrane lining of the middle ear and mastoid. By means of a small suction, exudate is removed from the ear canal as well as through the perforation. Following this step, the ear is carefully wiped with small, cotton-tipped wire applicators dipped in a corticosteroid otic suspension such as Cortisporin. All exfoliated skin and debris are removed by wiping the ear canal. Also by wiping the ear canal, the medication is applied to the skin of the ear canal. Following this, chloramphenicol (Chloromycetin) powder is gently insufflated into the ear canal and through the perforation. If the ear does not become dry, a mucous plug may be present in the eustachian tube. If this is suspected, the ear should again be suctioned to remove all excess mucus and debris. The patient then lies with the affected ear up, and the canal is filled with a corticosteroid solution such as Neodecadron. A pneumatic otoscope is then used to apply pressure and force the drops through the eustachian tube. The eustachian tube blockage may be caused by mucosal edema or scar tissue from a previous surgery.

Occasionally, a patient may also develop an allergy to certain medications, often the neomycin present in almost all ear drops. If an allergy is suspected, an ophthalmologic drop, such as dexamethasone (Decadron ophthalmic) is substituted. Systemic antibiotics are of limited benefit in a chronically draining ear; however, on the first visit, the ear discharge should be cultured and the appropriate systemic antibiotic administered.

SURGICAL TECHNIQUE

When a new technique such as the homograft tympanic membrane is first introduced, many physicians tend to attempt to use it to solve all their problem cases, such as wet and infected ears and previous failures. Unfortunately, if they do not understand the limitations and rationale of the new technique, and if sound physiologic principles are not followed, a poor result will ensue.

Except in extreme circumstances, one should not operate on an infected ear (see under Medical Treatment). Sometimes, the ear will not become dry, but there is distinct difference between a wet ear and an infected ear. In the wet ear, the secretions are clear and do not spill out above the rim of eardrum that remains. When the ear is suctioned clean, several hours or days will pass until the fluid reaccumulates. There is no pain, and a culture shows no growth for bacteria. An ear often remains wet because of blockage of the anteroinferior middle ear by adhesions beneath the malleus handle. This situation often follows a previous underlay fascial graft that undergoes retraction and adheres to the promontory. Polyps or polypoid mucosa in the eustachian tube orifice also produces a similar condition. The pathology described for these two cases will not respond to medical therapy, and the ear is usually wet at the time of surgery.

Preoperative Preparation

Before beginning the actual surgery, this author positions the patient on the operating table. The patient lies on a special four-inch-thick foam rubber pad, which is more comfortable for the patient and also makes possible the use of the Juers-Derlacki head holder. This head holder consists of a headrest mounted on a ball-and-socket joint to which the patient's head is secured with adhesive tape. The holder is then moved to the most comfortable and advantageous position for the surgeon and then locked in place.

Although similar in many ways, each ear canal is different in size, shape, and angulation on the skull. For the surgeon to accomplish his or her goal of grafting and ossicular reconstruction, the head must be positioned so that the ear canal can be viewed throughout its length while the surgeon is seated comfortably. In some ears, especially those with congenital abnormalities, the canal appears to angle toward the top of the patient's head rather than straight toward the opposite ear. To better visualize the eardrum, it is often necessary to place folded blankets or other padding beneath the patient's shoulders so that the head is lowered and the angulation of the ear canal straightened. When a high percentage of the surgeries are performed through the ear canal, as in my practice, the time spent positioning the patient at the beginning of the procedure is saved many times over by allowing the surgeon to have good visualization and to work in a relaxed manner.

The preparation of the ear for surgery consists of two stages: one before draping and the other after draping. After the head is positioned under microscopic vision, as described earlier, the head is secured in position by taping it to the headrest. First, a strip of one-inch adhesive tape is applied to the undersurface of the head holder and brought over the head above the ear to hold and cover the hair above the ear. Plastic tape is applied in a like manner both in front and behind the ear to hold the hair out of the field. If the surgery is to be performed transmeatally, the hair is not shaved but is fastened back with plastic tape. If a postauricular incision is anticipated, the head is shaved dry for an area of approximately 1 inch around the pinna. The loose hairs are removed by repeatedly dabbing the area with the adhesive side of two-inch plastic tape. The head is then taped to the Juers-Derlacki head holder with one-inch adhesive tape; this tape is used over the edge of the shaved area to hold and cover the hair. As stated previously, the shave is dry so that the tape will adhere properly. Plastic tape is then used in a like manner both in front and behind the ear to cover and hold the hair.

The ear is then scrubbed with Rondic sponges dipped in pHisoHex soap. The soap is removed with Ringer's lactate solution and the area rescrubbed with 70 per cent ethyl alcohol. The skin is dried with the Rondic sponges. Next, a 3M plastic drape with a round hole is applied over the previously placed tape. A large plastic body drape is then positioned over the patient and the ear located by feel through the drape. With a scissors, a round cutout is made approximately twice the size of the hole in the 3M drape. Over this, another 3M drape is placed, thus securing the body drape to the patient's head and ear. Next, the microscope is brought back into position and the ear canal visualized through a sterile speculum. The second part of the preparation is now accomplished. The canal is copiously irrigated with 70 per cent ethyl alcohol through the speculum with constant suction to remove all wax and debris and to further sterilize the ear canal and drum. After repeated washings, the alcohol is removed with repeated irrigations and suction with Ringer's lactate. The alcohol irrigation is used regardless of an open perforation and is in fact used to remove mucus and debris from the middle ear and margins of the perforation. If the perforation is dry and clean, the Ringer's lactate is used alone.

Tympanic Membrane Grafting with Homograft Dura

Central perforations are usually approached through the ear canal. If they are small, that is, less than 3mm in diameter, they are repaired with an underlay technique as follows (Fig. 13–3).

The undersurface of the remaining tympanic membrane around the perforation is scarified by the introduction of a scraper through the hole in the eardrum. Then, a small, right-angled pick is employed to remove the cuff of squamous epithelium and to freshen the edges of the perforation. Next, an incision is made approximately 8mm from, and parallel with, the eardrum to a point a few millimeters anterior to the perforation. Thus, if the perforation is posterior, the incision would extend to approximately 6 o'clock,

whereas if it lies in the anterior quadrant, the incision would extend to 8 or 9 o'clock.

The dissection is carried down to the middle ear, and the fibrous annulus is elevated with the drum, creating a high tympanomeatal flap (Fig. 13–4). It is folded over the manubrium of the malleus and tents against it. By means of a sharp sickle knife the periosteum over the midportion of the malleus handle is incised and a subperiosteal pocket created. If the perforation contacts the tip of the malleus handle, the subperiosteal dissection is continued down and off the tip of the malleus. This produces a situation in which the entire handle of the malleus is bare (Fig. 13–5). This maneuver makes it possible to place the graft completely over the lower half of the malleus, rather that just abutting the graft against it so that a recurrent perforation may occur. Additionally, the graft now has three-point suspension: the posterior superior bony wall, the anterior inferior bony wall, and the malleus tip (Fig. 13–6). The tympanomeatal flap is then replaced, and the graft can be seen shining through the perforation (Fig. 13–7). Fascia or perichondrium may be used for the graft; however, I prefer thin homograft dura, which is periosteal dura obtained from the middle fossa of the cadaver temporal bone. It has more body and stiffness than fascia and is very resistant to breakdown or infection. Its use also eliminates the need to make a separate incision to obtain the graft.

Canal Skin Tympanoplasty with Homograft Tympanic Membrane and Dura

For larger perforations or in situations in which the remaining tympanic membrane is thin or poorly epithelialized, an overlay technique using canal skin and dura or homograft tympanic membrane is employed. The canal skin technique is based on the premise that the skin covering the bony external auditory meatus is different than skin anywhere else on the body and is the only skin that will duplicate the tympanic membrane and retain its self-cleaning characteristics.

The first incision is made to outline the vascular strip and is carried up the tympanomastoid suture line (Fig. 13–8). The second incision is a vertical one that extends up the tympanosquamous suture line.

FIGURE 13–3. Small posterosuperior perforation, ideal for underlay technique.

FIGURE 13–4. Creation of a high tympanomeatal flap.

FIGURE 13–5. Tympanomeatal flap dissected off malleus handle.

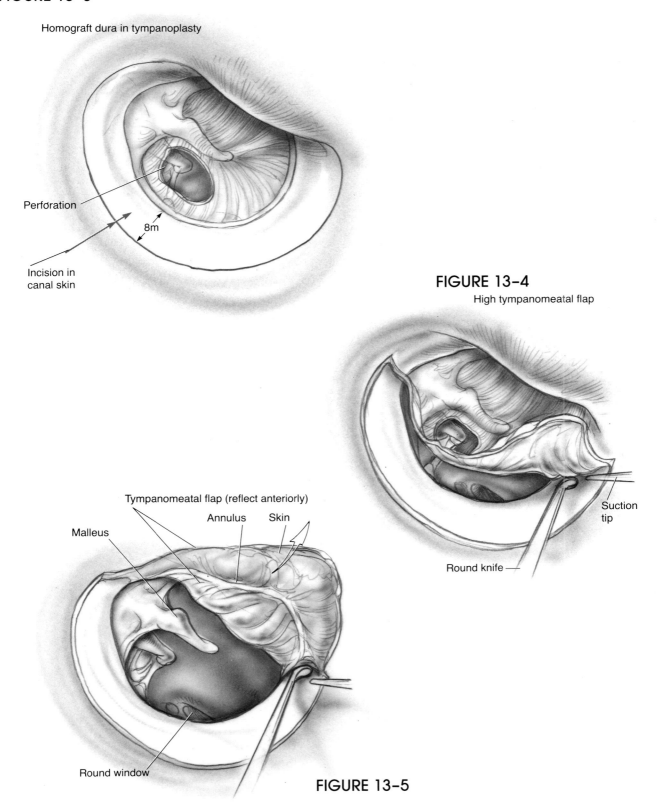

FIGURE 13-3

Homograft dura in tympanoplasty

Perforation

8m

Incision in
canal skin

FIGURE 13-4

High tympanomeatal flap

Suction
tip

Round knife

Tympanomeatal flap (reflect anteriorly)

Annulus   Skin

Malleus

Round window

FIGURE 13-5

FIGURE 13-6

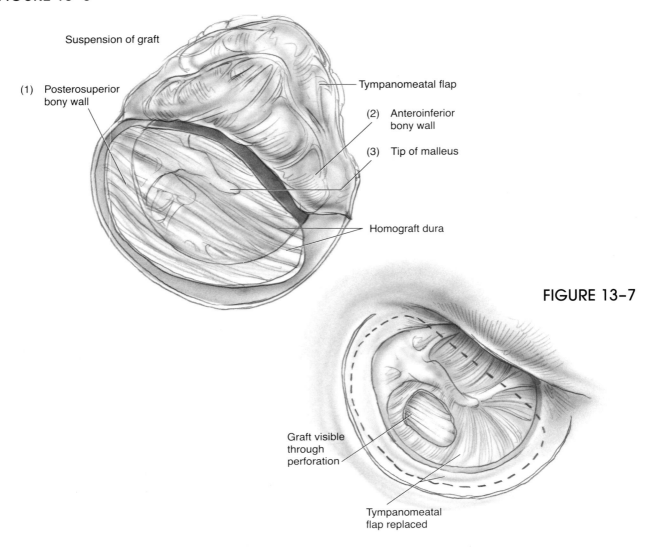

FIGURE 13-7

Suspension of graft

(1) Posterosuperior bony wall

Tympanomeatal flap

(2) Anteroinferior bony wall

(3) Tip of malleus

Homograft dura

Graft visible through perforation

Tympanomeatal flap replaced

FIGURE 13-6. Homograft dura graft in place over bare malleus handle.

FIGURE 13-7. Underlay graft seen shining through former perforation.

FIGURE 13-8. Initial incision for canal skin tympanoplasty in tympanomastoid suture line.

FIGURE 13-9. Second incision up the tympanosquamous suture line and circumferential incision at bony membranous junction.

FIGURE 13-10. Canal skin and epithelial layer dissected from drum remnant.

FIGURE 13-8

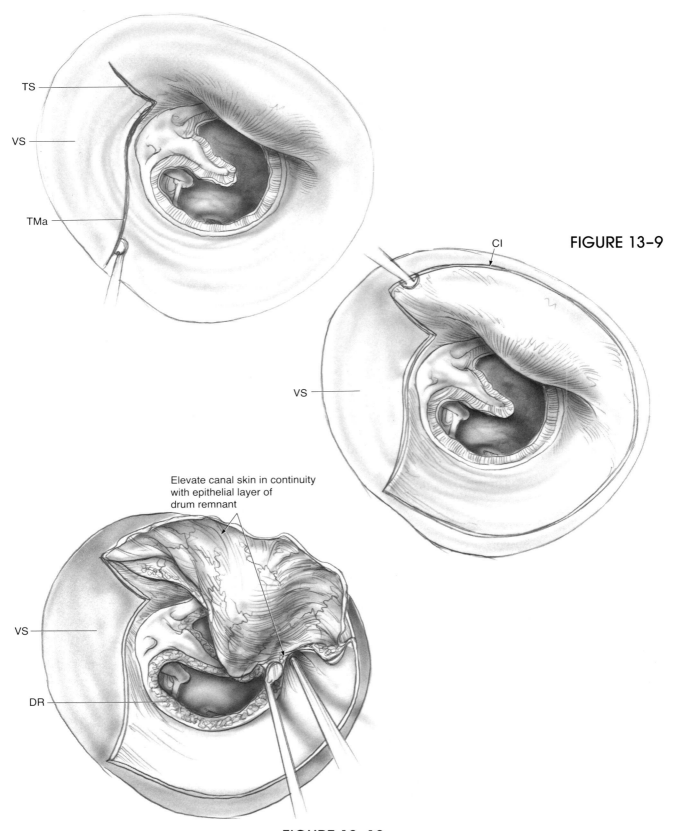

TS

VS

TMa

CI

FIGURE 13-9

VS

Elevate canal skin in continuity
with epithelial layer of
drum remnant

VS

DR

FIGURE 13-10

These incisions are then connected by a circumferential incision carried around at the bony ear canal just below its junction with the thicker membranous skin (Fig. 13–9). This thin canal skin is then elevated down to the tympanic membrane and elevated in continuity with the epithelial layer of the eardrum (Fig. 13–10). The dissection is carried to the edges of the perforation and followed to the undersurface of the drum until normal mucous membrane is encountered, thus eliminating the possibility of leaving squamous ingrowth beneath the drum remnant.

After removal of the canal skin, the ear is prepared for reconstruction and grafting. Advantages of the canal skin technique include excellent visualization of the entire bony ear canal. If anterior bony overhang obscures the anterior drum remnant, it is now drilled down with a diamond burr under constant irrigation. This procedure affords an excellent view of the anterior drum remnant so that the graft may be placed accurately. There is also good visualization of the posterosuperior quadrant. By removing some bony annulus with a curette, the status of the ossicular chain may be evaluated and reconstruction undertaken, if necessary (Fig. 13–11). Also, any middle ear adhesions may be removed and the condition of the middle ear mucosa and eustachian tube evaluated. Implants of thin silicone sheeting may be placed in the middle ear space to prevent adhesions. These were described previously[3] and have a cutout for the stapes and tensor tympani tendon, as well as an optional tongue, which may be placed under the bony annulus to the mastoid antrum.

The middle ear is now ready for reconstruction. If the ossicular chain is intact and mobile and the perforation is large or total, reconstruction will require the use of a homograft tympanic membrane to establish the cone shape of the drumhead and assure contact of the umbo to the tip of the patient's malleus (Fig. 13–12). The canal skin graft is now placed over the homografts (Fig. 13–13), thereby reinforcing the graft as well as affording rapid epithelialization over the nonliving tissue.

The canal skin was removed as a cylinder and must be trimmed so that it is replaced in a rectangular shape. The graft is placed on a tongue blade and trimmed of the thin epithelial elements covering the drum remnant. It is also turned about 180° so that the part that covered the bony anterior canal will extend over the anterior drum remnant. The graft contacts the vascular strip superiorly and extends to, but does not turn up, the anterior canal wall so that an acute angle, which is so important for a good hearing result, can be maintained. The graft does extend up the posterior and inferior canal walls (Fig. 13–14). This leaves considerable bare bone exposed; however, this area will epithelialize with canal type of skin in a few weeks. The ear canal is now packed with absorbable gelation sponge (Gelfoam) pledgets saturated in antibiotic solution. The entire canal is filled with this material because it is important to cover all the bare bone anteriorly and inferiorly. This packing is removed by suction in the office approximately 2 weeks postoperatively.

If ossicular discontinuity exists in addition to the perforation, it is repaired before grafting. The excellent exposure provided by the canal skin approach makes the reconstruction easier. The reconstruction is carried out with the ossicular replacement prosthesis of hydroxyapatite as described in Chapter 14. Following the ossicular work, the grafting is completed with homografts and canal skin, as described earlier.

In addition to discontinuity or erosion of the incus and stapes there may be involvement of the malleus as well. The manubrium may be softened or eroded so that it cannot be used in the reconstruction and must be removed. Also, one often sees squamous ingrowth below the malleus handle, around the tensor tympani or even around the neck and head. If this cannot be safely and totally removed, it is best to cut the tensor tympani tendon and remove the entire malleus.

In these cases, the reconstruction requires a homograft eardrum with malleus as well as the hydroxyapatite prosthesis. The head of the homograft malleus is placed in the epitympanum where the patient's malleolar head had been. In some instances, the homograft head will not fit and must be removed; however, it should be retained if possible. The notch of the

---

FIGURE 13-11. Note good visualization of both anterior and posterior aspects of middle ear after the canal skin has been removed.

FIGURE 13-12. Homograft tympanic membrane in place over patient's malleus.

FIGURE 13-13. Canal skin graft replaced over homografts.

FIGURE 13-14. Note canal skin graft unfolded so that it contacts the vascular strip and abuts the anterior bony canal wall.

FIGURE 13-15. Middle ear reconstruction in tympanomastoidectomy with homograft tympanic membrane and malleus.

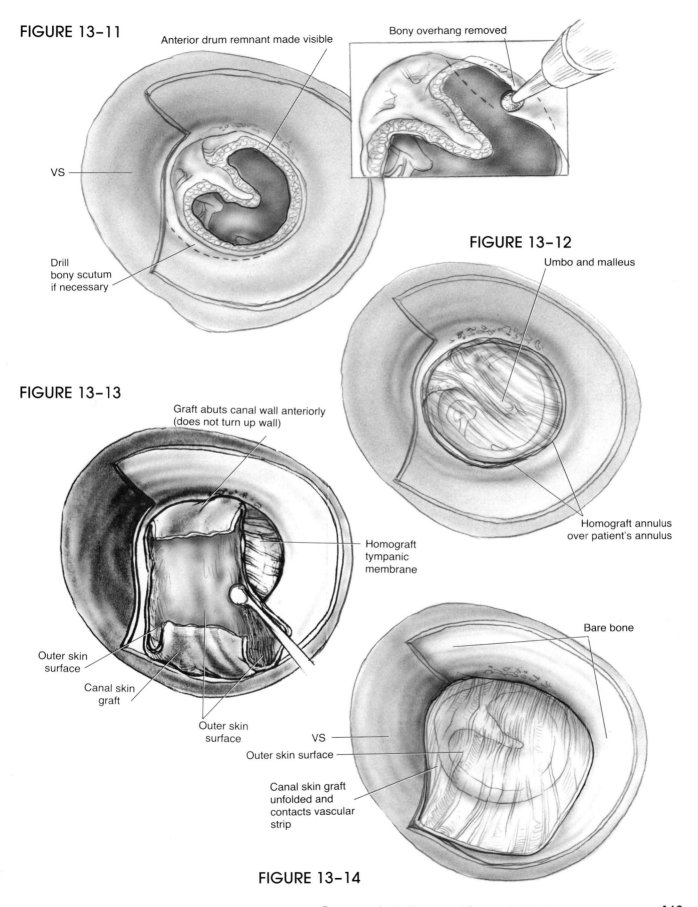

FIGURE 13-11

Anterior drum remnant made visible

Bony overhang removed

VS

Drill
bony scutum
if necessary

FIGURE 13-12

Umbo and malleus

Homograft annulus
over patient's annulus

FIGURE 13-13

Graft abuts canal wall anteriorly
(does not turn up wall)

Homograft
tympanic
membrane

Outer skin
surface

Canal skin
graft

Outer skin
surface

Bare bone

VS

Outer skin surface

Canal skin graft
unfolded and
contacts vascular
strip

FIGURE 13-14

replacement prosthesis goes just below the malleolar neck, and the head keeps it balanced with manubrium and the attached eardrum like a teeter-totter. This situation offsets the loss of the stabilizing effect of the tensor tympani tendon. Grafting is now carried out with the canal skin as described previously.

Tympanomastoidectomy with Homograft Tympanic Membrane and Dura

In cases of cholesteatoma or mastoid reconstruction, or in instances in which a postauricular approach is required, the canal skin should not be removed, because stenosis of the bony canal may occur. In these cases, the homograft tympanic membrane is covered with fascia or homograft dura.

In cases of tympanomastoidectomy for removal of cholesteatoma, the bony posterior canal wall is preserved if at all possible. If the cholesteatoma is attic or posterosuperior, the incus and head of the malleus must be removed. If the manubrium of the patient's malleus is still present, it is used, but if it is absent or diseased, the homograft tympanic membrane with its attached malleus becomes the main building block in the reconstruction. Usually, there is a rim of eardrum to support the homograft tympanic membrane anteriorly; posteriorly, it rests on the bony annulus. The head of the malleus is preserved and extends under the scutum where the patient's malleolar head had been. The sound pressure mechanism is rebuilt with a replacement prosthesis of hydroxyapatite, with the notch under the manubrium of the malleus and the cup over the head of the stapes or the shaft to the stapedial footplate (Fig. 13–15). If the bony wall cannot be preserved or is being reconstructed with the homograft knee cartilage, the head of the homograft malleus extends under this structure, and the hearing mechanism is restored as described earlier.

As canal skin is not available with this approach, the homograft tympanic membrane should be reinforced with facia or homograft dura. This reinforcement is used as an underlay graft in most instances. However, if the perforation extends to the malleus but the anterior drum is intact, the epithelial layer of the remaining drum is elevated and reflected anteriorly. The fascia graft is then put into place as an overlay graft, and the elevated epithelium reflected back over it to produce a sandwich graft.

Dressing

For procedures performed transmeatally, the dressing consists of a strip of 1/4-inch, selvage-edge gauze approximately two inches in length placed in the outer ear canal. A cotton ball is then used in the concha. When a postauricular incision has been employed, the incision is closed with a subcuticular suture of 4.0 plain catgut, then a standard mastoid dressing secured by three-inch Kling is applied. The patient is usually discharged the morning of the day following the surgery. The mastoid dressing is removed at this time.

Postoperative Care

The patient is instructed to change the cotton in the external ear approximately three times a day for a few days. When bleeding stops, the cotton should be left out altogether. Scratching or rubbing the ear is forbidden, and the patient is instructed to clean the ear by putting a damp washcloth over the index finger, tipping the head toward the affected ear, then gently cleaning the outer ear. Ear drops are not used routinely, but if the healing is slow or there is surface irritation, Cortisporin otic drops are recommended. The drops are used on a decreasing basis, usually beginning with two drops three times a day for 3 days, then twice a day for 2 days, and then at bedtime for a week. When the patient washes the hair approximately 5 days following surgery, it should not be done in a shower but rather in a tub or lavatory. Cotton saturated in white petroleum jelly is used in the outer ear to prevent contamination with water. The patient is seen for the first postoperative checkup approximately 2 weeks following the surgery. At this time, any remaining gelatin sponge packing is removed with gentle suction. The patient returns at 2-week intervals until the ear is healed, usually 6 weeks postoperatively. At that time, a postoperative audiogram may be obtained.

Complications

Fortunately, complications with the use of the homograft tympanic membrane are rare. When this author first began using these transplant materials, a marked inflammatory reaction or rejection was fully expected to occur. The middle ear and mastoid appear to be favored sites, and they accept and tolerate this tissue well. There is occasional breakdown and recurrent perforation; however, it appears to be a vascular phenomenon that is related to cases in which the canal skin is extremely thin and of poor character. If a recurrent perforation is encountered on the first or second postoperative visit, a paper patch is applied, usually without cauterization. If the perforation has not closed by the next visit, the edges are freshened and cauterized with trichloroacetic acid and another patch applied. If the perforation still fails to heal, the patient is cautioned as to aural hygiene and observed for 4 to

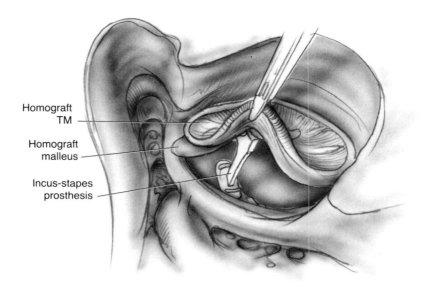

FIGURE 13-15. Middle ear reconstruction in tympanomastoidectomy with homograft tympanic membrane and malleus.

Homograft TM

Homograft malleus

Incus-stapes prosthesis

6 months. I believe that it is a mistake to attempt a revision immediately after surgery because there is still edema of the tissues and the healing is poor. After the ear has stabilized, the revision can be carried out in an orderly manner.

This procedure is usually performed through the ear canal, even if the initial procedure was a postauricular approach. If the recurrent perforation is central, the technique consists of freshening the edges of the perforation, elevating a tympanomeatal flap by use of an underlay graft of homograft dura, as described previously. Occasionally, the perforation recurs anteriorly, and there is considerable bony overhang, which may have contributed to poor visualization of this area and may account for the failure. In these cases, a canal skin tympanoplasty is performed so that the bony overhang may be removed with a diamond burr and the anterior drum remnant visualized. A new homograft tympanic membrane is then employed to close the perforation as previously described.

These techniques deal with alcohol-preserved material only. Based on my experience, the canal skin should not be placed over a tympanic membrane that was stored in formaldehyde, for even after adequate rinsing and preparation, all the preservative cannot be removed. In cases in which this was attempted, considerable reaction occurred, with granulation tissue and slow healing.

Complications with homograft dura are somewhat different, as it is thick and very resistant to breakdown. When it is used in conjunction with canal skin, the resulting graft is much thicker than that obtained with the homograft tympanic membrane, and the hearing results are not as good. A source of difficulty may be when large pieces of dura are used in reconstruction of the posterior canal wall. These ears are often involved in cartilage reconstruction in which dura was substituted for the absent temporal fascia. In these cases, there may be large areas of bare dura that continue to weep and granulate. It may be necessary at times to trim the dead edge and apply cautery to encourage healing. In some instances, it takes several months to get a dry ear.

References

1. Chalet NL: Tympanic membrane transplant. Harper Hosp Bull 22: 27–34, 1964.
2. Marquet J: Reconstructive micro-surgery of the eardrum by means of a tympanic membrane homograft. Preliminary report. Acta Otolaryngol (Stockh) 4: 459–464, 1966.
3. Brandow EC Jr: Homograft tympanic membrane transplant in myringoplasty. Trans Am Acad Ophthalmol Otolaryngol 73(5): 825–835, 1969.
4. Glasscock ME III, House WF: Homograft reconstruction of the middle ear: A preliminary report. Laryngoscope 78: 1219–1225, 1968.
5. Smyth GD, Kerr AG: Tympanic membrane homografts. J Laryngol Otol 83(11): 1061–1066, 1969.
6. Plester D: Tympanic membrane homografts in ear surgery. Acta Otorhinolaryngol Belg 24(1): 34–37, 1970.
7. Perkins R: Human homograft buffered formaldehyde preparation. Trans Am Acad Ophthalmol Otolaryngol 74: 278–282, 1970.
8. Wehrs RE: Homograft tympanic membrane in tympanoplasty. Arch Otolaryngol Head Neck Surg 98: 132–139, 1971.
9. Wehrs RE: Three years' experience with the homograft tympanic membrane. Trans Am Acad Ophthalmol Otolaryngol 76: 142–146, 1972.
10. Gagnon NB, Piche J, Larchelle D, Williams MI: Homografts of the middle ear. Privileged tissue or privileged site. Arch Otolaryngol Head Neck Surg 105: 35–38, 1979.
11. Lesinski SG: Homograft tympanoplasty in perspective. A long-term clinical-histologic study of formalin-fixed tympanic membranes used for the reconstruction of 125 severely damaged middle ears. Laryngoscope (Suppl 32):1–37, 1983.

14

Tympanoplasty: Ossicular Tissue and Hydroxyapatite

ROGER E. WEHRS, M.D.

FIGURE 14-1. Homograft incudi prostheses. A, Notched incus with short process. B, Notched incus with long process.

FIGURE 14-2. Hydroxyapatite prostheses. A, Incus replacement prosthesis. B, Incus stapes replacement prosthesis.

FIGURE 14-3. Hydroxyapatite prostheses with double notch. A, Incus replacement prosthesis. B, Incus stapes replacement prosthesis.

In the early and mid-1960s, repositioning of the patient's incus fragment emerged as the most reliable method of ossicular reconstruction in tympanoplasty.[1,2] In 1967, this author published an article suggesting the substitution of homograft incudi when the patient's incus was unusable.[3] They were first used as wedges between the patient's stapes and malleus in the same way that the autograft incus had been employed. They functioned well, with no tendency to extrude, and were invaded by blood vessels and covered with mucous membrane to become living tissue. To improve their stability and to improve hearing, prostheses were sculptured from these homograft incudi.[4] Two primary prostheses emerged: the notched incus with short process and the notched incus with long process. The first replaced the patient's incus and carried the sound pressure from the malleus to the intact stapes. The second replaced not only the incus but the stapedial superstructure as well and carried sound directly to the stapedial footplate (Fig. 14-1A and B).[5] Because two-point fixation occurred between the notch under the malleus handle and the stapedial head or footplate, these prostheses locked in place. They were stable, as the notch under the malleus prevented dislocation either forward or backward. The prostheses would not be displaced inferiorly because of the spring of the malleus, or superiorly, because of the tensor tympani tendon. Furthermore, sound pressure was thus carried to the fluids of the inner ear by direct columellar pressure. This design, therefore, produced excellent hearing and anatomic results.[6] However, there are disadvantages with the use of the human tissue; it can be difficult or impossible to obtain, has a limited shelf life, and carries the remote danger of disease transmission. Also, there cannot be any mass production of a standardized sterile prosthesis that would meet definite criteria.

It was deemed prudent and necessary, therefore, to develop an acceptable alternative for the homograft ossicles. This new material should be biocompatable, similar to bone in weight and physical characteristics, and able to be made into the same dimensions and shape as prostheses derived from homograft ossicles. The reasons for the design were that the notched incus with long and short process had evolved over time

into prostheses of proven reliability. They had consistently produced good anatomic and functional results with a minimum of complications. Hydroxyapatite most nearly met these specifications. It had a long history of excellent biocompatability, including use in the middle ear.[7] It had the same color and approximate appearance as bone. Furthermore, it could easily be shaped with a diamond burr into prostheses. The bony prostheses, known as notched incudi with short and long process, were used as patterns. Prostheses of hydroxyapatite were sculptured to have the same size and characteristics as those of bone (Fig. 14-2). The early prostheses were square and boxy and had sharp edges. Furthermore, their surfaces were smooth and slick, so they could not be picked up with a suction tip, as was done with their bony counterparts. These first prototypes functioned satisfactorily and proved that the concept of replacing a familiar and time-proven prosthesis with an identical one of a different material was valid.

The early prostheses were modified, making them thinner with rounded contours, even more like their predecessors of bone. By a process similar to sand-blasting, the surfaces were satinized so that they could be picked up with suction tips and maneuvered into position.

Further modification, again learned from the homograft prostheses, consisted of extra notches in the short process to accommodate an anteriorly placed malleus (Fig. 14-3). There is also variation in the height of the stapes and the distance from the footplate to the graft. Therefore, prostheses of different height were developed.

PATIENT SELECTION

All patients with a perforated eardrum are potential candidates for tympanoplasty with ossicular reconstruction. During the initial or preoperative exam, a significant conductive loss may be discovered. Erosion of the long process of the incus may also be seen. These findings indicate that the patient will require ossicular reconstruction. However, there may be only

FIGURE 14-1

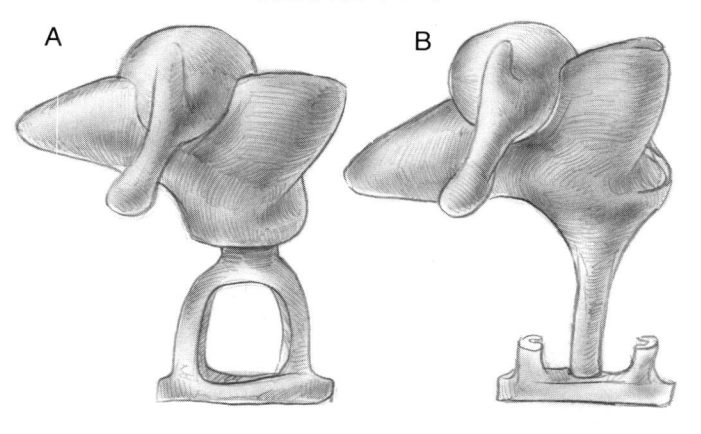

FIGURE 14-2

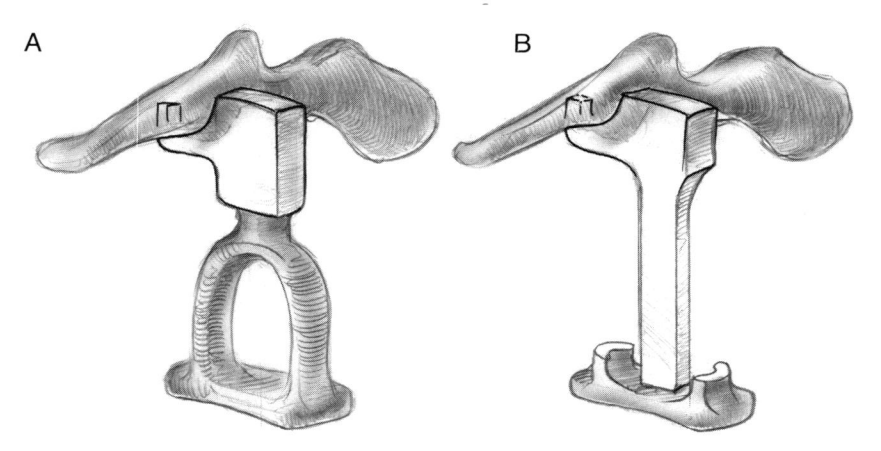

FIGURE 14-3

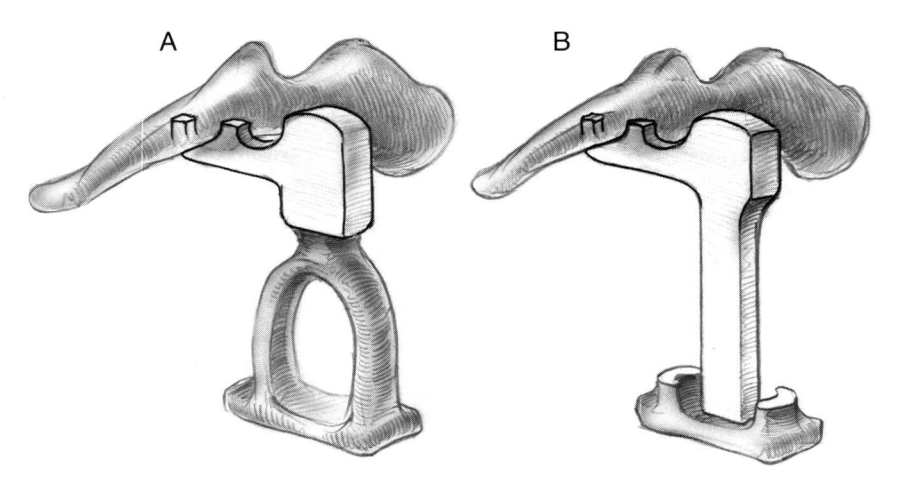

a slight retraction pocket over the long process of the incus with very little conductive component to the hearing loss. Not until the time of surgery is the long process of the incus discovered to be friable or stiff, and reconstruction will be required.

Other candidates for the procedure may present with an intact eardrum but a significant conductive component to their hearing loss. These may represent a congenital malformation of the ossicles or cases of revision, in which the reconstruction was delayed to a second stage.

A history of head injury especially correlated to distortion of the eardrum or healed fracture of the bony ear canal may indicate ossicular discontinuity and the need for reconstruction.

Patients with cholesteatoma are prime candidates for ossicular reconstruction, as the incus and head of the malleus usually need to be removed even if the ossicular chain is intact and there was a minimal air-bone gap before surgery.

Surgery is recommended when the ear is dry and clean often at the initial visit if no cholesteatoma or infection is present. As a general rule, the decision to use either the homograft bony prosthesis or the hydroxyapatite prosthesis is made at the time of surgery. Occasionally, a patient will express a specific desire for either artificial, manmade material or the homograft transplant, and these wishes are respected as much as possible. The use of total or partial ossicular replacement prostheses and other manmade materials are not discussed in this chapter, as they are not used by this author.

Preoperative Evaluation and Counseling

The patient is informed and brought into the surgical planning as much as possible. Today, most patients are sophisticated and well educated. They need to understand the rationale as well as the advantages and disadvantages of the procedure. This is especially true of the patients who have had one or more failures with previous ear surgery.

When the patient presents with a dry perforation and obvious ossicular discontinuity, they are informed that they have a 90 per cent chance of hearing improvement with a dry and grafted eardrum. They are further told that in some instances, the hearing may not improve but may actually get worse. In most instances, this loss would be conductive in nature, and a revision would be indicated. However, in rare instances, usually fewer than 1 per cent, the hearing could become worse as a result of deterioration of the nerve of hearing, and in extreme instances, they could lose all hearing in that ear.

Due to the fact that most of my surgery is performed though the ear canal, there is very little pain that acetaminophen or mild analgesics will not control. Also, bleeding is not a problem, and antibiotics are not used routinely.

The return of hearing acuity varies among patients and depends on several factors. If they have bilateral middle ear disease and a large conductive component in each ear, they may notice some improvement at the first postoperative visit 2 weeks following surgery; however, if the opposite ear exhibits normal hearing, then the patient is not aware of much improvement until 4 to 6 weeks following the reconstruction. The first postoperative hearing test is obtained when the ear is healed, approximately 6 to 8 weeks following surgery.

PREOPERATIVE EVALUATION

It is my firm opinion that any type of ear surgery will be more successful if the ear is dry or at least not infected at the time of surgery. When a patient is first seen seeking relief from infection and hearing loss, the ear must first be treated medically.

Medical Treatment

The first priority is to carefully clean the ear under microscopic vision so that the pathology can be more accurately evaluated and the proper medications can reach the skin of the ear canal and mucous membrane lining of the middle ear and mastoid. By means of a small suction, exudate is removed from the ear canal, as well as through the perforation. Following this procedure, the ear is carefully wiped with small cotton-tipped wire applicators dipped in a corticosteroid otic suspension, such as Cortisporin. All exfoliated skin and debris are removed by wiping the ear canal. Also, by wiping the ear canal, the medication is applied to the skin of the ear canal. Following this step, chloramphenicol (Chloromycetin) powder is gently insufflated into the ear canal and through the perforation. The patient is then instructed on aural hygiene, which consists of the following regimen.

The patient is instructed not to rub or press on the ear or to clean it with Q-tips. After the physician has cleaned the ear, the itching is usually less of a problem and may be controlled with acetaminophen or diphenhydramine (Benadryl). Also, rubbing the ear has often become a habit and part of a vicious cycle of itching, rubbing, and drainage. Once patients realize the importance of aural hygiene, they can leave the ear alone.

The only way the patient should clean the ear is with a finger in a damp wash cloth with the head tipped toward the affected side. They should also not wash their hair in a shower but use a cotton ball

saturated in white petroleum jelly in the outer ear when washing hair over a lavatory or tub.

Most people with a draining ear feel they should sleep on the ear so that it can "drain better." In my opinion, this is exactly the wrong thing to do, as the exudate should drain down the eustachian tube and not onto the external ear, where it causes irritation and crusting. The patient is instructed to place a large spiny hair curler in the hair just above the affected ear. This will remind him or her not to lie on the ear with the perforation.

The patient must be carefully followed up and is asked to return in a few days to 2 weeks, depending on the severity of the infection. On returning, the ear is usually dry and clean. If it is not, the reason for the persistent discharge must be ascertained. Often, this persistence is due to a mucous plug in the eustachian tube. If this condition is suspected, the ear should again be suctioned to remove all excess mucus and debris. The patient then lies with the affected ear up, and the canal is filled with a corticosteroid drop, preferably Neodecadron, as it is less viscid than Cortisporin. A pneumatic otoscope is then used to apply pressure and force the drops through the eustachian tube. One often feels a sudden release of pressure as the eustachian tube opens and the medication flows into the patient's nasopharynx. If the tube will not open easily, excess pressure should be avoided, as it may cause vertigo, and there is also a rare possibility of rupturing the dura over a dehiscent mastoid tegmen and producing meningitis or a brain abscess.

The eustachian tube blockage may be due to mucosal edema or scar tissue from a previous surgery. The occasional patient may also develop an allergy to certain medications, often the neomycin present in almost all otic drops. If an allergy is suspected, an ophthalmologic medication, such as Decadron ophthalmic solution, is substituted.

Systemic antibiotics are of limited benefit in a chronically draining ear; however, on the first visit, the ear discharge should be cultured and the appropriate systemic antibiotic administered.

PREOPERATIVE PREPARATION

Before beginning the actual surgery, this author positions the patient on the operating table. The patient lies on a special 4-inch-thick foam rubber pad, which is comfortable for the patient and also makes possible the use of the Juers-Derlacki head holder. This holder consists of a headrest mounted on a ball-and-socket joint to which the patient's head is secured with adhesive tape. The holder is then moved to the most comfortable and advantageous position for the surgeon and is then locked in place.

Although similar in many ways, each ear canal is different in size, shape, and angulation on the skull. For the surgeon to accomplish the goal of grafting and ossicular reconstruction, the head must be positioned so that the ear canal can be viewed throughout its length while the surgeon is seated comfortably. In some ears, especially those with congenital abnormalities, the canal appears to angle toward the top of the patient's head rather than straight toward the opposite ear. To better see the eardrum, it is often necessary to place folded blankets or other padding beneath the patient's shoulders so that the head is lowered and the angulation of the ear canal straightened.

When a high percentage of the surgeries are performed through the ear canal, as in my practice, the time spent positioning the patient at the beginning of the procedure is saved many times over by allowing the surgeon to have a good view and work in a relaxed manner.

The preparation of the ear for surgery consists of two stages: one before draping and the other after draping. After positioning the head under microscopic vision as described earlier, the head is secured in position by taping it to the headrest. First, a strip of 1 inch adhesive tape is applied to the undersurface of the head holder and brought over the head above the ear to hold and cover the hair above the ear. Plastic tape is applied in a like manner both in front and behind the ear to hold the hair out of the field. If the surgery is to be performed transmeatally, then the hair is not shaved but taped back with plastic tape. If a postauricular incision is anticipated, then the head is shaved dry for an area of approximately 1-inch around the pinna. The loose hairs are removed by repeatedly dabbing the area with the adhesive side of 2-inch plastic tape. The head is then taped to the Juers-Derlacki head holder with 1-inch adhesive tape, using this tape over the edge of the shaved area to hold and cover the hair. As stated previously, the shave is dry so that the tape will adhere properly. Plastic tape is then used in a like manner both in front and behind the ear to cover and hold the hair. The ear is then scrubbed with Rondex sponges dipped in pHisoHex soap. The soap is removed with Ringer's lactate solution and the area rescrubbed with 70 per cent ethyl alcohol. The skin is dried with the Rondex sponges. Next, a 3M plastic drape with round hole is applied over the previously placed tape. A large plastic body drape is then positioned over the patient and the ear located by feeling through the drape. With a scissors, a round cutout is made approximately twice the size of the hole in the 3M drape. Over this, another 3M drape is placed, thus securing the body drape to the patient's head and ear. Next, the microscope is brought back into position and the ear canal viewed through a sterile speculum. The second part of the preparation is now accomplished. The canal is copiously irrigated with 70 per cent ethyl alcohol through the speculum, with constant suction to remove all wax and debris and to further sterilize the ear canal and drum. After repeated washings, the alcohol is removed with repeated irrigations and suction with Ringer's lactate. The alcohol irrigation is used regardless of an open perforation and is in fact used to remove the mucus and debris from the middle ear and margins of the perforation. If the perforation is dry and clean, the Ringer's lactate is used alone.

SPECIAL INSTRUMENTS

As the canal skin tympanoplasty is often used to prepare the ear for ossicular reconstruction, special instruments are used in this procedure. These consist of canal skin knives, in which the blade is oval and longer than the 2mm or 3mm one usually employed. The blades are approximately 4mm and 5mm in length and are used to elevate the canal skin from under the bony overhang of the anterior bony canal wall. Special diamond burrs, 3mm to 4mm in diameter, have also been designed for the Skeeter drill to remove the bony overhang of the anterior canal wall after the canal skin has been removed.

The Smith Nephew Richards Company has designed implant accessories to assist in handling the Wehrs hydroxyapatite prostheses. The implant-holding fixture (Fig. 14–4) is a device that has grooved slots with a screw lock to secure the prosthesis while it is shaped or modified with the diamond burr. In addition to securing the prosthesis, there are millimeter markings along the grooves to assist in sizing the prosthesis. Another valuable instrument is the Posigator forceps, which is an alligator forceps with a spring design that keeps the jaws closed until they are opened by the surgeon. In this way, the prosthesis may be picked up by the scrub nurse and handed to the surgeon, who can place it in position without the danger of it being released by the forceps and dropping on the floor. Although not instruments, disposable templates are also made by the company. These templates are approximate replicas of the prostheses and can be used to determine the size and length of the replacement prosthesis prior to its placement in the ear.

SURGICAL TECHNIQUE

Most cases of ossicular reconstruction are approached through the ear canal. It is important to use a speculum holder so that both hands are free to hold the suction and instruments. Tapered speculums should also be employed; they hold the vascular strip out of the way, providing good anterior and inferior views.

Dry central perforations, retracted perforations, congenital ears with ossicular discontinuity, second-stage tympanoplasties, and cases of ossicular discontinuity due to trauma may be approached in this manner. Infected ears with mastoid disease, squamous ingrowth, or cases of cholesteatoma should be approached through a postauricular incision. Regardless of the approach used, the actual ossicular reconstruction is identical and will be described in detail.

OSSICULAR RECONSTRUCTION

There are three main categories of ossicular defects that prevent the transmission of sound pressure across the middle ear. These are loss of ossicular continuity, fixation of the ossicles, and a combination of the two.

As described in the introduction, sculptured prostheses made from homograft ossicles were used exclusively for many years. However, since 1986, the clones made of hydroxyapatite have enjoyed an increasingly prominent role in ossicular reconstruction. The homograft prostheses are still used occasionally when the stapes capitulum is eroded or fragile and when the patient prefers not to have manmade materials inserted. However, the bony and hydroxyapatite prostheses are completely interchangeable, and the following details of technique apply equally to both materials.

INCUS REPLACEMENT PROSTHESIS

This prosthesis is used to correct a break in the ossicular chain caused by a defect of the incus. It rebuilds the hearing mechanism between an intact and mobile stapes and manubrium of the malleus.

The lenticular process of the incus usually remains attached to the head of the stapes. If possible, the incudostapedial joint is separated and the lenticular process removed. In this way, any squamous epithelium on the tip of the long process or lenticular process is removed. The normal-sized head will assure that the hole in the prosthesis will fit over the capitulum of the stapes. If the incudostapedial joint is fused and replaced by bone, or if the stapes is extremely mobile, the lenticular process should not be removed, as the manipulations required could produce trauma to the inner ear, dislocation of the stapedial footplate, or both. Therefore, if the joint does not separate easily, it should be left attached. It is important, however, to remove all squamous epithelium, scar tissue, or mucous membrane from the lenticular process. Because the attached lenticular process makes the stapes higher, a shorter prosthesis will be required.

The distance between the head of the stapes and the malleus is evaluated. Unless the malleus appears to be directly over the stapes or extremely far forward, the single-notched prosthesis is chosen. Next, the height of the stapes to the malleus and posterior annulus is evaluated. In 80 per cent of cases, the stapes head will be 2mm to 3mm below the malleus handle, and the short-incus replacement prosthesis will be chosen.

The prosthesis is then introduced lying on its side on the promontory with the notch just off the tip of the malleus and the hole in the base near the stapes head (Fig. 14–5A). By means of a right-angle pick, the manubrium of the malleus is elevated, and the body of the prosthesis is engaged with a gentle curve pick and the notch slid up along the undersurface of the malleus (Fig. 14–5B). The hole in the prosthesis should then engage the stapedial head (Fig. 14–5C). The prosthesis is adjusted until it is vertical to the stapes and appears stable. It should be stable but loose. It should not be wedged tightly in place, as there may be insufficient movement, and the hearing results will not be as good. Also, there is danger of dislocation of the stapedial footplate and inner ear damage.

Gentle pressure on the body of the prosthesis should produce motion of the stapes (Fig. 14–5D). Motion can be determined by observing the stapedial footplate or tendon. Occasionally, a round-window reflex can be obtained.

INCUS-STAPES PROSTHESIS

The incus-stapes prosthesis is used to reconstruct the hearing mechanisms when the stapes superstructure is absent. Reconstruction is carried out between the stapedial footplate and the malleus handle.

The footplate should be evaluated to determine if it is mobile. If it is covered by thick mucosa or scar tissue, this should be removed prior to reconstruction. The mucosa should also be removed from the under-surface of the malleus handle.

Once the ear is prepared, the relationship of the malleus to the stapedial footplate is evaluated. The height from the stapedial footplate to the malleus determines the length of the prosthesis, whereas the distance from the center of the stapes footplate to the malleus determines the position of the notch. In my experience, the short, single-notch prosthesis will be used in 80 per cent of the cases.

The prosthesis is placed on the promontory with the shaft of the implant on the stapedial footplate and the notch off the tip of the malleus (Fig. 14–6A). With a right-angle pick, the manubrium of the malleus is elevated, and a gentle curve pick is placed under the implant (Fig. 14–6B). The notch is slid up on the malleus (Fig. 14–6C). One should be careful not to exert undue pressure on the stapedial footplate or to wedge the prosthesis tightly in place. It should fit loosely but not fall over without support. The long process should be centered on the stapedial footplate by advancing it toward the anterior crus (Fig. 14–6D). This maneuver has the effect of increasing the height of the prosthesis and making a loose fit more secure. On the other hand, if the prosthesis is slightly too long, it will tend to tip forward, and the long process will be at the posterior part of the footplate. If this is the case, the prosthesis should not be forced into place, as this could result in fracture or dislocation of the footplate and inner ear damage. The prosthesis should be pushed back down the malleus and removed. It is either replaced by a shorter prosthesis, or the long process may be drilled down with a diamond burr. If the oval window is narrow, it may be necessary to grind down and round the square shaft so that it will not contact the edges of the oval window. Occasionally, the tip of the malleus will be very close to the promontory. In these cases, the prosthesis fits tightly under the tip as it is elevated, but once in an upright position, it appears too loose. It may be tipped slightly toward the promontory and slid down the malleus to a point where it is more stable. Absorbable gelatin sponge (Gelfoam) may be packed around the long process and body to stabilize it in position until healing has taken place.

MALLEAR DEFECTS

The malleus head may be fixed in the epitympanum by a bony bridge or direct attachment. The ossicular chain is usually intact but moves poorly, if at all.

Management of these cases consists of first separating the incudostapedial joint to prevent any injury to the inner ear when the malleus is manipulated. Next, the mobility of the stapes is ascertained to be sure it was not the culprit producing the fixation. The incudomallear joint is engaged with a right-angle pick, and the incus's mobilized and removed. The malleus head is then exposed by curetting some of the bone over the epitympanum. Now the malleus head is engaged with a House Dieter malleus nippers just above the short process, and the mallear head is mobilized and removed. This usually is not difficult, but on occasion the bony connection is massive and cannot be fractured without damage to the surgical instruments. When this is the case, the lower part of the head may be drilled or curetted away, and silicone sheeting may be placed in the defect to prevent any reattachment of

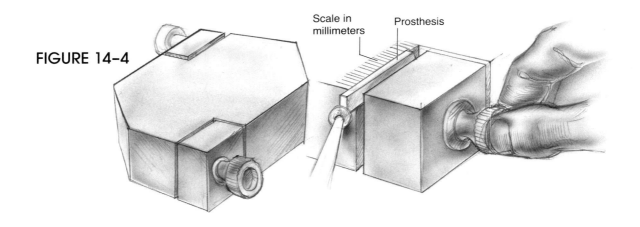

FIGURE 14-4

Scale in millimeters

Prosthesis

FIGURE 14-5

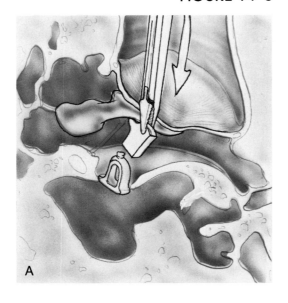

A

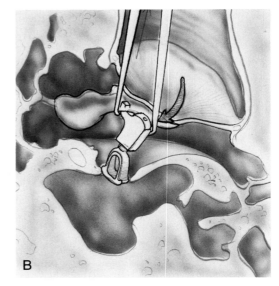

B

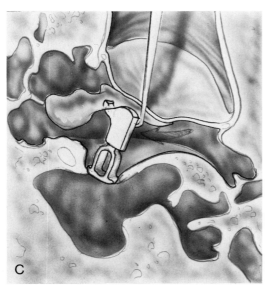

C

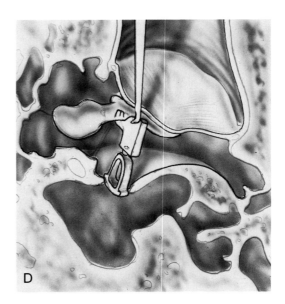

D

FIGURE 14-6

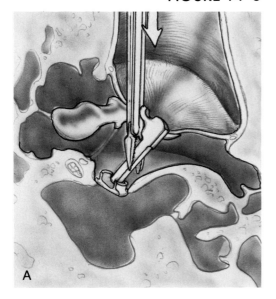

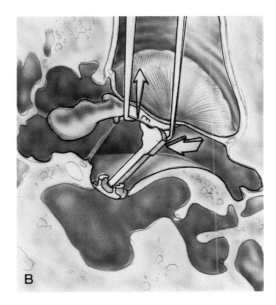

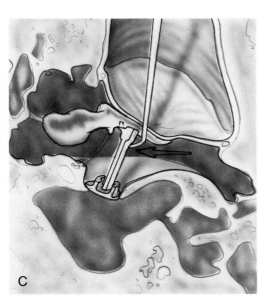

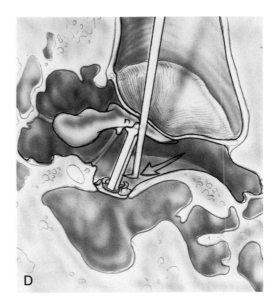

FIGURE 14-4. Wehrs implant-holding fixture.

FIGURE 14-5. *A,* Introducing the incus replacement prosthesis onto the promontory. *B,* Manipulating the incus prosthesis up under malleus. *C,* The hole in the prosthesis fits over the stapes capitulum, and it is brought up to a vertical and stable position. *D,* The motion of the stapes is tested by gentle pressure on the prosthesis with a right-angle pick.

FIGURE 14-6. *A,* Placing the incus-stapes prosthesis in the middle ear. *B,* The implant is manipulated with the notch under the malleus handle. *C,* The notch slides up the malleus to a vertical and stable position. *D,* Adjustment of the shaft so that the prosthesis is centered on the stapedial footplate.

the neck to the head. The ossicular chain is rebuilt with a incus replacement prosthesis of hydroxyapatite, as described under incus defects.

Another mallear defect is erosion and shortening of the manubrium of the malleus. Often, the incus is present and the remaining ossicular chain intact and mobile. In this instance, I recommend removal of the incus and the remaining head and neck of the malleus. Reconstruction is carried out with a homograft tympanic membrane and malleus. The head of the homograft malleus is placed into the epitympanum, into the space previously occupied by the patient's mallear head. The ossicular chain is rebuilt with the incus replacement prosthesis made of hydroxyapatite. This may be carried out in a single stage; however, due to the fact that the tensor tympani tendon is no longer present to stabilize the malleus, it is a good idea to postpone the reconstruction for a later date. At this time, the malleus has stabilized, and the reconstruction is easier and more successful.

If in the situations described earlier the stapedial crura are also absent, the reconstruction is carried out in a similar manner, but with the incus-stapes prosthesis to the stapedial footplate.

COMBINED DEFECTS OF MALLEUS AND OSSICLES

Erosion of the incus and loss of the stapes superstructure constitutes the most common multiple defect of the ossicular chain. This defect is corrected by removal of the incus and reconstruction with the incus-stapes prosthesis of hydroxyapatite in the manner previously described.

Another combination defect is constituted by an intact but fixed ossicular chain. The first step in this case would be separation of the incudostapedial joint. If the stapes is then found to be fixed but the incus and malleus are mobile, a stapedectomy is indicated. If the tympanic membrane is intact, stapedectomy should be performed immediately. However if there is a drum defect, it should be repaired first and the stapedectomy delayed for a second stage. When the stapes is mobile, the incus should be removed and the mobility of the malleus ascertained. If the malleus is found to be freely mobile, reconstruction should proceed with an incus replacement prosthesis as previously described. However, if the malleus head is fixed, it must be dealt with in the manner described under mallear defects.

The ultimate combination defect consists of loss of all ossicular tissue except the stapedial footplate. This may occur when there is a total perforation, extensive cholesteatoma, or when the ossicles have been removed and the drum grafted without any ossicular reconstruction. These cases are rebuilt with the homograft tympanic membrane and malleus as the main building block. The homograft eardrum maintains the malleus in anatomic position as well as reinforcing the graft. If the malleus head fits well in the epitympanum and there is good middle ear mucosa, the reconstruction may be carried out in a single stage. However, if the head of the malleus must be amputated or if poor mucosa is present, the reconstruction to the footplate should be delayed for a second stage.

DRESSING

For the procedures performed transmeatally, the dressing consists of a strip of 1/4-inch selvage edge gauze approximately 2 inches in length placed in the outer ear canal. A cotton ball is then used in the concha. When a postauricular incision has been employed, the incision is closed with a subcuticular suture of 4.0 plain catgut, then a standard mastoid dressing secured by 3-inch Kling bandage is applied. The patients are usually discharged the morning following the surgery. The mastoid dressing is removed at this time.

POSTOPERATIVE CARE

Patients are instructed to change the cotton in the external ear approximately three times a day for a few days. When there is no more bleeding, they should leave the cotton out altogether. Scratching or rubbing the ear is forbidden, and patients are instructed to clean it by putting a damp wash cloth over the index finger and tipping the head toward the affected ear, then gently cleaning the outer ear. Ear drops are not used routinely, but if the healing is slow or if there is surface irritation, then Cortisporin otic drops are recommended. The drops are used on a decreasing basis, usually beginning at two drops three time a day for 3 days, twice a day for 2 days, and at bedtime for a week. Patients should not wash their hair in a shower but rather in a tub or lavatory for approximately 5 days after surgery. Cotton saturated in white petroleum jelly is used in the outer ear to prevent contamination with water. The patient is seen back for the first postoperative check approximately 2 weeks following the surgery. At this time, any remaining gelatin sponge packing is removed with gentle suction. The patient then returns at 2-week intervals until the ear is healed, usually 6 weeks postoperatively. At that time, a postoperative audiogram may be obtained.

PITFALLS AND COMPLICATIONS

To date, there have been no serious complications with the use of these prostheses; however, as with any device, there are potential complications.

Intraoperative immediate complications would consist of using a prosthesis with too much height and forcing it into place. In the case of the incus prosthesis, this could result in fracture of the crura, dislocation of the stapes, or tear of the annular ligament with a resultant perilymph fistula and severe or total sensorineural hearing loss. In the case of the incus stapes prosthesis, it could fracture the stapedial footplate and be pushed into the vestibule, with similar results. To prevent these complications, the prostheses must be handled gently, and sudden undue pressure must be avoided. If the prosthesis does not slip into place easily, it should be removed and a shorter prosthesis used, or if it is the shortest prosthesis available, it may be modified with a diamond burr.

If there is a tear of the annular ligament or a crack in the stapedial footplate, then a tissue seal of fat or fascia should be placed over the affected area. Attempts at ossicular reconstruction should be postponed and the ear closed or grafted. At a second stage, definitive reconstruction could be instituted.

Immediate postoperative complications could consist of vertigo, which could be related to unrecognized trauma, as previously described. If the reconstruction was difficult, then the possibility of perilymph fistula should be considered. Exploration may be necessary if the patient does not respond to conservative therapy, such as antibiotics and antivertigo drugs. If one is sure that no excess force was used in the reconstruction, the patient's ear should not be re-explored but only observed.

The anatomic results following use of these prostheses have been good. The outline of the prosthesis is often seen through the graft. There has been minimal crusting, and in the first 2 years of use, no extrusion of a prosthesis. However, in the past year, there have been cases in which the tissue has thinned and crusted over the prosthesis, with resultant granulation tissue and breakdown with exposure of the prosthesis. In one instance, the patient underwent a revision with a canal skin tympanoplasty and ossicular reconstruction with a homograft ossicle. In another, a recurrent cholesteatoma was found at revision, but the implant was not removed and has continued to function well. In two cases, the prosthesis was removed through the perforation, and the ears subsequently healed and became dry. When a conductive component remains, revision surgery should be carried out. If the prosthesis is exposed but the hearing remains good, one may elevate a tympanomeatal flap and carry the elevation over the prosthesis. There would then be a perforation of the flap where the prosthesis had been. Fascia, homograft dura, or another tissue graft, such as perichondrium, should be placed over the prosthesis. Then, the tympanomeatal flap is replaced in the same manner as that used in an underlay tympanoplasty. If the hearing is poor, the prosthesis should be removed and replaced with a prosthesis that would correct the hearing problem.

If the graft is normal and the ear healed but there has been no improvement in hearing, a revision is usually not recommended until 6 months following the surgery. The reason for this delay is twofold. First, the hearing in many of these ears will improve after 3 to 4 months. Also, it is much better to allow the graft to thin and the ear to become completely healed and the middle ear to become less vascular before a revision is attempted. At the time of revision, the incisions for the tympanomeatal flap are more lateral than for a virgin ear, as the grafted flap, although thicker than the original canal skin, tends to shrink and may not close the defect. The flap is dissected off the prosthesis and folded forward on the malleus. One usually finds a good mucosal envelope formed around the hydroxyapatite prosthesis similar to those found around the bony prostheses. Once the flap has been elevated, the cause of the hearing failure should be determined. The cause may be simple dislocation of the prosthesis from the stapes head or malleus. Other causes may be that Silastic sheeting exists between the stapes head and the prosthesis, or that the prosthesis is not making contact for another reason. If a incus-stapes type of prosthesis had been used in the reconstruction, the footplate area should be inspected. Occasionally, the shaft has been dislocated from the stapedial footplate or is too short to make good contact. The shaft may not have been rounded, and the old square shafts tend to be hung up on the margins of the oval window.

After the cause of the failure has been determined, it is almost always necessary to completely remove the prosthesis from the ear and either modify it or use a new and different prosthesis. If the dislocation occurred because the prosthesis was too loose, a larger size would be indicated. If the stapedial head was eroded or absent, one may elect to rebuild directly to the stapedial footplate with an incus-stapes prosthesis. This may be accomplished without removing the superstructure of the stapes if it is leaning toward the promontory or is partially dislocated with an intact annular ligament. Here, one would place the rounded shaft of the incus-stapes prosthesis between the crura and on the footplate. This placement cannot be accomplished unless the stapes is already displaced. Another solution is removal of the stapedial crura to expose the footplate. When the stapes is intact and normal, it is difficult to remove the crura without dislocating the footplate. However, if one has access to a laser, then this can be more easily accomplished. Following vaporization and removal of the stapes superstructure, reconstruction would proceed in the usual fashion.

HEARING RESULTS

The hearing results have been good. In a study based on the hearing results of 86 patients operated on over a period of 3 years, 85 per cent of the incus replacement cases and 65 per cent of the incus-stapes replacement cases closed the air-bone gap to within 20dB of the preoperative bone conduction.

References

1. Wehrs RE: Management of chronic otitis externa. Trans Pacific Coast Otolaryngol Ophthalmol Soc 60: 297–303, 1979.
2. House WF, Sheehy JL: Functional restoration in tympanoplasty. Arch Otolaryngol Head Neck Surg 78: 304–309, 1963.
3. Wehrs RE: The borrowed incus in tympanoplasty. Arch Otolaryngol Head Neck Surg 85: 371–379, 1967.
4. Wehrs RE: The notched incus in tympanoplasty. Arch Otolaryngol Head Neck Surg 100: 251–255, 1974.
5. Wehrs RE: Incus replacement prostheses of hydroxyapatite in middle ear reconstruction. Am J Otol 10: 181–182, 1989.
6. Wehrs RE: Hearing results in tympanoplasty. Laryngoscope 95: 1301–1306, 1985.
7. Grote JJ: Tympanoplasty with calcium phosphate. Arch Otolaryngol Head Neck Surg 110: 197–199, 1984.

15

Tympanoplasty: Cartilage and Porous Polyethylene

JAMES L. SHEEHY, M.D.

Restoration of function in tympanoplasty requires an intact tympanic membrane, an air-containing mucosal-lined middle ear space, and a connection between the mobile tympanic membrane and the inner ear fluids. Obtaining this connection with porous polyethylene and cartilage, or cartilage alone, is the subject of this chapter.

It is difficult to consider management of ossicular problems separately from management of the mastoid, staging the operation, and use of plastic in the middle ear. In order not to confuse the issue, however, this chapter will discuss only the ossicular problem. Each of the other items are considered elsewhere in this book.

HISTORICAL ASPECTS

When tympanoplastic surgery was introduced by Wullstein[1] and Zollner,[2] little attempt was made to reconstruct the ossicular chain. They established a sound pressure differential between the oval and round windows by adapting the operation to the ossicular problem encountered. If the incus was missing, the graft was placed on the stapes capitulum (type III or columellar tympanoplasty). If both the incus and stapes crura were missing, the graft was laid on the promontory, leaving a mobile footplate exposed (type IV, oval window, or cavum minor tympanoplasty), thereby producing sound protection for the round window.

In most instances, the tympanoplasty resulted in a mastoid cavity and, because of what was mentioned in the previous paragraph, a shallow middle ear space. With more experience it became apparent that routinely creating a mastoid cavity was a drawback and that the results were better when the middle ear space was not narrowed. If a cavity was to be avoided and the eardrum reconstructed in its natural position, it became necessary to perform some type of reconstruction of the sound pressure-transfer mechanism.

Many prosthesis and techniques were used at the House Ear Clinic (HEC) beginning in the late 1950s, only to be discarded as better methods evolved. It became apparent that to obtain satisfactory long-term results, the middle ear space should not be narrowed and that whatever connection was used for sound pressure transfer, this connection should be under adequate tension. One also had to take steps to prevent extrusion.

The first prosthesis (used at HEC) was polyethylene tubing to the capitulum of the stapes or the mobile footplate.[3] In due time, one of two things happened: extrusion (if under tension) or separation from the stapes (if not under tension). The interposition of soft tissue between the polyethylene tubing and the tympanic membrane only delayed extrusion. Unfortunately, no one (at HEC) thought of using cartilage, as is done now.

In the early 1960s, ossicular transposition was used, and later, the fitted ossicular prosthesis.[4-7] The most common cause of failure there was separation of the ossicle from the stapes. A completely stable malleus and tympanic membrane were therefore a necessity, and this goal frequently required a two-staged procedure when it might not otherwise have been indicated. The use of a homograft tympanic membrane with a malleus attached resolved some of those problems, but the homograft tympanic membrane did not have a satisfactory graft take rate in the hands of the HEC doctors.[8]

The incus replacement prosthesis, developed successfully for use in stapedectomy in the fenestrated ear, was tried but quickly abandoned.[9] It often pulled off the mobile footplate or extruded. Homograft tympanic membrane with en bloc ossicles were also tried.[8] The conclusion reached was that other methods were simpler and usually yielded as good, if not better, results.

In 1967, the HEC doctors began using cartilage alone as a prothesis, following some thoughts by Shea and Glasscock.[10] Tragal cartilage had one significant advantage: it could be applied under tension without fear of extrusion. When used as a block to the capitulum of the stapes, the hearing results were stable. This technique is still used regularly in canal wall down procedures so that the middle ear space is not narrowed by placing the graft on the capitulum.[11] When cartilage was used as a strut to the footplate, the results were less stable because of the lack of stiffness of the cartilage; as a result, cartilage is no longer used as a strut to the footplate.[12, 13]

Porous polyethylene prostheses (total ossicular replacement prostheses [TORPs] and partial ossicular replacement prostheses [PORPs]) were introduced by John Shea in 1974.[14] Because of the extrusion experience with polyethylene tubes, these prostheses were not used at HEC. Then, in a 1976 personal communication, Coyle Shea suggested using tragal cartilage interposed between the platform and the tympanic membrane graft. Shortly thereafter, use of porous polyethylene with tragal cartilage became routine at HEC.[15]

PATIENT SELECTION, EVALUATION, AND COUNSELING

Patient selection, evaluation, and counseling were covered in detail in Chapter 10 (tympanic membrane grafting). Most of what was said on this subject in Chapter 10 applies equally here. The main difference is in regard to the hearing results. (Assume that this is a dry central perforation with good mucosa.)

In most cases, it is possible to know ahead of time that ossicular reconstruction will be necessary. One can see that the incus, the stapes, or both, are diseased or missing, or one concludes that there must be an ossicular problem based on a conductive deficit of greater than 25dB.

When one suspects a problem but cannot see for sure, tell the patient merely that the second ear bone will probably need to be replaced. What one says in regard to the final outcome from surgery depends on how much of a conductive deficit exists preoperatively and the surgeon's personal experience.

If the bone-air gap is 45dB or greater, the patient is told that there are seven out of ten chances that the hearing result will "make both of us happy." If loss is in both ears, one is justified in saying eight chances out of ten. Err on the conservative side.

If the deficit is 40dB or less, tell the patient that there are six chances out of ten for a good result. Again, if the other ear is similarly involved, "three chances out of four" would be a reasonable statement. The result, "making us both happy," depends on the overall situation, including the other ear, the bone conduction level, and whether the patient wears hearing aids already. A technical success may not be judged as a success by the patient, and this fact must be remembered when outlook is discussed.

SURGICAL TECHNIQUE

Management in the office, preoperatively and in surgery are the same as presented in Chapter 10.

TORPs and PORPs were used initially. The platform was modified to 3mm early on ("Sheehy's modification"). In the mid 1980s, total ossicular prostheses (TOPs) and partial ossicular prostheses (POPs) were developed. These have a rounded platform to better conform to the tenting of the tympanic membrane brought about by putting the prosthesis under slight tension. In addition, the stem of the TOP is oval (0.8mm by 1.0mm) to facilitate bypassing the stapedial crura when necessary.[16, 17]

The basic technique for using a TOP or a POP (or various individual variations of these) is the same.[11] Discussed here (and illustrated) will be the use of the TOP. To facilitate presentation, a planned second-stage procedure is described, that is, the tympanic membrane is intact, and no ossicles are present.

Exposure

A semilunar incision is made at the junction of the outer amd middle third of the ear canal. Flap eleva-

tion is from posteroinferiorly to anterosuperiorly (Fig. 15–1).

The reason for this type of incision and exposure is to keep the tympanic membrane stable in the area where the prosthesis and cartilage will contact the membrane and to avoid incisions near the bony annulus. One may better judge the proper prosthesis length to maintain slight tension and not have any tension to distract incision edges at the annulus.

Preparation of Cartilage

After any plastic material placed in the middle ear at the first stage is removed and the ear is inspected for residual disease, the middle ear and canal are packed temporarily to keep blood out of the middle ear.

An incision is made on the posterior surface of the tragus (to avoid retracted scars, which may develop if the incision is made over the dome), and a large piece of cartilage is removed. The perichondrium is removed by blunt dissection, using a Bard-Parker knife handle and holding the cartilage on a piece of gauze.

The cartilage is then placed on a moist tongue blade, trimmed to the appropriate size (about 5mm × 5mm), and thinned with a No. 11 Bard-Parker blade. This thinning process, particularly on the edges, results in cartilage that has a slight dome shape. Having this shape, the cartilage will conform more easily to the contours of the tympanic membrane when the prosthesis and cartilage are placed under slight tension.

Preparation of Prosthesis

Trimming the stem to the appropriate size is a matter of judgment and experience. No measuring device has been satisfactory. In cases with an intact canal wall and without a malleus handle, a 5mm length is usually correct for the TOP (and a 2mm length for a POP). If the manubrium is present, a 4mm length may be correct. In open-cavity cases, 3.5mm is usually the correct length.

Wet the prosthesis and cut it on a moist tongue blade using a No. 11 Bard-Parker blade. By having both the tongue blade and the prosthesis moist, one will find that the prosthesis tends to adhere to the tongue blade.

Placement of Prosthesis

After temporary packing is removed from the middle ear and canal, the middle ear is filled lightly with pieces of slightly moistened absorbable gelatin sponge (Gelfoam). This moistened gelatin sponge is placed to facilitate placement of the prosthesis and cartilage, to stabilize them temporarily, and to act as counterpacking for the packing that will be placed in the canal after replacement of the tympanomeatal flap. A small piece of perichondrium may be placed on the mobile footplate and will be commented on later.

The moistened TOP is most easily placed in position in the middle ear by using a No. 3 Barron suction on the platform as a prosthesis guide and holder. The prosthesis should fit perfectly without tension prior to placement of the cartilage (Fig. 15–2). If the prosthesis is slightly short, the length may be corrected, later by adding an additional piece of cartilage.

Because it may be difficult to slide the cartilage across the prosthesis without displacing it, the TOP is tipped posteroinferiorly first. The cartilage is placed on the flap, slid into the proper position, and then flipped onto the platform (Fig. 15–3). Then the assembly is moved into position (Fig. 15–4). There should be slight tension on, or tenting of, the tympanic membrane (Fig. 15–5). The flap is replaced, and gelatin sponge packing is used with a plug of cotton in the outer meatus. A mastoid dressing is not necessary.

Management of Ossicular Chain Fixation

Tympanosclerosis

Tympanosclerosis is a term used to describe a sclerotic or a hyalin change of the submucosal tissue of the middle ear. It appears to be an end product of recurrent acute or chronic ear infection. Hyalinized connective tissue develops under the mucous membrane, superficial to the bone. Calcification and ossification may occur.[11]

Tympanosclerosis is clinically significant only when it impedes motion of the ossicular chain. Plaques in the tympanic membrane remnant are not of significance but are usually removed at the time of grafting. Fixation of the malleus or incus, however, is of significance, and is usually a phenomenon that results from massive involvement in the epitympanum. It is best to remove the malleus and incus, bypassing the chain rather than trying to mobilize it.

Tympanosclerotic fixation of the stapes may be due to involvement of the tendon, to pressure on the crura from lesions on the fallopian canal and promontory, or to diffuse involvement of the oval window niche. Mobilization of the stapes by removal of the lesions is possible two thirds of the time. When the involvement is diffuse, it is best to graft the drum and perform a stapedectomy as a second-stage procedure.

Otosclerosis

Otosclerotic fixation of the stapes should, likewise, be corrected in a secondary procedure after the ear is free of infection and the perforation closed. When fixation is due to either tympanosclerosis or otosclerosis, a stapedectomy may be performed as a planned second stage. If the lateral chain is not available for use, we use a TOP, after covering the oval window with perichondrium.

POSTOPERATIVE CARE

The patient is given a postoperative instruction card just before entering the hospital. This is commented on, and appears as Appendix 2, in Chapter 10.

The patient is seen in the office in 7 to 10 days. The cotton plug is removed and the gelatin sponge packing aspirated. The patient is told that blowing the nose is permitted but that no water should be allowed into the ear. A second postoperative visit is scheduled for a month postoperatively, at which time the hearing is tested. It may take 3 months for the hearing to increase to its maximum, and the patient is told this at the first postoperative visit.

PREVENTIVE PROBLEMS

An early recognized problem was displacement of the lateral (platform) end of the TOP or POP, particularly

---

FIGURE 15–1. Elevation of tympanomeatal flap after semilunar incision at junction of outer and middle third.

FIGURE 15–2. Total ossicular prosthesis (TOP) between footplate and tympanic membrane, without tension.

FIGURE 15–3. Sliding cartilage into position.

FIGURE 15–4. Shifting of prosthesis and cartilage into position.

FIGURE 15–5. Final position, with slight tension.

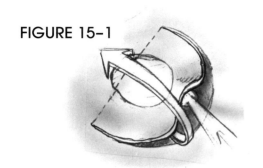

FIGURE 15-1

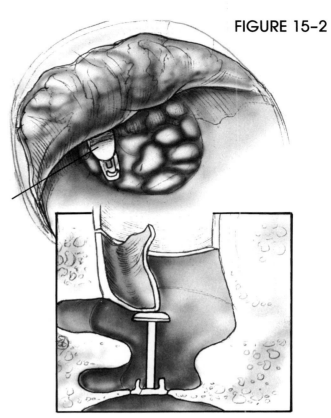

FIGURE 15-2

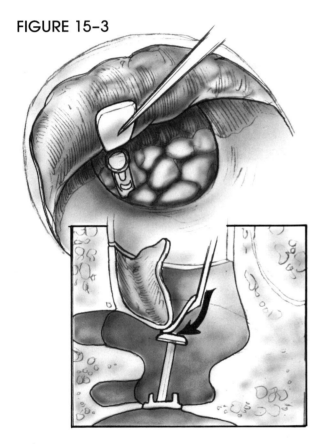

FIGURE 15-3

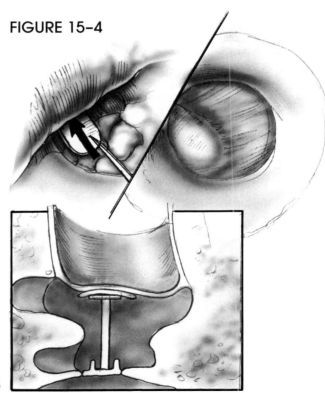

FIGURE 15-4

FIGURE 15-5

in ears with a normal malleus. This normal malleus maintains a cone-shape to the tympanic membrane, even when the perforation grafted was a total one. This tends to force displacement of the lateral end of the prosthesis, despite the presence of a piece of cartilage. Dislocation outward of the malleus handle is advisable at the time of surgery to prevent this problem and to produce a *flat* tympanic membrane.

Stabilizing the stem of the TOP (or TORP) on the mobile stapes footplate can be a problem. Covering the footplate with tissue (perichondrium or fascia) facilitates stability. It also prevents direct contact of the porous polyethylene with the footplate. There have been a few instances of resorption of the bone in the area of contact without any slippage into the vestibule.

The main concern of ear surgeons is prosthesis extrusion. This problem was common early on, before cartilage was used over the prosthesis platform. But it continued to occur in 5 per cent of cases, even with cartilage use. With the use of larger pieces of cartilage on a 3mm platform, and with rounded platforms, the incidence has been reduced further. Staging the operation is also important if there is a major mucous membrane problem, to prevent adhesions (see Chapter 21).

Despite all precautions, extrusion continues in a small percentage of cases. When this problem is analyzed, it appears to most often be related to middle ear space and mucous membrane problems: it occurs much more often in cases requiring a two-stage procedure in the first place, the "bad ears."[18]

Acknowledgment

Many of the illustrations are modified from *Otolaryngology,* Vol. 1, published by J. B. Lippincott Company.

References

1. Wullstein H: Theory and practice of tympanoplasty. Laryngoscope 66:1076–1093, 1956.
2. Zollner F: Principles of plastic surgery of the sound conducting apparatus. J Laryngol Otol 69:637–652, 1955.
3. House WF, Sheehy JL: Functional restoration in tympanoplasty. Arch Otolaryngol Head Neck Surg 78:304–309, 1963.
4. Sheehy JL: Ossicular problems in tympanoplasty. Arch Otolaryngol Head Neck Surg 81:115–122, 1965.
5. Farrior JB: Ossicular repositioning and ossicular prostheses in tympanoplasty. Arch Otolaryngol Head Neck Surg 69:661–666, 1959.
6. Hall A, Rytzner C: Autotransplantation of ossicles: Stapedectomy and biological reconstruction of the ossicular chain mechanism. Arch Otolaryngol Head Neck Surg 74:22–26, 1961.
7. House WF, Patterson ME, Linthicum FH: Incus homografts in chronic ear surgery. Arch Otolaryngol Head Neck Surg 84:148–153, 1966.
8. House WF, Glasscock ME, Sheehy JL: Homograft transplants of the middle ear. Trans Am Acad Ophthalmol Otolaryngol 873:836–841, 1969.
9. Sheehy JL: Stapedectomy with incus replacement prosthesis: Report of 50 cases. Laryngoscope 76:1165–1180, 1966.
10. Shea MC, Glasscock ME: Tragal cartilage as an ossicular substitute. Arch Otolaryngol Head Neck Surg 86:308–317, 1967.
11. Sheehy JL: Surgery of chronic otitis media. *In* English GM (ed): Otolaryngology. Philadelphia, Harper and Row, 1984.
12. Pulec JL, Sheehy JL: Tympanoplasty: Ossicular chain reconstruction. Laryngoscope 83:448–465, 1973.
13. Sheehy JL, Altenau MM: Tympanoplasty: Cartilage prosthesis. Laryngoscope 88:895–904, 1978.
14. Shea JJ, Emmett JB, Smyth GDL: Biocompatible implants in otology. ORL Digest 39:9–15, 1977.
15. Sheehy JL, Brackmann DE: Tympanoplasty: TORPs and PORPs. Laryngoscope 89:108–114, 1979.
16. Sheehy JL: Personal experiences with TORPs and PORPs: A report on 455 operations. Am J Otol 6:80–83, 1985.
17. Brackmann DE, Sheehy JL, Luxford WM: TORPs and PORPs in tympanoplasty: A review of 1042 operations. Otolaryngol Head Neck Surg 92:32–37, 1984.
18. Sheehy JL: TORPs and PORPs: Causes of failure. Otolaryngol Head Neck Surg 92:583–587, 1984.

16

Biocompatible Materials in Chronic Ear Surgery

JAN J. GROTE, M.D., Ph.D.

Since the introduction of closed techniques for the eradication of chronic middle ear disease and the use of homologous middle ear implants, we thought that the problems of cholesteatoma surgery were solved.[1] It was possible to remove the disease and preserve or restore the anatomy of the middle ear while avoiding the problems of a cavity. With homologous ossicles and even a total homologous middle ear, including ossicular chain and tympanic membrane, it was possible to reconstruct a sound-conducting system with a normal anatomy.[3] At the end of the 1970s, an increasing number of recurrent and residual cholesteatomas were reported,[3] and it was demonstrated that cholesteatoma microscopically invaded the ossicles and the surrounding bone, leading to residual disease. The defects in the bony annulus had to be reconstructed to avoid recurrent cholesteatoma. Also, in many cases, because of the local anatomy, a proper and safe way to eradicate cholesteatoma via a combined approach was not possible.

Because of the repeated interventions required, the possibilities of physiologic reconstruction diminished. During the first operation, the stapes superstructure was often present, but during a second look, resorption by the recurrent cholesteatoma was observed, indicating that the best chance for reconstruction is a safe and cholesteatoma-free middle ear. However, the problems of an open cavity and the uncertain results of tympanoplasties in these cavities are well known.

In addition to the controversy over closed versus open techniques for eradication, the use of homologous implants led to new doubts in the 1980s. The preservation of these implants was solved, but a major problem with these implants came with the possibility of virus inclusion and transplantation. However, there is no proof that HIV can be transferred via these implants. In many countries, using these implants is not allowed if they are not proved to be from HIV-free donors. Also, slow virus inclusions, such as Jakob-Creutzfeldt virus, entered the otologic discussion. Therefore, it looked as if we had to start again to find solutions in chronic otitis media surgery. "Once a cholesteatoma always a cholesteatoma" is more true now than ever.

In the 1970s, new developments in material science, cell biology, and reconstructive surgery gave rise to new implant materials and a better understanding of the interaction between these implant materials and the body. Biomaterial science became important for middle ear reconstruction.

For the reconstructive surgery with biomaterials, the surgeon must combine surgical criteria with biomaterial criteria. Only if a good combination of these criteria is made can reconstructive surgery be successful. This combination of criteria is necessary because of the different tissues involved in the wound healing.

The demands for the reconstructive surgery performed by an orthopedic surgeon are clearly different than those performed by an otologist. Even in the middle ear, different tissues are involved in wound healing; therefore, different materials must be used.

SURGICAL CRITERIA

The most important criterion for middle ear surgery in case of a cholesteatoma is a radical eradication of the disease. All the tissue that has been in contact with the cholesteatoma, whether the ossicular chain, the canal wall, or the mucosa of the middle ear and mastoid, must be totally removed and in continuity with a safe margin, without consideration of reconstruction. Definitive eradication of cholesteatoma is more possible with an open technique. Many patients with cholesteatoma have a sclerotic mastoid, and if it is eradicated by open technique, the patient is left with a small mastoid cavity. A tympanoplasty type III in this cavity often leads to good function, and the patient is well off with one operation. If indicated, reconstruction can be done in a second stage.

For the reconstruction of a functioning middle ear, a wide middle ear mastoid cleft must be made. This is possible if the annulus of the middle ear is more lateral than in the often narrow ears of cholesteatoma patients. The function of a reconstructed middle ear chain must be comparable to that achieved with a normal ossicular chain, i.e., the ossicular chain must have a lever mechanism and must have contact with the tympanic membrane by the handle of the malleus. The ossicular chain must have a good contact with the footplate or the stapes and the tympanic membrane. The ossicles must stay mobile and not be resorbed or extruded, even in an infected middle ear. For a lasting reconstruction of the canal wall, the new canal wall must be bone or must become bone.

BIOMATERIAL AND BIOCOMPATIBILITY CRITERIA

The selection of materials for reconstructive surgery is based on information derived from physical, chemical, biomechanical and surgical concepts. With the increasing number of implants on the market, it is essential that the otolaryngologist has a fundamental knowledge of biomaterial science, which can be related to his or her surgical aims.

The interaction of the human body and the implant is studied in terms of local and general reactions. The implant material must have no cytotoxicity. The influence of the body on the prosthesis is also important because these reactions can lead to degradation. The biocompatibility of an implant material determines the interface of the implant with the body, which ultimately leads to a good, permanent integration. This integration is dependent on the surface of the implant material and on the breakdown and remodeling of the implant by the body.

SURFACE ACTIVITY

An implant material is regarded as *bioinert* if the body does not react at all with the implant material, as *biotolerated* if the body regards the implant material as a foreign body but does not extrude the implant, and as *bioactive* if the body has an active surface integration with the implant material, which leads to a firm integration between the body and the implant. An implant material will always be placed in a wound, and the normal wound reactions will take place. A foreign body will be encapsulated by a fibrous capsule with a varying number of reactive cells, particularly foreign body giant cells. In case of a bioinert material, no significant reaction occurs on the surface, and although bone may be in contact with the implant, a bond does not occur. A biotolerated material has a fibrous capsule between the implant material and the bone. Cellular activity in the form of giant cell reactions can be present, even after longer postoperative periods, but the integration will be stable. Bioactive material will achieve a real bond with the surface of the surrounding bone tissue, which takes place via an active ion exchange, leading to a firm bond between the implant and the body.

STRUCTURE

In the 1970s, porous implant materials were developed.[4] This advance enabled the host tissue to grow into the porous part of the implants, resulting in better integration with the body. Macropores of 100μm allowed the ingrowth both of fibrous tissues and of bone tissue if they were adjacent to the implant material. Micropores of several micrometers seemed to be essential, especially if the implant material had to be resorbed and remodeled in living tissue. These pores can be a problem in materials that are not meant for degradation. The body will always react at the surface with the implant, and the material will be resorbed to some degree, depending on the surface activity. If the surface area is large, the response of the body to the implant material will be more extensive, with the production of large numbers of macrophages and giant cells. With this degradation, inclusions of toxic substances can be harmful for the body, and therefore a good understanding of the type of implant material is necessary to avoid long-term problems, either locally

or systemically. These problems of structure are comparable to those occurring with the homologous implant materials, in which in the case of bone chips or cartilage resorption can take place before remodeling occurs. Also, the use of mixtures of granules with blood or fibrinogen glue gives a very large surface area, which can lead to a resorption before remodeling occurs. This is the reason why initially good anatomic results are achieved, but after longer postoperative periods, resorption takes place, especially if an infection occurs. Therefore, the behavior of the implant material in infected surroundings should be taken into account. With the newer biomaterials, regulating the surface activity and the structure is possible.

Many implants are labeled with trade names that give no information on the capacity of the material. Therefore, the generic names of the material must be used and indicated. In addition to the generic names of the materials, the additives, which might be part of the implant materials and the trace elements present, should be noted.

In otology, three classes of biomaterials are used: metals, polymers, and ceramics. These different classes of biomaterials have advantages and disadvantages with regard to biocompatibility, integration capacity, and surgical application.

CLASSES OF BIOMATERIALS

Metals

Metals are used only in reconstruction of the middle ear in otosclerosis. Integrated into a mobile middle ear chain in a healthy middle ear, these implants are reliable. If mechanically fixed, they will not extrude, but if they are in contact with a mobile tympanic membrane, they will extrude.

Polymers

In 1952, Wullstein was the first to use a biomaterial in reconstructive middle ear surgery. He implanted a columella of Palavit in the middle ear for the reconstruction of the middle ear chain, and although the initial hearing results were good, the implants extruded. Then different polymers, such as polyethylene, polytetrafluorethylene (Teflon), and silicon rubber (Silastic) were used,[5] but in the end of the 1960s, the use of polymer implant materials in reconstructive middle ear surgery was abandoned because of their high extrusion rate. Silicone sheeting and Teflon are still used as a plastic sheeting, and Teflon is used in otosclerosis surgery. The concept of porous implant materials was applied to these polymers. The advantage of the pores was better integration in the body, and porous polyethylene has been especially widely used as total and partial ossicular replacement prosthesis (columella between the footplate and tympanic membrane or between the stapes superstructure and tympanic membrane).[6] The surface activity of the first porous plastic implants was biotolerated, but the surface activity was not favorable for integration, and an interface was necessary between the tympanic membrane and the implants. Even then, an increasing extrusion rate was reported. In recent years, special interest has focused on the development of polymers with a bioactive surface that can be used for the reconstruction of soft tissue. We developed the first bioactive polymer, which belongs to a group of copolymers (Polyactive).[7, 8] This new biodegradable polymer has shown its bioactivity at the surface, especially in contact with bone, but also enhances the ingrowth and the integration of collagen. The material has shown its bioactivity in tissue cultures as well as in long-term animal studies, and the first clinical trials have proved its bioactivity and integration in soft tissue defects. As with the other polymers, these new types of implant materials can also be made in different porosities, which will lead to better integration and predictable resorption and remodeling.

Ceramics

For the reconstruction of bone defects, especially in the middle ear, ceramics are the material of choice. Biologically, ceramics can be classified as bioinert materials (most oxide ceramics) and reactive materials (glass ceramics and calcium phosphate ceramics).

Aluminum oxide ceramic is a bioinert ceramic that is used in ossiculoplasty.[9] Its advantage is that it stays mobile in the middle ear chain, and there is no resorption and no reaction of the body. Because of its bioinertness, however, integration is less favorable.

The bioactive ceramics glass ceramics and calcium phosphate ceramics are used in otology. There are different types of glass ceramics, and every glass ceramic has its own distinct composition and reactivity with the surrounding tissue. They are mainly used for the reconstruction of the middle ear chain in the form of columella prostheses.[10] They can be difficult to shape, and long-term studies have shown that resorption occurs. Therefore, we studied calcium phosphate ceramics. Their composition resembles that of bone tissue. There are different types of calcium phosphates, and we have focused our interest on hydroxyapatite, which is the mineral matrix of living bone tissue. It has proved to be a bioactive material, which achieves a real integration with bone tissue without encapsulation. Hydroxyapatite can be made in porous as well as in dense forms, depending on the surgical requirements. The continuation of the remodeling of the porous forms is also controlled in infected surroundings. The interaction with epithelium and connective tissue is excellent, with a direct bond between the material and the tissue. The attachment of epithelium to the apatite surfaces has been shown to take place by means of hemodesmosomes, and the implants are not encapsulated by fibrous tissue. The disadvantage of hydroxyapatite is its brittleness and its insufficient tensile strength; therefore, only non–load-bearing defects in the bone can be repaired with it. The use of this ceramic in long-term clinical studies in middle ear surgery has validated its biocompatibility and usefulness.[11–17] Otologous and homologous materials are often considered ideal for the reconstruction of defects in the middle ear. However, after preservation, the remodeling of the body with these implant materials takes place in the same way as with the biomaterials, which we have chosen for our reconstructive procedures.

The advantage of the hydroxyapatite implant for bony reconstruction is that the material is readily available. Because of standard manufacturing procedures, resorption and remodeling are controlled. There is no possibility of transmission of diseases, and this material can be shaped according to individual demands. If used in combination with good surgical criteria, the body will remodel these implants in its own material or integrate the implants where needed, which will finally lead to a good lasting result. The usefulness of these materials is demonstrated also with retrieved implants that were removed in patients because of problems that will be discussed later. The histology of these implants proved their utility in reconstruction of the middle ear, and the results in the human body are comparable to those studied in vitro and in long-term animal experiments.[18–22]

SURGICAL TECHNIQUE

The development of new implant materials for a reliable and lasting reconstruction of defects in the middle ear makes it possible to separate eradication and reconstruction. This separation has the advantage that during the eradication, all the diseased tissue and adjacent bone can be removed. Only in cases in which the cholesteatoma is lateral of the ossicular chain, without ingrowth in the facial recess or sinus tympani, can the eradication and the reconstruction be done in the same stage. In more extensive cholesteatomas, an eradication is done first with an open technique, and reconstruction is done in a second stage, if indicated.

Eradication

The skin incision is made retroauricularly, and a cranial-based periosteal flap is mobilized. A lateral flap in the posterior skin of the ear canal is made, and after retraction of the flaps, the middle ear is inspected by mobilization of the tympanomeatal flap anteriorly. The remnants of the ossicular chain and the extent of the cholesteatoma in the middle ear is inspected. The ear canal is widened, and via endaural approach, the cholesteatoma is now exposed. The first landmark is the tegmen tympani, exposed by drilling away the remnants of the scutum and opening the epitympanic area up until the tegmen tympani is seen. The cholesteatoma is followed and exposed posteriorly. The next landmark is the sinodural angle. The posterior border is found by widening of the bony ear canal and exposure of the cholesteatoma. The facial recess is not opened in this stage. Along the tegmen tympani, the supratubal cells are opened anteriorly, and the cog is drilled away.

The surgical landmarks of the anterior epitympanum are superior to the tegmen tympani, anterior to the zygoma root, medial to the bone plate covering the geniculate ganglion, and inferior to the canal of the tensor tympani (Fig. 16–1). Via the anterior epitympanum, the eustachian tube is found. From there, the cholesteatoma can be mobilized posteriorly, and the landmark of the canal of the tensor tympani leads to the cochleariform process.

The head of the malleus and, if present, the incus, are removed, and superior to the cochleariform process, the horizontal part of the facial nerve is found. The cholesteatoma matrix is mobilized in continuity with the perimatrix, and the facial recess is now opened. The oval window niche is identified via the hypotympanum so as not to luxate remnants of the stapes superstructure. The cholesteatoma is further exposed by drilling away the cortex of the mastoid. The facial ridge is lowered and in this way, the total cholesteatoma is exposed and can be removed. A meatoplasty is performed, and the cranial-based periosteal flap covers the skin of the meatoplasty, forming a lateral lining of the cavity. Via this endaural approach for eradication, the patient has the smallest cavity possible. This is an advantage in sclerotic mastoids. If the stapes is present, a modified radical is made with a tympanoplasty type III. If the footplate is empty but mobile, plastic sheeting is put in the middle ear, and a myringoplasty is performed without trying to reconstruct the sound-transforming mechanism in this stage.

This stage enables the patient to have a safe ear without problems, especially in patients with a sclerotic mastoid. If necessary, a reconstruction of the middle ear can be done in a second stage. Residual cholesteatoma will be seen in cavities within 1 year postoperatively. To be sure that the reconstruction can be done in a cholesteatoma-free ear, it is therefore wise to delay the reconstruction for at least 1 year.

Reconstruction

The indications for reconstruction of a cavity are as follows:

1. The patient wishes to hear better.
2. The patient has recurrent infections of the cavity and wants a dry ear.
3. The patient wants to be able to swim.
4. The patient needs better canal conformation for fitting of a hearing aid.
5. The patient becomes dizzy if the ear is exposed to wind.
6. Any combination of the above.

Patient Selection

In general, I do not advise reconstruction in children if they still have frequent upper airway infections; I wait until the child is 7 to 10 years old. In cases of a cavity in both ears, the worst ear is always operated on first. If the main indication for operation is hearing improvement, better-hearing ear is taken into account. The best ear is never operated on, and the contralateral ear must be kept safe and dry. There is no use in gaining 20dB in the worst ear if the combination of both ears is not leading to better hearing. For the reconstruction, the ear must be as dry as possible or can be made dry during operation by excision of the diseased tissue.

Preoperative Care

It is important that the cavity is free of cholesteatoma. For a successful reconstruction, enough healthy epithelium for the covering of the new canal wall is necessary. Although in many cases of large infected cavities the only way to get a dry ear is to reoperate, it is still advisable to get the cavity as dry as possible with regular preoperative cleaning and local and sometimes systemic antibiotics prescribed based on a proper culture. Upper airway infections must be cured before reconstruction.

Canal Wall Reconstruction

For the reconstruction of the canal wall, a canal wall prosthesis, made of porous hydroxyapatite ceramic, chemical composition $Ca_{10}(PO_4)_6(OH)_2$, is used. The material has a macroporosity of 30 per cent, a pore size of approximately $100\mu m$, and a microporosity of less than 5 per cent (pore size, approximately 3μm). With this porosity, bone ingrowth will take place in about three quarters of a year, and it serves as the mineral matrix of bone.

A postauricular incision is made, the skin is elevated up to the concha, and the lateral lining of the cavity is kept intact. Posterior to the cavity, an incision is made in the periosteum, parallel to the skin incision. The periosteum is mobilized in the right plane, up to the border of the cavity without opening the cavity. Then, with a sharp knife, the periosteal flap is mobilized from the lining of the cavity, from inferior to superior. By mobilizing this periosteal flap and cutting it from the concha, a cranial-based periosteal flap is formed. This cranial-based periosteal flap is needed for the covering of the canal wall prosthesis at the end of the operation. Therefore, a cranial-based periosteal flap is mobilized because the undersurface of the periosteum is the bone-inducing surface, and the contact between this periosteal flap and the canal wall will stimulate new bone formation. If the epithelial lining of the cavity is not expected to be sufficient, a larger periosteal flap is needed. The soft tissue covering of the new canal wall prosthesis is very important.

Now, the lateral epithelial lining of the cavity is incised with a knife pointing anteriorly and not downward, especially in old cavities, because of the danger of cutting into an exposed sinus or an exposed dura. The lateral skin lining of the cavity is mobilized, and incisions are made at 12 o'clock and at 6 o'clock in the meatal skin. In this way, the lateral epithelium of the former ear canal is mobilized. In this stage, it is important to control whether a good meatoplasty is made. If not, part of the conchal cartilage has to be removed now. The new ear canal will be wider, and therefore, this epithelial flap must be in direct contact with the new ear canal. The cranial-based periosteal flap and the epithelial flap are very important for a successful integration of the canal wall of hydroxyapatite. With a large diamond burr, the lining of the mastoid cavity is mobilized, and with an elevator, this lining is further mobilized from posterior to anterior.

In case of a very thin epithelium in the cavity, the epithelial lining is mobilized carefully. In case of disruption of the continuity, the adjacent bone is drilled away. In this way, the tegmen tympani is identified, and the skin lining is mobilized along the tegmen tympani to the anterior epitympanic area and the zygoma root. In many old cavities, the anterior epitym-

panic area is not opened sufficiently, and the remnant of the cog has to be removed, as well as the anterior buttress, so that there is a complete overview of the anterior epitympanic area. Often in old cavities, residual cholesteatoma is present in this area. Reconstruction will not be performed in these cases, and an operation with a modified radical is done.

With the overview of the anterior epitympanic area the patient is turned away from the surgeon. The entrance of the eustachian tube can be found with identification of the canal of the tensor tympani. From there, the eustachian tube is inspected and although quite often granulation tissue or scar tissue can be present in the protympanum, surprisingly, in most cavities the eustachian tube itself has no disease. Now the epithelial lining is mobilized posteriorly along the canal of the tensor tympani. The cochleariform process is identified, and from there, the horizontal part of the facial nerve is found, and the skin is mobilized along the facial nerve, even if it is denuded. Care is taken that the epithelial lining is mobilized in continuity. The middle ear is not opened at the area of the oval window niche, so as not to luxate the stapes, if present.

Once the level of the facial nerve is identified, the mastoid epithelium is mobilized out of the mastoid tip, taking care to preserve much of the cortex in this place because this area will later provide stability for the canal wall prosthesis. Now, the whole lining of the cavity is put forward and outward. Via the hypotympanum, the middle ear cleft is entered, and from inferior and posterior, the oval window niche area is inspected. The epithelium and the remnants of the tympanic membrane are lifted off from the remnants of the stapes superstructure or, if the structure is not present, from the footplate. In this way, the whole tympanomeatal flap, including a large piece of skin lining of the cavity, is mobilized outward. If the tensor tympani is still present, it is cut to lateralize the tympanic membrane completely. Now a good inspection of the eustachian tube and the protympanum can be performed, and the mobility of the footplate and/or the stapes superstructure is tested with the round window reflex. Also in this stage of the operation, the skin of the tympanomeatal flap can be trimmed, taking care that there is enough skin lining for the canal wall and that the skin lining will fit exactly on the new canal wall prosthesis (Fig. 16–2). Also, the edges of a tympanic membrane perforation are freshed.

FIGURE 16–1. The landmarks of the attic.

FIGURE 16–2. The soft tissue flaps. Cranial-based periosteal flap, lateral skin flap, and tympanomeatal flap.

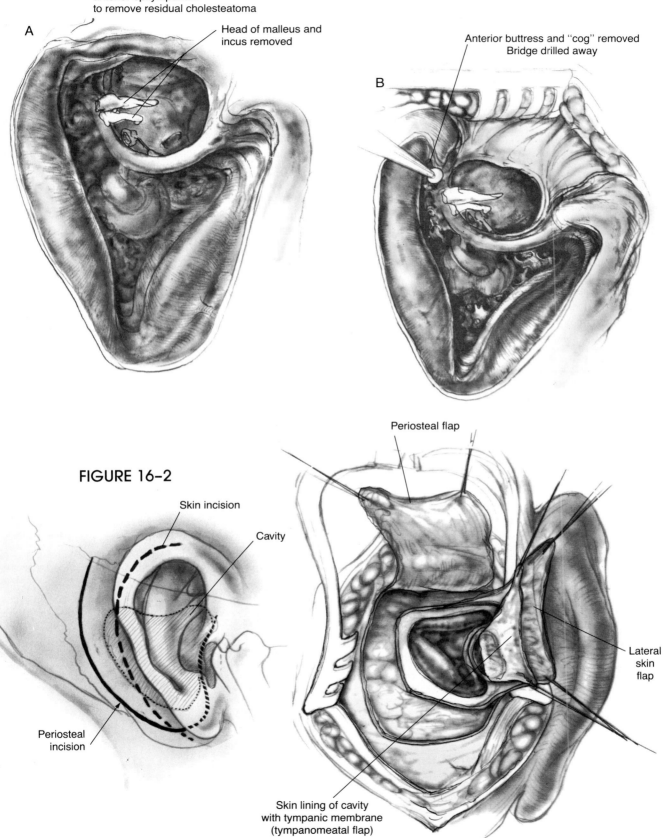

FIGURE 16-1

Remove old cavity and open
anterior epitympanum
to remove residual cholesteatoma

A

Head of malleus and
incus removed

Anterior buttress and "cog" removed
Bridge drilled away

B

Periosteal flap

FIGURE 16-2

Skin incision

Cavity

Periosteal
incision

Lateral
skin
flap

Skin lining of cavity
with tympanic membrane
(tympanomeatal flap)

Two grooves for the canal wall prosthesis are drilled. Anteriorly, the groove is made in the zygomatic root, just underneath the tegmen tympani, superior of the former location of the ear canal. Therefore, the tegmen tympani is drilled as flat as possible, and a groove is made in the zygomatic root. The reason for placing this anterior groove directly adjacent to the tegmen is so that with a new ear canal no epitympanic area will be left, so in cases of retraction of the tympanic membrane, recurrent cholesteatoma will not occur. The level of the new annulus can be chosen as far lateral as possible.

The posterior groove is drilled in the facial ridge, lateral of the facial nerve. The stability of the groove is especially important in the cortex of the mastoid. If there is no mastoid cortex left, the groove has to be drilled in the floor of the former ear canal, anterior of the facial ridge, to get a stable position for the canal wall prothesis (Fig. 16–3). This action, of course, yields a smaller ear canal, and it is preferable to have a wide round ear canal for self-cleaning. With a width measurement instrument, the width between the two grooves is measured, and with a depth measurement instrument, the depth of the posterior groove is measured (Figs. 16–4 and 16–5). The canal wall prosthesis is drilled with a large diamond drill with water, or with a diamond drill blade without water. The porous canal wall prosthesis is as brittle as bone but can be shaped easily. In the anteromedial part of the canal wall prosthesis, the annulus goes up and can therefore be drilled before the canal wall is placed. Depending on the width and depth, a large, medium, or small canal wall prothesis can be used. The canal wall prosthesis is placed into the two grooves with stability especially at the cortex of the mastoid tip and in the facial ridge (Fig. 16–6). The new annulus is far more lateral than the original and leaves a wide posterior tympanotomy opening, but there is no epitympanic area. Therefore, the retraction of the tympanic membrane can be done anteriorly but will then be part of the ear canal, or it can be done posteriorly through the wide posterior tympanotomy. Because of this wide opening, such a retraction is self-cleaning.

Obliteration of the mastoid cavity is not advisable. Even with good biomaterials, such as granules of hydroxyapatite, complete ossification of the mastoid cavity is not certain, and holes will stay under the obliteration. In addition, there is also a possibility of leaving epithelium or perhaps residual disease, which in case of an obliteration is not advisable. In reconstruction of the canal wall, residual disease will grow in the mastoid cavity and can come out and be noticed via the middle ear. In addition, the middle ear cleft will be smaller. There is no air reserve, which is a disadvantage for a good functioning middle ear. With the canal wall prosthesis in place, a strip of absorbable gelatin film (Gelfilm) is placed from mastoid through the posterior tympanotomy to the eustachian tube orifice, and in case of denuded promontory, a piece is also placed in the middle ear. A fascia graft is used as an underlay in case of a tympanic membrane perforation, with the support of some absorbable gelatin sponge (Gelfoam) anteriorly in the middle ear. The ossiculoplasty is now performed (as described later), and the tympanomeatal flap is placed in contact with the canal wall prosthesis. It is important that the canal wall prosthesis has a good contact anteriorly with the anterior canal wall. Then the cranial-based periosteal flap is turned into the new ear canal underneath the tympanomeatal flap. A skin defect will be present laterally, but the new ear canal is covered by soft tissue. The lateral skin defect is covered with the concha-based epithelium flap, which was the lateral skin lining of the cavity. When the pinna is turned backward, this skin flap falls in place (Fig. 16–7). It is important that the ear canal wall prosthesis is at the same level as the former cortex of the mastoid, so that this epithelial flap will not fall behind the new ear canal. Now, the tympanomeatal flap and the lateral skin flap are kept in place with gelatin sponge in the new ear canal, and loose oxytetracycline-soaked cotton wool is used the first week. The incision is stitched in one layer. The cotton wool is removed after 7 days, and in only a few cases, depending on the state of the skin lining of the new ear canal, is replaced for another week. If necessary, local antibiotic eardrops can be administered.

Postoperative Problems

More than 1200 reconstructions have been performed from 1980 to 1989, and although most of the patients

FIGURE 16–3. The anterior and posterior groove and the canal wall prosthesis.

FIGURE 16–4. Width measurement instrument.

FIGURE 16–5. Depth measurement instrument.

FIGURE 16–6. Porous hydroxyapatite canal wall prosthesis.

FIGURE 16–7. The different layers on top of the reconstruction.

FIGURE 16-3

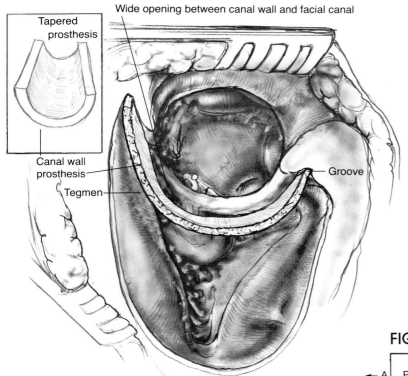

Tapered prosthesis

Canal wall prosthesis

Tegmen

Wide opening between canal wall and facial canal

Groove

FIGURE 16-6

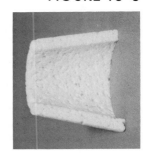

FIGURE 16-4

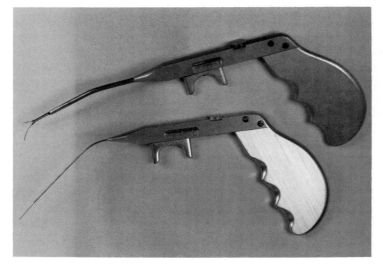

FIGURE 16-5

FIGURE 16-7

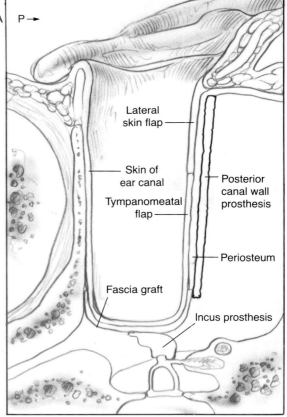

← A | P →

Lateral skin flap

Skin of ear canal

Tympanomeatal flap

Fascia graft

Posterior canal wall prosthesis

Periosteum

Incus prosthesis

have a dry ear and can swim, over the years different problems were encountered.

DEFECTS IN THE SKIN LINING. A skin defect can be present, mostly in the medial part of the canal wall, especially in cases of insufficient skin lining in the cavity or insufficient covering of a large, cranial-based periosteal flap. With high magnification, there is clearly a one-layer flat epithelium, but the borders of this skin defect can be vulnerable, and therefore the patients are not allowed to swim. In most cases, this skin defect heals gradually in several months. In cases of a persistent defect, the skin is mobilized after the total integration of the canal wall prosthesis, which is in about three quarters of a year, and then this defect can be closed with a skin graft.

DENUDED MEDIAL PART OF THE EAR CANAL PROSTHESIS. In some cases, the tympanomeatal flap is not sufficient and grows underneath the annulus of the new ear canal, leaving a denuded medial part of the canal wall prosthesis. These patients are not allowed to swim, and with local ear drops, the ear canal can be kept dry. After total integration after three quarters of a year, this medial part of the denuded canal wall prosthesis can be drilled away with a diamond drill. The skin lining comes into view and leaves a small cavity, although the mastoid tip is covered. In cases of continuous running ears postoperatively, there are different possibilities.

INFECTED LATERAL POCKET. If the meatoplasty was not wide enough, the lateral skin lining may not be in good contact with the canal wall prosthesis, and a pocket behind the lateral skin lining may be formed. This lateral pocket can then be infected, and although the medial part of the ear canal is normalized and integrated and the tympanic membrane can be completely normal without signs of infection of the middle ear and mastoid, this lateral pocket can have granulation and purulent discharge, which in most cases necessitates reoperation. Reintervention has to be done, preferably as late as possible so as not to interfere with the integration of the canal wall prosthesis after three quarters of a year.

RETRACTION AND ATELECTASIS OF THE MIDDLE EAR. Retraction and even atelectasis of the middle ear are possible. This problem results from the original disease, mostly the scar tissue. The retraction can take place anteriorly but will then be controlled and cleaned via the wide new ear canal. There is no epitympanic area. Retraction of the tympanic membrane may also occur posteriorly, through the posterior tympanotomy, but this is a very wide opening, and so far, this problem has led to recurrent cholesteatoma in

only a few patients over a postoperative period of 12 years. Patients with retractions are not allowed to swim, so as to avoid infection of this pocket.

RESIDUAL CHOLESTEATOMA. In cases of a residual cholesteatoma behind the lining of the former cavity, I advise not to reconstruct in the same stage. In cases in which I did reconstruct in the same stage, residual cholesteatoma recurred in half the cases. This problem, however, will be readily apparent because of the wide posterior tympanotomy and the wide new ear canal.

FRACTURE OF THE NEW EAR CANAL. In some cases with trauma caused by manipulation in the new ear canal, fracture of the brittle new ear canal prosthesis occurs. It takes three quarters of a year before this ear canal is completely integrated. Therefore, such trauma has to be avoided.

INFECTION OF MIDDLE EAR AND MASTOID. In cases of upper airway infections, some patients tend to develop middle ear infections again. These infections are treated in the usual way, with antibiotics, and the ear will run only temporarily. However, in some cases, a massive granulation takes place in the middle ear as well as in the mastoid. When reoperation is necessary, the canal wall prosthesis is removed. The retrieved canal wall prostheses have been examined histologically over the years and have revealed that hydroxyapatite is resistent to infection and that new bone formation has taken place, indicating the capacity of the material. If ossiculoplasty is not done in the same stage as the canal wall reconstruction, transcanal ossiculoplasty can be performed after 1 year. Via incision in the skin of the posterior canal wall, the tympanomeatal flap can be elevated in the usual way, as in the normal middle ear.

Results

Two hundred patients with a cavity had reconstruction surgery and were followed up for at least 10 years. For the reconstruction of the posterior canal wall, a canal wall prosthesis of porous hydroxyapatite was used. The indication for operation was in most cases a combination of hearing loss and running ear. A persisting running ear of the cavity was present in 77 patients (38.5 per cent), and after the reconstruction only eight patients had persistent otorrhoea (4 per cent). Recurrent otorrhoea was present in 53 patients (26.5 per cent), and postoperatively, 33 of these patients had a running ear after upper airway infections one or two times (16.5 per cent). The tympanic membrane was perforated preoperatively in 154 patients (77 per cent), and in 24 patients there was a perforation (12 per cent) postoperatively. Of the 200 patients, 25 (12.5 per cent) had a retraction pocket, but this pocket had such a large opening via the wide posterior tympanotomy that it was self-cleaning.

In 4 patients (2 per cent), reintervention was necessary because of a laterally infected new ear canal because the lateral skin of the new ear canal was not in touch with the canal wall prosthesis. Therefore, a meatoplasty had to be done to get a good alignment of the lateral skin of the new ear canal. The pocket between the skin and the new ear canal was infected and continued to drain.

Another problem was the denuded medial part of the canal wall prosthesis. In five patients, this problem resulted from the tympanomeatal flap being located behind the new ear canal; in these cases, reintervention was necessary. In the 200 patients, a residual cholesteatoma was found in 12 patients (6 per cent), and these were all cases in which I had done a reconstruction in a cavity with cholesteatoma. In this series, only one recurrent cholesteatoma (0.5 per cent) occurred, and the canal wall had to be removed. In all the cases of reintervention, the canal wall had to be removed, and histology showed living bone tissue.

The conclusion from this long-term follow-up is that it is possible to reconstruct a cavity with a new ear canal. The ear canal is ossified within three quarters of a year, and there is no resorption. The patients are allowed to swim if there is a closed tympanic membrane and no retraction pocket.

Ossiculoplasty

The most reliable way to perform an ossiculoplasty is to reconstruct the defect in the ossicular chain in such a way that the ossicular chain is moved via the tympanic membrane by its contact with the handle of the malleus and that the lever mechanism of the ossicular chain is part of the transmission, making a proper pistonlike function possible.

Different possibilities for a defect in the ossicular can be encountered:

1. Malleus present, stapes superstructure present, incus absent
2. Malleus present, stapes superstructure absent, incus absent
3. Malleus absent, stapes superstructure present
4. Malleus absent, incus absent, stapes superstructure absent, but a mobile footplate present

To overcome the defects in the ossicular chain, there are two approaches for the reconstruction: using a columella or bridging the defect in the ossicular chain.

For the columella there are two possible approaches. When the stapes superstructure is present,

a short columella from the stapes head to tympanic membrane can be used in the form of a partial ossicular replacement prosthesis. When the stapes superstructure is missing but a mobile footplate is present, a long columella connecting the mobile footplate with the tympanic membrane can be used. This is a total ossicular replacement prosthesis.

The use of a columella in the reconstruction of the ossicular chain has several disadvantages. Even with the use of a good biomaterial, the postoperative results are uncertain. The function of a columella depends on a good contact with the footplate or stapes superstructure and a good contact on a larger surface area, with the tympanic membrane. The healing process of the tympanic membrane is not predictable and can lateralize. There is also a possibility that the columella integrates in the tympanic membrane but lateralizes with no contact with the footplate or stapes. Another possibility is that the tympanic membrane will fold over the columella during time. This result is often blamed on a eustachian tube dysfunction or the implant material itself, but from animal experiments it is clear that a mobile tympanic membrane always tends to fold over something that is placed against it and even without effusion can eventually extrude the columella, even if it is made of homologous ossicles.

Therefore, bridging defects in the ossicular chain yields more predictable results with implanted ossicles that bridge such that the handle of the malleus, which is integrated in the tympanic membrane, drives the ossicular chain. Another advantage of this assembly technique is the restoration of the lever mechanism of the ossicular chain. With this technique, the function of the ossicular chain is independent of the level of the tympanic membrane, and because of good integration with the remnants of the ossicular chain, extrusion will not occur.

A set of dense hydroxyapatite prostheses is used for tympanoplasty. The dense hydroxyapatite is integrated in the ossicular chain and is covered by mucosa in a few days. The dense hydroxyapatite is not resorbed and resists infections of the middle ear.

Incus Prosthesis

In cases of a missing incus, a dense hydroxyapatite incus prosthesis is used to bridge the gap between the handle of the malleus and the mobile stapes (Fig. 16–8). The incus prosthesis has a corpus with a depression that fits on the stapes head. It overcomes the height difference between the stapes head and the handle of the malleus and a handle, which connects the stapes head with the handle of the malleus. The longest distance between stapes head and handle of the malleus is chosen, necessitating removal of half of the handle in most cases. The incus prosthesis can be shaped with a diamond drill, but the handle of the incus prosthesis can also be cut with a small chisel. At the neck of the malleus, there is a loose connective tissue connection between the tympanic membrane and the handle of the malleus, and therefore, it is easy to make a natural pocket between the tympanic membrane and the handle of the malleus, just inferior to the lateral process of the malleus. The distance between the stapes head and the handle of the malleus is measured with the width measurement instrument, and the incus prosthesis is cut to an individual length. The corpus of the incus prosthesis is placed with the niche on top of the head of the stapes, and the handle is placed on top of the handle of the malleus in the pocket, underneath the tympanic membrane (Fig. 16–9). The new incus is integrated in the ossicular chain via the contact at the malleus and stapes head. The incus prothesis can also be placed underneath the handle of the malleus, but this is a less stable position, and if there is a long distance between the stapes head and the malleus handle, the prosthesis can fall onto the promontory. The dimensions of the incus prosthesis are such that there is no contact between the annulus or facial ridge, thereby avoiding bony contact and fixation.

PROBLEMS WITH THE INCUS PROSTHESIS. It is important to establish the right distance between the stapes head and the handle of the malleus. If the handle of the incus prosthesis is too long, it may perforate the tympanic membrane. In such cases, there is a good integration of the incus prosthesis, but there can be crusts around the perforated tympanic membrane. If the handle of the incus is just on top of the malleus in the pocket, there is a good integration and no problem with the interface of the tympanic membrane and the new incus prosthesis.

Another problem can be the contact of the stapes head with the incus prosthesis: when a tendon of the stapedial muscle inserts at the top of the head of the stapes, the contact between the corpus of the incus prosthesis and the stapes head can be insufficient. Therefore, a groove must be drilled in the corpus of the incus prosthesis, or the tendon of the stapedial muscle has to be cut. A piece of gelatin sponge is placed underneath the bony annulus on top of the incus prosthesis to keep the incus prosthesis in good contact for the first few days, to secure good integration. There is a fibrous layer on top of the stapes head and mostly also a periosteum on the malleus; therefore, the contact between the incus prosthesis and the malleus and stapes head is fibrous.

To get predictable postoperative results, the stapes superstructure and the footplate must be inspected carefully. In cases of a missing anterior or posterior crus, which, in many cases, can be fibrous, it is advisable not to use an incus prosthesis but an incus stapes prosthesis between the remnants of the stapes on the footplate, in connection with the handle of the malleus. This will be described later.

In cases in which the stapes superstructure is bent to the promontory by scar tissue, the results with an incus prosthesis are also poor, because the transfer mechanism in this case is not pistonlike. In these cases, the use of an incus-stapes prosthesis is advised.

In cases of a missing lenticular process, the remnant of the long process of the incus is cut off, whereas the corpus of the incus, if mobile, is left in place. This prevents scar tissue formation in the epitympanic area. The incus prosthesis is used as a bridge between the stapes head and the handle of the malleus. The function and the mobility of the reconstruction is tested via the round window reflex.

RESULTS. In 200 patients with an incus prosthesis who have been followed up for at least 10 years, the air-bone gap closure was within 20dB in 80 per cent. Two patients had to be reoperated on because the incus prosthesis was too long and perforated the tympanic membrane. These patients were not allowed to swim, and the incus prosthesis was well integrated. The connection between the handle of the malleus and the stapes superstructure was fibrous. A shorter incus prosthesis was implanted. In ten cases of no improvement, incus prostheses were reinspected. In these cases, there was a problem with the stapes superstructure being partly fibrous or bending to the promontory, resulting in poor function. In these cases, an incus stapes prosthesis was used.

There were no extrusions, and good results remained constant. There were no signs of resorption or fixation.

Incus-stapes Prosthesis

In cases of a present malleus, an absent incus and stapes superstructure, and a present mobile footplate, an incus-stapes prosthesis of dense hydroxyapatite is used as a connection between the handle of the malleus and the mobile footplate (Fig. 16–10). The incus-stapes prosthesis consists of a shaft, with a dimension of 0.6mm of dense hydroxyapatite, and a handle. The handle is placed in the pocket, as described earlier. It is a natural pocket in the loose connective tissue between the tympanic membrane and the handle of the malleus, just inferior to the lateral process. The shaft of the incus-stapes prosthesis is placed in the middle of the mobile footplate. To secure the shaft in the middle of the footplate, gelatin sponge can be used. It is also possible to cut a small shaft of gelatin film. The shaft of gelatin film around the incus-stapes pros-

FIGURE 16–8

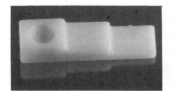

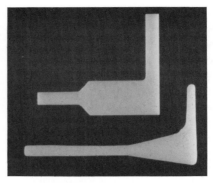

FIGURE 16–10

FIGURE 16–9

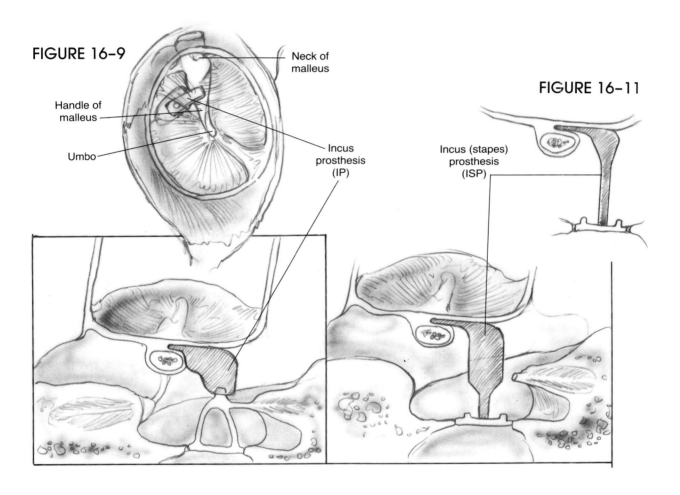

Neck of malleus

Handle of malleus

Umbo

Incus prosthesis (IP)

FIGURE 16–11

Incus (stapes) prosthesis (ISP)

FIGURE 16–8. Incus prosthesis of dense hydroxyapatite.

FIGURE 16–9. Schematic drawing of incus prosthesis between stapes head and malleus.

FIGURE 16–10. Incus-stapes prosthesis.

FIGURE 16–11. Incus-stapes prosthesis between footplate and malleus.

thesis is pushed in the oval window niche, keeping the incus-stapes prosthesis in the center of the footplate. There is no need for an interface between the prosthesis and the footplate, and only in cases of a hypermobile or fractured footplate is a vein graft placed on top of the footplate. The handle is cut to an individual length, and the incus-stapes prosthesis stands stable between the handle of the malleus and the footplate (Fig. 16–11). The mucosa on the footplate is not removed, resulting in a fibrous contact between the hydroxyapatite shaft and the footplate. A piece of gelatin sponge is put underneath the bony annulus to secure a good adaptation for the first days. The bioactive material induces a good integration within a few weeks. The mobility of the new ossicular chain is tested via the round window reflex. In cases of a remnant of a mobile stapes superstructure, an incus-stapes prosthesis with a 0.6mm shaft can be easily placed between the anterior and the posterior crus, securing the place of the incus-stapes prosthesis. In cases of overhang of the facial nerve, the shaft can also be drilled in a smaller dimension. A piece of gelatin film is placed between the incus-stapes prosthesis and the facial nerve.

RESULTS. Two hundred patients with an incus-stapes prothesis have been followed up for at least 10 years. In 118 patients, this prosthesis was used as an assembly that connected the malleus and the footplate. The air-bone gap closure was within 20dB in 74 per cent, and no improvement was found in 16 per cent. There was no extrusion in this long follow-up period.

Once a good result was established, it remained constant during the entire 10-year observation period; no resorption or fixation took place.

Since 1982, the incus-stapes prosthesis has also been used as a columella in 82 cases of a missing handle of the malleus. In these cases, the results were less good: air-bone gap closure within 20dB in 34 per cent, and no improvement in 64.7 per cent. Extrusion was observed in 4.7 per cent. The extrusion took place via the following mechanism. The tympanic membrane gradually folded over the columella. There was no erosion or granulation of the tympanic membrane, but finally the incus-stapes prosthesis was extruded. The experience with this incus-stapes prosthesis as a columella indicated that either the design of the prosthesis was not ideal for the columella technique or the columella gives less favorable results. Therefore, a tympanic membrane–malleus prothesis is preferred in cases of an absent malleus.

Total Alloplastic Middle Ear

In cases of a missing handle of the malleus, an incus or incus-stapes prothesis, which can bridge the gap in the ossicular chain, cannot be used. Therefore, the concept of the total homologous implant, including tympanic membrane, malleus, incus, and stapes, was used to make a total alloplastic middle ear (Fig. 16–12). In 1983, ten total middle ears were implanted in which the ossicular chain was connected to the canal wall with a joint. For biomechanical and biologic reasons, this situation was not ideal. It was shown that a tympanic membrane malleus prosthesis was necessary to obtain a complete equivalent of the normal-functioning middle ear. Therefore, in vitro and in vivo studies were performed to find a degradable bioactive polymer to serve as a substitute for the middle layer of the tympanic membrane and for the integration of the handle of the malleus. Myringoplasty yielded good results with fascia, but for the development of the tympanic membrane–malleus prosthesis, a soft tissue replacement biomaterial was necessary.

In vivo studies and long-term animal studies resulted in the selection of a new biomaterial for this purpose, a degradable copolymer (Polyactive). Polyactive is the first bioactive polymer showing a direct bond with the surrounding tissue. Exposed to bone, it enhances new bone formation, and in soft tissue, for instance in the tympanic membrane, it serves as a scaffold for the ingrowth of collagen and elastic fibers, forming a good middle layer. Polyactive has been used as an underlay, and a tympanic membrane–malleus prosthesis was developed to use in a total artificial middle ear, which includes the use of a canal wall prosthesis, a tympanic membrane malleus prosthesis as an underlay under the remnants of the tympanic membrane, and an incus or incus-stapes prosthesis connecting the stapes superstructure or the mobile footplate with the handle of the malleus in the artificial tympanic membrane.

This technique makes total reconstruction of an empty middle ear possible. There are several advantages to the combination of these prostheses. The eradication can be done in the first stage without any concessions to the reconstruction. All diseased tissue can be removed, and in a second stage, even an empty middle ear cavity can be reconstructed. The tympanic membrane–malleus prosthesis is placed underneath the remnants of the tympanic membrane in such a way that the pocket between the artificial tympanic membrane and the malleus is placed superiorly and in the same anatomic relation with the cochleariform process. The advantage of the canal wall prosthesis is that the level of the annulus can be chosen as far lateral as possible, thereby permitting the formation of a wide middle ear mastoid cleft. Then the incus or incus-stapes prosthesis is placed on the stapes or the footplate, as described before. It connects the new artificial handle of the malleus with stapes superstructure or footplate. With gelatin sponge, the prosthesis

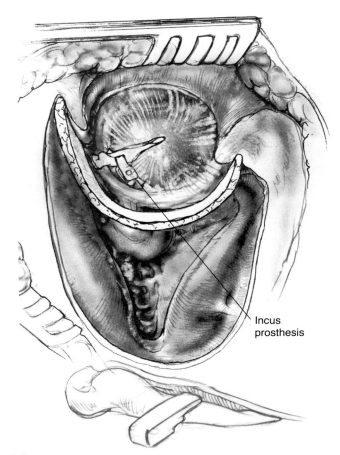

Incus
prosthesis

FIGURE 16-12. Total alloplastic middle ear.

is stabilized for the first few days, and gelatin film secures the drainage from the mastoid–middle ear cleft to the eustachian tube. It will take several weeks before the epithelium has completely covered the tympanic membrane material, and degradation of the new tympanic membrane scaffold takes place in half a year, and remodeling in collagen and elastic fibers continues in that period. The main problem with the new tympanic membrane material is infection. If a purulent middle ear infection occurs in the first month, this material will degrade even faster, and being a polymer, it will have more reaction.

RESULTS

In 20 patients in whom an empty cavity was reconstructed with a total artificial middle ear, tympanic membrane closure occurred in 80 per cent of the patients with sufficient epithelium, and an air-bone gap closure within 20dB occurred in 45 per cent.

Long term results, however, have to prove the utility of this new material. However, the concept of the assembly and the concept of a total middle ear, as was done with a total homologous middle ear, has proven to be a good concept and can be reproduced with a total artificial middle ear.

SUMMARY

I introduced hydroxyapatite for the reconstruction of the bony defects in the middle ear, and over the past 12 years, it has proved its usefulness. It is the mineral matrix of bone and it can be used in different forms, depending on the defect to be bridged and the demands of remodeling and resorption. This flexibility makes different prosthetic designs possible. It is my practice to stage eradication and reconstruction if cholesteatoma is present. With the new prostheses, we are no longer depending on the former anatomy. On the contrary, a new wide middle ear cleft can be made with a new round ear canal in which the epitympanic area is taken into the new ear canal, thereby avoiding future problems. Obliteration is not ideal, because of the possibility of burying diseased tissue that induces uncontrollable problems. For new middle ear function, it is also good to have a wide middle ear–mastoid cleft. For the reconstruction of the ossicular chain, the assembly technique gives the most predictable results. The hydroxyapatite ossicles bridge the gap in the ossicular chain, so that the tympanic membrane drives the ossicular chain via the handle of the malleus. The ossicular chain is moved with a lever mechanism and a pistonlike function on the footplate.

For the total empty middle ear, an equivalent of the total homologous middle ear implant was designed. A soft tissue replacement material for the tympanic membrane–malleus prosthesis was developed. This material is still in an experimental phase, although in vitro and in vivo studies and 2-year clinical studies are very promising. If the principles we learned from the homologous implants are used, more predictable and uniform ways of reconstruction are possible. The development of new materials in otology gives new possibilities for the future.

References

1. Jansen C: The combined approach for tympanoplasty (report of 10 years' experience). J Laryngol 82: 776–793, 1968.
2. Grote JJ: Tympanoplasty with calcium phosphate. Am J Otol 6: 269–271, 1985.
3. Smyth GDL: Chronic Ear Disease. New York, Churchill Livingstone, 1980.
4. Homsy CA: Biocompatibility in selection of materials for implantation. J Biomed Mater Res 4: 341–356, 1970.
5. Austin DF: Ossicular reconstruction. Arch Otolaryngol Head Neck Surg 94: 525–535, 1971.
6. Brackmann DE, Sheehy JL: Tympanoplasty with TORPS and PORPS. Laryngoscope 89: 108–114, 1979.
7. Bakker D, van Blitterswijk CA, Hesseling SC, et al.: The behavior of alloplastic tympanic membranes in *Staphylococcus aureus*–induced ear infection. II. Morphological study of epithelial reactions. J Biomed Mater Res 24: 809–828, 1990.
8. Grote JJ, Bakker D, Hesseling SC, van Blitterswijk CA: New alloplastic tympanic membrane material. Am J Otol 12(5): 329–335, 1991.
9. Jahnke K, Schmidt C: Histological studies on the suitability of Macor ceramic implants. *In* Grote JJ (ed): Biomaterials in Otology. Boston, Marinus Nijhoff Publishers, 1984, pp 74–79.

10. Reck R: Bioactive glass-ceramics in ear surgery: animal studies and clinical results. Laryngoscope 94: (Suppl 33): 1–54, 1984.
11. van Blitterswijk CA, Koerten HK, Bakker D, et al.: Biodegradation-dependent trace element accumulation: a study on calcium phosphate ceramics and polymers. *In* Wiliams KR, Lesser THJ (eds): Interface Medicine Mechanics. Trowbridge, England, Dotesios Printers, 1990, pp 110–119.
12. van Blitterswijk CA, Grote JJ: Biological performance of ceramics during infection and inflammation. Crit Rev Biocompatibil 5: 23–43, 1989.
13. van Blitterswijk CA, Grote JJ, Koerten HK, et al.: The biological performance of calcium phosphate ceramics in an infected implantation site. III. Biological performance of B-whitlockite in the non-infected rat middle ear. J Biomed Mater Res 20: 1197–1218, 1986.
14. van Blitterswijk CA, de Groot K, Daems WT, et al.: The biological performance of calcium phosphate ceramics in an infected implantation site. I. Biological performance of hydroxyapatite during *Staphylococcus aureus* infection. J Biomed Mater Res 20: 989–1002, 1986.
15. van Blitterswijk CA, Bakker D, Grote JJ, Daems WT: The biological performance of calcium phosphate ceramics in an infected implantation site. II. Biological performance of hydroxyapatite during short term infection. J Biomed Mater Res 20: 1003–1006, 1986.
16. van Blitterswijk CA, Grote JJ, Kuijpers W, et al.: Macropore tissue ingrowth: a quantitative and qualitative study on hydroxyapatite ceramic. Biomaterials 7: 137–143, 1986.
17. van Blitterswijk CA, Kuijpers W, Daems WT, Grote JJ: Epithelial reactions to hydroxyapatite: an in vivo and in vitro study. Acta Otolaryngol (Stockh) 101: 231–241, 1986.
18. Grote JJ, van Blitterswijk CA: Reconstruction of the posterior auditory canal wall with a hydroxyapatite prosthesis. Ann Otol Rhinol Laryngol 95(Suppl 123): 6–9, 1986.
19. Grote JJ, Kuijpers W, de Groot K: Use of sintered hydroxyapatite in middle ear surgery. ORL J Otorhinolaryngol Relat Spec 43: 248–254, 1981.
20. Grote JJ, van Blitterswijk CA, Kuijpers W: Reconstruction of the middle ear with hydroxyapatite implants. Ann Otol Rhinol Laryngol 95 (Suppl 123): 1–12, 1986.
21. Grote JJ: Tympanoplasty with calcium phosphate. Am J Otol 6: 269–271, 1985.
22. Grote JJ: Reconstruction of the ossicular chain with hydroxyapatite prostheses. Am J Otol 8: 396–401, 1987.

17

Surgery of Acute Infections and Their Complications

J. GAIL NEELY, M.D., F.A.C.S.

DEFINITION

Complications of suppurative ear disease, acute or chronic, manifest acutely and are medical and surgical emergencies. They are defined as a spread of infection beyond the confines of the pneumatized spaces and the attendant mucosa.

Complications are classified into two groups, aural and intracranial. Aural complications are 1) mastoiditis, 2) petrositis, 3) labyrinthitis, and 4) facial paralysis. Intracranial complications are 1) extradural abscess or granulation tissue, 2) dural venous sinus thrombophlebitis, 3) brain abscess, 4) otitic hydrocephalus, 5) subdural abscess, and 6) meningitis (Fig. 17–1).[1, 2]

ETIOLOGY AND PATHOGENESIS

Acute and chronic suppurative otitis media are common diseases, yet complications are relatively rare; this fact makes identifying the exact mechanisms involved in the formation of a complication very difficult.

Obstruction of the aditus ad antrum, congenitally preformed pathways through the oval or round window, or acquired pathways from fractures or chronic erosive infection, granulation tissue, or cholesteatoma, especially virulent organisms such as type B *Haemophilus influenzae,* and synergistic pathogenicity resulting from anaerobic organism microenvironmental changes may all play a role in the pathogenesis of complications (Fig. 17–2).[3–5] Clinically, however, several important observations have been made that help alert the physician to the possible occurrence of a complication and may reflect some of the pathobiology.

Signs and symptoms of possible impending complications are 1) persistent acute infection for 2 weeks, 2) recurrent symptoms of infection within 2 weeks, 3) acute, fetid exacerbation of chronic infection, 4) fetid discharge during treatment, 5) *Haemophilus influenzae,* type B, or anaerobes cultured from the ear, or 6) fever in the presence of a chronically perforated tympanic membrane, with or without cholesteatoma.

CLINICAL PRESENTATION

When the possibility exists that the patient has a complication from suppurative ear disease, the complete list of the ten complications and the fact that more than one complication is most likely can be somewhat overwhelming. Fortunately, the complications tend to manifest in some obvious or predictable clinical patterns.[5]

The three most obvious complications are facial paralysis, labyrinthitis, and meningitis. Facial paralysis is obvious, and if it occurs as a result of acute infection, it is usually the only complication. If it occurs as a result of cholesteatoma, a horizontal canal fistula may also exist.

Labyrinthitis presents in an obvious fashion, manifesting as ipsilateral sensorineural hearing loss, nystagmus toward the contralateral side, and vertigo. It is classified according to what enters the perilymphatic space: serous labyrinthitis toxins, suppurative labyrinthitis bacteria, or chronic labyrinthitis soft tissue, such as cholesteatoma. Suppurative labyrinthitis destroys all the hearing and rapidly progresses to meningitis. Labyrinthitis with some hearing, resulting from acute infection, is usually serous and isolated without other complications. Labyrinthitis with hearing, resulting from a cholesteatoma, may well be associated with a labyrinthine fistula of the horizontal canal and a dehiscence of the fallopian canal, with or without a facial paralysis.

Meningitis also presents in an obvious fashion. Meningitis associated with acute otitis media almost always is the result of hematogenous dissemination, and other complications are rare. Meningitis associated with chronic suppurative otitis media is usually the result of a dehiscence in the dura that allows continuity between an extradural abscess and the cerebrospinal fluid.

Less obvious complications follow. Subdural abscesses are extremely rare, usually devastatingly obvious, and easily seen by magnetic resonance imaging (MRI). If there is any doubt that a catastrophic intracranial lesion exists, the chance of a subdural abscess being present is remote. Otitic hydrocephalus characteristically presents with headache, some degree of lethargy, and severe papilledema. Almost without exception, otitic hydrocephalus is associated with occlusive sigmoid sinus thrombophlebitis and extradural abscess. Petrositis presents with retro-orbital pain; however, the patient may not volunteer this symptom. It is crucial to ask about retro-orbital pain to be assured of its absence. Petrositis is rarely, if ever, present without mastoiditis; however, intracranial complications are more frequent with petrositis.

The remaining four complications of suppurative ear disease are mastoiditis, extradural abscess or granulation tissue, dural venous sinus thrombophlebitis, and brain abscess. Unfortunately, these can be very silent, but extremely serious. Fortunately, they occur together in predictable patterns. Mastoiditis may occur alone but often results in a silent accumulation of extradural abscess or granulation tissue. The extradural infection may occur, in the case of cholesteatoma, in the middle fossa at the tegmen, but it characteristically occurs along the extraluminal surface of the lat-

INTRACRANIAL
COMPLICATIONS

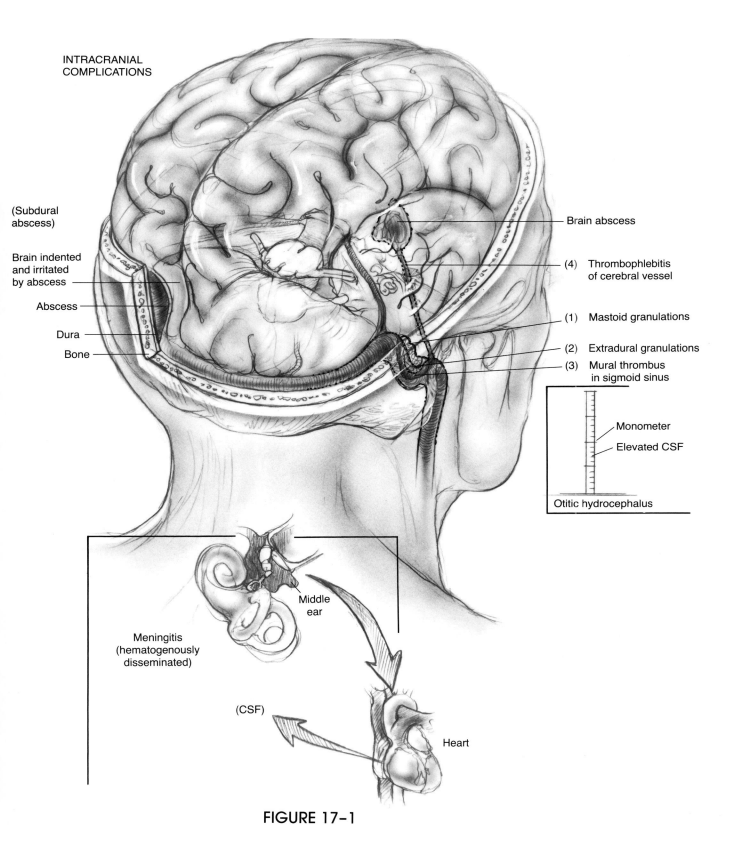

(Subdural
abscess)

Brain indented
and irritated
by abscess

Abscess

Dura

Bone

Brain abscess

(4) Thrombophlebitis
of cerebral vessel

(1) Mastoid granulations

(2) Extradural granulations

(3) Mural thrombus
in sigmoid sinus

Monometer

Elevated CSF

Otitic hydrocephalus

Middle
ear

Meningitis
(hematogenously
disseminated)

(CSF)

Heart

FIGURE 17-1

eral wall of the sigmoid sinus, creating an often-silent, nonoccluding phlebitis of the sinus wall and an induced mural thrombus, sigmoid sinus thrombophlebitis. In every case of suspected or operated mastoiditis, extradural granulation tissue and sigmoid sinus thrombophlebitis should be sought, preoperatively and intraoperatively. Brain abscess occurs as a result of retrograde thrombophlebitis of cerebral or cerebellar veins that are tributary to the inflamed sigmoid sinus or other adjacent dural sinuses. Brain abscesses have four stages:

1. Invasion stage, the initial onset of cerebritis. This stage creates vague symptoms of mild headache, lethargy, and malaise that last several days then resolve.
2. Localization stage, the stage of quiescence and latency. This stage is totally silent for weeks.
3. Enlargement stage, in which most abscesses manifest with seizures or focal neurologic signs.
4. Termination stage, in which the abscess catastrophically ruptures into the ventricle or subarachnoid space. Brain abscesses are very silent, take weeks from onset to be detectable, even with imaging, and can be devastating. It is prudent to look for brain abscesses in cases of mastoiditis initially and again 3 to 4 weeks later (Fig. 17–3). Thus, the pathophysiologic and diagnostic key to occult complications is mastoiditis.

Without the use of, and compliance with, adequate antibiotic dosages and durations and careful medical care, the classic presentation of acute coalescent mastoiditis with an associated subperiosteal abscess characterizes the clinical presentation of mastoiditis.[6] Masked mastoiditis, in patients with what seems to be adequate care, however, is much harder to diagnose, can be much more devastating, and is more often associated with intracranial complications.[7, 8] Patients with any of the signs and symptoms of impending complications, particularly with a recurrence of deep, not necessarily severe, pain may have masked mastoiditis. If bone destruction is present, the diagnosis is made. However, masked mastoiditis may exist without bone destruction being apparent. If pain persists, despite adequate, culture-guided, antibiotic administration, surgical exploration and treatment are indicated.

DIAGNOSIS

The most powerful, rapid, efficient, and useful diagnostic tools for diagnosis are the history and physical examination. In the history, look for

1. Symptoms suggesting impending complications
2. Symptoms of retro-orbital or deep, boring head pain
3. Symptoms of lethargy, headache, or both, currently and within the past 2 months

In the physical examination, look for

1. Signs suggesting impending complications
2. Signs diagnostic of obvious complications
3. Signs of catastrophic neurologic disease
4. Funduscopic examination for papilledema

If none of these signs are present, the chances are remote that a complication exists. The most important error in the investigation is a poor history with little attention paid to the details of previous symptoms and the associated time courses. Another error is to assume that the organisms cultured from the ear canal drainage accurately reflect the organism causing the complication; aspiration and intraoperative cultures from the complication and the involved tissues of the ear best reflect the responsible pathogens.

When a complication is suspected, high-resolution computed tomography of the temporal bone and associated brain, with and without infusion, is indicated. Computed tomography allows a good look at the bone and a reasonable look at the intracranial structures. If bone is eroded over the sigmoid sinus or at the tegmen, MRI is indicated to get a better appreciation of possible extradural, intradural, subdural, and intracerebral granulation; edema; and abscess. If mastoiditis, and particularly sigmoid sinus phlebitis, is surgically proved, repeat MRI is indicated 3 to 4 weeks postoperatively to detect the development of an occult brain abscess.

Complications are medical and surgical concerns. Careful surgical observations, through thin bone, of the dura at the tegmen, the sigmoid sinus, and the facial nerve are crucial for complete diagnosis (Fig. 17–4).

Diagnoses are made from the history, physical examination, and surgical exploration. Imaging is crucial to observe brain abscesses and subdural abscesses, but reliance on imaging modalities at the expense of these three elements, carefully done, will lead to serious errors.

TREATMENT

The treatment of all complications is admission to the hospital and adequate use of antibiotics that are culture guided from the ear and the complication. The surgical treatment is outlined below.

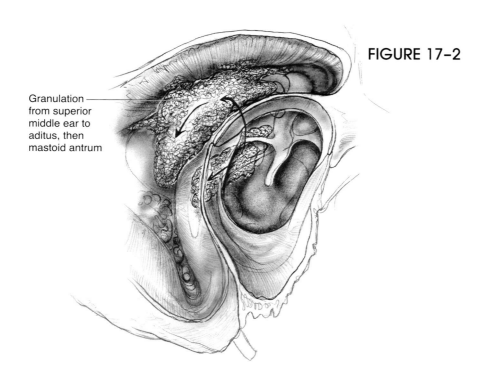

FIGURE 17-2

Granulation from superior middle ear to aditus, then mastoid antrum

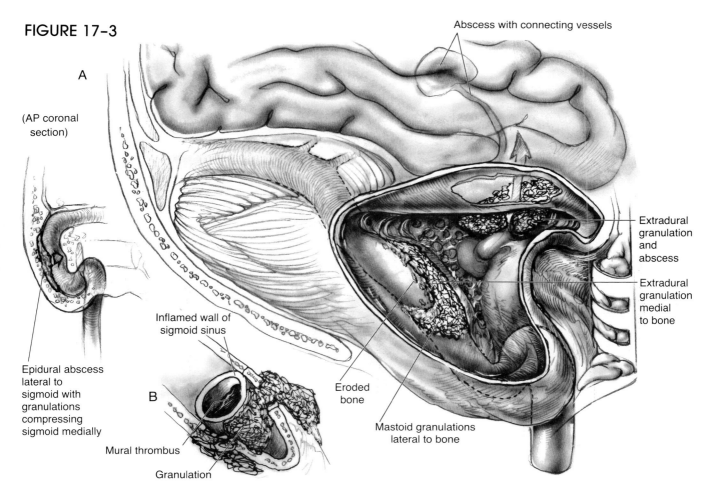

FIGURE 17-3

A

(AP coronal section)

Abscess with connecting vessels

Extradural granulation and abscess

Extradural granulation medial to bone

Epidural abscess lateral to sigmoid with granulations compressing sigmoid medially

Inflamed wall of sigmoid sinus

B

Eroded bone

Mural thrombus

Granulation

Mastoid granulations lateral to bone

The treatment of acute coalescent mastoiditis and masked mastoiditis, with or without subperiosteal abscess, is wide myringotomy, complete canal wall up mastoidectomy, and wide facial recess approach from the mastoid into the middle ear. The aditus ad antrum is obstructed and cannot be adequately maintained open. Sometimes the granulation tissue is severe in the middle ear and mastoid, and symptoms suggest petrositis; in these cases, total resection of the tympanic membrane with careful maintenance of the ossicles in situ and resection of the posterosuperior canal wall allows adequate drainage. Reconstruction of the tympanic membrane can be done at a later date in a healed ear (Fig. 17–5).

The treatment of most chronic mastoiditis is the same as for cases of chronic suppurative otitis media, with or without cholesteatoma. Most of these cases improve with reconstruction of the middle ear at the same setting, that is, with canal wall up or down procedures (see Chapters 18 and 19). Chronic mastoiditis is a diagnostic dilemma; the primary way to establish the diagnosis is to intraoperatively identify granulation tissue–induced erosion of bone, usually over the sigmoid sinus.

In all cases undergoing mastoidectomy for suppurative disease, inspection of the dura of the tegmen, sigmoid sinus, and the facial nerve through thin bone is crucial. Otherwise, granulation tissue in the middle and posterior fossa and along the facial nerve may go unrecognized and untreated.

The treatment of petrositis may require two stages, but the second stage is usually not necessary. The first stage is a radical mastoidectomy, or the modification of the radical procedure mentioned earlier in which the intact ossicular chain is left intact, the drum is removed, and the five tracts to the petrous apex are opened as far as possible.[9] The second stage, if the first doesn't resolve the infection, is a middle-fossa approach to the total exenteration of disease in the petrous apex and in the perilabyrinthine cells. This dissection is combined with the previous lateral approach, and all pneumatized spaces in the temporal bone are removed, sparing the vital structures of the inner ear, facial nerve, carotid artery, jugular bulb, sigmoid, and the contents of the internal auditory canal. The cavity is left open (Fig. 17–6).

The surgical treatment of labyrinthitis in acute infection is confined to myringotomy. The treatment of labyrinthitis in chronic infection, with or without cholesteatoma, is tympanoplasty and mastoidectomy following the surgeon's usual preference. If a fistula is identified in the cochlea, it is usually better to leave the cholesteatoma matrix on the fistula, close the ear, and return to remove it when the ear is well healed and sterile. This is a good technique for wide, deep fistulas in the vestibular labyrinth as well. For narrow, shallow fistulas in the semicircular canals, the cholesteatoma matrix may be carefully removed and the fascia placed over the fistula; if the matrix appears to be attached to the membranous labyrinth, dissection should cease and the matrix left, to be removed later. An important point to re-emphasize is that one cannot be sure prospectively if the labyrinthitis is toxic (serous) or suppurative nor can one be comfortable that a serous labyrinthitis may not become suppurative. Suppurative labyrinthitis is soon associated with meningitis. Thus, hospitalization and intravenous antibiotics need to be continued until the infection has been eradicated.

The surgical treatment of facial paralysis from acute infection is myringotomy. If subacute or chronic infection is present, mastoidectomy to eradicate disease and to explore the fallopian canal for invasive granulation tissue is indicated; this exploration can be done by thinning the bone of the canal to allow observation of the contents. Decompression may not be worthwhile. Opening the sheath and exposing the nerve in the face of infection is probably contraindicated. If invasive granulation tissue is found within the canal, the canal should be opened for at least the length of the extent of the granulation. Extraneural sheath granulations may be removed, but no attempt should be made to remove granulations from within the sheath; this tissue tends to infiltrate between fibers, and attempts to remove it will result in fiber destruction.

The treatment of preoperatively or intraoperatively discovered extradural granulation tissue or abscess is the wide exposure of the abnormal dura. Careful attempts to bluntly remove excess granulation tissue without penetrating the dura are indicated; removing every bit of the granulations is unnecessary. Abscesses should be completely drained into the mastoid. If an abscess is encountered, the canal wall should be taken down so that complete drainage is assured (Fig. 17–7).

Dural venous thrombophlebitis rarely requires additional surgical treatment beyond a complete mastoidectomy and management of the extradural granulations or abscess. In the rare case in which classic preoperative spiking fever and chills precede the discovery of a completely solidified sinus, careful opening of the sinus to explore for an intraluminal abscess may be indicated. Usually, a fibrotic, nonabscessing mural thrombus is found, for which no further intraluminal work should be done. If an easily identifiable intraluminal abscess is found, it should be drained into the mastoid. Bleeding can be controlled with an extraluminal piece of Surgicel, which is left in place at the conclusion of the procedure; a piece of fascia may be additionally placed lateral to this patch. The use of anticoagulants and thrombolytics is not usually required; their use is still somewhat controversial in

FIGURE 17-4

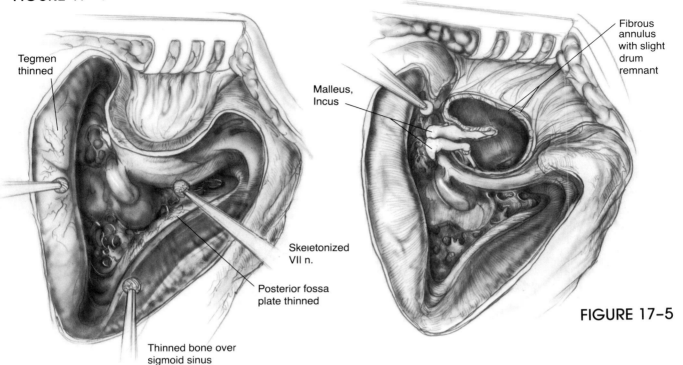

Tegmen
thinned

Skeletonized
VII n.

Posterior fossa
plate thinned

Thinned bone over
sigmoid sinus

A PETROSITIS—Lateral approach—Tracts to petrous apex
First stage

Malleus,
Incus

Fibrous
annulus
with slight
drum
remnant

FIGURE 17-5

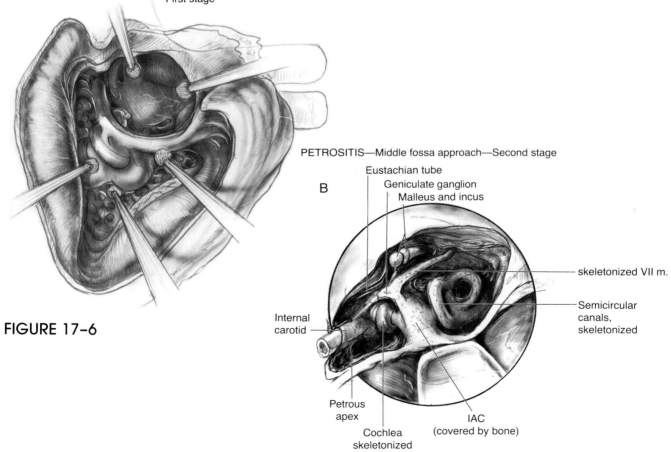

FIGURE 17-6

PETROSITIS—Middle fossa approach—Second stage

B

Eustachian tube
Geniculate ganglion
Malleus and incus

skeletonized VII m.

Semicircular
canals,
skeletonized

Internal
carotid

Petrous
apex

Cochlea
skeletonized

IAC
(covered by bone)

FIGURE 17-7

FIGURE 17-8

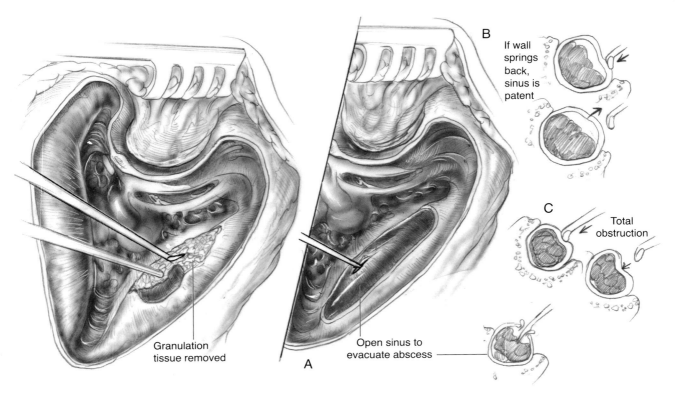

Granulation
tissue removed

Open sinus to
evacuate abscess

A

B
If wall
springs
back,
sinus is
patent

C
Total
obstruction

REMOVAL OF DEEP BRAIN ABSCESS

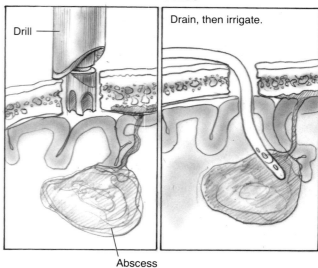

Drill

Drain, then irrigate.

Abscess

FIGURE 17-9

A INTERNAL AUDITORY CANAL (Lateral wall dehiscent in IAC)

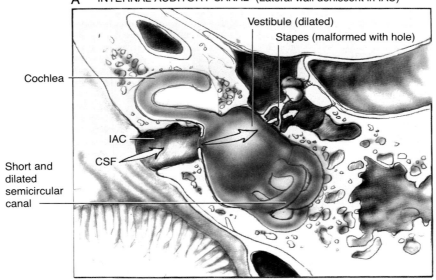

Vestibule (dilated)

Stapes (malformed with hole)

Cochlea

IAC

CSF

Short and
dilated
semicircular
canal

B INTRALABYRINTHINE OBLITERATION

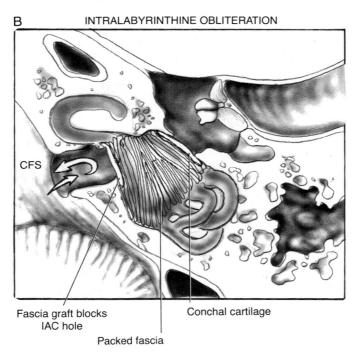

CFS

Fascia graft blocks
IAC hole

Conchal cartilage

Packed fascia

FIGURE 17-10

intracranial lesions. If they have a role, it is in cases associated with otitic hydrocephalus (Fig. 17–8).

The treatment of brain abscess is under the guidance of neurosurgery. When the abscess is under control, the ear should have surgery. Aspiration for culture through a sterile field distant to the ear with or without intra-abscess instillation of antibiotics is not always done; systemic antibiotics may be the only treatment required to resolve the brain abscess. Without a culture, however, the offending organism or organisms are unknown. Except for aspiration, these abscesses are usually not openly drained or resected, unless they fail to resolve. The ear usually can be operated on within several days of diagnosis. Mastoidectomy, a canal wall up or down procedure, and the management of extradural granulation tissue is usually the treatment required. Rarely is the brain abscess in direct continuity with the ear; if it is and it spontaneously drains into the mastoid, it can be drained through the ear (Fig. 17–9).

The surgical treatment of otitic hydrocephalus is the management of mastoiditis, extradural granulations, and sigmoid sinus thrombophlebitis. Care must be taken to follow up the patient's vision with an ophthalmologist and the long-term care of intracranial hypertension with a neurosurgeon or neurologist. Techniques of management of intracranial thrombophlebitis and chronic intracranial hypertension are controversial and rapidly evolutionary; optimal treatment is provided by a local team of expert consultants involved with the case. Ventricular shunting and optic nerve decompression may be required.[10] The main point of treatment is careful management of the ear and chronic intracranial hypertension. Blindness or brain herniation are the serious concerns.[11]

The treatment of a subdural abscess occurs under the guidance of neurosurgery. The surgical control of the mastoiditis, extradural granulations or abscess, and sigmoid sinus thrombophlebitis is crucial for recovery. Craniotomy and drainage of the subdural abscess are sometimes the neurosurgical treatments of choice. The two surgeries may be done at the same time or sequentially. Subdural abscesses are extremely rare from suppurative ear disease, tend to be very severe, and may have direct connections through the infected dura. My very limited experience with these lesions has sensitized me and my neurosurgical colleagues toward a very aggressive approach.

The treatment of meningitis from acute ear infection is predominantly medical, except for myringotomy. If a severe Mondini deformity with dehiscence of the medial wall of the vestibule is present on the infected side, intralabyrinthine obliteration is required after recovery of the meningitis (Fig. 17–10).[3]

Meningitis from chronic ear infection is a surgical and medical emergency because of the probability of a dehiscence in the dura and an ever-increasing flow of pus directly from the ear into the subarachnoid space. Radical mastoidectomy with exploration of all dural surfaces directly or through thin bone is necessary. When the extradural abscess is evacuated, care should be taken to identify the dural defect. When the defect is found, it may be repaired with fascia placed intradurally and extradurally. Wedging or suturing the graft is usually possible. Postoperative cerebrospinal fluid leak is often present but tends to close as the meningitis and excessive production of cerebrospinal fluid resolves.

SUMMARY

A detailed and time-specific history and physical examination are the most powerful tools of diagnosis. Imaging is the only way to detect brain abscess and subdural abscess. The complete diagnosis depends on carefully done intraoperative observations.

Complications of suppurative ear disease manifest in obvious or predictable patterns that help guide preoperative diagnosis and intraoperative diagnosis and treatment. Treatment of complications requires hospitalization, culture-specific intravenous antibiotics, if possible, and expedient surgical exenteration of the ear disease.

References

1. Neely JG: Complications of Suppurative Otitis Media, Part I: Aural Complications. A Self-Instructional Package from the Committee on Continuing Education in Otolaryngology. Washington, D.C., American Academy of Otolaryngology, a Division of American Academy of Ophthalmology and Otolaryngology, 1978.
2. Neely JG: Complications of Suppurative Otitis Media, Part II: Intracranial Complications. A Self-Instructional Package from the Committee on Continuing Education in Otolaryngology. American Academy of Otolaryngology–Head and Neck Surgery, Revised 1983.
3. Neely JG: Classification of spontaneous cerebrospinal fluid middle ear effusion: Review of 49 cases. Otolaryngol Head Neck Surg 93(5): 625–634, 1985.
4. Neely JG: Complications of temporal bone infections. In Cummings CW, et al. (eds): Otolaryngology–Head and Neck Surgery, Vol 4, 2nd ed. St. Louis, CV Mosby, 1993, pp 2840–2864.
5. Neely JG: Intratemporal and intracranial complications of otitis media. In Byron Bailey (ed): Head and Neck Surgery–Otolaryngology. Philadelphia, JB Lippincott, 1993, pp 1607–1622.
6. Hawkins DB, Dru D: Mastoid subperiosteal abscess. Arch Otolaryngol 109: 369, 1983.
7. Holt GR, Gates GA: Masked mastoiditis. Laryngoscope 93: 1034–1037, 1983.
8. Bluestone CD, Klein JO: Intratemporal complications and sequelae of otitis media. In Bluestone CD, Stool SE (eds): Pediatric Otolaryngology, Vol 1. Philadelphia, WB Saunders, 1983, pp 513–564.
9. Mawson SR: Diseases of the Ear, 3rd ed. Baltimore, Williams & Wilkins, 1974.
10. Horton JC, Seiff SR, Pitts LH, et al.: Decompression of the optic nerve sheath for vision-threatening papilledema caused by dural sinus occlusion. Neurosurgery 31(2): 203–211, 1992.
11. Gower DJ, Baker AL, Bell WO, Ball MR: Contraindications to lumbar puncture as defined by computed cranial tomography. J Neurol Neurosurg Psychiatry 50(8): 1071–1074, 1987.

18

Mastoidectomy: The Intact Canal Wall Procedure

JAMES L. SHEEHY, M.D.

There are two ways of handling mastoidectomy in cases of cholesteatoma. The canal wall down (CWD) technique will be discussed by Smyth and Toner in Chapter 19. The canal wall up (CWU) technique is dealt with here.

This chapter will cover not only the technique for CWU but also the evolution of the technique, controversies in regard to CWU versus CWD, indications for CWD procedures, a discussion of the facial nerve in surgery of chronic ear disease, and management of the labyrinthine fistula.

DEFINITIONS

The common mastoid operations performed for chronic ear infections are listed below. Technical surgical variations peculiar to each surgeon do not alter the fundamental classification.[1]

Radical Mastoidectomy

Radical mastoidectomy is an operation performed to eradicate middle ear and mastoid disease in which the mastoid antrum, tympanum, and external auditory canal are converted into a common cavity exteriorized through the external meatus. This operation involves removal of the tympanic membrane and ossicular remnants, with exception of the stapes, and does not involve any reconstructive or grafting procedure. Frequently, the surgeon will place a plug of soft tissue in the tubotympanum or may even lay soft tissue over the middle ear to assist in healing, but this does not alter the name of the procedure.

Modified Radical Mastoidectomy

Modified radical mastoidectomy is an operation performed to eradicate mastoid disease, in which the epitympanum, mastoid antrium, and external auditory canal are converted into a common cavity exteriorized through the external meatus. This technique differs from the radical operation in that the tympanic membrane, or remnants thereof, and ossicular remnants are retained to preserve hearing. (This operation *does not involve any reconstructive procedure.*)

Tympanoplasty with Mastoidectomy

Tympanoplasty with mastoidectomy is an operation performed to eradicate disease in the middle ear and mastoid and to reconstruct the hearing mechanism, with or without tympanic membrane grafting.

There are essentially three variations of this operation. The classic type of procedure involves permanent exteriorization of the epitympanum and mastoid,

a CWD procedure. One may do a CWD procedure and then obliterate the cavity or reconstruct the external auditory canal. Finally, there is the CWU procedure, the intact canal wall tympanoplasty with mastoidectomy, which is the subject of this chapter.

EVOLUTION OF TECHNIQUE

Prior to the mid 1950s there were essentially two operations for chronic otitis media with cholesteatoma: radical mastoidectomy and modified radical mastoidectomy. These are classic operations that are still indicated at times. Their object is to create a safe ear, by exteriorizing the disease, and preserve hearing, if possible.

When tympanoplasty was first introduced by Wullstein[2] and Zollner[3] exenteration of the mastoid was the rule. Two problems eventually became apparent. Moisture in the cavity had a deleterious effect on the full-thickness skin used to graft the tympanic membrane, and the narrowed middle ear space created in the classic type III and IV tympanoplasties was prone to collapse, nullifying any hearing improvement (see Chapter 15).

It became apparent that if satisfactory hearing results were to be obtained, some method of avoiding a narrow middle ear space would be necessary. Many felt that the best way of solving this problem was by not creating an exteriorized cavity, by reconstructing the tympanic membrane in a normal position and then inserting some type of tissue or prosthetic device to re-establish the sound pressure transfer mechanism (see Chapter 15). Although this concept led to better hearing results, many problems developed over the course of the years, some of which are still being seen.

It was learned that the harder one tried to obtain a good functional result, the more problems (and failures) one had. To avoid these problems, some surgeons still advocate the classic modified radical and radical mastoidectomy, nonreconstructive procedures.

The doctors of the House Ear Clinic (HEC) began performing the intact canal wall tympanoplasty with mastoidectomy in 1958, under the direction of William House.[4] By 1961, over half of all cholesteatoma cases were so managed at the HEC, but many revision operations were required for correction of recurrence of cholesteatoma due to retraction pockets. As a result, many at the HEC reverted to taking the canal wall down and then obliterating the cavity with muscle, based on a procedure suggested by Rambo.[5] In 1963, 50 per cent of cholesteatoma cases were so managed.

By 1964, it was realized that the technique of obliteration did not eliminate the cavity and the problems involved. In addition, the routine use of plastic sheeting through the facial recess in the intact canal wall procedure was reducing the number of cases that had to be revised because of retraction pockets (recurrent cholesteatoma). From that point on, the percentage of cases managed by a CWD technique gradually decreased to 10 per cent in 1970. Since then, there have been yearly fluctuations: 15 to 25 per cent CWD procedures over the last 10 years.

THE CONTROVERSY

The controversy over CWU versus CWD centers mostly on safety: safety of the operation procedure and safety over the ensuing years.[6] The consideration should—but rarely does—include the technical ability of the surgeon. In the surgery of aural cholesteatoma, be it CWU or CWD, judgment and technical ability are major factors in the outcome.

Let us assume that the technical ability and judgment are superior in the two groups. Why is there a difference in opinion as to what is best for the patient?

Are hearing results a factor? Not really. The HEC doctors do not find much difference. Of course, they are very careful not to narrow the middle ear space (see Chapter 15) and stage the operation almost as frequently as in CWU (see Chapter 21).

Is there a difference in the healing? Yes. CWU procedures, with lateral surface grafting (see Chapter 10) may well take 6 to 8 weeks to heal. Open cavities frequently require 3 to 4 months, and occasionally, 6 to 8 months, and there is a small percentage that are never free of minor moisture problems.

What about residual and recurrent disease? Most surgeons who use both CWU and CWD procedures find little difference in the incidence of middle ear residual disease, or disease left behind. They also find little difference in the incidence of staging the operation (see Chapter 21).

Recurrent cholesteatoma is a different matter. Recurrent cholesteatoma characteristically results from a posterosuperior retraction pocket,[7, 8] which occurs only in CWU procedures. Those who have reported a 20 to 40 per cent incidence of recurrent cholesteatoma have failed, with rare exceptions, to stage the operation when indicated (75 per cent of the time) and have failed to use plastic sheeting through the facial recess, even when the operation was being performed in one stage. Advocates of the CWU procedure, those who have had extensive experience, have less than a 5 per cent incidence of recurrent cholesteatoma.

Everyone knows when a cavity is created that it is usually necessary to clean (remove dead skin) every 6 to 12 months for the rest of the patient's life. One need see the CWU patient every 1 to 2 years for about 10 years.

Precautions relative to not getting water in the ear are necessary 50 per cent or more of the time in CWD cases, depending on whether the cavity is healed, how large it is, whether an adequately sized meatus was created, and whether the cavity is round, rather than bean shaped.

Finally, the adequate size meatus is relevant. If one creates a meatus large enough to have a trouble-free ear and allow water in the ear, the size can pose a problem with fitting a hearing aid, if and when there is a need for the aid in the future. The problem consists of getting a secure fit and preventing feedback. Fortunately, the behind-the-ear aid usually solves this problem and is the best aid anyway for use in an ear that may have some drainage from a cavity.

INDICATIONS FOR MASTOIDECTOMY

Mastoidectomy may be indicated in tympanoplasty surgery to eliminate disease, to explore the mastoid to ensure that there is no disease, to enlarge the air-containing middle ear–antral space, or on occasion, to create temporary postauricular drainage (with a catheter) in patients with compromised eustachian tube problems or uncontrolled mucosal infection.[9] By far the most common indication, however, is the treatment of cholesteatoma and the associated infection.

What about those who recommend at least a cortical ("simple") mastoidectomy in all tympanoplasties? The rationale appears to be that it is "good practice" and that "it's better to be safe than sorry." There are also arguments, mentioned earlier, that this practice can increase the middle ear cleft space, and that this is a good idea if there is compromised eustachian tube function.

In fact, the indication for mastoidectomy is made on the basis of the clinical history and the appearance of the ear in the doctor's office. The final decision is made during the surgery. There are some patients for whom a mastoidectomy is not done when it was thought necessary, or is done when the decision had not been realized preoperatively.

X-rays and imaging studies play little part in making the diagnosis, the decision to do the surgery, or management of the mastoid at surgery.

INDICATIONS FOR AN EXTERIORIZED MASTOID CAVITY

The HEC doctors prefer not to create a cavity but may do so at times. That decision may be made preoperatively, but more often than not, the operation is begun as a CWU procedure, and the decision to exteriorize the mastoid is made intraoperatively.[10]

Preoperative Decisions

The decision to perform a CWD procedure is made preoperatively in some cases. This decision is based on the consideration of the hearing in the involved ear, the status of the opposite ear, preoperative complications, the degree of posterior canal wall destruction by disease, and the age and health of the patient.

With rare exceptions, a cholesteatoma requiring mastoid surgery in an only hearing ear is managed with a CWD technique. Usually, the procedure is a classic modified radical mastoidectomy, leaving the middle ear and hearing the way they are. A classic modified radical mastoidectomy may be used in cases in which the affected ear has serviceable hearing and the opposite ear has a severe uncorrectable impairment. One does not wish to jeopardize the only serviceable ear.

In labyrinthine fistula cases, one may decide preoperatively to use a CWD operation if the mastoid is small or if the opposite ear has a cholesteatoma that will require surgery. If the hearing is serviceable, one will probably perform just a classic modified radical procedure, particularly for patients in poor health or in the elderly.[10–12]

A CWD operation may be decided on preoperatively if it can be seen that the cholesteatoma has destroyed a significant portion of the posterior canal wall. If the opposite ear already has a cavity, one may elect to create a cavity on the other ear at the time of surgery. In elderly patients or those in poor health, we are more likely to use a classic modified radical mastoidectomy; the less done, the better.

Intraoperative Decisions

Advocates of the CWU procedure will generally start the operation in this manner unless the decision has been made preoperatively. When one encounters a very contracted mastoid, particularly with an ear canal slanting up and forward, or if one encounters an unsuspected canal wall destruction, one would not hesitate to take the canal wall. Intraoperative decisions normally (at HEC) account for two thirds of the decisions for CWD.

PREOPERATIVE EVALUATION AND TREATMENT

How does one make the diagnosis of cholesteatoma, what tests are necessary, and how vigorously does one treat the chronically draining ear preoperatively?

The diagnosis of cholesteatoma is based on a well-taken history by the doctor and a careful examination of the ear under an operating microscope to confirm ingrowth of skin into the middle ear, at the epitympanum, or both.

The only routine testing is the hearing test. This test is not related to making the diagnosis but is to allow proper counseling. Occasionally, the hearing test will result in a change of approach to the surgery, as noted in the preceding section.

X-rays or imaging studies play very little part in making the diagnosis or directing the surgical approach. These tests are usually obtained if there is a complication or if one is considered likely, for example, semicircular canal fistula, facial paralysis, meningitis, or other intracranial complications.[12] Under these circumstances, imaging studies will rarely make a difference in the overall surgical approach but should allow the surgeon to predict any complications or sequelae. The patient and family can be counseled properly and forewarned of problems.

Treatment of the Chronically Draining Ear

How much, if any, treatment of the draining ear is indicated prior to surgery? Must the ear be dry before the surgery? If so, for how long? How vigorous should treatment be? Are cultures of the drainage indicated?

The HEC doctors rarely take cultures of draining ears unless there appears to be a subacute mastoiditis or a suspected complication. Then a culture may be indicated.

In the noncholesteatomatous ear, the benign central perforation, local treatment is indicated to obtain a dry ear prior to surgery (see Chapter 9). One would like to have the ear dry for 3 or 4 weeks prior to tympanic membrane grafting. If the ear is draining at the time of surgery, it is probably best to perform at least an antrotomy through the mastoid cortex and place a catheter drain (to ensure drainage while the tympanic membrane graft is healing).[9] Furthermore, it is more likely that a mucosal problem could dictate staging the operation if the ear is still draining at the time of surgery (see Chapter 21).

Many ears with cholesteatoma have only intermittant discharge, if any. These ears usually respond quickly to various local medications. If the cholesteatomatous ear has a history of almost continual drainage and there are no associated symptoms requiring treatment, it may be best to leave the ear alone. Certainly, if local treatment is started it should be effective quickly, if it is going to help at all. The exception to this course is the actively draining ear with polyps; these should be treated with local medication. Resolution of discharge despite the history is common.

PREOPERATIVE COUNSELING

(I will use the first and second person to describe the procedure at the HEC. Using a Chronic Ear Patient Discussion Booklet, I explain how a normal ear functions. I then show on a second drawing of the ear how skin grows into the ear and forms a cholesteatoma.)

Cholesteatoma is an ingrowth of skin into the mastoid. This forms a skin-lined cyst that we call a cholesteatoma. It is not a tumor or truly a growth. But it does tend to get larger as time goes on if the ear continues to drain.

There are three reasons why the ear should have surgery at some time. In the first place, it is potentially dangerous. If the drainage continues, we know that about 20 per cent of patients with these ears will eventually develop severe dizziness because the cholesteatoma breaks into the balance canal. There is about a 1 per cent chance that it may break into the nerve to the face or break into the covering of the brain.

Secondly, the longer the problem goes on, the more damage may be done to the hearing. If the cholesteatoma should break into a balance canal, one might then lose all hearing permanently.

Thirdly, there is the matter of the drainage.

The objectives of surgery are to get a safe, dry, and hearing ear. Getting a safe, dry, healed ear is almost certain. Unfortunately, to obtain a good hearing ear it is frequently necessary to do the operation in two stages. There is a 60 to 70 per cent chance of helping the hearing with the second operation.

There is nothing urgent about having the surgery. You certainly can have it done in a month or 3 months, but I wouldn't put it off indefinitely. It is like sitting on a keg of dynamite. It is not a very good place to sit; you are not quite sure whether the dynamite will ever explode and cause a serious problem.

I have made notations of all of this in the booklet. In the back of the booklet there is an area called Risks and Complications of Surgery. The only serious complication that happens with any degree of regularity, and it is serious, is a total, 100 per cent loss of hearing in the ear that had the operation. The likelihood of this happening is no more then a 1 to 2 per cent chance; all of the other things listed here are either very remote or are temporary. (The Risk and Complications sheet appears as Appendix 1 in Chapter 10)

If the patient has a labryinthine fistula, as between 5 and 10 per cent of our patients with cholesteatoma do, the patient is then told that there is a 10 per cent chance of a total loss of hearing and prolonged dizziness, which would eventually clear up.

PREOPERATIVE PREPARATION OF THE PATIENT

Preoperative preparation of the patient differs little from what was described under tympanic membrane grafting, (see Chapter 10). The operation is done under general anesthesia unless the patient requests otherwise.

SURGICAL TECHNIQUE

Just as the preparation prior to and in surgery is the same as that described for tympanic membrane grafting (see Chapter 10) the initial steps are identical: making canal incisions, elevating the vascular strip, turning the ear foreward, removing and dehydrating the temporalis fascia, removing canal skin, enlarging the ear canal by removing the overhanging bone anteriorly and inferiorly, and assuring that the remnant is de-epithelized.[13]

Removal of Middle Ear Disease

Cholesteatoma should be dissected in continuity to ensure total removal. All diseased tissue is dissected from the bone or mucosa, beginning in the anterosuperior quadrant, proceeding inferiorly, then posteriorly, and superiorly until the superior edge of the promontory, the lower edge of the oval window, is reached. Normal mucosa should not be sacrificed.

No attempt should be made at this time to remove cholesteatoma that surrounds the stapes or is in the oval window. Manipulations in this area should be postponed until the mastoidectomy has been completed and the facial recess is open. Removal of oval window disease should always be deferred until the end of the procedure, so that if a fistula develops inadvertently, the operation may be terminated expeditiously.

Before proceeding with the mastoidectomy, one must determine the status of the incudostapedial joint. If there is an intact chain, the incudostapedial joint should be separated at this time. This facilitates removal of the incus after the facial recess is opened and prevents possible trauma to the inner ear, which could occur should the drill inadvertently touch the incus when the epitympanum or facial recess is being opened.

Mastoid Exenteration

The mastoid is exenterated, under the microscope, using a drill with various-sized round cutting burrs. Continuous suction-irrigation during drilling is used to cool the bone, to keep the field clean at all times, and to prevent clogging of the burr by bone dust.

The initial burr cut is made along the linea temporalis. This marks the lowest point of the middle fossa dura in most cases. The second burr cut is along a line perpendicular to the one just described and tangent to the posterior margin of the ear canal (Fig. 18–1). These two burr cuts outline a triangular area, the apex of which is at the spine of Henle. Projected into the mastoid, parallel to the direction of the ear canal, the apex of this triangle is directly over the lateral semi-circular canal. The only structure of importance lying within this triangle as one proceeds with the exenteration is the lateral (sigmoid) sinus.

The deepest mastoid penetration is always at the apex of this triangle. This ensures that the antrum is entered and the lateral canal identified before deeper penetration in other areas. The dural plate is skeletonized superiorly and the lateral sinus skeletonized posteroinferiorly as the dissection proceeds. Uncovering the middle fossa or sigmoid sinus dura is not necessary but should not result in any problem. It is not considered a complication.

After the lateral semicircular canal has been identified and the cortical mastoidectomy has been completed, the zygomatic route is exenterated to allow access to epitympanum. The posterior bony canal wall is thinned at this time (Fig. 18–2).

I have certain "rules of thumb" that I use in teaching in regard to the initial approach to the mastoid. Let me comment on each of these.

Always keep the deepest area of penetration into the mastoid at the apex of the two initial burr cuts. The direction in which one proceeds is not necessarily perpendicular to the bone; it should be parallel to the ear canal. Following parallel to the ear canal will lead to the mastoid antrum.

Do not dig a "deep dark hole." One must remember to saucerize the margins, to open the exposure as one proceeds deeper. In this way, it is possible to see what one is doing and also to use the suction irrigation with the drill.

Always use the largest burr possible. If one should inadvertently uncover the middle fossa dura or the facial nerve or the sigmoid sinus, one is less likely to do serious damage with a large burr as opposed to a very small burr. Furthermore, if there is a problem, one will be able to see what was done.

Finally, "if lost on the way to the antrum, go high and forward." This is exactly what I say to students taking our temporal bone surgical dissection course. And this is in fact what I do when I sit down with one of them who has gotten halfway through the dissection and is lost. By going high, one identifies the middle fossa dural plate. By going forward, one then squeezes into the angle between the dural plate and the ear canal. Going medial in that direction leads to the epitympanum and avoids the matter of fenestrating the lateral semicircular canal or getting into other troubles should the mastoid antrum be filled with bone.

Opening the Facial Recess

The facial recess is one of the posterior recesses of the middle ear. It is bordered laterally by the chorda tympani, medially by the upper mastoid segment of the facial nerve, and superiorly by bone of the fossa incudis (Fig. 18–3). This recess is frequently the seat of cholesteatoma, particularly when cholesteatoma is associated with a perforation below the posterior malleal fold. Bone in this area may be cellular even in poorly developed mastoid.

The landmark for opening into the facial recess is the fossa incudis. One visualizes the triangular area that is inferior to the fossa and is bordered by bone of the fossa incudis superiorly, the upper mastoid segment of the facial nerve medially, and the chorda tympani laterally (Fig. 18–4). The bone is saucerized in this area with a large cutting burr. When the bony canal wall lateral to the recess has been thinned satisfactorily (care being taken not to perforate into the external canal), bone removal is continued with a smaller cutting burr. One should always stroke with a burr parallel to the direction of the nerve, never allowing the burr to pass the bone of the fossa incudis superiorly (Fig. 18–5).

The facial recess is opened from the mastoid to remove disease in the area, to gain additional access to the posterior middle ear (oval and round windows), to gain a better view of tympanic segment of the facial nerve, and to facilitate postoperative aeration of the mastoid. Opening into the middle ear through the facial recess is a key step in performing an intact canal wall tympanoplasty with mastoidectomy; with rare exceptions, it should not be omitted (Fig. 18–6).

FIGURE 18–1. Burr cuts to begin mastoidectomy. Note lateral semicircular canal ghosted in.

FIGURE 18–2. Exenteration of the mastoid is completed.

FIGURE 18–3. Horizontal cross-section of temporal bone, looking at the upper segment from below. Note facial recess (FR) and tympanic recess (TR).

FIGURE 18–4. Facial recess area outlined by triangle: borders are bone of the fossa incudis, upper mastoid segment of the facial nerve, and the chorda tympani.

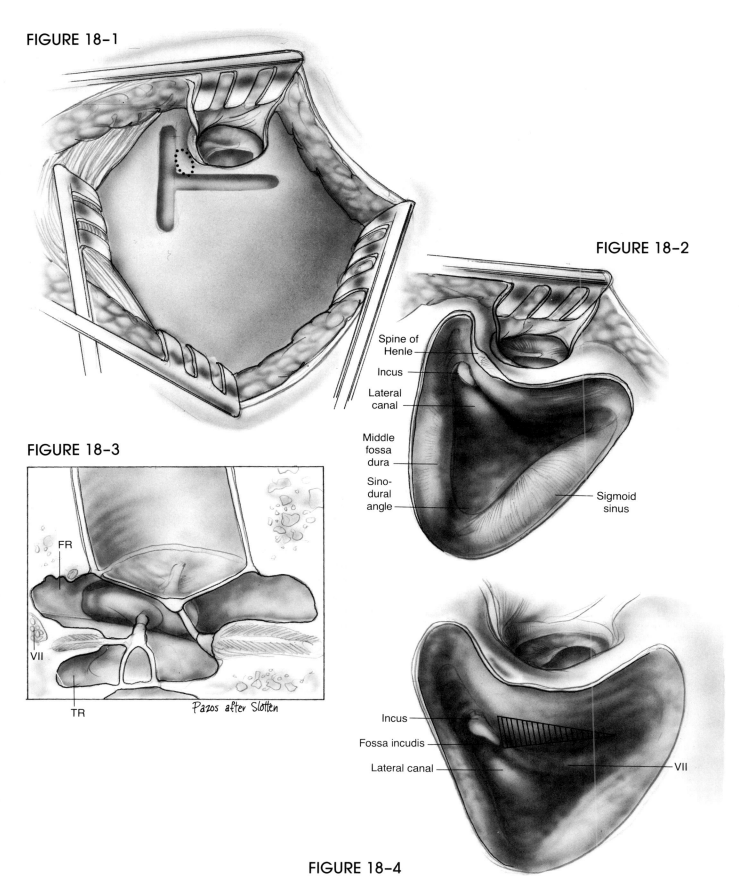

FIGURE 18-1

FIGURE 18-2

Spine of
Henle
Incus
Lateral
canal
Middle
fossa
dura
Sino-
dural
angle
Sigmoid
sinus

FIGURE 18-3

FR
VII
TR
Pazos after Slotten

Incus
Fossa incudis
Lateral canal
VII

FIGURE 18-4

There are two things one may notice when approaching the facial nerve in this area. Frequently, bleeding is encountered from one of the vessels intimately associated with, but lying outside, the bony canal of the nerve. Before actually uncovering the nerve one may note its white sheath showing through the thin bone. Often, this sheath is highlighted by the sight through the bone of one of the vessels on the sheath.

Identification of the facial nerve provides an additional landmark for opening into the facial recess. A small cutting burr is used to enter into the middle ear, just lateral to the nerve, and then the opening is enlarged to the extent possible with diamond stones. It is usually possible to obtain at least a 2mm opening.

It is not necessary to expose the nerve with this approach, but there is no harm in doing so. Fortunately, the facial nerve is quite resistant to gentle trauma.[14] One can use the cutting burrs when approaching the nerve in the region of the facial recess. Bone removal is quicker than with the diamond stone, and it is easier to determine when the nerve is exposed. To make this differentiation, the exposed area can be probed with a mobilizing needle. If the exposed area is nerve sheath, it rebounds immediately after release of the probe; it "bounces back." If what has been uncovered is mucosa or cholesteatoma, one may note that it will "come back at you" but that it doesn't bounce back or rebound. After the recess has been opened, the incus, if present, is removed along with bone of the fossa incudis. It is possible to see the pyramidal eminence, the oval and round windows, that part of the tympanic portion of the facial nerve lying posterior to the cochleariform process.

Elimination of Disease

As disease is encountered in the mastoid it is removed by dissecting it from *behind forward*. It is important to remove all cholesteatoma matrix in continuity so that no remnant of epithelium remains. The mastoid is exenterated to the extent indicated by the disease process and to the extent necessary to obtain adequate exposure. It is not necessary to remove normal-appearing cells, to exenterate all cells, as one would do in a CWD procedure.

From the mastoid approach, all mastoid and facial recess disease may be removed by elevating it and dissecting it toward the epitympanum and middle ear. Unless there is an unusually narrow angle between the tegmen and the superior wall of the ear canal it should be possible to remove all epitympanic disease. When the cholesteatoma has contacted the malleus head, as it frequently has, the entire malleus should be removed. This exposes the opening into the supratubal recess and facilitates dissection of disease from behind and through the ear canal simultaneously.

Posterosuperior middle ear disease is removed at this time through both the ear canal and mastoid (via the facial recess). The cholesteatoma matrix is dissected in continuity, if possible.

The areas that are most difficult to see with this or any other approach, even radical mastoidectomy, are the posterior middle ear recesses: infrapyramidal and tympanic recesses.[15] These are the areas posterior to and between the oval and round windows (Fig. 18–7). They extend for a variable distance medial to the pyramidal process and facial nerve (and lateral to the posterior semicircular canal). They are often the seat of cholesteatoma, particularly in cases associated with perforations below the posterior malleal ligament. The area must be cleaned with a right-angle dissector. Removal of the pyramidal process and adjacent bone with a diamond burr may be necessary at times to facilitate the cleaning but can only be done safely in a case where the stapes superstructure and tendon are missing. If the tympanic recess is deep and there is disease in it, it can be approached in a well-developed mastoid from the mastoid side, medial to the facial nerve and lateral to the posterior semicircular canal. This approach is not usually feasible, or necessary, but is to be kept in mind. It is an approach commonly used in connection with glomus tumor surgery.

FIGURE 18–5. Horizontal cross-section showing progressive saucerization and opening into the facial recess; compare with Fig. 18–3.

FIGURE 18–6. Facial recess is open and incus is removed.

FIGURE 18–7. View through the ear canal showing location of tympanic sinus, medial to the facial nerve.

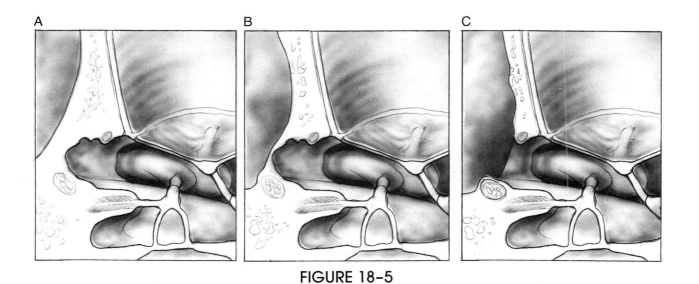

FIGURE 18–5

FIGURE 18–6

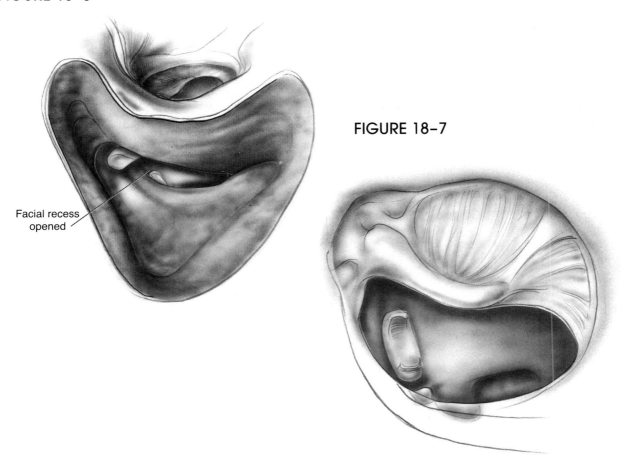

Facial recess
opened

FIGURE 18–7

Use of Plastic Sheeting

Plastic sheeting is used routinely in the intact canal wall procedure, regardless of the status of the middle ear mucosa, to prevent adhesions between the raw undersurface of the tympanic membrane graft and the denuded bone of the epitympanum and facial recess area. (Other uses of plastic sheeting are discussed in Chapter 21).

Before it was realized that plastic sheeting should be used through the facial recess, there were many cases of recurrence of cholesteatoma due to retraction of the tympanic membrane into the facial recess and epitympanum (Fig. 18–8). If the operation is not being staged, thin silicone sheeting is used through the recess. An opening can be created in the plastic to allow for reconstruction to the stapes capitulum (Fig. 18–9). When staging of the operation is indicated, as it usually is in cholesteatoma cases, either thick silicone sheeting or Supramid is used (see Chapter 21) (Fig. 18–10).

Completion of the Operation

The tympanic membrane remnant is grafted with rehydrated fascia, the ear canal skin is replaced on the denuded bone, packing is inserted, the vascular strip is replaced, and closure postauricularly is with subcutaneous suture, all as described for tympanic membrane grafting (see Chapter 10).

In the occasional case in which the mastoid is badly infected and this infection has broken out of the confines of the cholesteatoma, it is wise to irrigate the mastoid with antibiotic solution. In this situation, it is also wise to place a catheter drain to the antrum, bringing it out to a separate incision. The drain may be left until the first postoperative visit. The purpose of this procedure is to make sure that anything that can drain out will and will not interfere with the tympanic membrane graft take.

A superficial Penrose drain is occasionally indicated when oozing has been a problem. The drain extends from the area of the fascia removal and exits at the lower part of the incision. This drain may be removed on the first postoperative day.

Dressing and Postoperative Care

There is no difference between the dressing or postoperative care for this procedure and that for tympanic membrane grafting (see Chapter 10) except that it is much more common to keep the patient overnight with this procedure. The schedule and plan for office visits are the same.

THE FACIAL NERVE IN SURGERY OF CHRONIC OTITIS MEDIA

One of the greatest fears of the inexperienced surgeon is that there may be damage to the facial nerve during a mastoidectomy.[14] This fear may result in avoidance of the nerve rather than positive identification. This can result in inadvertent damage to the nerve that has not been identified. In CWD surgery, this fear certainly results in the inadequacy of some of the surgical procedures, leaving the posterior bony canal wall high, creating a "bean-shaped" cavity.

Familiarity with the facial nerve results in respect: respect for helping to guide one throughout the temporal bone and respect for its ability to withstand manipulations and minor trauma.

There are three segments to the facial nerve: labyrinthine, tympanic, and mastoid. In surgery of chronic otitis media, concern is with the tympanic and mastoid segments.

Tympanic Segment

The tympanic segment is that portion of the nerve extending from the geniculate ganglion to the exterior genu (adjacent to the pyramidal process). Landmarks for identification of the nerve in its tympanic course are the cochleariform process, the oval window, and the pyramidal process. From the mastoid approach, the lateral semicircular canal and the cog are useful. These will be discussed later.

The upper edge of the oval window is bordered by the facial nerve (Fig. 18–11). If this is not apparent, the cochleariform process may be identified. The facial nerve lies both posterior and superior to the cochleariform. One may also identify the pyramidal process and note that the facial nerve lies both above and behind this structure.

When none of these landmarks are apparent, the semicanal for the tensor tympani may be identified in the anterior middle ear and followed posteriorly. Its inferior border is continuous with the upper margin of the oval window, the facial nerve.

On rare occasions, one may need to identify the vertical groove on the promontory for the tympanic nerve. This groove is then followed superiorly to the cochleariform process or its remnants. The facial nerve is both posterior and superior to the cochleariform process.

From the mastoid approach, there are two landmarks to the tympanic course of the facial nerve: the lateral semicircular canal and the cog. The posterior half of the tympanic segment is immediately inferior to the lateral canal. The nerve course is anteriorly, passing superior to the cochleariform process and anterior to the cog.

The cog is a ridge of bone that extends inferiorly from the tegmen epitympani and partially separates the anterior tympanic compartment (supratubal recess) from the mesoepitympanum. The cog lies immediately superior to, and just slightly posterior to, the cochleariform process and anterior to the head of the malleus (Fig. 18–12). As the facial nerve runs between the cochleariform process and the geniculate ganglion, it courses under the base of the cog and anterior to it in the floor of the supratubal recess.

Mastoid Segment

In mastoidectomy, the initial landmarks within the temporal bone are the mastoid antrum and the lateral semicircular canal. Once the lateral canal is identified, the surgeon knows where the facial nerve is and is prepared to remove all the diseased tissue from the mastoid (Fig. 18–13).

The short crus of the incus is located inferior, and slightly lateral, to the anterior portion of the lateral canal bulge. The fossa incudis is at the tip of the short crus. The facial nerve lies medial to the fossa incudis and inferior to the lateral canal. As the nerve travels inferiorly in its course to the stylomastoid foramen, it travels in a slightly posterior direction, in most instances, and also travels laterally. (The reader would be well served by reading the article by Litton et al. on the relationship of the facial canal to the tympanic sulcus.)[16]

Two further landmarks to the mastoid segment of the facial nerve are the digastric groove and the posterior semicircular canal. Neither are usually involved (in facial nerve identification) in surgery of chronic otitis media because of the lack of cellular development in most cases of this type. The digastric groove leads to the stylomastoid foramen. The inferior portion of the posterior semicircular canal travels medial to the facial nerve.

MANAGEMENT OF THE LABYRINTHINE FISTULA

There is no way of knowing for certain preoperatively that a patient with cholesteatoma does not have a labyrinthine fistula; up to 10 per cent do.[11]

Each mastoid must be approached as if a fistula existed. When the cholesteatomal sac is encountered in the mastoid it should be opened, and the medial wall of the sac lying on the lateral semicircular canal should be palpated to detect any bony dehiscence.

Bony erosion may be obvious by flattening of the usual prominence of the lateral canal.

If there appears to be a fistula, a decision has to be reached as to management of the mastoid: continue as an intact canal wall procedure or create an open cavity? If an open cavity is to be created, the matrix may be left on the fistula permanently.[10]

If the operation is to continue as an intact canal wall procedure, carefully incise the matrix around the fistula. The rest of the matrix may be removed without removing the segment covering the fistula. If a decision has been reached that the operation is to be performed in two stages (see Chapter 21), leave the matrix over the fistula. It will be removed at the planned second stage when the ear is healed. If the operation is to be performed in one stage, complete the operation, including grafting, ossicular chain reconstruction, and packing of the ear canal. If you suspect that the fistula is small, it is reasonable to remove the matrix at this time and cover the fistula immediately with fascia. If on the other hand the fistula appears to be large or the ear is infected, it is probably best to leave the matrix and come back into the mastoid in 6 months to remove it.

REPAIR OF CANAL WALL DEFECTS

Defects in the posterior or superior bony canal wall need to be repaired to prevent recurrence of cholesteatoma from retraction pockets. Defects may be the result of the disease or the surgery.

Defects due to Disease

It is not unusual for cholesteatoma to erode some of the lateral epitympanic wall, but it may at times destroy a larger portion of the posterior canal wall. If the canal wall destruction is extensive, it is probably wise not to repair the defect but to change to a CWD procedure.

In most cases, canal wall destruction is limited to the lateral epitympanic wall (Fig. 18–14). If a second-stage procedure is planned (see Chapter 21), it is wise not to reconstruct the defect; the Supramid or thick silicone sheeting will prevent a retraction pocket between stages one and two. At stage two, after removing the plastic, one may see through the defect to detect any residual disease. The defect may be repaired at that time with bone paté or cartilage.

If a second-stage operation is not indicated, then the defect may be repaired in similar way after the graft has been tucked under the bony defect (Fig. 18–15).

FIGURE 18-8

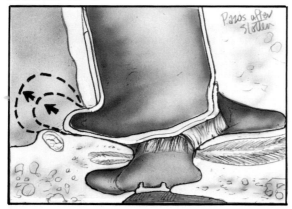

FIGURE 18-9

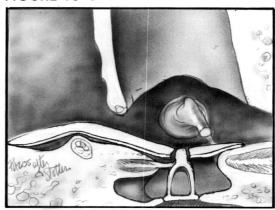

FIGURE 18-10

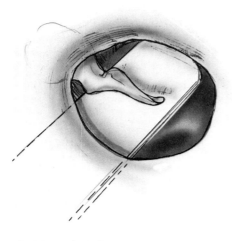

FIGURE 18-11

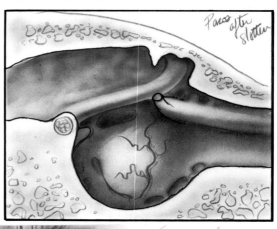

FIGURE 18-12

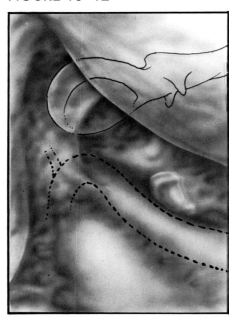

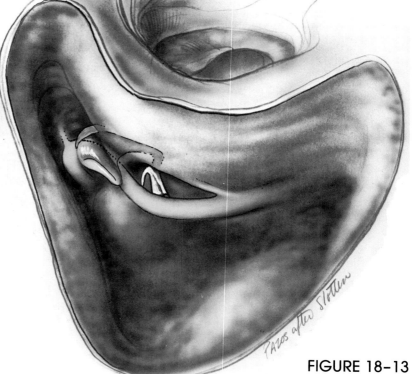

FIGURE 18-13

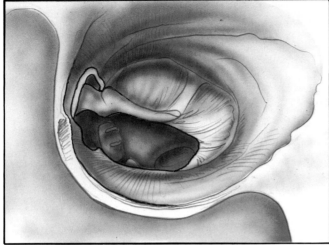

FIGURE 18-14

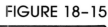

FIGURE 18-15

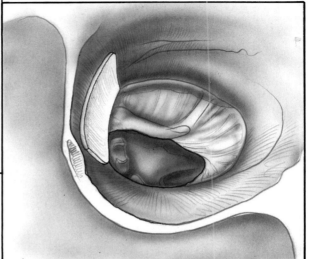

FIGURE 18-8. Retraction of new tympanic membrane into the facial recess, caused by scar tissue; plastic sheeting was not used. Arrows indicate development of recurrent cholesteatoma.

FIGURE 18-9. Thin plastic through the facial recess; capitulum is protruding through the opening to allow reconstruction.

FIGURE 18-10. Thick plastic sheeting extending from the mastoid into the middle ear through the facial recess.

FIGURE 18-11. Parasagittal section through the middle ear of the right temporal bone to show landmarks. Facial nerve lies superior to the oval window and posterior (also superior) to the cochleariform process. The nerve lies superior, and also posterior, to the pyramidal process and anterior to the cog in the floor of the supratubal recess. The cog is a ridge of bone extending inferiorly from the tegmen epitympani, above the cochleariform process (refer to Fig. 18-12). Note relationship of semicanal for the tensor tympani and a groove in the promontory for the tympanic nerve of Jacobson.

FIGURE 18-12. View from the mastoid into the epitympanum (facial recess has been opened). Malleus head has been ghosted in to show the relationship to the cog (compare with Fig. 18-11). The cog is a ridge of bone extending inferiorly from the tegmen epitympani, anterior to the malleus head, above the cochleariform process.

FIGURE 18-13. Facial nerve (labyrinthine, tympanic, and mastoid segments) has been ghosted in to show the relationship to the ossicles, facial recess opening, and lateral semicircular canal.

FIGURE 18-14. Defect in lateral epitympanic wall.

FIGURE 18-15. Repair of lateral wall defect with cartilage.

Defects due to Surgery

If one is using an intact canal wall technique, it is unwise to perform atticotomy. At times, however, it is necessary to do so, particularly anteriorly, if the middle fossa dural plate is low or the ear canal is angled in such a way that one cannot obtain adequate vision into the supratubal recess. The repair of these problems is the same as mentioned above.

At times, there will be an inadvertent opening made in the canal wall when the mastoid is drilled. To avoid this, the ear canal bone should be thinned as the final step in the procedure before the facial recess is opened. This procedure prevents inadvertently knocking a hole in the wall while drilling in the mastoid. Should such a defect occur, it may be repaired with a shaving of cartilage over the hole on the canal side prior to replacement of the ear canal skin.

Acknowledgment

Many of the illustrations are modified from *Otolaryngology*, Vol. 1, published by J. B. Lippincott Company.

References

1. Committee on Conservation of Hearing of the American Academy of Ophthalmology and Otolaryngology: Standard classification for surgery of chronic ear infection. Arch Otolaryngol Head Neck Surg 81:204–205, 1965.
2. Wullstein H: Theory and practice of tympanoplasty. Laryngoscope 66:1076–1093, 1956.
3. Zollner F: Principles of plastic surgery of the sound conducting apparatus. J Laryngol Otol 69:637–652, 1955.
4. Sheehy JL, Patterson ME: Intact canal wall tympanoplasty with mastoidectomy. Laryngoscope 77:1502–1542, 1967.
5. Rambo JHT: Further experience with musculoplasty. Arch Otolaryngol Head Neck Surg 71:428–436, 1960.
6. Sheehy JL: Intact canal wall tympanoplasty with mastoidectomy. *In* Snow JB (ed): Controversy in Otolaryngology. Philadelphia, WB Saunders, 1980.
7. Sheehy JL: Cholesteatoma surgery: Residual and recurrent disease. Ann Otol Rhinol Laryngol 86:451–462, 1977.
8. Sheehy JL, Robinson JV: Cholesteatoma surgery at the Otologic Medical Group: Residual and recurrent disease. A report on 307 revision operations. Am J Otol 3:209–215, 1982.
9. Sheehy JL: Chronic tympanomastoiditis. *In* Gates GA (ed): Current Therapy in Otolaryngology—Head and Neck Surgery, Vol 4. Philadelphia, BC Decker, 1990, pp 19–22.
10. Sheehy JL: Cholesteatoma surgery: Canal wall down procedures. Ann Otol Rhinol Laryngol 97:30–35, 1988.
11. Sheehy JL: Cholesteatoma surgery: Management of the labyrinthine fistula. Laryngoscope 89:78–87, 1979.
12. Sheehy JL, Brackmann DE, Graham MD: Complications of cholesteatoma: A report on 1024 cases. *In* McCabe B, Sade J, Abramson M (eds): Cholesteatoma, First International Conference. Birmingham, AL, 1977. Aesculapius Publishing Company.
13. Sheehy JL: Surgery of chronic otitis media. *In* English GM (ed): Otolaryngology. Philadelphia, Harper and Row, 1984.
14. Sheehy JL: Facial nerve in surgery of chronic otitis media. Otolaryngol Clin North Am 7:493–503, 1974.
15. Donaldson JA, et al: The surgical anatomy of the sinus tympani. Arch Otolaryngol Head Neck Surg 91:219–227, 1970.
16. Litton WB, et al.: The relationship of the facial canal to the annular sulcus. Laryngoscope 79:1584–1604, 1969.

19

Mastoidectomy: Canal Wall Down Techniques

GORDON D.L. SMYTH, M.D., F.R.C.S.

JOSEPH G. TONER, M.B., F.R.C.S.

Born in 1929, Gordon Smyth sadly succumbed to a short illness during the preparation of this chapter. He made a significant contribution to many aspects of otology over the past 30 years. His pioneering reports of combined-approach tympanoplasty in the early 1960s were followed by meticulous study of large surgical series. This enabled him to produce accurate statistical data regarding surgical outcomes. When these data demonstrated potential problems, he had the courage to voice these concerns. He published widely in international journals on many aspects of otology, delivered many eponymous lectures, and was given numerous academic honors, including honorary membership in the American Otologic Society.

INTRODUCTION

Disappointment with the long-term results of closed operations for ears with extensive cholesteatoma has led to a renewed preference for open techniques. Although the technical advantages provided by magnification and hypotensive anesthesia have reduced the numbers of unstable postoperative open mastoidectomy cavities, this problem has not been eliminated. This chapter will focus primarily on refinements of surgical technique designed to obtain optimum results in canal wall down tympanoplasty. Classical modified radical and radical mastoidectomy and mastoid obliteration techniques will also be discussed, as well as revision of old mastoidectomy cavities.

PATIENT SELECTION

Tympanoplasty with Canal Wall Down Mastoidectomy

When the extent of cholesteatomatous disease of the tubotympanic cleft is such that access through a transcanal approach is inadequate, mastoidectomy becomes necessary. Whether the osseous canal wall should be maintained or removed has become a matter of serious debate. It has been argued that by preserving the canal wall and thus avoiding an open surgical cavity, patients will be spared the burden of a need for life-long cavity care and have better hearing. Most proponents of intact canal wall tympanoplasty (ICWT) now advise that the procedure be carried out in two stages 6 to 12 months apart. The opposing view is that removal of the canal wall very considerably reduces the incidence of postoperative cholesteatoma with no worse hearing results, that refinements in surgical technique result in reliable cavity stability, and that open-cavity procedures significantly reduce the need for multiple operations.

Those who favor a canal wall down method pose the question, Why should patients be subjected to at least two operations when one procedure will achieve the same if not a better result in the long term? Therefore, for proponents, the main indication for taking the canal wall down is the presence of a cholesteatoma that extends quite a distance into the epitympanum, to the aditus or further. Nevertheless, although many surgeons routinely prefer canal wall down procedures for all ears with extensive cholesteatoma, many of those who continue to advocate maintenance of the canal wall do make exceptions when the ear in question is the only, or the overwhelmingly better-hearing ear, when there is preoperative evidence of facial nerve or labyrinthine involvement, when there is more than minor posterior canal wall destruction, or when the patient is infirm or elderly.

Classical Radical Mastoidectomy

This procedure was the first definitive procedure for chronic suppurative disease of the mastoid air cell system, and it continued to be used as the only available means of preventing the spread of ear infection intracranially until 80 years ago. The ear canal, middle ear, and the mastoid air cell system are converted into a single cavity that communicates with the exterior through the orifice of the external meatus. Remnants of the tympanic membrane and ossicles are removed. Because no reliable steps are taken to prevent the egress of infected nasopharyngeal secretions, postoperative otorrhea is to be expected. This operation is currently most often employed in developed countries only for ears affected by neoplastic disease.

Classical Modified Radical Mastoidectomy

Classical modified radical mastoidectomy was the forerunner of modern tympanoplasty. Observation of useful preoperative hearing led surgeons to preserve middle ear structures not involved in an irreversible pathologic process whenever possible in the hope that preoperative function would be maintained. Attempts to repair defects of the ossicular chain and tympanic membrane (tympanoplasty) did not begin until the 1950s. Although this operation is now rarely performed because of problems with cavity stability resulting from persistent tympanic membrane defects, it is appropriate for ears with an intact atelectatic tympanic membrane and reduced cochlear reserve, especially when there is good contralateral hearing.

Indications for Revising a Pre-existing Mastoid Cavity

Although the frequency of open-cavity instability is now certainly less than in the premicrosurgical era, the problem still exists, and even in centers of excellence, is reported in as many as 10 per cent of patients. Although persistent or frequently recurrent postoperative otorrhea usually results from inadequate surgical technique or lack of patient compliance, a small number of patients whose operations were correctly performed have cavity skin instability with a dermatologic basis. Such patients should be treated with appropriate topical medications. In the majority, surgical errors are identifiable, and these are usually either inadequate contouring of the mastoid bowl or insufficient ventilation of the cavity, often in combination. If the bowl is constricted by cortical bone overhangs remaining on its lateral margins, or the emigration of epithelial debris and cerumen is impaired in recesses because of inadequate removal of the facial ridge or anterior buttress, the integrity of the cavity epithelium is likely to be impaired, leading to the development of chronic dermatitis and the formation of granulation tissue. Similarly, inadequate ventilation of cavities whose communication with the exterior is inappropriate to their volume may result in atmospheric conditions conducive to the growth of bacteria and fungi. Frequently, the problem also results from contamination of the cavity by infected secretions passing from the nasopharynx through a residual tympanic membrane defect.

When such deficiencies in the original surgical procedure are evident, an appropriate revision operation is indicated.

PREOPERATIVE EVALUATION AND PATIENT COUNSELING

As the numbers of long-term reports on the results of tympanoplasty accumulate, awareness of the shortcomings of some current therapies for cholesteatomatous disease has increased.

Decision to Operate

If we are not always able to improve the lot of our patients, we must at least take every possible precaution to ensure that we make it no worse. Although the possibilities of success in tympanoplasty have improved, the threat of complications, such as severe hearing loss and incapacitating tinnitus and vertigo, nevertheless continues. Should we surgeons not more frequently ask what our patients do not ask—is this operation is really necessary? It is worth remembering that there may be more dead ears from surgery than from middle ear disease. Do we know for certain that a cholesteatoma without signs of acute inflammation or evidence of complications in a 55-year-old person necessarily requires major surgery instead of periodic toilet?

With so much at stake, the decision to operate must be preceded by a systematic analysis of all of the factors that may influence the outcome for each individual. Such an analysis plays a vital part in the treatment of every patient with middle ear disease.

The aims of treatment in chronic ear disease are, first, to eradicate disease; second, to restore function; and third, to maintain the health of the ear over time. Because of its nature, chronic otitis media is rarely cured by purely medical means, and the aims of treatment can generally be achieved only by surgery. The decision to operate is based on the threat of the disease and the functional need of the patient.

In evaluating the threat of disease, surgeons are influenced by the type and extent of disease, the general health of the patient, and the patient's age. Clearly, one would be more inclined to operate in cases of cholesteatomatous disease occurring in young people who are medically fit, whereas an elderly patient with circulatory disease might be better treated by more conservative means, such as suction clearance repeated at regular intervals.

The hearing status of the patient and the patient's need and potential for improvement will influence the decision as to whether ossiculoplasty is indicated, which will be based on the cochlear reserve, involvement and hearing status of the contralateral ear, and the age of the patient. In young patients, especially those with bilateral involvement, any hearing gain may be of value, whereas this might not be the case in the older patient who has managed well for many years with only one functional ear.

Preoperative Evaluation

Factors such as vertigo and persistent drainage over a long period suggest a disease process that is more extensive than one that can be reached by a purely transcanal technique. The visual evidence provided by clinical examination, especially when aided by the operating microscope, and the response to the fistula test may provide further evidence of the extent and type of the disease and help in deciding whether the disease process can be managed by a purely transcanal technique or whether a more extensive operation, with or without removal of the canal wall, is necessary. Patients with bilateral involvement pose a special problem because of the need to retain or improve auditory function in at least one ear, and in such a situation, the choice of operation may be difficult, depending on the anatomic status of the ear and the surgeon's experience. On the other hand, when the contralateral ear is normal and tests indicate little useful cochlear reserve in the diseased ear, the decision is less delicate, and a canal wall down operation, with repair of the tympanic membrane, will usually provide the best solution.

Audiology

The importance of correctly assessing the cochlear reserve cannot be overemphasized. The audiologic investigation begins not with the audiometrician but with the surgeon, who uses a tuning fork and Bárány noise box. It is obviously not justifiable to operate to improve hearing without first checking cochlear function, and for determining this, competent masking during speech testing and pure-tone audiometry is essential. When there is bilateral disease, it is prudent to operate first on the ear with worse hearing.

Operations on the Discharging Ear

Many of the standard textbooks warn against tympanoplasty in any ear that has not been dry for 3 to 6 months or even longer; the interval recommended varies from one author to another. However, many patients come to the operation with longstanding purulent discharge, and most comparisons of the results in "wet" and "dry" ears indicate that this factor plays little part in the final result. In view of the usual resistance of bacteria cultured from the chronically infected ear to all of the antibiotics that can be given systemically with safety, preoperative bacterial culture would appear to have limited practical value as an aid to routine therapy. Nevertheless, culture of secretions from the middle ear should be done preoperatively because this may provide invaluable information should an infective complication occur postoperatively.

Radiologic Examination

The principal benefit to be derived from "straight" mastoid X-rays lies in the predictive information they provide on the extent of pneumatization, which may influence the choice of procedure, that is, endaural as opposed to postaural. However, X-rays are positively dangerous if relied on as a means of excluding cholesteatoma or a labyrinthine fistula. Computed tomographic scans are essential if labyrinthine or intracranial extensions of the disease are suspected, and also in ears in which a perceptive hearing loss may be due to a coexisting acoustic schwannoma.

Evaluation of Eustachian Tube Function

Much has been said and written about evaluating eustachian tube function before deciding whether to operate. Elaborate tests have evolved, but unfortunately we do not yet know their prognostic relevance. The results certainly do not indicate the cause of any dysfunction. Consider how often at operation there is a polyp, cholesteatomatous cyst, or retracted membrane lying across the lateral end of a tube that is otherwise patent. One must also query the prognostic value of tests of tubal patency in infected ears, where the tubal mucosa is inevitably edematous preoperatively but can reasonably be expected to improve following eradication of inflammation distally.

Informed Consent

It is most important that the patient be given an easily understood verbal and written explanation of the reason for his or her operation and of the prospects for success or failure, including the risks to the cochlea and facial nerve. Although with modern microsurgical techniques and comprehensive training programs facial nerve trauma should be very rare, difficulties can arise when the nerve is dehiscent or abnormally located. Patients should always be aware that even in the most competent hands, postoperative facial dysfunction does occur, albeit very infrequently. Likewise, diminished cochlear function and dysequilibrium are well documented, but fortunately unusual, sequelae of uncomplicated operations (even myringoplasty). The risks are much greater when there is pathologic invasion of the labyrinth and should be discussed with the patient and relatives. It should be explained that a second operation may occasionally be necessary to ascertain that there is no residual disease in the mesotympanum and also that the ossicular mechanism can be reconstructed under circumstances that most enhance success.

Finally, the patient should be informed of the expected length of stay in the hospital and the frequency of postoperative review. The importance of the patient's responsibility to have periodic inspection and toilet of the surgical cavity, possibly indefinitely, must be emphasized.

SURGICAL TECHNIQUE

Preoperative Preparation

Preparation for all canal wall down operations is basically the same. Following admission on the day prior to the intended procedure, the patient's ears are examined under magnification, and debris and secretions are removed by the surgeon. The advice previously given regarding the intended operation, the duration of hospitalization, and the patient's expectations are reviewed, ensuring also, as far as possible, the patient's relatives' full comprehension. Pure-tone audiometric responses are confirmed, and infected aural secretions are submitted for laboratory analysis. Suitability of general health for anesthesia is ascertained. Arrangements are made for sedation and provision of any medication habitually used by the patient.

Prior to transfer to the operating room, hair is removed with scissors to expose an area of skin 4cm broad behind and above the ear, which is then washed with pHisoHex and povidone-iodine solutions, and a sterile gauze dressing is applied.

Surgical Site Preparation and Draping

Standard preoperative site preparation and draping are used. The skin is swabbed with chlorhexidine solution and then povidone-iodine solution. An adhesive disposable ear towel is applied to the prepared site and then a fenestrated surgical towel.

Special Instruments

Standard otologic instrumentation is sufficient to perform all the procedures that will be discussed.

Technique of Surgery

1. PRELIMINARY EXAMINATION OF MIDDLE EAR AND ASSESSMENT OF ITS PATHOLOGIC STATE

    After debridement of the ear canal and exposed areas of the mesotympanum, assisted by irrigation with Ringer's solution if necessary, the visible extent and location of keratinizing epithelium and granulation tissue is noted to confirm the previous clinical assessment.

2. EXPOSURE OF THE MESOTYMPANUM

    A wide triangular tympanomeatal flap is turned forward. Its apex should be 6mm and its limbs 2mm lateral to the sulcus tympanicus. Creating such a flap at this stage best ensures a viable margin of meatal skin around the tympanic membrane defect for use in its later repair.

    The exposed mesotympanum is inspected and its pathologic aspects and the status of the ossicular chain determined. If the incudostapedial joint is intact and disease involvement of any of the ossicles indicates that dissection resulting in excessive ossicular manipulation will be unavoidable, the joint should be disarticulated. At this stage, it is convenient and advantageous to remove keratinizing epithelium that has retracted into the sinus tympani and facial sinus. To this end, before elevating the tympanomeatal flap, it is frequently helpful to place a short-term ventilator in the anterior tympanic membrane. If the retracted epithelium has not yet become firmly adherent to mesotympanic structures, suction gently applied to the retracted tissue will pull it laterally as air enters the middle ear through the ventilator. An air-containing space can usually be located in the hypotympanum and with angulated excavators, cubes of porous plastic sponge can be manipulated into the plane between the epithelium and the medial and posterior walls of the mesotympanum. In this way, it is often possible to evert even a deep retraction pocket and bring it into full view, rendering its complete removal possible. As this dissection proceeds, care must be taken to avoid injury to the round window membrane and to avoid manipulation or dislocation of the stapes, and to this end, the oval window region and the stapes superstructure should be kept in the visual field at all times.

3. MEATOPLASTY

    In ears in which there is radiologic evidence of significant pneumatization and therefore a likelihood of an eventually sizeable mastoid bowl, it is expedient to perform a meatoplasty at this stage rather than later. The appropriate soft tissues can be most easily excised while still firmly attached to the mastoid cortex. This order of steps is more relevant to operations in which the surgeon plans to use a postaural incision to approach the mastoid than those in which an endaural incision (being appropriate to a sclerotic mastoid) is preferred. In such ears, the decision to include a meatoplasty should be left until the final dimensions of the mastoid bowl are known.

    Meatoplasty begins with elevation of the conchal skin using an incision around the posterior margin of the meatal orifice, which is extended posteriorly either from its upper and lower limits (Fig. 19–1A) or from its midpoint (Fig. 19–1B), according to the desired size of the meatoplasty. The conchal skin is then dissected off the underlying cartilage, which is excised together with all underlying soft tissue, leaving the mastoid cortex cleanly exposed. Later, at the conclusion of the operation, the skin flaps are rotated inward and secured to the soft tissue on the medial aspect of the concha with catgut sutures.

Mastoidectomy

Traditional methods of open mastoid surgery frequently inflict patients with cavities much larger than those required to control their disease. This is because much normal, mostly posteriorly located bone is removed when the first anatomic landmark sought is the mastoid antrum, as in the classical posterior-to-anterior procedure.

There is more than a little logic to support a renewal of interest in the alternative direction of operating proposed by Stacke in 1897[1] and revived 40 years later by Tumarkin,[2] whereby, instead of approaching the cholesteatoma from its posterior aspects, the cholesteatomal sac is exposed at its origin in the posterior mesotympanum or epitympanum and followed posteriorly, with removal of only that bone necessary for its complete exteriorization and a beveled, contoured cavity. Thus, because the mastoid process in many cholesteatomatous ears, especially in adults, is sclerotic, the size of the resultant cavity is smaller with the anterior-to-posterior method. Other advantages are greater safety because vital structures, including the ossicles, are identified early; less chance of missing a small antrum because of Körner's septum; and better orientation and judgment of depth in relation to the tympanic sulcus. For these reasons, the anterior-to-posterior route is easier to perform and safer to teach. An added benefit of the reversed-direction method is that it allows for the repair of a small surgical defect in the canal wall with tragal or conchal cartilage when a cholesteatomatous sac is found to be limited to the epitympanum.

Although the operation can be performed through an endaural incision, for routine use, especially in ears in which the extent of pneumatization is uncertain and complete access to the mastoid tip may be required, a postaural incision will accommodate all surgical requirements. This incision is curved, commencing 1cm inferior to the mastoid tip and terminating 1cm superior to the root of the zygoma. At its midpoint, it should lie 2cm behind the postaural fold to allow the development of a postaurally based soft tissue flap, should this be required to obliterate an extensive retrofacial cell system. If such a flap is not later required, it will be returned to its site of origin at the conclusion of the operation. Two or three self-retaining retractors are used to expose the linea temporalis and the mastoid tip. The remaining meatal skin is then reflected anteriorly to expose the inferior, posterior, and superior osseous ear canal. At this stage, with the mesotympanum in clear view, using cutting burrs and suction irrigation, the outer epitympanic wall and the bone overlying the aditus and facial recess are systematically removed, working superiorly and posteriorly from the medial margins of the meatus. Extreme care must be taken to avoid contact between a rotating burr and any part of the ossicular chain when this is intact (Fig. 19–2). If the chorda tympani is involved in the cholesteatoma, it should be sectioned and removed.

As bone removal proceeds, the cholesteatoma matrix is exposed and followed to its full extent. Bone removal should continue until there is a flat and upwardly sloping plane of bone between the cortex and the roof of the antrum and epitympanum. The removal of the superficial layer of cortex is extended well beyond the floor of the middle cranial fossa and posterior to the sigmoid sinus and sinodural angle. By this means, the boundaries of the surgical cavity are saucerized, leading to an eventual considerable reduction in its depth (Fig. 19–3).

When the cholesteatoma matrix lies superficial to an intact ossicular chain, the chain can often be preserved in continuity with the tympanic membrane remnants. When the matrix extends medial to the malleus head or incus, these must be removed to avoid persistence of the cholesteatomatous process. Removal of extensions of matrix into supralabyrinthine, apical, and retrofacial cells and into cells in the solid angle between the superior and posterior semicircular canals requires precise knowledge of the anatomy of the geniculate ganglion, the facial nerve, and the labyrinth.

When the cellular system is wider in its distribution than the cholesteatoma, bone removal should be continued sufficiently to allow the detection and removal of all granulation tissue and diseased bone. The overriding principle is the creation of a smooth and roundly contoured cavity. The most common error in this respect is failure to remove sufficient bone lateral to the vertical course of the facial nerve (the facial ridge) and from the area (anterior buttress) that separates the anterior epitympanum from the anterior mesotympanum.

By drilling, the facial ridge is lowered to the level of the fallopian canal using large-toothed and diamond burrs and working in parallel with the course of the nerve, never across it. In spite of the lowering of the facial ridge to the level of the fallopian canal, an extensive retrofacial cell system or pneumatization extending to the mastoid tip may result in an unavoidable "sump" posterior to the facial nerve. If so, the sump should be obliterated with bone pate covered with a layer of tragal cartilage with perichondrium. To remove the mastoid tip, it is skeletonized from its lateral aspect, fractured, and rotated away

---

FIGURE 19–1. Meatoplasty incisions. The posterior margin of the meatal orifice is incised down to conchal cartilage. A skin flap(s) is developed by extending this incision posteriorly for 1.0–1.5cm either as in (A) (Schuknecht 1964) or in (B) (Fisch 1980), after flap elevation underlying cartilage and soft tissue are widely excised (C). The skin flap(s) is rotated medially, sutured, and supported with a pack. (Redrawn from Fisch U (ed): Tympanoplasty and Stapedectomy. New York, Thieme-Stratton, 1980; and Schuknecht HF: Tympanoplasty video tape. Richards Manufacturing Company, No. 2413, File VA. 208.)

FIGURE 19–2. Bone removal starts at the scutum and posterosuperior sulcus tympanicus and proceeds posteriorly. (Redrawn from Dawes JDK: Epitympanotomy and tympanomastoidectomy. In Ballantyne J (ed): Robb & Smith's Operative Surgery, 3rd ed. London, Butterworth & Company, 1976.)

FIGURE 19–3. Bone overlying the middle and posterior fossa dura is removed extensively until dural shadow is visible. (Redrawn from Dawes JDK: Epitympanotomy and tympanomastoidectomy. In Ballantyne J (ed): Robb & Smith's Operative Surgery, 3rd ed. London, Butterworth & Company, 1976.)

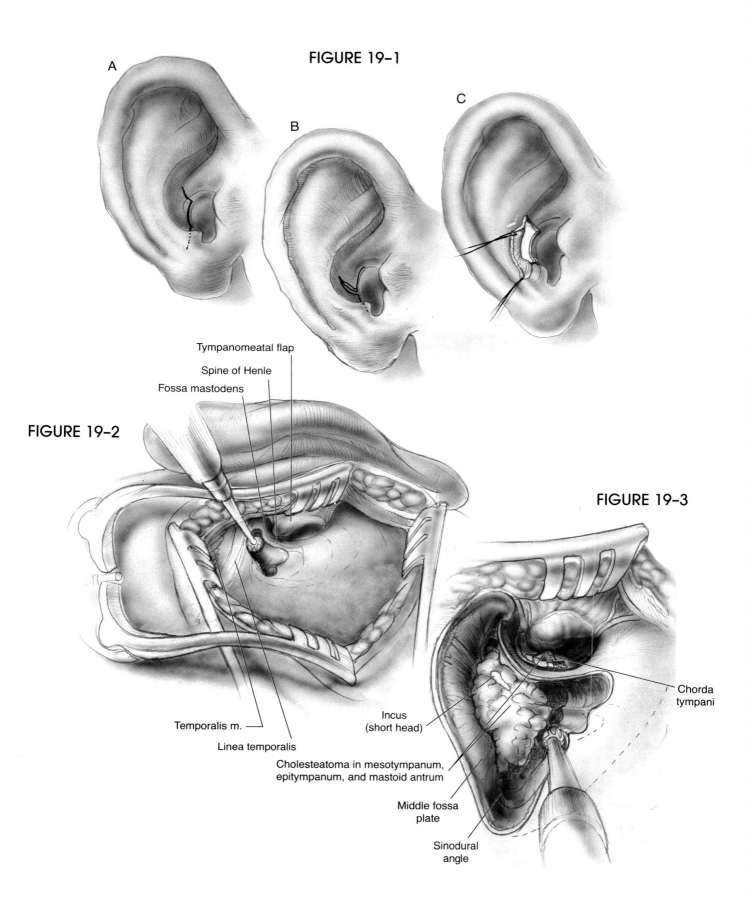

FIGURE 19–1

A

B

C

FIGURE 19–2

Tympanomeatal flap

Spine of Henle

Fossa mastodens

Temporalis m.

Linea temporalis

FIGURE 19–3

Incus
(short head)

Cholesteatoma in mesotympanum,
epitympanum, and mastoid antrum

Middle fossa
plate

Sinodural
angle

Chorda
tympani

from the stylomastoid foramen with a rongeur and then excised from its medial soft tissue attachments with curved scissors. The inferior meatal wall and the inferior aspect of the surgical cavity should finally be continuous and on a level plane. To eliminate the anterior buttress, bone is removed in the area of the root of the zygoma and the superior tympanic plate until the anterior epitympanum is continuous with the anterior mesotympanum. Frequently, a bony partition extending inferiorly from the roof of the epitympanum anterior to the malleus head separates the main epitympanic space from supratubal cells. This partition (the "cog") should be removed by drilling and all soft tissue removed from the cells, bearing in mind the proximity of the geniculate ganglion and the cochlea (Fig. 19–4). The desired final result is a rounded, kidney-shaped space in which the mastoid air cell system, mesotympanum, epitympanum, and ear canal are converted into a single smoothly contoured cavity, commencing with the exterior through a meatal orifice of at least twice the normal size (Fig. 19–5).

On completion of all the steps of mastoidectomy, the superior meatal skin is incised from lateral to medial close to its attachment to the squamotympanic suture, creating an inferiorly based flap, which is rotated onto the posteroinferior walls of the surgical cavity.

Finally, after elevating the margins of the remnant tympanic membrane to an appropriate extent, ossiculoplasty and tympanic repair with underlaid temporalis fascia or tragal cartilage with perichondrium is carried out.

The operation is concluded by filling the cavity and ear canal with half-inch gauze impregnated with bismuth iodoform paraffin paste or antibiotic ointment, working through the meatal orifice and viewing through the postaural incision to ensure a snug fit and to avoid displacement of the inferior skin flap. The incision is then closed in layers by using catgut sutures to approximate soft tissues and silk to suture the skin edges. A pressure dressing is then applied.

If obliteration of the cavity is considered necessary on grounds of size, prior to packing and suturing, the previously created musculoperiosteal flap is shaped to allow its rotation into the cavity without tension and covered on its anterior aspect with a layer of temporalis fascia (Fig. 19–6). The use of fascia in this situation prevents the formation of granulation tissue in the immediate postoperative phase.

Revision of Old Mastoidectomy Cavities

Unsatisfactory results from previous open-cavity operations are usually due to inadequate technique in the first instance. Factors such as inadequate ventilation, persistence of infection in residual air cells, and recurrence of cholesteatoma trapped in inadequately opened cell tracts in the epitympanum or behind a high facial ridge are frequently detected, often in combination.

Alternatively, recurrent contamination of the surgical cavity through a defect in the tympanic membrane may be the principal cause for cavity instability. To secure a better final result, revision mastoidectomy with or without tympanoplasty will usually be necessary. The skills required for successful revision mastoidectomy are as exacting as any operation on the tubotympanic cleft. The surgeon must presume all important temporal bone structures to be at risk. The difficulties are frequently compounded by uncertainty about what was previously done (prior surgical notes not available or lacking detail), and by the continuance of destructive effects of uncontrolled pathologic factors.

In revision mastoidectomy, a wide postaural incision is necessary, with the creation of an anteriorly based musculoperiosteal flap, which will be available for cavity obliteration should the need subsequently be indicated. The incision should provide unobstructed access to the middle and posterior fossa dural plates and to the mastoid tip. The skin of the mastoid bowl is dissected from posterior to anterior, preserving it as far as possible for later use. This dissection is assisted by the use of cubes of plastic sponge to sweep it off the walls of the cavity with minimal risk to unprotected dura mater and the sigmoid sinus. The dissection is advanced to the facial ridge and the posterior aspect of the lateral semicircular canal. It is pru-

FIGURE 19-4. *A*, Anatomic landmarks after opening the mastoid antrum and removing the canal wall. Note osseous spurs and overhangs in the anterior epitympanum and the high facial ridge. (Redrawn from Fisch U, Mattox D: Microsurgery of the Skull Base. New York, Thieme Medical Publications, 1988.) *B*, The cog originates from the roof of epitympanum, anterior to malleus handle.

FIGURE 19-5. After removal of anterior buttress and lowering facial ridge, a smoothly contoured, kidney-shaped cavity results. (Redrawn from Fisch U, Mattox D: Microsurgery of the Skull Base. Thieme Medical Publications, 1988.)

FIGURE 19-4

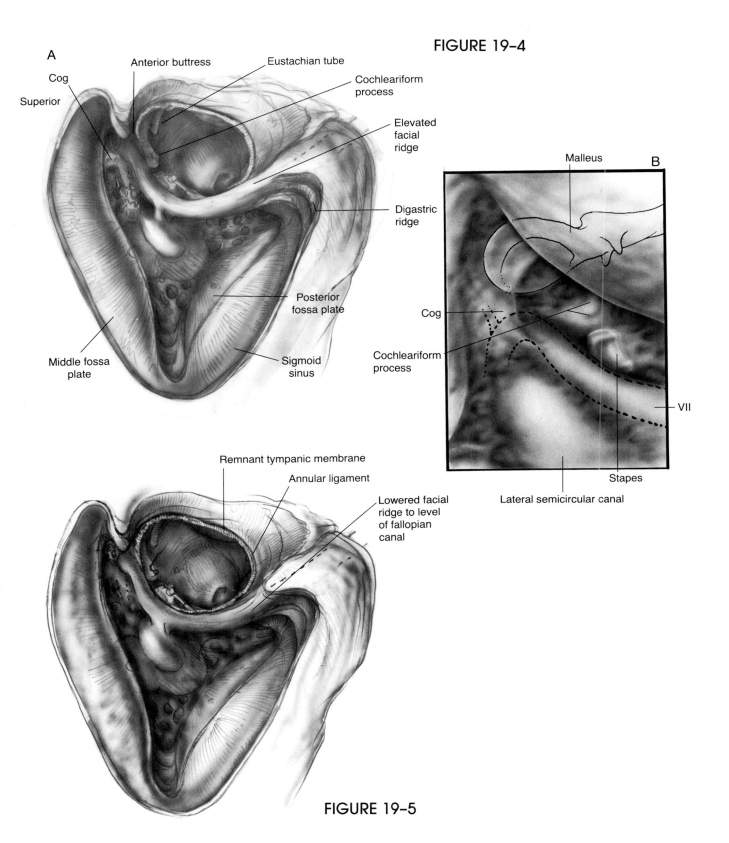

A

Cog

Superior

Anterior buttress

Eustachian tube

Cochleariform process

Elevated facial ridge

Digastric ridge

Middle fossa plate

Posterior fossa plate

Sigmoid sinus

Malleus

B

Cog

Cochleariform process

VII

Lateral semicircular canal

Stapes

Remnant tympanic membrane

Annular ligament

Lowered facial ridge to level of fallopian canal

FIGURE 19-5

dent to anticipate the presence of a labyrinthine fistula, which can usually be identified by visual inspection of the semicircular canals through their epithelial covering. When granulation tissue is present, great care must be taken to avoid inadvertent opening of a fistula, and its removal should be postponed until the completion of all other parts of the operation. If, as the aditus is approached, no orientating landmarks are apparent, the bone overlying the middle fossa dura is drilled just short of dural exposure. Followed medially and anteriorly, the status of the aditus and epitympanum can then be determined with minimal risk. As with the possibility of a labyrinthine fistula, possible dehiscence or pathologic involvement of the facial nerve should be assumed. Both hazards often occur in tandem. The site of facial nerve risk is usually between the first and second genu but can occur in the vertical segment as a result of prior surgical exposure.

When no reliable landmarks for the facial nerve are available, the risk of trauma can be minimized if a properly planned procedure is followed carefully. When the mesotympanum is completely filled with granulations or cholesteatoma, it is best to first find the landmark that is more resistant to disease than any other—the eustachian tube. From here it is safe to dissect posteriorly over the promontory as far as the grooves for the tympanic plexus. These grooves can then be followed superiorly to the base of the cochleariform process, which is adjacent to the junction of the labyrinthine and tympanic segments of the facial nerve. When the process has been destroyed, a useful alternative guide is the muscle belly of the tensor tympani, which, although exposed, usually persists in such cases (Fig. 19–7).

Dissection can then proceed posteriorly following the osseous canal of the tympanic segment of the nerve. Alternatively, dissection can be carried out in an inferior direction from the tegmen across the medial epitympanic wall and the lateral semicircular canal, approaching the tympanic segment of the nerve from its superior aspect. Should the fallopian canal be eroded, careful dissection will reveal the dehiscence and permit avoidance of trauma. Otherwise, a comparison of the rounded, faintly pink bone overlying the nerve with the characteristically dense, ivory white labyrinthine capsule will indicate the relative position of the nerve canal so that dissection can proceed safely over the canal in all directions. A fistula of the lateral semicircular canal should always alert the surgeon to the real possibility of a coexistent dehiscent facial nerve.

There are several abnormalities of the facial nerve in this region that may be a source of disastrous confusion if they are not recognized; the most common of these is the facial nerve, which overlies the footplate of the stapes. It is thus important to positively identify the facial nerve in its normal horizontal canal before removing soft tissue from the surface of the footplate. The importance of making detailed notes and drawings regarding any abnormality or problem with the nerve at all operations is obvious. Such information may well be instrumental in avoiding a disaster should a second operation prove necessary.

Small, exposed areas of the nerve require special management and should be further uncovered for several millimeters in both directions to avoid later neural herniation, which frequently occurs through minor osseous defects, leaving the nerve sorely threatened by any subsequent operation.

The Semicircular Canals

Most ear, nose, and throat surgeons who obtain unsatisfactory results from mastoidectomy already have considerable experience in this field. They are accustomed to opening the mastoid antrum and removing the bony partition between the ear canal and the mas-

---

FIGURE 19–6. Division of obliterative flap into two segments to create an L-shaped strip that permits the graft to reach the epitympanum. (Redrawn from Smyth GDL: Chronic Ear Disease. New York, Churchill Livingstone, 1980.)

FIGURE 19–7. Landmarks on the medial aspect of the tympanum that are frequently resistant to destruction by disease: eustachian tube, cochleariform process, and grooves for tympanic plexus. (Redrawn from Sheehy JL: Surgery of Chronic Otis Media. Otolaryngology, vol 1. New York, Harper & Row, 1977.)

FIGURE 19–8. Schematic drawing to indicate the average dimensions of the semicircular canals and their relation to the facial nerve (VII). A = 4.0mm, B = 4.6mm, C = 3.9mm, D = 4.7mm, E = 4.0mm. (Redrawn from Smyth GDL, Kerr AG, Dowe AC, Khajuria KC: A practical alternative to combined approach tympanoplasty. J Laryngol Otol 83: 1143, 1969.)

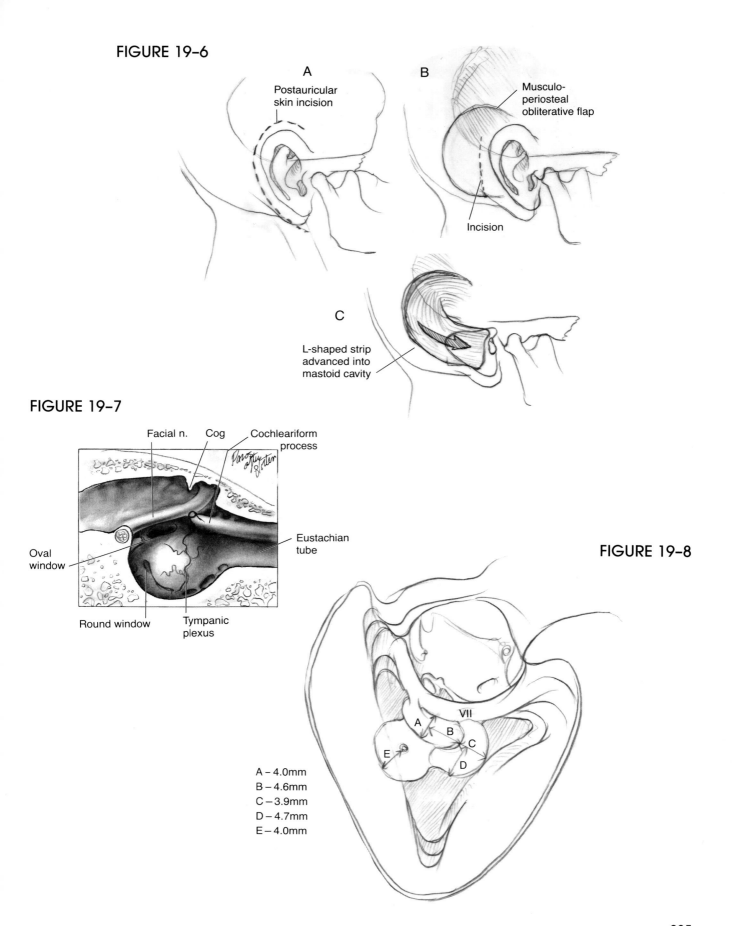

FIGURE 19-6

A

Postauricular
skin incision

B

Musculo-
periosteal
obliterative flap

Incision

C

L-shaped strip
advanced into
mastoid cavity

FIGURE 19-7

Facial n.   Cog   Cochleariform
process

Eustachian
tube

Oval
window

Round window   Tympanic
plexus

FIGURE 19-8

VII

A
B
C
D
E

A – 4.0mm
B – 4.6mm
C – 3.9mm
D – 4.7mm
E – 4.0mm

toid air cells. Usually, further education in the principles of temporal bone surgery is all that is required to substantially improve their results.

Although a loss of continuity of the epithelium between peripheral cells and the middle ear and eustachian tube has been blamed for contamination of the mastoid bowl, this explanation is not entirely satisfactory. Invariably, persistent postoperative discharge after mastoidectomy arises from unhealthy bone and granulations that remain in the mastoid process or from exposed mesotympanic mucosa. Granulation tissue may persist in any part of the mastoid bowl, but most frequently in the retrofacial region and around the semicircular canals. Such a complication usually represents an inadequate technique arising from the surgeon's lack of anatomic knowledge, resulting in a deep gutter behind the facial nerve that promotes the accumulation of debris and leads to dermatitis in the posterior parts of the mastoid bowl. This gutter and residual cells in Trautmann's triangle are errors commonly detected in the revision of unsatisfactory cavities.

Much has been written and said about the importance of the surgeon's acquaintance with the course of the facial nerve, and in most centers trainees are encouraged to acquire this knowledge by dissection of temporal bones. Less importance appears to be attached to understanding the anatomy of the labyrinth. The semicircular canals bear a very constant relationship to one another.

The transverse diameter of the horizontal canal is 4mm and is approximately equal to half its length, and the same relationship exists for the superior and posterior canals. Most importantly, it should be known that the middle third of the posterior canal lies immediately behind the posterior end of the lateral canal, where it straddles the latter squarely (Fig. 19–8). The distance from the lateral surface of the horizontal canal to the common crus is 6.5mm.[3] This knowledge enables the surgeon to locate each canal (particularly the posterior) at the time of operation, using a 4mm burr as a handy measuring device.

Cholesteatomatous Fistula of the Labyrinth

A longstanding controversy exists among otologic surgeons regarding the removal of a cholesteatoma matrix in open-cavity operations.[4, 5] On the one hand, the argument for removing the cholesteatoma membrane is based on the assumption that the matrix exerts, and will continue to exert, an osteolytic chemical effect on underlying bone. This is opposed by the view that the bone-eroding effect of a cholesteatoma matrix results primarily from the pressure exerted by a large cholesteatomal sac and that adequate exterior-

izing the sac is sufficient to avoid an environment within the cavity that would lead to secondary infection and a resurgence of bone-eroding potential. It has also been postulated that leaving some matrix on the medial wall of the mastoid cavity assists epithelialization.

The dimensions of this controversy as it applies to the management of the labyrinthine fistula are clearly demonstrated by the opposing opinions frequently expressed. On one hand, an open technique with preservation of the matrix over fistulae, which are not extending deeply into the labyrinth, has been recommended to avoid the risk of serious sensorineural hearing loss. On the other hand, removal of the matrix (as the *final* step in the procedure, to minimize the effects of suction on the labyrinth), followed by the application of a fascial graft, is also recommended in spite of the calculated risk to the cochlea.[4]

Alternatively, a staged closed technique (ICWT) has been advocated to protect the labyrinth by temporarily preserving a small area of cholesteatoma over and around the fistula,[5] which would not be removed until a second operation when the fistula would be covered with a fascial graft. Although removal of matrix from a superficial labyrinthine fistula obviously must always entail *some* risk of inner ear dysfunction, the risk must be extremely high in extensive fistula cases. Unless the fistula is considered not likely to be self-cleansing, surgical conservatism is surely prudent. Certainly for cholesteatomatous fistula without deep inward extension of keratinizing epithelium in the only hearing ear, the use of an open technique with preservation of the matrix is unquestionably an ethical obligation.

Management of Acquired Cholesteatoma in Children

The treatment of chronic suppurative otitis media (CSOM) in patients who have not yet achieved normal adult immunity to upper respiratory infections continues to be a contentious issue, and it is generally held that the problems of CSOM are more difficult to manage in younger patients, especially when there is cholesteatoma.[6]

The belief that childhood CSOM is a different disease than CSOM in adults, in the sense that the results of surgical therapy are significantly less satisfactory, is commonplace.

Notwithstanding this view, there are certainly no major dissimilarities in anatomic configuration or relationships within the middle ear cleft distinguishing one age group from another, apart from an almost invariably greater degree of pneumatization in the younger patient.

The relevance of nasal and paranasal disease in CSOM is not disputed, and it is sought and treated no less assiduously in children than in older patients. Treatment of the otologic disorder is frequently preceded by therapy of sinus infection, nasal allergy, and, on occasion, adenoid hypertrophy.

In managing childhood cholesteatoma, apart from the necessity of treating a potentially lethal disease,[7] there is the obvious advantage of eliminating unpleasant symptoms, such as recurrent or persistent discharge, and frequently, discomfort, and the possibility of maintaining or improving auditory function. Rehabilitation is particularly pertinent to the problem of children suffering from bilateral involvement. The aggressive nature of the disease must support the view that the earlier treatment is begun, the fewer will be the problems of functional restoration that confront the surgeon. All of the statistics on ossicular reconstruction confirm the view that it is far better to operate *before* the incudal long process or stapes arch has been lost.

Nevertheless, with rare exceptions, most comparisons between the results of closed cholesteatoma surgery in children and adults indicate less satisfactory control of the disease in younger patients. This is scarcely a surprise in view of their continued exposure to the presumed etiologic factors in the immediate postoperative period. With closed techniques, extensive involvement of the mastoid cell system is likely to make total removal of deeply invasive keratinizing squamous epithelium less certain. In spite of high rates of cholesteatomatous complications with ICWT, because of the difficulties in managing the large postoperative cavities, which the extent of pneumatization in ears developing cholesteatoma in early life usually renders unavoidable, staged closed techniques are often preferred to open-cavity operation by those who routinely use an open method for their adult patients. Possibly the best eventual result for children undergoing a two-stage procedure could be achieved by routinely converting a primary ICWT to an open-cavity operation, using bone pate and a musculoperiosteal flap at the second stage if there is then no evidence of residual cholesteatoma to avoid the risk of eventual retraction pocket formation. The surgical method must be strictly individualized according to the pathology of the patient. No single method is superior in all cases.

Postoperative Management

Although there is no unanimity of opinion regarding the necessity of antibiotic cover postoperatively, many surgeons routinely prescribe broad-spectrum antibiotics postoperatively in the belief that by so doing, healing is enhanced and wound infection prevented.

Immediate postoperative care consists of keeping the patient under careful observation and testing at least once daily for evidence of deterioration in labyrinthine function. Spontaneous nystagmus should be sought and tests of balance performed at the bedside. Bone conduction thresholds should be measured using the modified Rainville method[8] if there is any suspicion of inner ear dysfunction. The Rainville method employs the reverse masking principle and is performed by applying a bone conduction masker to the forehead and an air conduction stimulus to the test ear and measuring the degree of threshold shift. Prompt treatment with dexamethasone, for its anti-inflammatory and membrane stabilizing effects, and inhalation for 1 hour during alternate waking hours of 5 per cent carbon dioxide and 95 per cent oxygen, to increase inner ear oxygenation, has been advocated to reverse or contain the effects of surgical labyrinthine trauma.

On the first postoperative day, the postaural wound should be inspected and covered with a gauze dressing, which is renewed daily until the removal of sutures, usually on the fifth postoperative day. Usually the patient can leave the hospital on the first or second postoperative day. Packing is removed from the mastoidectomy cavity after ten days, and broad-spectrum antibiotic with steroid drops prescribed twice daily for 1 week. Thereafter, the ear is examined and cleansed at monthly, and eventually 6-monthly and yearly intervals, as appropriate. During the early postoperative period, any development of granulation tissue can be controlled by chemical cautery and application of gentian violet. Epithelialization of the mastoid bowl and ear canal is usually complete at 1 month. Periodic check-ups are especially important, both to detect residual cholesteatoma and also to remove accumulations of cerumen and keratin, which may threaten the stability of cavity epithelium.

Pitfalls of Surgery

The proximity and frequent involvement of vital and delicate neural and vascular anatomic components of the temporal bone by the diseased tissues, which the surgeon seeks to eliminate, are constantly at risk during any tympanoplastic procedure. An exact knowledge of normal anatomy and its variants is an essential prerequisite for all otologic surgeons. Equally important is an understanding of the distortions of that anatomy that are consequent on chronic disease and previous operative procedures. The surgeon does well to presume that all possible anomalies may exist in any ear on which he or she operates. However, in spite of following the guidelines already proposed to limit dangers to the facial nerve and labyrinth, risk to these structures is by no means eliminated. Nevertheless, should injuries occur, the consequences may be offset by prompt remedial action. For example, the immediate occlusion with bone wax of an iatrogenic fenestration of the labyrinthine capsule, coupled with administration of intravenous antibiotic and steroid therapy, may offset or diminish serious postoperative inner ear sequelae.

Facial nerve trauma demands immediate action. If the sheath remains intact and only an edematous re-action is anticipated, bone removal to decompress the nerve for 3mm in either direction may prevent long-term disability. Whether the sheath should also be opened in an infected ear is debatable. Antibiotic and steroid therapy should be commenced immediately, without waiting for a clinical assessment of nerve function. If disruption of nerve fibers has occurred to a significant extent, graft replacement will be re-quired. Whether this should be immediate or delayed for 3 to 4 weeks to take advantage of neural regrowth is undecided. When consequences of facial nerve trauma, unsuspected by the surgeon, are observed on recovery from anesthesia, the options depend on its degree. Partial loss of function presumed due to edema demands prompt administration of steroid therapy and daily clinical evaluation and measure-ment of response to electrical testing. Evidence of pro-gressive and severe loss of response is generally con-sidered to be an absolute indication for exploration and nerve grafting, if appropriate. On the other hand, immediate postoperative total facial paralysis must be presumed as indicative of potentially irreversible damage to nerve tissue and requires immediate explo-ration and appropriate remedial action, ranging from release of intersheath hematoma to removal of im-pinging bone fragments to nerve replacement.

Excessive hemorrhage from tears in the walls of large veins in the tegmen dura or from the sigmoid sinus of the jugular bulb can usually be easily con-trolled by the application of Surgicel strips. If, at the conclusion of the operation, there is uncertainty about reliable hemostasis, this should be ensured by addi-tional packing with antibiotic-impregnated gauze, which will be removed from the cavity 1 week later.

Tears in the dura resulting in a leak of cerebrospinal fluid are controlled and eliminated by firmly applied strips of temporalis fascia supported by absorbable gelatin sponge (Gelfoam). Postoperative cerebrospinal rhinorrhea is an absolute indication for reoperation to identify its source and effect a dural repair.

RESULTS

In the evaluation of the results of canal wall down tympanoplasty, only those reported by surgeons whose adherence to the essential principles of tech-nique already described are relevant. Because the cri-terion of success of any operation for chronic inflam-matory disease in the tubotympanic cleft is its ability to maintain the health of the ear over time, long-term observation of analyzable numbers of ears for no less than for 5 and ideally for 10 or more years is neces-sary to reach a reliable opinion of merit. Unfortu-nately, there are few reports that meet this require-ment, but those that do exist provide supportive evidence for the use of an open-cavity technique in the management of extensive cholesteatoma.

The principle criteria in evaluating the worth of tympanoplasty procedures are elimination of choles-teatoma, freedom from its recurrence, stability of the ear, and quality of hearing (which will also be dis-cussed elsewhere in this volume).

Postoperative Cholesteatoma

Although it has been suggested that epidermoids de-tected postoperatively develop from matrix not re-moved by the surgeon, the possibility that they may also originate from nests of keratin formation in gran-ulation tissue or from a subsequent metaplastic proc-ess cannot be discounted. Regardless of their etiology, they represent a major cause of surgical failure and may give rise to serious intracranial complications.[9]

In a recently completed study of cholesteatomatous complications in 85 canal wall down operations per-formed in the classical posterior-to-anterior route, the incidence of postoperative cholesteatoma in 83 pa-tients all followed up for 5 years was 2.5 per cent.[10] Similarly, in a subsequent group in which the ante-rior-posterior route was used, the incidence was 6 per cent in 43 patients, all followed up for 5 years.[11] In children, postoperative cholesteatoma has been re-ported in 2.8 per cent. These statistics are in striking contrast with those reported by 11 authors during the past 18 years in almost 3000 intact canal wall opera-tions in which the mean recurrence rate of cholestea-toma was 30 per cent.[12–22]

Postoperative Stability of the Ear

Although there is little published evidence to indicate the incidence of moisture or discharge following canal wall down operations, two 10-year studies show that improvements in surgical technique have reduced the frequency of this complication.[23] Moist cavities are re-ported in 3 per cent of ears having an open-cavity operation without obliteration and the same incidence in another group with cavity obliteration. In another study of 279 ears with cavity obliteration, there was a 4 per cent incidence of discharge after the first year.[24]

Excessive wax and epithelial debris formation in canal wall down ears can be anticipated in at least 6 per cent. It has been confirmed that the use of an obliterating flap resulted in a smaller cavity at 10 years, mean volume 1.8cm^3 as opposed to 2.4cm^3 when no flap was used (normal controls, 0.96cm^3)[23]: no relationship between cavity volume variance and stability has been shown so far.

Postoperative Hearing

The auditory status (0.5kHz to 2kHz) of 92 ICWT, 92 canal wall down operations with obliteration, and 74 canal wall down ears without obliteration was evaluated.[23] Long-term information on hearing status after the surgical treatment of cholesteatoma is scant. However, at 1 year postoperatively, ICWT patients had greater improvement in air conduction threshold than canal wall down ears. However, at final review (8 to 11 years), this advantage for the ICWT group was lost, with average hearing gain being similar for both groups. A separate analysis with an air-conduction average including 4kHz did not show any additional differences between either group. With the criteria for patient satisfaction in operations to improve hearing being a reduction of interaural difference to less than 15dB or an air-conduction average of less than 30dB,[25] it is salutory to note that neither technique meets these criteria despite substantial decreases in air-conduction thresholds.

References

1. Stacke L: Die operative Freilegung der Mittelohrraume. Tubingen, F Pietzcker, 1897, p 2.
2. Tumarkin A: A contribution to the study of middle ear suppuration with special reference to the pathology and treatment of cholesteatoma. J Laryngol Otol 53: 737, 1938.
3. Smyth GDL, Kerr AG, Dowe AC, Khajuria KC: A practical alternative to combined approach tympanoplasty. J Laryngol Otol 83: 1143, 1969.
4. Palva T, Karja J, Palva A: Opening of the labyrinth during chronic ear surgery. Arch Otolaryngol 91: 75, 1971.
5. Law KP, Smyth GDL, Kerr AG: Fistula of the labyrinth treated by staged combined approach tympanoplasty. J Laryngol Otol 89: 471, 1975.
6. Baron SH: Management of aural cholesteatoma in children. Otolaryngol Clin North Am 2:71, 1969.
7. Sheehy JL, Brackmann DE, Graham MD: Complications of cho-

lesteatoma: A report of 1024 cases. *In* McCabe B, Sade J, Abramson M (eds): Cholesteatoma, First International Conference. Birmingham, AL, Aesculapius, 1977, p 420.
8. Rainville MJ: Nouvelle methode d'assourdissement pour le releve des courbes de conduction osseuse. J Fr Otorhinolaryngol Lar 4: 851, 1955.
9. Fisch U: Intracranial complications of cholesteatoma. *In* Sade J (ed): Cholesteatoma and Mastoid Surgery. Amsterdam, Kugler, 1982, p 369.
10. Smyth GDL, Toner JG: Canal wall down tympanoplasty. Am J Otol 1993 [In press].
11. Smyth GDL, Brooker DS: Small cavity mastoidectomy. Clin Otolaryngol 17: 280, 1992.
12. Bellucci JR: Problems in surgical control of cholesteatoma. *In* McCabe B, Sade J, Abramson M (eds): Cholesteatoma, First International Conference. Birmingham, AL, Aesculapius, 1977, p 390.
13. Brown JS: A ten year statistical follow-up of 1142 consecutive cases of cholesteatoma: The closed vs the open technique. Laryngoscope 92: 390, 1982.
14. Cody DTR: Cholesteatoma recurrent or residual. *In* Shambaugh E, Shea JJ (eds): Shambaugh International Workshop. Huntsville, AL, Strode, 1980, p 88.
15. Deguine, quoted by Brandow EL: Implantation cholesteatoma in mastoid. *In* McCabe B, Sade J, Abramson M (eds): Cholesteatoma, First International Conference. Birmingham, AL, Aesculapius, 1977, p 253.
16. Glasscock ME, Miller GM: Intact canal wall tympanoplasty in the management of cholesteatoma. Laryngoscope 86: 1639, 1976.
17. Jansen C: Evaluation of surgery for cholesteatoma. *In* McCabe B, Sade J, Abramson M (eds): Cholesteatoma, First International Conference. Birmingham, AL, Aesculapius, 1977, p 352.
18. Kinny S: Intact canal wall tympanoplasty with mastoidectomy. Laryngoscope 92: 1395, 1982.
19. Smyth GDL: Postoperative cholesteatoma in combined approach tympanoplasty. J Laryngol Otol 90: 597, 1967.
20. Wright WK: A concept for management of otitis cholesteatoma. *In* McCabe B, Sade J, Abramson M (eds): Cholesteatoma, First International Conference. Birmingham, AL, Aesculapius, 1977, p 374.
21. Abramson M, Lechenbruch PA, Paress JHB, McCabe BF: Results of conservative surgery for middle-ear cholesteatoma. Laryngoscope 87: 128, 1977.
22. Austin DF: The significance of the retraction pocket in the treatment of cholesteatoma. *In* McCabe B, Sade J, Abramson M (eds): Cholesteatoma, First International Conference. Birmingham, AL, Aesculapius, 1977, p 379.
23. Toner JG, Smyth GDL: Surgical treatment of cholesteatoma: A comparison of three techniques. Am J Otol 11: 247, 1990.
24. Ojala K: Late results of obliteration in chronic otitis media. Acta Innversitatis Ouluensis Ophthalmol Oto Rhino Laryngol 5: 53, 1979.
25. Smyth GDL, Patterson CC: Results of middle ear reconstruction: Do patients and surgeons agree? Am J Otol 6: 276, 1985.

20

Canal Wall Reconstruction With Homograft Knee Cartilage

ROGER E. WEHRS, M.D.

In the early 1960s, this author embraced the concept of the intact wall type of tympanoplasty. By eliminating a cavity, a trouble-free ear was created that was more amenable to reconstruction of hearing. However, many patients still had draining cavities and were seeking a way to obtain a dry ear. In these early revisions, different methods of cavity obliteration, such as muscle flaps, were tried. The initial results were good, but over the longer term, atrophy and absorption of the muscle with breakdown occurred and a wet cavity recurred. In my opinion, these problems occurred because it is virtually impossible to remove every mastoid cell, and those that remained were trapped and would secrete and cause breakdown and a recurrent wet ear.

Also, in some cases of intact wall tympanoplasty, there was very little space between the dural plate and the bony ear canal. Therefore, preserving the intact bony canal wall was very difficult. Dehiscence of the canal wall was repaired with homograft nasal cartilage, which worked very well for small defects; however, these scraps of cartilage were not large enough to rebuild an entire canal wall. The use of homograft knee cartilage for this purpose was discovered quite by accident. The discovery involved a case with a huge open cavity. Different pieces of nasal cartilage were obtained, but none were large enough to close the defect. The nurse anesthetist noted my dilemma and commented that the orthopedic physician in the next room had just removed a knee cartilage from a football player, and it was too bad we could not use that. The use of knee cartilage in an ear had not occurred to me before, but we decided to look at the cartilage. In those days, the orthopedist removed large portions, and sometimes, as in this case, the entire meniscus. It was cleaned, soaked in penicillin, and brought into the field. When viewed under the operating microscope, its resemblance to the posterior bony wall was uncanny (Fig. 20–1). It had a gentle curve and thin lower edge that very much resembled the normal scutum of the bony canal wall. It was trimmed to size and used to create a new posterior canal wall. At that time, the cartilage's fate was unknown, but fortunately it was accepted by the host with no evidence of an adverse reaction. The ear healed well and the patient had an almost normal-appearing canal wall and good hearing.

Following this experience, a technique was developed that used homograft knee cartilages in mastoid reconstruction for primary cases as well as in revisions of open cavities. The orthopedic surgeons were very cooperative in saving the extracted menisci for use in reconstruction of the ear. The knee cartilages were preserved in the same way as were homograft ossicles and tympanic membranes: in 70 per cent ethyl alcohol. The first few cartilages were placed directly

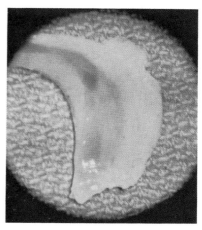

FIGURE 20–1. Homograft knee cartilage demonstrates a gentle curve and thin lower edge.

in the alcohol solution following their removal from the knee. However, the pathologists soon began to demand that the surgical specimen be examined and recorded. This step produced a potential snag in that the cartilages were placed in formalin before they were sent to the pathologist for examination and report, which had the effect of rendering them unfit for transplantation purposes. Therefore, a compromise was worked out in which the cartilage fragments were placed in the alcohol solution in the operating room and then sent to the pathologist, who would look at the specimen and report that they were indeed fragments of menisci and then replace the fragments in the alcohol container. These were then picked up routinely by the private scrub nurse and placed in a special bottle labeled "Knee Cartilage Bank." At the time of surgery, they were put through several washings of Ringer's lactate solution to remove the alcohol and then soaked in an antibiotic solution (usually penicillin) until needed at surgery.

In 1972, the first paper describing the technique was presented.[1] Fifteen ears had been reconstructed by that time, and detailed studies were presented on three of these cases, including their preoperative and postoperative audiograms. Satisfactory hearing and a dry cavity was reported for all ears. A follow-up paper was also published in 1978 that covered 79 ears and provided detailed anatomic and hearing results on 63 cases.[2] Satisfactory anatomic results were obtained on 57 per cent and serviceable hearing in 77 per cent of the cases. During the next decade, this technique continued almost unchanged. However, in the early 1980s, two events changed things dramatically: the introduction of the arthroscope and the HIV epidemic. The specimens from the orthopedic surgeons became smaller and less abundant, and we could no longer trust alcohol sterilization alone. Fortunately, at about this time, the American Red Cross became active in obtaining all types of transplant tissues from cadavers, including knee cartilage menisci. The donors were carefully screened for HIV, hepatitis, and other contaminants. The Red Cross produced an adequate supply of large, high-quality cartilage transplants so that this technique could continue.

PATIENT SELECTION

Three types of ears qualify for this operative procedure. The first is a chronically wet or draining ear that has not responded to conservative therapy or has frequent relapses. The second is an ear with a dry cavity but a 30dB or more conductive hearing loss. The third type is a dead ear with a chronically draining cavity.

Indications

The indications for surgery are based on hearing loss and drainage and have been divided into the following categories:

- The patient has had radical surgery on both ears, and they both drain. The ear with the worst hearing would be operated on first, followed by the second ear in 3 or 4 months.
- One ear is normal and the other has a draining cavity. The important consideration here is stopping the drainage. This procedure is indicated even if there is a total sensorineural hearing loss in the affected ear.
- The patient has undergone radical surgery on both ears, and both are dry. The indication for the surgery would be to improve the hearing. Assuming that the bone conduction, discrimination score, and eustachian tube function were good, the poorer-hearing ear should be operated on first unless the patient had been successfully wearing a hearing aid in it, in which case the better-hearing ear should be operated on first.
- One ear is normal with good hearing, and there is a conductive loss in the other but a dry cavity. Reconstruction would not be indicated unless the conductive component were large, the bone conduction excellent, and the patient highly motivated.

Contraindications

Some ears should remain open cavities so that they may drain and are accessible to cleaning from the outside. These include cases of extensive cholesteatoma, especially ears that have had several revisions. Patients with malignancy of the temporal bone or brain abscess would not be candidates for reconstruc-

tion, nor would patients in whom a large fistula of the horizontal canal or dehiscence of the facial nerve was encountered at the original surgery. It would be difficult and dangerous to elevate the epithelium over these structures, and even if successful, the new wall would impinge on them. There have also been cases in which the squamous epithelial lining of the cavity was intimately attached to the middle fossa dura or lateral sinus; if these could not be completely dissected off, the reconstruction was not completed.

PREOPERATIVE EVALUATION

For this operation to be successful, the ear must be dry or at the very least not infected at the time of surgery. On the initial visit, the ear is cleaned and evaluated under the operating microscope. All debris and mucus are suctioned or removed by cotton-tipped wire applicators dipped in Cortisporin otic suspension. Bleeding granulations are cauterized by means of a silver nitrate stick. The ear is then wiped dry and chloramphenicol (Chloromycetin) powder gently insufflated into the cavity. The patient is instructed on aural hygiene, which consists of sleeping with the affected ear toward the ceiling, not blowing the nose, and sneezing with the mouth open. In addition, the patients should not wash their hair in a shower but over a tub or lavatory, and they should saturate a large cotton ball with white petroleum jelly and place it in the concha. These patients have had itching from the drainage and are in the habit of rubbing and scratching the ear. They must be convinced that this behavior be terminated for the ear to dry. They are told that the itching is a mild type of pain and that the physician will do everything possible to help them leave the ear alone, including cleaning the ear as described previously as well as prescribing antipruritic and analgesic medications, such as diphenhydramine (Benedryl) and acetaminophen. The patients are then seen again about 2 weeks later, at which time the ear is usually dry and surgery can be scheduled.

RATIONALE OF PROCEDURE

The rationale of the procedure is explained to the patient. The goal of the surgery is to restore the ear to normal anatomic structure and function. In the normal ear, the mastoid is a honeycomb of air cells aerated through the eustachian tube. The mucus from the cells drains into the middle ear via the eustachian tube to the nasopharynx. The eardrum is supported by the posterior bony canal wall so that a normal middle ear space is maintained. The ossicular chain conducts the sound vibrations from the eardrum to the fluids of the inner ear. The external ear canal cleans itself by epithelial migration (Fig. 20–2).

Now let us consider what occurs after this bony wall has been removed. Support for the eardrum is lost, and it collapses against the medial wall of the middle ear. The middle ear space is compromised so that the ossicles, if they survived, cannot function normally, and the motion of the tympanic membrane is limited. The mastoid air cells that remain are trapped and cannot drain to the eustachian tube but keep the cavity wet. Due to the large cavity and rough contours, the patterns of epithelial migration are changed, allowing crusts and epithelial debris to collect in the cavity (Fig. 20–3).

Now let us look at a reconstructive procedure that restores as nearly as possible the ear to normal anatomic configuration and function. The posterior canal wall is reconstructed in anatomic position with homograft knee cartilage. The new drumhead is rebuilt with a homograft tympanic membrane and malleus. The sound-conduction mechanism consists of an incus-stapes prosthesis of hydroxyapatite between the stapedial footplate and the homograft malleus. The middle ear space is normal in size and function and is aerated through the former mastoidectomy cavity, which is now one large air cell. Mucus from the mastoid drains into the middle ear and down the eustachian tube. The external ear is of normal size and cleans itself by epithelial migration (Fig. 20–4).

The patient is told that he or she has an 85 to 90 per cent chance of a dry, trouble-free ear. The chance of hearing improvement is good, especially when the bone conduction and discrimination are normal. Patients are warned, however, that in this type of surgery we are trying to give them something rather than take it away, as occurs in most operations. Furthermore, there is a chance that the hearing may get worse instead of better, and there is always the chance of total deafness. They are further counseled that there is very little pain associated with this operation and that the pain can be controlled by mild analgesics, such as acetaminophen. Bleeding is not a problem, and transfusion will not be necessary. Subcuticular sutures are employed, and the patient is usually discharged the day following the surgery.

PREOPERATIVE PREPARATION

There is no special preoperative preparation except to have the ear as dry as possible. The patient is told that an area of approximately one inch will be shaved around the ear, and that a bun type mastoid dressing will be applied for 24 hours. They are told that because the new wall, eardrum, and implants cannot be sewed in position but depend on packing and gravity, it is important to keep the operated ear toward the ceiling. They are not to chew solid food the day of surgery and are not to sit up to eat. In addition, they should not blow their nose and should sneeze with the mouth open. Also, they should not rub the ear or neck.

The preparation of the ear for surgery consists of two stages: one before draping and the second after draping. After the head is positioned under microscopic vision, the head is secured into position by taping it to the head rest. First, a strip of one-inch adhesive tape is applied to the undersurface of the head holder and brought over the head above the ear to hold and cover the hair above the ear. Plastic tape is applied in a like manner both in front and behind the ear to hold the hair out of the field. As a postauricular incision is anticipated, an area of approximately one inch around the pinna is shaved dry. The loose hairs are removed by repeatedly dabbing the area with the adhesive side of a piece of two-inch plastic tape. The head is then taped to the Juers-Derlacki head holder with one-inch adhesive tape, which is also used over the edge of the shaved area to hold and cover the hair. As stated previously, the shave is dry so that the tape will adhere properly. Plastic tape is then used in a like manner both in front and behind the ear to cover and hold the hair. The ear is then scrubbed with Rondex sponges dipped in pHisoHex soap. The soap is removed with Ringer's lactate solution and the area rescrubbed with 70 per cent ethyl alcohol. The skin is dried with the Rondex sponges.

Next, a 3M plastic drape with round hole is applied over the previously placed tape. A large plastic body drape is then positioned over the patient, and the ear is located by feel through the drape. With a scissors, a round cutout is made approximately twice the size of the hole in the 3M drape. Another 3M drape is placed

FIGURE 20–2. Normal middle ear and mastoid. Note honeycomb of air cells and drainage.

FIGURE 20–3. Middle ear and mastoid after canal wall has been removed. Note collapse of drum to stapedial footplate and open cavity.

FIGURE 20–4. Middle ear and mastoid after reconstruction with homograft knee cartilage, tympanic membrane, and incus-stapes prosthesis of hydroxyapatite.

FIGURE 20-2

NORMAL ANATOMY

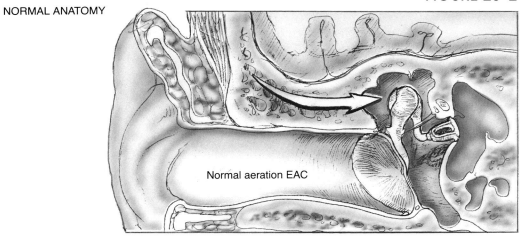

Normal aeration EAC

FIGURE 20-3

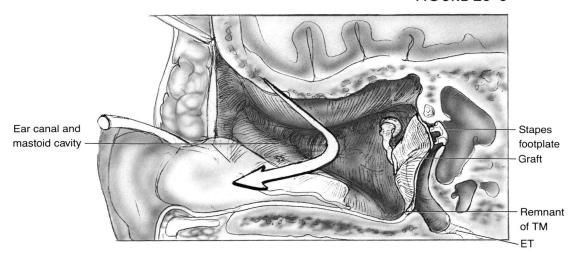

Ear canal and
mastoid cavity

Stapes
footplate
Graft

Remnant
of TM
ET

FIGURE 20-4

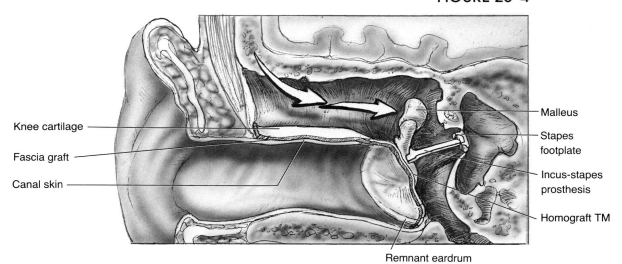

Knee cartilage

Fascia graft

Canal skin

Malleus

Stapes
footplate

Incus-stapes
prosthesis

Homograft TM

Remnant eardrum

over this drape, thus securing the body drape to the patient's head and ear. Next, the microscope is brought back in position and the ear canal visualized through a sterile speculum. The second part of the preparation is now accomplished. The canal and cavity are copiously irrigated with 70 per cent ethyl alcohol through the speculum with constant suction to remove all wax and debris and to further sterilize the cavity and drum. After repeated washings, the alcohol is removed with repeated irrigations and suction with Ringer's lactate. The alcohol irrigation is used regardless of an open perforation and is in fact used to remove the mucus and debris from the middle ear and margins of the perforation. If the perforation is dry and clean, then the Ringer's lactate is used alone.

SURGICAL TECHNIQUE

The procedure is carried out through an incision that falls in the postauricular sulcus. This location affords good access to the middle ear, in addition to producing a minimal scar in a skin fold. The incision is deepened slowly and deliberately to create subcutaneous flaps and not create an opening directly into the mastoidectomy cavity. Both anterior and posterior flaps are created so that there is wide exposure from the conchal cartilage to well behind the mastoid bowl.

Next, the posterior border of the mastoid cavity is palpated, and a new incision is made through the subcutaneous tissue and periosteum to the bone a few millimeters posterior to the bone edge. The lining of the cavity is elevated, and care is taken not to tear the epithelium as it is lifted off the bone. If air cells have been trapped, their secretions often macerate and erode the skin, thus creating a wet mastoid bowl. As the lining over these areas is removed, mucous cysts and mucosa-lined cells are encountered. Their lining need not be removed because one objective of this operation is to convert the previous mastoidectomy cavity into a large air cell. Residual cholesteatoma may also be found and of course must be meticulously and completely removed before any reconstruction can take place. Other complications encountered during the elevation include exposure of the lateral sinus, middle fossa dura, or facial nerve. Usually, the epithelial lining can be removed from these structures, but if this cannot be safely accomplished, the reconstructive effort must be abandoned.

The dissection is carried forward along the dural plate and over the facial ridge to the middle ear. If a remnant of eardrum remains, it will help in the reconstruction. The epithelial lining is removed from this remnant to obtain a bare bed and foundation for the homograft eardrum. Often, an air-containing space is found over the eustachian tube orifice. A mastoid Silastic implant (Xomed Treace) fills the middle ear, with a cutout for the oval window, and extends back into the mastoid.[3] This encourages mucous membrane to grow back into the cavity, producing aeration of the mastoid and preventing retraction.

After the middle ear is prepared, attention is turned to the task of rebuilding the posterior canal wall. A template is fashioned from the tinfoil of a suture packet to serve as a pattern for the new wall. It extends from the behind the facial ridge to the anterior part of the dural plate. Occasionally, grooves must be drilled in the facial ridge and dural plate to support the new cartilage wall. When the tinfoil appears to recreate the wall in an anatomic position, it is placed as a template over a piece of semilunar knee cartilage. With a scalpel, the template is traced, and a block of cartilage is outlined. Each end of the cartilage block is split into a thin and a thick sheet with a sharp scalpel (Fig. 20–5). The thicker part of the homograft cartilage will fit into the grooves for support, and the thin layer will overlap the facial ridge and dural plate to prevent formation of retraction pockets, which could lead to crusting (Fig. 20–6). The sculptured cartilage wall is temporarily put in place and modified if necessary. It is then removed and the middle ear reconstruction begun. If the patient's malleus is still present, it is used, but if it is absent or involved in disease, the homograft tympanic membrane with its attached malleus becomes the main building block in the reconstruction. Usually, there is a rim of eardrum to support the homograft tympanic membrane anteriorly;

FIGURE 20–5. Grooving of homograft knee cartilage. Thin flaps overlap facial ridge and dural plate, and thicker ones are for support.

FIGURE 20–6. Knee cartilage temporarily in place. Note position of thin and thick flaps.

FIGURE 20–7. *A*, Cartilage wall removed temporarily so that the hearing mechanism can be rebuilt. *B*, Homograft tympanic membrane and malleus with incus-stapes prosthesis of hydroxyapatite in place.

FIGURE 20–8. Homograft dura or fascia overlay the homograft tympanic membrane, malleus, and replacement prosthesis.

FIGURE 20-5

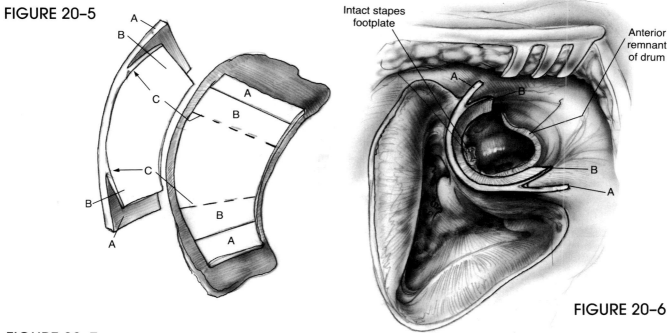

Intact stapes footplate

Anterior remnant of drum

FIGURE 20-6

FIGURE 20-7

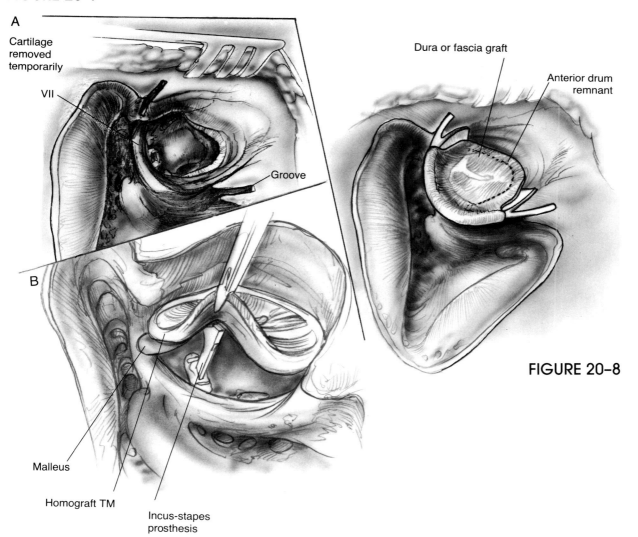

A

Cartilage removed temporarily

VII

Groove

B

Malleus

Homograft TM

Incus-stapes prosthesis

Dura or fascia graft

Anterior drum remnant

FIGURE 20-8

posteriorly, it rests on the knee cartilage. The head of the malleus is preserved and extends under the cartilage wall. The sound pressure mechanism is rebuilt with a replacement prosthesis of hydroxyapatite with the notch under the manubrium of the malleus and the cup over the head of the stapes or the shaft to the stapedial footplate (Figs. 20–7A and B).

The cartilage wall is replaced, and both it and the homograft eardrum are overlaid with fascia or homograft dura (Fig. 20–8). The redundant skin that had been elevated from the mastoidectomy cavity is trimmed and reflected back over the new posterior wall. These structures are held in place with moist absorbable gelatin sponge (Gelfoam) packing. The subcutaneous flap created at the beginning of the procedure is now replaced over the cartilage wall and cavity. It is then sutured to the perichondrium, and the tissues are closed tightly; in this way, subsequent postauricular depression is prevented. No drain is used, even in wet cavities, because the mastoid now has good drainage beneath the cartilage wall to the middle ear and down the eustachian tube. The skin incision is closed with silk, and a mastoid dressing is applied.

DRESSING

A piece of ¼-inch, selvage-edge gauze saturated with Cortisporin ointment is inserted into the external auditory meatus. A cotton ball is placed in the concha. A conventional mastoid-type of pressure dressing is applied that consists of fluffs and 4 × 4 gauze pads made into a bun and secured by wrapping the head with a 3-inch Kling dressing.

POSTOPERATIVE CARE

The absorbable gelatin sponge packing and the force of gravity are the main forces holding the homografts in place. Therefore, the patient should keep the affected ear uppermost for the first few hours following surgery and should not lie deliberately on the ear for 1 week.

The mastoid dressing is removed the morning after the surgery, and the patient is discharged from the hospital. Antibiotics are not used routinely but occasionally are prescribed when the operative time is prolonged or the ear wet preoperatively. The patient is cautioned to avoid rubbing or scratching the ear or neck. The hair may be washed 4 days following the surgery by plugging the external ear with a cotton pledget saturated with white petrolatum jelly. There are no restrictions on flying by airplane immediately following surgery. The patient is cautioned *not* to autoinflate the ear.

Two weeks following surgery, the patient is seen in the office. The postauricular incision should be well healed, and if the ends of the subcuticular sutures remain they are removed. By means of gentle suction, the gelatin sponge, blood clots, and debris are removed from the ear canal. Subsequent visits occur at 2-week intervals. The new canal wall and drum are usually epithelialized and dry 6 weeks following surgery. A hearing test may be performed at this time unless there is still edema or delayed healing.

ANATOMIC RESULTS

Once the ear has healed, the patient may resume all activities and is next seen approximately 6 months following the surgery. At that time, the ear is examined according to the following criteria, which were set up several years ago as representing a satisfactory result: normal contour of the ear canal and tympanic membrane, no crusts or retraction pockets, no wet areas or discharge, and no restrictions on swimming or showering. In a report covering a 10-year period, 57 per cent of the ears that had the operation met these criteria.

HEARING RESULTS

The overall hearing results have been good. In an earlier report, 72 per cent of the ears had closed the air-bone gap to within 20 dB of the preoperative air.

COMPLICATIONS

No serious complications have occurred with the use of homograft knee cartilage in more than 200 ears. When this technique was begun, some of the knee cartilages were expected to completely extrude. Fortunately, this did not happen; however, in one patient, the ear drained profusely postoperatively, and the bare cartilage could be seen through the external ear canal. The cartilage was removed through the ear canal under general anesthesia, and the ear healed with a dry but open cavity. One patient developed a wound infection 10 days following surgery, with breakdown of the incision and formation of a postauricular fistula. The fistula closed spontaneously a few months later, but the patient did not obtain good hearing. The knee cartilages should definitely not be preserved in formalin, as there may be poor healing with this type of storage.

Other complications include recurrent perforations, retraction pockets with crusts, recurrent discharge, and cholesteatoma with absorption of the cartilage. Other unfavorable outcomes result from a malfunctioning eustachian tube with serous otitis media.

Poor hearing results may occur as a result of dislocation or poor function of the ossicles used in the reconstruction. Poor hearing is especially likely if both a homograft malleus and a tympanic membrane were used because these materials create an unstable assembly owing to absence of the tensor tympani tendon.

Avoidance of Complications

Careful and meticulous surgery are the key to avoiding postoperative complications. The best way to prevent a complication is to review its cause and then attack the cause. For example, retraction pockets with subsequent crusts form because rough areas and poor support exist under the migrating canal skin. These usually form at the junction between the knee cartilage and the bone of the facial ridge or dural plate. To prevent this formation from occurring, it is necessary to groove the knee cartilage so that a thin sheet overlaps the bone and maintains a firm smooth contour for the new canal skin. Perforations occur because there has been a breakdown of tissue over the new middle ear because of a poor blood supply for the graft, and the cause of perforation may be poor preparation of the bed, or the homograft eardrum may not have been properly covered with fascia or homograft dura. The transplant drum is very thin, nonviable tissue. New skin must grow over it above and new mucosa below, and then it must be invaded and revascularized before it can again become living tissue. It is a race, therefore, between the invading tissues and the decaying ones. If the invaders win, a good intact graft results. If the decayers win, recurrent perforations will result. It is therefore to our advantage to do everything possible to help the invaders. This help consists of completely covering the thin transplant with the thicker and tougher fascia or dura, which will persist longer and resist breakdown until it has been revascularized.

Recurrent drainage means that the normal secretion from the mastoid cells has found its way under the skin rather than into the middle ear and down the eustachian tube. This problem is usually caused by failure to aerate the mastoid beneath the knee cartilage or failure to use silicone sheeting to prevent adhesions from blocking the egress of fluid from the mastoid. Occasionally, cells along the facial ridge are trapped, and these secretions are prevented from reaching the mastoid antrum.

For recurrent cholesteatoma, the only prevention is complete and meticulous removal. However, removal involves slow and tedious surgery. Unless one is willing to spend at least 2 or 3 hours on the task of removing the cholesteatoma in addition to the reconstructive surgery, one will have a high incidence of recurrence. If cholesteatoma recurs after two reconstructive procedures, it would probably be best to reconvert the ear back to an open cavity.

REVISIONS FOR HEARING

There are cases in which the wall is in a good position and the graft is clean and dry, but an air-bone gap with unserviceable hearing remains. Revision is carried out through the ear canal by the raising of a tympanomeatal flap, but one cannot cut over the knee cartilage with a canal skin knife. It is necessary, therefore, to begin the incision over the bone of the inferior or superior canal where bone still remains. The flap is extended to the cartilage wall, and then the elevation is completed over it with a sickle knife and scissors. The flap should be made larger than that used for stapedectomy because the graft shrinks considerably. The elevation is carried down to the middle ear cavity, and the mucosa is incised. At this stage one can determine the cause and extent of the defect and make repairs. Most frequently, the defect involves displacement of the incus prosthesis. Occasionally, an incus replacement prosthesis has been used on what appeared to be an intact stapes, but there had been erosion or absorption of the crura with only a phantom superstructure. In this instance, the floating stapes head and crura must be removed and reconstruction carried directly to the footplate by means of an incus-stapes replacement prosthesis.

On rare occasion, there may be absorption of the malleus handle, which must be replaced with a homograft tympanic membrane and attached malleus placed beneath the elevated flap. Reconstruction is then carried out with the appropriate incus prosthesis.

Occasionally, the cause of the conductive deafness is a malfunctioning eustachian tube and resulting serous otitis media. If this etiology is suspected, the patient should undergo a myringotomy preoperatively. If fluid is obtained, a temporary polyethylene tube is inserted for 24 hours and the audiogram repeated. When a good increase in the hearing occurs, the temporary tube is removed, and the patient is scheduled for a revision, with insertion of a permanent Silverstein or Jahn permanent aeration prosthesis.[4, 5] For this surgery, a tympanomeatal flap is raised and a hole drilled through the bony annulus just posterior to the round window for the Silverstein silicone sheeting tube. If there is insufficient space for the hole, a groove may be created in the bone of the posterior inferior canal for the Jahn hydroxyapatite prosthesis. The Silverstein tube should not be placed through the cartilage wall, because breakdown with a permanent perforation will occur.

ANATOMIC REVISIONS

Occasionally the ear heals well, the only defect being a recurrent perforation, which is best dealt with entirely through the ear canal by means of a canal skin tympanoplasty. The canal skin is removed in routine fashion except over the knee cartilage wall. Here, one cannot cut through the skin with a canal skin knife, but the skin must be elevated off the cartilage by means of a sickle knife and then cut with scissors. Another advantage of removing the canal skin is that any anterior bony overhang may be taken down with a diamond burr. This step is important because the bony overhang may have been responsible for poor exposure and placement of the original graft. Once the canal skin has been removed, the ossicular reconstruction may be carried out. The ear is then grafted with a homograft tympanic membrane and covered with the canal skin. If there was a hearing defect, it is also corrected at this time.

If the ear continues to have wet areas and drains after 2 or 3 months when healing should be complete, the cause may be trapped mucosa or blockage of mastoid air cells. This condition may occur along the facial ridge, as stated earlier. Another reason for drainage is blockage of the secretions from reaching the middle ear. The knee cartilage may have been placed too low or directly on the horizontal canal. Failure to use silicone sheeting under the new wall to the antrum will allow adhesions to form, with subsequent blockage and discharge.

Before revision, one should make sure that no allergy exists to eardrops or other topical medication that the patient may be using. Another cause of failure to heal may be the patient's scratching or rubbing; the patient must be cautioned against doing these activities. By careful, frequent cleaning and the use of drying powder, such as chloramphenicol, one can usually determine the site and probable cause of the drainage. If the drainage is at the junction of the cartilage and the bone of the facial ridge, the cause is probably trapped cells. However, if the drainage is high and just below the thicker membranous skin, the cause is probably blockage of the antrum. A recurrence of cholesteatoma may also be responsible for breakdown and drainage. In these cases, the wet area is most often over the grafted middle ear, and hearing loss and a foul odor are usually present as well. Because the new cartilage wall is much less resistant to the erosion of cholesteatoma than the walls of the bony cavity, breakdown will occur here first, eliminating any danger of trapped cholesteatoma and complications such as brain abscess or meningitis.

Operative revision is carried out through the usual postauricular incision. A subcutaneous flap is created to cover the cavity at the conclusion of the procedure. The cavity is exposed, and the cartilage wall is raised or replaced as need dictates. If trapped air cells are the source of the discharge, they must be completely removed or shunted to the mastoid antrum. Unless there is an associated hearing loss, the graft over the middle ear and ossicular reconstruction are not disturbed. If the antrum has been blocked for some time and has failed to aerate, there may be partial or complete absorption of the knee cartilage, which would necessitate complete replacement of the cartilage and aeration of the new cavity behind it.

Recurrent cholesteatoma may destroy the cartilage as well as the middle ear reconstruction. There must of course be complete and meticulous removal of all diseased tissue before a second reconstruction can be undertaken. On the rare occasions in which a cholesteatoma recurs after a cartilage wall revision, the ear should be converted to an open cavity.

References

1. Wehrs RE: Reconstructive mastoidectomy with homograft knee cartilage. Laryngoscope 82:1177–1188, 1972.
2. Wehrs RE: Results of reconstructive mastoidectomy with homograft knee cartilage. Laryngoscope 88:1912–1917, 1978.
3. Wehrs RE: Silicone sheeting in tympanoplasty. Laryngoscope 89:497–499, 1979.
4. Silverstein H: Permanent middle ear aeration. Arch Otolaryngol Head Neck Surg 91:313–318, 1970.
5. Jahn A: The Jahn Hydroxylvent Tube. Smith Nephew Richards Brochure. Memphis, TN.

21

Tympanoplasty: Staging and Use of Plastic

JAMES L. SHEEHY, M.D.

Elimination of disease and restoration of function are the two aims of tympanoplasty. In most teaching situations, one can separate the two aims, limiting the discussion to elimination of the disease or to restoration of function. The staging of the operation and the use of plastic in the middle ear, however, require that the discussion consider both objectives.

Staging the operation involves both disease and function, and it is not technique oriented, that is, staging does not vary significantly with the technique of tympanic membrane grafting or the technique of restoring the sound pressure–transfer mechanism, or even the management of the mastoid.

This chapter discusses the history of, and indications for, tympanoplasty, as well as techniques used in performing tympanoplasty in two stages. The controversies surrounding the procedure will be discussed at the end of the chapter.

HISTORICAL ASPECTS

In the mid 1950s, a persistent problem in obtaining satisfactory hearing results in tympanoplasty was the maintenance of an aerated middle ear space. When the space collapsed, eustachian tube malfunction was blamed.[1]

By the late 1950s, many recognized that although eustachian tube malfunction played a part in this collapse, a major contributing factor was surgical technique. Creating an open cavity and adapting the graft to whatever ossicular remnants remained resulted in narrowing of the middle ear space. As a result of this realization, many otologists stopped creating open cavities routinely, leaving the bony annulus and epitympanic plate intact (see Chapter 18). This procedure required that a prosthesis be used between the more normally positioned tympanic membrane and the stapes or stapes footplate (see Chapter 15). Although these efforts often led to successful results, collapse of the space continued to be a problem. This problem, however, was compounded by prosthesis extrusion and, at times, formation of a cholesteatoma resulting from retraction pockets into the epitympanum (recurrent cholesteatoma). Many investigators continued to blame collapse of the middle ear space on eustachian tube malfunction.

Rambo[2] recognized that much of the problem was caused by the formation of adhesions between the graft and the denuded medial wall of the middle ear. He recommended a two-stage procedure, the first stage of which involved filling the middle ear with paraffin. Paraffin maintained the space quite nicely, preventing adhesions and allowing normal mucous membrane to cover the denuded areas. For many reasons, Rambo's principle of staging the operation to obtain this mucous membrane–lined, air-containing middle ear space was not appreciated at the time.

The principle of staging the operation was refined by Tabb[3] in 1963, but he described a three-stage procedure. This seemed excessive to many otologists, who were still blaming eustachian tube malfunction for most of the problem. Nonetheless, from then on, staging the operation attracted more attention.

Various thin plastic sheetings (polyethylene, polytetrafluoroethylene [Teflon], silicone rubber) were used, but it was soon learned that this thin sheeting was ineffective in many of the worst ears.[4] The sheeting was pushed aside by fibrous tissue and, when pushed against the tympanic membrane, extruded.

By the late 1960s, some surgeons began using stiffer plastic in planned, two-stage procedures. Stiffer plastic maintained its position, accomplishing what Rambo had earlier accomplished with paraffin.[5-8]

INDICATIONS FOR STAGING

There are two reasons for staging the operation in tympanoplasty: obtaining a permanently disease-free ear and obtaining permanent restoration of hearing.[7-9] Whether one finds any indication for staging depends on how vigorously a good functional result is pursued in badly diseased ears.

The decision to stage or not to stage is made at the time of surgery. With experience, one usually can make this judgment preoperatively and thereby alert the patient to the possible necessity of a two-stage procedure. The decision is based on three factors: the extent of the mucous membrane problem, the certainty (or lack thereof) of removal of cholesteatoma, and the status of the ossicular chain. Taking these three factors into account, about 40 per cent of tympanoplasty operations are staged by House Ear Clinic (HEC) doctors: 10 to 15 per cent of ears without cholesteatoma and 75 per cent or more of ears with cholesteatoma.

Mucosal Disease Factors

There are frequently large areas of diseased or absent mucosa in the chronically infected middle ear. Groundwork is necessary to promote regrowth of normal mucosa. The first step is elimination of infection prior to surgery, if possible. The second step is removal of all squamous epithelium, granulations, and irreversibly diseased mucosa at the time of surgery. The middle ear is then sealed with a graft to prevent squamous epithelium from migrating back into the middle ear. This sealed middle ear space will fill with a blood clot, and this clot supports fibroblastic invasion with eventual formation of scar tissue or adhesions between the denuded surfaces. To prevent these adhesions from forming, and to allow mucosa to migrate in, plastic sheeting is used over the denuded areas.

A two-stage operation is indicated, both to obtain the best hearing results and to prevent recurrence of cholesteatoma (retraction pocket), in patients with extensive mucous membrane destruction. The object of the two-stage procedure is to obtain a well-healed ear with a mucosa-lined pneumatized middle ear cleft so that ossicular reconstruction may be performed later under ideal circumstances.

Ossicular Chain Factors

There has been an increase in the incidence of sensorineural hearing impairment in patients in whom the inner ear has been opened during actual or potential infection. Because of this result, a fixed stapes should not be removed at the time of tympanic membrane grafting. In cases of otosclerosis, a two-stage procedure is almost always indicated. When the fixation is due to tympanosclerosis, it may be possible to mobilize the stapes, depending on the area of fixation. If the oval window is *diffusely* involved, the procedure should be staged.

Residual Cholesteatoma Factor

It may seem quite illogical to leave behind epithelial disease, removing it at a planned second-stage procedure, but this is exactly what is done under certain circumstances.

Removal of cholesteatoma in the middle ear may be questionable, at times, in an acutely inflamed ear in which differentiating between granulation tissue and matrix is difficult. Differentiating becomes a particular problem when granulations fill the oval and round windows. Excessive manipulation in these areas could result in an inner ear complication.

The surgeon may have torn the matrix when removing it from the tympanic recess and may not be certain of complete removal, which presents a considerable problem under the pyramidal process, an area hidden from view regardless of the technique of surgery, whether it is an open- or closed-cavity technique. Removal of the pyramidal process with a diamond burr may or may not resolve the problem.

It is much easier to be certain of cholesteatoma removal from the mastoid, especially in a small apneumatic one. Extensive cholesteatoma in a pneumatized mastoid poses a problem. In using the intact canal wall procedure, one should usually revise the mastoid in such cases within 1 to 2 years to be certain not to leave disease behind.

The mastoid and epitympanum are often re-explored in patients in whom excessive bleeding oc-

curred at surgery. Unexpected residual disease in the epitympanum has been noted in some cases of this type in the past.

Timing the Second Stage

The second-stage operation may be performed in 6 to 9 months if the primary indication for staging was an ossicular or a mucous membrane problem. The middle ear should be well healed by that time.

If the primary reason for staging is reinspection of the mastoid and epitympanum for possible residual cholesteatoma, it is best to wait 9 to 18 months. The delay allows time for any residual disease to have grown to a 1mm or 2mm cyst so that it may be identified with greater ease. The only exception to this rule is if this disorder occurs in children or if serous otitis media develops; a residuum may grow faster under these circumstances.

PREOPERATIVE EVALUATION AND COUNSELING

The ability to predict the need for staging the operation depends on one's experience and philosophy regarding the badly diseased ear.

At HEC, the doctors have a section in the *Patient Discussion Booklet* dealing with planned second-stage procedure. Furthermore, the second-stage operation is mentioned as a possibility under the section on tympanoplasty without mastoidectomy and a probability under that on tympanoplasty with mastoidectomy.

If the patient has dry central perforations with normal mucosa, then the possibility of a second-stage operation need not be mentioned unless there is reason to believe that the stapes is fixed (otosclerosis or tympanosclerosis). When fixation is suspected or there is a major mucous membrane problem, staging is likely.

I think the outlook for obtaining a healed, dry ear is excellent—90 to 95 per cent chance. But it may be necessary to perform a second operation for hearing improvement. That depends on whether it is necessary to replace the third ear bone; it is not safe to do that at the same time as I graft the ear drum. (Or I say "that depends on how badly diseased the middle ear is").

If it is necessary to do the operation in two stages, the hearing will probably be worse between step 1 and step 2, for a period of 6 to 12 months.

In cases of cholesteatoma in the middle ear, and in any case requiring mastoid surgery, the patient should be told that a two-stage operation is probable.

The outlook for obtaining a healed, dry, safe ear is excellent: 90 per cent or better chance. Unfortunately, it is usually necessary to do a second operation to improve the hearing and to make sure that all the skin growth is out. Your hearing will be worse for 9 to 12 months, until I perform the second surgery.

There is no need to further elaborate on this preoperatively unless the patient asks for more information. If details are necessary, be frank. There is nothing to hide. Elaborate.

When the decision is made at surgery that a second stage is needed, one should explain at the time of the first postoperative visit exactly why this was done. Use a diagram, explain in simple terms, and record a note in the chart that this counseling has been done.

PLASTIC IN THE MIDDLE EAR

The commonest middle ear indication for staging the operation is a mucous membrane problem. To avoid confusion, the following discussion will be limited to that problem. The techniques are the same when there are other indications.[10]

Plastic Sheeting

Polyethylene film was used initially, then Teflon film. Since 1964, various thicknesses of silicone sheeting have been used and, at times, Supramid.

Silicone sheeting will be referred to here as "thin" and "thick." The thin sheeting is 0.005 inch; the thick sheeting is 0.040 inch. Silicone sheeting is distributed by Invotec International, Inc., Jacksonville, Florida.

Thin silicone sheeting is malleable. It adapts easily to the middle ear space and does not tend to curl when exposed to body temperature. Thick silicone sheeting is stiff and is not deformed by fibrous tissue that may develop in the middle ear. Although stiff, it is malleable enough to be withdrawn from the mastoid and middle ear through a tympanotomy exposure.

Supramid Extra is the trade name for a medical-grade nylon 6. The sheeting thickness of Supramid Extra Foil is 0.3mm. Because it is thinner than thick silicone sheeting, it is easier to insert. It is not malleable, however, and this quality prevents it from being extracted from the mastoid without a mastoid re-exploration.

Mucous Membrane Indications

When the mucous membrane problem is limited, there is no need for staging (Fig. 21–1). Adhesions form between denuded bone of the middle ear and the tympanic membrane graft but usually do not pose a long-term problem. Nonetheless, thin silicone sheeting is frequently placed over the denuded areas to prevent adhesions (Fig. 21–2). The silicone sheeting may be left indefinitely. Alternatively, one may use absorbable gelatin film (Gelfilm), if desired.

In more diseased ears one may find that normal mucosa remains only in the tubotympanum, facial recess, and epitympanum (Fig. 21–3). Reconstruction of this ear without regard to the mucous membrane problem usually results in a fibrosed middle ear.

When thin silicone sheeting was used in such cases in the early 1960s, the results were frequently disappointing. The silicone sheeting was rolled up or deformed by advancing fibrous tissue. If the silicone sheeting contacted the tympanic membrane, extrusion often occurred. To obtain the best hearing results in such cases, it was necessary to perform the reconstruction in two stages. At the initial operation, the tympanic membrane was grafted over a piece of thick silicone sheeting that filled the middle ear (Fig. 21–4). Six months later, the thick silicone sheeting was removed, and a suitable prosthesis was inserted.

In badly infected ears, there may be no mucosa remaining in the middle ear cleft except for the tubotympanum (Fig. 21–5). Some believe that nothing can be done to reconstruct such an ear; radical mastoidectomy has been advised. Ears of this type can be reconstructed by staging the tympanoplasty, as long as some mucosa remains in the tubotympanum and the plastic sheeting can reach the area to prevent eustachian tube closure.

In cases of extensive or total mucous membrane destruction, it may be wise to perform an intact canal wall mastoidectomy even though there may not be other indications for a mastoid exploration. The mastoid is opened into the middle ear through the facial recess for insertion of a sheet of Supramid or thick silicone sheeting (Fig. 21–6). This process ensures that the plastic will not roll up, thus no fibrous tissue. During revision, the plastic is removed, and a suitable prosthesis may placed between the stapes capitulum or footplate and the mobile tympanic membrane in a well-healed normal middle ear.

Canal Wall Down Procedures

The principles and indications involved in staging the operation in canal wall down procedures are the same as in canal wall up procedures, but the technique is different. Many who use both techniques in tympanoplasty have stated that their hearing results are less satisfactory in canal wall down cases. The probable reason for these results is the narrowing of the middle ear space, which should not be allowed to occur in canal wall down procedures (see Chapter 15).

In staging the operation in canal wall down procedures, a wide middle ear space is obtained by extending the thick silicone sheeting on to the fallopian ca-

FIGURE 21-1

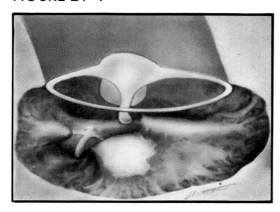

FIGURE 21-2

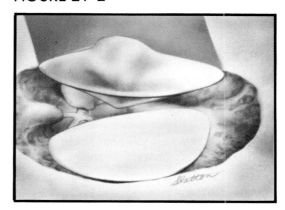

FIGURE 21-3

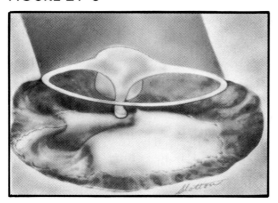

FIGURE 21-4

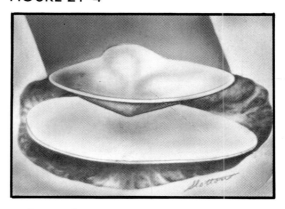

FIGURE 21-5

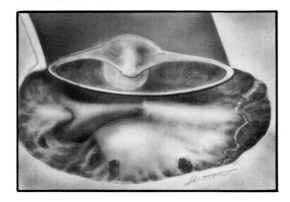

FIGURE 21-6

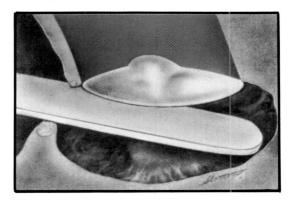

FIGURE 21-1. Absence of mucosa over promontory.

FIGURE 21-2. Silicone sheeting has prevented adhesions between tympanic membrane graft and denuded promontory.

FIGURE 21-3. More extensive mucous membrane destruction and absence of the stapes. Good mucosa remains in the recesses and the epitympanum.

FIGURE 21-4. Stiff plastic sheeting holds its position and prevents adhesions between the tympanic membrane graft and the raw areas of bone.

FIGURE 21-5. Mucous membrane destruction is extensive. Note a few islands, here and there, of mucosa and some in the tubotympanum.

FIGURE 21-6. Thick silicone or Supramid sheeting will not be displaced by fibrous tissue. Mucosa should regrow over all denuded bone and the undersurface of the graft.

nal. It is important to bevel the superior edge of the plastic to help delay extrusion; the graft rests on that edge.

Plastic Extrusion

There is no question that plastic material placed in the middle ear may extrude if an edge of the plastic comes in contact with the tympanic membrane. At HEC, where surgeons have used the techniques described herein over the past 25 years, extrusion has occurred in less than 0.5 per cent of the cases. Those who have reported a major problem with extrusion are probably using thin silicone sheeting in situations in which they should have used thick plastic and staged the operation.

It might be of interest for me to mention two patients, each of whom had plastic in the ear for over 20 years between stage one and stage two. I performed a canal wall down operation on a 6-year-old child and staged the operation, leaving in thick silicone sheeting. The patient returned at age 26, having had no further problem, and decided that it was time to have the second stage. There had been no ill effect from the thick silicone sheeting.

A second example is a patient in his mid-40s in whom cholesteatoma matrix was left over the lateral semicircular canal fistula. An intact canal wall procedure was performed, and a 1.2cm sheet of Supramid was placed through the facial recess. The patient came in for initial follow-up and made it clear that he was going to do nothing further and was lost to follow-up. He returned 21 years later and said that he wanted his second-stage procedure. Not only was the Supramid in good condition, as was the rest of the ear, the matrix that had been left over the fistula had disappeared, and the fistula was closed by bone.

THE CONTROVERSY

There is considerable difference of opinion among experienced otologists in regard to staging the operation. The major difference of opinion occurs over the more diseased ears, usually with cholesteatoma, and the difference is not related to the management of the mastoid, canal wall up or down, but instead to the surgeon's philosophy.

The following quotation is taken from the article "Tympanoplasty: To stage or not to stage."[9] The quotation is from a well-known otologist who stages "sometimes":

My hunch is that there might be a slight edge to those with a planned second stage, as you describe. However, this advantage, I think, would be overshadowed by the significant number that initially look like they needed a second stage,

but heal amazingly well and end up with an excellent result in spite of the massive pathology in the tympanic cavity. With a philosophy of a planned second stage procedure, these patients might be denied the opportunity to have had success with the first operation, thus requiring a needless second procedure. My inability to predict the frequent, excellent healing response makes me go all out in attempting to reconstruct the conductive mechanism the first time, hoping for a good healing and a good initial result.

Quoted here, from the same article, is the opinion from another highly regarded otologist who feels that there is essentially no indication to stage the operation:

I do not believe that staging should be a routine procedure. Every effort should be made to eliminate disease and maximize hearing results at the first operation. Should the hearing results be unsatisfactory, and if the postoperative status regarding pneumatization of the middle ear, etc., is satisfactory, a revision operation can be done. In most cases revisions are not necessary and, therefore, the staging procedure is avoided.

The HEC doctors believe that the great divergence of opinion on staging that one encounters is related to two factors. How hard does the individual pursue a good functional result in the most severely diseased ear? What does one accept as a satisfactory functional result? Certainly, in the ear with no remaining mucosa except in the tubotympanum, the HEC doctors have seen that unless the operation is staged, one cannot usually obtain a satisfactory functional result. Staging the operation has resulted in a satisfactory functional result in 50 to 60 per cent of cases—not perfect, but nonetheless good.

Acknowledgment

Many of the illustrations are modified from *Otolaryngology*, Vol. 1, published by J. B. Lippincott Company.

References

1. Sheehy JL: Testing eustachian tube function. Ann Otol 90:562–564, 1981.
2. Rambo JHT: Use of paraffin to create a middle ear space in musculoplasty. Laryngoscope 71:612–619, 1961.
3. Tabb HG: Surgical management of chronic ear disease with special reference to staged surgery. Laryngoscope 73:363–383, 1963.
4. House HP: Polyethylene in middle ear surgery. Arch Otolaryngol Head Neck Surg 71:926–931, 1960.
5. Austin DF: Types and indications of staging. Arch Otolaryngol Head Neck Surg 89:235–242, 1969.
6. Smyth GDL: Staged tympanoplasty. J Laryngol 84:757–764, 1970.
7. Sheehy JL: Plastic sheeting in tympanoplasty. Laryngoscope 83:1144–1159, 1973.
8. Sheehy JL, Crabtree JA: Tympanoplasty: Staging the operation. Laryngoscope 83:1594–1621, 1973.
9. Sheehy JL, Shelton C: Tympanoplasty: To stage or not to stage. Otolaryngol Head Neck Surg 104:399–407, 1991.
10. Sheehy JL: Surgery of chronic otitis media. *In* English GM (ed): Otolaryngology. Philadelphia, Harper & Row, 1984.

22

Management of Complications of Chronic Otitis Media

RICHARD J. WIET, M.D.
STEVEN A. HARVEY, M.D.
GEORGE P. BAUER, M.D.

Chronic otitis media can present a formidable challenge to the otologic surgeon. Competent operative management requires a thorough knowledge of the anatomy of the temporal bone as well as the pathologic subtleties of the disease. Because avoidance of complications is a major goal, steps toward prevention should begin with a thorough history and physical examination. In addition to the benefits of surgery, specific complications and their possible outcome must be discussed with the patient. Even the most experienced surgeon, however, will at some point in his or her career confront an intraoperative complication. When this does happen, the surgeon first must recognize that a complication has indeed occurred. Second, he or she must be capable of handling the complication in a way that minimizes subsequent morbidity. This ability to properly manage such complications requires a careful blend of knowledge and judgment.

This chapter emphasizes the management of complications from surgery for chronic otitis media, including otic capsule fistulas due both to the disease process and to the surgical treatment. Fistulas due to disease are discussed because improper management can lead to further morbidity. Other topics are sensorineural hearing loss from various causes, iatrogenic facial nerve trauma, and dural and vascular injury. Specific surgical techniques to prevent or deal with these problems will be mentioned as appropriate.

PREOPERATIVE COUNSELING

It is essential that the patient understand the goal of the surgery. The principal goal of ear surgery for chronic otitis media is elimination of infection. Correction of hearing loss is the secondary goal, often accomplished in a second procedure.

Preoperative counseling depends on a complete history and thorough examination. A history of vertigo or sensorineural hearing loss would be important findings with respect to counseling. The location of the tympanic membrane perforation may help in counseling the patient and in planning treatment. Central perforations are usually not associated with cholesteatoma, whereas marginal perforations are often more problematic. Those located in the attic are most often associated with secondary acquired cholesteatoma. Usually, hearing loss of greater than 30dB to 35dB implies erosion of the ossicular chain. Many times in the presence of cholesteatoma in the posterior superior quadrant, hearing is normal. The patient must be forewarned that sound transmission is occurring *through* the cholesteatoma, and hearing will probably decrease after surgery. Hearing improvement often requires a second-stage procedure. Management

of the patient with an only-hearing ear often necessitates a more conservative approach than the patient with bilateral hearing. Management of the diseased better-hearing ear may require immediate postoperative aural rehabilitation with a bone conduction aid.

We not only explain the procedure to the patient in simple layman's terms but also describe to the patient his or her medical diagnosis. The probability of surgical success is often explained in simple ratios, such as "eight or nine times out of ten we succeed in closing the perforation with a subsequent gain in hearing." The risks and the benefits of the procedure are discussed in detail. Our group follows the example outlined by Sheehy.[1] We then explain the potential risk of partial or total sensorineural hearing loss, dizziness, facial weakness, and other complications related to mastoid surgery.

An appropriate discussion of postoperative care and follow-up is outlined to the patient before discharge from the outpatient or inpatient setting. This discussion includes proper aural hygiene, water precautions, activity limitations, and the use of antibiotics, when deemed necessary.

If a complication requiring management occurs, the surgeon who is involved should freely consult with other experts for advice. This is especially true if the surgeon has managed very few complications resulting from disease or an iatrogenic cause. An example may be unwanted immediate onset of facial paralysis in primary cholesteatoma. It is considered good practice to consult with another physician when in doubt about a management decision.

LABYRINTHINE FISTULA SECONDARY TO CHRONIC OTITIS MEDIA

Labyrinthine fistulas are well-known complications of chronic otitis media. They are an unusual, but by no means rare, clinical entity and assume a significant risk. The inexperienced surgeon may not be prepared for the possibility of a fistula, and some cases of postoperative dead ears may result from the opening of an undiagnosed fistula. The incidence of labyrinthine fistulas secondary to chronic otitis media in the modern literature varies from a low of 3.6 per cent, reported by Palva et al.[2] to a high of 12.9 per cent, reported by Sanna et al.[3] Although the incidence of other complications due to chronic otitis media such as meningitis, sigmoid sinus thrombosis, and intracranial abscess have greatly decreased over the years, labyrinthine fistulas have had a remarkably stable rate of occurrence of about 10 per cent.[4]

The most common location for labyrinthine fistulas to occur is the lateral semicircular canal in all reported series (see Fig. 22–1). Most authors have reported the incidence of isolated lateral canal fistulas to be about 80 per cent, but this figure ranges from 57 to 90 per cent[5, 6] and is indicative of the fact that the lateral semicircular canal is the most exposed (to cholesteatoma) of the three canals. The remainder of fistulas in most series generally involved the lateral canal along with one or several other sites.

Distinction should be made also between a bony erosion and a fistula. Erosion is present when the endosteal layer of bone remains intact and may appear as a blue or gray line under the operating microscope and does not represent a true fistula.[5] When the endosteal bone layer is eroded, only the endosteal membrane separates the cholesteatoma matrix from the perilymphatic space. In this manner, direct pressure can be transmitted to the membranous labyrinth and is seen in most instances of described fistulas.

Many authors describe fistulas as small or large without quantifying the terms. Sanna et al., however, have classified fistulas as small (0.5mm to 1mm), medium (1mm to 2mm), and large (greater than 2mm) according to intraoperative findings.[3] They found that large fistulas made up the majority (74 per cent), followed by medium (18.4 per cent) and small (7.6 per cent) ones. Gacek also has classified fistulas as either small or large and uses 2mm in greatest dimension as the cutoff point.[5] Although he states that 2mm was chosen as an arbitrary dividing point, he points out that in fistulae smaller than 2mm, the bony margin of the opening is able to support the cholesteatoma matrix and separate it from the underlying endosteal membrane by a layer of connective tissue. This allows for safe removal of the matrix from the fistula.

Although the surgeon should be prepared to deal with a possible fistula in any ear with chronic otitis media, the length of symptoms may heighten suspicion. Sheehy and Brackmann, reporting on 97 cases of labyrinthine fistulas, noted that over 50 per cent had a history of chronic otitis media for 20 years or longer.[7] Ritter also noted that many of his patients had suffered from lifelong otorrhea, often dating back to childhood.

Vestibular symptoms also increase the possibility of a labyrinthine fistula. Sheehy and Brackmann noted that almost two thirds of patients experienced dizziness, and it was of a constant nature in 12 per cent.[7] Ritter noted that 76 per cent of patients complained of vertigo, which was usually of a brief nature, lasting several seconds to minutes.[8] Ostri and Bak-Pedersen,[9] reporting on 20 fistula cases, and Gormley,[10] on 35 cases, both noted frank vertigo in 65 per cent of patients. In cases of chronic otitis media without a fistula, dizziness has been noted much less commonly. One review found this figure to be 15 per cent in such cases and more related to age rather than duration of disease.[11] McCabe noted the highest incidence of ves-

TABLE 22–1. Site of Labyrinthine Fistula

SITE OF FISTULA	EYE MOVEMENTS
Lateral canal, postampulla	Horizontal, toward normal ear
Lateral canal, preampulla	Horizontal, toward fistulous ear
Vestibule	Rotary, horizontal, toward fistulous ear
Superior canal	Rotary, toward fistulous ear
Posterior canal	Vertical, with an arc

Adapted from McCabe BF: Labyrinthine fistula in chronic mastoiditis. Ann Otol Rhinol Laryngol 93(Suppl 112):138–141, 1983.

tibular symptoms (90 per cent) of any larger series, reporting on 79 cases of fistula.[4] In addition, a higher incidence of positive results on fistula tests (72 per cent) was noted.[4] McCabe has given an excellent, detailed description of the test along with the expected eye movements based on the location of the fistula (Table 22–1).

A positive result on a fistula test in the case of a postampullary lateral canal fistula (the most common site) is denoted by conjugate deviation (*not* nystagmus) of the eyes to the opposite ear with compression of air in the external canal. In this instance, endolymph and therefore the cupula are deviated anteriorly. If the positive pressure is sustained, nystagmus then results toward the diseased (test) ear. Subsequently, if the air pressure is pulsed, deviation to the opposite ear initially occurs, and as the pressure is released, the eyes drift back toward the midline. If the fistula is located at the junction of the lateral canal ampulla and vestibule (preampullary region), positive pressure will lead to posterior displacement of the cupula and subsequent conjugate deviation of the eyes toward the diseased ear. Positive pressure on a fistula of the vestibule will lead to deviation of the horizontal and superior canal ampullas and the associated rotary-horizontal eye movements noted in Table 22–1.

Dizziness may result from several factors. Extension of infection into the perilymph from the middle ear would be expected to lead to purulent labyrinthitis and complete loss of vestibular function. Serous labyrinthitis would be expected when only toxic byproducts and inflammatory cells gain entrance to the labyrinth, with subsequent vertiginous attacks.[8] Also, pressure changes transmitted from the middle ear into the perilymphatic space, the basis of the fistula test, may lead to cupular displacement and subsequent vestibular symptoms.

The level of preoperative hearing may serve as a clue to a possible labyrinthine fistula. Sheehy and Brackmann found a sensorineural impairment in over half of their fistula cases, compared with only 20 per cent of nonfistula cases.[7, 11] Sensorineural levels were more commonly diminished in patients with extensive fistulas at sites other than the lateral canal. Preoperative anacusis was found in 12 per cent of such cases.[7] Ritter also found decreased sensorineural levels in his series—70 per cent of patients had a loss of bone conduction, which averaged 26dB.[8] A discrimination score below 80 per cent was seen in 20 per cent of patients, and 30 per cent were deaf. Farrior has reported nonserviceable hearing preoperatively in 13 per cent of 31 fistula cases.[12] Ostri and Bak-Pedersen found anacusis in 15 per cent of their patients.[9]

Preoperative facial nerve weakness, although rare in fistula cases, is more common than in nonfistula cases: 4 per cent versus 1 per cent.[7] All series, however, report a high incidence of facial nerve dehiscence in fistula cases, including Gormley[10] (27 per cent), Ritter[8] (36 per cent), Sheehy and Brackmann[7] (50 per cent), and Ostri and Bak-Pedersen[9] (55 per cent). Thus, intraoperative facial nerve trauma, dealt with in another section of this chapter, represents a significant potential risk in these patients.

INTRAOPERATIVE MANAGEMENT OF LABYRINTHINE FISTULAS

Removal of cholesteatoma matrix versus leaving it in situ and performance of intact canal wall versus canal wall down mastoidectomy is a longstanding controversy in the management of labyrinthine fistulas that has not been resolved to this day. This controversy was first brought into sharp focus by Walsh and Baron in 1953. In a symposium regarding management of cholesteatoma matrix, Walsh advocated removing the matrix in all cases, feeling that this tissue had a chemical osteolytic effect on underlying bone.[13] Baron presented his views that bone erosion from cholesteatoma resulted mainly from a pressure effect and that exteriorization of the sac was sufficient.[14] Since that time, various techniques have been advocated.

Several general comments regarding the management of labyrinthine fistulas secondary to cholesteatoma are universally advocated by all authors. First, when a cholesteatoma sac is found in the mastoid, it should be opened and the contents evacuated (Fig. 22–1). The medial wall of the sac should be carefully palpated to detect any bony erosion, especially on the

dome of the lateral canal. Once a fistula is identified, matrix should be left over the site to protect it (even if eventual removal is planned) while the remainder of the ear is cleared of disease. This will protect the area from subsequent bone dust and irrigation solution. If removal of matrix is planned at that operative setting, it should be the last maneuver performed prior to completing the operation and closing the ear. When the fistula is exposed, it should be quickly covered with a tissue seal (e.g., fascia, vein, or perichondrium) (Fig. 22–2). Most authors advocate leaving matrix over extensive fistulas involving other semicircular canals, the vestibule, or cochlea (Fig. 22–3) because of the high incidence of postoperative sensorineural impairment. Sheehy and Brackmann reported a postoperative severe or total sensorineural hearing loss of 56 per cent in their cases of extensive fistulas when the matrix was removed.[7] Gacek reported a partial or profound hearing loss in all three cases in which matrix was removed from a cochlear fistula.[5] He states that the membranous semicircular canals and ampullas have thicker, more rigid walls than Reissner's or the basilar membrane of the cochlea and thus are less likely to rupture with removal of cholesteatoma matrix. Also, the cochlear duct occupies the outermost portion of the bony cochlea, thus allowing it to more readily come in contact with overlying matrix. Other authors who normally advocate matrix removal also feel that it should be left in situ in cases of multiple fistulas or those involving the vestibule or cochlea.[3, 10] A promontory cochlear fistula is considered one of the few absolute indications for radical mastoidectomy.[15]

With regard to the isolated lateral canal fistula, some authors feel that matrix always should be left undisturbed because of risk to the inner ear.[8, 16, 17] Ritter recommends performing a canal wall down mastoidectomy and leaving the matrix intact over the fistula site.[8] He reported that a decrease in hearing was noted in 47 per cent of cases in which the matrix was removed as opposed to 22 per cent in which matrix was left undisturbed. However, in his series of the cases in which matrix was removed, 80 per cent were not covered over with a tissue seal, which could lead to a significant increased risk of inner ear damage.

FIGURE 22-1. Cholesteatomatous fistula of the lateral semicircular canal. Facial recess has been opened.

FIGURE 22-2. Fascia placed over lateral semicircular canal fistula after removal of cholesteatoma matrix.

FIGURE 22-3. Cochlear promontory fistula secondary to cholesteatoma. Posterior canal wall is taken down in this dissection.

FIGURE 22-1

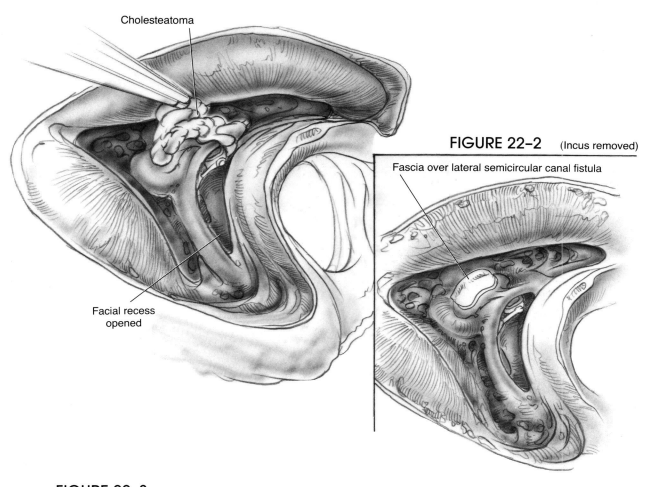

Cholesteatoma

Facial recess
opened

FIGURE 22-2 (Incus removed)

Fascia over lateral semicircular canal fistula

FIGURE 22-3

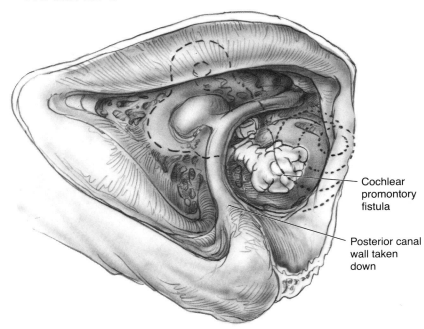

Cochlear
promontory
fistula

Posterior canal
wall taken
down

The first author (RJW) agrees with Ritter and Gacek regarding this opinion, especially when the fistula appears to be greater than 2mm on computed tomographic scan.

Other surgeons advocate performing a canal wall down tympanomastoidectomy along with removal of the fistula matrix in cases of isolated lateral canal fistula. Farrior prefers this method in a single-stage operation but cautions against matrix removal from an acutely inflamed or better-hearing ear.[12] He recommends a classic modified radical mastoidectomy in many cases of better-hearing ears with fistulas. Palva et al. likewise prefer a canal wall down tympanomastoidectomy with matrix removal at a single operation.[2] They base this preference on the finding of periodic otorrhea and continued vertigo on fistula manipulation postoperatively in cases in which matrix was left intact. All cases in which matrix was removed from the fistula and the area sealed with tissue subsequently healed with no further otorrhea or symptoms of vestibular upset.

Gacek feels that the decision to remove matrix should be based on several factors:[5]

1. Ability and experience of the surgeon. If the surgeon does not feel confident in his or her ability to remove the matrix over the fistula atraumatically, then it is wise to leave it undisturbed.
2. Location and size of fistula. In lateral canal fistulas less than 2mm in diameter, Gacek states that removal of matrix can be undertaken safely, as there is minimal risk to the inner ear. In canal fistulas larger than 2mm, only an experienced surgeon should attempt removal, and if the matrix appears to be adherent to the underlying membranous labyrinth, it is better left alone.
3. Function of the fistulous ear and relationship to the contralateral ear. In a fistulous ear with profoundly depressed function, the risk of underlying disease in the labyrinth takes precedence, as there is no risk to further hearing loss. Thus, the matrix should be removed and a labyrinthectomy considered. In the significantly better- or only-hearing ear with a fistula, no attempt should be made to remove matrix if the opening is over 2mm in size. Only in the case of a very small canal fistula should an experienced surgeon attempt removal in this situation.
4. Mechanism of bone erosion by the cholesteatoma. In cases in which the osteolysis appears to be secondary to pressure from an expanding cholesteatoma sac, one may elect only to exteriorize the disease, allowing for decompression, and leave the matrix intact over the fistula. This situation may be seen with noninfected or "dry" cholesteatomas, in which the keratin debris does not liquefy but remains impacted within the sac. On the other hand,

if the bone destruction appears to be secondary to a biochemical effect of the matrix, it may be more beneficial to remove this source of osteolysis. This situation may occur when granulation tissue is present in conjunction with cholesteatoma. The enzyme collagenase, which can lead to bone resorption, is present in cholesteatoma matrix and granulation tissue. When these two are present together, the activity of this enzyme is considerably increased.[18–20]

Sheehy and Brackmann take an eclectic approach to the problem of lateral canal fistulas also. They consider all of the factors mentioned by Gacek, except for number four above, in the decision-making process.[7] They do not feel that the mechanism of bone erosion by cholesteatoma plays an important part in the decision regarding fistula management. They prefer the intact canal wall tympanomastoidectomy approach with removal of the matrix over the fistula at a second-stage operation 4 to 6 months later once the infection is cleared and the ear well healed. Only in the case of a small lateral canal fistula (they do not define "small") in a noninfected ear with normal bone conduction do they feel it is reasonable to remove the matrix at the first stage.

When a fistula is found in a much better-hearing or only-hearing ear, Sheehy and Brackmann,[7] like Farrior,[12] advocate a classic modified radical mastoidectomy to avoid further risk to the ear or a second-stage operation. They do feel that when the mastoid is exteriorized, matrix should be left over the fistula rather than removed.

Sanna et al.[3] and Gormley[10] (reporting on Smyth's series of labyrinthine fistulas) both take a similar approach to that of Sheehy and Brackmann.[7] They prefer a staged intact canal wall tympanomastoidectomy with matrix removal from the fistula at the second-stage operation when the opposite ear is normal. In the presence of an only-hearing ear, a large posterior canal wall defect, multiple fistulas, or an elderly patient, Sanna et al. recommend exteriorizing the mastoid and leaving matrix over the fistula.[3]

Ostri and Bak-Pedersen advocate removal of the matrix over a fistula (even large fistulas) in conjunction with an intact canal wall mastoidectomy in a single-stage procedure.[9] They cite improvement in hearing in the majority of cases and a low incidence of postoperative anacusis as justification for this approach.

A wide variety of surgical procedures have been advocated for the management of labyrinthine fistulas, including at one extreme always exteriorizing the mastoid and leaving matrix over the fistula to removing the matrix over even large fistulas in a closed mastoid at one operation.[8, 9] Other authors take an approach between these diametrically opposed viewpoints.[3, 5, 7, 10, 12, 21]

Several technical points deserve mention for removal of cholesteatoma matrix from a fistula. As already stated, this procedure should be the last part of the operation prior to closing the ear. On elevating matrix, a determination should be made about whether the underlying membranous labyrinth is attached, and if so, attempts at further elevation should be aborted.[5] However, Bellucci feels that matrix does not become attached to the underlying endosteal membrane or membranous labyrinth and, therefore, can always be elevated under high magnification.[22] He states that damage to the labyrinth is secondary to suction or instrumentation. Farrior supports this concept and feels that instrumentation or suction should not be applied directly to the fistula site.[12] He recommends using strips of cellulose sponge applied to the matrix to help with dissection in a blunt fashion. This material has a slightly abrasive quality and helps to scrub the bony surface, ensuring complete removal of matrix. Irrigation should be gentle and is important for preventing contamination of the fistula by infected debris.

Preservation of sensorineural hearing levels is certainly a desirable goal in the management of labyrinthine fistulas. Postoperative hearing results vary among authors. However, direct comparison is impossible, as each series was managed by differing surgical approaches, and the extent of disease varied. Gormley[10] reported a 3.3 per cent incidence of anacusis postoperatively in ears that were functioning preoperatively. Ostri and Bak-Pedersen[9] reported a 5 per cent incidence of anacusis, whereas Sanna et al.[3] divided their results based on whether an open (9.5 per cent) or closed (2.6 per cent) mastoidectomy was performed. Gacek had a 14 per cent incidence of anacusis, all in ears in which matrix removal from a cochlear fistula was attempted.[5] Sheehy and Brackmann noted severe or total loss of hearing in 8 per cent of lateral canal fistulas and in 56 per cent of fistulas involving other sites (predominantly cochlear fistulas).[7] Law et al. noted postoperative anacusis in 22 per cent of patients.[21]

A decrease in sensorineural levels or discrimination scores without total hearing loss postoperatively has been reported as follows: Sanna et al.[3] (4 per cent—closed mastoidectomy, 6.4 per cent—open mastoidectomy), Gacek[15] (7 per cent), Ostri and Bak-Pedersen[9] (17 per cent), and Ritter[8] (37 per cent). Thus, the potential for postoperative sensorineural hearing loss is very real, and this possibility must be discussed preoperatively with any patient suspected of harboring a fistula.

Extensive destruction of the labyrinth does *not* invariably lead to loss of hearing, however. Phelps discussed a patient with an extensive cholesteatoma involving the vestibule along with the basal and middle turns of the cochlea who retained hearing preoperatively (destroyed after surgery).[23] Bumstead et al. reported on four cases of extensive labyrinthine destruction in which vestibular function was destroyed but hearing preserved (both preoperatively and postoperatively).[24] They theorized that the inflammatory response walled off the cochlea on an acute basis, allowing for preservation of hearing. They proposed four anatomic sites where this walling off may have occurred: 1) ductus reuniens, 2) saccular duct, 3) utricular duct, and 4) utriculoendolymphatic valve. At least one other report documents a case of labyrinthine fistula with preoperative anacusis and a significant gain in hearing postoperatively.[25] The preoperative hearing loss was thought to result from serous labyrinthitis that resolved after surgery.

IATROGENIC LABYRINTHINE FISTULA

It has classically been taught that the accidentally opened labyrinth will necessarily lead to a dead ear. Although the labyrinth is at risk during surgery for chronic otitis media, this is, thankfully, a relatively infrequent complication. The three sites that are most at risk for injury during surgery for chronic otitis media are the lateral semicircular canal, the promontory, and the oval window.[26] Injury to the membranous labyrinth does not always lead to loss of hearing, as evidenced by the number of case reports during the fenestration era describing accidental tearing of this structure with preserved sensorineural levels.[27–30]

Palva et al. reported iatrogenic injury to the lateral canal in the absence of a cholesteatomatous fistula in 0.1 per cent of chronic otitis media cases (two of 2192).[31] One of these had approximately a 20dB loss in bone conduction for the speech frequencies, and the other had no change in hearing thresholds. Jahrsdoerfer et al. described two cases of accidental drilling into the lateral canal with no subsequent postoperative loss of cochlear function.[32] A more recent review by Canalis et al.[33] reported a 0.08 per cent incidence of this mishap, similar to the figure given by Palva et al.[31] They made several interesting observations regarding this injury.[33] Noted in cases with an ultimately favorable outcome was a moderately severe sensorineural loss that occurred acutely; however, it returned to near preoperative levels over a period of 3 to 6 weeks. Permanent high-frequency losses of a mild nature were common, but speech discrimination scores returned to normal, and tinnitus was a rare complaint. Acute vertiginous symptoms and nystagmus were expected; however, these symptoms commonly continued well beyond the usual period of central compensation. Patients may demonstrate unsteadiness and positional vertigo along with spontaneous nystagmus 1 to 2 years following surgery, which is in keeping with a partial labyrinthine injury in which continued active impulses are generated.

Canalis et al. felt that opening the lateral canal at its posterior limb away from the ampullary end in a previously normal inner ear was associated with a better outcome.[33] In this situation, symptoms may result from hemorrhage and serous labyrinthitis rather than from the chemical injury of endolymph contamination of the perilymphatic space. The latter effect may be more common with injury near the ampullary end and may lead to permanent cochlear damage. They postulated that the cochlear protection seen in their cases was due to local changes at the site of the fistula. The walls of the membranous labyrinth possibly collapse due to loss of fibrovascular support from the periotic tissue within the perilymphatic space. This, along with a sudden loss of endolymph and decreased pressure, may lead to collapse of the membranous walls and sealing off of the endolymphatic space from the surrounding perilymph.

Jahrsdoerfer et al. present a somewhat different theory on cochlear preservation.[32] They postulate a sealing off of the pars superior from the pars inferior at the level of the utriculoendolymphatic valve. With an acute loss of endolymph from the vestibular labyrinth, the utricular wall collapses, sealing off the valve area and protecting the cochlea from fluid decompression. They advocated sealing iatrogenic fistulas with a fascia plug. Bone wax[34] and muscle plugs[33] have been suggested also for sealing off iatrogenic fistulas.

Accidental fistulization of the inner ear appears to occur more commonly at the oval window than the lateral canal. Palva et al. reported a 1.4 per cent incidence of accidentally opening the labyrinth, and of their 12 cases, 11 occurred at the oval window.[2] Even though infection was present at the time of surgery, none of the ears developed total sensorineural hearing loss in the immediate postoperative period. However, three did subsequently exhibit depressed bone conduction thresholds several months after surgery. The loss was assumed to result from serous labyrinthitis

with subsequent fibrosis. Of their 11 cases, two had complete avulsion of the footplate, three had dislocation, and the remaining six suffered fracture without dislocation. In a follow-up report 5 years later, they added a single case of oval window fistulization in an additional 1362 cases of chronic otitis media, for an overall incidence of 0.5 per cent.[31] This is still higher than the reported rates of lateral canal fistulization mentioned above.

This relative retention of sensorineural hearing in the majority of patients supports the findings of an earlier report by Weichselbaumer.[35] He described 27 cases of accidental fistulization at the oval window but no postoperative dead ears. Only two patients developed a postoperative decrease in bone conduction (each by 20dB). Of his cases, complete footplate avulsion occurred in 11, partial avulsion in 12, and footplate perforation in the remaining five cases. Likewise, Sheehy and Brackmann, in their report on labyrinthine fistula secondary to cholesteatoma, noted inadvertent fistulization of the oval window from surgical manipulation (not cholesteatoma) in 11 cases—none of which resulted in a sensorineural impairment.[7]

Several guidelines can be offered to minimize the possibility of oval window fistulization secondary to surgical manipulation. Cholesteatoma should be removed from the oval window–stapes region by dissecting parallel to the stapedius tendon, which stabilizes the stapes and prevents inadvertent mobilization (Fig. 22–4).[12] Manipulation in a superior-inferior direction, along with depression of the stapes, must be strictly avoided to prevent disruption of the annular ligament (Fig. 22–5). In situations in which remnants of cholesteatoma cannot be safely dissected from the stapes, one may try laser with a mildly defocused beam. Otherwise, it is safer to reconstruct the tympanic membrane, seal the ear, and perform a second-stage operation 6 to 9 months later. At that time, surrounding inflammation has subsided, and an epithelial pearl is usually found that can be easily removed, followed by ossicular reconstruction. If fistulization occurs at the second stage, there is less risk of contamination to the inner ear and subsequent senso-

FIGURE 22–4. Correct method for removal of cholesteatoma from stapes. Dissection should be from posterior to anterior, allowing stapedius tendon to stabilize stapes.

FIGURE 22–5. Incorrect method for removal of cholesteatoma from stapes. Stapes is not stabilized by stapedius tendon and is thus at risk for inadvertent dislocation or subluxation.

FIGURE 22–6. Inadvertent contact between mastoid burr and intact incus. This situation could lead to dislocation of the incus or vibratory transmission to stapes if incudostapedial joint is intact.

FIGURE 22-4

CORRECT

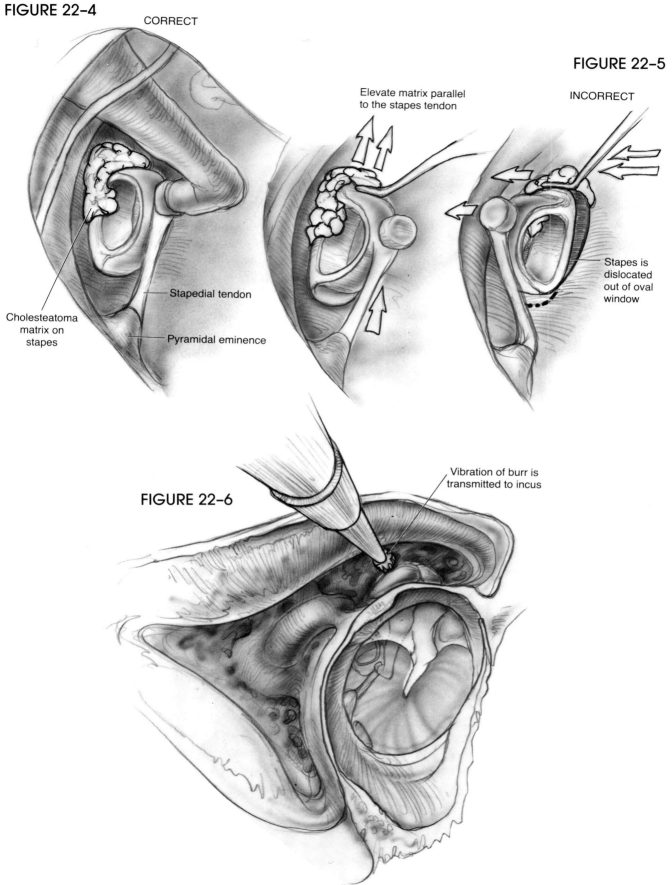

Cholesteatoma
matrix on
stapes

Stapedial tendon

Pyramidal eminence

FIGURE 22-5

Elevate matrix parallel
to the stapes tendon

INCORRECT

Stapes is
dislocated
out of oval
window

FIGURE 22-6

Vibration of burr is
transmitted to incus

rineural depression.[12] Should opening into the oval window occur, it should immediately be sealed with fascia that has already been prepared. Palva et al. recommend delaying ossicular reconstruction until a stable tissue seal has formed over the area.[31] Absolute avoidance of suction is also necessary.

If granulation tissue and thickened mucosa surround the stapes, the surgeon should be very conservative in their removal, as this will quickly resolve once the remainder of the middle ear cleft is cleared of disease and sealed with tympanic membrane reconstruction.[36] The laser has proved useful in atraumatically clearing disease from the stapes and oval window region.[37, 38]

SENSORINEURAL HEARING LOSS

Postoperative sensorineural hearing loss in patients with chronic otitis media may obviously result from either cholesteatomatous or iatrogenic fistulization of the labyrinth, as already discussed. However, it may also occur from excessive manipulation of the ossicular chain (without fistulization) or other unidentifiable factors. Smyth reviewed his personal series of 3000 chronic ear disorder operations and found the overall incidence of cochlear damage to be 2.5 per cent from all causes.[39] He defined significant sensorineural depression as a 10dB drop from 500Hz to 4000Hz or a 10 per cent reduction in speech discrimination.

In reviewing his tympanoplasty procedures (without mastoidectomy), he found the incidence of cochlear injury to be twice as high when the ossicular chain was disarticulated (2.6 per cent) compared with when it was left intact (1.3 per cent). This difference was attributed to intentional disarticulation during the process of removing tympanosclerotic plaques. In cases of intact canal wall tympanomastoidectomy with a facial recess approach (combined-approach tympanoplasty), the incidence of sensorineural impairment was reversed: higher for intact-chain cases (5.6 per cent) than for disarticulated chain cases (2.5 per cent). Loss of hearing in the intact-chain situations resulted equally from contact of the drill with the incus and excessive manipulation of the malleus in removing cholesteatoma from its medial surface (Fig. 22–6). In the case involving a disarticulated ossicular chain due to either disease or intentional sectioning, the majority of losses are theorized to develop after excessive manipulation of the stapes during disease removal or reconstruction of the ossicular chain. When a canal wall down procedure with cavity obliteration was performed, there was a higher incidence of sensorineural loss when the ossicular chain was left intact (50 per cent) but no losses when it was disarticulated.

Palva et al. reported their incidence of sensorineural hearing loss following chronic ear surgery to be 4.5 per cent in 1680 cases.[36] They noted that the majority of hearing losses were high frequency, in the range of 4000Hz to 8000Hz (57 per cent). Only 8 per cent occurred across all test frequencies, and all ears demonstrated some recovery during the first 3 months postoperatively. Following that time, there was no appreciable change for better or worse in hearing thresholds. Discrimination scores remained above 80 per cent if the hearing loss occurred at 2000Hz or greater. If low frequencies were affected, discrimination varied between 50 and 80 per cent. They found that the majority of losses occurred in ears with an intact ossicular chain (81 per cent) and when considerable disease was cleaned from the epitympanum.

These studies allow one to make several generalizations about minimizing the incidence of postoperative sensorineural impairment. When squamous epithelium is removed from the malleus handle, dissection should be parallel, not perpendicular, to this structure and in a slow, deliberate manner, which allows the stapes to move across its longitudinal diameter, disturbing inner ear fluid movements the least.[31] Slow dissection allows time for the perilymph to pass through the helicotrema toward the round window without damaging the organ of Corti.[39] Cholesteatoma should be dissected off the lateral surface of the incus in a posterior-to-anterior direction and parallel to the long process. This process allows for partial stabilization of the incus by its posterior and lateral suspensory ligaments and by the malleus head.[12] If dissection in the epitympanum is required, it is safest to disarticulate the incudostapedial joint first (working parallel to the stapedius tendon) and remove the incus.[36] Careful drilling in the region of the antrum and aditus along with raising and lowering the irrigant level to allow early identification of the incus (the so-called water sign) helps prevent vibratory transmission to this ossicle or its dislocation.[2]

Management of disease in the stapes and oval window region is as detailed in the previous section. Additionally, caution in attempts to remove significant tympanosclerotic plaques must be advised. Although delaying stapedectomy until a second stage decreases cochlear risk from acute inflammation, many patients may be better served with a hearing aid in this situation.[39]

Using many of these guidelines, Palva et al., in a 3-year follow-up report on an additional 512 procedures for chronic otitis media, noted no further cases of high-frequency sensorineural hearing loss.[31] They did report a 0.2 per cent incidence of unexplained deafness in the postoperative period that could not be attributed to a specific factor. Noise from the drill and suction-irrigation may play a role. Even low-intensity noise can lead to spasm of the vessels in the zona arcuata of the basilar membrane in laboratory animals.[40] The greater metabolic needs of hair cells in the presence of noise may lead to ischemia and subsequent damage.[39]

FACIAL NERVE INJURY

The literature[22, 41–43] supports the precept that the best precaution for preventing facial nerve injury is a thorough knowledge of temporal bone anatomy, specifically, the landmarks used for identification of the facial nerve. This knowledge is acquired only by repeated, meticulous dissection in the temporal bone laboratory combined with careful, attentive dissection in surgery and years of clinical experience. The useful landmarks to accurately identify the facial nerve are the mastoid antrum and the prominence of the lateral semicircular canal. Once the lateral canal is identified, the fossa incudis is located at the tip of the short process of the incus. The facial nerve lies medial to the fossa incudis and immediately inferior to the horizontal semicircular canal.[43]

The incidence of iatrogenic facial paralysis from otologic surgery has been reported to range from 0.6 to 3.6 per cent, and is as high as 4 to 10 per cent in revision cases.[26, 43] In one large series of 958 operations for chronic otitis media, only two patients had a transient postoperative facial palsy after radical mastoidectomy.[42] In one case, a dehiscent tympanic segment was present. There was no apparent dehiscence in the other case. Both of these nerves recovered to full function several weeks following surgery. The authors re-emphasized the need for thorough knowledge of temporal bone anatomy combined with careful surgical dissection when operating for chronic otitis media, as normal facial nerve landmarks may be destroyed.[42]

Transection of the mastoid segment of the facial nerve with the cutting burr is the most frequently encountered injury (Fig. 22–7).[41] Special care is needed in revision cases because of altered anatomy. Drilling under continuous suction-irrigation to prevent thermal injury to the nerve is necessary.[43] Furthermore, cool irrigation has a hemostatic effect on the bleeding encountered from the inflammatory response of chronic mastoiditis and cholesteatoma and allows for better visualization.

If facial nerve injury is recognized during surgery, the facial canal should be opened proximally and distally to ensure continuity of the nerve. Paparella et al.[44] recommend preserving the nerve sheath unless discontinuity of the nerve is suspected because this condition will invite fibrous proliferation and reduction of nerve regeneration. Other authors[22, 43] recommend decompression of the edematous segment (if there is no nerve substance loss) by opening the nerve sheath until normal-appearing nerve is found proximal and distal to the site of injury.

If the surgeon is unaware of a facial nerve injury and the patient awakens with a facial paralysis, several reasons should be considered. If intramastoid ear packing has been used, it could be in direct contact with the facial nerve, producing the paralysis from pressure. The surgeon should loosen the packing.[43] Also, the use of a local anesthetic could lead to a temporary facial nerve paralysis.[43] The effects of the local anesthetic must be allowed to wear off. If enough time has elapsed, the packing has been loosened, and the patient still has facial paralysis, the decision concerning re-exploration must be entertained.

FACIAL NERVE GRAFTING

Because results of early repair of facial nerve transection are more favorable, the clinician must carefully consider the clinical situation, using objective studies and historical information provided by any previous surgeon. If a first surgeon identified the nerve and is confident that it was not transected, neuropraxia is likely the problem. An expectant course based on electrical study can be maintained. If, however, electrical silence is observed beyond 3 days after the event and doubt exists regarding the degree of trauma, inspection is warranted. Most authors feel that if the diameter of the nerve is disrupted by one third or greater, ultimately better return of facial function can be obtained with resection of the segment and grafting (Figs. 22–8 and 22–9).[45–49]

If resection and reanastomosis or grafting are required, several factors affect the timing of repair, including 1) connective tissue proliferation, 2) proximal neuroma formation, 3) distal glioma formation, and 4) axoplasmic flow.[48] Connective or fibrous tissue formation is evident within several days of neural injury and is capable of infiltrating distal endoneural tubules to the exclusion of regenerating axons. The main source of this fibrosis is not surrounding connective tissue but rather the epineurium itself.[41, 50, 51] Approximately 10 to 14 days following injury, Schwann cells proliferate, which in the proximal nerve stump intermingle with connective tissue and axonal filaments, leading to neuroma formation. Distally, the Schwann cells and connective tissue lead to glioma formation at the nerve stump.[48] Multiple studies have shown that maximal axonal regenerative ability is present 21 days following injury.[52–54]

Previous studies have advocated delaying repair for several weeks to allow maximal axonal regeneration and subsequently push the axons across the anastomotic site.[55, 56] However, more recent literature supports *early repair* within several days of injury and certainly within 30 days.[57–59]

Once the decision has been made to resect the injured portion of the facial nerve, it must be determined whether end-to-end anastomosis or interposition cable grafting is better suited for reconstruction. Rerouting of the labyrinthine and tympanic segments (in a nonhearing ear) to gain additional length can be performed by sectioning the greater superficial petrosal nerve. A gap width of up to 1cm has been proposed as the cutoff point for attempted rerouting and primary anastomosis.[45] The first author (RJW) has not found this method of repair to be successful. Some authors feel that if tensionless end-to-end anastomosis can be obtained, the results are ultimately better than those of interposition grafting. However, in rerouting procedures, the blood supply is necessarily disrupted, and this fact must be taken into consideration.[45, 60, 61] Others feel that interposition grafts yield results equal to those of end-to-end anastomosis.[62] This has been our experience also.

For interposition cable grafting, the ipsilateral greater auricular nerve is the donor site of choice.[43, 45] This nerve can be used for grafting segments up to 10cm in length. The proximal-distal orientation of the graft is reversed to prevent regenerating facial nerve axons from growing into endoneural tubes that leave the donor nerve trunk prior to the end of the graft.[63] The graft length should exceed that of the gap to be repaired by 3mm to 5mm both proximally and distally to allow for tensionless reapproximation.[64]

The use of epineural versus perineural coaptation in grafting is controversial.[65] Fisch and Lanser, however, advocate removal of 3mm to 4mm of epineurium from the end of the graft and nerve stump site.[63] This recommendation is based partly on the work of Millesi and Berger[50, 51] and also on the ability to better assess the true anastomotic cross-section of the graft end. The greater auricular nerve has a fascicular pattern of axonal location, whereas the facial nerve changes from a mono- to multifascicular pattern as it is followed from the geniculate region to the stylomastoid foramen.[63]

A clean, oblique cut should be made on both the nerve stumps and the cable graft. This allows for increased contact surface area and permits a greater number of regenerating axons to cross the anastomotic site.[45, 66, 67] Determination of the site for freshening the proximal nerve stump can be difficult, and no adequate guidelines are available. Axonal sprouting by the proximal facial nerve stump can take place up to at least 10mm proximal to the site of injury in experimental animals.[57]

Sutureless reapproximation is the preferred anastomotic technique, as no motion is present within the temporal bone, in contrast to the situation with extratemporal nerve grafting.[45, 48] Also, the fallopian canal provides an excellent cradle for the interposition graft.[47] The use of fibrin glue has been advocated to stabilize the anastomosis, as has the placement of bovine collagen membrane (Cargile) over the site (Fig. 22–10).[45, 63] This material is reabsorbed within 4 to 6 weeks and helps protect the repair site from fibrous tissue infiltration during this time period. The material has increased the number of regenerating neurofibrils across the anastomosis in animal experiments.[63] Other materials that have been used to cover the anastomotic site include topical thrombin, absorbable gelatin sponge (Gelfoam), gold foil, and skin grafts.[44, 47] Brackmann recommends splinting the anastomosis with clotted blood without the use of any other supporting material.[46] Other authors also rely on natural tissue adhesiveness for intratemporal facial nerve grafting.[45, 48]

In conjunction with interposition grafting, another proposed technique is peripheral ligation of the zygomatic and buccal branches of the facial nerve so that selective rerouting of regenerating neurofibrils can be directed to the more important fronto-orbital and marginal mandibular branches.[63] This effect has occurred in experimental studies.[68]

In spite of careful, tensionless approximation, epineurial stripping, and wrapping with absorbable collagen, only 20 to 50 per cent of the original facial nerve fibers will traverse the graft site to innervate

FIGURE 22–7. Injury to mastoid segment of facial nerve with drill. Complete transection of the nerve occurs most commonly at this location.

FIGURE 22–8. Partial disruption of facial nerve involving less than one third of total diameter.

FIGURE 22–9. Complete transection of facial nerve.

FIGURE 22–10. Greater auricular interposition graft. Ends of graft and facial nerve are beveled to increase available surface area for coaptation. Epineurium is stripped back 3mm to 5mm to prevent fibrous proliferation at anastomotic site. Area sealed with bovine collagen membrane and fibrin glue.

FIGURE 22-7

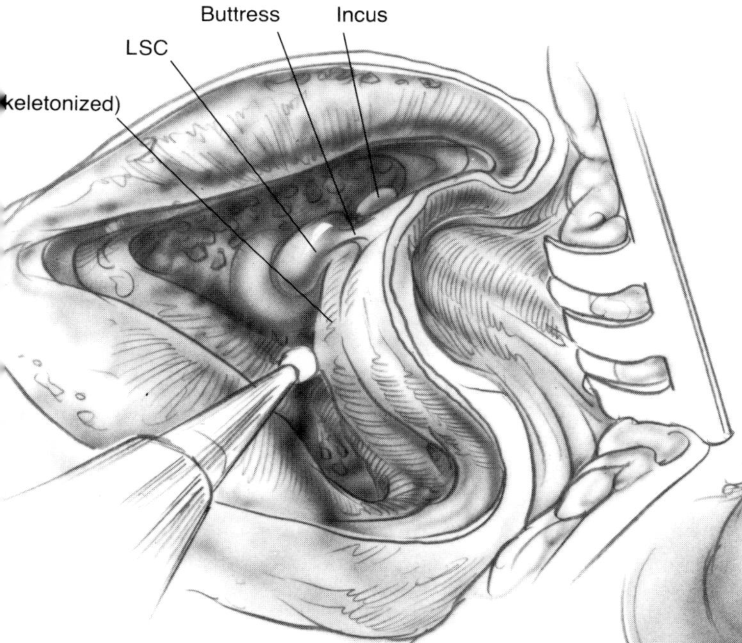

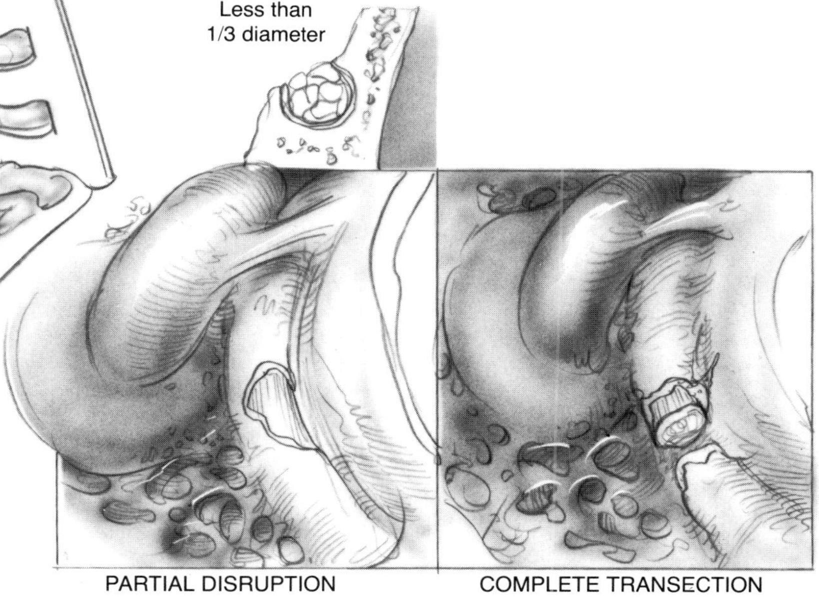

Buttress
Incus
LSC
(skeletonized)

FIGURE 22-10

Less than
1/3 diameter

PARTIAL DISRUPTION

COMPLETE TRANSECTION

FIGURE 22-8

FIGURE 22-9

Fallopian
canal

Epineurium
sutures

(Great auricular n.)
graft

LSC

Sutures

Epineurium

Epineurium
stripped back
3–4mm

Cargile membrane
(bovine collagen)

Fallopian
canal

Fibrin glue

Beveled end
of nerve

Nerve graft

Epineurium

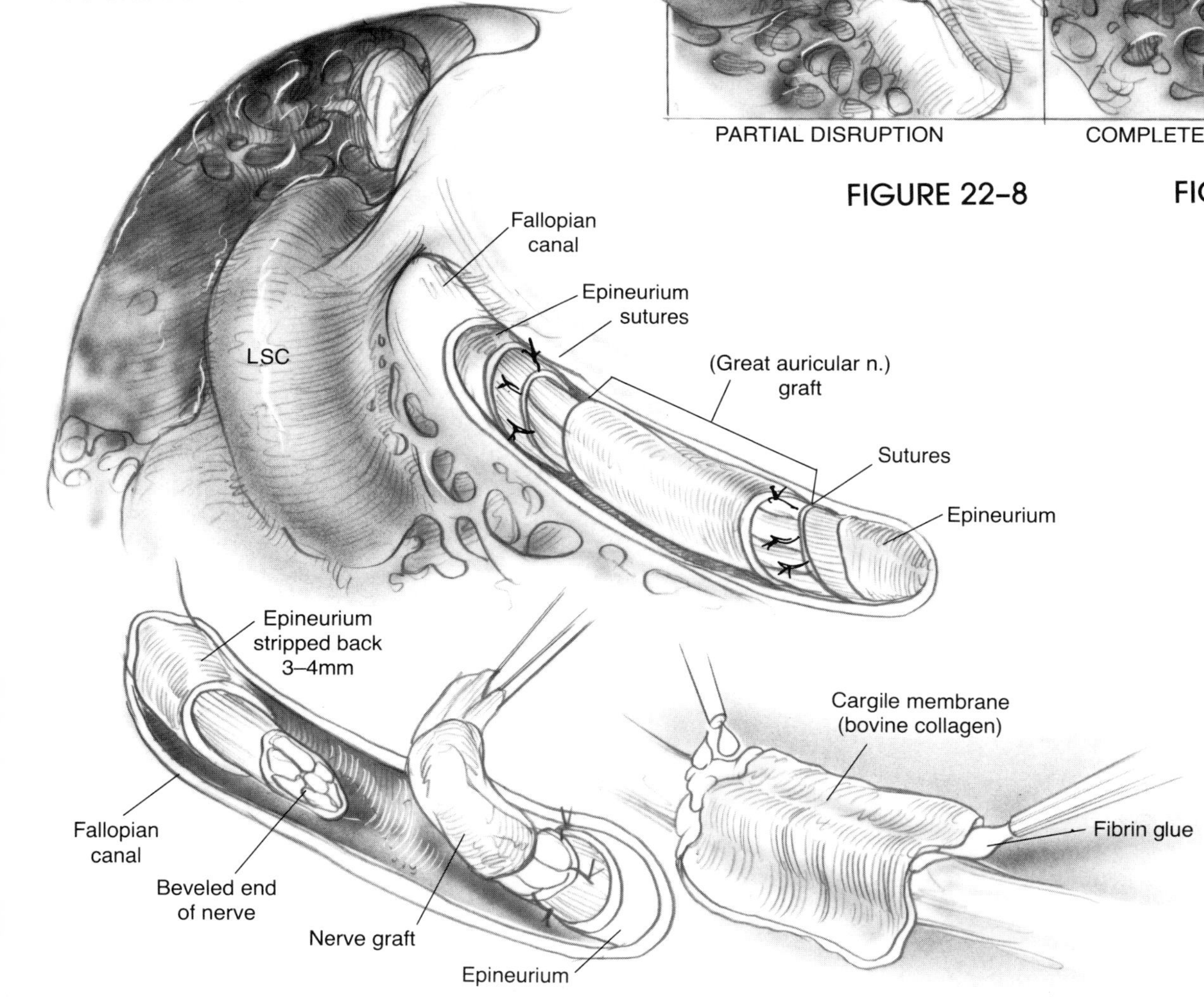

motor endplates.[63, 69] Fisch and Lanser state that maximal restoration of facial movement following grafting does not exceed 75 per cent of normal, which corresponds to a grade III on the House-Brackmann scale.[63] Farrior also states that 60 to 80 per cent recovery of facial function can be expected with meticulous repair.[12] Synkinesis is always a problem because of sprouting of the regenerating fibers and intermixing secondary to disruption of endoneural tubes in the graft and peripheral nerve stump.[64] One may expect some return of facial nerve function within 5 to 7 months following repair of the tympanic or mastoid segment of the nerve.[61]

DURAL INJURY

Inadvertent exposure of the dura usually presents no serious problems.[44] Normal dura, composed of two layers—an inner thin (meningeal) layer that covers the brain and an outer thick layer composed of collagen bundles serving as the endosteum for the skull, is quite capable of supporting the cerebrum without bony support. In most cases, simple dural exposure without injury requires no therapy.

With the use of the otologic microscope and general improvements in operative techniques, the incidence of dural injury has decreased.[70] Dural injury is often caused by indiscriminate cauterization of bleeding dural vessels and can usually be prevented with either the use of bipolar cautery or lower-power settings with unipolar cautery. Another mechanism of injury is direct trauma caused by the rotating burr or the curette.[22] Once the dura is injured, cerebrospinal fluid can be seen leaking from the site of dural penetration (Fig. 22–11).

If dural injury with cerebrospinal fluid leakage is noted at the time of surgery, repair should be undertaken immediately. Small leaks from the middle cranial fossa dura may close spontaneously because of the presence of abundant arachnoid tissue at this location.

With middle cranial fossa dural injury, Paparella et al. recommend removal of surrounding bone to expose normal dura 5mm circumferentially.[44] A fascial graft can then be placed between the normal dura and surrounding bone to ensure repair (Fig. 22–12). We have found that macerated muscle gently placed in

the defect will stop most leaks. If the dural defect is more in the form of a slit, it may be repaired by suture.

Posterior fossa dural injury is more problematic because of the decreased arachnoid tissue available to aid in spontaneous repair. More profuse cerebrospinal fluid leaks are likely. Repair involves again exposing normal dura for approximately 1cm in each direction by removing bone.[44] A fascia graft can then be applied. Postoperatively, the patient may require a few days of bed rest with the head elevated to help reduce the intracranial cerebrospinal fluid pressure and to facilitate healing. If the cerebrospinal fluid leak persists, serial lumbar punctures or the placement of an indwelling lumbar drain may be needed to reduce the cerebrospinal fluid pressure.[22, 44]

Materials other than temporalis fascia can be used to repair large middle fossa defects (Fig. 22–13). Bellucci recommends using fascia, skin, or bone and emphasizes the use of tight intramastoid packing to secure the tissue graft in firm contact with the dura.[22] Neely and Kuhn described the use of a cartilage-perichondrial graft to repair the defect.[71] Silicone sheeting can be used to repair a defect of middle cranial fossa dura but should not be used in the presence of infection. Larger defects may require rotational flaps, fat obliteration, or pedicled or free muscle flaps to support the fascia during healing.[72] Kamerer and Caparosa further recommend the use of surgical packing in the mastoid cavity to support the repair.[72] Packing should remain in place postoperatively for up to 3 weeks. They also recommend intraoperative and postoperative antibiotic coverage.[72]

VASCULAR INJURY

The three major vascular structures at risk during surgery for chronic otitis media are the sigmoid sinus, jugular bulb, and internal carotid artery. Iatrogenic injury to these structures is more likely in cases of anatomic variation, in poorly pneumatized mastoids, and in revision surgery. Venous injury is relatively more common than arterial injury.[22]

Sigmoid Sinus

The sigmoid sinus is commonly encountered during mastoidectomy (Fig. 22–14). It may be identified by a

---

FIGURE 22-11. Laceration of exposed middle cranial fossa dura by mastoid drill with subsequent cerebrospinal fluid leak.

FIGURE 22-12. Repair of dural and tegmental defect with bone graft–fascia sandwich placed via middle cranial fossa approach.

FIGURE 22-13. Repair of dural and tegmental defect with bone graft–rotation temporalis muscle flap placed via middle cranial fossa approach.

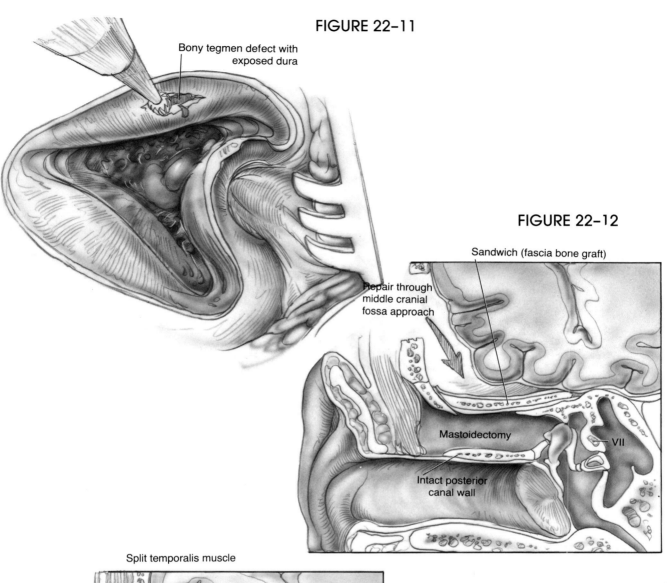

FIGURE 22–11

Bony tegmen defect with exposed dura

FIGURE 22–12

Sandwich (fascia bone graft)

Repair through middle cranial fossa approach

Mastoidectomy

VII

Intact posterior canal wall

Split temporalis muscle

Temporalis m.

Bony-fascia graft

FIGURE 22–13

bluish coloration beneath an intact bony plate, or by a change in pitch of the rotating drill bit to a higher frequency on contacting the compact bone overlying the sinus. The most common anatomic anomaly of the sigmoid sinus is anterior displacement into the mastoid cavity.[26] The sinus is intradural, as are all of the intracranial sinuses, enclosed by two layers that split to envelop this structure. The outer layer (toward the mastoid cavity) is the thinner of the two layers, being approximately half the thickness of the inner or intracranial portion.[73] The wall of the sinus has no contractile muscular elements and cannot collapse unless overlying bone is removed. Laceration of the sigmoid sinus may be prevented by initially identifying this structure in the sinodural angle superiorly and then following it down from there to the mid- and inferior portions of the sinus.[26] When the sinus is displaced far anteriorly, obscuring more medial structures, such as the labyrinth, it can be collapsed with a self-retaining retractor once all of the overlying bony plate is removed.

The mastoid emissary vein enters the sigmoid sinus in its upper third and on the posterolateral aspect. Multiple veins may occasionally be found. This structure may be lacerated or avulsed during mastoidectomy. To prevent or control bleeding, the vein should be skeletonized first with a cutting burr and then completely exposed with a diamond burr. It can then be coagulated with bipolar cautery and divided. The distal bony foramina are then obliterated with bone wax.[74, 75]

Bleeding from the sigmoid sinus may be either minimal or profuse, depending on the nature of the injury. Oozing may occur from small dural veins overlying the sinus, and small lacerations of the sinus wall itself may be produced by the edge of a bone fragment. These can often be controlled with gelatin sponge soaked in thrombin or with bipolar cauterization. Long segments of the sinus should be coagulated in a stripping fashion rather than a spotting one.[75]

Larger lacerations require either extraluminal or intraluminal packing. Prior to packing, however, bone must be completely removed circumferentially around the site of hemorrhage. The simplest method of packing is to obliterate the sinus extraluminally by placing a large sheet of Surgicel between the bone and wall of the sinus distal to the laceration. The sinus can

also be obliterated intraluminally distal to the site of hemorrhage. In either case, a large sheet of Surgicel (4cm × 4cm) should be used to prevent embolization (Fig. 22–15).[75]

Another method is to place a bolus of Surgicel directly over the laceration and then cover it with bone wax to secure it in place. This packing can also be held in place with through-and-through dural sutures on both sides of the sinus.[75] The advantage of packing over the sinus is that it prevents total obstruction of the lumen.

In severe hemorrhage, the sinus must be obliterated both above and below the laceration. First, the internal jugular vein must be ligated in the neck to prevent embolization. Then, inferior to the laceration, the sinus is occluded intraluminally while bleeding above is controlled with extraluminal compression by packing Surgicel between bone and the sinus wall. Another method of control requires exposure of dura in front of and behind the sinus both above and below the laceration. The dura is punctured, and large hemoclips are placed to obliterate the sinus lumen (Fig. 22–16).[76]

Superior Petrosal Sinus

The superior petrosal sinus may occasionally be lacerated when the posterosuperior cell tract is drilled out in a well-pneumatized mastoid. Usually, this problem can be managed with bipolar cautery. If not, control must be gained by isolating the sinus both medial and lateral to the laceration. Medially, the lumen can be obliterated by an intraluminal or extraluminal technique.[75]

Jugular Bulb

The jugular bulb may show great anatomic variation. The average dimensions of the bulb are 15mm wide by 20mm high; however, the latter figure may vary as much as 10mm.[73, 77] In most individuals, the right jugular bulb is slightly larger than on the left side. The dome of the bulb is generally covered by bone and resides in the hypotympanum. However, the more anteriorly placed the sigmoid sinus, the higher the dome of the bulb lies.[73] One study[78] has shown a 6 per cent incidence of the jugular bulb lying above the

FIGURE 22–14. Large laceration of sigmoid sinus during mastoidectomy.

FIGURE 22–15. Large sheets of Surgicel placed intralumenally for sigmoid sinus obliteration.

FIGURE 22–16. Vascular clips placed proximal and distal to large sigmoid sinus laceration. Dural exposure is required anterior and posterior to sinus for intradural placement of clip.

FIGURE 22-14

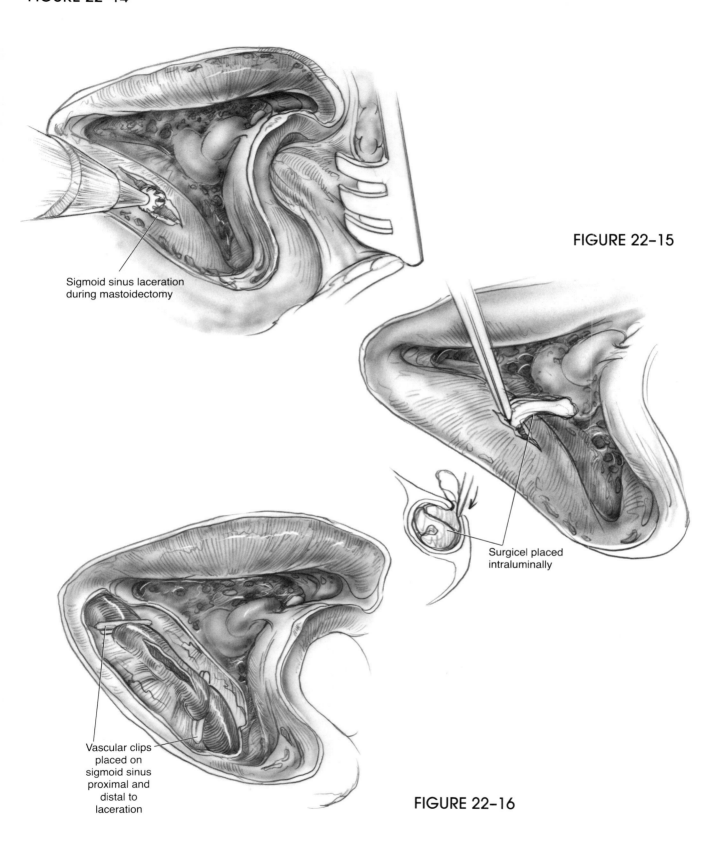

Sigmoid sinus laceration
during mastoidectomy

FIGURE 22-15

Surgicel placed
intraluminally

Vascular clips
placed on
sigmoid sinus
proximal and
distal to
laceration

FIGURE 22-16

level of the inferior tympanic annulus, and another, quoted by Graham,[73] has shown a 7 per cent incidence of dehiscent bone over the bulb. Injury to an exposed jugular bulb may occur during dissection of cholesteatoma from either the hypotympanic or retrofacial air cells. Also, elevation of a tympanomeatal flap has been reported to cause massive hemorrhage due to entering an exposed bulb.[73, 79, 80] An exposed bulb is especially prone to injury, as the vessel wall is extremely thin in this area. The sigmoid sinus wall superiorly gains support from the dura that ends as the sinus leaves the posterior fossa. Inferiorly, once the jugular vein leaves its foramen, a heavy adventitial layer surrounds the vessel. These extra layers of support are missing in the region of the jugular dome.[73] High-resolution computed tomography is the most sensitive means of diagnosing a high or dehiscent jugular bulb.[81]

Bleeding from the bulb can be managed in several ways. Small openings may be occluded with bone wax or gelatin sponge that is pressed into place with a cotton applicator or neurosurgical cottonoid.[74] Larger lacerations may be controlled by packing Surgicel between the bony defect and the bulb.[75] This material may be held in place with bone wax if further dissection in the area is required. Care should be taken not to overpack the area, as unwanted pressure on cranial nerves IX, X, and XI could result. If this procedure does not control the hemorrhage, the jugular vein should be ligated in the neck to prevent embolization, then the bulb and proximal sigmoid sinus lumen should be obliterated with packing.

Should hemorrhage from a high bulb occur with elevation of a tympanomeatal flap, the flap should be replaced and the external auditory canal packed firmly with petrolatum gauze,[73] which should be left in place for 1 week, then slowly advanced over several days to a week.

Carotid Artery

Carotid artery injury is rarely encountered in chronic ear surgery. However, it is closely related to several anatomic structures within the middle ear and may be exposed either congenitally or secondary to disease. The vertical portion of the petrous carotid normally lies slightly medial and anterior to the basal turn of the cochlea. At the genu where the artery turns into the horizontal segment, it lies anteroinferior to the cochleariform process, medial to the eustachian tube orifice, and anterior to the cochlea.[82] Usually, the petrous carotid artery is well covered by bone; however, the bone may be less than 0.5mm thick in the area of the eustachian tube orifice and in 1 per cent of cases is dehiscent.[49, 83]

Quite rarely, the petrous carotid artery may take an anomalous course through the temporal bone. Normally, the artery is found medial to the vestibular line, which is a vertical plane that runs through the lateral aspect of the vestibule and approximates the level of the promontory.[70, 84] The anomalous vessel can be lateral to this line, and the carotid foramen may be seen opening into the posterior hypotympanum.[84, 85]

An exposed artery must be kept in mind whenever dissection in the anterior mesotympanum and eustachian tube is undertaken. The lack of pulsations in the petrous carotid artery makes positive identification more difficult.[22] Often, bleeding from this area is from the vasa vasorum within the wall of the artery, rather than the artery itself. A true rupture of the carotid wall is exceedingly difficult to manage through the limited exposure afforded by the usual approaches for chronic otitis media. Small lacerations can repaired with No. 7 to No. 10 Prolene suture if temporary proximal and distal vessel occlusion can be obtained in time.[74] Larger lacerations can be controlled with temporary balloon occlusion until the damaged area is resected and grafted, or if adequate collateral circulation via the circle of Willis is present, simple ligation can be performed.[86, 87] However, these maneuvers first require greater exposure of the carotid artery within the temporal bone.

SUMMARY

Specific surgical complications in the management of chronic otitis media have been discussed. Thankfully, these problems do not arise commonly. Largely because of this, however, an added element of difficulty is present when complications do occur, as the surgeon may be unfamiliar with subsequent proper management. Varied manifestations of chronic otitis media and the subtle differences found in temporal bone anatomy from patient to patient also must be considered. This combination of factors leads to the creation of a unique situation in every operative case that requires thoughtful judgment. Thorough knowledge and careful technique guide the surgeon in his or her quest for that most important goal first stated by Hippocrates, "Above all, do no harm."

Acknowledgement

The authors gratefully acknowledge the work of Ann Hileman in the manuscript preparation.

References

1. Sheehy JL: Surgery of chronic otitis media. *In* English GM (ed): Otolaryngology, Vol I. Philadelphia, Harper & Row, 1985, pp 1–86.
2. Palva T, Kårjå J, Palva A: Opening of the labyrinth during

chronic ear surgery. Arch Otolaryngol Head Neck Surg 93: 75–78, 1971.

3. Sanna M, Zinni C, Gamoletti R, et al: Closed versus open technique in the management of labyrinthine fistula. Am J Otol 9: 470–475, 1988.

4. McCabe BF: Labyrinthine fistula in chronic mastoiditis. Ann Otol Rhinol Laryngol 93(Suppl 112): 138–141, 1983.

5. Gacek RR: The surgical management of labyrinthine fistulae in chronic otitis media with cholesteatoma. Ann Otol Rhinol Laryngol 83(Suppl 10): 3–19, 1974.

6. Wayoff MR, Friot JM: Analysis of one hundred cases of fistulas of the external semicircular canal. In McCabe BF, Sadé J, Abramson M (eds): First International Conference on Cholesteatoma. Birmingham, AL, Aesculapius Press, 1977, pp 463–464.

7. Sheehy JL, Brackmann DE: Cholesteatoma surgery: Management of the labyrinthine fistula—A report of 97 cases. Laryngoscope 89: 78–87, 1979.

8. Ritter FN: Chronic suppurative otitis media and the pathologic labyrinthine fistula. Laryngoscope 80: 1025–1035, 1970.

9. Ostri B, Bak-Pedersen K: Surgical management of labyrinthine fistulae in chronic otitis media with cholesteatoma by a one-stage closed technique. ORL J Otorhinolaryngol Relat Spec 51: 295–299, 1989.

10. Gormley PK: Surgical management of labyrinthine fistula with cholesteatoma. J Laryngol Otol 100: 1115–1123, 1986.

11. Sheehy JL, Brackmann DE, Graham MD: Complications of cholesteatoma: A report of 1024 cases. In McCabe BF, Sadé J, Abramson M (eds): First International Conference on Cholesteatoma. Birmingham, AL, Aesculapius Press, 1977, pp 420–429.

12. Farrior JB: Surgery for cholesteatoma. In Wiet RJ, Causse JB (eds): Complications in Otolaryngology—Head and Neck Surgery, Vol 1. Philadelphia, BC Decker, 1986, pp 69–76.

13. Walsh TE: Why I remove the matrix. Symposium on the surgical management of aural cholesteatoma. Trans Am Acad Ophthalmol Otolaryngol 57: 687–693, 1953.

14. Baron SH: Why and when I do not remove the matrix. Symposium on the surgical management of aural cholesteatoma. Trans Am Acad Ophthalmol Otolaryngol 57: 694–706, 1953.

15. Glasscock ME: The open cavity mastoid operations. In Glasscock ME, Shambaugh GE Jr. (eds): Surgery of the Ear. Philadelphia, WB Saunders, 1990, pp 228–247.

16. Freeman P: Fistula of the lateral semicircular canal. Clin Otolaryngol 3: 315–321, 1978.

17. Ruedi L: Acquired cholesteatoma. Arch Otolaryngol Head Neck Surg 78: 252–261, 1963.

18. Abramson M: Collagenolytic activity in middle ear cholesteatoma. Ann Otol Rhinol Laryngol 78: 112–125, 1969.

19. Abramson M, Gross J: Further studies on a collagenase in middle ear cholesteatoma. Ann Otol Rhinol Laryngol 80: 177–185, 1971.

20. Abramson M, Huang CC: Localization of collagenase in middle ear cholesteatoma. Laryngoscope 87: 771–791, 1977.

21. Law KP, Smyth GDL, Kerr AG: Fistulae of the labyrinth treated by staged combined approach tympanoplasty. J Laryngol Otol 89: 471–478, 1975.

22. Bellucci R: Iatrogenic surgical trauma in otology. J Laryngol Otol 8(Suppl): 13–17, 1983.

23. Phelps P: Preservation of hearing in the labyrinth invaded by cholesteatoma. J Laryngol Otol 83: 1111–1114, 1969.

24. Bumstead RM, Sadé J, Dolan KD, McCabe BF: Preservation of cochlear function after extensive labyrinthine destruction. Ann Otol Rhinol Laryngol 86: 131–137, 1977.

25. Sheehy JL: Dead ear? Not necessarily. A report of three cases of chronic otitis media. Am J Otol 4: 238–239, 1983.

26. Wiet RJ, Herzon GD: Surgery of the mastoid. In Wiet RJ, Causse JB (eds): Complications in Otolaryngology—Head and Neck Surgery, Vol 1. Philadelphia, BC Decker, 1986, pp 25–31.

27. Cawthorne T: The effect on hearing in man of removal of the membranous lateral semicircular canal. Acta Otolaryngol 78(Suppl): 145–149, 1948.

28. Jonkees LBW: On the function of the labyrinth after destruction of the horizontal canal. Acta Otolaryngol (Stockh) 38: 505–510, 1950.

29. Sadé-Sadowsky N: The damage to the membranous labyrinth

during fenestration and its influence upon hearing. J Laryngol Otol 69: 753–756, 1955.

30. Thomas R: Fenestration operation. Experience of first ninety-six (consecutive) cases. J Laryngol Otol 65: 259–274, 1951.

31. Palva T, Kårjå J, Palva A: Immediate and short-term complications of chronic ear surgery. Arch Otolaryngol Head Neck Surg 102: 137–139, 1976.

32. Jahrsdoerfer RA, Johns ME, Cantrell RW: Labyrinthine trauma during ear surgery. Laryngoscope 88: 1589–1595, 1978.

33. Canalis RF, Gussen R, Abemayor E, Andrews J: Surgical trauma to the lateral semicircular canal with preservation of hearing. Laryngoscope 97: 575–581, 1987.

34. Cullen JR, Kerr AG: "How I do it." Iatrogenic fenestration of a semicircular canal: A method of closure. Laryngoscope 96: 1168–1169, 1986.

35. Weichselbaumer W: The opening of the vestibule during tympanoplasty. Z Laryngol Rhinol Otol 44: 457–464, 1965.

36. Palva T, Kårjå J, Palva A: High-tone sensorineural losses following chronic ear surgery. Arch Otolaryngol Head Neck Surg 98: 176–178, 1973.

37. McGee TM: Argon laser in chronic ear and otosclerotic surgery. Laryngoscope 93: 1177–1182, 1983.

38. Parkin JL: Lasers in tympanomastoid surgery. Otolaryngol Clin North Am 23: 1–5, 1990.

39. Smyth GDL: Sensorineural hearing loss in chronic ear surgery. Ann Otol Rhinol Laryngol 86: 3–8, 1977.

40. Lawrence M: In vivo studies of the microcirculation. Adv Otorhinolaryngol 20: 244–255, 1973.

41. May M, Wiet RJ: Iatrogenic injury—prevention and management. In May M (ed): The Facial Nerve. New York, Thieme, 1986, pp 549–560.

42. Vartiainen E, Kårjå J: Immediate complications of chronic ear surgery. Am J Otol 7(6): 417–419, 1986.

43. Wiet RJ: Iatrogenic facial paralysis. Otolaryngol Clin North Am 15: 773–780, 1982.

44. Paparella MM, Meyerhoff WL, Morris MS, DaCosta SS: Mastoidectomy and tympanoplasty. In Paparella MM, Shumrick DA, Gluckman JL, Meyerhoff WL (eds): Otolaryngology, Vol II, 3rd ed. Philadelphia, WB Saunders, 1991, pp 1405–1439.

45. Adkins WY, Osguthorpe JD: Management of trauma of the facial nerve. Otolaryngol Clin North Am 24: 587–611, 1991.

46. Brackmann D: Otoneurosurgical procedures. In May M (ed): The Facial Nerve. New York, Thieme, 1986, pp 589–618.

47. Kamerer DB: Intratemporal facial nerve injuries. Otolaryngol Head Neck Surg 90: 612–616, 1982.

48. McCabe BF: Symposium on trauma in otolaryngology. I. Injuries to the facial nerve. Laryngoscope 82: 1891–1896, 1972.

49. Myerson MD, Ruben H, Gilbert JG: Anatomic studies of the petrous portion of the temporal bone. Arch Otolaryngol Head Neck Surg 20: 195–210, 1934.

50. Berger A, Millesi H: Nerve grafting. Clin Orthop 133: 49–55, 1978.

51. Millesi H: Healing of nerves. Clin Plast Surg 4: 459–473, 1977.

52. Grafstein B: The nerve cell body response to axotomy. Exp Neurol 48(Part II): 32–51, 1975.

53. McCabe BF: Facial nerve grafting. Plast Reconstr Surg 45: 70–75, 1970.

54. Sunderland S: Some anatomical and pathophysiological data relevant to facial nerve injury and repair. In Fisch U (ed): Facial Nerve Surgery. Birmingham, AL, Aesculapius Press, 1977, pp 47–61.

55. Ducker TB, Kauffman FC: Metabolic factors in surgery of the peripheral nerves. Clin Neurosurg 1: 406–424, 1977.

56. McQuarrie IG, Grafstein B: Axon outgrowth enhanced by previous nerve injury. Arch Neurol 29: 53–55, 1973.

57. Barrs DM: Facial nerve trauma: Optimal timing for repair. Laryngoscope 101: 835–848, 1991.

58. May M: Facial reanimation after skull base trauma. In May M (ed): The Facial Nerve. New York, Thieme, 1986, pp 421–440.

59. May M: Management of cranial nerves I through VII following skull base surgery. Otolaryngol Head Neck Surg 88: 560–575, 1980.

60. Harker L, McCabe BF: Temporal bone fractures and facial nerve injury. Otolaryngol Clin North Am 7: 425–431, 1974.

61. Johns M, Crumley R: Facial Nerve Injury, Repair and Rehabilitation (SIPac), 2nd ed. Alexandria, VA, American Academy of Otolaryngology, 1977, p 9.
62. Fisch U, Rouleau M: Facial nerve reconstruction. J Otolaryngol 9: 478–492, 1980.
63. Fisch U, Lanser MJ: Facial nerve grafting. Otolaryngol Clin North Am 24: 691–708, 1991.
64. Fisch U: Facial nerve grafting. Otolaryngol Clin North Am 7: 517–529, 1974.
65. Orgel MG: Epineurial versus perineurial repair of peripheral nerves. Clin Plast Surg 11: 101–104, 1984.
66. Yamamoto E, Fisch U: Experiments on facial nerve suturing. ORL J Otorhinolaryngol Relat Spec 36: 193–204, 1974.
67. Yasargil MG, Fisch U: Unsere Ertahrungen in der mikrochirurgischen exstirpation der akustikusneurinome. Arch Ohrenheilk 194: 243, 1969.
68. Mattox DE, Felix H, Fisch U, Lyles CA: Effect of ligating peripheral branches on facial nerve regeneration. Otolaryngol Head Neck Surg 6: 558–563, 1988.
69. Ashur H, Vilner Y, Finsterbush A, et al.: Extent of fiber regeneration after peripheral nerve repair: Silicone splint vs. suture, gap repair vs. graft. Exp Neurol 97: 365–374, 1987.
70. Glasscock ME, Dickins JR, Jackson CG, et al.: Surgical management of brain tissue herniation into the middle ear and mastoid. Laryngoscope 89: 1743–1764, 1979.
71. Neely JG, Kuhn JR: Diagnosis and treatment of iatrogenic cerebrospinal fluid leak and brain herniation during or following mastoidectomy. Laryngoscope 95: 1299–1300, 1985.
72. Kamerer DB, Caparosa RJ: Temporal bone encephalocele—Diagnosis and treatment. Laryngoscope 92: 878–881, 1982.
73. Graham MD: The jugular bulb: Its anatomic and clinical considerations in contemporary otology. Laryngoscope 87: 105–125, 1977.
74. Leonetti JP, Smith PG, Grubb RL: Control of bleeding in extended skull base surgery. Am J Otol 11: 254–259, 1990.
75. Moloy PJ, Brackmann DE: "How I do it." Control of venous bleeding in otologic surgery. Laryngoscope 96: 580–582, 1986.
76. Hotaling AJ, Rejowski JE, Kazan RF, Wiet RJ: "How I do it." Control of sigmoid sinus in glomus jugulare tumor resection. Laryngoscope 95: 481–482, 1985.
77. Glasscock ME, Dickins JR, Jackson CG, Wiet RJ: Vascular anomalies of the middle ear. Laryngoscope 90: 77–88, 1980.
78. Overton SB, Ritter FN: A high-placed jugular bulb in the middle ear. A clinical and temporal bone study. Laryngoscope 83: 1986–1991, 1973.
79. Hough JVD: Congenital malformations of the middle ear. Arch Otolaryngol Head Neck Surg 78: 335–343, 1963.
80. West JM, Bandy BC, Jafek VW: Aberrant jugular bulb in the middle ear cavity. Arch Otolaryngol Head Neck Surg 100: 370–372, 1974.
81. Lo WWM, Solti-Bohman LG: High-resolution CT of the jugular foramen: Anatomy and vascular variants and anomalies. Radiology 150: 743–747, 1984.
82. Leonetti JP, Smith PG, Linthicum FH: The petrous carotid artery: Anatomic relationships in skull base surgery. Otolaryngol Head Neck Surg 102: 3–12, 1990.
83. Goldman NC, Singleton GT, Holly EH: Aberrant internal carotid artery. Arch Otolaryngol Head Neck Surg 94: 269–273, 1971.
84. Valvassori GE, Buckingham RA: Middle ear masses mimicking glomus tumors: Radiographic and otoscopic recognition. Trans Am Otol Soc 62: 85–91, 1974.
85. Lapayowker MS: Presentation of the internal carotid artery as a tumor of the middle ear. Radiology 98: 293–297, 1971.
86. Andrews JC, Valavanis A, Fisch U: Management of the internal carotid artery in surgery of the skull base. Laryngoscope 99: 1224–1229, 1989.
87. DeVries EJ, Sekhar LN, Janecka IP, et al.: Elective resection of the internal carotid artery without reconstruction. Laryngoscope 98: 960–966, 1988.

23

Dural Herniation and Cerebrospinal Fluid Leaks

MALCOLM D. GRAHAM, M.D.
LARRY B. LUNDY, M.D.

The otologic surgeon may have occasion to manage dural defects in the temporal bone that manifest as brain herniation into the middle ear or mastoid or as cerebrospinal fluid escaping from a temporal bone defect. Appropriate management depends on proper diagnosis, which can range from the obvious to the very difficult, and the application of a few fundamental principles for surgical repair. There are several different causes of dural herniation and cerebrospinal fluid leakage (Table 23–1).

Two major categories of defects, dural herniation and cerebrospinal fluid leak, are covered in this chapter. Dural or brain herniation associated with chronic otitis media can result directly from the disease process or from a postsurgical defect. Spontaneous cerebrospinal fluid leaks arising from the temporal bone may have childhood onset or adult onset. This chapter describes the characteristics, diagnostic techniques, and surgical management of the two major categories. Post-traumatic, neoplastic, congenital, and miscellaneous causes are well recognized but are beyond the scope of this chapter. However, surgical repair of these defects still follows the basic principles that are elaborated herein.

CHRONIC OTITIS MEDIA–RELATED ENCEPHALOCELE

The successful management of dural and brain herniation and cerebrospinal fluid leakage via the temporal bone depends on a fundamental understanding of the pathophysiology, accurate preoperative diagnosis, and appropriate surgical techniques for repair of the lesion.

Protrusion of brain and dura out of the cranial cavity into the mastoid and middle ear has been variously called brain hernia, brain prolapse, cerebral hernia, brain fungus, endaural encephalocele, fungus cerebri, encephalocele, and meningoencephalocele. The clinical spectrum of presentations include herniation associated with a space-occupying lesion (brain abscess or tumor),[1, 2] temporal lobe seizures,[3–10] recurrent meningitis,[11–16] spontaneous cerebrospinal fluid otorrhea,[13, 17, 18] and rhinorrhea.[13, 19] The character and circumstances under which these occur have changed with the evolution of otology.[20]

Around the turn of the century, brain herniation was frequently related to otitis media and brain abscess.[21] Acute or chronic otitis media was a primary source of brain abscess, and the only treatment was surgical drainage. Not surprisingly, in this preantibiotic, preimaging, and premicrosurgical technique era, the mortality under such dire circumstances was extremely high, primarily because of purulent menin-

TABLE 23–1. Dural Herniation and Cerebrospinal Fluid Leak

Related to chronic otitis media	Neoplastic
Direct inflammation	Congenital neural tube defects
Postoperative	Miscellaneous
Spontaneous	Post XRT
Adult onset	Infectious
Childhood onset	Degenerative
Post-traumatic	

gitis and the brain abscess itself.[21] Faced with a patient who a possible brain abscess and a draining ear, the surgeon would trephine through the infected mastoid and dura, and with a finger probe enter into the brain in an attempt to locate and drain the abscess.[22, 23] Frequently, a delayed, secondary brain hernia would develop that was infected from the abscess or was prolapsing through the infected mastoid. In 1910, Dean[22] significantly altered this standard management of brain abscess by advocating exploratory trephination through a clean field unless there was an actively discharging sinus. Rand, as quoted by Hall,[1] concurred with this change of basic principle, and both noted a dramatic drop in brain hernia as well as mortality. In 1939, Hall[1] noted that "The important clinical point is that this complication of abscess surgery, which was common many years ago, has become very rare during the past 25 years." He also noted that "brain hernia is a rare complication in mastoid surgery . . . and in the majority of cases, an avoidable complication."

Although the incidence of brain hernia into the mastoid is a rare complication of mastoid surgery (Fig. 23–1), it still exists.[1, 4, 9, 12, 24–32] In 1961, Alberti and Dawes[24] clearly documented the relationship of chronic otitis media with cerebrospinal fluid leak and meningitis. They reported on six patients: two had meningitis, two had prior ear surgery, and five had cholesteatoma. Brain hernia can also occur in chronic ear disease without prior surgery.[5, 24, 33–35] In 1963, Blatt[36] noted one case of cerebrospinal fluid leakage and brain hernia 11 weeks after a radical mastoidectomy as well as two cases of exposed brain found at the time of surgery for active chronic otitis media. In 1960, Schurr[9] reviewed three cases of postmastoidectomy endaural cerebral hernia, two of which had known dural penetration at the time of initial surgery, and the third had dural exposure. In 1969, Stout et al.[32] reported a case of postmastoidectomy dural herniation, which recurred after repair with Silastic sheeting. In 1969, Baron[25] reported on three patients with brain herniation into the mastoid cavity. Baron noted that none of the three had cerebrospinal fluid leakage and that brain hernia can easily be mistaken for a blue dome or chocolate cyst.

In 1970, Dedo and Sooy[20] added 11 cases to the 30 cases published from 1934 to 1970 (i.e., after the antibiotic era had begun). Only three of these cases were associated with brain abscess, and in those, drainage of the abscess occurred through the mastoid. Twenty-six of these 41 cases resulted from known dural perforation at the time of surgery, with the most common site being the tegmen antri or the tegmen tympani. They mentioned that if dural defects are noted during surgery, herniation can be prevented by covering the defect with temporalis fascia or temporalis muscle, or both, and supporting it with packing in the mastoid bowl with iodoform gauze for 10 days in closed mastoid bowls, then 6 to 12 weeks in open mastoid bowls. In 1971, Levy et al.[37] described a case of what they believed to be spontaneous herniation of dura and cerebral tissue into the middle ear with a 30-year history of conductive hearing loss and no prior history of significant ear disease. In 1977, Fernandez-Blasini and Longo[28] reported on four cases of postmastoidectomy dural herniation into the mastoid cavity.

Although rare, dural exposure with resultant herniation and cerebrospinal fluid leakage can occur as a result of chronic otitis media with or without cholesteatoma.[24, 27, 35, 38] Paparella et al.,[35] in 1978, and Glasscock, et al.,[5] in 1979, added ten cases and 11 cases, respectively, to this number. Paparella et al.[35] reported on ten cases of brain hernia, all of which had chronic otitis media, six of which had not had prior surgery. Dural prolapse is typically found incidentally at the time of surgery and can be mistaken for granulation tissue. Paparella et al. speculated that in the present era of antibiotics, brain herniation could be an abortive attempt at brain abscess formation when mastoiditis is present. They noted the chronic low-grade infection involving the mastoid and middle ear likely led to destruction of tegmen with extension to dura, followed by involvement of adjacent brain and herniation. In their cases, only two patients had cholesteatoma, whereas all had granulation tissue.

Eight of the 11 cases presented by Glasscock et al.[5] were associated with chronic otitis media and prior surgery. They noted that granulations from infection on exposed dura compromised the integrity of dura. Therefore, the dura was no longer a protective barrier and allowed local cerebritis to occur.

Glasscock et al.[5] noted that one contributing factor to the decreased incidence of brain herniation was the progression of surgical techniques to include the operating microscope and high-speed drills rather than chisels, gouges, and curettes. Both groups note, as others have, that herniated tissue is functionless and should be excised.[4, 5, 7, 10, 13, 27, 28, 31, 35, 38–41] Several authors stress the importance of sending supposed granulation tissue for histologic confirmation.[5, 8, 10, 35, 37, 42]

In the 1980s, 111 cases of brain herniation and cerebrospinal leaks were identified, 71 of which occurred postoperatively.[3, 4, 6–8, 10, 26, 29, 31, 38, 39, 41, 43–53]

SPONTANEOUS CEREBROSPINAL FLUID LEAKAGE

Spontaneous cerebrospinal fluid otorrhea is a rare but potentially life-threatening condition with two different subtypes—children with otic capsule defects and sensorineural hearing loss and adults with meningoencephaloceles. The two subtypes have distinctly different manifestations.

The concept of spontaneous cerebrospinal fluid leakage was first positively established by Thomson[19] in 1899. He quoted Escat (1897) as reporting the first case of spontaneous cerebrospinal fluid otorrhea in a 10-year-old girl. The source was identified as a fine white line in the inner one third of the external auditory canal. Escat reported that this flow ceased after applying galvanocautery to it; however, follow-up lasted only 2 months. In 1933, Kline[18] reported on a 54-year-old man with spontaneous cerebrospinal fluid otorrhea that occurred after stooping. The patient subsequently died 8 days later from fulminant meningitis. An autopsy revealed a 2.5mm defect in the floor of the middle cranial fossa and dural herniation in a fistulous tract, which was considered the duct of a congenital cyst.

In 1987, Wetmore et al.[52] reviewed the literature on spontaneous cerebrospinal fluid otorrhea and added four cases of their own to total 87 cases. Of these 87 cases, 63 (72 per cent) were of the childhood type, with the median age of onset of 4 years. Seven of these 63 were diagnosed as adults. Subsequently, three authors[54–56] have added ten additional cases to the literature, one of which had bilateral oval window fistulas. By combining these data for the childhood-onset type, a high incidence of certain features is noted. Meningitis occurred in 93 per cent, profound sensorineural hearing loss in 82 per cent, and a Mondini defect in 83 per cent. These numbers are likely higher for sensorineural hearing loss and Mondini's defects because audiograms and accurate imaging were not always reported in some of the earlier literature. The most common site of the cerebrospinal fluid leakage was the otic capsule (92 per cent).[14, 52, 56–59] The stapes footplate and oval window area account for approximately 75 per cent of the fistulas[51, 54–60] frequently associated with a Mondini-type defect (Fig. 23–2).[51, 56, 58, 61] Other miscellaneous sites include the round window,[61, 62] the eustachian tube area,[61] the promontory,[14] Hyrtl's fissure,[63] the hypotympanum,[52] and the fallopian canal.[64]

The secondary major subtype of spontaneous cerebrospinal fluid leakage from the temporal bone occurs in adults[17] and has distinctly different characteristics and presentations. The site of the defect and leak is usually (88 per cent) in the floor of the middle cranial fossa (Fig. 23–3), occasionally in the posterior fossa

FIGURE 23-1

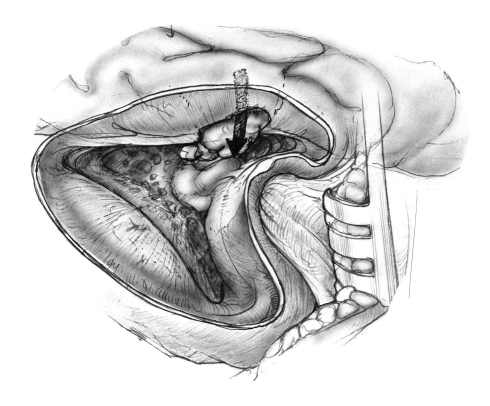

FIGURE 23-1. Temporal lobe herniation into the mastoid cavity through tegmen defect.

FIGURE 23-2. Meningocele filling a Mondini defect and protruding through the oval window.

FIGURE 23-3. Spontaneous encephalocele through tegmen.

FIGURE 23-2

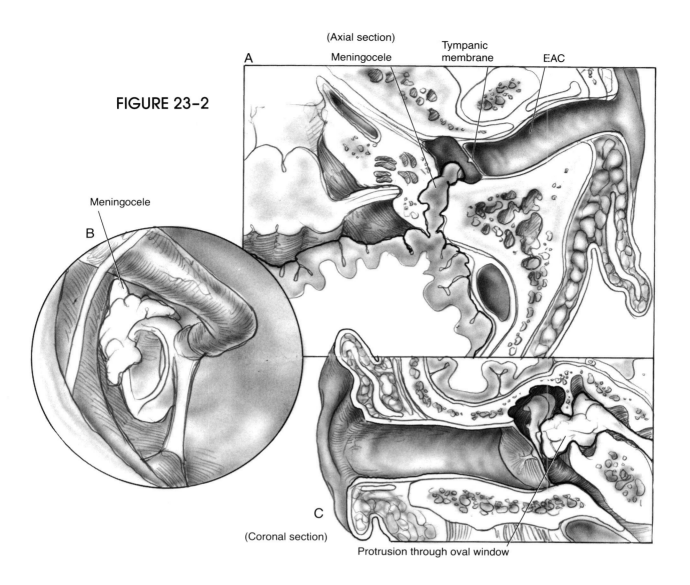

Meningocele

A

(Axial section)
Meningocele   Tympanic membrane   EAC

B

C

(Coronal section)

Protrusion through oval window

FIGURE 23-3

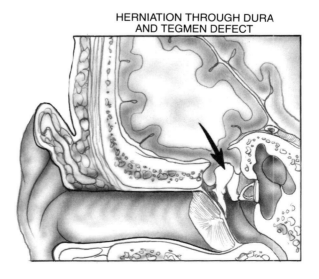

HERNIATION THROUGH DURA
AND TEGMEN DEFECT

wall.[44, 45, 52, 65] Leakage occurs in two primary areas in the floor of the middle cranial fossa:[17, 48] anteromedially or the tegmen tympani or mastoideum (Fig. 23–4). Of the 30 cases reported in the literature,[66] 40 per cent had two or more defects. A common presentation is that of serous otitis media.[17, 42–45, 48, 67, 68] In this disorder, clear, watery, thin fluid escapes and continues to drain on myringotomy. Alternatively, cerebrospinal fluid can drain through a patent eustachian tube to present as cerebrospinal fluid rhinorrhea, and this source is commonly mistaken for the anterior cranial fossa and cribriform plate area.[53]

Meningitis occurs in up to 36 per cent of adult-onset patients.[45] Profound sensorineural hearing loss, Mondini's malformation, and otic capsule fistulas are not associated with adult-onset spontaneous cerebrospinal fluid leaks (Table 23–2).

The pathophysiologic mechanism for adult-onset cerebrospinal fluid leaks is not completely understood. In 94 consecutive autopsies, Ahren and Thulen[69] noted a 6 per cent incidence of multiple (five to ten) bone defects in the tegmen tympani. In 15 per cent of the autopsy specimens, there were fewer than five perforations. An additional 16 per cent had only a thin, transparent cortical bone covering the pneumatic air cells of the tegmen tympani and, "when demonstrated, the bone defects were mainly found bilaterally and similarly distributed."[69] Ferguson et al.[45] found a 22 per cent incidence of tegmen defects in 27 preserved, dried temporal bones examined, usually with four to ten defects, 0.5mm to 2.0mm in diameter.

The high incidence of middle cranial fossa floor bony defects associated with the rarity of spontaneous cerebrospinal fluid leaks is difficult to reconcile. Congenital bony defects have also been implicated in cerebrospinal fluid rhinorrhea. In addition to congenital defects of the cribriform plate, numerous small "pit holes" have been noted in the anterior medial portion of the middle cranial fossa, independent of any history of spontaneous cerebrospinal fluid rhinorrhea.[70] If these pits appear juxtaposed to sphenoid or ethmoid air cells, cerebrospinal fluid rhinorrhea may occur.[53, 70–72] Kaufman et al.[70] speculate that these defects result from normally occurring arachnoid villi

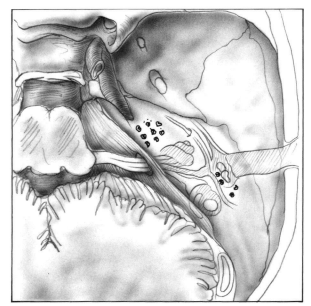

FIGURE 23–4. View of middle cranial fossa floor demonstrating frequent sites of bony defects.

and draining veins that penetrate the middle cranial fossa floor and enlarge as a response to normally occurring elevations of cerebrospinal fluid pressure. A commonly accepted premise is that decades of cerebrospinal fluid pulsations in the region of the bony defect are necessary before meningoencephalocele or meningeal dehiscence can occur.[73] Increased intracranial pressure is a possible contributing factor, but four cases in which a computed tomographic scan was obtained preoperatively showed normal-sized ventricles, a finding that questions the concept of increased intracranial pressure playing a significant role.[43, 52]

Gacek[64] further elaborated on adult-onset cerebrospinal fluid leaks. He reported on a case of aberrant arachnoid granulation tissue on the posterior mastoid dural surface of the temporal bone responsible for cerebrospinal fluid leakage. A subsequent examination of 188 temporal bones revealed that 9 per cent had posterior fossa mastoid plate dural arachnoid granulations.[64]

Arachnoid granulations are macroscopic enlargements or distentions of minute projections of arachnoid mater, termed *arachnoid villi*. Arachnoid granulations project into the intradural venous sinuses, and the centers of the arachnoid granulations are filled with cerebrospinal fluid. Cerebrospinal fluid passes from the center of the arachnoid granulations into the intradural venous sinuses, providing for resorption of cerebrospinal fluid into the blood-stream.[74]

The concept of bony pits associated with arachnoid tissue is not new. In 1870, Von Recklinghausen reported on the first case of multiple cerebral herniations, and in 1898, Beneke reported on two others.[2] In

TABLE 23–2. Spontaneous Cerebrospinal Fluid Leak

	CHILDHOOD TYPE	ADULT TYPE
Meningitis	93%	36%
Profound sensorineural hearing loss	82%	—
Otic capsule defect	83%	—
Cerebrospinal fluid otorrhea or rhinorrhea	—	very common
Dural defect	—	always

1908, Wolbach[2] reported on nine autopsy cases of increased intracranial pressure: six resulted from tumors, two, acquired internal hydrocephalus, and one, massive cerebral hemorrhage. Wolbach noted numerous pits in the skull bone and gave Beneke credit for the concept that these pits were partly preformed by arachnoid villi. Wolbach also noted that "the most striking anatomical relationship is that to the vessels of the dura. This was particularly marked about the middle meningeal vessels and their branches in the middle fossa. It is probable that the distribution of minute arachnoid villi is far more widespread than has been believed."[2]

Arachnoid granulations are not limited to the intradural venous sinuses, but are "disseminated over a considerable area; they increase in number and size as age advances. They cause absorption of bone and so produce the pits or depressions . . ."[75]

Schuknecht and Gulya[76] recently called attention to the structures on the middle fossa and posterior fossa surfaces of the temporal bone. The size and location of arachnoid granulations, as well as the degree of pneumatization of the mastoid air cell system, could create an opportunity for communication between cerebrospinal fluid and the mastoid air cell system. The same scenario could apply to the sphenoid and ethmoid sinuses, thereby producing cerebrospinal fluid rhinorrhea. Infection from suppurative otitis media can also ascend into the subarachnoid space, producing meningitis. As support for the clinically relevant role of temporal bone arachnoid granulations, Gacek[67] reported on seven patients with temporal bone arachnoid granulations, one of which had meningitis. Arachnoid granulations can be suggested by computed tomographic scans and magnetic resonance imaging, depending on their size and location.

DIAGNOSIS

The diagnosis of dural herniation and cerebrospinal fluid otorrhea is primarily clinical, with supplemental information provided by various imaging tests. History and physical examination quite often provide all the necessary information for a diagnosis. As discussed previously, brain herniation related to chronic otitis media can occur alone or with cerebrospinal fluid leak.

In an ear with chronic otitis media without prior surgery, typical presentations can range from clear watery discharge,[17, 29, 43–45, 48, 67, 68] conductive hearing loss,[29, 37, 67, 77] seizures,[3–7, 9, 10, 48] or meningitis,[5, 6, 9, 18, 21, 33, 34, 36, 39, 46, 48, 78] in addition to the characteristic signs and symptoms associated with chronic otitis media. The same applies for a prior intact canal wall mastoid procedure. In these circumstances, if suspicion is

aroused, high-resolution computed tomographic scan with bone windows may provide additional information, although it is seldom conclusive.[45, 48] In a radical or modified radical mastoid cavity, the same symptoms can manifest, as can the presence of a mass.[6] Baron[25] noted that these encephaloceles can mimic a blue dome cyst. A key point in differentiation between the two is that the encephalocele will pulsate and enlarge with the Valsalva maneuver, whereas the blue dome cyst will not.[25, 27] Computed tomographic scans can assess bony integrity, and recently, magnetic resonance imaging has proved to be of benefit in differentiating brain versus cholesteatoma.[3, 79]

Spontaneous cerebrospinal fluid leakage from the temporal bone is primarily a clinical diagnosis but it can be quite difficult to make if the quantity of the fluid is limited. Also, if cerebrospinal fluid presents as rhinorrhea, the diagnosis and preoperative localization become more difficult. Cerebrospinal fluid in sufficient quantities has a clear, watery, thin appearance. Cerebrospinal fluid leakage in children can be assessed by the history of meningitis (especially recurrent), severe-to-profound sensorineural hearing loss, and computed tomographic evidence of otic capsule abnormality. Middle ear exploration may be ultimately required as a diagnostic measure. In adults, cerebrospinal fluid flow will increase with Valsalva maneuvers, pressure occlusion of the jugular vein, and a dependent head position.

Glucose testing with commercially available test papers has been of little clinical value, especially if the result is negative. Immunoelectrophoretic identification of β_2-transferrin is pathognomonic for cerebrospinal fluid.[80] This test can be of great value if the quantity of suspected fluid is small and contaminated. However, this sophisticated test is not always readily available in clinical laboratories. Computed tomographic scan with metrizamide contrast[49, 61, 81] can demonstrate extracranial extravasation of cerebrospinal fluid for diagnosis and location. The main limitation is with very small sites of leakage or intermittent leakage, both of which can make the tests falsely negative. Other techniques used to demonstrate cerebrospinal fluid leakage include injection of colored dyes into the subarachnoid space (fluorescein, methylene blue, indigo carmine, and toluidine blue) or radioactive isotopes[16, 23, 40, 45, 82–86] (radioactive sodium, ^{111}In-DTPA, ^{99m}Tc-DTPA [diethylenetriamine pentaacetic acid], [99m]TcHSA [human serum albumin]). With these techniques (dye or tracer), pledgets are placed at the suspected site to absorb with the dye or tracer, then visually inspected or submitted for radiation counting techniques. Methylene blue (methylthionine chloride) has been abandoned as an intrathecal injection technique to detect cerebrospinal fluid leaks because of severe reactions, including transverse myelitis.[27] Fluorescein is usually safe[27, 43, 44, 68, 82, 87–89] to use intrathecally, although transient paraplegia and seizures were reported once[90] when it was used in high concentration. Schuknecht et al.[68] recommend using 0.5ml of 10 per cent fluorescein mixed with 9.5ml of cerebrospinal fluid removed by lumbar puncture. The entire 10ml mixture is injected intrathecally via the lumbar spinal needle slowly over 5 minutes. Suspected ear fluid is examined 2 hours later visually or with the aid of a Wood lamp.

SURGICAL MANAGEMENT

As expected, surgical management techniques depend on the type of defect as well as the location. Substances used for repair need only be strong enough to withstand normal intracranial pressure (less than 200mm of water) and be compliant enough to form a seal. For a temporal lobe herniation through the floor of the middle cranial fossa into a radical or modified radical cavity, the herniation is usually broadbased. The favored technique (Fig. 23–5) consists of a combined mastoid-temporal craniotomy with fascia-bone-fascia support.[6, 48]

A wide mastoidectomy is performed and the extent of dural and temporal lobe herniation determined. Fibrous adhesions between the dura and adjacent soft tissues are separated; however, reduction of the temporal lobe is not attempted. A middle cranial fossa temporal skin incision is then made, and a large piece of temporalis fascia is acquired and dried for future use. A temporal craniotomy is then fashioned with the cutting drill and suction irrigation. Dura is elevated off the floor of the middle cranial fossa, and the herniated temporal lobe is elevated and supported by the House-Urban middle fossa retractor. A portion of the squamous temporal bone removed at craniotomy is then fashioned to lie on the floor of the middle cranial fossa, bridging the tegmen defect. Two layers of dry temporalis fascia are then placed over and under the bony plate. The dural defect should be closed with sutures, if possible. If the defect is too large to close primarily, it should be covered by fascia to prevent cerebrospinal fluid leak. The dura middle fossa retractor is removed and the temporal lobe allowed to re-expand slowly. The wound is then closed in layers without drainage. Canfield,[21] in 1913, and Dandy,[11] in 1944, corrected dural defects with prolapse of the temporal lobe following mastoidectomy by suturing dura and fascia into the dural defect. Hall[1] described a case of brain hernia into the mastoid cavity and reviewed the literature to that date. In 1963, Blatt[36] described dural defect repair with fascia and bone graft and amputation of the herniated dura. In 1969, Baron[25] described three patients with dural and temporal lobe herniation; one condition resulted from fenestration surgery, and two, mastoid surgery. In 1970, Dedo and Sooy[20] reviewed nine cases and described the surgical method of correction by temporalis muscle flap rotation to the mastoid cavity to seal the defect after the brain herniation had been excised, the flap being held in place by packing. In 1977, Fernandez-Blasini and Longo[28] described four cases of temporal lobe herniation through the radical mastoid defect and the successful correction by middle fossa temporal parietal osteoplastic craniotomy. They also described dural hernia and bony defect repair by pedicled temporalis muscle and fascia graft. In 1977, Bhatnager[91] described an instance of temporal lobe herniation following intact canal wall tympanoplasty with mastoidectomy. The prolapse eroded through the posterior bony canal wall postoperatively; the defect was successfully closed by temporalis fascia. In 1978, Iliades[30] described a case occurring 19 months after radical mastoidectomy that was followed by *Pseudomonas* infection. This defect was not repaired. In 1978, Paparella et al.[35] used a temporalis fascia graft to cover a defect on the mastoid side and used a split-thickness skin graft carefully placed to line the remaining cavity. A firm pack held the graft in place for 2 weeks. In 1979, Glasscock et al.[5] discussed in depth the problem of brain tissue herniation into the middle ear and mastoid cavity and reviewed methods of repair, that is, from below via mastoidectomy and by a combined intracranial and mastoid approach.

The surgeon should be prepared to deal with an encephalocele encountered incidentally during surgery for chronic otitis media. Typically, the mass is pedunculated through a small opening. This her-

FIGURE 23–5. *A*, Tegmen defect covered by fascia-bone-fascia technique via a temporal craniotomy approach. *B*, Temporal lobe herniation reduced and supported by fascia-bone-fascia technique.

FIGURE 23–6. Fascia "dumbbelled" through small dural defect.

FIGURE 23-5

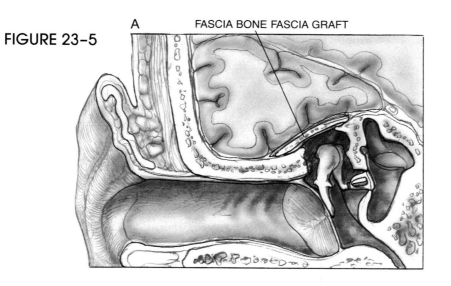

A   FASCIA BONE FASCIA GRAFT

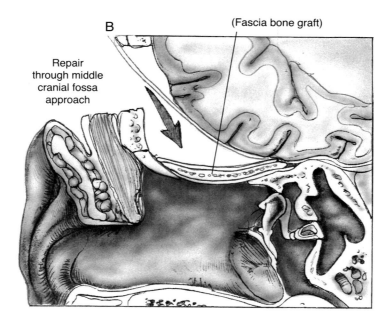

B   (Fascia bone graft)

Repair
through middle
cranial fossa
approach

FIGURE 23-6

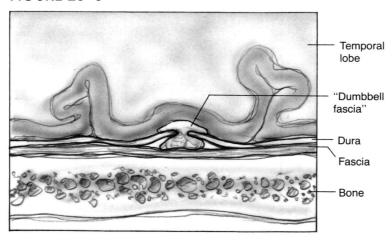

Temporal
lobe

"Dumbbell
fascia"

Dura

Fascia

Bone

niated tissue is functionless and should be amputated.[4, 5, 7, 13, 27, 28, 31, 35, 38–41] The surgeon must decide whether this problem can be repaired from below (mastoid approach) or from above (middle cranial fossa approach).

Various options for transmastoid repair include temporalis fascia or fascia lata[3, 11, 24, 41] inserted intracranially but extradurally with or without firm support, such as conchal cartilage graft[4, 31, 38, 39] or cortical bone.[4, 6, 26, 48] Another option includes rotating pedicled temporalis muscle flap[3, 17, 24, 25, 27, 28, 32, 34, 39, 40, 42–45, 47, 63, 92] for additional support or abdominal fat graft[52, 68, 89] in the mastoid cavity. Some authors[3, 5, 27, 32, 40 46, 50] have used synthetic material (silicone sheeting, Marlex, stainless steel mesh, Vivosil, acrylic, methyl methacrylate) for bony defect closure, but there is a higher incidence of infection, recurrence, and extrusion with these materials.[3, 5, 32] Others[3, 5, 12, 14, 24, 27, 28, 36, 39] have advocated packing the cavity (open or closed) until healing is well under way, then removing it. For temporal craniotomy, an intradural temporalis fascia or fascia lata graft can be placed and provides a better anatomic seal. A combined mastoidectomy-minicraniotomy approach has been successfully used.[4, 8, 38]

For children with otic capsule defects, the oval window is by far the most common site because there is almost always no functional hearing; therefore, a total stapedectomy is performed, with soft tissue obliteration of the vestibule.[14, 51, 54–60, 82, 93, 94] For the rare miscellaneous sites of otic capsule defects, a radical mastoidectomy with obliteration of the eustachian tube, middle ear, and mastoid, and blind sac closure of the external auditory canal are recommended.[14, 52, 68, 95, 96] This procedure will provide the best chance of permanent closure of cerebrospinal fluid fistula and control over recurrent meningitis, while maintaining cochlear function.

Probably the most challenging issue is the adult onset of spontaneous cerebrospinal fluid leakage. As noted earlier, the source can be posterior fossa mastoid dural surface, middle fossa dural surface, or, very rarely, the middle ear. Multiple sources of cerebrospinal fluid leaks are frequently encountered.[8, 11, 17, 25, 36, 43, 45, 48, 52, 53, 62, 70–72] Therefore, a combined mastoid–subtemporal craniotomy approach is recommended.[6, 48] The dural surfaces of the mastoid and posterior fossa should be thoroughly explored, as should the middle ear. The final portion of the procedure is the subtemporal craniotomy with wide exposure of the entire middle cranial fossa floor, especially the anteromedial portion. Experience has shown that the multiple small sites would easily be missed from a mastoid-alone approach. If the dural defects are small, an oversized piece of fascia can be "dumbbelled" into the opening, and then an extradural fascia graft can be done (Fig. 23–6).

SUMMARY

Dural or brain herniation and cerebrospinal fluid leakage from the temporal bone is a widely recognized, but infrequently encountered, challenge for the otologic surgeon. Two major categories are reviewed in this chapter: dural herniation secondary to chronic otitis media and spontaneous cerebrospinal fluid leaks. Dural herniation secondary to chronic otitis media can result from the chronic otitis media itself or from surgery for chronic otitis media. Spontaneous cerebrospinal fluid leakage from the temporal bone has two recognized subtypes: childhood onset and adult onset. Each has distinctly different characteristics and presentations.

Regardless of the underlying cause, a break in the integrity of the intracranial-extracranial barrier poses significant risk of complications, such as meningitis[5–7, 9, 12, 14–16, 18, 21, 33, 34, 36, 39, 42, 46, 52, 55–60, 77, 78, 82, 83, 93, 94, 96, 97] and seizures.[3–10] The diagnosis and management of these disorders were discussed.

References

1. Hall C: Brain hernia: A postoperative complication in otology. Ann Otol Rhinol Laryngol 48: 291–309, 1939.
2. Wolbach SB: Multiple hernias of the cerebrum and cerebellum due to intracranial pressure. J Med Res 19: 153–173, 1908.
3. Bowes AK, Wiet RJ, Monsell EM, et al.: Brain herniation and space occupying lesions eroding the tegmen tympani. Laryngoscope 97: 1172–1175, 1987.
4. Feenstra L, Sanna M, Zini C, et al.: Surgical treatment of brain herniation into the middle ear and mastoid. Am J Otol 6: 311–315, 1985.
5. Glasscock ME, Dickins JRE, Jackson CG, et al.: Surgical management of brain tissue herniation into the middle ear and mastoid. Laryngoscope 89: 1743–1754, 1979.
6. Graham MD: Surgical managment of dural and temporal lobe herniation into the radical mastoid cavity. Laryngoscope 92: 329–331, 1982.
7. Hyson M, Andermann F, Olivier A, Melenson D: Occult encephaloceles and temporal lobe epilepsy: Developmental and acquired lesions in the middle fossa. Neurology 34: 363–366, 1984.
8. Iurato S, Ettorre GC, Selvini C: Brain herniation into the middle ear: Two idiopathic cases treated by a combined intracranial mastoid approach. Laryngoscope 99: 950–954, 1989.
9. Schurr PH: Endaural cerebral hernia. Br J Surg 47: 414–417, 1960.
10. Williams DC: Encephalocele of the middle ear. J Laryngol Otol 100: 471–473, 1986.
11. Dandy WE: Treatment of rhinorrhea and otorrhea. Arch Surg 49: 75–85, 1944.
12. Lillie HI, Spar AA: Escape of cerebrospinal fluid into the wounds of operations on the temporal bone. Arch Otolaryngol Head Neck Surg 46: 779–788, 1947.
13. Mosberg WH: Spontaneous cerebrospinal fluid rhinorrhea and otorrhea. Md Med J 8: 62–65, 1959.
14. Nenzelius C: Spontaneous cerebrospinal otorrhea due to congenital malformations. Acta Otolaryngol (Stockh) 39: 314–328, 1951.
15. Precechtel A: The problem of recurrent meningitis in ORL. Acta Otolaryngol 45: 427–430, 1954.
16. Spitz EB, Wagner S, Sataloff J, et al.: Cerebrospinal fluid otorrhea and recurrent meningitis. J Pediatr 59: 397–400, 1961.
17. Dysart BR: Spontaneous cerebrospinal fluid otorrhea—A report on a case with successful surgical repair. Trans Am Laryngol Rhinol Otol Soc 62: 381–387, 1959.

18. Kline OR: Spontaneous cerebrospinal otorrhea. Arch Otolaryngol Head Neck Surg, 18: 34–39, 1933.
19. Thomson St. C: The Cerebro-spinal Fluid: Its Spontaneous Escape from the Nose. New York, William Wood & Company, 1899.
20. Dedo HH, Sooy FA: Endaural brain hernia (encephalocele) diagnosis and treatment. Laryngoscope 80: 1090–1099, 1970.
21. Canfield RB: Some conditions associated with the loss of cerebrospinal fluid. Ann Otol Rhinol Laryngol 22: 604–622, 1913.
22. Dean LW: Operative procedure for brain abscess of otitic origin. Ann Otol Rhinol Laryngol 19: 541–556, 1910.
23. DiChiro G, Ommaya AK, Ashburn WL, Briner WH: Isotope cisternography in the diagnosis and followup of cerebrospinal fluid rhinorrhea. J Neurosurg 28: 522–529, 1968.
24. Alberti PWRM, Dawes JDK: Cerebrospinal otorrhea and chronic ear disease. J Laryngol Otol 75: 123–135, 1961.
25. Baron SH: Herniation of the brain into the mastoid cavity: Postsurgical, postinfectional, or congenital. Arch Otolaryngol Head Neck Surg 90: 127–133, 1969.
26. Bartels L, Luk LJ, Balis G, Bald C: Endaural brain hernia: Repair using mastoid cortical bone. Am J Otol (Suppl): 121–125, 1985.
27. Dedo HH, Sooy FA: Endaural enchephalocele and cerebrospinal fluid otorrhea: A review. Ann Otol Rhinol Laryngol 79: 168–177, 1970.
28. Fernandez-Blasini N, Longo R: Surgical correction of dural herniation into the mastoid cavity. Laryngoscope 87: 1841–1846, 1977.
29. Gavilan J, Trujillo M, Gavilan C: Spontaneous encephalocele of the middle ear. Arch Otolaryngol Head Neck Surg 110: 206–207, 1984.
30. Iliades CE: Brain hernia: A postoperative complication in otology. Ear Nose Throat J 57: 39–43, 1978.
31. Neely JG, Kuhn JR: Diagnosis and treatment of iatrogenic cerebrospinal fluid leak and brain herniation during or following mastoidectomy. Laryngoscope 95: 1299–1300, 1985.
32. Stout JJ Jr., Trowbridge WV, Ruggles RL: Surgical repair of dural herniation into the mastoid bowl. Arch Otolaryngol Head Neck Surg 89: 72–77, 1969.
33. Mealey J Jr.: Chronic cerebrospinal fluid otorrhea—Report of a case associated with chronic infection of the ear. Neurology 11: 996–998, 1961.
34. Moore GF, Nissen AJ, Yonkers AJ: Potential complications of unrecognized cerebrospinal fluid leaks secondary to mastoid surgery. Am J Otol 5: 317–323, 1984.
35. Paparella MM, Meyerhoff WL, Oliviera CA: Mastoiditis and brain hernia (mastoiditis cerebri). Laryngoscope 88: 1097–1106, 1978.
36. Blatt IM: Surgical repair for cerebrospinal otorrhea due to middle ear and mastoid disease—A report of six cases. Laryngoscope 73: 446–460, 1963.
37. Levy RA, Platt N, Aftalion B: Encephalocele of the middle ear. Laryngoscope 81: 126–130, 1971.
38. Adkins WY, Osguthorpe JD: Mini-craniotomy for management of CSF otorrhea from tegmen defects. Laryngoscope 93: 1038–1039, 1983.
39. Jahn AF: Endaural brain hernia: Repair using conchal cartilage. J Otolaryngol 10: 471–475, 1981.
40. Jahrsdoerfer RA, Richtsmeier WJ, Cantrell RW: Spontaneous CSF otorrhea. Arch Otolaryngol Head Neck Surg 107: 257–262, 1981.
41. Ramsden RT, Latif A, Lye RH, Dutton JEM: Endaural cerebral hernia. J Laryngol Otol 99: 643–651, 1985.
42. Kramer SA, Yanagisawa E, Smith HW: Spontaneous cerebrospinal fluid otorrhea simulating serous otitis media. Laryngoscope 81: 1083–1089, 1971.
43. Adams GL, McCoid G, Weisbeski D: Cerebrospinal fluid otorrhea presenting as serous otitis media. Minn Med 65: 410–415, 1982.
44. Briant TDR, Bird R: Extracranial repair of cerebrospinal fluid fistula. J Otolaryngol 11: 191–197, 1982.
45. Ferguson BJ, Wilkins RH, Hudson W, Farmer J Jr.: Spontaneous CSF otorrhea from tegmen and posterior fossa defects. Laryngoscope 96: 635–644, 1986.
46. Hicks GW, Wright JW Jr., Wright JW III: Cerebrospinal fluid otorrhea. Laryngoscope 80(Suppl 25): 1–25, 1980.
47. Kamerer DB, Caparosa RJ: Temporal bone encephalocele—Diagnosis and treatment. Laryngoscope 92: 878–882, 1982.
48. Kemink JL, Graham MD, Kartush JM: Spontaneous encephalocele of the temporal bone. Arch Otolaryngol Head Neck Surg 112: 558–561, 1986.
49. Myer CM, Miller GW, Ball JB: Spontaneous cerebrospinal fluid otorrhea. Ann Otol Rhinol Laryngol 94: 96–97, 1985.
50. Richardson GS: Brain herniation into the mastoid antrum. Am J Otol 2: 39, 1980.
51. Weider DJ, Geurkink NA, Saunders RL: Spontaneous cerebrospinal fluid otorhinorrhea. Am J Otol 6: 416–422, 1985.
52. Wetmore SJ, Herrmann P, Fisch U: Spontaneous cerebrospinal fluid otorrhea. Am J Otol 8: 96–102, 1987.
53. Yeates AE, Blumenkopf B, Drayer BP, et al. Spontaneous CSF rhinorrhea arising from the middle cranial fossa: CT demonstration. AJNR Am J Neuroradiol 5: 820–821, 1984.
54. MacRae DL, Ruby RRF: Recurrent meningitis secondary to perilymph fistula in young children. J Otolaryngol 19: 222–225, 1990.
55. Phillipps JJ: Bilateral oval window fistulae with recurrent meningitis. J Laryngol Otol 100: 329–331, 1986.
56. Quiney RE, Mitchell DB, Djazeri B, Evans JNG: Recurrent meningitis in children due to inner ear abnormalities. J Laryngol Otol 103: 473–480, 1989.
57. Barr B, Warsall J: Cerebrospinal otorrhea with meningitis and congenital deafness. Arch Otolaryngol Head Neck Surg 81: 26–28, 1965.
58. Bennett RJ: On subarachnoid tympanic fistula—A report of two cases of the rare indirect type. J Laryngol Otol 80: 1242–1252, 1966.
59. Biggers WP, Howell NN, Fisher ND, Himadi GM: Congenital ear anomalies associated with otic meningitis. Arch Otolaryngol Head Neck Surg 97: 399–401, 1973.
60. Tschiang HH, Harrison MS, Ozsahinaglu CAN: Cerebrospinal otorrhea. J Laryngol Otol 87: 475–483, 1973.
61. Park TS: Spontaneous cerebrospinal fluid otorrhea in association with a congenital defect of the cochlear aqueduct and Mondini dysplasia. Neurosurgery 11: 356, 1982.
62. Brodsky L: Spontaneous cerebrospinal fluid otorrhea and rhinorrhea co-existing in a patient with meningitis. Laryngoscope 94: 1351–1354, 1984.
63. Gacek RR, Leipzig B: Congenital cerebrospinal otorrhea. Ann Otol 88: 358–365, 1979.
64. Gacek RR: Arachnoid granulation cerebrospinal otorrhea. Ann Otol Rhinol Laryngol 99: 854–862, 1990.
65. Finsnes KA: Lethal intracranial complication following insufflation with a pneumatic otoscope. Acta Otolaryngol 75: 436–438, 1973.
66. Wilkins RH, Radtke RA, Burger PC: Spontaneous temporal encephalocele: A case report. J Neurosurg 78: 492–498, 1993.
67. Gacek RR: Evaluation and management of temporal bone arachnoid granulations. Arch Otolaryngol Head Neck Surg 118: 327–332, 1992.
68. Schuknecht HF, Zaytoun GM, Moon CN: Adult onset of fluid in the tympanomastoid compartment. Arch Otolaryngol Head Neck Surg 108: 759–765, 1982.
69. Ahren C, Thulin CA: Lethal intracranial complications following inflation in the external auditory canal in treatment of serous otitis media and due to defects in the petrous bone. Acta Otolaryngol 60: 407–421, 1965.
70. Kaufman B, Yonas H, White RJ, Miller CF: Acquired middle cranial fossa fistulas, normal pressure, and non-traumatic in origin. Neurosurgery 5: 466–472, 1979.
71. Brisman R, Hughes JEO, Mount LA: Cerebrospinal fluid rhinorrhea. Nerolology 22: 245–252, 1970.
72. Kaufman B, Nulsen FE, Weiss MH, et al.: Acquired spontaneous non-traumatic normal pressure cerebrospinal fistulas originating from the middle fossa. Radiology 122: 379–387, 1977.
73. Ommaya AK: Cerebrospinal fluid rhinorrhea. Neurology 15: 106–113, 1964.
74. Weed LH: The absorption of cerebrospinal fluid in the venous system. Am J Anat 31: 191–221, 1923.
75. Warwick R, Williams PL (eds): Gray's Anatomy, 35th British ed. Philadelphia, WB Saunders, 1973, p 991.
76. Schuknecht HF, Gulya AJ: Anatomy of the Temporal Bone with

Surgical Implications. Philadelphia, Lea & Febiger, 1986, pp 125–126.

77. Koch H: Meningocele of the temporal bone. Acta Otolaryngol (Stockh) 38: 59–61, 1950.

78. Feenstra L, Blom ER: Mastoid approach for brain herniation into the middle ear. Clin Otolaryngol 8: 187–190, 1983.

79. Kaseff LG, Seidenwurm DJ, Neiberding PH, et al.: Magnetic resonance imaging of brain herniation into the middle ear. Am J Otol 13: 74–77, 1992.

80. Irjala K, Suompaa J, Laurent B: Identification of CSF leakage by immunofixation. Arch Otolaryngol Head Neck Surg 105: 447–448, 1979.

81. Loew F: Traumatic spontaneous and postoperative CSF rhinorrhea. Adv Tech Stand Neurosurg 11: 169, 1984.

82. Harris HH: Cerebrospinal otorrhea and recurring meningitis: report of three cases. Laryngoscope 88: 1577–1585, 1978.

83. Kaseff LG, Neiberding PH, Shorago GW, Huertas G: Fistula between the middle ear and subarachnoid space as a cause of recurrent meningitis: Detection by means of thin section, complex motion tomography. Radiology 135: 105–108, 1980.

84. Ommaya AK, DiChiro G, Baldwin M, Pennybacker JB: Nontraumatic cerebrospinal fluid rhinorrhea. J Neurol Neurosurg Psychiatry 31: 214–225, 1968.

85. Ray BS, Bergland RM: Cerebrospinal fluid fistula: Clinical aspects, techniques of localization, and methods of closure. J Neurosurg 30: 399–405, 1969.

86. Rotillio A, Andrioli GC, Scanarini M, et al.: Concurrent spontaneous CSF otorrhea and rhinorrhea. Eur Neurol 21: 77–83, 1982.

87. Kirchner FR: Use of fluorescein for the diagnosis and localization of cerebrospinal fluid fistulas. Surg Forum 12: 406–408, 1961.

88. Kirchner FR, Proud GO: Method for identification and localization of cerebrospinal fluid, rhinorrhea and otorrhea. Trans Am Laryngol Rhinol Otol Soc 70: 786–796, 1960.

89. Montgomery WW: Surgery for cerebrospinal fluid rhinorrhea and otorrhea. Arch Otolaryngol Head Neck Surg 84: 92–104, 1966.

90. Mahaley MS Jr., Odom GL: Complications following intrathecal injection of fluorescein. J Neurosurg 25: 298–299, 1966.

91. Bhatnager HN: Meningoencephalocele of the mastoid. Ear Nose Throat J 56: 20–28, 1977.

92. Andrew WF: Temporal lobe herniation through traumatic defect in tegmen of temporal bone with cerebrospinal fluid otorrhea. Ann Otol Rhinol Laryngol 60: 622–626, 1951.

93. Gundersen T, Haye R: Cerebrospinal otorrhea. Arch Otolaryngol Head Neck Surg 91: 19–23, 1970.

94. Herther C, Schindler RA: Mondini's dysplasia with recurrent meningitis. Laryngoscope 95: 655–658, 1985.

95. Neely J, Neblett CR, Rose JE: Diagnosis and treatment of spontaneous cerebrospinal fluid otorrhea. Laryngoscope 92: 609–612, 1982.

96. Schindler RA: Congenital deafness, recurrent meningitis, and neural tube defects. Transpac Coast Oto Ophthalmol Soc 82: 275–282, 1976.

97. Hall GM, Pulec JL, Hallberg OE: Persistent cerebrospinal fluid otorrhea. Arch Otolaryngol Head Neck Surg 86: 43–47, 1967.

24

Total Stapedectomy

HOWARD P. HOUSE, M.D.
JED A. KWARTLER, M.D.

The goal of stapes surgery is to re-establish sound transmission through an ossicular chain stiffened due to otosclerosis. Various techniques have been used to accomplish this goal, including stapes mobilization, fragmentation, small fenestration, and partial as well as total stapes footplate removal.

The history of surgery for otosclerosis is a fascinating story that began to unfold in the latter part of the nineteenth century. A group of pioneering surgeons, including Kessel,[1] Boucheron,[2] Miot,[3] Faraci,[4] and Passow,[5] began to mobilize the stapes. At about this time, Jack[6] reported on a series of cases in which he removed the stapes entirely.

Despite the relatively immediate good hearing results, the unacceptably high rate of inner ear injury and infection led to the abandonment of stapes surgery. As stated in Goodhill's book[7] "it was probably Siebenmann[8] along with Moure[9] who closed the door on further stapes surgery at the turn of the century."

Surgery for otosclerosis was reactivated in 1923, when Holmgren[10] bypassed the stapes area by creating a fenestra in the horizontal canal to stimulate inner ear fluids in response to sound, and the fenestration operation was reborn. In 1937, Sourdille[11] presented a series of fenestration cases before the New York Academy of Medicine. It was Lempert,[12] however, who in 1938 introduced his unique one-stage fenestration technique using his endaural approach and a dental drill to create the fenestra. Surgeons throughout the world beat a path to his door to learn his technique, which became the standard. He will forever be known as the father of otosclerosis surgery.

In 1952, Rosen[13] reintroduced stapes mobilization for otosclerosis. For a brief time, this technique was widely used and threatened to replace the Lempert procedure. It was soon realized that refixation of the footplate often occurred. Fortunately, Shea[14] introduced his technique of total stapedectomy. After removing the total stapes, he covered the oval window with a vein graft and introduced an artificial stapes made of polytetrafluoroethylene (Teflon) by Harry Treace to make the connection with the incus. This reactivation of stapedectomy by Shea replaced both Lempert's fenestration procedure and Rosen's mobilization operation and, with modification, is now used universally throughout the world. We indeed are greatly indebted to Shea for his tremendous contribution to otosclerosis surgery.

PATIENT COUNSELING

All patients should be told that even though their hearing loss is hereditary, their children or grandchildren will not necessarily have a similar problem. They should be assured they are not going to become to-

tally deaf, and that their hearing may be stabilized with the use of fluorides.[15] The mechanics of the hearing loss should also be explained in detail, preferably by use of a suitable illustration.

Patients who are suitable for stapes surgery should be told that they have the option of wearing hearing aids, and if there is any doubt about the decision to have surgery, they should be encouraged to have a trial period with hearing aids unless they are already wearing them.

The expected hearing result as well as all possible risks, such as further or even total hearing loss, taste disturbance, dizziness, the effect on tinnitus, if present, and the very remote possibility of a partial or total facial paralysis, should be clearly understood.

Hearing improvement is in direct proportion to the preoperative bone conduction level, and the patient must understand the degree of improvement to be expected.

SELECTION OF PATIENTS FOR STAPES SURGERY

All patients who are suitable for stapes surgery should be thoroughly informed of both the advantages and the possible complications of the operation. For some, serviceable hearing will be restored with no need for a hearing aid. In others, the hearing will be improved so they may need a hearing aid only for distant conversation. In still others, the hearing will be improved, and they may be able to convert their postauricular aid to an all-in-the-ear aid or from an all-in-the-ear aid to an intracanal aid. With proper fitting, less power is required, and the likelihood of feedback is diminished.

Occasionally, patients will have a totally blank audiogram and still be suitable for stapes surgery. This situation occurs when the bone conduction level exceeds the capability of the audiometer. There may be a 75dB or 80dB bone conduction level but a 40dB to 50dB air-bone gap. Typically, when the patient is initially evaluated, he or she is hearing surprisingly well with a powerful hearing aid and possesses excellent speech quality. On examination, one may note a positive Schwartze sign, but the 512 tuning fork is not helpful. Following surgery, these patients are most grateful because they can now wear the less powerful hearing aids with fewer feedback problems.

Indications for Stapes Surgery

The patient should understand the details of the operation, including the operative procedure itself, and all admission and discharge procedures.

1. The patient should be in reasonably good health, especially if general anesthesia is contemplated.
2. The age of the patient is not a factor in the decision to perform surgery. The youngest in my series was 7 years of age, and the oldest was 98.
3. The poorer-hearing ear, based on the patient's statement and not necessarily on the audiogram, should be chosen for surgery. In children, the poorer-hearing ear should be operated on so that the hearing aid can be eliminated before they enter school. Surgery for the second ear should be delayed until they are old enough to make their own decision.
4. Tuning forks should be used to confirm the audiometric findings. If bone conduction is heard louder than air conduction with a 512 or a 1024 tuning fork, the individual is a suitable candidate for surgery. If one reverses the 2048 fork, he or she is an excellent candidate. The minimum air-bone gap should be 15dB, as averaged in speech frequencies.
5. Speech discrimination is not a great factor in determining stapes suitability. If the patient understands sentences and answers questions correctly using a speaking tube while masking the opposite ear with a Bárány apparatus, he or she is suitable, providing the above criteria are met. The improvement the patient receives with a cochlear implant substantiates the value of any sound that helps patients hear and react better to their environment.
6. Indications for stapes surgery are essentially the same whether the hearing loss is unilateral or bilateral. Surgery in the opposite ear can occur 6 months later, provided it is then the poorer-hearing ear.

Contraindications of Stapes Surgery

Stapes surgery is contraindicated in patients

1. In poor physical health
2. With a current balance problem, such as active Ménière's disease or a fluctuating type of hearing loss
3. With pre-existing tympanic membrane perforation
4. With active external or middle ear infection
5. With an inadequate air-bone gap confirmed by an audiogram and the 512 tuning fork

SURGICAL TECHNIQUE

STEP 1. Stapes surgery may be performed either with a local or a general anesthetic. My preference is local anesthesia with adequate sedation that may be supplemented during the procedure with intravenous midazolam (Versed) or diazepam (Valium), if necessary. I prefer local anesthesia because there is less bleeding, and the surgeon is alerted if any vertigo occurs while working on the footplate, inserting the prosthesis, or removing the prosthesis, in a revision case.

STEP 2. During surgery, the patient's vital signs are monitored by electrocardiography, blood pressure, and oxygen saturation. The auricle and the surrounding area is cleaned, and povidone-iodine (Betadine) is applied. A small amount of hair is shaved, plastic drapes and folded towels are applied. A final head drape with an opening exposing the ear is placed over the head and rested on a metal support to help prevent the feeling of claustrophobia.

STEP 3. The operating table is placed in Trendelenburg's position and rotated slightly toward the surgeon so he or she may look directly down the ear canal from the sitting position without bending over the patient. This position does not cause further bleeding.

STEP 4. The ear canal is washed with warm saline solution to remove the povidone-iodine, and local anesthesia containing 2% lidocaine fortified by 1:20,000 of epinephrine is infused. If the patient is elderly or has hypertension or arteriosclerotic heart disease, the epinephrine additive is reduced. The initial injections are made with a 30-gauge needle around the periphery of the entrance to the ear canal. Approximately 2.5ml to 3ml of this solution is injected, and a drop or two is placed in the vascular strip just external to the tympanic membrane. This helps reduce the bleeding at the time of the incision. The tissue to be used, whether vein, fascia, perichondrium, or fat, may be obtained before or after the canal surgery is started.

Several sizes of speculums, both oval and round, should be on the tray, and the largest one that can be seated into the canal is used. The shaft of the instruments entering the speculum are in firm contact with the middle finger, which in turn is stabilized against the speculum and the speculum stabilized by the other fingers against the head. A fixed speculum holder is not used. The advantage of not using a fixed speculum holder is flexibility of the speculum for viewing purposes and for allowing the patient to move his or her head, if desired. The speculums as well as all instruments should be plain metal, because black speculums and instruments absorb much-needed light. The shafts of the needles and hooks should be malleable so that they can be bent slightly to reach difficult areas.

The inferior and superior vertical incisions are

made at 6:30 and 11:30 o'clock positions (Fig. 24–1). The point of the sickle knife is started 1mm from the edge of the tympanic membrane to prevent a possible tear. It is extended externally approximately 8mm, and this distance can be confirmed when the curve of the incision knife strikes the edge of the properly inserted speculum. If one extends the incisions further externally, the skin becomes thicker, and more bleeding occurs. Several sweeps are made to be certain that one cuts through the periosteum.

The horizontal incision begins by elevation of the skin from the depth of the suture indentation and then continues inferiorly in short increments toward the inferior vertical incision to avoid tearing of the skin toward the eardrum. Several clean sweeps of the knife are again made to ensure that the periosteum that connects to the inferior vertical incision has been cut through. A similar superior incision is made in increments halfway to the superior vertical incision. Again, several sweeps are made on this partially completed incision. The knife is inserted beneath the remaining skin to elevate it. Scissors are then used to connect with the end of the superior vertical incision. Scissors crush the vessels in the vascular strip and help reduce the bleeding.

Following these incisions, a broad separator is used to elevate the skin flap in a uniform manner toward the eardrum. Considerable pressure is applied on the instrument, especially inferiorly, to stay under the periosteum until it enters the middle ear area posterior to the ligament. Scissors are used to sever the 1mm remaining when the first superior vertical incision was started.

A curved needle is used superiorly to elevate the eardrum and identify the position of the chorda tympani nerve (Fig. 24–2). Once the nerve is identified, the needle is inserted superiorly to the nerve and carried forth to contact the malleus. This action provides the superior exposure. The needle is then used inferior to the chorda tympani to identify the beginning of the tympanic membrane ligament. An elevator is used to lift the ligament inferiorly and to identify the round window. At this point, a cotton ball soaked in the lidocaine-epinephrine solution is placed on the raw surface of the skin flap to lessen the bleeding for a moment. The entire skin flap is then elevated anteriorly, and a few drops of lidocaine-epinephrine are dropped onto the mucosa of the middle ear for anesthesia and to control any mucosal bleeding later as work is done in the stapes area.

At the upper limit of exposure superiorly, one should observe the lower half of the transverse portion of the fallopian canal (Fig. 24–3). If one can see the beginning of the curve of the body of the incus, a subsequent retraction pocket may develop. The posterior exposure is limited to observation of the stapedial tendon and the beginning of the pyramidal process. If more bone is removed, a posterior retraction pocket may develop. This exposure is usually done with curettes, but a diamond burr may be necessary to expose the posterior portion of the chorda tympani. On completion of this exposure, a square area is created posterosuperiorly. When the curette or the burr is used, the patient under local anesthesia should be forewarned of the noise that will be created so there will be no surprise to the patient.

If the footplate area appears to be thin, a sharp needle is used to make a small perforating hole in the thinnest area. This perforating hole will later provide a small opening in which an obtuse hook can be later inserted if the footplate is inadvertently mobilized at the time the crura are fractured.

A small, round, right-angled knife is used now to separate the incudostapedial joint (Fig. 24–4). The intact stapedial tendon helps prevent an inadvertent mobilization from occurring. In this manipulation, a mild pressure and "jiggling" of the knife blade back and forth is used because if strong direct pressure is applied, dislocation of the incus may occur when the joint is suddenly separated.

FIGURE 24–1. The inferior and superior vertical incisions.

FIGURE 24–2. Elevating the skin flap.

FIGURE 24–3. Middle ear exposure.

FIGURE 24–4. Separating the incudostapedial joint.

FIGURE 24–5. Adequate exposure.

FIGURE 24-1

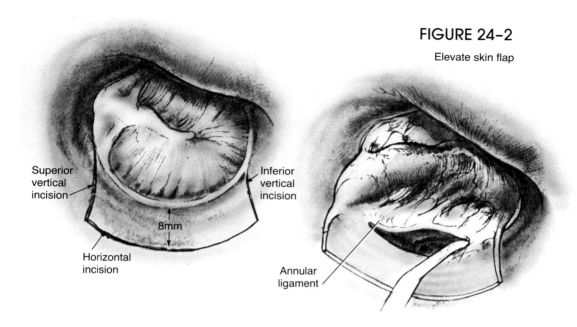

FIGURE 24-2

Elevate skin flap

Superior
vertical
incision

Inferior
vertical
incision

8mm

Horizontal
incision

Annular
ligament

FIGURE 24-3

FIGURE 24-4

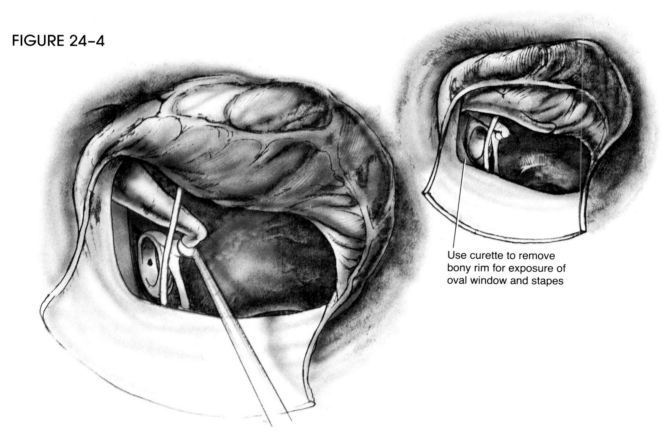

Use curette to remove
bony rim for exposure of
oval window and stapes

The necessary limits of exposure are the round window inferiorly, the lower half of the fallopian canal superiorly, the majority of the stapedial tendon, and some of the pyramidal eminence posteriorly and the malleus anteriorly (Fig. 24–5).

The malleus is now checked to determine its mobility. One in 200 patients has a fixed malleus. If fixed, alternative techniques must be used (to be described later).

The stapedial tendon is cut; then the patient is forewarned that a loud sound is forthcoming. The Rosen mobilizing needle is placed on the superior side of the stapes arch near the neck, and the superstructure is sharply fractured toward the promontory and removed (Fig. 24–6).

The distance from the top of the incus to the thin, fixed footplate is measured (Fig. 24–7). Some surgeons measure from the inferior surface of the incus, and the prosthesis length is made accordingly. The prosthesis length should be checked before it is inserted. The measurement from the outer portion of the incus to the footplate is usually 4.5mm but may vary from 3.5mm to as much as 5.5mm. One half of a millimeter is added to this distance to determine the prosthesis length.

The membrane is left intact over the footplate because it helps prevent bony chips from dropping into the vestibule. Obtuse, right-angled hooks and finally the Hough hoe is used to remove the posterior and then the anterior portion of the footplate, thereby effecting a total removal (Fig. 24–8).

Great caution must be used to avoid suction of the perilymph when blood is suctioned from around the oval window. During footplate removal, bone chips or blood entering into the vestibule are left undisturbed.

The previously prepared tissue of choice, measuring about 5mm × 5mm, is grasped with a nonserrated alligator forceps and slipped over the oval window so that it covers all the edges and is positioned superiorly over a portion of the fallopian canal (Fig. 24–9). The prosthesis is then inserted with a nonserrated forceps into the center area of the oval window and over the incus (Fig. 24–10). A crimper is used to close the loop on the incus, and the wire is moved toward the lenticular process.

The skin flap is then placed back in its normal position, and a small gauze wick is inserted into the hypotympanic area. A cotton pledget is placed over the opening of the external ear canal, and an adhesive bandage or two holds the cotton in position, thereby completing the procedure.

In our experience, whether one totally or partially removes the footplate or uses the small fenestra technique or whether one uses the diamond burr or the laser to create the small fenestra, the end result is quite similar. More surgeons are using the small fenestra technique, and the postsurgery imbalance is less noticeable because perilymph disturbance is minimal.

It is not the technique, the instruments, or a particular prosthesis that leads to a successful result, but rather the hands and mind behind the instruments. If one is closing the air-bone gap in 90 per cent of the cases and encountering no more than a 1 per cent severe sensorineural loss, one should stay with that technique.

POSTOPERATIVE CARE

Patients may have some dizziness for a few hours following surgery. They are cautioned not to blow their nose hard. If patients sneeze, they should do so with their mouth open, and they should avoid excessive straining for 2 weeks. If operated on in the morning, the patient usually can go home that night and remove the adhesive bandage, cotton, and gauze wick the following morning. Patients are allowed to travel by air 3 days after surgery and are instructed to use a nose spray and swallow frequently on descent.

Most patients hear immediately after surgery, but their hearing level may drop back somewhat a few hours later. Barring complications, patients should have their first hearing test 3 weeks after surgery, at which time most have recovered their hearing. In others, the hearing will improve over the next 3 months. The hearing they have at this time is what they will keep. We do not do revision surgery on any patient until 4 months have passed. All patients are routinely placed on a sodium fluoride and calcium carbonate supplement (Florical), 8mg three times a day, and are followed up routinely on an annual basis.

FIGURE 24–6. Fracturing the crura from footplate.

FIGURE 24–7. Measuring for the prosthesis.

FIGURE 24–8. Removing the footplate.

FIGURE 24–9. Placing tissue over the oval window.

FIGURE 24–10. Placing the prosthesis.

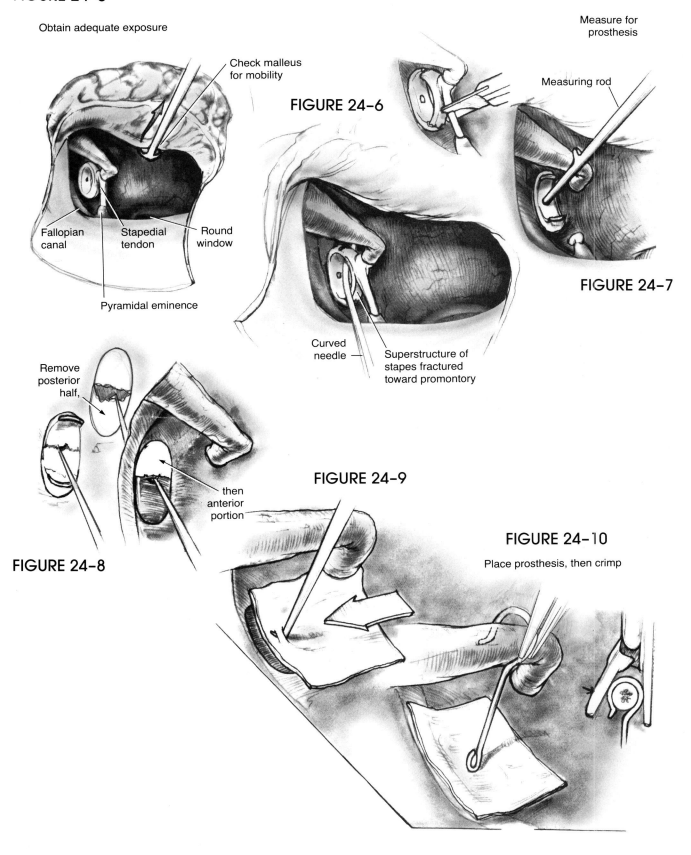

FIGURE 24-5

Obtain adequate exposure

Check malleus for mobility

Fallopian canal

Stapedial tendon

Round window

Pyramidal eminence

FIGURE 24-6

Measure for prosthesis

Measuring rod

FIGURE 24-7

Curved needle

Superstructure of stapes fractured toward promontory

Remove posterior half,

then anterior portion

FIGURE 24-8

FIGURE 24-9

FIGURE 24-10

Place prosthesis, then crimp

INTRAOPERATIVE PITFALLS

Chorda Tympani Nerve (Fig. 24–11)

During the procedure, the chorda tympani nerve may be enlarged or may be in a position to interfere with proper visualization of the stapes area. The chorda tympani may be gently moved superiorly and inferiorly. If it is stretched to the point of a partial tear, it should be severed rather than left partially functioning—the patient has less taste disturbance than when a partially functioning chorda is left intact. One should not sever the chorda if the opposite ear is operated on, as a dry mouth and a severe taste disturbance may result.

Ear Drum Perforation

If a small perforation of the tympanic membrane occurs during surgery, it will often heal if the edges are placed together. If a larger tear occurs, tissue is used with an underlay technique.

Malleus Fixation (Fig. 24–12)

If the malleus is fixed and the stapes is mobile, further stapes surgery is abandoned. The incudostapedial joint is carefully separated, and the incus is removed. The head and neck of the malleus are further exposed anteriorly, and the Lempert snipper is used to sever the neck. Fixation usually results from tendon ossification, and tapping with a small chisel on the head of the malleus will free it, thereby enabling removal. Continuity between the mobile stapes and the eardrum then may be re-established by reconstruction.

If the stapes is also fixed, an incus replacement prosthesis (IRP) is used. Incisions are made to separate the periosteum from the middle one third of the malleus, and an incus replacement wire prosthesis is inserted through the opening. A right-angled hook is used to rotate the loop portion and placed on the surface of the footplate to determine if the length is proper. The usual length is 5.5mm. Following this step, the loop is elevated away from the footplate, and the head and neck of the malleus are removed. The footplate is removed, and the loop of the prosthesis is placed into the oval window. The shaft of the prosthesis is grasped with a nonserrated alligator forceps to stabilize it, and with the right hand, it is tightened on the malleus by use of a right-angled hook. Fat or absorbable gelatin sponge (Gelfoam) centers the loop in the oval window.

Other types of prostheses, such as clamp-on plastic pistons, are available, and for some surgeons, these are more easily attached and inserted into the oval window.

Facial Nerve Abnormalities

The facial nerve is often dehiscent in its tympanic segment, but the dehiscence is rarely seen because it often occurs on its undersurface. If the dehiscence is extensive, a prolapse covering half of the footplate area may occur. In this case, the facial nerve may be carefully elevated superiorly, and an opening may be made in the footplate for insertion of the prosthesis. If the shaft of the prosthesis needs to be bent, it usually does not provide a satisfactory hearing result. If the prosthesis rubs on the prolapsed facial nerve, it will not disturb facial nerve function.

A marked prolapse covering the entire oval window requires a prosthesis from the malleus. In these cases, the incus is removed, and the facial nerve is elevated slightly superiorly so the inferior part of the footplate can be visualized and then fragmented for insertion of the incus replacement prosthesis with the loop in the fragmented area.

Floating Footplate

The most difficult complication in otosclerosis surgery is the solid floating footplate. When one encounters either this or the large prolapsed facial nerve, it is best to terminate the case and send it to your worst enemy! This is the most complicated and difficult procedures encountered in stapes surgery and should be managed only by highly experienced surgeons.

In this problem, a small cutting burr is used posteroinferiorly on the promontory of the oval window to gain room. The drilling stops 1mm from the floating footplate. Straight and obtuse needles are used to enter the vestibule along the side of, but at no time touching even the edge of, the floating footplate.

A right-angled hook is inserted into the opening and then rotated to the undersurface of the footplate. It is elevated outward and anteriorly toward the fallopian canal. Blood adhesiveness allows the plate to remain there after the hook is removed and reinserted under the edge of the footplate to then slip it up and over the fallopian canal, where it can be grasped. Only then can the surgeon take his or her first breath with a sigh of relief!

FIGURE 24–11. Superior retraction of chorda tympani for visualization.

FIGURE 24–12. Incus replacement prosthesis.

FIGURE 24-11

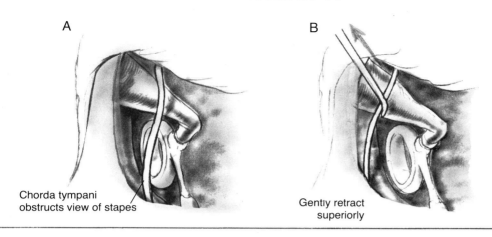

A

Chorda tympani
obstructs view of stapes

B

Gently retract
superiorly

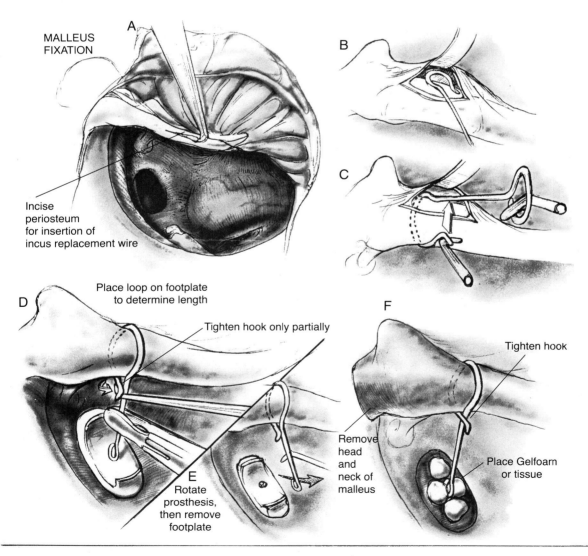

A

MALLEUS
FIXATION

Incise
periosteum
for insertion of
incus replacement wire

B

C

D

Place loop on footplate
to determine length

Tighten hook only partially

E

Rotate
prosthesis,
then remove
footplate

Remove
head
and
neck of
malleus

F

Tighten hook

Place Gelfoam
or tissue

FIGURE 24-12

The Solid or Obliterated Footplate

(Fig. 24–13)

By observation, the surgeon cannot determine whether the footplate is minimally fixed at the edges or is obliterated. In each instance, it is necessary to use a cutting burr with a gentle paintbrush-type stroking motion anteroposteriorly. If the slightest give is felt with the drill, minimal fixation and a floating footplate exist. Perilymph escape is noted around the edges. The technique to be used is the same as for the solid floating plate.

The Obliterated Footplate

With an obliterated footplate, a cutting burr is used anteroposteriorly and around the edges to develop a thin blue area. The burr is then used to enlarge the opening sufficiently to cover the area with a graft and to insert the prosthesis of choice. The edges will always be jagged because there is no demarcation between the attachment of the footplate to the surrounding bone as there is in the solid footplate. These patients respond well either to the small fenestra, the subtotal footplate, or the total removal technique. The floating footplate does not occur in obliterated cases.

Round Window Closure Due to Otosclerosis

A round window closure due to otosclerosis is a rare occurrence that is best left undisturbed. In these cases there is always a fibrous band leading to the round window that is apparently sufficient to produce the necessary relationship between the opening of the oval window and the round window. Complete drilling out of the round window has not given the desired result and may make the hearing worse.

Perilymph Gusher

When the cochlear aqueduct is widely patent, it may result in an excessive perilymph flow after the surgeon perforates the footplate. If it is a massive gusher, like a broken fireplug, one should not proceed with the removal of the stapes. It would be best to scrape the membrane of the footplate and the surrounding oval window area with suction in one hand, followed by the placement of small pieces of fascia or perichondrium in the arch of the stapes that will help hold them in place. On one such occasion, we proceeded to remove the stapes and its footplate. The tissue placed over the oval window floated away, and it needed to be held in place with a suction tip in one hand until the prosthesis was inserted onto the incus. We packed the middle ear solid with gelatin sponge and replaced

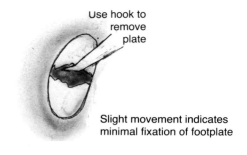

Use hook to remove plate

Slight movement indicates minimal fixation of footplate

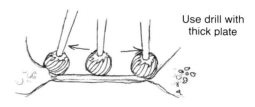

Use drill with thick plate

FIGURE 24–13. A minimally fixed solid footplate.

the flap only to note the flap being elevated by the flow of perilymph. The ear canal was tightly packed to hold the flap in place, and the patient was elevated to a sitting position. The mastoid dressing was changed repeatedly. After 24 hours, a spinal tap was inserted, which reduced the flow. Fortunately, the patient's hearing improved, and excessive vertigo did not occur.

Intraoperative Vertigo

When the patient is under local anesthesia, his or her response to sudden vertigo is immediately noted by the operating surgeon. This may occur more often in revisions if the covering tissue membrane is inserted too deeply into the vestibule or if the prosthesis is too long. If the cause is tissue, it should be very carefully removed and replaced. If the prosthesis is too long, it should likewise be removed and replaced with a shorter one. In revision, the incidence of further sensorineural loss is slightly more common than in a primary case.

The Deep Oval Window

In some cases, the oval window niche will be very narrow and very deep. If this condition results from otosclerotic encroachment on the sides of the oval window, it can be enlarged by use of a cutting burr. If there is another cause, a broad posterior crus located in the deep narrow niche may be difficult to fracture from the footplate. In this instance, after a small perforating hole has been made in the footplate, a tiny cutting burr or a laser may be used to cut through the posterior crus, thereby making removal of the superstructure of the stapes possible.

SUMMARY

Training surgeons is difficult because of the scarcity of suitable otosclerotic patients, and it is most difficult for residents to obtain sufficient experience to assure good hearing results in their patients.

We again emphasize that if a surgeon is obtaining the results being reported in the literature, namely, 90 per cent closure of the air-bone gap within 10dB and no more than 1 per cent further sensorineural loss, there is no need to change technique. I stress again— it is not the instruments or technique that ensure success, but rather the minds and the hands in control of the instruments.

References

1. Kessel J: Uber das Mobilisieren des Steigbugels durch Ausschneiden des Trommelfelles, Hammers und Amboss bei undurchgagikeit der Tuba. Arch Ohrenheilkd, 13: 69–88, 1878.
2. Boucheron E: La mobilisation de l'etrier et son procede operatoire. Union Med Can, 46: 412–416, 1888.
3. Miot C: De la mobilisation de l'etrier. Rev Laryngol Otol Rhinol (Bord) 10: 49–54, 1890.
4. Faraci G: Importanza acustica e funzionale della mobilizzazione della staffa: Risultati di una nuova serie di operazioni. Arch Ital Otol Rinol Laringol 9: 209–221, 1899.
5. Passow KA: Operative anlegung einer offnung in die mediale paukenhohlenwand bei stapesankylose. Ver Dtsch Otol Ges Versamml 6: 141, 1897.
6. Jack FL: Remarkable improvement of the hearing by removal of the stapes. Trans Am Otol Soc 284: 474–489, 1893.
7. Goodhill V: Stapes Surgery for Otosclerosis. New York, Paul B. Hoeber, 1961.
8. Siebenmann F: Traitement chirurgical de la sclerose otique. Cong Int Med Sec Otol 13: 170, 1900.
9. Moure EJ: De la mobilisation de l'etrier. Rev Laryngol Otol Rhinol (Bord) 7: 225, 1880.
10. Holmgren G: Some experiences in surgery of otosclerosis. Acta Otolaryngol (Stockh) 5: 460, 1923.
11. Sourdille M: New technique in the surgical treatment of severe and progressive deafness from otosclerosis. Bull NY Acad Med 13: 673, 1937.
12. Lempert J: Improvement in hearing in cases of otosclerosis: A new, one stage surgical technic. Arch Otolaryngol Head Neck Surg 28: 42, 1938.
13. Rosen S: Restoration of hearing in otosclerosis by mobilization of the fixed stapedial footplate, an analysis of results. Laryngoscope 65: 224–269, 1955.
14. Shea J Jr: Fenestration of the oval window. Ann Otol Rhinol Laryngol 67: 932–951, 1958.
15. Shambaugh GE Jr, et al: Sodium fluoride for arrest of otosclerosis. Arch Otolaryngol 80: 263–270, 1964.

25

Stapedectomy: Use of Natural Material

J. V. D. HOUGH, M.D.

MICHAEL McGEE, M.D.

R. STANLEY BAKER, M.D.

GRAHAM BRYCE, M.D.

INTRODUCTION

After over 30 years, there is still no universally accepted surgical technique for restoration of hearing in patients with stapedial otosclerosis. In view of the amazing, even perplexing, anatomic and pathologic differences the surgeon encounters in and around the oval window, it is perhaps best that we not adopt a single strategy. Fortunately, today's popular techniques, properly done, give similar excellent results. The total stapedectomy, partial stapedectomy, and stapedotomy techniques are at the forefront of today's surgical armamentarium. These three accomplish the essential requirements for long-term success; that is, they first open the oval window by removing enough of the footplate for unimpeded sound entry into the inner ear, and they provide effective sound conduction from the incus to the labyrinth by using an artificial prosthesis or by preserving the stapedial crura in a functional state. Each of these techniques seems to have unique and distinctive advantages applicable in certain circumstances, and under diverse anatomic and pathologic conditions.

The authors use all three of these techniques but predominantly perform a stapedectomy with preservation of the posterior crus while using a tragal perichondrial graft to seal the opening of the oval window. This method eliminates the need for an artificial prosthesis and the resultant complications caused by a foreign body.

The first stapedectomy with preservation of the posterior crus was done by the senior author quite by accident in 1956 while doing a stapes mobilization using the improved Fowler anterior crurotomy procedure.[1]

In this patient, as prescribed by the technique, the footplate had been transected and the anterior crus cut, thus liberating the posterior footplate, bypassing the anterior otosclerotic focus. But while a portion of the stump of the anterior crus was being removed, the entire anterior half of the footplate came out. Because there was no trauma to the labyrinth, the hearing result was excellent and remained so. From a surgical perspective, these results seemed good: the involved anterior portion of the footplate had been removed and the normal portion of the stapes preserved.

Total stapedectomy was also introduced during that year, but it required routine removal of the crural arch, necessitating the use of a prosthesis between the incus and the oval window. Since that time, much effort and frequent changes have been made by many surgeons trying to find the proper prosthesis to insert between the incus and the oval window. Thirty-five years later, the proper choice of prosthesis to rebuild the ossicular chain is still debated.

Also during this time, the authors and others had been trying to find better techniques and instrumentation that allowed more frequent preservation and use of the posterior crus. The authors are now able to avoid using an artificial prosthesis by preserving the posterior crus in over 80 per cent of ears. The authors also believe that a diverse-technique approach is preferable to make use of the advantages of other methods in ears for which the posterior crus cannot be preserved.

PATIENT SELECTION

The object of stapedial surgery is to improve the patient's hearing. This simple statement has important implications and, if applied, broadens the indications for stapedectomy. A surgeon should not withhold a chance for the patient to obtain improvement in hearing, provided that improvement is beneficial, and the procedure is not deleterious to the patient's well-being. The following conditions would *not* be exclusions or contraindications unless other medical, psychological, or physical constraints make it impractical or unreasonable to do the surgical procedure.

1. Unilateral conductive impairment. (Binaural hearing is important!)
2. Age.
3. Profound hearing loss (i.e., speech reception threshold of over 90dB or discrimination of less than 10 per cent) with a significant detectable air-bone gap. (Many of these patients' hearing can be restored to acceptable levels with a hearing aid.)
4. Mild-to-moderate hearing loss. (e.g., a 30dB to 35dB speech reception threshold with a 12dB to 15dB air-bone gap in a patient requiring better hearing for job performance.)
5. Moderately severe hearing impairment with a good air-bone gap, but bone conduction indicating that the patient will still require hearing aids for good socially adequate hearing. (Functionally, many of these patients can be improved dramatically.)

SURGICAL TECHNIQUE

Surgical Preparation Room

Preoperative Medications (Use Routine Orders)

Sedation should be given 30 minutes prior to the surgical intervention. The authors use an analgesic, barbiturate, and atropine combination.

Surgical Preparation

The ear is not instrumented or cleaned before surgery. A hearing aid mold should not be used in the ear for 1 week prior to surgery. The ear is prepared with a povidone-iodine solution, or its equivalent, 20 minutes before surgery. The ear canal should be filled and the scalp scrubbed along with the face and neck in an area three inches in diameter around the ear canal. The ear is allowed to soak until draped and is irrigated later in the operating room.

During this time, an intravenous line is started with 5 per cent dextrose and Ringer's lactate solution. The hair is not shaved but is retracted to expose the ear and surrounding area for sterilization. The patient's clinic chart, as well as the hospital record, is with the patient and is carefully checked to verify the identifying information, such as correct ear for surgery, name, and allergies.

Operating Room Procedures

The patient is moved to the operating room and properly placed on the surgical table. It is very important that the surgical table be an adjustable, motor-driven table. The controls should be on a panel at the head of the table, with control buttons easily palpable by the surgeon's fingers through the drapes. The table should be movable in three dimensions:

1. Up and down
2. Head up or down
3. Rotated from side to side (away from or toward the surgeon).

The latter direction is extremely important in allowing good visualization of the tympanic cavity anteriorly and posteriorly to accommodate the large variety of ear canal configurations encountered.

The patient's head is placed on a small, two-inch-thick flat foam pillow with a three-inch neck roll edge, which provides stability and comfort. Electrodes are attached, and cardiovascular and respiratory monitoring is established. Properly trained personnel are in constant attendance to observe the vital signs throughout the procedure. During this time, if the patient is observed to be unusually anxious, 5mg of diazepam (Valium) is given intravenously at least 5 minutes before the first injection of the local anesthetic. Later, during the procedure, the dose may be repeated in 2.5mg increments, up to a total of 10mg for an adult.

Draping

The patient is draped in the usual fashion with a complete body drape followed by a regional ear drape, leaving only the external ear exposed. The face of the patient should remain exposed under a canopy provided by a semicircular adjustable gooseneck arch, which is placed lateral to, and in front of, the head. This allows an attendant seated in front of the patient and opposite the surgical side of the table to see the patient's face, monitoring their reactions and reassuring them by verbal communication.

The patient's head should be almost flush with the end of the table, and the arm on the side toward the surgeon stretched slightly toward the knee to bring the shoulder down, thus increasing access to the ear.

Suction tubing is provided from a constant central vacuum source and passes through a surgeon-controlled foot pedal valve system (Hough-Cadogen foot pedal control) placed conveniently on the floor under the surgeon's foot. This allows the suction to be immediately stopped and the line exhausted. It also allows various degrees of intensity of the suction to be controlled by the foot pedal.

Preference in microscope design, flexibility and lens distance is variable. The authors prefer a light, highly maneuverable microscope with a 200mm lens for stapes surgery and a 225mm lens for all other temporal bone surgery. When the microscope is brought into the field, it should be finally set so that the surgeon is in a very comfortable position. The table, the microscope, and the rest of the materials should be brought to the surgeon so that he or she is not in an awkward position or stretching or reaching for the patient.

Anesthetic

Local anesthetic is preferred for all patients except children and unusually tense adults. In these, a general anesthetic is used.

The solution of local anesthetic is composed of 2% lidocaine hydrochloride (Xylocaine) with 1:30,000 epinephrine with hyaluronidase (Wydase) added for perfusion. This mixture is administered through a 1ml Luer-Lok syringe firmly attached to a two-inch 25-gauge needle.

The first injection is introduced into the soft tissue just inside the superior canal area between the helix and the tragus, depositing approximately 0.2ml. Another injection is made in the inferior area of the canal just medial to the conchal cartilage.

The ear is then irrigated copiously to remove all antiseptic solution and debris. By the time this step is accomplished, the discomfort of the next two injections is much less noticeable. The next injection is more medial in the ear canal, superiorly in the vascular strip. This area is infiltrated with approximately 0.1ml. The infiltration should be seen lifting and slightly blanching the soft tissue to near the tympanic

membrane. The last canal injection is inferiorly in the external canal just exterior to the junction of the thicker skin at the external orifice and the very thin skin over the bony external canal. This juncture is always clearly visible. The needle should penetrate the thicker skin near the juncture and be inserted to the bone so that blanching caused by subperiosteal infiltration can be clearly seen advancing deep toward the tympanic membrane. The placement of these last two injections is extremely important if good anesthesia and hemostasis is to be obtained for successful surgery. Lastly, the dome of the tragus is injected subcutaneously with approximately 0.1ml.

The total anesthetic solution used ranges from 0.6ml to 0.9ml. The remainder of the solution in the syringe can be used later for topical anesthesia of the mucous membranes of the tympanic cavity.

A spatula can then be used to mold the flexible canal to facilitate insertion of the speculum. After the incision and flap elevation, the canal tissues will frequently be dilated enough by the speculum to allow the use of a larger speculum for more complete exposure of the tympanic cavity.

Incision and Elevation of the Tympanomeatal Flap

The incision is made with a Hough modification of the Rosen knife. The modification is simply a rounding off of the very acute–angle tip of the original Rosen knife. The incision is made by the sharp sides or leading edge of the knife and is done in a sweeping motion, or occasionally in a guillotine-like cutting fashion. Because of the angle of the knife, the semilunar incision line is made with the limbs of the incision closer to the tympanic membrane both superiorly and inferiorly. The arch of the incision is made just medial to the area where there is a clear distinction between the thick lateral canal skin and the thin skin nearer the tympanic membrane. It is very important to make the incisions completely through the skin, subcutaneous tissue, and periosteum.

Elevation of the tympanomeatal flap is usually made by carefully dissecting the periosteum off the bone, which is successfully done by using the same knife to scrape the periosteum off the bone down to the annular rim. A commercially prepared No. 3 preformed dental cotton ball rested against the elevated flap is very helpful in protecting the flap and in maintaining a dry, clean field. If the tympanomeatal flap is dissected hard against the bone, the annulus of the tympanic membrane is not in danger of being overrun. Once it is identified, it should be elevated out of the sulcus tympanicus (at about the 9 o'clock position in the right ear and the 3 o'clock position in the left ear). The mucous membrane of the tympanic cavity

usually separates at this point, but if not, it is incised with a pick in a sweeping motion, staying hard against the bone of the annulus. The tympanomeatal flap and tympanic membrane are elevated inferiorly to the 6 o'clock position and superiorly all the way to the notch of Rivinus (12 o'clock position).

Removal of the Posterosuperior Canal Bone to Expose the Oval Window

Usually, it is necessary to remove bone from the posterosuperior bony canal wall to properly visualize the oval window. The No. 3 dental cotton ball is again helpful and is placed inferiorly, holding the tympanomeatal flap anteriorly, and being in position to catch bone chips. With a serrated Hough curette, the edge of the curette is engaged along the bony margin. The notch of Rivinus usually makes an easy beginning point. With care taken to stay well above and away from the chorda, the bone is curetted by twisting motions counterclockwise, and the cutting pressure is directed posteriorly. If the bone is thick and dense, it is prudent to gradually thin it superiorly before finally cracking it off just superior to the chorda tympani. Contrary to initial perception, the chorda tympani is best preserved by curetting the bone with counterclockwise twists to crack the fragments against the nerve rather than elevating the nerve and curetting upward. Enough bone should be removed to visualize the stapedius tendon at its entry into the pyramidal eminence. In approximately 5 per cent of cases, the nerve must be sacrificed for exposure.

All bone chips are now removed, and the cotton ball previously placed inferiorly is removed. The tympanic cavity is now properly exposed. A drop or two of lidocaine is now applied to the mucosa of the oval window and provides instant topical anesthesia.

Examination of the structures of the middle ear is now done in a systematic fashion. Vascular structures, nerve elements, and ossicular variations, as well as the pathology producing the hearing impairment, must be carefully evaluated to allow proper choice of surgical techniques and possible variations.

The mobility of the ossicular chain should be tested, beginning with the malleus. Experience provides assurance in determining mobility or fixation. The lack of mobility of the incus may be misleading if the stapes is firmly fixed. Careful observation of the movements of the mucous membrane at the incudostapedial joint is helpful.

Evaluation of the Oval Window

The oval window is examined. Commonly seen primitive mesenchymal strands and cicatricial bands need to be removed. Frequently, mucosal vessels cross the

footplate. These need to be severed so that adequate time for natural hemostasis can occur early in the procedure. However, mucous membrane should not be stripped from the footplate, because it later provides a natural holding blanket to keep the footplate fragments from falling into the labyrinth. More profuse bleeding can occur from larger blood vessels in the mucous membrane anterior to the oval window, and it is sometimes advantageous also to cut these vessels early.

A dehiscent facial nerve is commonly present superior to the oval window. Other than being careful not to penetrate or scrape it with sharp picks, it may be ignored. More rarely, the nerve bulges over the oval window to obscure portions of the field. Usually, it can be partially retracted or worked around for successful completion of the task.

Choice of Stapedial Procedures

Pathology and Anatomy of the Oval Window and Stapes

In approximately 80 per cent of ears, the otosclerotic pathology will be confined to the anterior footplate. In approximately 18 per cent, circumscribed otosclerosis will involve most of the footplate (biscuit-type otosclerosis with areas of the annular ligament still identifiable). In approximately 2 per cent, there will be diffuse obliterative otosclerosis (the oval window will be covered, and no identifiable annular ligament margins exist).

In the authors' hands, all of the first group and most of the second are candidates for stapedectomy with preservation of the posterior crus. The diffuse obliterative otosclerosis group and some of the circumscribed, biscuit-type otosclerosis group may be primary candidates for a stapedectomy with a piston technique or the use of a nonossicle homograft stapes replacement technique.[2]

Before the oval window is opened or the superstructure of the stapes is cut or removed, the distance between the footplate and the incus is measured. This step prepares for any variation in the usual technique that might necessitate employing a prosthesis or a homograft bone transplant.

Certain anatomic restrictions may also make preservation of the posterior crus unwise, such as

1. An extremely narrow oval window niche. Frequently, on first observation this condition may seem to be an impossible barrier. The picture may change dramatically, however, once the stapedial arch is out of the oval window and the footplate is removed. Regardless of how narrow the oval window niche is, attempting to preserve the posterior crus does no harm. It can always be removed later

during the procedure if it cannot be used. The authors *always* try to preserve the posterior crus until it is determined to be useless.

2. A stapes that lies at an acute angle against the promontory, making it difficult to reposition the posterior crus so that it will not be too adherent to the oval window margins or the promontory.

Stapedial Surgery for Preservation of the Posterior Crus

Opening the Footplate

Usually, a thin portion of the footplate can be visualized. This area is opened by barely thrusting a fine pick through the bone in several places, preferably joining them with a fracture line (Fig. 25–1).

NOTE. This step should be done *before* cutting the tendon, cutting the crus, or otherwise manipulating the superstructure because any of these maneuvers may cause complete mobilization of the stapes, producing a floating footplate, whereupon further attempts to open the footplate with any downward pressure with instruments could be dangerous. Although rare, a floating footplate requires a surgical decision. One can abandon further attempts and terminate the operation as a completed stapes mobilization, or one can attempt to remove the superstructure and drill out a pothole entry into the labyrinth on the promontory side of the oval window for removal of the footplate, or one can now very successfully use the laser to safely open the oval window.

If the footplate has circumscribed, biscuit-type otosclerosis (annular ligament can be identified), and it is palpated to be impenetrable by the pick, the superstructure can be lifted out of the oval window and the entire footplate visualized for safer instrumentation. Usually, however, even when the footplate is thick, enough of it is visualized around the arch to allow the use of a small burr in one or more places even before removal of the superstructure.

Cutting the Anterior Crus

The anterior crus is sectioned high, preferably about one third of the distance from the stapedial head to the footplate. This is done with specially designed angulated bone-cutting forceps (crural nippers). In the past, sectioning had been done with scissors, whirlybirds, and motor-driven saws, but all of these are not nearly as uniformly successful or as safe as the nippers (Fig. 25–2).

NOTE. When the crural nippers are used, after the cut has been made, the tendency is to bring the forceps out laterally and inferiorly, which may fracture the

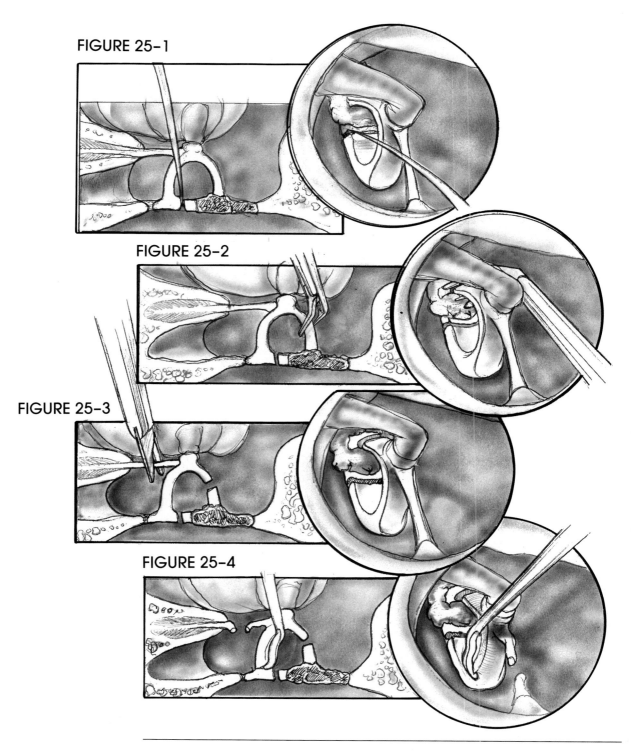

FIGURE 25-1

FIGURE 25-2

FIGURE 25-3

FIGURE 25-4

FIGURE 25-1. Opening the footplate.

FIGURE 25-2. Anterior crurotomy.

FIGURE 25-3. Cutting the stapedial tendon.

FIGURE 25-4. Cutting the posterior crus with a whirlybird.

FIGURE 25-5. Lifting the incus.

FIGURE 25-6. Lifting the posterior crus out of the oval window arch to the promontory.

FIGURE 25-7. Removing the footplate.

FIGURE 25-8. Sealing the oval window with perichondrial graft.

FIGURE 25-9. Replacing the posterior crus in the oval window.

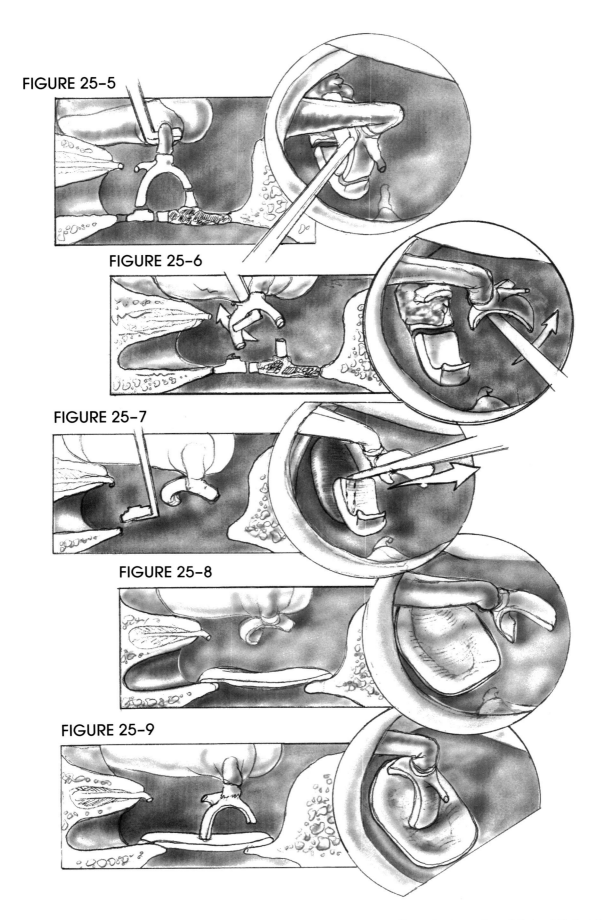

FIGURE 25-5

FIGURE 25-6

FIGURE 25-7

FIGURE 25-8

FIGURE 25-9

remaining stapedial arch. Remember to move the instrument medially, anteriorly, and then inferiorly before bringing it out, which will fracture the anterior stump attached to the footplate but will not disturb the remaining arch.

Inadvertent fracture of the neck, arch, or posterior crus seems to occur most often as the anterior crus is being manipulated while being transected. One of the authors has found that this problem can be managed by using the HGM Argon Laser-Otoprobe to cut the crus. The 0.2mm laser fiber can be custom shaped to blindly palpate the anterior crus while it is transected with laser energy.

Cutting the Stapedial Tendon

Cutting the stapedial tendon may also be done with the laser but is usually done with Bellucci's scissors. The scissor blades should not reach downward and engage the posterior crus—often, the tendon is resting on the posterior crus (Fig. 25–3).

The primitive mesenchymal strands, heavy sheets of mucous membrane, and scar bands should now be removed with the laser or with curved and right-angle picks in a gentle, sweeping motion parallel to the posterior crus. This tissue may, if left alone, later cause fracture of the posterior crus or joint separation during manipulation.

Occasionally, a portion of the posterior crus may be hidden by the overhang of the pyramidal eminence. The pyramidal eminence may be easily shaved away with fenestration excavators for better exposure.

Cutting the Posterior Crus at the Footplate

The earlier steps have all been taken in systematic order for specific reasons. Until now, it has been important that the arch remain attached to the footplate to prevent floating, and that it not be twisted so that the posterior crus could be prematurely fractured in the wrong place, making it too short.

Now the posterior crus is to be separated from the footplate. The whirlybird instrument is placed under the crural arch in the obturator foramen. According to the patient's anatomy, it may be inserted either on the facial nerve side or on the promontory side of the arch. The blade of the instrument is passed inside the arch and onto the footplate. It is moved along the footplate posteriorly until it encounters the posterior crus (Fig. 25–4). This portion may or may not be visualized. With the blade of the whirlybird flush against the footplate and pushing firmly in a posterior direction against the posterior crus, a twisting motion is made, which will fracture the posterior crus at the footplate. The posterior crus can be easily palpated and cut, even blindly, by this maneuver. Fortunately,

the posterior crus has its weakest, most cancellous bone at the footplate and is therefore most likely to fracture at the desired point. Even if it should fracture so that the posterior crus is only three fourths its normal length, it can still be used very successfully. Long-term results with a shortened crus are still highly successful, as will be discussed later.

Lifting the Posterior Crus and Resting It on the Inferoposterior Promontory

This is the most delicate maneuver of the technique and is perhaps the reason most surgeons do not attempt the procedure. Once mastered, however, it quickly becomes a worthwhile routine.

Before attempting to lift the crus out of the oval window, it is important that all adhesions and binding mucous membrane be removed from the posterior crus. A right-angle excavator (Hough's hoe) is now placed under the incus and lifted laterally to test the stiffness of the incudal joints and ligaments (Fig. 25–5). Watching the posterior crus, the surgeon lifts the incus slightly laterally to cause some flexibility in joints that have been chronically out of use. Be careful that binding mucous membrane does not hold the stapedial arch down, causing a separation of the incudostapedial joint during this maneuver. The right-angle excavator is then placed in the obturator foramen under the neck of the stapes. Depending on the anatomy, it may be engaged under the arch, either on the superior or inferior surface of the arch. With firm, steady, continuous pressure, the arch is then lifted out gently and rotated so that the posterior stapedial crus clears the promontory and rests on its posterior slope (Fig. 25–6).

The exposure of the oval window is now excellent. Because the incus has been retracted slightly laterally and the arch is completely out of the oval window, the exposure of the oval window and footplate is definitely more complete than with any other stapedectomy or stapedotomy technique.

There are three advantages to preserving the arch in this fashion:

1. Provides better visualization of the entire oval window
2. Provides practice in performing this useful maneuver
3. Provides the possibility of using the posterior crus rather than employing a prosthesis

Obtaining the Perichondrial Graft

Rationale

The use of tragal perichondrium to seal the oval window has been an excellent contribution to stapedial

surgery since Goodhill described it in 1961.[3] It has been used by the authors in thousands of ears, and its record of successful results has been repeated by many other otologists. Of significance is the fact that the authors have not encountered a single incident of long- or short-term postoperative fistulas when it has been used. Some of the advantages of its use in stapedial surgery are

1. It is already in the field. One does not need to change to another body site to obtain a graft. Therefore, the procedure saves time and reduces the chances of contamination.
2. It is histologically akin to the normal inhabitants of the oval window.
3. It forms a natural little "boat" that nestles down in the oval window for an excellent fit.
4. Because of its boat or "tray" edges in the oval window, it naturally centers the posterior crus so that it will not drift or adhere to the bony margins of the oval window, thus preventing refixation.
5. It can be made extremely thin for ears with a very narrow oval window niche. The graft can easily be thinned with scissors and placed in an absorbable gelatin sponge (Gelfoam) press. Also, it can be left thick for ears in which the preserved posterior crus fractures high and is short (not quite full length).

Surgical Technique for Removal of Perichondrium

If the tragus is pushed forward with the thumb, the dome of the tragus is outlined through the skin. With a scalpel, an incision is made over the dome of the tragal cartilage. The edge of the incision is grasped with thumb forceps and retracted forward. With curved scissors, the soft tissue is dissected to the dome of the tragal cartilage. If the scissors are used in a penetrating, spreading fashion, soft tissue is dissected away from the perichondrium on both sides of the tragus, approximately 1cm. The tragus is then grasped in the thumb forceps while the dome of the tragal cartilage with its perichondrium is removed with curved iris scissors. To prevent hematoma, the external wound is closed with only one silk suture.

The cartilage and perichondrial tissue are placed on a polytetrafluoroethylene (Teflon) disk. With the whirlybird, the cartilage is broken away in pieces and cleanly removed from the perichondrium. With curved scissors, the graft is cleared of all useless soft tissue, thinned, and cut for the size of the oval window. If the niche is narrow, the graft may be pressed in a House gelatin sponge press, which will facilitate the use of the posterior crus or a prosthesis in a narrow space.

The graft is usually placed on the promontory at this time, to be ready for closing the oval window once the procedures in the oval window have been accomplished.

Removal of the Footplate of the Stapes

A small, right-angle 0.3mm pick is inserted through the fracture line of the footplate. It should be inserted only deep enough to engage the medial surface of the footplate. Usually, the pick can be visualized through the bone. The point of the pick is usually turned to point posteriorly. A fragment of bone is then lifted out. If only a small segment of bone is removed, a right-angle excavator (Hough's hoe) is then used to remove the remainder of the footplate. This instrument has a flat surface and is not sharp on the tip or along its edges, thus making it the safest instrument to use below the footplate.

Occasionally, the entire half of the posterior footplate is removed cleanly from the oval window in one piece (Fig. 25–7). Even though the entire posterior edge of the oval window may not be visible, the rim of the footplate is identifiable as it is removed, and one is assured of clean and complete removal. Removal of as much of the footplate as can be easily extracted is accomplished using this instrument. Remember not to insert the instrument deeper than is necessary to engage the medial surface of the footplate. Also, do not pick at the edges of the footplate, as this may cause it to loosen en masse and to tumble into the labyrinth. Rather, try to remove as much as will easily lift out of the window by engaging the full right-angled surface of the excavator. On occasion, a very hard, trapped anterior portion of the footplate may be left in place so that the labyrinth is not traumatized by attempted forceful removal. Fragments of the footplate that have been lifted out of the oval window are then extracted by the use of forceps or suction. The variable on/off control of suction is extremely important in removing fluid, blood, and footplate fragments in the oval window niche. This can be done safely only by using suction that is controlled by the surgeon's foot, that is, the foot-pedal suction control (i.e., Hough-Cadogen foot-pedal suction).

Sealing the Oval Window With the Use of the Perichondrial Graft

After the oval window has been cleared of footplate fragments, the perichondrial graft is moved into the niche from its anterior end. This perichondrial dome of the tragus makes a perfect boat that nestles down to seal the oval window. Fortunately, its tray edges also center the posterior crus in the window, preventing refixation (Fig. 25–8).

Replacing the Posterior Crus in the Oval Window

With a right-angle excavator, the posterior crus is carefully lifted back into the oval window niche and placed in the center, or the widest portion, of the oval window. It is lifted back just as it was lifted out with the excavator under the arch (Fig. 25–9). The crus can then be moved toward the center by placing the excavator under the bony projection provided by the insertion of the stapedius tendon on the posterior rim of the crus.

Occasionally, the graft may be tucked behind the crus to prevent it from drifting posteriorly. The incudostapedial joint may become somewhat loose during the various proceeding manipulations, and occasionally it is necessary to lift the incus and the stapedial arch simultaneously in a two-handed maneuver.

The techniques the authors use when the posterior crus fractures too high or the incudostapedial joint is completely disrupted are discussed later.

Replacement of the Tympanic Membrane and Canal Packing

The tympanic membrane and tympanomeatal flap are replaced so that the incision lines are reapproximated. Gelatin sponge strips soaked with physiologic solution (Physiosol) are placed over the incision lines, and an expandable cellulose wick (a Pope wick) is placed in the ear canal. A cotton ball covered with cortisone ointment is then used to occlude the ear canal, and another cotton ball is placed in the concha. No other head dressing need be used.

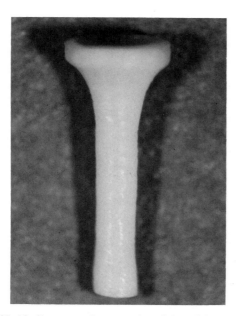

FIGURE 25–10. Stapes replacement sculptured from nonossicular homograft cortical bone.

Conditions in Which the Posterior Crus Cannot Be Preserved

1. FRACTURE OF THE POSTERIOR CRUS CAUSING A SHORT CRUS.

   In the authors' experience, the posterior crus is anatomically not reasonable to use, or is fractured too high to remain useful in 9 per cent of ears. However, if it is two thirds to three fourths its normal length, it is not always considered useless. When the arch is rotated forward toward the center of the oval window, it gains length by its rotation and can usually be used. Furthermore, the perichondrial graft can be left somewhat thicker so that the membranous oval window is higher postoperatively. Our statistical results among these patients indicate that there is no sacrifice of benefit and that hearing perception is equal to that of patients with normal-length crura.[4, 5]

2. INCUDOSTAPEDIAL JOINT SEPARATION OR PROBLEMS CAUSING DELIBERATE REMOVAL OF THE STAPEDIAL SUPERSTRUCTURE.

   Unfortunately, incudostapedial joint separation from manipulation of the arch or anatomic conditions causing removal of the arch can occur, necessitating treatment alternatives. These conditions occur in approximately 4 per cent of ears.

For years, the senior author resorted to artificial prostheses of various types in these cases, but only if the loose stapes and the joint could not be replaced. However, once the incudostapedial joint was dislocated, it was difficult to manipulate the posterior crus and the head of the stapes back in position.

The Use of Homograft Transplants in Stapedial Surgery

Both the problems of joint separation and fracture of the stapedial arch have now been solved by the use of a sculptured homograft bone transplant. During the past several years, when irreparable joint separation or undesirable crural fracture occurs, a sculptured bone implant has been used. Since the technique of sculpturing homograft bone was developed by McGee[5] and refined by Bryce, this transplant is now used more often. The convenience and usefulness of this sculptured homograft has accelerated the use of natural materials in recent years.[2, 5]

With either very dense homograft labyrinthine capsular bone or other hard homograft cortical bone (e.g., femur), a stapes replacement implant in the shape of a Robinson piston can be easily used (Fig. 25–10).

Dense labyrinthine capsular bone or other cortical bone (e.g., femur) can be purchased from the American Red Cross bone banks. These materials form the basis of this replacement prosthesis. From tiny sec-

tions of this bone, the piston-shaped implant is microscopically sculptured using a lathe and a drill with a diamond burr. This sculpturing produces a precisely designed and measured natural tissue implant to be kept in the operating room bone bank ready for use.

These precision-shaped, carefully measured transplants are easily inserted after the oval window has been covered with the perichondrial graft. The tip of the implant shaft is placed in the center of the oval window, and the implant is rotated so that the cup rests under the proximal portion of the long process of the incus (near the body of the incus). With a pick, the cup end of the homograft transplant is then depressed slightly into the oval window as the cup is moved inferiorly. Finally, it is fitted into place with the cup securely under the lenticular process of the incus. Gelatin sponge is not required to hold it in place.

This use of homograft bone has allowed the authors to use almost no artificial foreign material in stapedial surgery, except in diffuse obliterative otosclerosis (in approximately 2 per cent of ears). In these, a stainless steel piston is used.

Management of Extensive Stapedial Otosclerosis

Circumscribed Otosclerosis (Biscuit-type)

Circumscribed biscuit-type otosclerosis is distinguished by very thick, sometimes soft, biscuit-like otosclerosis confined to the footplate and involving the oval window margin only in a restricted area. The annular ligament area is usually clearly identifiable around the bulging footplate. The authors have found that the footplate can be transected with a pick or a fine drill in most of these ears. The biscuit footplate frequently rolls out completely in two large pieces, and the technique of posterior crus preservation can usually be carried out as routinely planned, or the sculptured homograft procedure discussed earlier is used. Regrowth and refixation are rare in patients with this pathology.[2, 4, 6]

Diffuse Obliterative Otosclerosis

Diffuse obliterative otosclerosis occurs in approximately 2 per cent of ears in North America. This pathologic process produces massive involvement of the entire footplate, annular ligament, and surrounding labyrinthine capsule. In contradistinction to circumscribed biscuit-type otosclerosis, diffuse obliterative otosclerosis leaves no annular ligament visible, even when the bone in the area is drilled away.

In the early history of stapedectomy, most surgeons re-created the oval window with a massive drill-out procedure, followed by the use of a prosthesis. Due to

excessive labyrinthine trauma and bone regrowth, results were very unsatisfactory.

The use of a metal piston prosthesis is now the procedure of choice. In the authors' view, this condition is the only one for which the use of an artificial prosthesis in performing primary stapedectomy procedures is preferred.

The procedure begins the same as described earlier. After laying aside the crural arch with the crus on the promontory, the incus is held slightly laterally. When diffuse obliterative otosclerosis is identified, a shaft of 0.7mm in diameter is slowly drilled into the labyrinth. The drill must be a microdrill designed for work in the tympanic cavity (e.g., Skeeter's or Kerr's drill). A diamond burr measuring 0.7mm in diameter is used. The shaft or the hole into the labyrinth should be placed slightly inferiorly and posteriorly to the center of the footplate. If the bone is thicker than 1mm to 1.5mm, the operation should be terminated because the anatomic position of the labyrinthine structures may be obscure. The authors commonly use a 0.6mm stainless steel piston long enough to extend 0.25mm into the labyrinth. Soft tissue is used to surround the shaft of the oval window.[2, 4, 6]

Postoperative Care

The inner cellulose wick and gelatin sponge are removed from the canal 5 days to 1 week postoperatively. Usually, the blood clot and gelatin sponge adhere to the wick, and the extraction is easily done. Suction may be used along the anterior canal wall to remove excessive fluids, but it is unnecessary to remove all the gelatin sponge. The hearing is then tested, and the patient is instructed to return for evaluation at 6 weeks, 6 months, and then every 2 years thereafter.

Results Using the Posterior Crus Preservation Technique

Over the past 30 years, results using the posterior crus preservation technique in several large series have been reported by the senior author.[1, 2, 4, 5, 7] Good results with few complications have been the consistent findings. Results at 6 months or longer postoperatively show that

1. Approximately 90 to 95 per cent of patients closed the air-bone gap to within 10dB of the preoperative bone conduction threshold in the three speech frequencies.
2. Eighty per cent overclosed or totally closed the air-bone gap.

Overclosure simply represents recapture of the Carhart notch and probably does not represent actual improvement in inner ear cochlear function. Nevertheless, overclosure is important. In the authors' opinion, this represents an added physiologic advantage in the preservation of normal tissues, which allows:

    a. The maintenance of the normal incudostapedial joint

    b. A firm normal tissue attachment of the stapedial crus to the soft tissues over the oval window.

3. The hearing was made worse from a slight 10dB loss to profound loss of hearing in all the series in fewer than 1 per cent of cases. The total loss of useful hearing (loss of discrimination of 50 per cent or more) occurred an average of less than 0.25 per cent. These results are unsurpassed by any other stapedectomy or stapedotomy technique reported.

The Use of Homograft Replacements

When the posterior crus cannot be used, the authors believe the use of natural human materials is still the best option. The results from the use of refined sculptured homograft bone transplants have been equally gratifying. Closure of the air-bone gap to within 10dB of the preoperative bone conduction still occurs in over 90 per cent of cases, and overclosure of the air-bone gap is approximately 5 to 10 per cent less, but still equal to or better than that of other procedures using artificial materials.[2, 6]

SUMMARY

Depending on dexterity, effort, and experience of the surgeon, human material can be used to reconstruct the ossicular chain in over 95 per cent of ears requiring stapedectomy. The benefits are

1. No foreign body reaction, thus preventing soft tissue reaction in the oval window and bone erosion of the incus caused by artificial materials.
2. Better exposure. Excellent surgical exposure of the oval window is obtained without removal of the normal stapedial arch.
3. Better healing. More physiologic healing occurs at the oval window, and the normal incudostapedial joint is maintained.
4. Good results. In thousands of ears and in repeated series of cases reported, the short-term and long-term results with this technique are not excelled, and usually not equalled, by other techniques reported in the scientific literature.
5. Once mastered, the authors find that this technique can be accomplished more rapidly, and with less effort.
6. Cost effectiveness. Because this technique seldom requires expensive adjunct equipment, such as drills and lasers, and seldom uses an artificial prosthesis, it is always more cost-effective.

References

1. Hough JVD: Partial stapedectomy. Ann Otol Rhinol Laryngol 69: 571, 1960.
2. Hough JVD: A critique of stapedectomy. J Laryngol Otol 90(1): 15, 1976.
3. Goodhill V: Tragal perichondrium as oval window graft. Laryngoscope 71: 975, 1961.
4. Hough JVD: Otosclerosis: The method of JVD Hough, MD. *In* Gates GA (ed): Current Therapy in Otolaryngology—Head and Neck Surgery, 1982–83. BC Decker, 1982, pp 24–30.
5. McGee M: Non-ossicle homograft bone prosthesis in the middle ear. Part 2. Laryngoscope 100 10 (Pt 2) (Suppl 51): 1990.
6. Hough JVD: Operative treatment for otosclerosis: Stapedectomy with preservation of the posterior crus and the use of perichondrial graft over the oval window. *In* Snow JB (ed): Controversy in Otolaryngology. Philadelphia, WB Saunders, 1980, pp 266–280.
7. Hough JVD: Ten year results with stapedectomy. Panel presentation, Annual Meeting of the American College of Surgeons, San Francisco, CA, October 9, 1969.

26

Laser Stapedotomy

RODNEY PERKINS, M.D.

A new era in the treatment of otosclerosis was opened in 1956 when the stapedectomy procedure was introduced by John Shea.[1] Since then, variation from the original technique has occurred in three major areas: the design of the prosthesis, the nature of the oval window seal, and the small fenestra technique. One only need look in an otologic prosthesis catalogue to see the wide variation in design and materials used in prostheses for connecting the incus with the perilymphatic fluids of the vestibule. The literature from the past three decades is replete with reports of various biomaterials (e.g., vein, perichondrium, fascia, absorbable gelatin sponge [Gelfoam], and fat) that have been used to seal the oval window area. Although these variations in prosthesis design and seal material have contributed to improvement of the original procedure, the development of the small fenestration concept has probably been the most important variant of the stapedectomy procedure for otosclerosis.

The small fenestra technique was primarily championed by European otologists during the 1970s. This technique involved careful manual dissection of a small hole in the footplate and the subsequent placement of a piston-type prosthesis in the created fenestra. The primary advantage of this procedure was that it minimized iatrogenic trauma to the inner ear and reduced the incidence of the prosthesis becoming malpositioned as a result of postoperative healing dynamics or of being engulfed by scar tissue, which commonly fills the oval window niche after manual stapedectomy. However, the technique had problems: it required an excellent technician to effect the procedure successfully, and it was not always possible to create a uniform circular fenestra because of the tendency of the footplate to crack and therefore, in some cases, force removal of the entire footplate.

As a result of observing the small fenestra technique performed by many skilled European otologists (Fisch, Marquet, and Smyth), I began to develop a technique to facilitate making a fenestra atraumatically and, in September 1978, performed the first laser stapedotomy.[2] This procedure has proved to be exceptionally safe and efficacious and, although it has been refined, is performed similarly today.

PREOPERATIVE PREPARATION

The laser stapedotomy procedure is done under local anesthesia on an outpatient basis. To perform otologic surgery successfully with the patient under local anesthesia, the surgeon, the patient, and the operating room must be properly prepared.

Surgeon Preparation

In addition to being familiar with the classic techniques of otosclerosis surgery, the surgeon must become familiar with the laser, its biologic characteristics, beam manipulation to achieve various surgical effects, and safety measures that protect the patient and operating room personnel. Otologists planning to use the laser in otosclerosis surgery and other otologic surgery should take an appropriate training course and practice using the laser on temporal bone specimens prior to clinical application.

Microscope Preparation

It is of critical importance to set up the operating microscope and the laser in the following manner prior to laser stapedotomy when a microscope-mounted beam delivery system, such as the Microbeam device from Laserscope, is used. The following procedure makes the microscope parfocal, allowing the focus of the optical plane to remain the same when magnification is changed. When this procedure is followed by the laser preparation described later, the focus of the laser beam and that of the optical plane remain the same through changes in magnification. Otherwise, the laser spot will not be in focus at the optical plane, and the energy will not be appropriately delivered. In addition, these procedures ensure that the laser beam will have diminished energy density after the focal point, giving increased safety to the procedure.

Parfocal Procedure

- Position the microscope above a flat, stationary surface.
- Using a pen or pencil, make a dot on a piece of white paper to serve as a focus target and place it in the center of the illuminated field of the microscope.
- After adjusting both eyepiece diopter settings to "0", set the microscope fine-focus controls so that they are at the approximate midpoint of the fine-focus range.
- Advance the microscope to its highest magnification setting and focus, using the fine-focus control until a sharp image of the dot is obtained.
- Being careful not to shift microscope position, change the magnification setting to its lowest position. Focus left and right eyepieces, *one at a time*, with the opposite eye closed, by turning the diopter rings. When these settings can be repeated to within one-quarter diopter, you may wish to record these settings for future use with this microscope.

Laser Preparation

- Identify the spot-size adjustment knob on the right side of the Laserscope Microbeam microscope adapter. Turn it fully counterclockwise (toward the user) to the minimum spot setting.
- Check that the system status on the video display screen is "ready" and that power and duration are at the minimum setting.
- Press the foot switch halfway down to activate the aiming beam.
- Identify the focus adjustment knob on the back of the adapter. Look through the microscope, turn the focus adjustment knob either clockwise or counterclockwise until the aiming beam spot is as small as possible.
- The microscope and the laser are now parfocal together.

Patient Preparation

There are two components of patient preparation for otologic surgery performed under local anesthesia: psychologic and pharmacologic.

Psychologic

To reduce anxiety and create rapport, the surgeon should give the patient a full explanation of the procedure, its objectives, benefits, and risks. In addition, a surgical nurse or medical assistant should explain what will happen to the patient in the operating room by describing such things as the operating room environment, use of an intravenous line for medication delivery, placement of monitor electrodes, and draping. By informing the patient of these things and making him or her part of the process, the physician and nurse will reduce anxiety and ensure cooperation and less bleeding. Beyond the technical advantages achieved by such preparation, there is an ethical responsibility to inform the patient. In addition, the likelihood of the patient becoming litigious as a result of a poor outcome is markedly reduced if he or she has been informed of the procedure, the risks and benefits, and has had an opportunity to discuss them with the surgeon prior to the surgery.

Pharmacologic

The chemical preparation of the patient can be achieved in many ways. The pharmaceutical agents that I have employed have worked for me, but many premedication regimens will achieve a similar result.

In the average adult, I give pentobarbital (Nembu-tal), 150mg, orally 1 hour prior to surgery. One half hour prior to surgery, meperidine (Demerol), 75mg, and diazepam (Valium), 10mg, are given by intramuscular injection. An intravenous catheter is started in the arm opposite the operative ear before the patient arrives in the operating room, and dextrose, 5%, in Ringer's solution is started with a Volutrol. Unless the patient appears very sedated, an additional 25mg of meperidine is placed in the Volutrol and infused slowly over 30 to 45 minutes. In addition, patients receive penicillin VK, 250mg, or another appropriate antibiotic 1 hour before surgery.

General anesthesia is contraindicated in otosclerosis surgery in mentally competent adult patients for four primary reasons. First, the surgeon should avoid unnecessarily exposing the patient to the risks of anesthesia. Second, in the fully anesthetized patient, there is no indication of cochleovestibular trauma occurring during the procedure, whereas, in the sedated but awake patient, stimulation of the vestibular system during the procedure evokes nausea or subjective dizziness, which is usually reported by the patient immediately. This is a valuable early warning to desist from whatever manipulation is evoking the response. Third, vomiting in the postoperative period is more likely under general anesthesia. Although vomiting may have no effect on the ultimate outcome of the procedure, the increased spinal fluid pressure and intracochlear pressure that would likely accompany vomiting may force a perilymphatic fistula. However, this concern is higher in conventional manual stapedectomy than in the laser stapedotomy procedure described here because there is an extremely good fit of the prosthesis in the fenestra and an excellent biologic seal. A fourth consideration is the cost of general anesthesia. In this procedure, general anesthesia is unnecessary and hence an additional financial burden on an already expensive health care system.

Site Preparation

The auricle and periauricular area are scrubbed with povidone-iodine (Betadine) solution. A plastic drape is placed over the area, with the auricle exteriorized through the opening in the drape. This drape is placed over an L-shaped bar that is fixed in the rail attachment of the operating table (Fig. 26–1). Attached to the bar is a small, low-volume office fan that provides a gentle cooling breeze to the patient's face during the procedure. The plastic drape forms a canopy, allowing the patient to see from under the drape and reducing the feeling of claustrophobia. In addition, a foam ear piece from a speaker is inserted into the opposite ear. This ear piece is connected to a com-

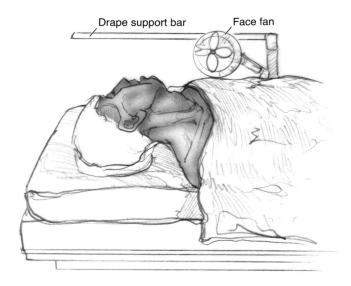

FIGURE 26-1. The drape support bar and face fan.

pact disk player and input microphone that allows the patient to listen to relaxing music and provides a pathway to converse with the patient if desired. The dorsum of the ipsilateral hand is scrubbed with povidone-iodine solution and draped in preparation for the harvest of a vein graft later in the procedure.

Analgesia

It is important not only to achieve analgesia but also to maximize canal hemostasis with injections into the external auditory meatus. By using 2% lidocaine (Xylocaine) with 1:20,000 epinephrine solution in a ringed syringe with a 27-gauge needle, a classic quadratic injection is made such that each injection falls within the wheal of the previous injection. Another injection that I have found useful is an anterior canal injection, which is made with the bevel of the needle parallel to the bony wall of the external meatus (Fig. 26–2). After the needle is inserted, it is advanced a few millimeters, and a few drops of the solution are injected extremely slowly. The solution infiltrates medially along the anterior canal wall and adds to the hemostasis in the anterior extent of the tympanomeatal incision.

OPERATIVE TECHNIQUE

The ear canal is cleansed of wax and epithelial debris and irrigated with povidone-iodine solution. Through as large an oval-beveled speculum as possible, incisions for a tympanomeatal flap are created. The initial incision is made with a sickle knife just lateral to the inferior annulus of the tympanic membrane at the 6 o'clock location and brought laterally along the floor of the canal approximately 4mm. A second incision is made with a 2mm round canal knife beginning at the lateral extent of the initial incision and extending in a curvilinear fashion, first posteriorly and then anterosuperiorly until it terminates about 2mm above the pars flaccida. This second incision is made in multiple small segments. Each segment is composed of an initial crushing application of the knife into the canal skin and a subsequent cutting action that connects that small segment with the previously cut segment. The crushing portion of this action seems to impart additional hemostasis. An additional advantage of making this incision in multiple small segments is that it eliminates the tendency of the tissue to tear, especially in patients in whom the superior medial canal skin is thick.

Through the use of a small round or lancet knife, the described skin flap is elevated progressively and equally toward the annulus. While the knife edge is kept tight to the bone, the fibrocartilaginous annulus is elevated from the bony sulcus. The investing tympanic cavity mucosa is torn with a blunted curved needle, and care is taken to identify and preserve the chorda tympani nerve. The tympanomeatal flap is then folded anteriorly, revealing the posterior tympanic cavity (Fig. 26–3). The superior portion of the manubrium of the malleus should be visible.

The malleus is palpated with a blunt, curved needle to assess the mobility of the malleus and incus and to rule out fixation of these ossicles as a cause for the conductive impairment. The stapes is palpated as a preliminary confirmation of the diagnosis. The middle ear is inspected, with particular attention to the round window area, which may be obliterated in cases of extensive otosclerosis. A small amount of 2% lidocaine with 1:20,000 epinephrine is infused into the middle ear and then immediately aspirated. This infusion provides analgesia to the sensory distribution

FIGURE 26-2. The anterior canal injection.

FIGURE 26-3. The tympanomeatal flap is reflected.

FIGURE 26-4. Curettage begins away from scutum edge.

FIGURE 26-5. A groove is created, facilitating removal of the thinned scutum edge.

FIGURE 26-6. The chorda tympani nerve is separated from the malleus.

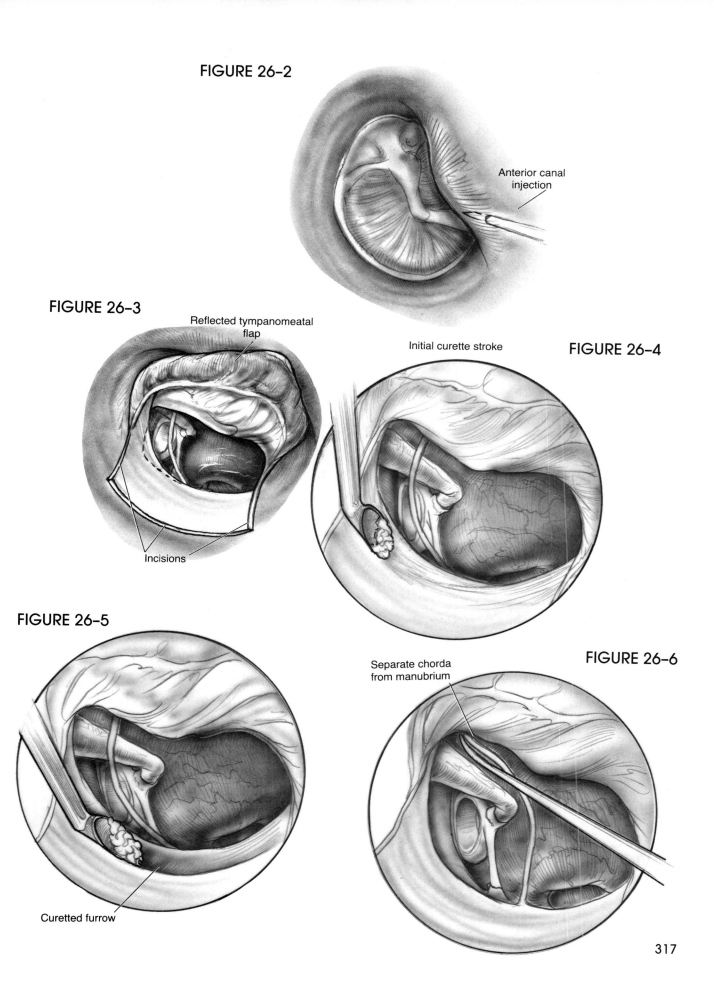

FIGURE 26-2

Anterior canal injection

FIGURE 26-3

Reflected tympanomeatal flap

Incisions

Initial curette stroke

FIGURE 26-4

FIGURE 26-5

Curetted furrow

Separate chorda from manubrium

FIGURE 26-6

317

in the middle ear space, and the rapid aspiration of the excess mitigates its potential absorption through the round window membrane, which might cause a temporary paresis of vestibular function and vertigo.

A sharp double-ended curette is used to remove an adequate amount of the posterosuperior medial canal wall bone (scutum) to give a satisfactory view of the stapes and the pyramidal process. In laser stapedotomy, it is sometimes advisable to curette slightly more bone than in conventional stapedectomy to provide an unobstructed pathway for the laser beam. The initial curettage should be lateral to the edge of the scutum (Fig. 26–4). Creating a furrow lateral to the edge of the scutum allows the surgeon to protect the incus from inadvertent disarticulation during the portion of the curettage when more pressure is applied to the curette (Fig. 26–5). Adequate scutum removal has been attained when the pyramidal process can be seen.

The stapes is inspected and palpated, and the diagnosis of otosclerosis is confirmed. The chorda tympani nerve is separated from the medial surface of the manubrium of the malleus with a curved needle or joint knife (Fig. 26–6). This maneuver allows any stretching of the chorda tympani nerve that might be necessary to be distributed along the full course of the intratympanic chorda tympani rather than only between the manubrial attachment and the iter chordae posterius, through which it emerges into the tympanic cavity. Any dehiscence in the bony covering of the facial nerve immediately above the stapes is noted. If mucosal adhesions are present between the promontory or facial nerve and the stapes, they are vaporized by slightly defocusing the minimally focused beam, using 100 millisecond bursts of about 2W of the potassium titanyl phosphate crystal (KTP)/532 laser. Although these adhesions could be interrupted with a small pick, the laser is less likely to excite bleeding because of its coagulating characteristics.

A measurement is made of the distance between the footplate and the medial surface of the lower portion of the long process of the incus to select a prosthesis of appropriate length (Fig. 26–7). Although some surgeons make this measurement after the superstructure of the stapes has been removed, it is more accurately made before disarticulating the incudostapedial joint because this is the undisturbed natural position of the incus. To accommodate the entrance of the prosthesis slightly into the vestibule, 0.25mm to 0.5mm should be added to this measured distance for prosthesis length. If there appears to be reasonable access to the footplate, a stainless steel bucket-handle prosthesis with a piston diameter of 0.8mm is selected (Fig 26–8). However, if large facial nerve overhang or a narrow niche or other anatomic variation exists that compromises the surgeon's ability to see a large amount of footplate, selecting a 0.6mm diameter prosthesis may be advisable.

The tympanomeatal flap is placed back into position loosely to decrease mucosal drying and to prevent blood from entering the middle ear while a segment of vein is harvested from the hand. Attention is turned to the prepared dorsum of the ipsilateral hand, and the povidone-iodine residue is removed with a moist sponge. If the superficial venous structure is not readily visible, the surgeon may bring these into view by tightly grasping the patient's wrist to obstruct venous return. A venous segment is identified within 2cm of the knuckles. Care is taken to avoid an incision too close to the knuckle fold because slower healing may occur in that dynamically moving area. The larger veins found more superiorly on the hand may be too thick for this application. The flat bevel of a 27-gauge needle is placed immediately over the desired vein, and a 1cm intradermal wheal of 2% lidocaine with 1:20,000 epinephrine is created. While this wheal is still elevated, a No. 15 scalpel is used to make a 0.75cm incision through the dermis and subcutaneous

---

FIGURE 26–7. A measuring instrument is used to determine the length of the prosthesis.

FIGURE 26–8. Stainless steel bucket-handle prosthesis.

FIGURE 26–9. A vein segment is placed over a hole in the Teflon block. The prosthesis is inserted into the hole, dragging the vein with it.

FIGURE 26–10. The incudostapedial joint is sectioned with the joint knife.

FIGURE 26–11. The stapedial tendon is vaporized with the KTP/532 laser, and the smoke and vapor plume is aspirated.

FIGURE 26–12. Adequate stapedial tendon vaporization brings into view the posterior crus of the stapes.

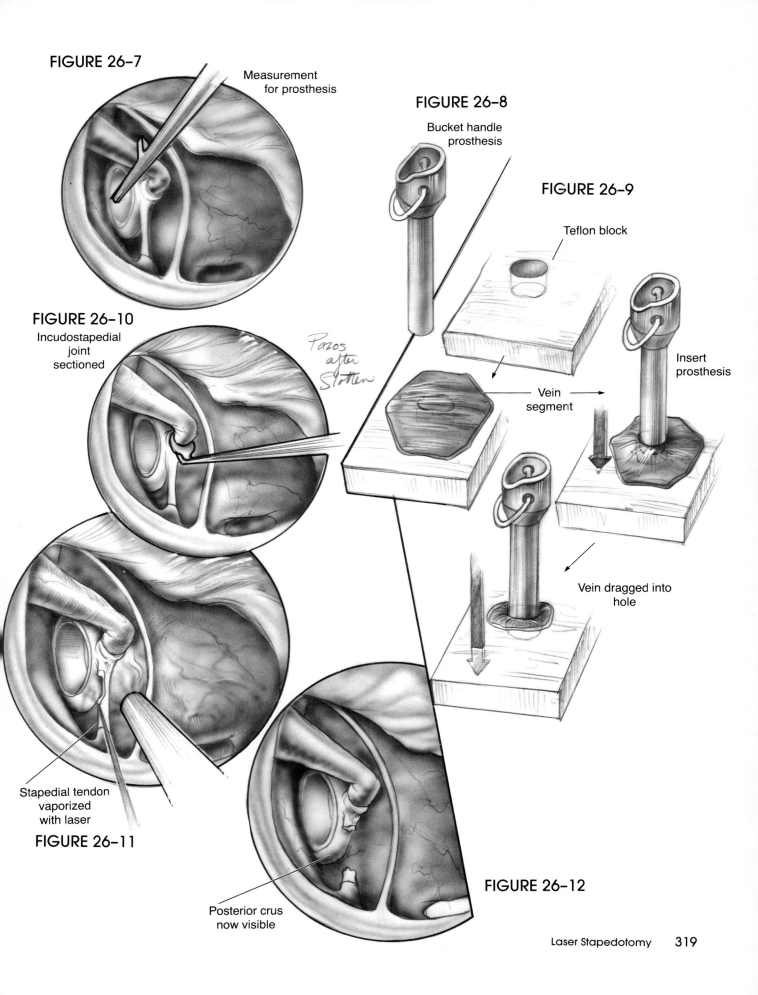

FIGURE 26-7

Measurement for prosthesis

FIGURE 26-8

Bucket handle prosthesis

FIGURE 26-9

Teflon block

Vein segment

Insert prosthesis

Vein dragged into hole

Pazos after Slotten

FIGURE 26-10

Incudostapedial joint sectioned

Stapedial tendon vaporized with laser

FIGURE 26-11

Posterior crus now visible

FIGURE 26-12

tissues. Through the use of two mosquito clamps that have been honed to have narrow sharpened tines, tissues adjacent to the vein are separated by expansion of the tines parallel to the vein. The closed mosquito clamp is then passed beneath the vein and brought to the surface. The desired segment of the vein is then clamped at both ends with mosquito clamps, and the vein is grasped with a fine hand forceps and cut at the clamp site with a clean No. 15 blade that has not been used on the skin. The delivered vein segment is placed in a moist sponge and the ends of the vein are tied with 4.0 polyglactin 910 (Vicryl) suture and the wound closed with 6.0 Dermalon. An adhesive bandage is applied parallel to the incision.

On a separate side table, the vein is prepared. Small, sharp-pointed scissors are inserted into the venous lumen, and the vein is stretched slightly by opening the tines. Excess adventitial tissue is removed by grasping this tissue with small sharp jeweler's forceps and tearing it from the vein. With a No. 15 scalpel, the stretched vein is incised longitudinally, and the adventitial side is placed over a hole (0.8mm to 1.0mm in diameter, depending on the thickness of the vein) in a polytetrafluoroethylene (Teflon) block (Fig. 26–9). Excess venous tissue is cut away with the scalpel, leaving a disk of vein that is approximately 2.5mm to 3.0mm in diameter. The previously selected stainless steel bucket-handle prosthesis is then placed into the hole in the block, dragging the wet vein in with it (Fig. 26–9). Any flange of vein remaining on the block is smoothed onto the piston shaft. This prosthesis-vein assembly is then left to air dry until needed.

The tympanomeatal flap is then reopened and the stapes area brought into view. Through use of the incudostapedial joint knife, the joint is sectioned (Fig. 26–10). Because it is sometimes difficult to be sure of the exact location of the joint, it is advisable to shift the incus slightly in an anteroposterior direction while observing for the light reflex of the joint capsular ligament. The joint knife is first used to incise this ligament superiorly and inferiorly prior to insinuating it into the joint capsule with a slight rotating motion. After separation of this joint, the laser phase of the procedure is begun. Prior to using the laser, the speculum should be fixed in place with an articulated speculum holder. Usually, a larger speculum that increases visibility and enhances canal hemostasis can be used at this point.

The smallest spot size, 100-millisecond pulses (2W to 2.5W) of the (KTP)/532 laser are used to vaporize the stapedial tendon, and the smoke and vapor plume is aspirated with a 24-gauge suction tip (Fig. 26–11). Initial vaporization is enhanced by the placement of the aiming beam on a vessel on the tendon. The tendon removal should be adequate to allow a good view of the posterior crus (Fig. 26–12). Continuing with the same laser parameters, the posterior crus is vaporized (Fig. 26–13). The char created is picked away with a 30° stapes pick (Fig. 26–14). Sometimes, portions of the crus remain unvaporized, and it is necessary to continue with additional pulses into these intact bone remnants. The posterior crus must be vaporized to as near the footplate as possible to allow a clear beam pathway to the footplate (Fig. 26–15).

Attention is then turned to vaporization of the anterior crus of the stapes, which is accomplished by use of a small mirror that has special optical coating to reflect the laser wavelength. First, the focused beam is placed on the anterior oval window niche area between the incus and the stapes. Then, with a No. 24 suction tip in the left hand and the mirror in the right hand (opposite if the surgeon is left-handed), the beam is directed into the anterior crus (Fig. 26–16). Should the previously warmed mirror fog with condensate, placing the suction tip near it will usually clear the surface. The anterior crus is vaporized just below the neck of the stapes (Fig. 26–17). Multiple pulses are placed into the anterior crus until char is created along 1mm or 2mm of the crus. The superstructure of the stapes is removed by a blunt right-angle hook (Fig. 26–18).

The topography of the footplate surface is now

FIGURE 26–13. The posterior crus is vaporized.

FIGURE 26–14. Char residue is removed with a 30° stapes pick.

FIGURE 26–15. Further vaporization of the posterior crus base allows a beam pathway to the footplate.

FIGURE 26–16. The anterior crus is vaporized by a special optically coated miniature mirror.

FIGURE 26–17. The anterior crus is vaporized just below the neck of the stapes.

FIGURE 26–18. The head, neck, and upper crura are removed with a blunt pick.

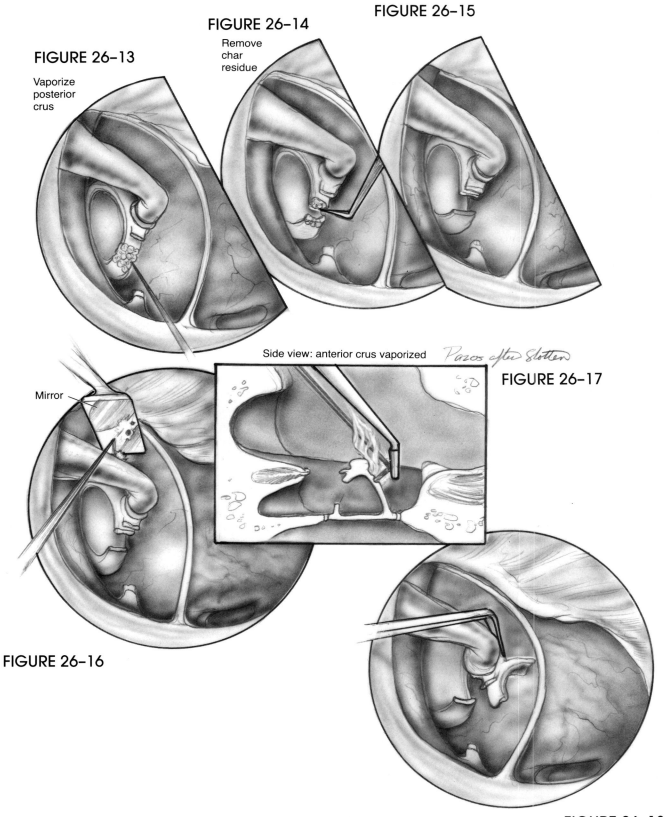

FIGURE 26-13

Vaporize posterior crus

FIGURE 26-14

Remove char residue

FIGURE 26-15

Side view: anterior crus vaporized

Pazos after Slattery

FIGURE 26-17

Mirror

FIGURE 26-16

FIGURE 26-18

studied (Fig. 26–19). Bony ridges, thick areas of otosclerosis, and blood vessels are noted. By use of a 0.6mm or 0.8mm (preferable)–diameter measuring instrument, the target zone for the laser fenestra is identified (Fig. 26–20). The KTP/532 laser is set at the smallest spot size, 100-millisecond pulse, and 2W. Ridges or areas of thickened bone are vaporized first. The rationale is to lower these areas to the same thickness as the thinner areas before perilymph comes onto the surface. The presence of perilymph makes vaporization slightly more difficult because it reflects some of the beam and becomes a surface heat sink. For the first pulse, it is frequently advantageous to start on a small blood vessel. The hemoglobin provides excellent absorption of the KTP/532 beam. The aim beam should be overlapped onto the char of the previous hole as the progressive rosette pattern of holes is being made (Fig. 26–21). The dark char is a chromophore that absorbs the wavelength very well and optically "catalyzes" the next hole. Once the first hole is made, a small amount of perilymph will come onto the surface of the footplate. Small No. 26 and No. 28 suction tips placed away from the holes, but on the footplate surface, safely remove this perilymph, facilitating the vaporization process (Fig. 26–22). After the rosette is completed, a central segment of bone may be unvaporized and can be vaporized in a similar fashion. This process is continued until a completed rosette pattern of holes has been created that results in a fenestra of appropriate diameter (Fig. 26–23). The adequacy of the size of the fenestra is assessed with the measuring instrument (Fig. 26–24). It is not necessary to remove the charred bone lattice within the fenestra prior to placement of the prosthesis.

The prosthetic piston-vein assembly is then carefully removed from the Teflon block to keep the vein clad on the piston (Fig. 26–25). With the bucket-handle wire resting opposite the notch in the cup for the long process of the incus, the prosthesis is carried into the field and placed on the footplate. A 30° pick and a No. 24 suction tip help insert the prosthesis assembly into the stapedial fenestra, and the bucket-cup portion is manipulated onto the lenticular process of the incus. Slight lateral displacement of the long process of the incus with the pick while guiding the piston into position with the suction tip facilitates this maneuver. The bucket-handle wire is then brought over the lateral surface of the inferior long process (Fig. 26–26). Optionally, autogenous fibrin glue or a small piece of vein may be placed over it to improve stability of the bucket-handle position.

Inspection of the footplate area should be done at this time to confirm that the vein has now hydrated and its flange lies on the footplate (Fig. 26–26). If it does not surround the piston or looks as though an edge has been carried into the vestibule, consideration should be given to removing the piston, repositioning the vein over the fenestra, and reinserting the prosthesis. Palpation of the incus should confirm an easy motion of the prosthesis. If motion is difficult, the prosthesis may not be in the fenestra. This can be checked by gently pushing the shaft of the prosthesis anteriorly. If the piston is in the fenestra, it will not displace anteriorly, but if it is residing on the surface of the footplate, it will slip anteriorly when the pressure is applied. Gently checking for a round window reflex is desirable. However, if a good round window reflex is not seen, the prosthesis may still be in good position. Persistent movement of the prosthesis to elicit a round window reflex should be avoided because the increased iatrogenic trauma is undesirable.

The tympanomeatal flap is placed back into ana-

FIGURE 26–19. The topography of the footplate is studied and a target zone identified.

FIGURE 26–20. A measuring device is used to confirm the adequacy of the target zone.

FIGURE 26–21. The aimed beam slightly overlaps the previous hole.

FIGURE 26–22. Suctioning distal to rosette aspirates perilymph, facilitating vaporization.

FIGURE 26–23. The rosette of small vaporization holes creates a fenestra of appropriate diameter.

FIGURE 26–24. The measuring instrument is used to assess the adequacy of the fenestra.

FIGURE 26–25. The dried vein remains clad on the prosthesis after removal from the Teflon block.

FIGURE 26–26. The vein-clad piston in place with optional fibrin glue and vein-stabilizing bucket handle.

FIGURE 26-19

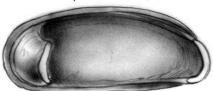

Footplate without crura

FIGURE 26-20

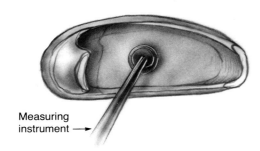

Measuring instrument

FIGURE 26-21

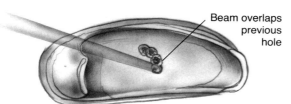

Beam overlaps previous hole

FIGURE 26-22

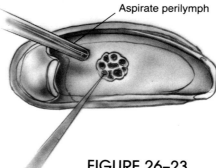

Aspirate perilymph

FIGURE 26-23

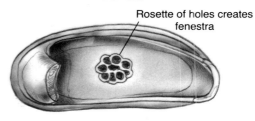

Rosette of holes creates fenestra

FIGURE 26-24

Check diameter of fenestra

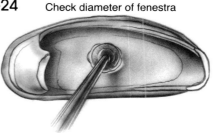

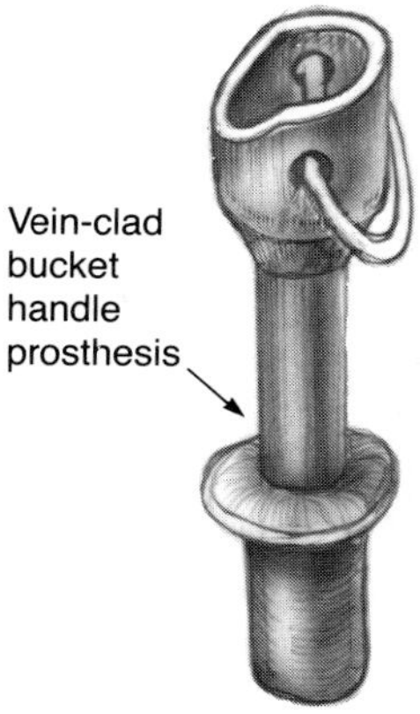

FIGURE 26-26 Piston in place

FIGURE 26-25

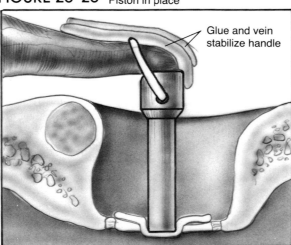

Vein-clad bucket handle prosthesis

Glue and vein stabilize handle

AZOS after Stotter

tomic position, and one or two small pledgets of absorbable gelatin sponge are placed over the incision. Alternatively, if available, a small amount of autogenous fibrin glue can be placed on the bony canal wall under the flap.

It is worthwhile to give a whisper test to the patient by having him or her repeat numbers spoken by the surgeon with decreasing intensity. The results may give some credence to good placement of the prosthesis in the absence of a round window reflex. However, variation in the alertness of the patient and the lack of control of the test make it difficult to ascribe any accurate objectivity to it.

After the drapes are removed, the patient can be evaluated for dizziness and nystagmus. The lack of nystagmus is a very good sign, but the presence of slight nystagmus does not mean that a good result will not be obtained.

A mastoid-type dressing is applied by the nurse, and the patient is taken to his or her room. Patients are routinely discharged the afternoon of the surgery. However, should they have significant vertigo, it is best to hospitalize them overnight rather than have them drive home or to their hotel.

SPECIAL CONDITIONS

The previous description depicts the technique employed in the majority of cases. However, certain conditions call for special techniques to surmount unusual anatomic or pathologic problems.

Overhanging Facial Nerve

Usually, almost the entire width of the middle portion of the footplate is seen by the surgeon. This visibility allows access of the beam to create the fenestra and allows for the placement of the preferable larger-diameter prosthesis. However, one occasionally encounters a facial nerve whose bony covering is dehiscent in the area of the oval window, and the protruding nerve prevents direct observation of all but the inferior portion of the footplate. Two techniques that are helpful in these circumstances are the facial nerve displacement technique and the partial promontory fenestra technique.

Facial Nerve Displacement Technique

The overhanging facial nerve is a problem for both conventional manual stapedectomy and for laser stapedotomy techniques. Although facial nerve displacement technique may be used in both, it is more satisfactory in laser stapedotomy because of the lower incidence of bleeding in the oval window area with laser stapedotomy compared with conventional manual stapedectomy. This technique can be used with both the dehiscent and nondehiscent overhanging facial nerve. Most overhanging facial nerves are dehiscent, but if a bony covering is present, it can be picked off and thus converted to a situation similar to a dehiscent facial nerve.

Facial nerve displacement is first employed during the assessment of the footplate stage of the operation and then during the creation of the laser fenestra. It involves displacement of the nerve for short periods, which can be done without causing damage. The side of a No. 24 suction tip is placed on the inferior edge of the dehiscent facial nerve adjacent to the midpoint of the stapes. With the application of slight pressure superiorly, the facial nerve will compress and provide an improved view of the footplate. This pressure is applied for short durations of up to 5 seconds and released. After 10 to 15 seconds, the process is repeated until an assessment of the footplate and the target zone for the fenestra has been completed. During creation of the fenestra, the displacement process is repeated. While the nerve is displaced and the footplate is visible, the laser is pulsed. This is repeated until the rosette has been completed. In this situation, it is sometimes necessary to use a wire-type prosthesis, which attaches to the long process of the incus. The wire may be bent to curve around the dehiscent nerve. When selecting such a prosthesis, it is advisable to add 0.50mm to 0.75mm to the selected length to accommodate the additional distance needed because of the bend around the nerve.

Partial Promontory Fenestra Technique

When the facial nerve obstructs observation and obstructs the pathway of a prosthesis, the partial promontory fenestra technique may be employed alone or in combination with the facial nerve displacement technique. The KTP/532 laser (4W; 100-millisecond pulses) vaporizes the superior extent of the promontory, which forms the inferior wall of the oval window niche. The bone residue is removed with an oval window rasp, and this process is repeated until the removal is at the level of the footplate. In this situation, care should be taken not to pulse the laser too frequently because the higher energy level used here may cause rapid deposition, absorption of heat in the bone, and transient vertigo. Then, the rosette pattern is created such that the fenestra is partially in the inferior footplate and partially in the inferior wall of the oval window niche. The vein-clad prosthesis is placed in the usual fashion. Again, a wire prosthesis may be bent to accommodate the facial nerve obstruction, although with this technique, the prosthesis pathway is less likely to be obstructed.

Obliterated Footplate

Footplates that are thick or obliterated can be effectively managed with a variant of the laser technique described above. The laser is used to progressively vaporize several layers of the footplate until the perilymph is reached. This step is accomplished by starting with a rosette pattern that is a millimeter or so wide, removing the char that is created with a pick, and then vaporizing another rosette. The char is again removed and the process is continued until perilymph comes into the created hole by capillary action. Once this occurs, it is more difficult to lase successfully, and a portion of the fenestra sometimes has to be removed with a small stapes pick. Alternatively, one could use a microdrill to thin the footplate and then make the entering fenestra with the laser. It is sometimes necessary to use a 0.6mm-diameter prosthesis without the vein clad on it. If so, a small amount of venous blood should be infused into the oval window niche or minute pieces of gelatin sponge should be packed around the piston to provide a temporary seal. This blood may be obtained from an antecubital vein with a conventional syringe and infused with a blunted No. 22 spinal needle.

Floating Footplate

A floating footplate is not likely to be created when the laser stapedotomy technique is used. However, should it be created during the course of a conventional manual stapedectomy, the operation should be halted if no laser is available. After 4 months' healing, the patient should be reoperated using the laser. At this time, the rosette pattern is created, and a vein-clad prosthesis is installed, thereby avoiding the high risk of iatrogenic trauma that is attendant to manual management of the floating footplate.

POSTOPERATIVE CARE

Surgical Facility

The patient remains in the outpatient surgical facility for 2 or 3 hours after the procedure and is then driven home or to other appropriate accommodations by a relative. The marked reduction in iatrogenic vibratory trauma attendant to the laser procedure compared with manual procedures results in less postoperative dizziness and nausea and makes possible the management of otosclerosis as an outpatient procedure. Even with a smooth and uneventful procedure, an occasional patient will have nausea and vomiting and will be kept overnight. Patients who have dysequilibrium, vertigo, or vomiting are given diazepam, 5mg to 10mg intramuscularly, every 4 hours as needed for vestibular suppression. It is also worthwhile to give patients diazepam, 10mg orally, about 45 minutes before discharge to reduce the potential of vestibular disturbance initiated by the automobile ride to their destination.

Office

Patients from the local area are seen at 1 week, 1 month, 4 months, and 1 year after surgery. Patients from outside the area may travel by land or air the day following surgery.

On the first visit, any gelatin sponge that has been placed in the canal is removed. Usually, no eardrops are prescribed unless there is evidence of a developing external otitis.

Medications

Patients are given a prescription for penicillin VK, 250mg, three times a day, to be taken for 5 days after the surgery. An additional prescription for acetaminophen with codiene (30mg) is given with the instructions to fill only if their pain is not alleviated by their usual over-the-counter pain remedy.

RESULTS

Patients who have laser stapedotomy experience far less labyrinthine disturbance in the postoperative period than patients having manual stapedectomy. In fact, this is the primary reason that the procedure can be routinely performed on an outpatient basis.

In the most recent study of results, a comparative study of three prosthesis-seal combinations, a postoperative air-bone gap in speech frequencies of less than 10dB was achieved in 90 per cent of patients who had laser stapedotomy with the vein-clad prosthesis.[3] The average postoperative air-bone gap in the speech frequencies was 4.5dB. None of the patients in my series have had catastrophic hearing impairment in the operative or perioperative period in the 14 years since the first laser stapedotomy.

In addition to the reduced morbidity and risk of adverse effect, laser stapedotomy will likely result in better high-frequency hearing compared with conventional manual stapedectomy. In 1969, in a small unpublished study, I compared my last 15 manual stapedectomy patients with the first 15 laser stapedotomy patients and found better results at both 2000Hz and 4000Hz in the latter group. This better efficacy has continued to be my clinical impression. I believe that the improvement derives from the reduction in iatrogenic vibratory trauma to the nearby hair cells in the high-frequency area of the basilar turn when laser stapedotomy is performed.

DISCUSSION

The Vein-Clad Bucket-Handle Prosthesis

In the first laser stapedotomy in 1978, I used a vein-clad stainless steel wire piston in the first 15 or 20 cases.[2] Subsequently, the procedure was changed to employ an autogenous blood seal in the oval window, along with a special platinum wire–Teflon piston. However, over time and a larger number of cases, the wire prosthesis occasionally eroded the long process of the incus. Also, the hearing result with this platinum wire–Teflon piston–blood seal combination did not seem to be quite as good as those of the initial small number of cases in which the vein-clad wire piston prosthesis was employed. Therefore, I have returned to the vein-clad prosthesis and am now employing this concept with a bucket-handle piston prosthesis.

The vein-clad bucket-handle piston prosthesis appears to have numerous actual and theoretical advantages over other prostheses. By cladding the vein on the end of the piston, one can easily, atraumatically, and simultaneously place the prosthesis and tissue seal into the fenestra. This is a much easier procedure than first manipulating the vein into position on the footplate and then searching for the location of the fenestra beneath a previously placed vein segment. When the dehydrated vein enters the footplate fenestra, it immediately hydrates and provides a moderate resistance to the entry of the piston into the vestibule. This action prevents the piston from dropping into the vestibule when it is displaced medially to manipulate the bucket receptacle up onto the lenticular process. Also, tissue material between the piston and the edge of the fenestra would be expected to form a superior seal.

The normal annular ligament is an important part of the middle ear transducer function. The elastic nature of vein may provide a pseudoannular ligament or "biogasket" that could mimic the acoustic function of the annular ligament of the stapes (Fig. 26–27). This concept has been studied by Causse et al. and believed by them to be important.[4]

The bucket-handle prosthesis will likely evoke a lower frequency of erosion of the incus than metal wire prostheses attached to the incus long process. Also, theoretically, force transmission would be expected to be slightly better from the medial surface of the lenticular process than from the inferior portion of the long process of the incus, as is the case with wire or Teflon prostheses that attach to the inferior portion of the long process (Fig. 26–28).

KTP/532 Versus Argon Versus Carbon Dioxide Lasers

KTP/532, argon, and carbon dioxide lasers have all been used in performing laser stapedotomy. Visible-light lasers such as KTP/532 and argon, have far greater target accuracy than carbon dioxide because their aiming beam is an attenuated version of the surgical beam. The spot size and the beam location of the aiming beam are exactly where the surgical beam will hit the target when released. This is not as important in gross applications of the laser, but in the oval window area, the accuracy and small beam size are important. The carbon dioxide laser, being invisible, requires a separate second laser to act as an aiming beam. This is usually a red helium-neon beam, which has an ill-defined fuzzy perimeter, and its central axis may not be in alignment with the axis of the surgical beam. These factors make the actual spot size at tissue level difficult to determine. All of these factors tend to decrease precision and could increase the risk of damage to adjacent nontargeted structures.

KTP/532 and argon lasers are very similar in their biosurgical effect. KTP/532 is somewhat better absorbed in hemoglobin, but the observable clinical difference in these two lasers in stapedotomy application is negligible. Consideration should be given to the cost of operation and maintenance, higher in argon lasers because of tube degradation and tube replacement costs, which are unnecessary in the solid-state KTP/532 laser.

FIGURE 26–27. The pseudoannular ligament may mimic the acoustic function of the normal annular ligament.

FIGURE 26–28. A more normal force vector is present with a prosthesis driven by the lenticular process.

FIGURE 26–29. Stapedotomy performed using microdrill with diamond burr.

FIGURE 26–28

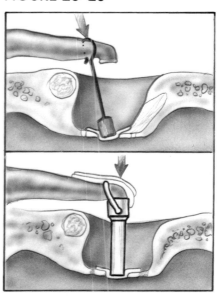

FIGURE 26–27

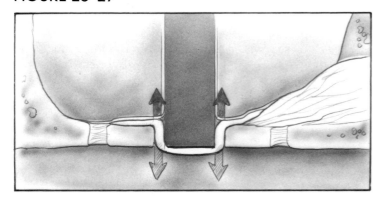

FIGURE 26–29

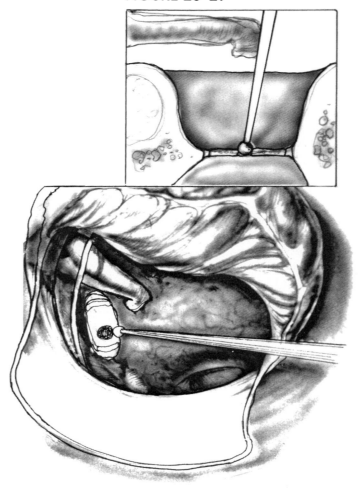

Beam Versus Probe

A laser stapedotomy can be performed with a beam directed from a device mounted under the microscope or from a beam emitting from the end of a hand-held quartz fiber optic wave guide. I prefer the microscope-mounted delivery for stapedotomy, although I use the hand-held probe in all other otologic and neurotologic applications. By placing the finely focused aiming beam on the footplate, one can see exactly where the hole will occur, whereas with the microprobe, the instrument itself tends to obscure the field of vision. Also, unless the probe is touching the footplate, the size of the hole tends to vary, and the completeness of vaporization is erratic because of the varying spot size coming from the probe at differing attack distances. When contact vaporization is done with the probe, there is some risk of physically penetrating a thin footplate. The exquisite focus and the target accuracy of the focused spot coming from the KTP/532 Microbeam device mounted on the microscope results in extremely accurate spot placement and uniformity in the vaporization hole.

Vestibular Safety

When the laser stapedotomy procedure was conceived, one of the obvious considerations was the potential effect that the laser might have on the vestibule. Would the thermal energy of the laser cause stimulation of the vestibular neural endings because of movement of vestibular fluids created by the thermal effect? Another consideration was the potential direct damage that laser energy might cause to the saccule or the macula of the utricle.

This proposition was considered by Gantz et al. in an article in which cats were used as experimental animals.[5] They found that with the beam parameters that were recommended with an argon laser for laser stapedotomy, the cat saccule was damaged by beaming a laser pulse into the vestibule in some cases. This finding was of interest because I had tried to make an opening in the saccule in hopes of finding a means of treating Ménière's disease by creating a shunt from the endolymphatic system to the perilymphatic system. In fact, I found it very difficult to do this because the saccular membrane is transparent and contained no chromophores to absorb the energy of the argon wavelength. It was also interesting to note that cat footplate is considerably thinner than that of the human, and the distance between the footplate and the saccule is much less. This laboratory finding was inconsistent with my experience in the laboratory in human temporal bones and completely insupportable by clinical results from hundreds of laser stapedotomies by myself and other clinicians. In a later study,

Lesinski attempted to discredit visible-wavelength lasers in stapedotomy.[6] He reported the results of beaming a visible wavelength laser into the vestibule of temporal bones, measuring the heat and drawing conclusions adverse to the use of visible wavelength lasers in stapedotomy. This experiment reflected a lack of understanding of the basic physics of laser absorption. It was flawed because the dark thermocouple used to measure the heat is itself a chromophore and absorbed the energy, whereas in the normal vestibule there is no such chromophore. In fact, and quite to the contrary, the lack of intraoperative vestibular effects resulting from the KTP/532 and argon lasers in stapedotomy has been extremely remarkable.

The lack of significant thermal effect seems to result from several factors. Probably most of the heat is dissipated in the vaporization of the bone and pulled off by the suction. The energy is delivered, not in one large pulse, but in a series of pulses over time, allowing any heat build-up to be removed by the vasculature within the vestibule. In addition, the beam is in focus on the lateral surface of the footplate and immediately defocuses as it goes beyond the focal point. Engineering calculations suggest that the energy density of the defocusing beam is significantly decreased from its strength at the footplate by the time it arrives at the saccule some 1.8mm medially. Although these calculations are rough and may have some error, they do underscore the fact that the beam below the footplate has less power density than the spot focused on the surface.

However, even though the safety of the KTP/532 laser is well established, caution should be used to prevent beam penetration into an open vestibule when blood has entered the vestibule. In this situation, the hemoglobin of blood in the perilymph or perhaps lying on the saccule acts as a chromophore and will absorb the beam energy and create heat. This could cause thermal damage and perhaps a shunt between the endolymph and the perilymph.

Facial Nerve Safety

Concern often arises over damage to the facial nerve if a pulse hits the bone overlying it or the sheath of a dehiscent nerve. When the suggested laser parameters are used, pulses will not penetrate the bony covering over the nerve or the sheath in the case of a dehiscent nerve sufficiently to cause damage to the neural structures beneath. The bone of the fallopian canal is much thicker than the footplate, and the white neural sheath tends not to absorb much of the beam energy. However, one should always assess the location and status of the facial nerve before lasing in any case. An anatomic variant, such as a bifid facial nerve with a portion of it traveling inferior to the oval window niche, may be present. If this is not identified and the partial promontory technique described earlier is employed, the unidentified aberrant nerve could be damaged by the repeated laser pulses.

SUMMARY

The laser stapedotomy procedure has been proved to be safe and effective for the treatment of otosclerosis. It represents part of the continuum of development and refinement of the surgery for otosclerosis. The low level of iatrogenic vibratory trauma attendant to this procedure reduces the chances of catastrophic loss of hearing and vestibular disturbance postoperatively, and provides the basis for the outpatient surgical treatment of otosclerosis on a routine basis. Fourteen years' experience with laser stapedotomy has proved it to be a safe and effective procedure of choice for otosclerosis.

EDITORIAL COMMENT

Microdrill Small Fenestra Stapedotomy

Although this editor preferentially uses a laser to perform small fenestra stapedotomy, similar to the method described in this chapter, a laser is not required for this technique. A small fenestra can easily be created using one of the microdrills that are now available from several manufacturers.

To make the footplate opening, a 0.7mm diamond burr is used, which allows sufficient clearance for a 0.6mm piston prosthesis. After the stapes superstructure has been removed, the burr is lightly placed on the footplate (Fig. 26–29). Pressure is not exerted against the footplate, and a light touch is used. The drill motor is activated, and when the fenestration is completed, the surgeon will sense a subtle resistance change. The appropriate prosthesis can then be placed.

This technique results in quick and reliable fenestration of the footplate and yields results similar to those obtained with other techniques.

C.S.

References

1. Shea JJ: Fenestration of the oval window. Ann Otol Rhinol Laryngol 67: 932–951, 1958.
2. Perkins RC: Laser stapedotomy for otosclerosis. Laryngoscope 91: 228–241, 1980.
3. Perkins RC, Curto FS Jr.: Laser stapedotomy: A comparative study of prostheses and seals. Laryngoscope 102: 1992.
4. Causse JB, Causse JR, et al.: The Annular Ligament of the Stapes Footplate: Reconstitution of its Function in Otosclerosis and Dysplasia Surgery. International Workshop on Otosclerosis, Rome, April 25–27, 1989.
5. Gantz BJ, Jenkins HA, Fisch U, Kishimoto S: Argon laser stapedotomy. Ann Otol Rhinol Laryngol 91: 25–26, 1982.
6. Lesinski SG: Lasers for otosclerosis: CO_2 vs. argon and KTP-532. Laryngoscope 99 (6 Pt 2 Suppl 46): 1–8, 1989.

27

Partial Stapedectomy

MENDELL ROBINSON, M.D., F.A.C.S.

Many surgeons prefer a partial stapedectomy technique for the surgical treatment of otosclerosis. However, a partial stapedectomy is endorsed by the author only when the surgeon follows certain basic principles in stapedial footplate surgery. This chapter covers those surgical principles and the manner in which they apply to the partial stapedectomy technique. Additionally, this chapter addresses the application of these principles to the total stapedectomy and the stapedotomy techniques.

HISTORY

In 1958, Shea advocated total stapes footplate removal when using the polyethylene strut prosthesis and a vein graft to seal the oval window.[1] Shortly thereafter, Schuknecht advocated the use of a wire and fat prosthesis, and House advocated the use of a wire with absorbable gelatin sponge (Gelfoam) prosthesis.[2, 3] The use of the wire-Gelfoam or wire-fat necessitated a total footplate removal for the wire prosthesis to function satisfactorily. Other methods that could be considered a partial stapedectomy technique included the shattered footplate procedure with the use of a polyethylene strut and the subluxated footplate procedure, both of which necessitated removal of the superstructure of the stapes.[4] The two techniques quickly fell into disrepute because of the associated sensorineural hearing loss due to either surgical trauma or a perilymphatic fistula. In 1961, the piston concept was introduced in which a cup-piston prosthesis was used with a connective tissue graft of vein to seal the oval window.[5] The introduction of the piston prosthesis no longer required a total removal of the stapes footplate. Thus, the concept evolved of "removing only that part of the footplate which comes out easily."[11] As a result, this newly introduced surgical technique produced more successful hearing results and fewer inner ear complications. The same technique could be used for the thin blue footplate with minimal otosclerotic involvement, or for the obliterative footplate, in which only a stapedotomy opening ("drill-out") could be created. Measurement of the distance between the long process of the incus and stapes footplate was eliminated because a 4mm prosthesis would protrude into the vestibule 0.2mm to 0.3mm in virtually every case. This slight protrusion would create its self-centering effect. By interposing a vein graft between the prosthesis and vestibule, there was rarely a regrowth of otosclerotic bone, including the obliterative type. Also, because of this protrusion, migration of the piston in subsequent years was virtually unknown.

Because of the unique design of the cup-piston, the surgeon was permitted a choice of a total stapedec-

tomy or partial stapedectomy or stapedotomy. The classic cup-piston prosthesis was fabricated of 316L stainless steel, an alloy that is inert in living tissue and is also nonmagnetic. Its design enhanced the self-centering effect because of the cup attachment to the lenticular process of the incus (the true physiologic point of attachment), and also because of the axially placed stem protruding minimally through the footplate opening. The four holes in the cup and the hole on the distal end of the piston encouraged tissue and vascular ingrowth to secure the prosthesis and to allow capillaries to vascularize the lenticular process, thereby eliminating the avascular necrosis that so frequently occurred with the polyethylene strut. The 4mm length is used in virtually every stapedectomy case whether it is a drill-out stapedotomy, a partial footplate removal, or a total footplate removal. Any connective tissue can be used with this prosthesis, but the author's preference is a vein graft that outlines the oval window opening and ensures a complete immediate seal of the oval window. Moon advocates the cup-piston with areolar tissue.[6] The cup-piston prosthesis is radiopaque and easy to localize and identify on routine mastoid X-ray views. Comparison of impedance studies of various stapes prostheses has shown the stainless steel cup-piston to be the closest in compliance to that of a normal mobile stapes.[7] Hearing results reported by otologic surgeons who have used this technique have consistently confirmed a 96 per cent air-bone gap closure to within 10dB.[8–10] Similarly, the complete closure (and overclosure) rate has been repeatedly confirmed at the 80 per cent level, which the wire-tissue prosthesis and wire-pistons have yet to attain.

Because the stapes does not increase in size with age, the 4mm cup-piston prosthesis has been used in children as young as the age of 5 as well as in adults and the elderly.

All patients who demonstrate an air-bone gap and normal results on otologic examination are candidates for stapedectomy surgery if stapedial fixation is found at the time of the middle ear exploration. Approximately 22 per cent of otosclerotic patients have a diminished cochlear reserve with a Shambaugh preoperative bone conduction classification of D or E. These patients have very severe mixed hearing losses, and in many, only a partial footplate removal can be obtained. These also are the patients who most frequently show complete closure and overclosure of the air-bone gap. For these, the extra 10dB of hearing gain is very crucial because of their mixed hearing loss. Approximately 74 per cent of the patients undergoing surgery have a partial or total footplate removal that doesn't necessitate drilling. The remaining 26 per cent require drilling to create a fenestra 0.8mm in diameter or larger to accept the vein graft and cup-piston prosthesis.[11]

In 1980, Austin compared the results of total stapedectomy and partial stapedectomy, tissue seal and no tissue seal, and the small fenestra of Smyth. His statistical analysis, using chi-square tables for success or failure, sensorineural hearing loss, fistula, and complete air-bone gap closure, was computed. He concluded that a tissue seal provides a better success rate, a significantly lower risk of fistula, and a better hearing result in terms of complete closure or overclosure of the air-bone gap. He also noted that in addition to the increased risk of sensorineural complications and fistulas the small-diameter pistons used in stapedotomies did not provide as good a hearing result.[12]

SURGICAL TECHNIQUE

Stapedectomy footplate surgery follows a very basic principle—*be as atraumatic as possible in removing the footplate of the stapes.* This principle is contingent on removal of "only that part of the footplate which comes out easily."[11]

The routine stapedectomy is divided into three stages. The first stage is exposure of the middle ear, incus, stapes, and footplate area. The second is removal of the stapes superstructure. The third is removal of the stapes footplate. If the opening is 0.8mm or larger, the piston will function satisfactorily. The new fenestra must be sealed with a tissue graft, and a self-centering 4mm cup-piston will then bridge the gap from the oval window membrane to the incus (Figs. 27–1 through 27–5).

Footplate surgery can be classified as follows: 1) total footplate removal, in which a blue footplate with all oval window margins is visualized; 2) partial footplate removal, in which absent margins are in part of the circumference of the footplate, but where there is a blue area for perforating; 3) total footplate removal with drilling, in which a thick footplate with margins and without a blue center exists for perforating the footplate (biscuit footplate); 4) partial footplate removal with drilling, in which absent margins are in part of the circumference of the footplate, and there is no blue area for perforating the footplate; and 5) the drill-out for obliterative otosclerosis, in which no margins of the oval window and thick-mounding otosclerotic bone exist.

The technique used in this method involves the use of the cup-piston stainless steel stapes prosthesis and a vein graft to seal the re-created oval window. The vein graft is usually taken from the dorsum of the opposite hand by an assistant surgeon at the same time the ear is being operated on. After the vein is opened, it is thinned and as much of the adventitia is removed as possible. It is then trimmed to a final size of 4mm × 8mm. The graft is placed in a small bowl of intravenous saline until it is ready for insertion. The vein is folded over the tip of a smooth-jawed microalligator forceps, umbrella style, and it is inserted into the middle ear, avoiding contamination by not touching the ear speculum or the wall of the external auditory canal. The vein is placed over the oval window opening with its adventitial surface facing the vestibule. It is indented slightly into the vestibule with a fine, curved needle so that the exact location of the oval window is visualized. Measurement of the distance between the long process of the incus and the oval window is not necessary, as the 4mm-length prosthesis is used in virtually every case. If there is a drill-out, a 4.5mm prosthesis may optionally be used to ensure the self-centering effect by protruding 0.7mm into the vestibule. This will also retard formation of new otosclerotic bone. The prosthesis is grasped at its cup end with a small, smooth alligator forceps and targeted into the dimpled portion of the vein graft. It is then engaged on the lenticular process of the incus by slightly depressing the socket with the curved needle and then allowing the prosthesis to rise up and lock onto the lenticular process. The wire loop is rotated over the long process of the incus. The wire is not crimped, because the fit is precise. Mucosa will grow over the wire loop and secure its position. Before the middle ear is closed, the malleus is gently palpated to be certain that there is mechanical transmission of vibration from the malleolar handle to the prosthesis. The vein graft is inspected to be certain that the edges of the graft overlap the entire oval window area and that there is no inversion of any of the edges toward the vestibule; otherwise this problem may predispose to a perilymphatic fistula. The tympanomeatal flap is replaced, and the ear canal is packed with a strip of silk and an expandable methyl cellulose otowick and saturated with Neosporin (neomycin and polymyxin B) solution. The canal packing is removed in 1 week. Prophylactic antibiotics are used preoperatively and postoperatively (tetracycline), and steroid-antibiotic eardrops (Cortisporin otic suspension) are used in the ear canal for 1 week to maintain sterility of the ear canal and to prevent the otowick from drying out.

This prosthesis, because of its unique design, is a "smart" prosthesis—it can be fitted to the incus under many circumstances. It can fit an angled lenticular process, an extra-large lenticular process, an extra-long long process, a short long process, or a fractured, atrophic, or necrotic long process. When a narrow oval window niche or a prolapsed facial nerve is present, the prosthesis easily self-centers into the vein graft. When there is only a partial footplate removal or a drill-out for obliterative otosclerosis, the vein graft and prosthesis align perfectly because of the self-centering feature.[8]

MODIFICATIONS OF THE CUP-PISTON STAPES PROSTHESIS

Infrequently, an anatomic variation in the middle ear may result in a prosthesis that performs less than optimally. For these infrequent situations, a cup-piston prosthesis with an offset shaft will compensate for a short long process of the incus, a prolapsed facial nerve, and an abnormally high rise of the promontory.

When the lenticular process of the incus is absent or there is erosion of the long process of the incus, the modified Robinson-Moon-Lippy stapes prosthesis will compensate for the absent lenticular process. A cutout is in the cup of the prosthesis to accept the eroded long process of the incus, and the shaft is offset in a way similar to the Moon modification. The length of this prosthesis should be 4.5mm to compensate for the fact that the long process is in the socket rather than above it.

The standard dimension of the cup is 0.875mm, inside diameter, and 0.6mm, stem diameter, with a 4mm length. The cup-piston prosthesis is available with a large well (1.0mm) and a narrow stem (0.4mm) for the large lenticular process or the narrow oval window niche.

INDICATIONS FOR THE CUP-PISTON PROSTHESIS

The partial or total stapedectomy technique described in this chapter is used for stapes fixation due to otosclerosis, tympanosclerosis, and osteogenesis imperfecta. It is also used for congenital stapes anomalies and stapedial injuries, including fracture or dislocation of the stapes.

POSTOPERATIVE RESULTS

The postoperative hearing results with this partial-total stapedectomy technique have been consistent and repeatable since first reported in 1961. Subsequent reports by this author and others have repeatedly shown a success rate of closure to within 10dB of the air-bone gap to be 96 per cent. A partial success rate of 3 per cent exists in closure to within 20dB, leaving only 1 per cent unsuccessful.

Delayed hearing losses have been infrequent. In a 21-year period, the incidence of delayed conductive losses was 1.6 per cent, and cochlear losses of more than 10dB was 1.2 per cent. Thus, the total continued long-term success rate is 93 per cent. These data were derived from a 20-year study of 4815 stapedectomy cases.[13] The causes of a delayed conductive loss and their incidence are as follows: otosclerotic regrowth, 3/1000; tympanofibrosis, 2/1000; malleus fixation, 1/1000; postoperative tympanic membrane perforation, 1/1000; incus necrosis, 1/1000; prosthesis migration, 1/3000; prosthesis extrusion (preoperatively healed perforation), 3/1000; and perilymphatic fistula (first vein graft too small), 1/1000.

Delayed cochlear losses resulted primarily from perilymphatic fistula (vein graft too small), 1/2000; cochlear otosclerosis, 1/1000; presbycusis, 4/1000; and viral labyrinthitis, 2/1000.

DISCUSSION

Comparison with Wire-Stapes Prosthesis

With wire prostheses, design, fabrication, and measurement are not standardized. Wires attach to the incus on its long process and not at the physiologic site where the capitulum of the stapes is attached to the incus. Wires are at a disadvantage when there is a short incus, an eroded incus, or a prolapsed facial nerve. Over a long period of time, there is usually notching of the long process of the incus and occasionally a necrosis of the long process from the notching. Wire-tissue prostheses require a total footplate removal, which can be traumatic, and wires are not self-centering and frequently develop a delayed conductive hearing loss due to migration and impingement on the margin of the oval window.

Wire-piston prostheses also exhibit some of the same disadvantages, including the lack of standardization and the incus attachment problems mentioned earlier. The oval window opening must be precise, as an exact fit is mandatory for the stapedotomy technique. The length must be precise; the piston must protrude 0.2mm into the vestibule. When a stapedotomy opening is created, microfractures of the footplate may occur, increasing the risk of a perilymphatic fistula.

Results with wire prostheses vary greatly: success rates range from 80 to 95 per cent. With wire-piston stapedotomy procedures, there frequently is a residual, small, air-bone gap in the low frequencies. Complete closure reports are sparse, but the wire-fat complete closure rate has been reported at 15 to 20 per cent, and the wire-piston stapedotomy procedure complete closure rate has been reported at not more than 50 per cent. However, the cup-piston complete

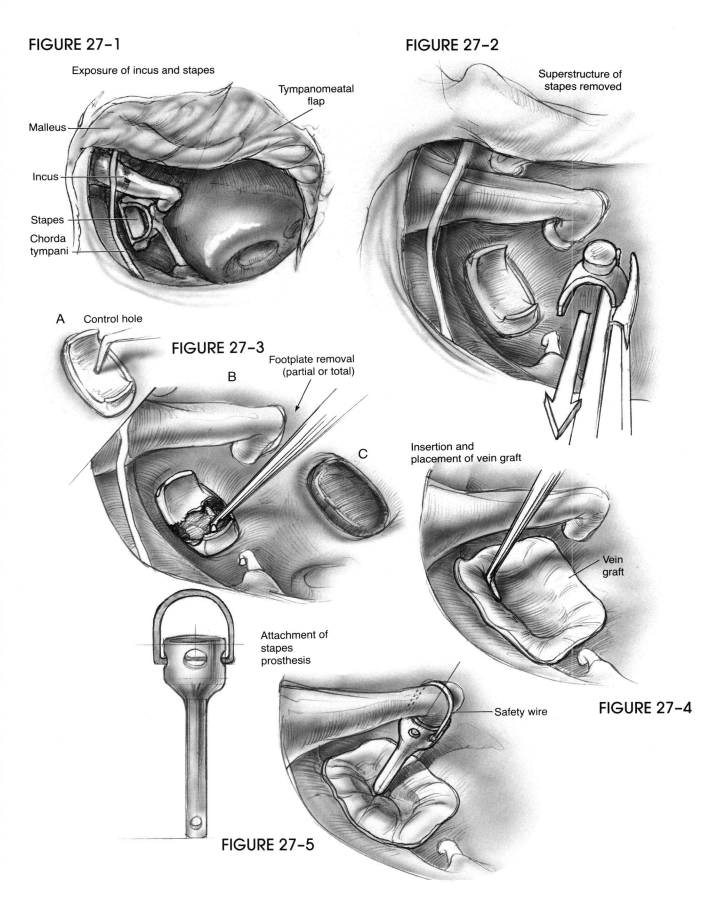

FIGURE 27-1

Exposure of incus and stapes

Malleus

Incus

Stapes

Chorda tympani

Tympanomeatal flap

FIGURE 27-2

Superstructure of stapes removed

FIGURE 27-3

A   Control hole

B   Footplate removal (partial or total)

C

Insertion and placement of vein graft

Vein graft

Attachment of stapes prosthesis

Safety wire

FIGURE 27-4

FIGURE 27-5

closure rate has consistently been at the 80 per cent level. Impedance studies have shown that wires have a very high compliance, whereas cup-piston prostheses have a compliance similar to that of a normal mobile stapes. This high compliance of wire prostheses reflects the less-than-perfect attachment to the incus because the wire is crimped over the long process and eventually loosens slightly when the notching of the incus occurs. Notching and loosening do not occur with the cup-piston prostheses.[7]

Stainless Steel Prostheses Versus Teflon Prostheses

Many materials have been used and advocated for the fabrication of stapes prostheses. Polytetrafluoroethylene (Teflon) has many advocates because of its inertness and lack of tissue reaction. The stainless steel cup-piston, which is fabricated of 316L stainless steel, has also shown lack of tissue reaction. The main difference between both materials is the weight. A Teflon cup-piston prosthesis weighs 3.3mg, and a stainless steel cup-piston weighs 12.5mg. An intact stapes freshly removed from the ear weighs 6mg. Bluestone first reported that by loading a polyethylene stapes prosthesis with a steel core, he would obtain a 10dB increase in hearing at 4000Hz and 8000Hz compared with that of the control group.[14] This author reported a study comparing the hearing results in patients with a Robinson stainless steel cup piston prosthesis and vein graft in the first ear and a Robinson Teflon cup-piston prosthesis and vein graft in the second ear.[15] This study eliminated all variables except the difference in weight of the prosthesis. The preoperative hearing level in each ear was the same, as was the footplate pathology in both ears. The design of the prosthesis was exactly the same, and only the weight differed. The stainless steel prosthesis weighed almost four times that of the Teflon prosthesis. The results demonstrated that the high-frequency gains in hearing were slightly better for the stainless steel ear (14dB) than for the Teflon ear (11dB). The rate of complete closure and overclosure of the air-bone gap was significantly greater in the stainless steel ear (80 per cent) than in the Teflon ear (52 per cent), even though the overall closure of the air-bone gap to within 10dB was 97 per cent in the stainless steel ear and 96 per cent in the Teflon ear. Impedance studies of this group again showed that the compliance of the stainless steel stapes prosthesis most resembled that of the normal mobile stapes, whereas the Teflon prosthesis showed a slightly reduced compliance (high impedance), but as a cup-piston, its compliance curves were more within the range of the mobile stapes than any of the wire prostheses.

This study proved that the heavier prosthesis resulted in a much greater complete closure and overclosure of the air-bone gap, and that there was a small but significant hearing advantage in postoperative results when a metallic prosthesis was used (6dB). In the mixed-type hearing loss, this increased hearing can have a significant effect on the patient's reaching a serviceable postoperative hearing level.[15]

Juvenile Otosclerosis

Otosclerosis is usually considered to be a disease of young and middle-aged adults, but juvenile otosclerosis occurs in 15.1 per cent of stapedectomy cases before the age of 18. The author presented an in-depth study of 610 patients out of a total of 4014 who developed clinical otosclerosis before the age of 18 and underwent stapedectomy.[16] Of these 610 patients, 35 underwent surgery before the age of 18, and 574 underwent surgery after the age of 18, but their hearing loss had developed during their juvenile years. The youngest patient was aged 5 years, and the average age of onset was 11.5 years.

The surgical technique performed on all 610 patients consisted of a partial or total footplate removal, as described in this chapter. All the patients under 18 received general anesthesia, whereas all the patients over age 18 had local anesthesia (lidocaine [Xylocaine] 2% with 1:30,000 epinephrine). The surgical footplate pathology varied considerably between those under 18 and those over 18. In the juvenile group, 66.7 per cent had a thin blue footplate, which was totally removed, whereas in those over 18, only 45.1 per cent had similar pathology. Partial footplate removal was performed in 5.5 per cent of the juveniles and 9.7 per cent of the group over 18. More significantly, drilling of the footplate because of diffuse otosclerosis involvement was necessary in 27.8 per cent of the juveniles and in 45.2 per cent of those who waited beyond the age of 18 years. Obliterative otosclerosis, which required drill-outs, was 5.6 per cent in the juvenile group and 12 per cent in their older counterparts. This result is in contrast to 3 per cent prevalence of obliterative otosclerosis for all stapedectomies.

The hearing results were more favorable in those who underwent surgery before the age of 18. One hundred per cent had an air-bone gap closure of 10dB or less, and 77.6 per cent complete closure or overclosure of the air-bone gap. Those who waited until after the age of 18 had a very successful closure rate, but only 93.6 per cent had their air-bone gap closed to within 10dB. Similarly, 77.3 per cent had complete closure or overclosure. A postoperative delayed conductive hearing loss occurred in only one patient (20dB) 5 years after the initial surgery in the juvenile group. The postoperative hearing level in all juveniles (4000Hz) remained the same or improved.

This study also revealed a very high incidence of bilateral otosclerosis (92 per cent) when the hearing loss appeared before the age of 18. Eighty per cent of juvenile otosclerotics had excellent cochlear reserve and did not show a deterioration of sensorineural function following stapedectomy. The longer the hearing loss existed, the greater the degree of footplate pathology that occurred. The probability of requiring a drill-out for obliterative otosclerosis increased fourfold when surgery was deferred to over the age of 18. Deferring a stapedectomy procedure in a juvenile may not be in the best interest of the patient because of the progressive nature of the footplate pathology and the increased necessity of drilling the footplate.[16]

SUMMARY

Stapedectomy and stapedotomy for the correction of hearing loss due to otosclerotic bony fixation of the stapes are surgical procedures that have evolved almost entirely in the "golden era" of otologic surgery (1955–1985). This golden era has passed, and even the most popular of the nationally known stapedectomists have experienced a dramatic decrease in the caseload for stapedectomy. This, in addition to the dispersion of patients to a larger number of trained otolaryngologists, has to some degree compromised the position of the otologic surgeon not only in developing skills and judgment but also in maintaining the acquired skill necessary to perform the more complicated and precise techniques. General otolaryngologists as well as otologists should, therefore, adopt a technique that is uncomplicated, relatively easy to perform, predictable, and safe for the patient. This technique should be standardized so that it can be performed in the same way for all stapedectomies. Reducing the variables and making one technique work for all cases of stapes fixation will allow the general otolaryngologist to gradually develop the high degree of skill necessary for this procedure. The technique adopted should have minimal risks and complications, either immediate or delayed and, if at all possible, should have the lowest incidence of revision, as revisions demand more skill, judgment, and knowledge than do primary stapedectomies.

More than 200,000 stapedectomies have been performed in the United States with the technique and prostheses described in this chapter. Despite the overall drop in the number of stapedectomy procedures performed annually, the number of Robinson cup-piston stapes prostheses used each year continues to increase, indicating the popularity of this simpler and safer technique.

References

1. Shea JJ Jr.: Fenestration of the oval window. Ann Otol Rhinol Laryngol 57: 932, 1958.
2. Schuknecht H: Stapedectomy and graft prosthesis operation. Acta Otolaryngol (Stockh) 51: 241–243, 1960.
3. House HP, Greenfield EC: Five year study of wire-loop absorbable gelatin sponge technique. Arch Otolaryngol Head Neck Surg 89: 420–421, 1969.
4. Goodhill V: Stapes Surgery for Otosclerosis. St. Louis, Paul B Hoeber, 1961, p 136.
5. Robinson M: The stainless steel stapedial prosthesis: One year's experience. Laryngoscope 73: 514, 1962.
6. Moon C: Stapedectomy connective tissue graft and the stainless steel prosthesis. Laryngoscope 78: 798–807, 1968.
7. Feldman A: Acoustic impedance measurement of post-stapedectomized ears. Laryngoscope 79: 6, 1132–1155, 1969.
8. Schondorf J, et al.: Der Einflub des Prosthesentyps auf das Langzeitergebnis der Stapedektomie. HNO 28: 153–157, 1980.
9. Elonka D, Derlacki E, Harrison W: Stapes prosthesis comparison. Otolaryngol Head Neck Surg 90: 263–265, 1982.
10. Girgis T: Stapedectomy: Robinson Stapes Prosthesis vs. Wire Prosthesis. American Society of Otology, Rhinology, and Laryngology. Middle Section Meeting. Chicago, January 1985.
11. Robinson M: A four year study of the stainless steel stapes. Arch Otolaryngol Head Neck Surg 82: 1965.
12. Austin DF: Stapedectomy with tissue seal. In Snow JB Jr. (ed): Controversy in Otolaryngology. Philadelphia, WB Saunders, 1980.
13. Robinson M: Total footplate extraction in stapedectomy. Ann Otol Rhinol Laryngol 90(6): 630–632, 1981.
14. Bluestone CD: Polyethylene stainless steel core in middle ear surgery. Arch Otolaryngol Head Neck Surg 76: 303, 1962.
15. Robinson M: Stapes prosthesis: Stainless steel vs. Teflon. Laryngoscope 84(11): 1982–1995, 1974.
16. Robinson M: Juvenile otosclerosis. Ann Otol Rhinol Laryngol 92(6): 1983.

28

Laser Revision Stapedectomy

T. MANFORD McGEE, M.D.

LARRY B. LUNDY, M.D.

This chapter is dedicated to T. Manford McGee, whose untimely death on April 14, 1992 occurred before he and I had completed this chapter. I had the privilege of working with Ted for 2 years and can speak for all who knew him, and there are many, in saying that he was an excellent surgeon, a superb physician, an outstanding role model, and most importantly, a wonderful friend. This unique combination of qualities embodied in T. Manford McGee is unequaled. He is, and will be, truly missed by all of us who knew him.

In recent years, the safety and efficacy of revision stapedectomy has come under scrutiny. Experienced surgeons report that the results of revision stapedectomy are often worse than results of primary stapedectomy, and that the risk of sensorineural hearing loss, tinnitus, and vertigo are increased. With the application of laser technology to revision stapes surgery, less traumatic and more precise techniques can be applied, thereby allowing better results and diminished risks, as compared with those of revision stapedectomy without lasers. This chapter reviews the clinically relevant principles of laser technology, compares results of revision stapedectomy with and without laser application, defines candidates for surgery, and reviews surgical technique.

LASER PHYSICS AND PRINCIPLES

Laser energy is derived from the release of energy (photons) occurring when stimulated electrons return to their resting orbital. As proposed by Einstein in 1917, when photons of the appropriate wavelengths strike excited atoms, a second additional photon is released as the electron returns to its ground state (Fig. 28–1). In this stimulated emission situation, both photons that are emitted from the excited atom have exactly the same frequency, direction, and phase as the incident photon, providing laser energy that is collimated, coherent, and monochromatic.

Lasers are typically named by the active medium, or the source of atoms that are excited and undergo stimulated emission of photons. The active medium can be either a liquid, solid, or gas. Common gas lasers include carbon dioxide, argon, and helium-neon. An example of solid state lasers are the Nd:YAG (neodymium:yttrium-aluminum-garnet) and the potassium titanyl phosphate crystal (KTP). The KTP laser is simply a Nd:YAG laser beam that passes through a KTP crystal, which halves the wavelength and doubles the frequency of the laser beam (Table 28–1).

The wavelength of the emitted photons, or laser beam, has important characteristics for tissue interaction. Lasers whose wavelengths fall into visible spectrum (380nm to 700nm) and infrared (700nm to 1mm) of the electromagnetic spectrum are considered thermal lasers. Interaction of these lasers with normal biologic materials is mediated by a photothermal process. On contact with tissue, the laser energy is converted to thermal energy, resulting in a rapid rise in tissue temperature. The laser-tissue interaction depends as much on the tissue type and its composition (e.g., bone, muscle, cartilage, or nerve) as it does on the laser energy.

Visible-spectrum laser (argon and KTP) energy absorption by tissue is partially dependent on tissue color. For soft tissue work, chromophores of hemoglobin and melanin absorb most of the energy. Lighter color tissues will reflect most of the laser energy. Energy absorption from the invisible carbon dioxide laser is primarily by intracellular and extracellular water, which is instantaneously converted to steam.

For any laser, the magnitude of the laser-tissue interaction can be regulated by the laser's power output, the power density at the point of impact, and the energy fluence. Every surgeon who uses a laser should thoroughly understand these fundamental concepts. Power is the time rate at which energy is emitted and is expressed as watts. The power output is directly adjusted by the control panel on the laser console. Laser energy is delivered through a focusing lens. Power density is a measure of the intensity, or concentration, of the laser beam spot size (Fig. 28–2). It is the ratio of power to surface area of the spot size and is expressed in terms of watts per square centimeter:

$$\text{Power density} = \frac{\text{Power (watts)}}{\text{Area of spot size (cm}^2\text{)}}$$

where area of spot size is πr^2, and
where r = spot size radius in centimeters.

Power density is inversely proportional to the square of the radius of the spot size. Consequently, for any specific power output, changes in the spot size can have a tremendous effect on power density (Fig. 28–3).

The third fundamental, practical concept is that of fluence, which is simply the power density × time. This is the total amount of energy delivered to the tissues:

$$\text{Fluence (joules)} = \frac{\text{Power (watts)} \times \text{exposure time (seconds)}}{\text{Area of spot size (cm}^2\text{)}}$$

As fluence increases, the volume of affected tissue also increases. The thermal energy having an impact on tissue rises dramatically as the time of exposure increases. If power density $\frac{W}{cm^2}$ is held constant and the exposure time is doubled, the energy delivered is doubled. However, the thermal effect of the tissue increases significantly because the rise in temperature is continuous. For example, assume the laser power is set at 2.0W, the spot size is 0.2mm², and exposure time is 0.2 seconds. Is this the same as delivering two separate impulses at 0.1 seconds each? Yes and no. Yes, it is the same in terms of energy delivered *from* the laser. But no, it is not the same in terms of thermal energy imparted *to* the tissue, because during the time between the two separate 0.1-second pulses, no matter how brief, the tissue is cooling down (Fig. 28–4).

TABLE 28–1. Characteristics of Laser Types

Characteristic	Argon	KTP-532	Carbon Dioxide
Medium	Gas	Crystal	Gas
Wavelength	488nm–514nm	532nm	10,600nm
Color	Blue-green	Green	Invisible
Smallest spot size	0.150mm	0.150mm	0.150mm
Delivery	Hand piece or micromanipulator	Hand piece or micromanipulator	Micromanipulator
Absorption	Pigment	Pigment	Water

FIGURE 28–1. According to the Bohr atomic model, an electron can absorb a photon, and the electron makes a transition to a higher energy level from its normal ground state. The electron will eventually return to the ground state by the spontaneous emission of a photon. In the condition of stimulated emission, a photon of appropriate energy interacts with the electron already in its excited state, thereby causing the release of two photons. (From Weisberger EC: Lasers in Head and Neck Surgery. New York, Igaku-Shoin, 1991.)

FIGURE 28–2. Illustration of planes of focus with spot size and power density.

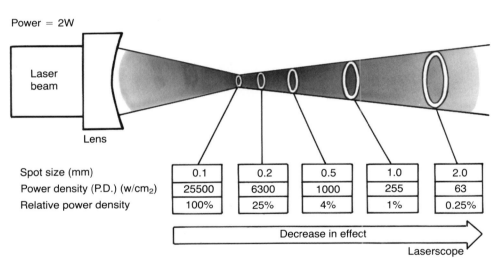

Power = 2W

Laser beam

Lens

Spot size (mm)	0.1	0.2	0.5	1.0	2.0
Power density (P.D.) (w/cm$_2$)	25500	6300	1000	255	63
Relative power density	100%	25%	4%	1%	0.25%

Decrease in effect

Laserscope

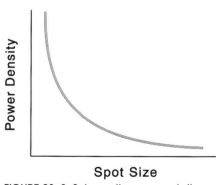

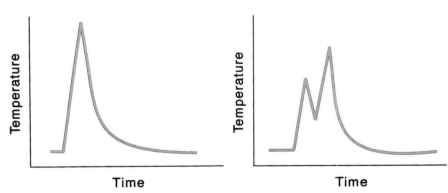

FIGURE 28–3. Schematic representation of relationship between spot size and power density.

FIGURE 28–4. Schematic representation of temperature–time of exposure relationship for a single pulse versus two separate pulses.

Granted, other factors come into play, such as the absorption characteristics of the damaged tissue in the center of the laser spot as well as dissipation of heat, but the important concept is that of the rise and fall of the temperature.

HISTORY OF REVISION STAPEDECTOMY

Several issues arise in the application of laser technology to otologic-neurotologic surgery, including some that are unique to revision stapedectomy. Are equal or better results obtained with conventional techniques or laser techniques for revision stapes surgery? Is there a difference in unfavorable results or complications with conventional techniques compared with laser techniques? What are the potential and real hazards of laser revision stapedectomy as compared with those of conventional techniques for revision stapedectomy? Which laser should be used? Which modality should be used—hand-held fiberoptic instrument or micromanipulator delivery? What are the advantages and disadvantages of laser usage in revision stapedectomy? Who is a candidate for its use?

The use of the laser in temporal bone surgery was the object of experiments as early as 1967 by Sataloff [1] and in 1972 by Stahle et al.[2] The evolution of laser otologic surgery has been based on a mixture of clinical, experimental animal, and laboratory observations. In 1977, Wilpizeski et al.[3] examined argon and carbon dioxide lasers on monkeys by performing a myringotomy, ossicular amputation, stapes fenestrations, lysis of stapedial tendon, and crurotomy. They noted damage to the organ of Corti in monkeys after using "excessive power." Escudero et al.[4] was the first to use a laser in human otologic surgery in 1977. They used the argon laser with a fiberoptic handpiece to tack temporalis fascia to tympanic membrane perforations. Perkins,[5] in 1979, presented a preliminary report of argon laser stapedotomy with excellent initial results in 11 patients. In 1980, DiBartolomeo and Ellis[6] expanded argon laser applications in 30 patients for middle ear and external ear soft tissue and bony problems. In ten patients, otosclerosis was corrected, including one revision case. In 1983, McGee[7] reported on the use of argon laser in over 500 otologic cases, 100 of which were primary stapedectomies. There were no laser-related complications in his study. This has held true over time, as in 1989 McGee[8] reported an update on 2500 tympanomastoid procedures, of which 510 were primary stapedectomies. By comparing 100 consecutive laser stapedectomies with a previous 139 small fenestra stapedectomies using instruments, McGee found that the laser technique permitted much shorter hospital stay, less vertigo, and excellent hearing results (93 per cent air-bone gap clo-

sure within 10dB at 6 months). Laser settings were 1.5W, 0.1 seconds, and a spot size of 120μm (250mm lens). This large study indicated the safety of argon laser use for stapedectomy and yielded comparable hearing results and less vertigo. This clinical evidence is not consistent with experimental animal studies, in which temporary changes of cochlear microphonics and saccular perforations were noted.[7, 9, 10] Clinical experience from several centers has illustrated the safe use of lasers in ear surgery; however, arguments and opinions persist regarding the best type of laser.[11-15]

In recent years, the potential use of laser technology for revision stapedectomy has been appreciated. Revision stapedectomy possesses a different set of challenges than primary stapedectomy. Stapedectomy failure can manifest as recurrence of conductive hearing loss, sensorineural hearing loss, or dizziness and vertigo. Sensorineural hearing loss can be related to progression of otosclerosis or to other unrelated reasons (e.g., presbycusis, acoustic trauma, or cerebellopontine angle tumor). Likewise, the evaluation of dizziness in a poststapedectomy patient requires the assessment and elimination of the usual causes. Ménière's disease, labyrinthitis, trauma, medications, and chronic illnesses all must be considered in the differential diagnosis. Revision stapedectomy is not indicated in these circumstances. In cases in which dizziness and sensorineural hearing loss are suspected to be the result of a perilymph fistula (e.g., a polyethylene strut stapedectomy), exploration and revision stapedectomy are reasonable options.

By far the most common manifestation of stapedectomy failure is reaccumulation of the conductive hearing loss. There are several causes of this, including prosthesis migration at the oval window, prosthesis displacement at the incus, oval window bony reclosure, oval window fibrous closure, incus necrosis, incus or malleus fixation, and a short prosthesis. These different causes can be identified only at the time of surgery.

Two primary issues are involved in revision stapedectomy—the potential benefit of hearing improvement of the conductive component versus the potential risk of inner ear damage (sensorineural hearing loss and prolonged vertigo). The resolution of these issues depends on the pathology encountered, and the key factor is the management of the oval window. Glasscock et al.,[16] Sheehy et al.,[17] and Lippy and Schuring[18, 19] advocate leaving the neomembrane intact and undisturbed, if possible, in revision cases to reduce the risk of severe sensorineural hearing loss, even though it may result in fewer patients with postoperative hearing improvement. Feldman and Schuknecht,[20] Pearman and Dawes,[21] and Derlacki[22] reported opening the neomembrane to identify the vestibule and ensure correct prosthesis placement. For revision stapedectomy with mechanical instruments, air-bone gap closure to within 10dB is achieved in fewer than half of patients.[16, 17, 20, 22–24] The incidence of significant sensorineural hearing loss is 3 to 30 per cent, and up to 14 per cent have profound sensorineural hearing loss.[16, 17, 20, 22–24] These results for revision stapedectomy are substantially different from the accepted standard for primary stapedectomy of greater than 90 per cent closure of air-bone gaps to 10dB or less, maintenance of good speech discrimination, and less than 1 per cent incidence of significant sensorineural hearing loss.

Removing the prosthesis from a fibrous oval window and opening the oval window into the vestibule with instruments presumably traumatize the inner ear, resulting in sensorineural hearing loss or vertigo. Temporal bone studies[25, 26] on poststapedectomy patients demonstrated fibrous adhesions between the prosthesis or neomembrane of the oval window and the saccule and utricle. The use of laser energy at the oval window is more precise and less traumatic than mechanical instruments for removing the prosthesis from the oval window.

The success of a revision stapedectomy depends on the cause of failure. In approximately two thirds of cases of failed standard primary stapedectomies, the cause of failure is prosthesis migration. After the tympanomeatal flap is elevated, the cause of initial failure is identified. The surgeon must assess the mobility and integrity of the ossicular chain, the status of the oval window, and the precise relationship of the existing prosthesis to the oval window. A common situation is that of a prior total footplate removal stapedectomy with a fat or fascia graft in the oval window and a prosthesis that has migrated. The existing tissue graft obscures the lateral margins and depth of the oval window. The surgeon's ability to see the precise relationship of the prosthesis to the vestibule is compromised by the attendant risk of sensorineural hearing loss with manipulation of these structures. Herein lies the elegant advantage of laser technology—atraumatic, precise vaporization of tissue obliterating the oval window, thereby allowing identification of underlying structures and their anatomic relationships as well as underlying pathology (e.g., bony regrowths, fibrous vestibule, and inappropriate prosthesis length).

TECHNIQUE

The vast majority of stapedectomies, either primary or revision, are performed with the patient under local anesthesia with intravenous sedation. Typically, 1ml to 2ml of fentanyl citrate plus 1mg to 2mg of midazolam are administered intravenously before the ear is prepared and draped. A short-acting barbiturate (50mg to 100mg of thiopental) is administered intravenously just prior to infiltration of the ear canal. This agent allows a brief somnolence, thereby allowing painless infiltration of the local anesthetic. One per cent lidocaine (Xylocaine) with 1:15,000 dilution of epinephrine is used to infiltrate the ear canal skin with a 27-gauge needle. Typically, only 0.3ml to 0.5ml of this solution is used. The relatively high concentration of epinephrine is not necessary for adequacy of vasoconstriction but is used for a more rapid onset of vasoconstriction. During the surgical procedure, if the patient is restless and appears inadequately sedated, additional medication can be given. Caution must be exercised, as an impatient surgeon or an inexperienced anesthetist can overmedicate, which paradoxically increases restlessness and movement.

A transcanal tympanomeatal-stapedectomy flap is raised with the patient under local anesthesia with vasoconstriction and intravenous sedation. On entry into the middle ear, the cause of the conductive hearing loss is assessed (Fig. 28–5). The malleus and incus are inspected and gently palpated to rule out fixation. Any obstructing middle ear fibrous adhesions are lysed with the laser. The chorda tympani nerve, if present, is frequently adhered to the tympanomeatal flap and can be sharply dissected with the laser. At the appropriate setting, the obliterating tissue of the oval window surrounding the prosthesis is vaporized until the exact oval window margins and depth are identified. For the KTP laser, the spot size is 0.150mm, the power setting is 1.2W to 1.4W, and the pulse duration is 0.1 seconds. For the carbon dioxide laser on the superpulse mode, the spot size is also 0.150mm, the power setting is 0.8W to 1.0W, and the pulse duration is 0.1 seconds. The attachment of the prosthesis at the incus is freed or loosened with a right-angled hook. The prosthesis may be removed at this point or may require further lysis at its base (Fig. 28–6). A series of laser "hits" are applied to the oval window neomembrane in a nonoverlapping rosette pattern (Fig. 28–7). A minimum of 2-second intervals between bursts is necessary to minimize heat build-up of the neomembrane and perilymph. A 0.6mm stapedotomy is created and is incomplete until the vestibule and clear perilymph are identified. The stapedotomy size is confirmed by use of a 0.5mm McGee-Farrior rasp. If the incus long process is satisfactory, a McGee 0.5mm stainless steel piston with a platinum ribbon is used. A length of 4.25mm is used in 90 to 95 per cent of cases. If the lenticular process is unsatisfactory, a McGee 0.6mm stainless steel piston with a large hook is used from the malleus to the fenestra. The most commonly used length for this instrument is 4.50mm to 4.75mm. After crimping, the ossicular chain is gently palpated to ensure freedom of movement and

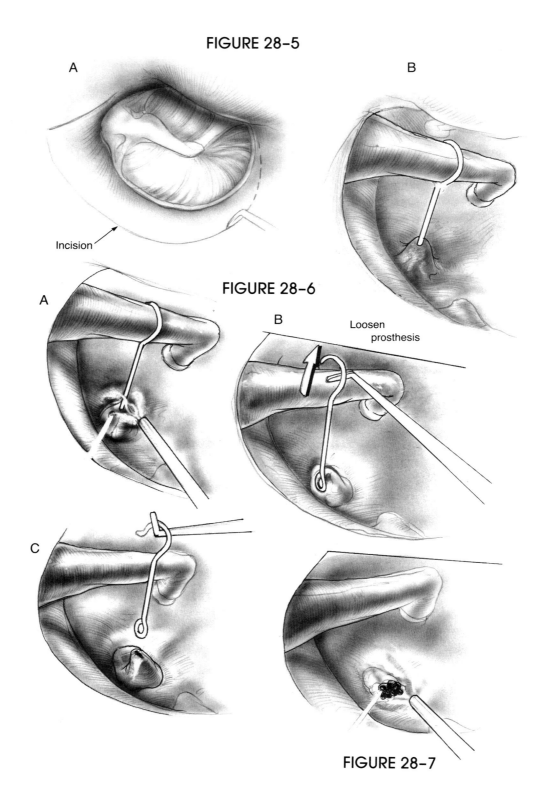

FIGURE 28-5

A

B

Incision

FIGURE 28-6

A

B

Loosen
prosthesis

C

FIGURE 28-7

FIGURE 28-5. *A*, Elevation of tympanomeatal flap. *B*, Migrated prosthesis with oval window obliteration.

FIGURE 28-6. *A*, Dissection of distal stapes prosthesis. *B*, Loosening of prosthesis at the incus. *C*, Removal of prosthesis.

FIGURE 28-7. Opening of vestibule.

appropriateness of prosthesis length. The oval window is sealed with areolar fascia or absorbable gelatin sponge. The tympanomeatal flap is returned to its anatomic position and secured with saline-moistened absorbable gelatin sponges.

RESULTS

The senior author[27] reported on 185 KTP laser revision stapedotomy cases, of which 77 involved actual removal of an existing prosthesis from the oval window, creating a new fenestra, and placing a new prosthesis. Of these 77 cases, 80.5 per cent had air-bone gap closure to within 10dB and 92.3 per cent had air-bone gap closure to within 20dB. Two of 77 (2.6 per cent) had a sensorineural hearing loss of 10dB or more at 4000Hz. Seventy of 77 (90.9 per cent) had no change in speech discrimination, six of 77 (7.8 per cent) had improvement of discrimination greater than 10 per cent, and one of 77 (1.3 per cent) had a loss of 24 per cent of discrimination. There were no dead ears. No patients reported an increase in their tinnitus, if it had been present preoperatively. Dizziness and vertigo were not a problem, as all patients were discharged to home within 23 hours, the majority within a few hours after completion of the surgery.

Lesinski[13] reported on his experience with the carbon dioxide lasers in 59 patients, in whom closure of the air-bone gap to within 10dB was obtained in 66 per cent, to within 20dB in 89 per cent. No patients experienced significant sensorineural hearing loss in the speech range (500Hz, 1000Hz, 2000Hz, and 3000Hz). Two of 59 (3 per cent) lost more than 15dB at 4000Hz. No patient experienced perioperative dizziness or vertigo.

Comparison of Lasers

Like any tool or instrument, each type of laser has advantages and disadvantages. The visible-wavelength lasers (argon and KTP) have the practical advantage of precision because the aiming beam and the working beam are one and the same. The blue-green (argon) or green (KTP) aiming beam has clear, crisp margins, which allows extreme precision. The carbon dioxide laser beam is invisible; therefore, a separate aiming beam (helium-neon) is required. This aiming beam is coaxial and focuses in a different plane from the carbon dioxide laser beam because of the differences in wavelength of the helium-neon and carbon dioxide lasers. Therefore, with these lasers, there is more potential for misalignment and a greater margin of error than with the KTP. It is critical that the carbon dioxide laser and its helium-neon aiming beam be calibrated precisely and checked frequently during the procedure to ensure maximum accuracy.

The tissue absorption of the visible-laser energy is color dependent, and for the argon and KTP lasers, peak absorption is dark red. For lightly colored tissues, such as a neomembrane or bone, a significant amount of laser energy is reflected rather than absorbed. A practical solution involves placing a minute quantity of blood in the field, or applying several bursts (*not* in rapid succession) to get a dark char, thereby increasing the laser energy absorption. With the carbon dioxide laser, this absorption is not a problem, because the laser beam is invisible, and absorption by water and tissue is not color dependent.

The visible-wavelength laser beam can be carried by thin fiberoptic cables, which allow two modes of delivery: a micromanipulator attached to the microscope or a hand-held probe (Fig. 28–8). The hand-held

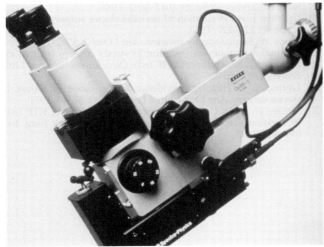
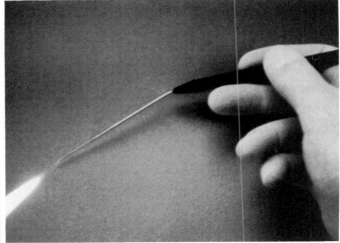

A   B

FIGURE 28–8. *A*, Micromanipulator delivery system. *B*, Hand piece delivery system.

As the incidence of surgery for otosclerosis declines, fewer surgeons acquire adequate experience in stapedectomy surgery. Even fewer treat the unusual problems of either complicated or unsuccessful stapedectomy. This chapter defines and illustrates unusual intraoperative problems and solutions. The solutions are presented in a logical, safe, stepwise manner to avoid irreversible difficulties.

Before the technical aspects of the chapter begin, some practical and philosophical points should be presented. When surgery is scheduled, a significant family member or friend should accompany the patient so that another person fully understands the goals and risks of the proposed surgery. During surgery, the surgeon should terminate the procedure if he or she encounters a problem that might further jeopardize the patient's hearing. Both patient and surgeon can more easily accept termination rather than a bad result. Do not be a compulsively neat surgeon during stapedectomy. For example, do not search for the superstructure should it fall into the hypotympanum; do not remove pieces of footplate floating in the perilymph; do not force on a wire keeper that is excessively tight. Remember, that second-stage procedures can be done.

This chapter reviews the technique of stapedectomy and the principles that prevent misadventures and discusses solutions to unusual problems. In addition, revision techniques for failed stapedectomy are detailed. Finally, cases of advanced otosclerosis with little or no testable hearing are discussed.

INTRAOPERATIVE AUDIOMETRY

In the past, surgeons demonstrated the success of stapedectomy when the patient under local anesthesia heard a sound ranging from a soft whisper to a loud voice. More sophisticated methods are now applied with great success. By using a portable audiometer in the operating room, the surgeon can precisely measure a patient's hearing before and after surgery. Such improved assessment benefits both surgeon and patient.

A portable audiometer from any manufacturer may be used. One of the earphones is removed from the headset and inserted into a sterile plastic sleeve, which is available as a disposable orthopedic drill sleeve. The surgeon holds the sterile earphone to the patient's ear or speculum (Fig. 29–1). Testing begins at an easily heard threshold for the patient. Threshold progressively descends until the patient cannot hear most tones. The frequency with the greatest air-bone gap is usually used for single-frequency testing, but multiple frequencies can easily be tested. Circulating nurses can easily learn to operate the audiometer.

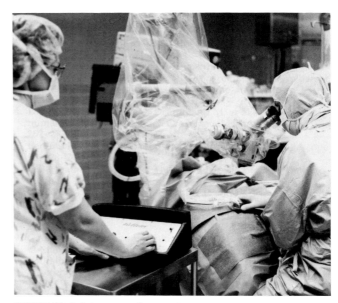

FIGURE 29–1. Intraoperative audiometer set-up.

Hearing is tested at the beginning and the end of the operation to measure the hearing gain. In spite of the disturbed eardrum and blood in the middle ear and in the perilymph, the hearing will usually be within 15dB and often as close as 5dB of the final hearing result.

Use of an audiometer in the operating room offers several advantages. First, the surgeon and the patient have instant and accurate feedback on the success of the operation. Second, the improvement of hearing defines the end point of surgery. Third, in revision cases, by repositioning the prosthesis in various locations in the oval window and then testing the hearing, the surgeon can explore the footplate without dissecting the tissue over the oval window. Finally, in difficult cases, different solutions can be attempted to determine the best prosthesis and best placement for optimum hearing.

ROUTINE STAPEDECTOMY

The basic technique of our standard stapedectomy, which has remained unchanged for 30 years, illustrates the principle of a safe approach. Use of this technique and the application of the principles described earlier have closed the air-bone gap in 96 per cent of 12,000 cases. Nonhearing ears developed in only 0.7 per cent.

Before surgery, our private surgical nurse carefully explains what to expect to each patient. This knowledge helps an otherwise anxious patient be calm and cooperative. In the holding area before surgery, the ear canal and tympanic membrane are treated by ionophoresis for 10 minutes with 5ml of 4 per cent lidocaine and 1ml of epinephrine 1:1000. The anesthesiologist or nurse anesthetist begins an intravenous infusion and then monitors the patient during the stapedectomy.

The operation begins with the injection of four quadrants of the ear canal with a mixture of 0.5ml of epinephrine 1:1000 solution and 4.5ml of 2 per cent lidocaine. This solution results in maximal control of bleeding and minimal cardiovascular changes or symptoms. If the patient remains anxious, intravenous medication is administered in a dose that keeps the patient comfortable but awake enough to permit intraoperative audiometry.

Each step of the operation should be completed carefully and exactly. Precision in one step makes the next step easier and results in perfection.

The speculum holder, which is always used, is positioned to see each portion of the tympanomeatal flap incision as it is made. The flap should be elevated carefully to prevent damage to the skin and tympanic membrane. As the middle ear is entered, an absorbable gelatin sponge (Gelfoam) pledget soaked in the anesthetic solution is placed into the middle ear to anesthetize the middle ear mucosa. As the drum is pushed back, the manubrium of the malleus and incus can be seen and palpated. Any fixation should not preclude completion of the operation but should be noted so that the patient can later be advised if the hearing result is suboptimal.[1]

A sharp, strong curet simplifies the task of curetting the ear canal. Enough of the scutum should be removed to see the origin of the stapedius tendon, the facial nerve, and the entire footplate area.

A control hole is placed in the footplate at the junction of the anterior one third and the posterior two thirds of the footplate. The hole facilitates later removal of the footplate. It also permits early detection of a rare perilymph gusher, when it can be more easily controlled. In addition, should the footplate come out with the superstructure, the hole will reduce the sudden change of pressure in the vestibule.

After the incudostapedial joint is severed, the superstructure is fractured toward the promontory and removed to expose the entire footplate. The control hole can be extended across the footplate, and then the footplate posterior to the hole is removed. A vein from the forearm, previously harvested, pressed, and prepared, can be immediately placed across the oval window with the adventitial side down to protect the vestibule.

The Robinson stainless steel prosthesis is then placed by use of a two-handed technique. One hand lifts the incus with an incus hook while the other gently directs the prosthesis with a strut guide. A prosthesis with a large well, narrow stem, and length of 4mm is suitable in 99 per cent of cases, thus eliminating the need to measure. Because this prosthesis centers itself in the oval window opening, middle ear packing is not used. The patient's hearing can be tested immediately after the tympanic membrane is replaced. If the wire keeper does not easily swing over the lenticular process, it is not necessary to employ it. Forcing it may displace the prosthesis from the center of the oval window (Fig. 29–2).

Intraoperative Problems

TYMPANOMEATAL FLAP TEARS. To avoid tearing the flap as it is lifted, the speculum is repositioned frequently for better vision, especially when dissection is near the annulus, where most tears occur. A torn flap need not stop the operation: it can be repaired by approximation or with tissue, such as vein, fascia, or perichondrium, whatever tissue is used to seal the oval window. Placement of the tissue underneath the tear gives the best result. Enough tissue should have been previously harvested both to cover the oval window and to repair any tears or perforations.

TYMPANIC MEMBRANE PERFORATION. Tears that involve the tympanic membrane are repaired in the same manner as are tympanomeatal flap tears. When a perforation develops centrally as a result of manipulation, a piece of tissue is placed under the perforation and packed against the tympanic membrane with absorbable gelatin sponge. The edges of the perforation are not treated.

ATROPHIC TYMPANIC MEMBRANE. Future problems should be anticipated in a patient with a thin tympanic membrane, signs of a healed perforation, or an atrophic or necrotic incus. As in treatment of a perforation, the intact tympanic membrane is reinforced from the underside of the tympanic membrane with tissue. This procedure should thicken the tympanic membrane and protect the incus by providing a better blood supply.

OSSICULAR DISLOCATION. During stapedectomy, the incus may be inadvertently loosened in several situations. Loosening may occur when the scutum is curetted away, when a wire is tightened on the incus, or when an instrument strikes the incus. The practical solution is to attach a rigid stapes prosthesis to the lenticular process that will help hold the incus in place. Surprisingly, two thirds of these cases will be successful; only a small number of unsuccessful cases will need a revision with a different solution.

FIXED MALLEUS. The malleus must always be routinely palpated with the same instrument under the

TABLE 29–1. Malleus-Incus Fixation and Otosclerosis Hearing Results (n = 102)

DEGREE OF FIXATION	AIR-BONE GAP (%)			
	Overclosed	*Within 10dB*	*Worsened Conduction*	*Sensorineural Loss*
Slightly (*n* = 40)	70	96	0	0
Moderately (*n* = 28)	29	97	0	0
Totally (*n* = 34)	24	68	9	0

surgeon's direct vision from the underside of the tympanic membrane. The malleus may be slightly fixed, moderately fixed, or totally fixed. If slight or moderate, the final result of stapedectomy will be as if the malleus were not fixed at all. The success rate will be the same (96 to 97 per cent), but the overclosure rate will be substantially reduced.[1, 2] Thus, partial malleus fixation should be ignored. When the malleus (and probably the incus) is totally fixed, a stapedectomy should be completed. Most of the footplate should be removed to create a large enough oval window opening for a second future procedure (malleus or tympanic membrane to oval window technique). Sixty-eight per cent of the totally fixed malleus cases will be successful to within 10dB, and the air-bone gap will be closed to within 10dB to 20dB in an additional 15 per cent. Cases with an air-bone gap of 20dB or more should be considered for a second-stage procedure. Applying this simple solution over the past 20 years, we have enjoyed surprisingly good hearing results, and no patient with otosclerosis and a fixed malleus has had a further sensorineural loss (Table 29–1). A more complex or possibly traumatic procedure can be postponed until an oval window tissue seal is present. Procedures to free the head of the malleus are usually nonrewarding on a permanent basis.

PARTIAL ABSENCE OF THE INCUS. When a partial absence of the long process of the incus is found in a patient with otosclerosis, a stapedectomy is still done. In place of the standard prosthesis, the Lippy-modified Robinson prosthesis is used. The fenestra should be somewhat larger than usual because the prosthesis will not self-center.[2, 3] The technique of prosthesis placement is important to success. The lower business end of the prosthesis is placed on the vein graft; the upper end with the open well, toward the eroded

incus. The prosthesis is then guided onto the remaining incus from the direction of the promontory. When a modified prosthesis is used, the hearing success rate is 80 per cent. If the lenticular process comes to a pointed rather than a blunted end, a microscissors can be used to square the end. One must be extremely careful not to displace the incus with this maneuver. If the incus cannot be cut easily, the modified prosthesis should still be placed under the pointed incus. Over the years, the prosthesis may erode through the pointed terminal end of the incus, leaving a blunt end. A revision procedure with the modified prosthesis can be performed with an even greater chance of success (Figs. 29–3 and 29–4).

DEHISCENT FACIAL NERVE. In otosclerosis surgery, the facial nerve rarely interferes with a stapedectomy except in a congenitally deformed middle ear or when the facial nerve canal is completely dehiscent. If any part of the footplate is visible, a stapedectomy usually can be accomplished. A hole should first be made in the visible part of the footplate. Often, a large portion of the footplate can be removed from underneath the dehiscent nerve by retraction of the facial nerve with the shaft of the same instrument used to extract the footplate. If the footplate cannot be removed, the technique is to shatter the footplate with a pointed pick—even blindly, if necessary. After a vein graft is placed across the open oval window, the prosthesis is inserted by compressing the facial nerve with the prosthesis. In our experience, this technique of compressing the facial nerve has never caused permanent facial nerve paralysis. However, the success rate is slightly lower for these cases.

OBLITERATIVE OTOSCLEROSIS. An obliterative footplate is saucerized with a 0.5mm-diameter carbide

FIGURE 29–2. Routine stapedectomy.

FIGURE 29–3. The Lippy-modified Robinson prosthesis.

FIGURE 29–4. Modified 4.5mm Robinson prosthesis in place on vein graft covering oval window.

FIGURE 29–5. Robinson prosthesis in place on mobilized footplate.

FIGURE 29–6. Revision stapedectomy wire prosthesis is pushed aside.

FIGURE 29–2

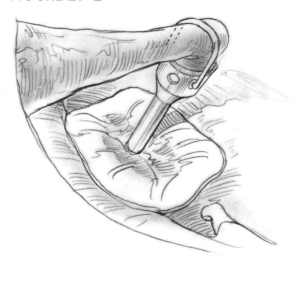

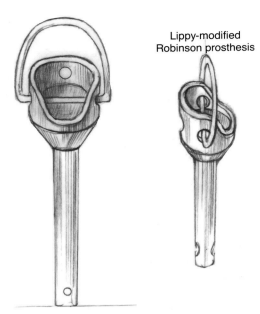

Lippy-modified
Robinson prosthesis

FIGURE 29–3

FIGURE 29–4

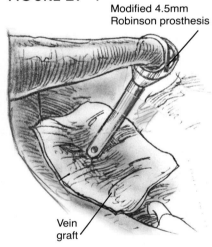

Modified 4.5mm
Robinson prosthesis

Vein
graft

FIGURE 29–5

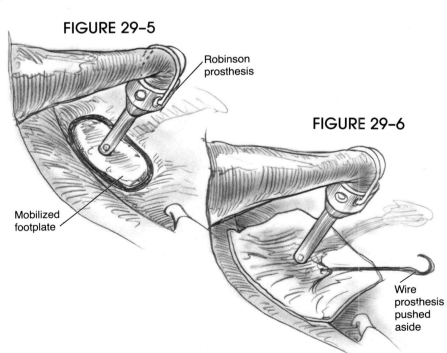

Robinson
prosthesis

Mobilized
footplate

FIGURE 29–6

Wire
prosthesis
pushed
aside

TABLE 29–2. Prosthesis on Mobilized Footplate

| | FOOTPLATE | |
HEARING	Thick White (n = 56) (%)	Thin Blue-Mixed (n = 92) (%)
Successful	52	95
Conduction worse	7	2
Sensorineural loss worse	0	0
Successful after revision	76	—

burr. As large an area as possible is drilled to saucerize the footplate. A small opening of the footplate should be avoided until a wide area is saucerized because enlargement of a small footplate opening surrounded by thick, hard footplate may be impossible. The aim is to develop a blue, eggshell appearance over as large an area of the footplate as possible, without penetrating the footplate. Occasionally, only the membrane under the footplate remains after drilling. It is helpful to drill off a small portion of the promontory adjacent to the footplate when the oval window niche is too narrow. The bit rests on the footplate, and several gentle outward strokes from the footplate are made. The footplate is then opened with a needle, and the pieces are removed with picks. Generally, more footplate is removed in this procedure than in routine stapedectomy in an attempt to prevent otosclerosis regrowth. If mobilization of the footplate occurs, the drilling is terminated and a prosthesis placed (see under *Floating Footplate*).

In the 1960s, 30 per cent of the footplates were drilled, in the 1970s, 9 per cent, and in the 1980s, 11 per cent. Fifty-five per cent of the cases overclosed, 80 per cent were successful, and 0.2 per cent were worse. Although the results of drill-out cases are certainly acceptable, they are not as good as non–drill-out cases.

FLOATING FOOTPLATE. The footplate can mobilize when the surgeon is drilling a hole in the fixed footplate, fracturing the stapes superstructure, or extracting the fixed footplate. Once the footplate is mobilized, regardless of whether it is solid (white) or diffuse (blue), a vein graft is placed on top of the mobilized footplate, followed by placement of a rigid stapes prosthesis that attaches to the lenticular process (Fig. 29–5).[2, 4] This conservative method gives excellent long-term results. If the mobilized footplate is mostly blue with diffuse otosclerosis, the hearing success rate is 95 per cent. If the footplate is thick, white, or biscuit-shaped, the hearing success rate is 52 per cent. If the thick, white footplate later refixes, it can be revised during a routine stapedectomy. If we add the results of the unsuccessful cases that required revisions to the initially successful cases, the final success rate is 76 per cent. If the footplate again mobilizes

during the revision procedure, no future surgery should be planned. Following this protocol, none of 147 cases of a floating footplate in a series of 8000 cases developed a further sensorineural loss (Table 29–2).

REVISION STAPEDECTOMY

Our experience is based on over 1000 cases. Cases are devided into two major categories: sensorineural hearing loss and conductive hearing loss. These cases should be further divided by the type of prosthesis and oval window covering used in the primary surgery.

We do not revise our cases (Robinson-vein) during the first 6 weeks after surgery. Previously, when we attempted early revision, tissue reaction was found throughout the middle ear, hindering our effort to analyze the problem. Furthermore, no patient gained improved hearing and many lost further hearing.

SENSORINEURAL HEARING LOSS. In patients with delayed sensorineural hearing loss after stapedectomy with an oval window tissue seal, revision is indicated only for a history of trauma or dizziness. In 27 such cases, 79 per cent had negative findings and no evidence of a surgical problem or oval window fistula. Only one case had a fistula.[5] We revise only an occasional case with unexplained persistent dizziness or cases in which a rare fistula is highly suspected. Twenty per cent of patients who are dizzy before revision gain at least some relief after revision. Parenthetically, we have never been able to improve a sensorineural hearing loss.

In cases with a delayed or immediate sensorineural hearing loss and without an oval window tissue seal, the findings at revision surgery are most dramatic. Most cases had a wire prosthesis with either absorbable gelatin sponge or a blood clot as an oval window seal. Fifty per cent of the cases had oval window fistulas. These cases were revised with an oval window tissue seal and a Robinson prosthesis. Hearing improved in a few cases, and dizziness improved in 75 per cent. The next most common findings were cases with negative findings and prostheses that were too long when placed. Table 29–3 illustrates findings in the cases with sensorineural hearing loss by comparing those with and without a tissue graft.

In summary, the surgeon should seriously consider a revision stapedectomy in patients with a sensorineural hearing loss without an oval window tissue seal. If a tissue graft was used to seal the oval window, the surgeon should be reluctant to do a revision.

CONDUCTIVE HEARING LOSS. The deciding factor for revision of conductive hearing loss is the hearing

TABLE 29–3. Surgical Findings in Revision of Sensorineural Cases

SURGICAL FINDINGS	TISSUE SEAL (n = 29) (%)	NO TISSUE (n = 42) (%)
Negative findings	79	24
Fistula	4	50
Long prosthesis	0	21
Tissue reaction	10	5
Lateral vein	7	0

history after the primary procedure.[6, 7] The most appropriate surgical candidates have hearing improvement postoperatively and then another conductive hearing loss. Cases with the same or worse hearing postoperatively have a low revision surgery success rate (Table 29–4).

The operative experience of the previous surgeon is another factor. The greater the surgical experience, the less likely a reversible problem will be found. Patients whose first surgeon was an experienced stapes surgeon and whose hearing did not improve are usually poor candidates for revision.

The type of prosthesis used and whether an oval window tissue graft was used are also important. For example, incus erosion is common with wire prostheses and can be revised with good results. Partial stapedectomy, in which the crus is mobilized into an opened oval window, is a procedure that is usually revised with a good result. Another successful revision occurs with conductive loss with distorted hearing or the feeling of vibrations because of a prosthesis that is too short. The symptoms may be eliminated by the addition of a vein graft and the placement of a new prosthesis of proper length.

Finally, patients with a negative attitude might not be candidates for revision. Because the risks are higher in revision than in primary surgery, the patient must be prepared to accept a potentially poor result.

Technique

Intraoperative testing is an important tool in revision surgery, allowing surgeons to obtain the most information with the least amount of trauma to the labyrinth. The patient must be under local anesthesia and should be instructed to inform the surgeon of any dizziness.

TABLE 29–4. Audiologic Patterns and Hearing Results

AIR-BONE GAP	SUCCESSFUL HEARING (%)
Delayed conduction	70
No change in hearing	35
Increased conduction	25

The surgical technique includes removing the previously placed prosthesis without disturbing the oval window seal and then placing a vein graft and a Robinson prosthesis. In cases with a wire prosthesis in which the patient experiences dizziness, the end of the wire that is attached to the incus is detached and pushed aside, leaving the distal end of the wire in the oval window seal (Fig. 29–6). A vein graft is then placed over the oval window area with a slit cut in the graft to accommodate the wire. A piston is then placed. At this point, the tympanomeatal flap is replaced, and the hearing is tested. If the hearing improves, the surgical procedure is finished.

If the hearing is not improved, the surgeon should consider other causes, such as previously inadequate footplate removal, otosclerosis regrowth, or a misdirected stapes prosthesis. The bottom of the prosthesis should first be moved slightly to find an opening into the oval window. In the routine stapedectomy technique, the prosthesis is always self-centering. However, in a revision, because the tissue graft is present and therefore less compliant, adjustment may be necessary. Should repositioning of the prosthesis not improve hearing, further dissection of the oval window niche may be necessary.

Surgical Findings

INCUS EROSION. This is the most common finding with wire prostheses. The pressure of the wire around the long process of the incus causes necrosis and erosion. If the only problem is a loose wire, the prosthesis can be crimped again. With prostheses that attach to the lenticular process of the incus, like the Robinson, incus erosion most often results from a previous infection, manifested by a healed perforation or an atrophic tympanic membrane and incus. For these types of cases, the success rate of revision with the Lippy-modified Robinson prosthesis is 70 per cent.

PROSTHESIS MALFUNCTION. Prosthesis malfunction in cases with a piston prosthesis on an oval window tissue seal is uncommon because of the self-centering ability of the prosthesis. A lenticular process that is too large can misdirect the piston from self-centering. This unusual problem can be avoided in the original procedure by using a 4mm polytetrafluoroethylene (Teflon) prosthesis with a large well. This well is 0.2mm larger than that of the Robinson prosthesis with a large well. This prosthesis accommodates the occasional extra-large lenticular process without causing misdirection. Malfunction is likely to occur in cases in which the stapes prosthesis becomes fused to the incus lenticular process and directed out of its self-centering position. If the fused prosthesis cannot be removed from the lenticular process, it may be left in place. A Bailey prosthesis should then be placed under the incus and over the oval window area.

A prosthesis that is too short and used with a tissue graft may give a good result at first. However, a conductive loss will develop as the tissue graft thins out. These problems can be corrected by revision. Wire prostheses, which lack rigidity, are more likely to migrate. The distal looped end of the wire commonly rests on the promontory or is fixed to a margin of the oval window. In addition, a loose attachment of the wire prosthesis on the long process of the incus may occur with incomplete crimping or gradual erosion of the incus. Lastly, short wire prostheses are frequently found, resulting from either improper measurement or inadvertent shortening when the prosthesis is crimped to the incus. Revision stapedectomy will correct these problems.

NEGATIVE FINDINGS. An interesting situation occurs when no problem can be recognized, the so-called negative finding category. In cases with an oval window tissue seal and a piston prosthesis, a revision stapedectomy did not improve hearing. However, hearing improved in 60 per cent of cases in which a wire prosthesis without a tissue seal was replaced by a Robinson piston on a vein (Table 29–5). The reason for this disparity appears to be the efficiency of the piston prostheses. The heavier and more rigid piston prosthesis more closely resembles the stapes than does the wire prosthesis and is, therefore, more efficient.

MALLEUS FIXATION. Malleus and incus fixation are discussed under intraoperative problems. Malleus fixation may have been present but ignored at the initial surgery, or it may have progressed in the interim. The totally fixed cases can be revised with a footplate-to-drum prosthesis or a malleus-to-footplate prosthesis when an oval window tissue seal is present.

OTHER FINDINGS. Adhesions that are dense enough to impede the prosthesis are extremely rare. Adhesions are often found during revision, but the hearing rarely changes when they are removed. Intraoperative audiometry allows the surgeon to evaluate the importance of such adhesions when they are removed.

Tissue graft lateralization, which is uncommon, can be revised by placing a new tissue graft on top of the old one, followed by a rigid piston prosthesis.

Otosclerosis regrowth is rare. Regrowth should not be removed, because the chances of further regrowth or further sensorineural loss are very high.

FISTULA. We have found only four fistulas in our cases with a piston prosthesis and a tissue seal. All four were women with smaller-than-usual vein grafts in

TABLE 29–5. Hearing Results in Negative-Findings Cases

| | HEARING RESULTS (%) | |
PROSTHESIS	Successful Hearing	Worse Hearing
Wire–no tissue	60	0
Robinson–tissue	0	9

whom fistulas occurred years after the original procedure. Each patient had a sudden hearing loss following descent either in a car or an airplane. The fistulas were found at the margin where the facial nerve canal adjoins the oval window. We now take a larger vein in women and attempt to remove some of the mucosa from the facial nerve canal or the facial nerve to create a surface to which the tissue seal will adhere and not slide toward the promontory. Fistulas were fairly common in conductive cases without tissue grafts.

SMALL FENESTRA. In revision stapedectomy of cases that have had a small fenestra technique, the most common surgical finding is displacement of the prosthesis from the small fenestra. The revision technique is to ignore the previous small fenestra to avoid manipulating adhesions that have formed in the vestibule. Often, a larger fenestra can be placed in the remaining portion of the footplate. Both fenestrae are covered by a tissue graft and a piston prosthesis placed in the new larger opening.

Recommendations

In cases of revision stapedectomy, the following are recommended:

1. Local anesthesia should be used both to monitor any dizziness and to permit intraoperative audiometry.
2. Intraoperative audiometry should be performed. A hearing gain is evidence of a successful technical solution. The surgeon need not further explore the oval window area. If hearing is not improved, the prosthesis should be moved. If the hearing is still not improved, then more tissue over the oval window should be removed, to find an intact otosclerotic footplate or otosclerosis regrowth.
3. A tissue seal should be used over the oval window whether or not it was opened for three reasons. First, tissue provides a seal of the oval window to prevent fistulas. Second, fistulas of the oval window, if present, are not always evident, because they can be minute or temporarily closed. Thus, the tissue graft seals the oval window. Third, the seal produced by absorbable gelatin sponge or mucosa will not safely support a rigid piston prosthesis.

4. The oval window should not be routinely re-opened. When the oval window is reopened, the incidence of hearing loss increases. Three factors are responsible: first, routine stapedectomy can cause vestibular adhesions from indentation of the oval window seal by the prosthesis. Therefore, re-opening the oval window can cause vestibular trauma because manipulation of the adhesions damages the membranous labyrinth. Second, the most critical part of stapedectomy is removing the footplate. Reopening the oval window in the absence of the footplate as a landmark is more technically difficult and thus carries the risk of greater surgical trauma. Third, delayed sensorineural hearing loss, which occurs rarely and inexplicably after stapedectomy, is probably related to a labyrinthine tissue reaction. Thus, the less trauma to the labyrinth, the less chance of a delayed sensorineural hearing loss. Again, the oval window seal should not be opened routinely.

5. Otosclerosis regrowth should not be removed. When it is encountered, the surgical procedure should be terminated. The reasons for not reopening the oval window seal are further supported by the difficult task of drilling and removing the otosclerosis regrowth. Even when the otosclerosis regrowth is successfully removed, the hearing gain is temporary in most patients. The incidence of a greater hearing loss is more than 50 per cent in our experience.

6. The distal loop of the wire prosthesis should be left in place in many cases. If the distal loop appears deep within the oval window seal, or if the patient experiences dizziness, the loop in the oval window seal is not removed. Removal may reopen the oval window, which will increase the likelihood of a hearing loss or dizziness. However, if the patient's main problem is significant incapacitating dizziness, the wire must be removed even if hearing is possibly sacrificed.

7. If the problem cannot be identified (negative findings), the case with a tissue seal should not be revised. On the other hand, cases without a tissue seal should be revised with good results.

FAR-ADVANCED OTOSCLEROSIS

Far-advanced otosclerosis is defined as no measurable air or bone conduction or, at best, air conduction no better than 95dB and bone at 55dB to 60dB at one frequency only. The history may include a family member with otosclerosis, previous audiograms showing a conductive hearing loss, and progressive hearing loss. The patient may be wearing a hearing aid successfully or may have previously worn an aid.

Findings would also include better-than-expected speech patterns and a softer voice than expected with a severe sensorineural hearing loss.

Most important is the ability to hear, not just feel, the 512Hz tuning fork on the upper teeth. This practical test gives up to 10dB more gain than when the tuning fork is placed on the mastoid. Edentulous patients are tested on their dentures or on their gums if they have no dentures.[8] In some patients, this test is the only one to yield measurable hearing evidence of far-advanced otosclerosis. Patients with some of these findings should be considered for a stapedectomy.

Technique

In far-advanced otosclerosis, the surgical techniques are the same as in the routine stapedectomy, but the surgical findings are different. Fifty per cent of the patients will have obliterative otosclerosis; therefore, the surgeon must be prepared to drill the footplate extensively, as recommended previously.

Results

Success is measured by improved air conduction, improved speech discrimination, and more benefit from a hearing aid. In our surgical experience with 72 far-advanced otosclerosis patients, the average hearing gain was 20dB, and 70 per cent benefited more from a hearing aid. In addition, there is a high correlation of success between ears: the patient who gained hearing after surgery in one ear also did well in the other; the patient who did not achieve a good result in the first ear did not do well in the second ear.

The results of stapedectomy for far-advanced otosclerosis are often dramatic. They will reinforce the surgeon's resolve to double-check patients with no measurable hearing.

References

1. Lippy WH, Schuring AG, Ziv M: Stapedectomy for otosclerosis with malleus fixation. Arch Otolaryngol Head Neck Surg 104: 338–389, 1978.
2. Lippy WH, Schuring AG: Solving ossicular problems in stapedectomy. Laryngoscope 93: 1147–1150, 1983.
3. Lippy WH, Schuring AG: Prosthesis for the problem incus in stapedectomy. Arch Otolaryngol Head Neck Surg 100: 237–239, 1974.
4. Lippy WH, Schuring AG: Treatment of the inadvertently mobilized footplate. Arch Otolaryngol Head Neck Surg 98: 80–81, 1973.
5. Lippy WH, Schuring AG: Stapedectomy revision following sensorineural hearing loss. Otolaryngol Head Neck Surg 92: 580–582, 1984.
6. Lippy WH, Schuring AG: Stapedectomy revision of the wire-Gelfoam prosthesis. Otolaryngol Head Neck Surg 91: 9–13, 1983.
7. Lippy WH, Schuring AG, Ziv M: Stapedectomy revision. Am J Otol 2: 15–21, 1980.
8. Lippy WH, Rotolo AL, Berger KW: Bone conduction measurement: Mastoid versus upper central incisor. Trans Am Acad Ophthalmol Otolaryngol 70: 1084–1088, 1966.

30

Avoidance and Management of Complications

MANSFIELD F. W. SMITH, M.D., M.S.
JOSEPH B. ROBERSON, Jr., M.D.

The reliable surgical correction of conductive hearing loss secondary to otosclerosis requires experience, precision, and discipline. The technical skills and judgment necessary to perform stapes surgery are among the most refined in the surgical disciplines.

The learning curve in stapes surgery suggests that a significant number of operations are required before a surgeon has appropriate surgical skills to match published results of recognized competent stapes surgeons.[1] This number may be greater than the training cases performed during residency.

A 1990 survey of otologic training in US residency programs revealed that 74 per cent of residents performed from zero to ten stapes surgeries, with an average for all residents of eight surgeries.[2] Frequently, a significant portion of these surgeries are performed by the attending surgeon. The surgical results in otosclerosis surgery obtained by residents within the residency training program are acceptable but not exceptional: approximately 68 per cent of the patients in this study achieved an air-bone gap of 10dB.[1] At our institution, 73 per cent of cases showed less than a 10dB air-bone gap postoperatively. (The measurement of air-bone gap is the difference between the postoperative air conduction and postoperative bone conduction measured at 500Hz, 1000Hz, and 2000Hz.) Outside the training institution, the occasional inexperienced surgeon may obtain even poorer results.

MATERIALS

Material for this chapter was compiled from information provided by a national symposium on otosclerosis by experienced otosclerosis surgeons,[3] a review of the literature on otosclerosis surgery complications from 1960 to 1992, and an analysis of the senior author's experience from 1960 to 1992. Potential complications are highlighted regarding the history, physical examination, hearing tests, informed consent, operating room, surgical procedure, and postoperative care. In addition, principles of a safe surgical approach are outlined for 1) the initial otosclerosis procedure, 2) identification and correction of surgical complications, and 3) revision procedures.

HISTORY—POTENTIAL RISK FACTORS

A history checklist is useful to avoid overlooking an important medical feature. It also is helpful to have a family member present during the interview, as he or she may remember things that the patient does not, such as prior ear surgery. Patients are occasionally defensive or secretive about prior operations that may

be of critical importance. The family member also may reinforce the information that the surgeon provides to the patient.

If the patient has had recent otitis externa, the patient must be treated appropriately to ensure that he or she is free of infection for at least 6 months. Fluctuating hearing loss or episodic vertigo may indicate endolymphatic hydrops. Because patients with hydrops who undergo stapes surgery have a higher rate of sensorineural hearing loss and chronic dizziness, this condition may be a contraindication to surgery.[3]

Imbalance may occur following otosclerosis surgery in spite of a well-done surgical procedure and an excellent hearing result. Professional dancers, athletes, high-wire artists, ice skaters, and other individuals dependent on maximum balance might be best advised to avoid surgery until completion of their careers. The elderly patient with a balance problem may be a poor candidate for surgery and may derive more benefit from amplification.

People whose careers depend on their sense of taste, such as professional chefs, wine tasters, and coffee tasters, should avoid stapes surgery until they have finished their careers, because a significant number of patients, possibly as high as 10 per cent, may lose some taste finesse provided by the chorda tympani fibers.

A patient with severe motion sickness or a particularly stormy vertiginous course following a first procedure would be considered at increased risk for long-term vertigo following subsequent otosclerosis surgery.

Lifelong hearing loss in one ear should alert the surgeon to the possibility of a congenital footplate fixation. This abnormality may have associated perilymph (cerebrospinal fluid leak). Footplate fixation is different from otosclerosis and has a great potential for a poor surgical result.[4] A history of claustrophobia or neuropsychiatric disease would suggest that the patient have a general anesthetic.

PHYSICAL EXAMINATION

Findings that may portend difficulties during otosclerosis surgery include

- A small ear canal, which would require enlargement of the external canal or postauricular incision.
- Exostosis of the external canal, common in cold water swimmers and divers. An initial procedure may be required to correct the exostosis and create an adequately sized canal and an intact external canal skin and tympanic membrane prior to a stapes procedure.

- Limited neck rotation in individuals with cervical disease or other types of neck problems may require that surgery be done with the patient under a general anesthetic with a surgical table that rotates 35° off the midline.

Microscopic examination in the office often helps the surgeon evaluate the anatomic difficulties and anticipate problems that may occur during the procedure. This preparation leads to better planning for the case. For example, a very obese patient may have special problems, or a large head may be an indication of Paget's disease, which has signs and symptoms consistent with otosclerosis. Another problem could be a preauricular sinus or other auricular or periauricular anomaly, which may indicate anomalies of the middle ear.[3]

HEARING EVALUATION

Voice tests and tuning fork tests still have an important place in determining the type of hearing loss. Bone conduction greater than air conduction at 256 and 512 cycles per second is an important indicator of a conductive loss. A patient with severe hearing loss but good voice quality, a history of hearing loss relatively early in life, and a suspected history of conductive hearing loss in the family may have otosclerosis. The diagnosis of otosclerosis may be missed in such patients.

PATIENT COUNSELING

Talk to the patient[3] to learn the patient's expectations for surgery, which may be unrealistic. Advise the patient of the risks, the rewards, and the alternatives, and inform the patient that the greatest potential problem is a profound sensorineural hearing loss, which may occur in 1:200 to 300 operations done by the best of surgeons. The patient should also be told about the potential for vertigo, taste disturbance, and strange sounds in the ear, such as a metallic sound or "cracked-speaker cone" sound distortion, intensification of recruitment phenomena, and diplacusis. Giving a list of complications is not recommended, but it may be helpful to indicate the major complications and state that some complications are listed for the patient, but that the list is not all-inclusive. It is always helpful to give the patient individualized written information describing in lay terms the surgeon's findings, details of the procedure, and potential risks. Such written information is an important part of a proper informed consent as well (see *Appendix*).

Patients should be told about the use of sodium fluoride and why you may or may not recommend its use. This step also is part of the informed consent process. Most US surgeons do not recommend the use of sodium fluoride, but a few enthusiasts still exist.

INFORMED CONSENT FOR REVISION OTOSCLEROSIS SURGERY

Revision stapes surgery requires more specific informed consent because the results are not as good as those of primary stapes surgery, and the potential for complications is greater. For example, the chorda tympani nerve often adheres to the flap and is more likely to be damaged in revision surgery. In addition, bilateral chorda tympani loss represents a greater hazard to the patient and puts the patient at increased risk when both ears have been operated on previously. Revision stapedectomy provides hearing improvement in 50 to 80 per cent of patients and hearing reduction in 2 to 10 per cent of patients, and patients should be informed of these statistics in preoperative counseling.[5] Patients undergoing revision surgery for relief of vertigo are in a poor prognostic class; they should be advised that the goal of surgery is alleviation of the vestibular symptoms. In many cases, hearing will be worse postoperatively,[6] but use of surgical lasers may improve these statistics. However, long-term data on this method are unavailable.

Neuropsychiatric patients need a very special form of informed consent, and a member of the family should be present at the time consent is obtained. Consent should include a detailed discussion of the risks, potential rewards, and all available options. A written summary of the discussion should be sent to the patient, family member, referring physician, and, if appropriate, the patient's psychiatrist. The summary report should include the history, physical examination, laboratory data, and informed consent information.

With the patient's permission, the second surgeon should call the first surgeon, discuss the case with him or her, and obtain all pertinent prior records, including operative reports. The second surgeon should always be aware that important information may be lacking from these records.

SURGICAL TECHNIQUE

OPERATING ROOM. Reproducible good results in otosclerosis surgery require trained assistants. The otologic surgeon must not be inconvenienced by having to look away from the microscope to determine the correct instrument or prosthesis. This step slows the surgery and may lead to complications. The surgeon needs an assistant who can hand these instruments correctly and can anticipate the needs of the surgeon and thus the needs of the patient. Use of an appropriately focused video monitoring system greatly aids the operating room personnel in anticipating the surgeon's needs.

The many details of the operating room, including the operating table, with appropriate room for the knees and rotation, the inventory of equipment, and the prosthesis, are the responsibility of the surgeon and the assistants. Preparation for the surgical procedure and the attitude in the operating room are very dependent on the attitude, enthusiasm, discipline, and attention to detail of the surgeon. Lack of attention to these elements may lead to complications in otosclerosis surgery.

PREPARATION OF THE SURGEON. The surgeon should never be surprised by any findings at the time of surgery. He or she should have available the necessary equipment, corrective devices, and a definite plan of action to accomplish the procedure. The surgeon should know exactly when not to continue with a procedure. Findings at the time of operation may preclude otosclerosis surgery because of increased risk to the patient.

A SMALL EXTERNAL AUDITORY CANAL OR MEATUS. These anatomic anomalies may require enlargement of the meatus or canal. One technique for this is the use of the Lempert speculum at the time of surgery. Several surgeons have recorded the use of an ear mold that was made for the external canal and gradually enlarged over 6 months to a year.[3] It is very unusual for competent surgeons to use an endaural or postauricular incision, but, according to many surgeons, this incision may be necessary in approximately one of 300 cases.

Lasers

Safe laser applications in otosclerosis surgery require that the surgeon understand the basic properties of laser light and how it interacts with tissue. A detailed comprehension of the significance of wavelength, power density, beam quality, and pulse format, and their affect on tissue cutting, vaporizing, and coagulating are central in establishing a full grasp of safe and effective laser surgical technique.[6] The primary clinical effect of the laser interaction on tissue results from absorption. The visible-spectrum lasers (argon, potassium titanyl phosphate crystal [KTP], and neodymium:yttrium-aluminum-garnet [Nd:YAG]) are largely transmitted through water and absorbed by chromophores (melanin and hemoglobin). The carbon dioxide laser is primarily absorbed by water. Once laser light is absorbed by tissue, it is immediately converted to heat. In otosclerosis surgery, an absolute minimum of laser energy is required to minimize thermal damage and preserve function. It is a paradox, but a critically important one, that minimal thermal damage occurs at high-power densities and vice versa. "The idea of working at low power in the interest of safety and precision may produce exactly the opposite result. Precise removal of tissue with minimal thermal damage to surrounding structures can only be accomplished by using a laser at high power density for a short time, rather than low power density for a longer time. For safe and precise work requiring clean oblation, a pulsed laser is useful."[6]

Carbon dioxide laser energy is absorbed by water, which composes 60 per cent of bone. At the high-power density setting, the pulsed laser vaporizes bone and releases heat and tissue into the vapor plume. Because the carbon dioxide laser energy is absorbed by water, it will not penetrate and be absorbed into neural tissue of the utricle and saccule. The visible-light-spectrum lasers (argon and KTP) depend on a char to begin the rosette or creation of a cylinder in the footplate, and the char absorbs the laser energy and creates heat. The laser energy can pass through either directly or by scatter and injure the neural tissue of the utricle and saccule.[5]

Instrumentation

A mirror-based carbon dioxide laser micromanipulator delivery system (Reliant Technologies Unimax 2000) produces a spot size of 0.1mm and provides continuous coincident spot sizes, so that the visible helium-neon aiming beam and invisible carbon dioxide laser beam are coincident.

The following instruments are recommended for laser otologic surgery:

- Carbon dioxide laser system pulsed and the (Reliant Technologies) micromanipulation
- Speculum holder (Treace Medical)
- Microdrill (Treace Medical, Skeeter Catalogue No. 5628) with appropriate burrs and a 0.8mm trephine
- Microbipolar cautery
- Standard otosclerosis instruments, including a micromirror for deflecting the carbon dioxide laser

Before surgery, all of the operating equipment should be analyzed, as should the availability of the various types of prostheses. The operating microscope should be parfocal and appropriately adjusted, and a biologic test of the laser microequipment must then be carried out to make certain that it is in working order and safe.

ANESTHESIA

Local Anesthesia

Many patients with otosclerosis have the surgical procedure done under local anesthesia. Using a minimal number of drugs preoperatively, thus reducing the risk of a drug reaction, is preferred. If a reaction occurs when this method is used, it can be more clearly ascribed to one drug. The senior author prefers using diazepam (Valium) intravenously preoperatively, which may be augmented during surgery. A local injectable anesthetic is 2% lidocaine (Xylocaine) with 1:40,000 epinephrine. These three drugs function well in most cases involving local anesthesia. Local anesthesia with an anesthesiologist on standby can provide a monitoring advantage in addition to the other advantages of a local anesthetic.

To reduce pain during surgery, the local anesthetic should be warm and should be injected with a 30-gauge needle that is quickly placed through the skin. Once a wheal has been raised, the next injection should stay within the wheal. Observing these features will often allow for a nearly pain-free administration of a local anesthetic.

The otologic surgeons surveyed in the 1984 symposium used various lidocaine and epinephrine solutions with similar results; thus the type of anesthesia-adrenalin solution mixture seems to make little difference.[3]

General Anesthesia

Reasons for using general anesthesia are patient's limited neck rotation, back pain, or claustrophobia, or when general anesthesia is the patient's choice. In addition, the medical problems of some patients can best be monitored under a general anesthetic administered by a well-trained anesthesiologist.

General Comments

A hand tremor is a handicap for an otosclerosis surgeon. The surgeon should drink no alcohol within 24 hours of the procedure and no coffee the day of surgery. In addition, there should be some type of arm and hand support for the surgeon to prevent or reduce a tremor. The use of sharp knives, such as sharp, disposable blades, are recommended for making the canal incision. An excellent blade is the sharp lancet knife made by the Beaver Company (Beaver ear blade Catalogue #7200). The canal incision is a single incision horizontal to the tympanic membrane that starts inferiorly on the right ear at approximately 6 o'clock and then extends superiorly to approximately 12 o'clock. Vertical incisions do not need to be made. The incision should be kept satisfactorily lateral to the tympanic membrane, particularly superiorly. The knife blade must be purposely brought more lateral as the surgeon extends the incision superiorly. A long flap in a small ear canal should be avoided because it may preclude satisfactory visualization of the middle ear. Complete hemostasis of the bone and soft tissue of the external auditory canal is important for continued visualization throughout the procedure.

Unipolar electrical coagulation is not recommended because it may be very uncomfortable for the patient: it can produce pain and alarm the patient, and in addition, can stimulate the facial nerve. Some bipolar miniature coagulation units can provide superb coagulation for ear surgery.

An ear speculum holder may provide increased visualization and assist the surgeon in better continuity of exposure. It may also provide a fulcrum for support of the microsurgical instruments.

To save time, use two independent suctions. When one suction tip is stopped or plugged, the surgeon can immediately be handed the second one, which is already prepared and of the same size.

Maximum preservation of chorda tympani function and the integrity of the incus result by directing a curet inferiorly toward the chorda tympani nerve. Many surgeons are now using the microdrill diamond burr to drill away portions of the posterior osseous canal, then using a curette for the remainder of the bone. The middle ear is then inspected, and determination of the mobility of the stapes, incus, and malleus is made. Confirmation of otosclerosis or footplate fixation is made. By use of the incudostapedial joint knife, the incus is separated from the stapes. Pressure is directed anteriorly, which is less likely to produce unexpected and inappropriate mobilization of the stapes. The stapedial tendon is cut with the laser. The posterior crus is also cut with the laser, and the crus is removed down close to the level of the footplate to allow adequate visualization for placement of the cylinder through the footplate.

The removal of the lateral portion of the anterior crus can often be accomplished by minimal displacement of the incus posteriorly or the use of an optical miniature mirror to deflect the laser onto the anterior crus. If the laser is not available, the anterior and posterior crus can be cut with a slow-rotation diamond knife (Treace Medical, Skeeter Catalogue #5621). The principle is to not break the crura or remove the crura by putting pressure either anteriorly or inferiorly because of the potential for mobilization of the footplate or possible displacement of the footplate into the vestibule. An additional precautionary measure is to make a small aperture in the footplate of the stapes prior to applying pressure on the footplate or the crura.

The thin, bluish or slightly thickened otosclerotic

footplate is an ideal situation for a carbon dioxide laser–created cylinder through the central portion of the footplate. The cylinder measures 0.8mm, into which a 0.6mm piston can be placed. There are three types of stapes replacement prostheses, and many modifications of each type:

1. A metal or some type of alloplast piston, with a wire or ribbon, often of platinum, shaped like a shepherd's crook, which can be crimped over the long process of the incus
2. The bucket prosthesis of the Robinson type, in which the incus fits into various sizes of buckets, and a loop flips over the incus to hold the whole apparatus in place
3. The continuous piece of polytetrafluoroethylene (Teflon), which is the piston, joining a circular piece of Teflon, which can be separated, and which grasps the end of the incus.

Our preference is for the McGee piston, which is stainless steel. There is a Teflon insert into the piston, and the platinum ribbon inserts into the Teflon. The flat aspect of the platinum shepherd's crook allows for stabilization against the incus, and a lack of memory of platinum tends to hold the shepherd's crook in close continuity to the incus.

No perfect all-purpose prosthesis exists; problems occur with all types of prostheses, as is demonstrated by the great variety of prostheses on the market. For example, the piston-shepherd's crook–type prosthesis may be complicated by long-term incus erosion, which produces a loose-wire syndrome.[7] A further problem with the piston-shepherd's crook wire or platinum ribbon is that occasionally a prosthesis is pushed off the incus by soft tissue formation, apparently in the oval window at the site of the stapedotomy. If the piston-shepherd's crook–type prosthesis is displaced, replacement with a Lippy-Robinson prosthesis, which has a 0.6mm piston, is recommended.

Measurement for the Prosthesis

Prosthesis measurement is very critical and must be done with great care. We recommend use of a prosthesis of the same type that the surgeon plans to use to make the measurement between the medial aspect of the incus to the footplate. (All stapes prostheses are measured from the medial aspect of the incus to the footplate as a result of the consensus of the 1984 Otosclerosis Symposium[3] and endorsement by the American Academy of Otolaryngology/Head and Neck Surgery.) Further, the McGee prosthesis has a marker at the 0.5mm mark that gives the surgeon more infor-

mation on the length of the prosthesis. The calculated projection of any prosthesis into the vestibule should be approximately 0.25mm and not more than 1.0mm (Fig. 30–1).[8–10]

The stapedotomy cylinder site can be sealed with blood or fat around the prosthesis and/or by placement of a thin vein over the stapedotomy and then placement of the piston. *It is very important that this vein be of adequate size* to completely cover the oval window area. It also must be thin, so that a small suction needle placed at the perimeter of the vein will cause the vein to suction down, clearly revealing the stapedotomy site. It is best to take the vein from the distal portion of the hand, where the veins tend to be thinner.

COMPLICATIONS

Anatomic Abnormalities

The stapes surgeon faces anatomic structures that are fortunately consistent, including the chorda tympani nerve, the oval window niche, and the vestibule and its contents. The amount of bony external canal overhang in the posterior superior quadrant, however, varies markedly. Bone can be removed from this portion of the external auditory canal with a curette directed away from the incus and toward the chorda tympani nerve. Some surgeons prefer to use a powered hand piece to remove this bone. In either case, great care should be taken to avoid dislocating the incus, fracturing the stapes superstructure, or stretching or tearing the chorda tympani nerve.

The facial nerve can provide obstruction to completing successful stapes surgery. Recognition of an aberrant or dehiscent facial nerve will prevent injury. Twenty-five to 40 per cent of temporal bones include dehiscence of the bony fallopian canal. Strategically located dehiscences may be sites of trauma due to surgical instrumentation. Local anesthetic agents may also penetrate these areas more readily, causing postoperative facial paralysis. The facial nerve has been reported to be entirely on the promontory side of the footplate, to be split with a portion on either side of the footplate, and to pass through the arch of the stapes.[11, 12]

A facial nerve overhanging the oval window niche will be regularly encountered. Successful stapedotomy can be performed if sufficient working space is present to allow insertion of a prosthesis without manipulation of the unusually dehiscent nerve. The prosthesis can be bent around the nerve to provide reconstruction. Occasionally, the nerve's encroachment into the oval window niche is great enough to produce

FIGURE 30-1

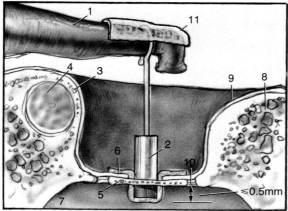

1. Incus
2. Piston
3. Bone of the facial nerve ridge
4. Facial nerve
5. Stapes footplate
6. Tissue seal
7. Vestibule
8. Promontory
9. Mesotympanum mucosa
10. Annular ligament
11. Tissue overlay

FIGURE 30-2

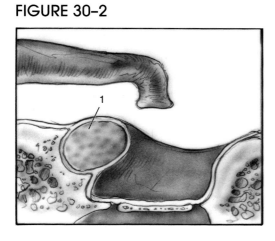

1. Dehiscent overhanging facial nerve

FIGURE 30-3

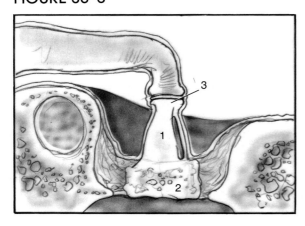

1. Posterior stapedial crura
2. Thickened footplate with obliterative otosclerosis
3. Incudostapedial joint

FIGURE 30-4

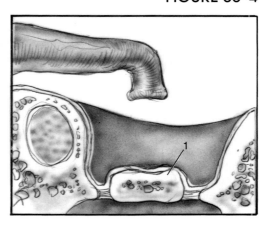

1. Biscuit footplate

conductive hearing loss. Prudent judgment may indicate termination of the procedure if iatrogenic injury to the facial nerve is a possibility (Fig. 30–2).

A persistent stapedial artery that courses from the fallopian canal through the arch of the stapes into the internal carotid artery may be encountered. If the vessel is small, fine bipolar cautery may be used to remove the vessel from the field, thereby allowing completion of the procedure. With larger arteries, it may be prudent to stop the procedure.

On entering the mesotympanum, the source of ossicular fixation is occasionally identified within the malleus-incus complex. Almost always, the source of problem comes from bony fixation of the head of the malleus in the roof of the epitympanic space. The incus, however, can be fixed at the posterior process. Exposure of the ossicular complex through a mastoidectomy extended into the epitympanum allows division of the bony bridge with the laser. If a drill is used, the incudostapedial joint should be disarticulated to prevent sensorineural hearing loss.

Obliterative otosclerosis with extreme thickening of the footplate and obliteration of the oval window niche is best managed using a slow rotation-per-minute microdrill trephine to create a 0.8mm diameter cylinder (Treace Medical, Skeeter 0.8mm trephine, Catalog #5628) (Fig. 30–3). Laser use in this situation creates a potential risk to the patient because of the heat transfer to the perilymph of the vestibule and subsequently to the utricle and saccule.

The microdrill must be in good working order to ensure no hesitation of the trephine rotation or possible surges in speed. The trephine needs to be replaced on a regular basis so that it is sharp and will cut easily and reliably. A thickened footplate and oval window area should not be drilled out using a diamond cutting burr because of reactivation and reformation of otosclerosis, which is associated with poorer hearing results.[13, 14] Drill-out of the oval window area is also associated with a high rate of sensorineural hearing loss.

The exact nature and position of the otosclerotic focus or foci should be appreciated prior to removal of the stapes superstructure. Occasionally, a very thickened footplate with tenuous attachments to the rim of the oval window niche (commonly known as a "biscuit footplate") will be encountered (Fig. 30–4). Such a footplate is at risk for mobilization under the slightest pressure, causing sensorineural hearing loss. In this setting, the laser is invaluable to remove the stapes superstructure and to perform a stapedotomy without risking mobilization of the footplate.

One may discover ossicular fixation secondary to tympanosclerosis of the stapes footplate. Stapedotomy may be performed safely with the laser in this situa-

tion. Excellent early results may be achieved, with some attrition over time.[15–17]

Surgical Trauma

Sensorineural hearing loss is perhaps the most disappointing and devastating complication for both the surgeon and the patient. Complete sensorineural hearing loss can result from the most meticulously and appropriately performed stapes procedure. Most cases, however, are probably due to surgical trauma. Intraoperative electronystagmographic studies performed during stapedectomy in the prelaser area implicate suctioning over the vestibule, drilling near the footplate or oval window niche, and manipulation of the footplate as the great offenders for vestibular and presumably for cochlear damage.[18]

It is of paramount importance for the surgeon to understand the relationship of the vestibular contents to the stapes footplate (Fig. 30–5). If possible, a posterior central or posteroinferior location for stapedotomy should be selected. Almost all patients have a minimum safe distance of 1.0mm between the medial surface of the footplate and the utricle and saccule. Penetration of the vestibule by more than 1.0mm with footplate instruments or prostheses may perforate the utricle or saccule, inducing sensorineural hearing loss, vertigo, or both.[9, 10] In patients with endolymphatic hydrops, the saccule may extend to contact the medial surface of the footplate, thereby placing these patients at high risk for complications from this procedure.

The "gusher" is a dramatic complication of stapes surgery. The smallest control hole of the footplate can produce a perilymph leak (cerebrospinal fluid) so profuse that it fills the middle ear and internal auditory canal within seconds.[19] Management of the stapes gusher is the same as management of a cerebral spinal fluid leak. Once the surgeon notes the onset of fluid leaking from the aperture in the stapes footplate, leakage may be controlled with a small piece of Surgicel and then tamponaded with cotton. General anesthesia should be induced at this point. A lumbar subarachnoid drain will allow effective diversion of cerebral spinal fluid, thereby decreasing the pressure of the perilymph. A vein graft is harvested from the hand. The surgeon removes the cotton and Surgicel from the oval window area, creating an 0.8mm or greater stapedotomy. The vein is then placed over the stapedotomy, providing a watertight seal for either a 0.4mm- or 0.6mm-diameter piston of the appropriate length. The bucket-type of prosthesis is recommended because of the possible cerebrospinal fluid pressure extrusion of a piston-shepherd's crook–type prosthesis (Fig. 30–6).

Postoperatively, the lumbar subarachnoid drain is removed. The head of the bed is elevated approximately 30°, and daily fluid intake is restricted to 1500ml to 1800ml. Oral acetazolamide (250mg, four times a day) is prescribed for the patient for 2 weeks. Acetazolamide is a potent carbonic anhydrase inhibitor that decreases cerebrospinal fluid production. Discharge is usually accomplished on the first or second postoperative day, with restricted activity, including bed rest at home, for another 5 days.[20] Direct communication between the internal auditory canal and vestibule allows high cerebrospinal fluid pressure to be transmitted to the perilymph.

Tympanic membrane perforations occurring at the time of surgery are not an indication to abort the procedure. These can be repaired using autologous fascia with good success.

Incus dislocation, however, precludes routine stapedectomy. The surgeon may elect to terminate surgery in hope that the incus and malleus will reattach and allow the standard technique to be used at a future time. Alternatively, the incus may be removed and a malleus-to-footplate prosthesis inserted.

Approximately one fourth of patients complain of dysgeusia in the postoperative period. Chorda tympani nerve dysfunction is usually transient, and fewer than 5 per cent of patients experience permanent deficits. Revision cases (in which the nerve has adhered to the posterior surface of the tympanic membrane), and "second ears" (in which chorda dysfunction may be present preoperatively on the contralateral side) deserve special attention.

Footplate mobilization rarely occurs when a laser is used, as very little force is applied to the footplate. If mobilization occurs, a stapedotomy can be performed safely by laser. If a laser is unavailable, the surgery should be terminated and the footplate allowed to refix before the procedure is done.

Footplate fragmentation will occasionally occur. Free-floating surface fragments should be removed and the surgery converted to a partial or complete stapedectomy. A tissue seal is mandatory in this setting.

Intraoperative vertigo, dizziness, or nausea does not always correlate with sensorineural hearing loss. These symptoms should, however, raise the surgeon's awareness that injury may have occurred to the vestibular apparatus, cochlea, or both. For this and other reasons, we prefer to perform stapedectomy with the patient under local anesthesia with intravenous sedation, as the surgeon is afforded feedback information.

Postoperative Complications

Prosthesis displacement is the most common postoperative complication, accounting for 50 to 70 per cent of revision surgeries (Fig. 30–7).[21–26] The hearing deterioration may be acute, as the prosthesis becomes dislodged, or chronic, as it is gradually displaced out of position. This complication may be encountered many years after stapes surgery. The diagnosis is definitively made at reoperation but may be suspected based on tuning fork and audiometric tests.

Fibrosis of the oval window niche with its coincident lateralization of the oval window membrane can displace a prosthesis or provide an impediment for transmission of sound vibration to the fluids of the inner ear. Removing the prosthesis and creating a fenestration using the carbon dioxide laser will allow reinsertion of a prosthesis and reconstitution of the sound-conducting mechanism. Results with this complication are poorer than expected.[23, 27]

Perilymph fistula is a cause of postoperative disequilibrium and sensorineural hearing loss. The signs and symptoms of perilymph fistula may be indistinguishable from normal postoperative findings.[43, 44] Oval window granuloma and too long a prosthesis impinging on elements of the vestibule may also cause disequilibrium and sensorineural hearing loss.

As with perilymphatic fistula, postoperative granuloma can be a source of disequilibrium, vertigo, or progressive sensorineural hearing loss. Granuloma may occur any time within the first 8 weeks postoperatively. High-dose steroids (prednisone, 60mg orally every day for 4 days, 40mg orally every day for 4 days, and 20 mg orally every day for 4 days) may decrease the inflammatory response and its effects on the inner ear. Progressive sensorineural hearing loss and unremitting disequilibrium and vertigo are indications for re-exploration. If encountered, the granuloma should be vaporized with a laser after the prosthesis is removed. The tissue seal should be placed over the oval window fossa. After healing, the patient may be returned to the operating room for a third procedure.

Foreign body reaction is the suspected etiology of postoperative granuloma. Glove starch, Teflon fragments, and refractile particles found in irrigating solution have all been implicated.[28, 29] For this reason, direct glove-prosthesis contact should be avoided. It may also be prudent to rinse the prosthesis prior to its insertion.

Prosthesis loosening due to erosion or notching of the incus and prosthesis displacement due to necrosis of the incus also occur (Figs. 30–8 and 30–9). With removal of the stapes arch, the blood supply to the long process of the incus is divided as it courses over the incudostapedial joint. Collateral vessels exist from the body of the incus and maintain the viability of the remaining bone. Circumferential overtightening of a prosthesis can remove the blood supply to the tip of the incus.

Incus notching and prosthesis loosening may be remedied by repositioning and tightening the prosthesis during revision surgery. If the lenticular process is missing, revision can be accomplished with the Lippy modification of the Robinson bucket-handle prosthesis. When much of the long process of the incus is missing, the malleus-to-footplate arrangement is the most suitable choice (Shea large-head-malleus–attached piston or Sheehy malleus to oval window prosthesis).[30–32]

When confronted with the patient complaining of postoperative conductive hearing loss and speech distortion, the clinician should suspect prosthesis loosening. Frequently, the symptoms improve with self-insufflation of the middle ear space.[7]

Almost all patients have some degree of phonophobia postoperatively; reassurance is adequate treatment.[33] Diplacusis binauralis occurs in approximately one third of patients. It is seldom problematic and fades by 6 weeks postoperatively.[34] Acute otitis media occurs in the postoperative period in patients who have had stapes surgery. The infection is usually successfully treated without sequelae. Entrance of pathogenic organisms into the perilymph can produce sensorineural hearing loss. Progression into the cerebrospinal fluid has been reported with meningitis.[35–39] Patients should be advised to seek medical attention early in the course of suspected middle ear infections. Foreign bodies introduced into the perilymph at the time of surgery may come to rest in the lymphatic-containing structures, and positional vertigo may result. Every effort should be made to prevent introduction of material into the vestibule. The surgeon should not, however, "fish out" fragments of materials from the vestibule.

A small number of cases of delayed facial nerve paralysis have occurred. Typically, the onset of paralysis occurs 7 to 10 days after surgery and is associated with pain. Treatment with a tapered dose of steroids has brought about resolution in all cases. Immediate facial nerve paralysis may result from use of local anesthetics. If there is any doubt as to the integrity of the facial nerve, the patient should be re-explored to rule out iatrogenic injury.[40]

Occasionally, material introduced in the area of reconstruction can bring about a return of conductive hearing loss. Introduced squamous cells can produce a cholesteatoma,[41] and perichondrium has been known to stimulate the formation of cartilage.[42]

REVISION OTOSCLEROSIS SURGERY

Although exact numbers are lacking, approximately 25 per cent of all otosclerosis surgery will require revision. Urgent re-exploration may be necessary if perilymph fistula, postoperative granuloma, too long a prosthesis, or iatrogenic facial nerve injury is suspected.

MANAGEMENT
If the surgeon seeing the patient is not the original operating surgeon, the operating surgeon must be called (with the patient's permission) so that all the information surrounding the surgery can be obtained, including preoperative evaluation, surgical details, and postoperative course. It is very important not to be critical of the operating surgeon and to attempt to refer the patient back to the original surgeon as soon as possible.

PACKING AND DRESSING
Absorbable gelatin sponge strips moistened with chloramphenicol (Chloromycetin) (or any other topical antibiotic of the surgeon's choice) are placed against the tympanomeatal flap, creating pressure on the flap by layering in an anterior direction. Sterile cotton is then placed at the meatus.

HOSPITAL POSTOPERATIVE CARE
The patients are instructed to avoid excessive head movement, and to move their head as if they are balancing a book on top of their head, thus reducing the amount of head motion. If the patient is nauseated, intravenous droperidol is administered. Most patients may go home within a few hours after surgery. It is preferable to have the patient remain quiet and in the hospital for approximately 4 hours after surgery. He or she may then go home with a much lower chance of being nauseated.

HOME POSTOPERATIVE CARE
The patient is instructed verbally on postoperative care and is given postoperative instructions printed on thick paper. Colored thick paper or cardboard is much less likely to be lost by the patient or family. The instructions include

- Please do not fly for _____ days (surgeon's choice) following surgery.
- Avoid rapid changes in head position for 2 weeks after surgery.
- Expect some dizziness on head movement for 2 weeks after surgery.
- Expect ear noises, such as voices seeming too loud, gurgling, popping, plugged sensation, and decreased hearing.
- Expect some taste disturbance, such as a metallic taste or a difference in taste.
- Change the cotton plug three times a day, use sterile

FIGURE 30-5

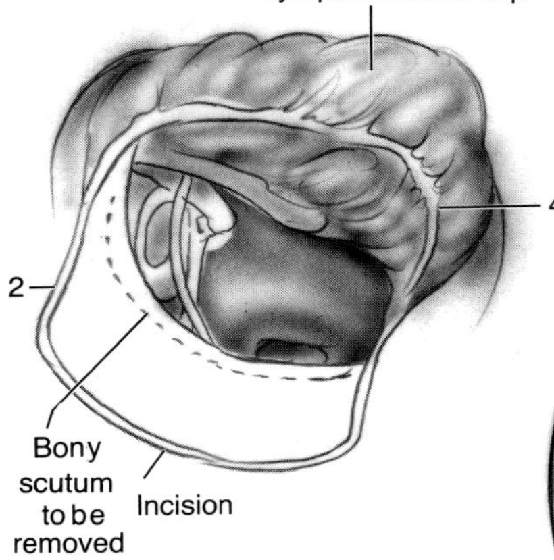

Tympanomeatal flap

4

2

Bony scutum to be removed

Incision

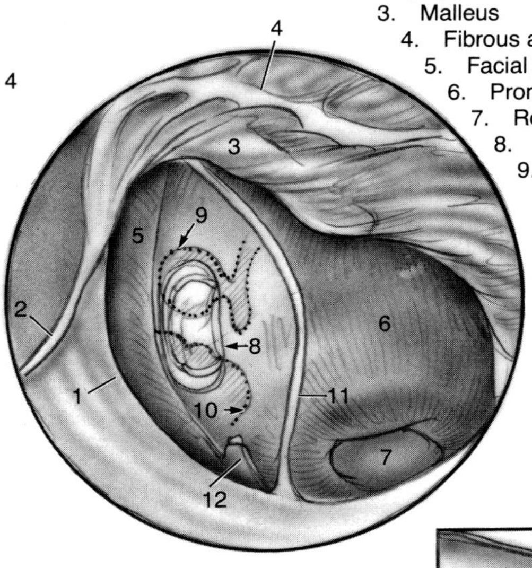

1. Bone of scutum (partially removed for exposure)
2. Tympanomeatal flap incision
3. Malleus
4. Fibrous annulus (elevated out of its sulcus)
5. Facial nerve ridge
6. Promontory
7. Round window niche
8. Stapes footplate
9. Saccule
10. Utricle
11. Chorda tympani nerve
12. Pyramidal eminence

4

3

9

5

2

8

1

6

10

11

7

12

FIGURE 30-6

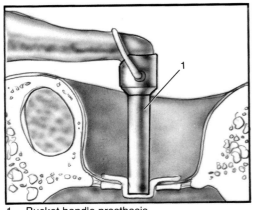

1. Bucket handle prosthesis
   (Lippy modification of Robinson prosthesis)

FIGURE 30-7

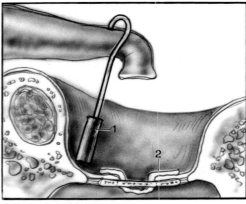

1. Displaced prosthesis
2. Tissue seal preventing perilymph fistula

FIGURE 30-8

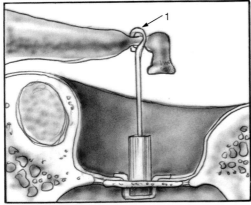

1. Incus erosion

FIGURE 30-9

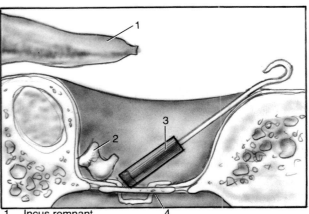

1. Incus remnant
2. Necrotic lenticular process
3. Displaced prosthesis
4. Tissue seal preventing perilymph fistula

cotton balls, and always wash hands prior to changing cotton.

- When shampooing the hair, sterile cotton moistened with baby oil may be placed in the opening of the ear canal.
- If there is any sign of ear infection, such as increased ear pain, yellow discharge, or fever, call the office immediately.
- If there is an increase in dizziness or vertigo, call the office immediately.
- Bloody or watery discharge of the ear may occur during the 3-week healing period, and you should not be concerned.
- Ear drops may be prescribed for the postoperative period. Use these on a daily basis as instructed.
- Your postoperative appointment is on _____.
- In case of emergency day or night, call the emergency number, which is _____.

SUMMARY

The principles of safe surgical techniques for otosclerosis management and thus avoidance of complications are as follows:

1. A surgeon who is carefully trained and disciplined in all aspects of otosclerosis surgery.
2. Special nurse or surgical technician who is thoroughly familiar with the operating room and can serve as an expert assistant to the surgeon.
3. Complete instrumentation and availability of prostheses for every type of otosclerosis problem. Carbon dioxide pulsed laser with a 0.1mm spot size and absolute coincidence of the aiming beam and laser beam. Use of the limited fenestra, that is, a stapedotomy prosthesis diameter of 0.4mm to 0.8mm, with approximate intrusion into the vestibule of approximately 0.25mm.
4. Reliable seal between the piston and stapedotomy cylinder.

References

1. Hughes FB: Learning curve in stapes surgery. Laryngoscope 101: 1280–1284, 1991.
2. Harris JP, Osborne E: A survey of otologic training in U. S. residencies programs. Arch Otolaryngol Head Neck Surg 116: 342–345, 1990.
3. Smith MFW, Hopp ML: 1984 Santa Barbara State-of-the-Art Symposium on Otosclerosis. Results, conclusions, consensus. Ann Otol Rhinol Laryngol 95: 1–4, 1986.
4. Olson NR, Lehman RH: Cerebrospinal fluid otorrhea and the congenitally fixed stapes. Laryngoscope 78: 352–360, 1968.
5. Glasscock ME, McKennan KX, Levine SC: Revision stapedectomy surgery. Otolaryngol Head Neck Surg 96: 141–148, 1987.
6. Smith MFW, McElveen JT: Neurological Surgery of the Ear. St. Louis, Mosby Yearbook, 1992, pp 131–162.
7. McGee TM: The loose-wire syndrome. Laryngoscope 91: 1478–1483, 1981.
8. Donaldson JA, et al.: Surgical Anatomy of the Temporal Bone, 4th ed. New York, Raven Press, 1992, p 201.
9. Anson BJ, Bast TH: Anatomical structure of the stapes and the relation of the stapedial footplate to vital parts of the labyrinth. Ann Otol Rhinol Laryngol 67: 389–399, 1958.
10. Pauw BKH, Pollack AM, Fisch U: Utricle saccule and cochlear duct in relation to stapedotomy. A histological human temporal study. Ann Otol Rhinol Laryngol 100: 966, 1991.
11. Leek JH: An anamolous facial nerve: The otologist's albatross. Laryngoscope 84: 1535–1544, 1974.
12. Willis R: Conductive deafness due to malplacement of the seventh nerve. J Otolaryngol 6: 1–4, 1977.
13. Derlacki EL: Revision stapes surgery: Problems with some solutions. Laryngoscope 95: N47, 1985.
14. Farrior D: Abstruse complications of stapes surgery: Diagnosis and treatment. In Henry Ford Hospital International Symposium on Otosclerosis. Chicago, Little Brown Company, 1962, pp 509–521.
15. Tos M, Lau T: Tympanosclerosis of the middle ear. Late results of surgical treatment. J Laryngol Otol 104: 685–689, 1990.
16. Gormley PK: Stapedectomy in tympanosclerosis. Am J Otol 8: 123–130, 1987.
17. Giddings NA, House JW: Tympanosclerosis of the stapes—Hearing results for various surgical treatments. Otolaryngol Head Neck Surg 107: 644–650, 1992.
18. Majoras M: Electronystagmography during stapedectomy. Int Surg 47: 323–327, 1967.
19. Glasscock ME: The stapes gusher. Arch Otolaryngol Head Neck Surg 98: 82–91, 1973.
20. Smith MFW, McElveen JT: Neurological Surgery of the Ear. St. Louis, Mosby Yearbook, 1992, pp 123–124.
21. Sheehy JL, Nelson RA, House HP: Revision stapectomy: A review of 258 cases. Laryngoscope 91: 43–51, 1981.
22. Feldman BA, Schuknecht HF: Experiences with revision stapedectomy procedures. Laryngoscope 80: 1281–1291, 1970.
23. Glasscock, ME, McKennan KX, Levine SC: Revision stapedectomy surgery. Otolaryngol Head Neck Surg 96: 141–148, 1987.
24. Pearman K, Dawes JDK: Post-stapedectomy conductive deafness and results of revision surgery. J Laryngol Otol 96: 405–410, 1982.
25. Bhardwaj BK, Kacker SK: Revision stapes surgery. J Laryngol Otol 102: 20–24, 1988.
26. Farrior J, Sutherland A: Revision stapes surgery. Laryngoscope 101: 1155–1161, 1991.
27. Mawson LR: Management of complications of stapedectomy. J Laryngol Otol 89: 145–149, 1975.
28. Dawes JDK, Curry AR, Rannie I: Post-stapedectomy granuloma of the oval window. J Laryngol Otol 87: 365–378, 1973.
29. Burtner D, Goodman ML: Etiological factors in poststapedectomy granulomas. Arch Otolaryngol Head Neck Surg 100: 171–173, 1974.
30. Alberti PWRM: The blood supply of the long process of the incus and the head and neck of stapes. J Otolaryngol Otol 79: 964–970, 1965.
31. Lippy WH, Schuring AG: Solving ossicular problems in stapedectomy. Laryngoscope 93: 1147–1150, 1983.
32. Sheehy JL: Stapedectomy: Incus bypass procedures. A report of 203 operations. Laryngoscope 92: 258–262, 1982.
33. Mathisen J: Phonophobia after stapedectomy. Acta Otolaryngol (Stockh) 68: 73–77, 1969.
34. Bracewell A: Diplacusis binauralis—A complication of stapedectomy. J Laryngol Otol 80: 55–60, 1966.
35. Gristwood RE: Acute otitis media following the stapedectomy operation. J Laryngol Otol 80: 312–317, 1966.
36. Brown JS: Meningitis following stapes surgery. The pathway of spread to the intra-cranial cavity. Laryngoscope 77:1295–1303, 1967.
37. Clairmont AA, Nicholson WL, Turner JS: Pseudomonas aeruginosa meningitis following stapedectomy. Laryngoscope 85: 1076–1083, 1975.

38. Snyder BD: Delayed meningitis following stapes surgery. Arch Neurol 36: 174–175, 1979.
39. Palva T, Palva A, Karga J. Fatal meningitis in a case of otosclerosis operated upon bilaterally. Arch Otolaryngol Head Neck Surg 96: 130–137, 1972.
40. Althaus SR, House HP: Delayed post-stapedectomy facial paralysis: A report of 5 cases. Laryngoscope 83: 1234–1240, 1973.
41. Von Haacke NP: Cholesteatoma following stapedectomy. J Laryngol Otol 101: 708–710, 1987.
42. Benecke JE, Gadre AK, Linthicum FH: Chondrogenic potential of tragal perichondrium. A cause of hearing loss following stapedectomy. Laryngoscope 100: 1292–1293, 1990.
43. Moon CN: Perilymphatic fistulas complicating the stapedectomy operation: A review of 49 cases. Laryngoscope 80: 515–535, 1970.
44. Lippy WH, Schuring AG: Stapedectomy revision following sensorineural hearing loss. Otolaryngol Head Neck Surg 92: 580–582, 1984.

Appendix

The booklet is entitled *Facts on Otosclerosis* and it can be on the individual physician's or physician's and audiologist's clinic stationery and/or could be stored in a computer database and be prepared for each individual patient. The booklet should be filled out for each patient.

Otologist

An otologist is first a Doctor of Medicine, and second, a medical and surgical specialist in diseases of the ear and related structures.

Audiologist

An audiologist has a Master's Degree or a Doctor of Philosophy Degree and performs hearing testing procedures to define hearing loss and provide or recommend rehabilitation programs for those having hearing loss. Some audiologists also have additional training to fit and dispense hearing aids.

Function of the Normal Ear

The ear is divided into three parts: the external ear, the middle ear, and the inner ear. Each part performs an important function in the process of hearing. Sound waves pass through the canal of the external ear and vibrate the eardrum. The eardrum separates the external ear from the middle ear. The three small bones in the middle ear act as a transformer to transmit energy of the sound vibrations in the air to the fluids of the inner ear. Vibrations in the inner ear fluid stimulate the approximately 16,000 inner ear hair cells of the hearing nerve, which then carries the sound impulses to the brain, where they are interpreted. A portion of the inner ear is involved in balance.

Types of Hearing Impairment

There are three types of hearing loss:

1. CONDUCTIVE
   A conductive loss may occur if there is a problem in the external or middle ear.
2. NERVE
   A nerve loss occurs when a problem lies in the inner ear or along the auditory pathways.
3. MIXED
   A mixed loss is the result of a combination of conductive and nerve losses.

Otosclerosis

Our clinical diagnosis of your hearing impairment is otosclerosis. Otosclerosis implies a fixation of the stapes or stirrup bone of the middle ear. Much evidence indicates that otosclerosis is a hereditary disease of unknown cause and is passed down in families, although some generations may be skipped.

Otosclerosis can exist for many years before it interferes with hearing ability. The hearing impairment grows worse gradually, but very rarely does otosclerosis cause total deafness. The hardening or fixation process may cease, in which event the hearing remains at a constant level throughout life. In some cases, the otosclerosis process involves the inner ear. This loss of nerve function, once it develops, is permanent. The amount of hearing loss due to fixation of the stapes, and the degree of nerve damage present, can be determined only by carefully administered hearing tests.

Head noises (tinnitus) may be present. These noises may be perceived as ringing, roaring, or buzzing in the ears or head. The amount of head noise is not necessarily related to the degree of hearing impairment. This head noise may be produced by either the fixation of the stapes or by involvement of the inner ear, or both.

Finding Causes

How is otosclerosis diagnosed? Diagnosis is based on your history, physical examination, and results of hearing testing.

Hearing Tests

One hearing test will be a measure of the softest level at which you are able to hear sounds of different pitches; another will measure the softest level at which you can hear speech. In addition, your ability to understand speech will be assessed.

Treatment of Otosclerosis

Medical

There is no local treatment to the ear itself, such as massage or inflations or any medication, such as drugs, vitamins, minerals, or diet that will have a permanent influence on the otosclerotic process.

Sodium fluoride has been used for the treatment of otosclerosis. However, the physicians at this institution do not use sodium fluoride in the treatment of otosclerosis because of limited scientific evidence to indicate its usefulness and because of potential complications. If you would like to pursue this issue further, we would be glad to discuss it with you in more detail.

Hearing Aids

Because hearing loss from otosclerosis is a loss of loudness, a hearing aid can be used successfully.

The Stapes Operation

Stapes surgery is frequently recommended for patients with otosclerosis. This operation is performed under local or general anesthesia and usually requires a short period of outpatient hospitalization. Convalescence lasts approximately 1 week.

In stapes surgery, an operating microscope is used. The eardrum is carefully elevated and the middle ear inspected. By use of a surgical laser or other method, a small hole is created in the stapes. Rarely, it is necessary to remove the entire stapes bone. Many techniques can then be used to connect the remaining middle ear bones with the inner ear. The eardrum is then replaced. This stapes operation allows the sound vibrations to pass again from the eardrum through the middle ear to the inner ear.

The patient having stapes surgery may return to work 6 or 7 days later. There may be slight dizziness with sudden head motion for several weeks. There may also be a taste disturbance immediately following surgery that usually subsides within 2 or 3 weeks. However, in a small percentage of patients, taste impairment is permanent. Fortunately, there is usually little postoperative discomfort.

Patients who reside a long distance from this office should plan to be in the area for a total of 5 days, including the day of surgery. Air travel is permissible 3 days following surgery (this varies from surgeon to surgeon and clinic to clinic).

Hearing Improvement Following Surgery
Hearing improvement may or may not be noticeable at the time of the operation. If the hearing improves at the time of surgery, it usually regresses in a few hours due to blood clot formation in the middle ear and packing in the external canal. Improvement in hearing will usually be apparent within 3 weeks following surgery. Maximum hearing is obtained in approximately 4 months.

If stapes surgery is not successful, the hearing usually remains the same as before the operation. In most instances, the ear may be reoperated on with a good chance of a successful result. In 2 per cent of the cases, the hearing may be further impaired in the ear that had surgery. In fewer than 1 per cent, there may be a severe loss of hearing in the ear. In this situation, the head noise may be more pronounced, and dizziness may persist for some time. For this reason, the poorer-hearing ear is usually selected for surgery. There are risks involved in stapes surgery, as in all surgery: drug reactions, postoperative infections, and injury to adjacent structures.

If you do not desire to have stapes surgery performed at this time, or do not choose to use a hearing aid, you should have your hearing retested in 1 year.

Should any questions arise regarding your hearing impairment, please do not hesitate to call or write to our office.

The Findings in Your Case
Our hearing tests reveal that your hearing loss approximates:

Right ear _____ dB Left ear _____ dB

( ) You have good hearing nerve function and are a very suitable candidate for the stapes operation.

( ) Your hearing nerve has been damaged slightly. If the stapes operation is successful, serviceable hearing will be restored to you.

( ) Your hearing nerve has been damaged to some extent. If the stapes operation is successful, you will be able to hear in many situations without a hearing aid but may need one for distant hearing.

( ) Your hearing nerve has been damaged by the otosclerotic process. If the stapes operation is successful, you will gain more benefit from the use of your hearing aid.

( ) Your hearing nerve has been severely damaged. For this reason, the chances of surgery improving your hearing are reduced. If surgery were successful, your hearing would improve to the extent that you may be able to use a hearing aid.

( ) You have such far-advanced otosclerosis that we do not recommend surgery at this time.

In your instance, you have approximately _____ out of 10 chances that surgery will give a permanent satisfactory hearing improvement to you.

The principles of an informed consent are careful explanation to the patient of the risks, rewards, and alternative courses of action. This informed consent is documented, and the consultation is dictated in the presence of the patient.

_____

Your signature on this informed consent form indicates that you have read the booklet on otosclerosis and that you wish to proceed with surgery.

_____   _____
Signature of the Patient   Date

_____   _____
Witness   Date

31

Perilymphatic Fistula

GEORGE T. SINGLETON, M.D.
WILLIAM H. SLATTERY, M.D.

Perilymphatic fistulas (PLFs) undoubtedly exist in association with stapedectomies and other invasive procedures of the cochlea. Likewise, severe head injury, abdominal blows, and rapid shifts in environmental pressure are accepted as causes of true PLF. Dissent remains, however, with regard to idiopathic PLF. Controversy stems from the interpretation of histopathologic findings of temporal bones in the region of the fissula antefenestrum and round window niche, the confusion of PLF with Ménière's disease, multiple tests that likely misidentify Ménière's disease as PLF, and the incidence of PLF in congenital forms of deafness. Some surgeons are doing large numbers of PLF operations based on these conjectural criteria; however, a recent national survey indicated that PLFs are uncommon.[1]

True PLF most commonly occurs as a result of external trauma to the head or abdomen or from rapid pressure shifts in the environment. Congenital defects of the middle ear space account for approximately 20 per cent of PLFs, if abnormally placed round window membranes are included. Complications resulting from invasive procedures of the cochlea, including stapedectomy, the "tack" procedure, and cochleosacculotomy for the treatment of Ménière's disease, may result in persistent PLF.[2] Acute and chronic mastoiditis with erosion into the labyrinth as well as chronic granulomatous diseases, such as syphilis and tuberculosis, is of historical interest only in the development of PLF.

Homeostasis of the pressure differentials between endolymph and perilymph is maintained by the presence of both a patent endolymphatic duct and sac located in the dura of the posterior fossa and the cochlear aqueduct that leads from the scala tympani of the cochlea to the posterior fossa. In children and some young adults, this aqueduct is open. With maturity, the duct is normally criss-crossed with arachnoid strands; thus, it functions as if sealed with a semipermeable membrane. Increased cerebrospinal fluid pressure in the normal adult results in equally increased pressures in the perilymphatic and endolymphatic space. Thus, damage to the endolymphatic membrane structure is unlikely.[3] The only outlet from increased intracochlear pressure is a tear of the round window membrane or annular ligament, which occurs most frequently anteroinferiorly, rarely superiorly, and never posteriorly around the stapes footplate. Congenital deformities of the stapes may occur and result in PLF. These deformities most commonly involve the posterior crus and posterior half of the footplate or occur as central perforations of the footplate. The round window membrane tears far less frequently; in the author's series, only twice has a normal round window membrane torn.[27] In both instances, there was a severe blow to the head, resulting in PLF at both the round and oval windows. The remaining tears to the round window membrane have occurred when its position was 45 degrees to the promontory and there was little or no overhanging promontory. In these cases, the round window membrane was directly visible when the middle ear was viewed transtympanically (Fig. 31–1A).[4, 5] This anomaly is probably associated with an abnormally patent cochlear aqueduct.[6] The cochlear aqueduct opens into the scala tympani adjacent to the round window.

The cribriform areas at the depths of the internal auditory canal are another source of potential transmission of increased cerebrospinal fluid pressure to the perilymphatic space. In rare instances, these areas are wide open, with direct connections of cerebrospinal fluid to perilymph. This is particularly true in Mondini deformities of the cochlea, which lead to gushers with any invasive operative procedure of the cochlea in these patients.

Goodhill coined the terms *implosive* and *explosive* pressure changes that result in PLF.[7] By implosive, he states that increased pressure from the tubal tympanic region is directed via the ossicles to the perilymphatic space, resulting in a tear in the annular ligament or the round window membrane. This problem may occur with inadequate equalization of the middle ear or with blast injuries. The explosive route results from increased intracranial pressure due to a blow to the head or abdomen. Increased intra-abdominal pressure is transmitted via the vertebral veins to increase the cerebrospinal pressure, thus causing an increase of intracranial pressure. Pressure is placed on both the

FIGURE 31–1. *A,* Right middle ear: surgeon's view with tympanomeatal flap and drum folded forward. *B,* Abnormal round window membrane at 45-degree right angle to promontory and no overhanging lip. *C,* Normal round window membrane hidden from view in depths of niche, with lip of bone overhang. Mucosal folds frequently appear to seal niche partially, with hole in center.

FIGURE 31-1

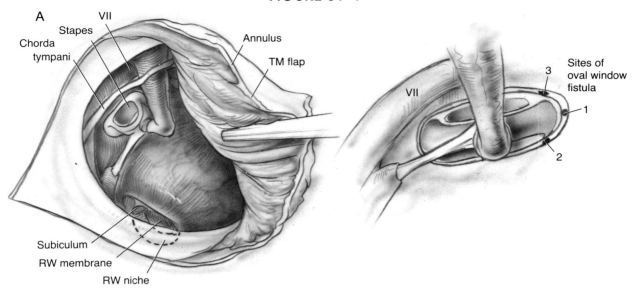

A

Chorda tympani
Stapes
VII
Annulus
TM flap

Subiculum
RW membrane
RW niche

VII

Sites of oval window fistula
3
1
2

Cross section

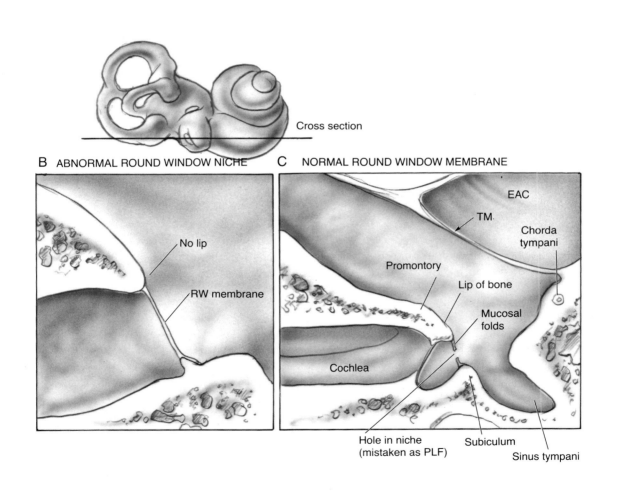

B ABNORMAL ROUND WINDOW NICHE

No lip
RW membrane

C NORMAL ROUND WINDOW MEMBRANE

EAC
TM
Chorda tympani
Promontory
Lip of bone
Mucosal folds
Cochlea
Hole in niche (mistaken as PLF)
Subiculum
Sinus tympani

endolymphatic and perilymphatic systems, as outlined earlier, with rupture from inside out of either the annular ligament or the round window membrane.[7]

Early stapedectomy procedures were more likely to result in PLF than the methods practiced today. A pointed polyethylene strut prosthesis placed over absorbable gelatin sponge (Gelfoam) or a thin tissue seal was a common culprit when the patient was subjected to a change in barometric pressure, that is, ascent or descent in the mountains or in airplanes. Various wire procedures with a gelatin sponge seal had a similar plight. Piston procedures, when used without interposed tissue, commonly resulted in fistula development. The current small fenestra, small-piston, tissue seal techniques have dramatically lowered the incidence of PLF.[8–12]

Invasive procedures of the stapes footplate, including the Fick procedure and the tack procedure for Ménière's disease, were ultimately abandoned because of the relatively high incidence of sensorineural hearing loss. Later exploration of many of these ears revealed a persistent PLF. Likewise, the 20 per cent sensorineural hearing loss associated with cochleostomy or cochleosacculotomy as it was originally described is, in most instances, probably related to a persistent round window PLF; surgeons did not remove the scutum, roughen the surface of the round window membrane, and seal the fistula they had made with the pick prior to closing the ear.[2]

Microfissures of the otic capsule may lead to PLF, although this hypothesis has never been confirmed in any patent or temporal bone.[13] Kohut et al., in temporal bone studies, has suggested that microfissures around the round window niche may result in leaks if there is no dense collagen plug on the middle ear side.[14] This study also demonstrated an intact inner ear lining, endosteum, periosteum, and middle ear mucosa in the temporal bones with these fissures. These investigators also reported that there are likely leaks through the fissula ante fenestram where no bony or cartilaginous plug exists.[14] Again in these cases, multiple layers seal this area, and no leak has been demonstrated. Kohut et al. reported seeing fluid in the area of the fissula ante fenestram after the mucosa in this area was destroyed with a pick or other instrument.[15] A follow-up study by Shazly and Linthicum has shown that the fissures do occur, and that the changes in the fissula ante fenestram as described by Kohut et al. are present. However, they demonstrated that there is absolutely no association between these findings and sudden sensorineural hearing loss and no evidence of a perilymphatic fluid leak.[16]

Numerous authors have added confusion to the issue of idiopathic PLF by describing the symptoms of PLF as exactly the same as those of Ménière's disease, that is, fluctuant sensorineural hearing loss, tinnitus, episodic vertigo, and pressure feeling in the involved ear. These authors use the same criteria to diagnose Ménière's disease and PLF. These criteria include the use of hyperosmolar solutions, such as Renografin, urea, and glycerine, to demonstrate an improvement in hearing exactly as would be expected in Ménière's cases (Weider and Johnson, unpublished data).[17] These same tests were used for predictive evaluation of Ménière's cases before endolymphatic shunt procedures were performed.

Numerous authors have touted electrocochleography as an effective technique for the differentiation of Ménière's disease from PLF.[18, 19] Results from a recent study suggest that electrocochleographic techniques are not valid for separating Ménière's patients from normal patients.[20] Meyerhoff describes electrocochleographic changes after patching windows without PLF and attributes this phenomenon to a change in fluid dynamics.[19] One must question this interpretation; electrocochleographic changes most likely represent normal changes seen in Ménière's disease.

A surprising number of re-exploration procedures by this author have been done on patients who have had previous PLF surgery. These patients have an absolutely classic history of Ménière's disease. The initial surgeon's operative record describes a hole in the round window membrane. In every case explored, a perfectly normal round window membrane was found lying deep in the niche with no evidence that the round window had been touched. The first surgeon simply sealed the mucosal folds that surround the round window niche (Fig. 31–1B).

For a time, patients with congenital deafness that exhibited fluctuating hearing loss were thought to have PLF. Studies by Riley, Parnes and McCabe, Pappas et al., and Bluestone have made it very clear that PLF associated with congenital sensorineural hearing loss is quite uncommon.[21–24] When a PLF is truly present and corrected, the associated dizziness is frequently improved, although the hearing is rarely improved, and only about half the time is it stabilized.[21–24] The Bluestone study is fairly typical. In this group of 244 children with congenital hearing loss, only 6 per cent had a PLF; 36 per cent of the 44 ears selected for exploration had a fistula present. Only 23% were improved by the operative intervention. Bluestone concluded that for a diagnosis of PLF in a case of congenital hearing loss to be correct, the patient had to have labyrinthitis, meningitis, additional sensorineural hearing loss following acute otitis media, or hearing loss made worse by trauma. The author's success in identifying PLF in congenital hearing loss cases has not occurred in those with fluctuating sensorineural hearing loss. However, in patients who have demonstrated positional nystagmus compatible with PLF, a positive eyes-closed-turning test result, a positive fistula test result, or a Tulleo response, a fistula has been identified without exception.[6]

PATIENT SELECTION

The typical patient with a PLF presents with a sudden onset of hearing loss, or mild vertigo or disequilibrium, or both, associated with a traumatic event. The onset is sudden in 94 per cent of proven PLF, and in 89 per cent of cases, trauma is related to the onset of symptoms. Trauma includes invasive inner ear surgical procedures, abdominal blows, head blows, blast injuries, or severe changes in environmental pressure, particularly in the presence of an upper respiratory infection or an acute allergic attack. Unsteadiness or dizziness is present in 90 per cent of cases, and the dizziness is usually positional in nature. Seventy-five per cent of patients will have a history of tinnitus, irrespective of whether a hearing loss is present.[6] Hearing loss is present in 53 per cent of patients and is not fluctuant in nature. PLF is *not* characterized by fluctuant hearing loss associated with episodic vertigo, tinnitus, and a full feeling in the ears, as some purport. That condition is Ménière's disease.

Significant physical findings in PLF include a characteristic positional nystagmus in 94 per cent of patients, a positive eyes-closed-turning test result to the side of the lesion in 89 per cent, a hearing loss in 53 per cent, a positive fistula test result in 25 per cent, and a positive Tulleo phenomenon in 4 per cent. The characteristic positional nystagmus may have a very short or no latency and a relatively long duration, and minimal or no fatigue is evident on repeated testing. Also, this nystagmus does not reverse direction on changing from the inducing position to the sitting position. It is not nearly as violent as that seen with benign paroxysmal postural vertigo. The nystagmus occurs with the involved ear undermost in 80 per cent of the cases, and it beats toward the involved ear in only 60 per cent. The nystagmus is rarely rotatory: from most to least frequent, it may be horizontal, diagonal, or vertical.[23, 24]

The hearing loss is usually sensorineural but may be predominantly conductive in the case of a slipped stapes prosthesis. When not associated with a slipped stapes prosthesis, the hearing loss is a sensorineural loss that may be flat, downsloping, or upsloping. The speech reception threshold is usually worse than one would anticipate from the pure tones, and the discrimination score is usually lower than expected.[6]

Identification of the involved ear is sometimes quite difficult. If hearing loss is associated with the traumatic event that created the PLF, then the involved side is obvious. The side is also obvious in cases with a positive fistula test result or in the presence of a Tulleo phenomenon. As indicated earlier, positional nystagmus occurs with the involved ear undermost in only 80 per cent of cases. The direction of the nystagmus is of no diagnostic value in determining which ear is involved. The eyes-closed-turning test result is positive in 90 per cent of patients with PLF and is highly specific to the side of involvement with only a 1 per cent error. The eyes-closed-turning test is performed by having the patient walk in a straight line with the eyes closed. The examiner taps the subject's shoulder, indicating to the patient to turn 180° either right or left and stop in a position of attention with the eyes still closed (Fig. 31–2). A positive test result is readily recognized by the patient's swaying or having a tendency to lose balance when he or she has turned to the side of the lesion. Patients with significant central nervous system lesions are unable to perform the test; therefore, these patients are not at risk of misdiagnosis as PLF.[25, 26]

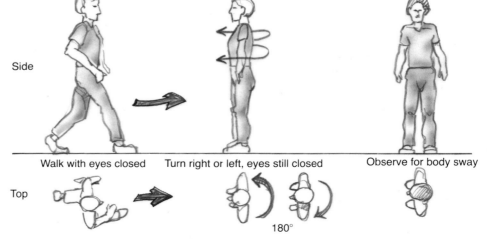

FIGURE 31–2. Eyes-closed-turning test. Patient walks with eyes closed, turns quickly right or left, then stops in position of attention with eyes still closed. A positive test result consists of staggering or swaying on turn to the involved side.

Side   Walk with eyes closed   Turn right or left, eyes still closed   Observe for body sway

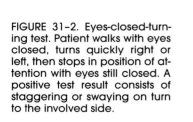

Top   180°

The Quix test has been recommended for identification of the involved side of the lesion; however, the result is positive only in about 20 per cent of cases.[27] This test involves having the patients stand erect with their feet together, their eyes closed, and arms outstretched. The examiner looks for a deviation of the arms to the side of the lesion. No specialized audiometric or electronystagmography test has been of any value in identifying a PLF or the side of the lesion. Flood et al. recommended a test in which the involved ear is placed uppermost in an attempt to get air into the vestibule and thus convert a neurosensory loss to a combined conductive neurosensory loss.[28]

We have been unsuccessful in 25 cases of proven PLF to see this phenomenon develop.

Black et al. reported posturography as being highly specific and highly sensitive in detecting PLF.[29] This finding has not been corroborated by others, and a critical look at this study suggests that there is probably confusion with Ménière's disease in the study population. In this study, the identification of probable fistulas took place after mucosa of the middle ear had been significantly disturbed.[29]

Silverstein advocated the use of twin cruciate myringotomy incisions over the oval and round windows of the suspected ear and micropipette collection of fluid from the oval window recess and the round window niche.[30] This procedure has not gained much favor because of technical difficulties and the fact that false-negative results occasionally occur.

PREOPERATIVE EVALUATION AND PATIENT COUNSELING

Patients should have the usual preoperative evaluation required for local anesthesia, with monitored anesthetic care in an ambulatory surgical setting. Healthy young adults receive only a hematocrit test preoperatively; older patients will receive more extensive evaluation, as will those who have systemic diseases. Patients are advised to stop aspirin and nonsteroidal analgesic therapy 10 to 14 days before their surgical date. Patients are instructed to wash their hair the night before surgery and to put nothing on their hair. They are told that three-fourths inch of hair will be shaved from around the ear. Patients are advised that if PLF is found, a small incision will be made either over the tragus or above and behind the ear for obtaining a graft.

Patients are informed that if a leak is found, they will be on bed rest for 5 days with bathroom privileges only. They are advised that when they get up, they are to roll onto their side and push up with their arms so that they do not tighten their bellies. They are advised that they will be placed on sedatives, and that

they will have stool softeners given to them so that they do not strain to have a bowel movement. They are to sleep either in a recliner chair or in a bed that has the head elevated four to six inches. For 9 days after the 5 days of bed rest, they may get up and walk around the house but may do no heavy lifting and have no sexual activity. At 2 weeks, they may return to work if they have a sedentary job; if they are manual laborers, they are not allowed to work for 3 months. They are advised that they will be seen in the clinic 2 weeks postoperatively for follow-up.

SURGICAL PROCEDURE

Preoperative Preparation

Patients will have an intravenous line started in the preoperative holding area. They are asked to go to the bathroom immediately before coming back to the operative suite. If they are unusually nervous, they may receive a small amount of midazolam (Versed) before coming back to the operating room. Patients are placed backwards on a standard operating table that is double-mattressed except at the head, thereby allowing room for the surgeon's legs. During surgical site preparation, the head is kept level on a folded towel or blanket. Approximately three-fourths inch of hair is shaved from around the ear, and all loose hair is removed with wide adhesive tape. The remaining hair is held back by brushing it with K-Y jelly so that it stays clear of the operative field. The anesthesiologist places the electrocardiographic monitors, chest stethoscope, and pulse oximeter on the patient. An automatic blood pressure cuff is placed on the arm opposite the ear to be operated on. This action prevents accidental movement of the surgeon's arm during insufflation. The skin is prepared with povidone-iodine (Betadine) soap, wiped clean, painted with povidone-iodine solution and dried, and the solution is wiped from around the ear. Skin around the ear is prepared with Mastisol adhesive. A 3M adhesive drape with a two-inch hole is placed over the ear. The drape is folded so that it does not fall over the patient's mouth and nose. A disposable, lint-free, paper, ear draping pack is used to cover the patient and the remaining portion of the operating field. No towels or other lint-bearing materials are used. The front of the drape is held up on an intravenous line pole so that the patient can see the anesthesiologist, and, if the patient wishes, can watch the television monitor.

Surgical Instruments

A standard tympanostomy setup is used. Disposable, straight, and angled Beaver ear blades are used for flap incisions. A Skeeter Micro Drill with 1mm to

1.4mm diamond burrs is used for removing scutum. A 0.5mm sharp 90-degree pick is altered slightly by bending its shaft 20-degrees two inches from the end to allow better visualization of the tip. An angled handle straight pick is used for work around the stapes footplate and to place grafts.

Surgical Technique

The folded blanket is removed from under the patient's head, and a single towel is placed between the patient's head and the table mattress. A four-quadrant injection of the ear canal with small amounts of 1% lidocaine (Xylocaine) with 1:50,000 epinephrine is used to prevent the speculum from hurting the ear. The area of the tragus and the area above and behind the ear over the temporalis muscle are also injected for potential harvesting of graft tissue. The local anesthetic from the four quadrants is disbursed with a spreading speculum. The ear canal is then irrigated copiously with normal saline to remove the povidone-iodine, cerumen, and hairs. A 1.5-inch 27-gauge needle is then used to inject the vascular strip area. Care is taken to produce no excessive injection or blisters. The inferior injection is placed posteroinferiorly at the bony cartilaginous junction, and care is taken to place the bevel of the needle against bone and under the periosteum. The injection is a very slow, deliberate process, with the surgeon watching carefully for blanching and making sure that it goes all the way to the annulus inferiorly. The surgeon now completes the removal of the desquamated epithelium from the ear canal with a small suction.

The inferior incision is made first by use of the No. 1 or straight Beaver blade. A cut is made from the 6 o'clock position and is angled to about 1cm lateral to the annular ring on the posterior ear canal. The No. 2, or angled, Beaver blade is used to make an incision superiorly from 2mm lateral to the short process of the malleus to join the tip of the other incision in the posterior ear canal. A duckbill elevator is used to elevate the skin of the posterior canal down to the annulus. If problems arise with fibers sticking in the suture line, a House No. 2 knife is used to separate these. Hemostasis is completed with the 20-gauge suction placed on the bleeder and touched with a Valley Lab cautery set between five and seven o'clock. Hemostasis must be obtained before the middle ear is opened. The middle ear is opened at the notch of Rivinus by use of a Rosen needle. The chorda tympani nerve is then identified, and the beginning of the annular ring is raised with the Rosen needle. The entire posterior portion of the annular ring may be elevated with the Rosen needle, or a drum elevator may be used. The chorda tympani is gingerly dissected free of the tympanic membrane, and the posterior half of the tympanic membrane and the ear canal flap are folded forward so that the middle ear may be inspected (see Fig. 31-1).

Frequently, clear fluid is seen in the oval window recess and in the round window niche. This fluid is usually local anesthetic that has seeped into the middle ear space, and a 24-gauge suction is used to remove it. The patient is then asked to perform a Valsalva maneuver to observe if fluid reaccumulates. If fluid does reaccumulate and it is unclear whether a fistula is present, the fluid may be checked to determine if it is perilymph in two ways. A simple way is to put a small piece of absorbable gelatin sponge on an angled straight pick, soak up the solution, and then place it on a Clinistrip for glucose testing. If the glucose reading is approximately 100 mg/dl and if no blood has been allowed in the middle ear, the surgeon can be sure that the fluid is perilymph. Another technique is to use the Xomed Treace kit for measuring protein. This technique has been described by Silverstein: a micropipette is used to pick up the fluid, which is placed on indicator paper. The color change is compared with a standard. Again, the presence of protein in the absence of blood in the middle ear space identifies the fluid as perilymph.[30] Note that the scutum has not been removed and that the mucosa in the middle ear has not been touched except with the 24-gauge suction to remove the fluid that may have been present when the middle ear was opened. The round window niche has not been disturbed, nor has the lip of the promontory overlying it.

If the round window membrane is immediately visible when the middle ear is opened, that is, at about a 45-degree angle to the plane of the promontory, then the surgeon should become suspicious of a probable PLF in the round window membrane.[29-31] Only after checking for the recurrence of fluid in these recesses does the surgeon remove the scutum and get complete exposure of the oval window area. If fluid was not present earlier and fluid did not appear on Valsalva maneuver, the surgeon can place a straight pick on the lenticular process of the incus and press gently, looking for the accumulation of fluid around the annular ligament or in the round window niche. If no fluid accumulates in either place with both Valsalva maneuver and pressure on the stapes, no repair is performed. The authors believe that there is risk for creating some degree of conductive hearing loss and a possibility of injuring the inner ear by patching a round window or oval window with no PLF.

Most PLFs at the oval window are located directly anterior to the anterior crus or immediately below it; a few are superior to the anterior crus (Fig. 31-3). Generally the surgeon can see this area and can actually see the hole. Leaks in this area are best repaired by teasing away the surface mucosa either with the straight pick or with the tiny right-angled pick. A graft of adventitia is obtained from over the temporalis fascia. This graft is compressed and cut into the shape of a small set of trousers, about 3mm long and 1.5mm wide, and a 2mm slit is made up the middle longways to form the pant's legs (Fig. 31–3A). The graft is then draped around the anterior crus and packed in place with gelatin sponge (Fig. 31–3B) soaked in Ringer's solution. This material is placed to the level of the tympanic membrane, and a sheet of absorbable gelatin film (Gelfilm) is placed over the gelatin sponge to prevent adhesions to the tympanic membrane.

If there is a congenital defect of the stapes footplate, the hole may be in the middle of the footplate or it may incorporate the entire posterior half of the footplate (Fig. 31–4). In these cases, the mucosa must be denuded all the way around the footplate. With larger perforations, the authors use perichondrium from the tragus because it is thicker and easier to handle to effect a seal. The area between the crura is packed full with gelatin sponge to hold the graft in place.

If the round window membrane has a fistula, the membrane will be in clear sight with no overhang of the round window niche. As a general rule, the tear will be readily visible somewhere around the annular ring of the membrane. Occasionally, it is in the center, particularly if it was made by a myringotomy knife or by a foreign body introduced into the ear. If the fistula is less than 2 weeks old, a fibrin clot or granulation tissue will be seen around the leak. The area around the perforation is roughened by use of the tiny right-angled pick. A thicker graft of perichondrium from the tragus is used. The graft is held in place with absorbable gelatin sponge packed all the way to the level of the tympanic membrane, and then a sheet of absorbable gelatin film is placed to prevent adhesive bands from forming between the tympanic membrane and the round window seal. The tympanic membrane is replaced to its normal position, the skin flap in the canal is laid flat, and a 0.25-inch × 1.5-inch strip of Owen's Non-adherent Surgical Dressing is dampened in saline and laid over the tympanic membrane and the flap. The graft site is then closed with suitable sutures.

Dressing and Postoperative Care

A cotton ball is placed in the ear canal. The patient is returned to the recovery room in a semisitting position. If a PLF was found, the patient is sent home with instructions for absolute bed rest except for bathroom privileges for the first 5 days. The patient should sleep with the head of the bed elevated or in a reclining chair. The patient is advised to roll on his or her side and push up with the arms rather than sit up so that the abdominal muscles are not tightened, which would increase cerebrospinal fluid pressure and float the graft out. The patient is kept on small doses of diazepam (Valium), 5mg, three times per day, and flurazepam (Dalmane), 30mg at bedtime. The sedatives are prescribed during the first 5 days of bed rest. A stool softener, such as bisacodyl (Dulcolax), is used for the first 2 weeks. The patient removes the cotton ball from the ear canal on the first postoperative day. This action will also remove the rayon strip and any blood clot in the ear canal. The patient is advised to sneeze with the mouth open only, and to not blow the nose for 2 weeks.

Pitfalls

There are two potential pitfalls of PLF surgery. The first is an inability to obtain adequate hemostasis and anesthesia, particularly in the lower portion of the flap. The second is obtaining adequate visualization of the oval window area without removing the scutum. Finally, some patients are quite uncomfortable when the surgeon begins to denude the area around the stapes or over the round window membrane in preparation for graft placement. We avoid putting 4% lidocaine in the middle ear as is routinely done when the middle ear is opened for a stapedectomy, singular neurectomy, or other middle ear procedures performed under local anesthesia. If the lidocaine gets into the inner ear, the patient will become violently dizzy and lose all hearing in the ear for a short period of time.

Adhesive bands must not form between the tympanic membrane and a graft over the round window membrane. If the bands do form, the patient will have

FIGURE 31–3. Details of oval window fistula sites in order of occurrence. Sites 1–3 are in the annular ligament site. *A*, Pants graft of areolar tissue 3mm × 1.5mm with legs 2mm long. *B*, Pants graft in place over denuded mucosa around perilymphatic fistula.

FIGURE 31–4. Congenital defects in posterior footplate.

FIGURE 31-3

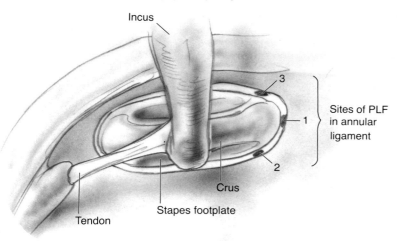

Incus

3

1 } Sites of PLF in annular ligament

2

Crus

Stapes footplate

Tendon

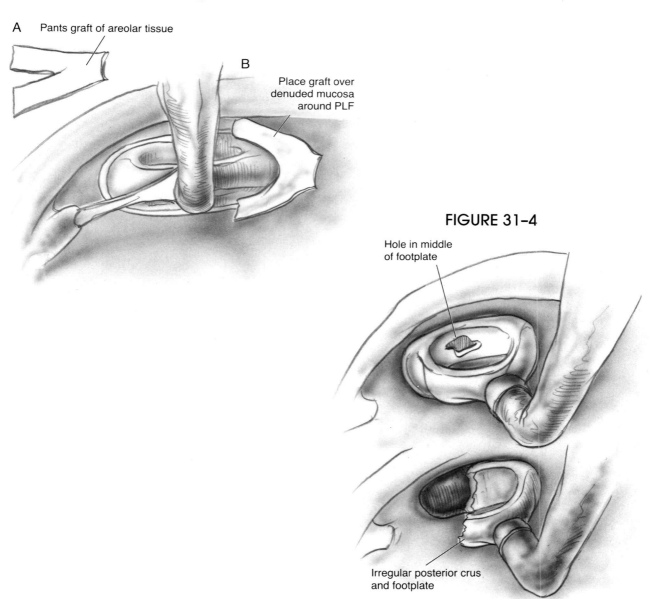

A   Pants graft of areolar tissue

B

Place graft over denuded mucosa around PLF

FIGURE 31-4

Hole in middle of footplate

Irregular posterior crus and footplate

an apparent sensorineural hearing loss combined with a conductive loss, both of which will clear when the adhesion is lysed. Fat should be avoided as a graft material, as the failure rate will exceed 50%.[25]

Revision PLF Repair

If instability and mild vertigo persist after the repair has healed, and if the turning or fistula test results are still positive, re-exploration should be considered. Failure occurs most frequently in cases with rather deep recesses of the oval window where one cannot get good access in front of the anterior crus to denude the bed and get the graft packed tightly enough into the area of the fistula tract. The procedure is identical to that used originally. Six weeks is allowed for the wound to completely heal before any revision is undertaken. The surgeon should attempt to re-repair a fistula at the oval window niche at least three times before considering doing a stapedectomy to close the fistula. For some reason, these PLF ears seem more sensitive than others to stapedectomy. In the author's hands, high-frequency sensorineural hearing loss has occurred every time a stapedectomy has been done for a PLF, whereas it rarely occurs with a small-window stapedotomy. If a stapedectomy is required to close a leak, one should use a perichondrial or fascial graft held in place with a 1mm piston prosthesis.

RESULTS

There is a negative exploration rate of 40 to 50 per cent with our current diagnostic armamentarium. A better than 90 per cent first-time closure rate of round window membrane fistulas can be expected. The success rate with oval window fistulas, particularly if the recess is quite deep and narrow, is considerably lower: the first-time oval window failure rate is 20 to 30 per cent.

ALTERNATIVE TECHNIQUES

Patients seen in the first week after the development of a PLF should be treated with bed rest. The best recovery of hearing loss occurs with this group of patients. Only after bed rest for 5 to 7 days should surgical intervention be considered. If hearing loss is present, waiting more than 2 weeks from the onset of PLF significantly reduces the likelihood of improving the hearing with operative intervention. Therefore, these patients must be seen early and followed up carefully with audiometric testing. Positional testing should be avoided early in the convalescent period, as this may reopen the fistula.

Syms et al. have developed a new technique that involves injecting fluorescein intravenously in the patient approximately 20 minutes prior to the start of the operation.[31] By use of a special interference filter on the light source of the microscope to produce 490nm light, the surgeon is able to see fluorescence from a PLF.[31] It has been argued that all the surgeon is seeing is increased uptake of dye in the blood vessels on the promontory. If one looks at the clearance of the blood, particularly in experimental animals, most of the dye is gone very quickly: the dye seems to be concentrated in perilymph in experimental animals, reaching its peak in about 20 minutes. The animal study by Applebaum measured the dye through an intact round window membrane with blood vessels.[32] However, in the experimental animal groups, the dye is of such low concentration that it cannot be seen with the usual Wood's light techniques with the eye. Fluorescein does not accumulate in cerebrospinal fluid, so if one is dealing with a cerebrospinal fluid leak through a congenital defect, then the fluorescein is probably of little or no value.[32] The experience with this technique is somewhat limited and controversial. A repeat of the Syms study by Poe et al., who carefully avoided blood loss, failed to demonstrate fluorescein in perilymph.[33]

References

1. House JW, Morris MS, Kramer SJ, et al.: Perilymphatic fistula: Surgical experience in the United States. Otolaryngol Head Neck Surg 105: 51–61, 1991.
2. Singleton GT: Perilymph fistulas. Adv Otolaryngol Head Neck Surg 2: 25–38, 1988.
3. Allen GW: Endolymphatic sac and cochlear aqueduct. Arch Otolaryngol Head Neck Surg 79: 322–327, 1964.
4. Pullen FW: Round window membrane rupture: A cause of sudden deafness. Trans Am Acad Ophthalmol Otolaryngol 76: 1444–1450, 1972.
5. Rybak LP: "How I do it"—Otology and neurotology. Laryngoscope 90: 2049–2050, 1980.
6. Singleton GT: Correlation of clinical symptoms of vertigo and/or hearing loss with anatomic site of surgically confirmed PLF. Third International Symposium on Surgery of the Inner Ear [In press].
7. Goodhill V: Sudden deafness and round window rupture. Laryngoscope 81: 1462–1474, 1971.
8. Douek E: Perilymph fistula. J Laryngol Otol 89: 123–130, 1975.
9. Goodhill V: Stapedectomy revision commandments: Posterior arch stapedioplasty. Trans Pac Coast Oto-ophthalmol Soc 55: 35–59, 1974.
10. Harrison WH, Shambaugh GE, Derlacki EL, et al.: Perilymph fistula in stapes surgery. Laryngoscope 77: 736–849, 1967.
11. Hemenway WG, Hildyard VH, Black FO: Post stapedectomy perilymph fistulas in the rocky mountain area: The importance of nystagmography and audiometry in diagnosis and early tympanotomy in prognosis. Laryngoscope 78: 1687–1715, 1968.
12. House HP: The fistula problem in otosclerotic surgery. Laryngoscope 77: 1410–1426, 1967.
13. Kamerer DB, Sando I, Hirsch B, Takagi A: Perilymph fistula resulting from microfissures. Am J Otol 8(6): 489–494, 1987.
14. Kohut RI, Hinojosa R, Ryu J: Sudden-onset hearing loss in eleven consecutive cases: A temporal bone histopathologic study with identification of perilymphatic fistulae. Trans Am Otol Soc 77, 1989.

15. Hinojosa R, Kohut RI, Lee JT, Ryu JH: Sudden hearing loss due to perilymphatic fistulae. II: Quantitative temporal bone histopathologic study. Trans Am Otol Soc 78: 121–127, 1990.
16. Shazly MA, Linthicum FH: Microfissures of the temporal bone: Do they have any clinical significance? Am J Otol 12: 169–171, 1991.
17. Lehrer JF, Poole DC, Sigal B: Use of the glycerin test in the diagnosis of post-traumatic perilymphatic fistulas. Am J Otolaryngol 1: 207–210, 1980.
18. Arenberg IK, Ackley RS, Ferraro J, Muchnik C: ECoG results in perilymphatic fistula: Clinical and experimental studies. Otolaryngol Head Neck Surg 99(5): 435–443, 1988.
19. Meyerhoff WL, Yellin MW: Summating potential/action potential ratio in perilymph fistula. Otolaryngol Head Neck Surg 102(6): 678–682, 1990.
20. Campbell KCM, Harker LA, Abbas PJ: Interpretation of electrocochleography in Ménière's disease and normal subjects. Ann Otol Rhinol Laryngol 101: 496–500, 1992.
21. Reilly JS: Congenital perilymphatic fistula: A prospective study in infants and children. Laryngoscope 99: 393–397, 1989.
22. Parnes LS, McCabe BF: Perilymph fistula: An important cause of deafness and dizziness in children. Pediatrics 89(4): 524–528, 1987.
23. Pappas DG, Simpson LC, Godwin GH: Perilymphatic fistula in children with pre-existing sensorineural hearing loss. Laryngoscope 98: 507–510, 1988.
24. Bluestone CD: Otitis media and congenital perilymphatic fistula as a cause of sensorineural hearing loss in children. Pediatr Infect Dis J 7(11): S141–S145, 1988.
25. Singleton GT, Karlan MS, Post KN, et al.: Perilymph fistulas: Diagnostic criteria and therapy. Ann Otol Rhinol Laryngol 87(6): 797–803, 1978.
26. Singleton GT: Perilymph fistula. In Sharpe JA, Barber HO (eds): The Vestibulo-ocular Reflex and Vertigo. New York, Raven Press, 1993.
27. Hart CW: The evaluation of vestibular function in healing and disease. In Otolaryngology. Hagerstown, MD, Harper & Row, 1972, pp 1–63.
28. Flood LM, Fraser JG, Hazell JWP, et al.: Perilymph fistula: Four-year experience with a new audiometric test. J Laryngol Otol 99: 671–676, 1985.
29. Black FO, Lilly DJ, et al.: Quantitative diagnostic test for perilymph fistulas. Otolaryngol Head Neck Surg 96(2): 125–134, 1987.
30. Silverstein H: Rapid protein test for perilymph fistula. Otolaryngol Head Neck Surg 105: 422–426, 1991.
31. Syms CA, Atkins JS, Olsson JE, Murphy TP: The use of fluorescein for intraoperative confirmation of perilymph fistula: A preliminary report [Submitted for publication].
32. Applebaum EL: Fluorescein kinetics in perilymph and blood: A fluorophotometric study. Laryngoscope 92: 660–669, 1982.
33. Poe DS, Gadre AK, Rebeiz EE, Pankratov MM: Intravenous fluorescein for detection of perilymphatic fistulas. Am J Otol [In press].

FIGURE 32–4

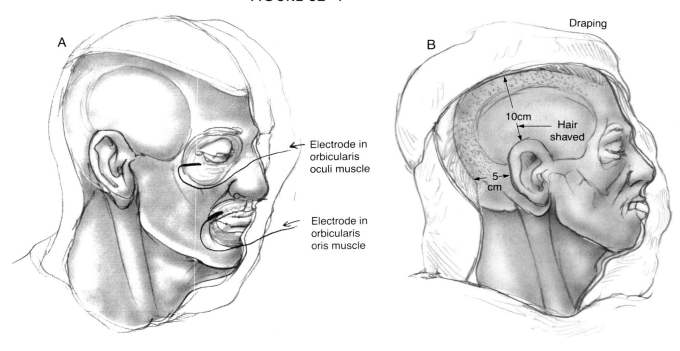

A

Electrode in
orbicularis
oculi muscle

Electrode in
orbicularis
oris muscle

B

Draping

10cm

Hair
shaved

5
cm

FIGURE 32–5

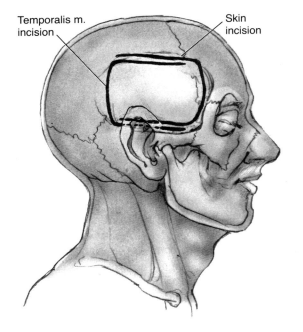

Temporalis m.
incision

Skin
incision

BRUCE J. GANTZ & MIRIAM I. REDLEAF

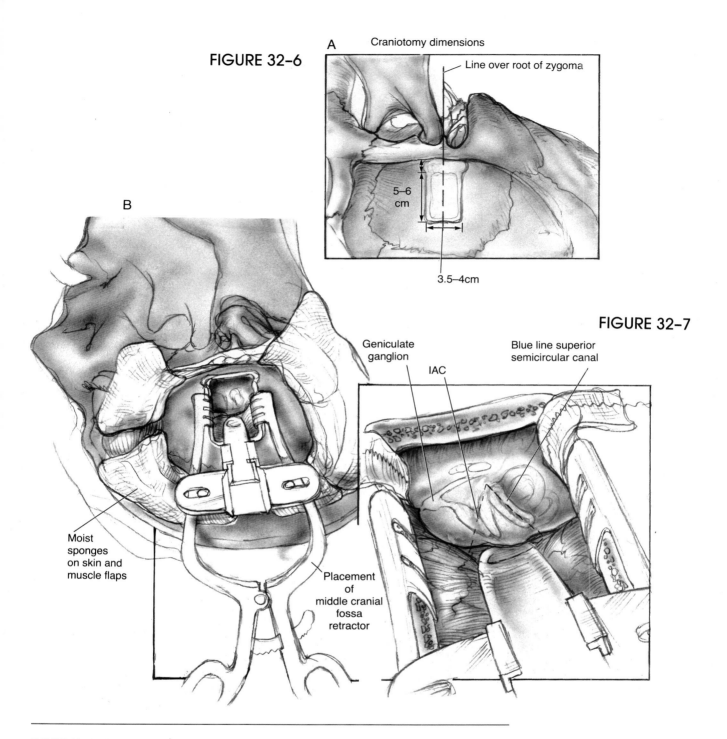

FIGURE 32-6

A Craniotomy dimensions

Line over root of zygoma

5–6 cm

3.5–4cm

B

Moist sponges on skin and muscle flaps

Placement of middle cranial fossa retractor

FIGURE 32-7

Geniculate ganglion

IAC

Blue line superior semicircular canal

FIGURE 32-4. *A*, Electrode placement for intraoperative electromyography. *B*, Draping with exposure of half the face for visual monitoring of facial movement.

FIGURE 32-5. Skin incision for middle cranial fossa approach. Mastoid exposure can be obtained by extending incision postauricularly. Incision of anteriorly based temporalis muscle flap is offset to keep suture lines from being directly in line.

FIGURE 32-6. *A*, Craniotomy for middle cranial fossa exposure. Inferior expansion of craniotomy allows more exposure during dural elevation. Vertical margins must be parallel for stability of retractor. Craniotomy should be centered on the temporal root of the zygoma *(dotted line)*. *B*, Placement of House-Urban middle cranial fossa retractor.

FIGURE 32-7. Exposure of superior semicircular canal blue line and position of internal auditory canal 60 degrees anterior to a line through the blue line. Superior canal blue line almost always is perpendicular to petrous ridge.

Surgical Technique

The skin incision is marked as shown in Figure 32–5. As the skin incision is being made, the anesthesiologist is instructed to ventilate the patient to a PCO_2 of 25mm Hg and to administer mannitol, 0.5g per kg body weight, to relax the brain. The skin incision is carried to the level of the temporalis fascia. The posteriorly based skin flap is elevated at the level of the temporalis fascia. A 4cm × 6cm piece of temporalis fascia is harvested and set aside in a moist gauze for use at the time of closure. An anteriorly based temporalis muscle flap is designed by placing the superior and inferior horizontal incisions 1cm to 2cm inferior to the corresponding skin margins. Staggering the incisions prevents dural exposure if wound dehiscence occurs. The temporalis muscle flap is elevated anteriorly along with the periosteum. The zygomatic root of the temporal bone is next exposed by elevation of the anteroinferior margin of the muscle. The zygomatic root identifies the floor of the middle cranial fossa and is the central landmark of the craniotomy. The skin and muscle flaps should be wrapped with moist sponges and secured with temporary retraction stitches.

The craniotomy should be approximately 4cm in anteroposterior dimension and 5cm to 6cm cephaladcaudal (Fig. 32–6A). The anteroposterior margins must be kept parallel for stability of the middle cranial fossa retractor. The craniotomy can be created using a 2mm cutting burr or craniotomy saw (Midas Rex). The bone flap should be elevated with care by use of a blunt dural elevator. Occasionally, the middle meningeal artery will be imbedded within the bone, requiring bipolar coagulation to free it. The bone flap is wrapped in a moist gauze and set aside for use at closure.

Dural elevation from the floor of the middle cranial fossa is accomplished with a Freer elevator, always in a posterior-to-anterior direction, which prevents injury to the greater superficial petrosal nerve and geniculate ganglion. The petrous ridge is identified at the posterior margin of the craniotomy, and the dura is slowly elevated over the arcuate eminence and meatal plane. Dural reflections are cauterized and sharply transected to allow elevation to the petrous ridge anterior. The hiatus of the facial canal with the greater superficial petrosal nerve and artery is the anterior margin of elevation. Further anterior elevation exposes the foramen spinosum and the pterygoid plexus of veins, which can cause troublesome oozing throughout the procedure. Following dural elevation, cottonoid sponges can be placed at the anterior and posterior margins of the elevation to help retract the dura during placement of the self-retaining middle cranial fossa retractor (Fig. 32–6B).

Prior to the bony exposure of the facial nerve, the Stenvers projection X-ray is re-examined to determine the depth of the superior semicircular canal in the temporal bone. The superior semicircular canal is the first structure to be located. Once its blue line is identified, the remaining intratemporal structures have consistent anatomic locations. Landmarks of the middle cranial fossa floor can be quite subtle. The arcuate eminence may not be apparent, and in many instances, is not parallel with the superior semicircular canal. One constant anatomic feature to remember is that the plane of the superior semicircular canal is almost always perpendicular to the petrous ridge (Fig. 32–7). If the arcuate eminence is not initially apparent, then drilling is begun posterior to the superior semicircular canal, slowly removing the tegmen mastoideum with a moderate sized diamond burr. The whitish color of the membranous temporal bone can be distinguished from the yellow dense otic capsule bone of the superior canal. Once the superior canal is identified, drilling in a parallel direction with the canal will gradually expose the blue line.

When the location of the superior canal is confirmed, an anterior line 60 degrees to the blue line locates the position of the internal auditory canal. The depth of the internal auditory canal is variable, but drilling medially near the petrous ridge provides a safe route to the canal. Drilling laterally near the anterior ampulla of the superior semicircular canal places the geniculate ganglion, labyrinthine segment of the facial nerve, and cochlea at risk. Once the blue line of the internal auditory canal is exposed, bone is removed in a lateral direction until Bill's bar is found (Fig. 32–8). Bone can now be removed over the geniculate ganglion and tegmen tympani.

The labyrinthine segment of the facial nerve is the narrowest portion of the fallopian canal and lies in an anterosuperior plane from Bill's bar to the geniculate

FIGURE 32–8. Middle cranial fossa exposure of cranial nerve (CN) VII and surrounding anatomy. Bone removed from tegmen tympani to expose tympanic segment of CN VII. Note edema of internal auditory canal segment CN VII, frequently found in Bell's palsy.

FIGURE 32-8

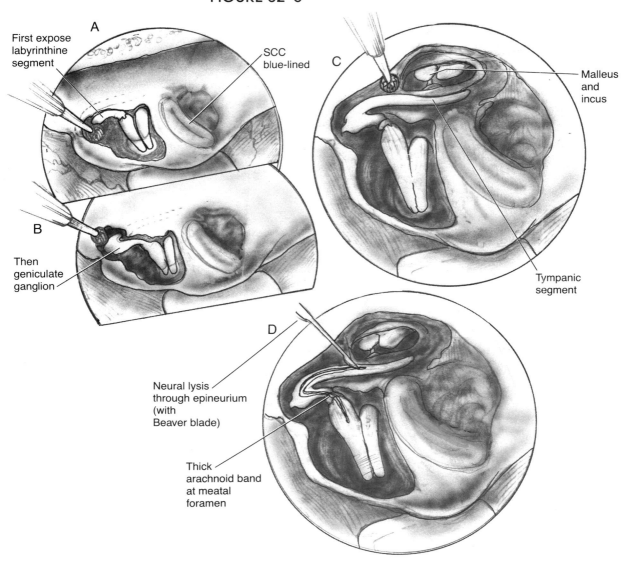

A First expose labyrinthine segment

SCC blue-lined

B Then geniculate ganglion

C Malleus and incus

Tympanic segment

D Neural lysis through epineurium (with Beaver blade)

Thick arachnoid band at meatal foramen

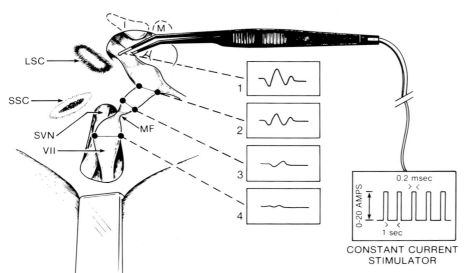

FIGURE 32-9. Intraoperative evoked electromyography to identify site of nerve conduction block. If conduction block is medial to geniculate ganglion, stimulation of tympanic segment results in motor unit potential (1); stimulation of internal canal segment (3) results in no response. Usually, conduction block is at meatal foramen (MF).

ganglion. A 1mm diamond burr is used to remove bone over the labyrinthine segment while the area directly anterior to the segment is closely observed for the blue line of the basal turn of the cochlea. The final layer of bone is removed with thin, angled hooks and blunt microelevators. At this point, marked swelling of the nerve in the internal auditory canal, labyrinthine segment, and geniculate ganglion is usually observed. Further swelling is apparent following neurolysis. A disposable microscalpel (Beaver No. 59-10) is used to slit the periosteum and epineural sheath.

Intraoperative electromyography is now used to localize the region of the nerve conduction block. Direct stimulation of the most distal exposed tympanic segment of the nerve is performed with monopolar or bipolar microforceps (Fig. 32–9). If the conduction block is medial to the point of stimulation and the nerve is not completely degenerated, a motor unit potential will be observed. Stimulating more medially toward the internal auditory canal will fail to elicit a motor unit potential if the conduction block is at the meatal foramen.

On completion of the decompression and confirmation of the site of conduction block, the opened internal auditory canal is covered with a piece of temporalis muscle and oxidized cellulose (Oxycel). The previously harvested temporalis fascia is placed over the opened floor of the middle fossa after bone waxing opened mastoid cells. The dural retractor is removed, and the anesthesiologist is asked to reestablish a normal P_{CO_2}.

A corner of the craniotomy bone flap is harvested and placed superior to the fascia to prevent herniation of the temporal lobe dura into the attic and internal auditory canal. The temporal lobe is allowed to re-expand into the middle cranial fossa floor. The remainder of the craniotomy flap is placed on the dura, and the temporalis is closed, creating a watertight seal with interrupted absorbable sutures. Skin is closed with a deep layer of interrupted absorbable sutures and an outer layer of nylon interrupted sutures. A mastoid-type dressing is applied. No drains are used.

Postoperative Care

Postoperative care includes intensive care observation overnight, limitation of fluids (1500ml to 1800ml per day), dexamethasone (Decadron) (6mg every 6 hours for 36 hours), broad-spectrum antibiotics for 36 hours, routine neural checks, and limitation of analgesia to codeine. There is little postoperative pain, and stronger narcotics may mask intracranial complications. The patient is transferred to a routine postoperative floor the next morning, encouraged to begin ambulation, and started on a diet as tolerated. Daily observations for cerebrospinal fluid rhinorrhea are made by asking the patient to lean forward with the head between the knees. If cerebrospinal fluid rhinorrhea occurs, bed rest, elevation of the head, and acetazolamide (Diamox) are used for 24 to 48 hours. If the leak persists, a spinal drain must be placed for 4 to 5 days. Following this regimen, only three patients in over 200 who underwent middle fossa procedures for acoustic neuromas, vestibular nerve sections, and facial nerve decompressions required surgical closure of their leak. Patients are usually discharged from the hospital in 5 to 7 days. No intracranial complications, including intracranial hemorrhage, aphasia, or seizures, occurred in this series.

Limitations and Special Considerations

The anatomy of the middle cranial fossa floor is quite variable and presents some difficulty in identification of landmarks. The surgeon must have a precise knowledge of the three-dimensional anatomy of the temporal bone. Many hours in the temporal bone dissection laboratory are required to attain the delicate microsurgical skills necessary for this type of surgery.

Dural elevation can be difficult, especially in patients over 65 years of age. If a dural tear occurs, a temporalis fascia repair must be performed. Hearing loss can occur from contact of the rotating burr with an intact ossicular chain or by entrance into the cochlea or labyrinth. Vestibular dysfunction can occur in a similar fashion. If the membranous labyrinth is violated, immediate placement of a small amount of bone wax may preserve auditory and vestibular function.

Correct positioning of the craniotomy and maintaining parallel vertical margins is essential. Meticulous hemostasis must be maintained with bipolar cautery, oxidized cellulose, and pressure. Maintaining a dry field is critical for microscopic dissection of subtle landmarks and prevention of complications. If large apical air cells are opened, they must be plugged with temporalis muscle to prevent cerebrospinal fluid leaks.

References

1. Adour KK, Byl FM, Hilsinger RL Jr, et al.: The true nature of Bell's palsy. Laryngoscope 88: 787–801, 1978.
2. Citron D, Adour KK: Acoustic reflex and loudness discomfort in acute facial paralysis. Arch Otolaryngol Head Neck Surg 104: 303–306, 1978.
3. May M, Schlaepfer WW: Bell's palsy and the chorda tympani nerve. Laryngoscope 85: 1957–1975, 1975.
4. McCormick DP: Herpes simplex virus as a cause of Bell's palsy. Lancet i: 937–939, 1972.
5. Weber T, Jurgens S, Luer W: Cerebrospinal fluid immunoglobulins and virus-specific antibodies in disorders affecting the facial nerve. J Neurol 234: 308–314, 1987.
6. Marsh MA, Coker NJ: Surgical decompression of idiopathic facial paralysis. Otolaryngol Clin North Am 24: 675–689, 1991.
7. Blatt IM: Detection of virus in Bell's palsy patients. In Graham M, House W (eds): Disorders of the Facial Nerve. New York, Raven Press, 1982, p 255.
8. Fisch U: Surgery for Bell's palsy. Arch Otolaryngol Head Neck Surg 107: 1–11, 1981.
9. Adour KK: Medical management of idiopathic (Bell's) palsy. Otolaryngol Clin North Am 24: 663–673, 1991.
10. Schwaber MK, Larson TC, Zealear DL, Creasy J: Gadolinium-enhanced magnetic resonance imaging in Bell's palsy. Laryngoscope 100: 1264–1269, 1990.
11. Fowler EP: The pathologic findings in a case of facial paralysis. Trans Am Acad Ophthalmol Otolaryngol 67: 187–197, 1963.
12. Proctor B, Corgill DA, Proud G: The pathology of Bell's palsy. Trans Am Acad Ophthalmol Otolaryngol 82: ORL 70–80, 1976.
13. Fisch U, Esslen E: Total intratemporal exposure of the facial nerve. Arch Otolaryngol Head Neck Surg 95: 335–341, 1972.
14. Fisch U: Total facial nerve decompression and electroneuronography. In Silverstein H, Norrell H (eds): Neurological Surgery of the Ear. Birmingham, AL, Aesculapius, 1977, pp 21–33.
15. May M, Klein SR: Differential diagnosis of facial nerve palsy. Otolaryngol Clin North Am 24: 613–645, 1992.
16. Esslen E: Electromyography and electroneuronography. In Fisch U (ed): Facial Nerve Surgery. Birmingham, AL: Aesculapius, 1977, pp 93–100.
17. Gantz BJ, Gmuer AA, Holliday M, Fisch U: Electroneurographic evaluation of the facial nerve. Ann Otol Rhinol Laryngol 93: 394–398, 1984.
18. Blumenthal F, May M: Electrodiagnosis. In May M (ed): The Facial Nerve. New York, Thieme, 1986.
19. Fisch U: Prognostic value of electrical tests in acute facial paralysis. Am J Otol 5: 494–498, 1984.
20. Peitersen E: The natural history of Bell's palsy. Am J Otol 4: 107–111, 1982.
21. Katusic SK, Beard M, Wiederholt WC, et al.: Incidence, clinical features, and prognosis in Bell's palsy, Rochester, Minnesota, 1968–1982. Ann Neurol 20: 622–627, 1986.
22. Adour KK, Wingerd JW, Bell DN, et al.: Prednisone treatment for idiopathic facial paralysis. New Engl J Med 287: 1276–1282, 1972.
23. Wolf SM, Wagner JH Jr, Davidson S, Forsythe A: Treatment of Bell's palsy with prednisone: a prospective, randomized study. Neurology 28: 158–161, 1978.
24. May M, Wette R, Hardin WB Jr, Sullivan J: The use of steroids in Bell's palsy. Laryngoscope 86: 1111–1122, 1976.
25. Fisch U: Surgery for Bell's palsy. Arch Otolaryngol Head Neck Surg 107: 1–11, 1981.
26. Peitersen E: Spontaneous course of Bell's palsy. In Fisch U (ed): Facial Nerve Surgery. Amstelveen, Netherlands, 1977.
27. Devriese PP, Moesker WH: The natural history of facial paralysis in herpes zoster. Clin Otolaryngol 13: 289–298, 1988.
28. Dickens JRE, Smith JT, Graham SS: Herpes zoster oticus. Laryngoscope 98: 776–779, 1988.
29. May M, Klein SR, Taylor FH: Idiopathic (Bell's) facial palsy. Laryngoscope 95: 406–409, 1985.

33

Traumatic Facial Paralysis

HERMAN A. JENKINS, M.D.
GREGORY A. ATOR, M.D.

The facial nerve may be injured by many blunt and penetrating mechanisms. Common causes include motor vehicle accidents, stab or gunshot wounds to the face (frequently seen in urban areas), and iatrogenic injuries during head and neck surgical procedures. Primary mechanisms of injury include stretching, compression, and transection of the nerve.

The course of the nerve from the brainstem to the facial musculature can be divided into three segments: intracranial, intratemporal, and extratemporal or peripheral (Fig. 33–1). The pathophysiology of facial nerve disorders varies according to the segment of the nerve involved and will be discussed individually.

INTRACRANIAL INJURY TO THE FACIAL NERVE

The intracranial facial nerve, extending from the brainstem to the fundus of the internal auditory canal, is rarely damaged by penetrating trauma because of the excellent protection afforded by the petrous bone and the cranial vault, but with severe trauma, stretch and shock wave–type injuries may still occur. Penetrating trauma to this region will likely be accompanied by extensive central nervous system pathology, which must first be evaluated and treated. Evaluation of the injured nerve begins with a careful examination of motor function as soon as possible after the injury is sustained. If the nerve is functional at presentation and becomes progressively paretic, a complete transection injury is unlikely. If the nerve manifests any motion, regular clinical observation can be used to follow up the status of the nerve. After the onset of complete paralysis, surgery is contemplated if the nerve shows electrical signs of near-total degeneration (see under *Timing of Surgery*).

INTRATEMPORAL INJURY TO THE FACIAL NERVE

The intratemporal facial nerve, extending from the internal auditory canal fundus to the stylomastoid foramen, is frequently damaged from blunt trauma to the skull that leads to a temporal bone fracture. Fractures produced by blunt trauma have been traditionally grouped into longitudinal and transverse varieties, although almost any type of fracture can be encountered. Two main groups of fractures are typically seen: longitudinal and transverse. Fractures with the main component parallel to the long axis of the petrous pyramid are classified as longitudinal (Fig. 33–2), whereas fractures perpendicular to the long axis (see Fig. 33–5) are considered to be transverse

fractures. Longitudinal fractures are produced by trauma to the lateral aspects of the skull in the temporoparietal region and comprise 80 per cent of fractures in most series.[1] Transverse fractures are produced by trauma to the occipital or frontal regions of the skull and comprise about 20 per cent of fractures. Many fractures are oblique or combine elements of longitudinal and transverse fractures.[2] Severely comminuted and complex fractures of the temporal bone are commonly produced by penetrating gunshot wounds of the temporal bone.[3]

A longitudinal fracture (Fig. 33–2B and 33–3) is suspected when a step-off is present in the external auditory canal and is frequently accompanied by blood in the external auditory canal. A perforation or tear of the tympanic membrane may be present, and cerebrospinal fluid (CSF) otorrhea is occasionally seen. Sterile instruments should be used during the examination of the external auditory canal to avoid introducing contamination into the area and producing retrograde meningitis. A conductive hearing loss will usually be present and can have numerous causes. Perforation of the ear drum, hematoma in the middle ear cleft, disruption of ligaments supporting the ossicles in the attic region, and disruption of the ossicular joints can all lead to varying degrees of conductive hearing loss (see under *Ossicular Damage*). Facial paralysis is seen in only 20 per cent of longitudinal fractures but is the most common cause of facial paralysis in blunt trauma of the temporal bone because of the relative infrequency of transverse fractures. The facial nerve is involved in the perigeniculate region in 90 per cent of cases[4, 5] and less commonly in the mastoid segment by fractures of the posterior external auditory canal (Fig. 33–4). The pathology of the facial nerve injury in blunt temporal bone trauma, in decreasing order of occurrence, consists of intraneural hemorrhage, bony fragment impingement, and nerve transection.[6]

A transverse temporal bone fracture is suspected when a patient presents with sensorineural hearing loss and vertigo accompanied by facial paralysis. The external canal is frequently intact and no evidence of canal wall discontinuity and hemotympanum may be present (Figs. 33–5B and 33–6). These patients have a 50 per cent incidence of facial paralysis, which occurs from damage to the geniculate ganglion region (Fig. 33–7).[7] The causes of injury are the same as for longitudinal fractures, and intraneural hemorrhage is the most common.

Gunshot wounds to the temporal bone region typically produce extensive damage, the degree of which is determined by the velocity of the projectile. Low-velocity civilian projectiles have relatively low energy and produce mainly locally destructive manifesta-

Text continued on page 404

FIGURE 33-1

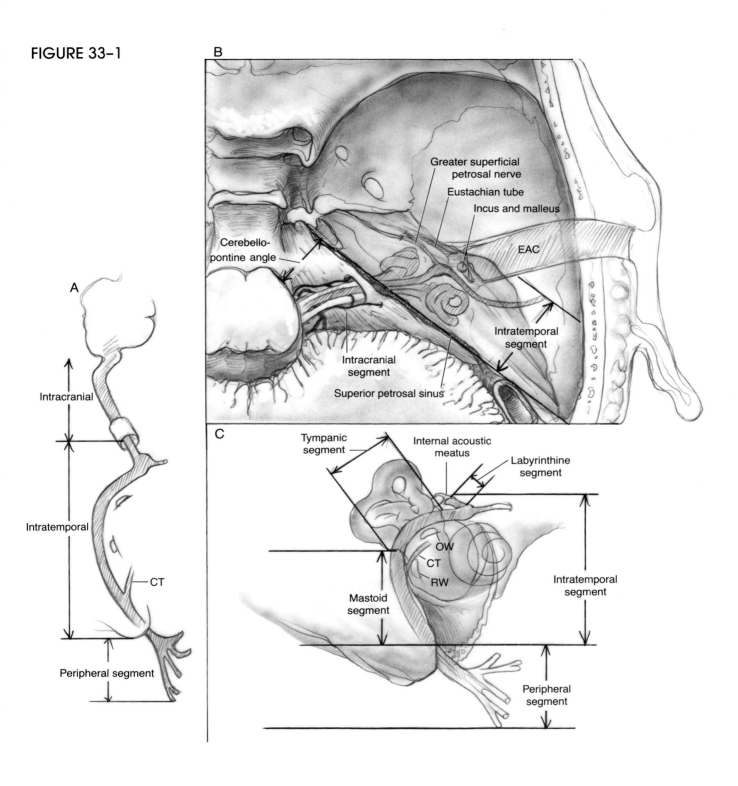

FIGURE 33-1. *A*, Schematic of facial nerve anatomy. *B*, Axial view. *C*, Lateral view.

FIGURE 33-2

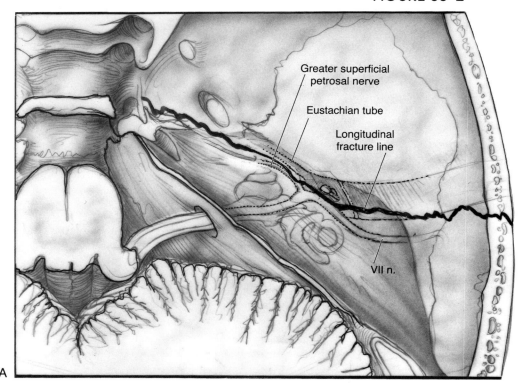

Greater superficial
petrosal nerve

Eustachian tube

Longitudinal
fracture line

VII n.

A

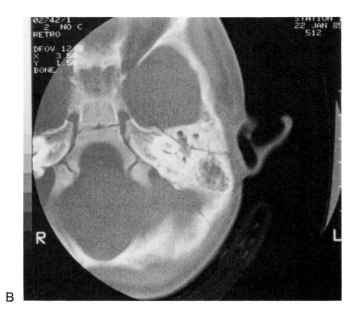

B

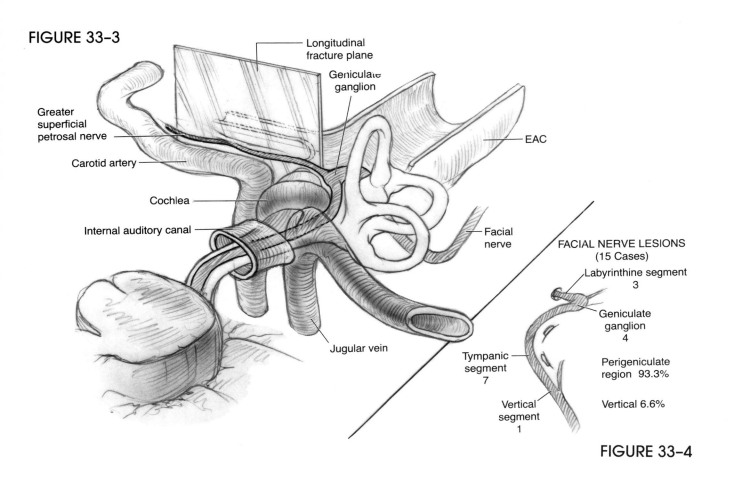

FIGURE 33-3

Longitudinal fracture plane

Geniculate ganglion

Greater superficial petrosal nerve

Carotid artery

Cochlea

Internal auditory canal

EAC

Facial nerve

Jugular vein

FACIAL NERVE LESIONS
(15 Cases)

Labyrinthine segment
3

Geniculate ganglion
4

Perigeniculate region 93.3%

Tympanic segment
7

Vertical 6.6%

Vertical segment
1

FIGURE 33-4

FIGURE 33-2. Longitudinal fracture of the temporal bone. *A,* Fracture line is parallel to the long axis. *B,* Computed tomographic scan.

FIGURE 33-3. Longitudinal fracture of the temporal bone.

FIGURE 33-4. Location of lesion to facial nerve in 15 cases of longitudinal fractures. (From Coker NJ, Kendall KA, Jenkins HA, Alford BR: Traumatic intratemporal facial nerve injury: Management rationale for preservation of function. Otolaryngol Head Neck Surg 97: 262–269, 1987.)

FIGURE 33-5

A   TRANSVERSE FRACTURE

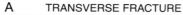

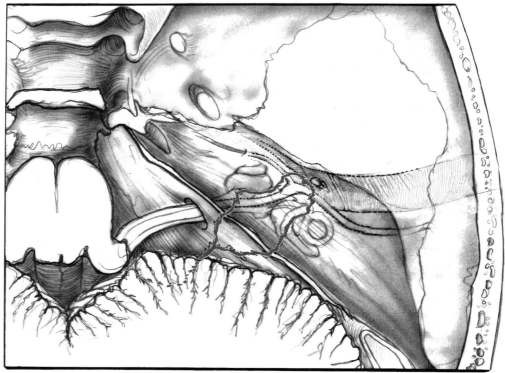

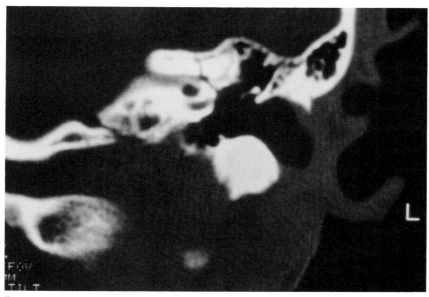

B

FIGURE 33-6

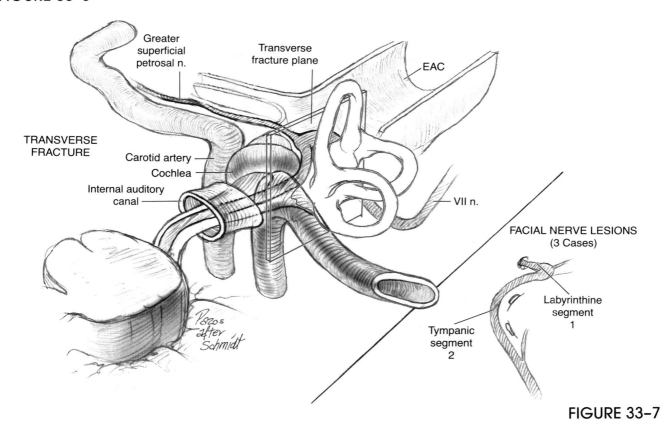

FIGURE 33-6

FIGURE 33-7

FIGURE 33-5. Transverse fracture of the temporal bone. *A,* Fracture line is perpendicular to the long axis. *B,* Radiograph of transverse fracture.

FIGURE 33-6. Transverse fracture of the temporal bone.

FIGURE 33-7. Location of lesion in three cases of transverse temporal bone fracture. (From Coker NJ, Kendall KA, Jenkins HA, Alford BR: Traumatic intratemporal facial nerve injury: Management rationale for preservation of function. Otolaryngol Head Neck Surg 97: 262–269, 1973.)

tions. On the other hand, high-velocity military weapons, which are increasingly being seen on city streets, are capable of widespread destruction, with extensive local and regional manifestations produced by the concomitant shock wave. People receiving low-velocity gunshot wounds to the intratemporal portion of the facial nerve have a 50 per cent incidence of facial nerve injury, with frequent injury to intracranial and extracranial structures. In a series of 22 cases of civilian gunshot wound injuries, Duncan et al.[3] found immediate onset of paralysis to be the most common presentation and violation of the facial nerve in vertical segment the most common site of injury. Other sites of injury were the tympanic portion in five cases; the stylomastoid foramen in two; and the labyrinthine segment in one. Treatment consisted of interposition grafts in five cases; transmastoid decompression in two; and rerouting with primary anastomosis in one. In summary, gunshot wounds of the temporal bone frequently result in loss of a segment of the nerve, usually in the tympanic portion, requiring interposition grafting for repair.[3] Associated central nervous system and vascular complications (32 per cent) are frequently present, and arteriography is recommended for evaluation of suspected damage to vascular structures of the temporal bone in these cases.[4]

EXTRATEMPORAL INJURY TO THE FACIAL NERVE

Facial paralysis after laceration or iatrogenic injury to the parotid region is best repaired primarily and as soon as the patient's condition permits. If no loss of nerve substance has occurred, the nerve should be repaired by direct anastomosis. When nerve substance loss has occurred, an interpositional graft should be used.

PATIENT EVALUATION

Electrical Prognostication

The presentation of facial nerve injuries greatly affects their management. The presence of a tightly enclosing fallopian canal around the intratemporal facial nerve makes the nerve much more susceptible to all types of trauma. Lack of any space to accommodate edema, which inevitably accompanies soft tissue trauma, leads to further neural injury. An injured nerve may not manifest significant clinical dysfunction initially, but later, once sufficient edema has occurred to prevent axoplasmic flow, the injury manifests. Fisch and others have shown that the area of the fallopian canal with the least expansion room for neural swelling is

in the region of the meatal foramen.[6, 8–10] Because most injuries to the facial nerve occur in the perigeniculate area just distal to the meatal foramen, the edema produced in facial nerve injury is quite critical in the pathophysiology of this disorder. Precise analysis of facial nerve function must be made at the earliest opportunity after trauma has occurred, prior to the onset of edema. A nerve with diffuse weakness in all branches can be observed clinically, and if some function persists, expectant management can be employed. If this situation deteriorates to total paralysis, electrical testing should be used to follow up the nerve to ensure that total degeneration does not occur.

Fisch and Esslen have postulated that surgery can facilitate return of facial nerve function if performed prior to complete degeneration. A level of 90 per cent degeneration, as determined by electroneuronography (ENoG), has been correlated with a uniformly good prognosis for return of function.[11] If the nerve is nonfunctional at the initial examination, the chance of a complete transection is high and will likely require surgery. Patients with complete facial paralysis at the initial examination are screened daily with nerve excitability testing. This test uses direct transcutaneous stimulation of the nerve on each side of the face and determines a stimulation threshold that produces perceptible movement. The normal side is used as a control. If the threshold difference between the normal and dysfunctional sides exceeds 2.5mA, ENoG is performed regularly thereafter. ENoG uses transcutaneous supramaximal stimulation of the facial nerve, while simultaneously recording the evoked potential from anterograde stimulation in the periphery of the face.[12] The maximal evoked response of the nerve is measured on each side by use of a nonfixed recording electrode technique. A side-to-side comparison is made, with the normal side serving as the control. The percentage of degeneration is calculated as the difference between the two sides. Recent data have shown that a correlation exists between ENoG and nerve excitability testing: a 90 per cent degeneration score on ENoG correlates to about a 3.5mA difference on nerve excitability testing.[13]

In a nonacute injury, ENoG can be relied on for up to 3 weeks, but after this period, a desynchronization (deblocking) of electrically evoked facial nerve discharge can occur, preventing a single unified discharge of all neurons in the trunk. This effect occurs because of the differing time courses over which recovering neurons re-establish electrical conductivity and the capability to conduct an action potential. At this stage, it is no longer possible to compare the diseased, asynchronously discharging side to the unaffected, synchronously discharging side, making accurate determination of the severity of degeneration by this technique alone impossible.

Electromyography (EMG) may be employed to establish whether recovering axons are present. Voluntary motor units and polyphasic potentials indicate that regeneration is in progress. Lack of the foregoing and fibrillation potentials indicate a fully degenerated nerve without evidence of ongoing recovery.

Radiologic Evaluation

Thin-cut computed tomographic (CT) examination of the temporal bone is routinely required for evaluation of trauma to the facial nerve. Evaluation of bone detail often establishes the anatomy of the fractures and allows prediction of neural segment damage. The geniculate ganglion region is most frequently involved in blunt trauma, and nondisplaced fractures across the tegmen may be difficult to recognize on CT scan. If facial nerve injury is suspected, special temporal bone views are necessary, as the resolution in standard brain CT scans is not sufficient to delineate the intricate bony features of the fallopian canal.

Carotid arteriography is indicated if major vascular injury is suspected, particularly in gunshot injuries to the temporal bone. Traumatic pseudoaneurysms and arteriovenous fistulas are occasional sequelae and are readily identified by arteriography.

Timing of Surgery

Timing and even the necessity of surgery in some cases of facial nerve injury remains controversial. McCabe suggested that exploration and repair be accomplished at 21 days after injury based on studies of motor neuron proteosynthetic activity levels and maximal repair activity at a neural anastomosis.[14] Recent evidence does not support this theory but does show a trend toward lower regeneration rates with increasing time after onset of injury.[15]

Facial nerve paresis arising from blunt trauma to the peripheral portion of the facial nerve should be managed expectantly. If no recovery is evident at the end of 6 months, reconstitution of the dysfunctional portion of the nerve may be required. Facial paralysis ensuing after laceration or iatrogenic injury to the parotid region is likely a transection and is best repaired primarily and as soon as the patient's condition permits. If a divided nerve cannot be repaired as soon as possible after the injury, then at least limited exploration of the wound should be performed to identify the severed ends of the nerve for subsequent repair. The use of an electrical nerve stimulator can be helpful for up to 48 hours after injury for stimulation of the distal ends of the severed nerve. The regional twitching of facial musculature then can be used as an aid to nerve identification.[4]

The role of surgery in delayed facial nerve injuries following blunt trauma remains controversial. However, significant sequelae from the injury exist in these patients. The present authors managed these injuries similarly to those of patients with Bell's palsy. Surgery is performed once a significant level of degeneration of the facial nerve is evident, that is, 90 per cent on ENoG. The reasoning behind this strategy is to prevent conversion of the neural injury from a Sunderland class II to a class III. The latter has pronounced synkinesis in a large percentage of cases. The goal of surgery is to relieve the pressure on the nerve, thereby permitting the nerve to expand, and to decrease damage to the endoneural tubules from the external constriction.

ASSOCIATED TRAUMA

Other structures in the vicinity of the facial nerve may be injured from the trauma. These injuries may require either immediate or delayed management, depending on the circumstances.

Ossicular Damage

Trauma to the ossicular chain frequently occurs in concert with damage to the intratemporal facial nerve. The ossicles are most often damaged in longitudinal temporal bone fractures as the fracture line passes through the vicinity of the attic and posterosuperior external auditory canal wall. Ossicles may be damaged by dislocation brought about by relative movement of supporting structures or by inertial factors associated with sudden movements of the supporting structures.[16] Many different types of injury to the ossicles can occur, but the most frequent are dislocation of the incudostapedial joint, fractures of the stapes crura, and subluxation of the stapes footplate.[17] The malleus is rarely injured, but occasional fractures of the long process of the malleus are seen.

The treatment of ossicular trauma depends on the nature of the injury. Fractures of the distal long process of the malleus near the umbo are treated by excision of the fractured segment and reconstruction of the drum with temporalis fascia. More proximal fractures near the head of the malleus must be treated by removal of the malleus and incus and placement of a partial or total ossicular replacement prosthesis if the stapes is not normal.

Dislocation of the incus can be from incudostapedial disarticulation, incudomalleolar disarticulation, or both. Two approaches have been advanced for treatment of this condition. The traditional approach is an incus interposition, in which the incus is shaped into a strut with the former incudomalleolar joint area transformed into a notch for the malleus handle, engaging it near the region of the insertion of the tensor tympani. The tip of the former short process of the incus is fashioned into a cup to fit over the stapes capitulum. The overall length of the incus strut is determined by trial and error, and care is taken to ensure a slight amount of tension exists after placement between the malleus handle and stapes capitulum to enhance retention of the prosthesis and to promote good sound conduction. Bone dust from the shaping operation should be allowed to remain on the incus remnant to encourage fixation of the prosthesis in good position. An alternative approach is to reduce the dislocation at the malleus and stapes with careful packing of the incus in reduction from the mastoid and middle ear aspects. Good results are obtained by some authors using this approach, particularly when the joint is not completely separated. However, we favor incus interposition in most of these cases.

Fractures of the crura of the stapes render the ossicle ineffectual as a conductor of sound to the inner ear, and a stapes replacement procedure of some type must be undertaken to restore acoustic function. Stapedectomy or stapedotomy, at the surgeon's preference, can be performed in cases of a normal footplate, but if the footplate is fractured or subluxed, stapedectomy may be required. Fenestration of the footplate, or indeed most ossicular reconstruction, should not be performed in the presence of an infected middle ear cleft, and consideration should be given to using a staged reconstruction approach.

The choice between autograft versus prosthetic ossicular reconstruction methods is usually resolved in favor of autograft because of extrusion problems and the greater incidence of long-term tolerance problems with prosthetic materials. However, when the incus is not available, an incus-stapes replacement prosthesis can be used quite effectively to reconstruct the ossicular chain. In cases in which the entire long process of the malleus is missing, a total ossicular replacement prosthesis or partial ossicular replacement prosthesis made of hydroxyapatite with a platform is used. The incidence of extrusion is greatly reduced by cartilage reinforcement of the platform surface at the interface with the tympanic membrane.

Traumatic Otorrhea

The presence of CSF drainage from the ear or nose of a patient with head trauma is not unusual and represents a defect in the dural covering of the brain.[18] The incidence of meningitis in patients with CSF leaks lasting longer than 2 weeks is approximately 36 per cent,[19] and the mortality may be as high as 10 per cent in traumatic cases.[20] Only otologic sources will be considered in the chapter, but an anterior or middle cranial fossa defect in the sinus region should always be considered in the differential diagnosis of CSF rhinorrhea, especially in traumatic injuries. Fluid originating from a posterior or middle fossa fracture defect may enter the mastoid and middle ear and drain into the nose or the oropharynx. CSF otorrhea is frequently associated with longitudinal temporal bone fractures because the fracture defect may result in a dural tear, whereas a step-off in the external ear canal provides a direct channel for egress of the fluid from the middle ear.

Clear fluid in the ear should alert the examiner to the presence of CSF, and the diagnosis should be straightforward. The diagnosis of CSF rhinorrhea, however, is typically confounded by the appearance of clear nasal secretions frequently accompanying nasal trauma. An informal test to make this differentiation is the halo test, whereby the fluid is placed on filter paper and allowed to diffuse. Blood in the sample will be left behind, and a ring of clear fluid will surround the red ring of blood products. The glucose levels in nasal secretions have also been used to identify CSF; high levels (greater than 50mg per 100ml) are considered to be indicative of CSF. The most sensitive and specific method of differentiation appears to be protein electrophoresis of the sample: the β-2 fraction of transferrin is specific to CSF.[21]

Potential help in localizing the source of the leak can be obtained from contrast-enhanced CT, radioisotope studies, and intrathecal dye instillation. Intrathecal dye methods are used infrequently because of potential adverse reactions, whereas radioisotope studies are more useful in studies of the anterior skull base. The metrizamide-enhanced CT scan provides the best localization for otorrhea because of the good detail of the bony defect usually accompanying the dural defect.

Pneumocephalus is a dreaded, potentially treacherous complication of a defect in the dural protective barrier of the brain.[22] It occurs when air is introduced into the cranial cavity via a fistula in the dura. Frequently, pneumocephalus will be accompanied by CSF leakage, but it may occur in the absence of clinical evidence of fluid leakage. The major difficulty in this entity is the potential formation of a tension pneumocephalus from a ball-valve defect in the dura. Continued accumulation of air may induce intracranial hypertension, with resultant brain herniation. Aggressive management is required in CSF fistulas accompanied by persistent pneumocephalus.

The treatment of CSF otorrhea must take into account the natural history of the entity, and in particular, the incidence of meningitis. Conservative management is possible because of the high probability that the condition will heal spontaneously and because of the efficacy of present-generation antibiotics in meningitis. In a series of anterior cranial fossa CSF fistulas

35 per cent resolved by 24 hours, and 85 per cent healed by 1 week.[23] The most common organisms isolated from post-traumatic meningitic cases are *Pneumococcus* species, and antibiotics are quite effective against them. Several measures may be implemented to aid spontaneous closure of CSF fistula. The most important treatment is bed rest and avoidance of activities that increase intracranial pressure, such as straining, lifting, or constipation. Placement of an indwelling lumbar subarachnoid drainage catheter may be useful in resistant cases. A closed drainage system allows removal of fluid daily and permits regular monitoring of CSF cell counts to allow early identification of meningitis. Avoidance of the need for repeated spinal taps is also a major benefit with these systems.

The indications for operative management of CSF fistula include persistent leakage despite adequate conservative measures, recurrent meningitis, and persistent pneumocephalus.[24] These cases may be approached via the middle ear, mastoid, or middle fossa, depending on the extent and localization of the defect. In general, the defect should be identified and repaired with some form of soft tissue reinforced by bone, where possible. Discrete defects in the dura of less than 1cm should be closed and the area reinforced with fascia. If a mastoid tegmen defect is identified, the dural defect is repaired, followed by soft tissue reinforcement, and finally bone graft support to stabilize the repair in the face of continuous CSF pulsation pressure and gravity.

SURGICAL TREATMENT

Preoperative Preparation

Patients with traumatic facial paralysis are often quite ill because of the multiple sequelae of severe head trauma. Trauma sufficient to produce fracture of the base of the skull and resulting facial nerve injury often damages intracranial contents as well as other structures throughout the body. Assessment of the entire patient must be made, with particular emphasis on the cervical spine, airway, and circulation. A thorough neurologic examination to rule out intracranial pathology, such as hematoma or parenchymal injury to the brain, must be performed and treatment rendered in a timely manner. Increased intracranial pressure is frequently seen as a result of head injury. High-dose steroids, hyperventilation, and head elevation are frequently required for pressure control, and intracranial pressure may be monitored by placement of an intraventricular catheter. Neurosurgical consultation should be obtained early in the treatment of these disorders. After stabilization of the overall neurologic status and treatment of any acute medical problems, the patient can be prepared for surgery to treat the facial nerve.

Patient Positioning

The patient is placed on the operating room table in supine position with anesthesia located away from the head and neck region, down at the side. In addition to the standard postauricular access, the head of the table must be available in case a middle cranial fossa approach is required. The head is placed on a head holder with a recess that allows positioning of the opposite ear without compression. The entire table, and not the head, is moved during the course of the procedure to prevent flexion vascular compromise to the opposite auricle should the ear be folded when the patient's head alone is moved. Approximately half of the scalp is prepared and the hair shaved after the patient is asleep. The entire hemifacial area to the midline is included in the preparatory area, and the lower neck and face are included if vascular control will be required. Prophylactic antibiotics are given at this time, and 1:100,000 epinephrine solution is injected subcutaneously into the line of incision. If intraoperative EMG is to be used, the skin lateral to the angle of the mouth and the area inferior to the inner canthus is prepared with povidone-iodine (Betadine) swabs. Bipolar electrodes are placed in the muscles and the electrodes gently tapped while recording to ensure that a discharge is elicited. A characteristic audio signal (pop) is elicited by this maneuver, which is used as a check for proper electrode and recording system function. The electrodes are sutured in place using sterile technique, and the rest of the preparation and draping are performed. Care is taken to drape the entire half of the face out into the sterile field so that direct observation of the face can be used to confirm electrophysiologic events.

No special instruments are employed in these procedures.

Technique

Intratemporal Nerve Segment

The surgical technique for mastoid facial nerve exploration is discussed in Chapter 18. Details specific to post-traumatic treatment for paralysis are presented here. Surgery for intratemporal traumatic facial paralysis centers on exposure of the damaged segment of the fallopian canal, thereby facilitating surgical repair and providing the nerve room to expand. In treating damage to the nerve in the intratemporal segment, several factors must be taken into account: status of individual nerve fibers, percentage of nerve loss, and

FIGURE 33-8

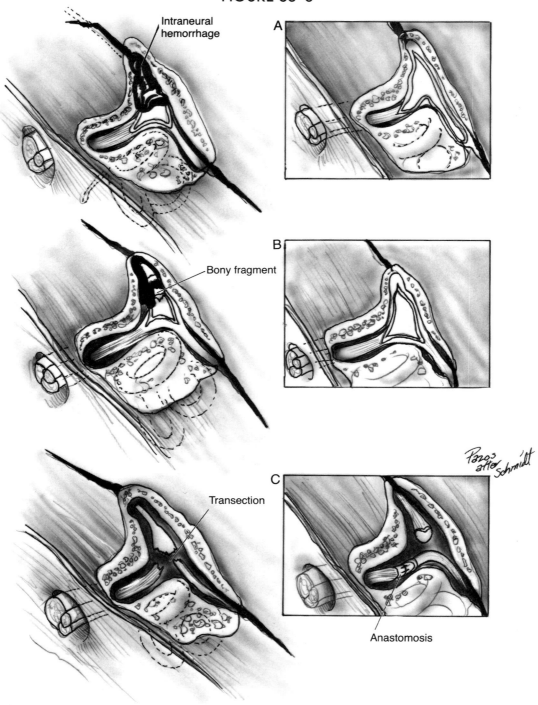

FIGURE 33-8. Surgical management of common facial nerve injuries in the perigeniculate region. *A*, Intraneural hemorrhage. *Inset*, After opening nerve sheath. *B*, Bony fragment impingement. *Inset*, After fragment removal and opening of nerve sheath. *C*, Perigeniculate transection. *Inset*, Direct anastomosis after section of the superficial petrosal nerve.

FIGURE 33-9. *A*, Loss of nerve length in the vertical segment in a nonhearing ear. A trough is created based on the fallopian canal, which helps maintain the graft and nerve in position and minimizes the need for suture fixation. *B*, Extensive loss of tympanic and proximal vertical segment of the facial nerve with rerouting from the internal auditory canal to the vertical segment in a nonhearing ear. The superficial petrosal nerve is sectioned.

FIGURE 33-9

A LOSS OF NERVE LENGTH IN VERTICAL SEGMENT

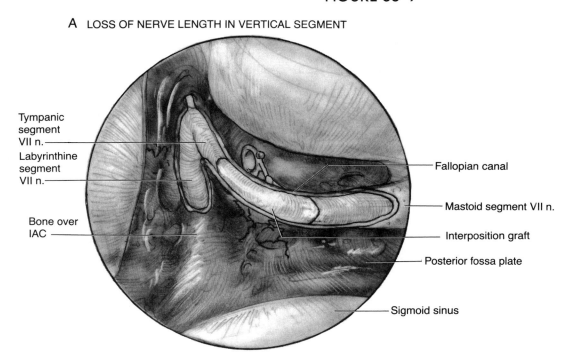

Tympanic segment VII n.

Labyrinthine segment VII n.

Bone over IAC

Fallopian canal

Mastoid segment VII n.

Interposition graft

Posterior fossa plate

Sigmoid sinus

B
EXTENSIVE LOSS OF TYMPANIC AND PROXIMAL VERTICAL SEGMENT

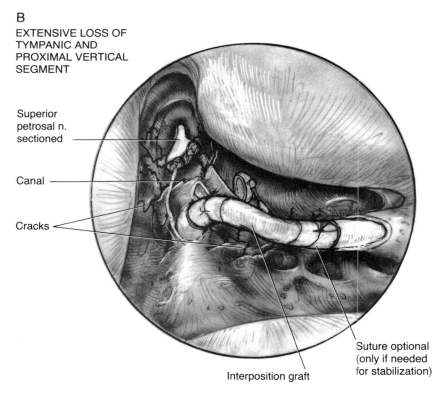

Superior petrosal n. sectioned

Canal

Cracks

Interposition graft

Suture optional (only if needed for stabilization)

length of nerve trunk loss. The repair techniques used for the repair of common lesions are shown in Figure 33–8. In injuries to the fallopian canal, the bone fragments may be in good reduction, betraying the true extent of injury to the nerve. In these cases, an intraneural hematoma can be produced by free blood within the intact nerve epineurium. Blood staining is frequently observed, but in some cases, the nerve will appear diffusely enlarged without areas of visible sheath staining. The nerve sheath should be incised using sharp, atraumatic technique and taking special care to preserve all underlying nerve fascicles (Fig. 33–8A). The Ziegler ophthalmic knife (Storz) is useful for incising the nerve sheath.

After the nerve sheath has been opened, degree of nerve loss is assessed. If a significant portion of the nerve fibers appears to be divided, clean division of the remaining trunk followed by an interposition graft should be considered. Bony fragments impinging on the nerve sheath should be atraumatically removed and the nerve assessed for intraneural hematoma and treated as above (Fig. 33–8B). Complete transection situations can be repaired using nerve rerouting, when the anatomy permits, to avoid the need for an interposition graft (Fig. 33–8C). Gunshot wounds to the temporal bone with a tympanic or labyrinthine segment injury and a dead ear are the typical situation (Fig. 33–9).[6] The interposition graft should be performed with a donor nerve graft of the appropriate diameter. In many situations, creation of a bony channel can enhance nerve and graft alignment without the need for multiple stabilization sutures and attendant postoperative inflammation (33–9A).[5] In all cases, the nerve should be widely decompressed until nonedematous nerve is encountered. In situations in which the loss of mastoid segment nerve tissue is minimal, the nerve can be dissected from the stylomastoid foramen region and the parotid facial nerve mobilized proximally to obviate an interposition graft.

Electrical monitoring of the facial nerve is helpful in determining when surgical trauma is occurring to the nerve. Obviously, if the nerve is completely transected, this technique will be of no value, but if the injury has occurred within 3 days, use of intraoperative facial nerve EMG can be helpful because the nerve will remain electrically active distally even though complete transection has taken place. In general, if the results of ENoG do not reveal 100 per cent degeneration, facial nerve monitoring may have some value because a few neurons will be able to produce discharge in the facial musculature, although this activity is not detectable clinically. Facial nerve EMG monitoring is performed by placing a pair of transcutaneous needle electrodes in the orbicularis oculi and oris muscles. The electrodes are connected directly by a short length of wire to a preamplifier and sent to the main recording unit. Processing and display options vary among commercially available units, but all process the signal to provide audio output of the signal and perhaps a visual record of the actual action potential or at least a visual indication of the amplitude of the response. The output signal is usually filtered, and artifact rejection mechanisms may eliminate signals produced by electrocautery and other electrical noise sources in the operating room. We employ a Nicolet Compact Four (Nicolet Biomedical Instruments, Madison, WI) evoked potential unit, which requires a technician for operation and set-up as well as for monitoring and recording the waveforms during the operative case. Audio output is available to the surgeon throughout the procedure, and care is taken to ensure that the same filter settings are used at all times so that the sound of facial nerve discharge can be identified consistently. Occasional discharges of the nerve are not considered as significant as prolonged trains of discharge: the latter usually indicate a more severe, potentially nonreversible insult to the nerve. The face is always exposed via a clear plastic drape so that visual confirmation and correlation of electrophysiologic events can be obtained.

The most common area of damage to the intratemporal segment is in the perigeniculate region, but location of the precise area of damage should be ascertained on preoperative CT scans. The middle fossa approach to decompression is used when labyrinthine function must be preserved. If clinical suspicion is confirmed by preoperative CT scans and intraoperative findings warrant, decompression of the mastoid segment of the facial nerve can be performed via a mastoid approach (see Chapter 18). During middle fossa decompression of the proximal facial nerve, the condition of the distal nerve can be determined by examination of the tympanic portion as it is exposed. If the nerve appears to be in good condition with no hemorrhage or edema evident, and no other indications exist for exploration of the mastoid portion of the nerve, exploration need not be performed.[4]

In many cases of transverse fractures and gunshot wounds of the temporal bone, the patient will have minimal or no residual hearing on audiometric testing. In these cases, a translabyrinthine approach to expose the entire facial nerve is possible without resorting to middle cranial fossa surgery. The labyrinth is removed and the internal auditory canal exposed. The nerve is identified in the tympanic segment adjacent to the lateral semicircular canal and in the labyrinthine segment distal to the internal auditory canal, and in this fashion, the entire intratemporal facial nerve is exposed.

During exposure of the nerve in the vertical and tympanic segments, surgical trauma to an already diseased nerve should be minimized. Minimal nerve trauma is produced because a thin shell of bone is left over the nerve throughout the decompression. At the conclusion of the gross exposure, a dissector is used to lift off the thin shell of bone as a large piece, thus avoiding contact of the diamond burr with the nerve sheath. At times, small fragments of the shell may be left in place without harm, and the goal of nerve decompression is still attained.

Repair should be performed at all anastomoses by use of neuroscopic technique, atraumatic handling of tissues, exact end-to-end anastomosis, tension-free closure, and the use of monofilament 9.0 or 10.0 suture.[5] Interposition grafts are employed when nerve tissue loss would produce tension in a direct anastomosis or when diseased nerve segments must be excised. The greater auricular nerve is adequate for defects less than 7cm, and the sural nerve can bridge defects as long as 30cm. The superiority of perineurial over epineurial repair has not been demonstrated, but meticulous techniques are clearly useful in reconstitution of the facial nerve.[25]

Extratemporal Nerve Segment

Establishing a functionally intact nerve in the frontal and marginal mandibular distribution of the face is important because of the limited anastomotic interconnection from adjacent branches of the facial nerve in these regions. Conversely, small branches in the midface region do not require extensive procedures to reestablish continuity, because of the rich anastomotic network that already exists. This quality leads to a much higher probability of a favorable outcome. Details of neural anastomosis techniques can be found in Chapter 34.

The technique for exposure of the peripheral nerve is based on techniques commonly used in parotid surgery. Penetrating trauma to the nerve at the stylomastoid foramen region may prevent identification of the nerve proximally, and the nerve will need to be found in the periphery and traced back proximally. Finding a branch of the marginal mandibular or frontal distribution is frequently useful.[26] If the exploration is performed within 2 days of the injury, the distal branches of the nerve will be able to be stimulated by electrical current, and observation of facial musculature twitching can help find the distal stump.

POSTOPERATIVE CARE

A modified mastoid dressing is applied, extending superiorly to apply pressure over the midfossa incision, if needed. The dressing is changed daily and the wound examined for signs of infection or CSF collection in the wound. A dressing is left in place for 2 to 3 days in the case of midfossa surgery, and for 1 day for mastoid surgery in which the dura is not violated.

Intravenous antibiotics are continued for 24 hours postoperatively. The dressing is left in place for 24 hours and then removed and the wound left exposed to allow easy observation. Any evidence of CSF collection in the wound is treated with pressure dressing and daily or twice daily observation to ensure that the fluid has not recurred. Needle aspiration is performed if indicated. Patients are asked to walk on the evening of surgery or the first day after surgery. Total hospital stay is 4 to 5 days.

PITFALLS OF SURGERY

The primary area of pathology in intratemporal injuries of the facial nerve is the labyrinthine segment. Frequently, the nerve must be exposed in this area if surgical intervention is required. If preservation of hearing is a goal, a middle fossa surgical approach will be required. Middle fossa surgery is a difficult technique because the anatomic approach is unfamiliar and the indications for its use are infrequent. These factors contribute to the difficulty in mastering this technique. However, the lack of good alternative procedures to address the anatomic region of greatest interest, the labyrinthine and meatal segment in the patient with intact hearing, makes maintenance of skills in middle fossa surgery a necessity for every active neurotologist.

RESULTS

The postoperative result depends largely on the severity of injury to the nerve and the timing of intervention to a lesser extent. Recovery is excellent for Sunderland's neurapraxic (1·) or axonotmetic (2·) lesions, which both involve intact endoneurial tubules. Primary anastomosis or interposition is required for neurotmesis (5·) injuries because complete separation of the nerve has occurred.[27] The best surgical result in this condition is a grade III or grade IV (AAO-HNS), with the latter being more typical. Crush and compression injuries are Sunderland 3· or 4· lesions, with varying degrees of endoneurial and perineurial disruption and no gross disruption of the nerve. These injuries present varying degrees of recovery, but grades III to V are usually attainable. The decision to resect and perform an anastomosis or to simply decompress is left to the surgeon; few physiologic data on which to base such a decision exist.[27] The best prognosis is obtained with early intervention in the acute phase of degeneration and prior to the onset of

Tumors of the facial nerve are rare causes of facial paralysis.[1–5] The two most common tumors are facial nerve neuromas, which are intrinsic to the nerve, and facial nerve hemangiomas, which are extraneural in origin. This chapter focuses on these two types of facial nerve tumors, although the techniques discussed can also be applied to other facial nerve neoplasms.

Because of their subtle presentation, facial nerve tumors may be very difficult to diagnose and require a high degree of clinical suspicion.[6, 7] The presenting symptoms vary with the tumor location, size, and histology. Facial nerve neuromas that arise in the internal auditory canal and cerebellopontine angle may present with a progressive sensorineural hearing loss similar to that caused by an acoustic tumor,[8] and the true diagnosis may be established only at surgery.[9, 10] In a patient with a suspected acoustic tumor, the presence of coexisting facial nerve symptoms (rare with acoustic tumors) should warn the surgeon that a facial nerve tumor may be present.[11, 12]

Facial nerve neuromas usually do not cause symptoms until they are fairly large and may present initially with hearing symptoms.[12–14] Tumors arising in the middle ear may contact the ossicles and cause a conductive hearing loss.[15] In such cases, when a mass behind the tympanic membrane is not visible, the patient may be thought to have otosclerosis, and the correct diagnosis is made during tympanotomy for stapedectomy.[6] When a middle ear mass is encountered in such a situation, a biopsy must not be done because a facial nerve paralysis will likely develop postoperatively (see *Pitfalls of Surgery*).[1, 6, 13, 16, 17]

Should the tumor erode into the labyrinth (typically, the lateral semicircular canal at the external genu), the patient may present with dizziness.[3] On examination, the fistula test result may be positive.

Facial nerve hemangiomas characteristically cause severe symptoms when very small.[18, 19] Like facial nerve neuromas, hemangiomas can occur in the internal auditory canal and present as acoustic tumors.[20] They usually cause a relatively severe sensorineural hearing loss for the size of the tumor. Hemangiomas of the geniculate ganglion can cause severe facial nerve symptoms when of extremely small size.[21, 22] Hemangiomas are extraneural and cause paralysis by compression,[23] but the small size of the tumor can make diagnosis by imaging studies very difficult; therefore, a high degree of clinical awareness is required.[24]

Patients with either tumor type may present with facial nerve symptoms. Typically, these patients have recurrent Bell's palsy, although the facial nerve recovery is less complete with each episode.[14] Facial nerve twitching can be present in some patients, and others may suffer facial paralysis with no recovery, or a slowly progressive facial paralysis.[25, 26] When evaluating a patient with atypical facial nerve symptoms, one must always suspect facial nerve neuroma.

Electrical testing can be helpful in establishing the diagnosis of a facial nerve tumor. Electroneuronographic results may be abnormal in patients with facial nerve tumors, even in the face of clinically normal function. Facial electromyography may show a pattern of simultaneous denervation and reinnervation in patients with tumors.[18] This pattern is seen in slowly progressive, pathologic processes and would not be expected with a rapid insult to the facial nerve, such as seen in Bell's palsy.

High-resolution magnetic resonance imaging with gadolinium may sufficiently detect most facial nerve tumors (Fig. 34–1). Imaging of a facial nerve neuroma generally reveals a mass lesion and enlargement of the fallopian canal. However, small facial heman-

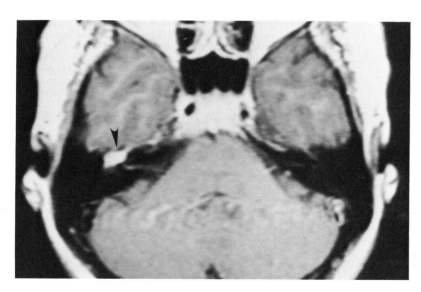

FIGURE 34–1. Magnetic resonance image of facial neuroma.

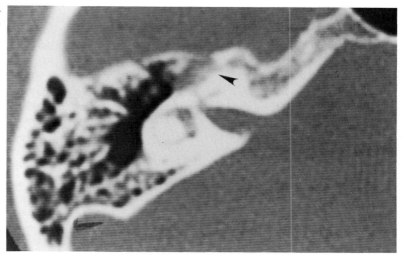

FIGURE 34-2. Computed tomographic scan showing hemangioma at geniculate ganglion with "honeycomb" bone.

giomas at the geniculate ganglion may require high-resolution computed tomographic scan (Fig. 34–2). These tumors exhibit characteristic bony changes termed *honeycomb* bone.[27] The medial extent of tumors arising at the geniculate ganglion can best be assessed with gadolinium-enhanced magnetic resonance imaging. This medial extension has important ramifications regarding selection of surgical approach.

PATIENT SELECTION

The timing of surgery is perhaps the most difficult aspect of planning. Many patients with facial nerve tumors have normal or nearly normal facial function. The best anticipated facial function after a facial nerve graft is a House-Brackmann grade III to IV.[16] However, waiting too long to remove the tumor can adversely affect the ultimate facial nerve results. Patients with a long-standing facial nerve paralysis achieve worse results after facial nerve grafting than those who have grafting when they have normal facial function.[9, 13] Extraneural tumors, such as facial nerve hemangiomas, can be removed with preservation of facial nerve continuity; therefore, early surgery in such cases may offer the best hope for excellent facial nerve function. Labyrinthine fistula can develop from bony erosion by the tumor and can lead to deafness and dizziness if the tumor is neglected too long.[13, 28]

For an older patient in poor health who has a small tumor and good facial function, observation may be the best strategy. Younger patients with good facial function may also be followed up, but they must be aware of the possible risk to the ultimate facial nerve outcome and to their hearing if surgery is delayed.[12] In some cases, we follow up patients until they show greater than 50 per cent denervation by electroneuronography. Once they reach this degree of denervation, we are concerned that facial nerve grafting after further loss of neural "firepower" will ultimately result in poor facial function.

Facial nerve neuromas in the internal auditory canal may be recognized during surgery for what was presumed to be an acoustic tumor.[29] (We counsel our acoustic tumor patients preoperatively about this unlikely possibility). Usually, the tumor is resected and a nerve graft placed. In a few patients with a facial neuroma, tumor decompression is carried out, giving the patient several additional years of good facial function before definitive surgery is required.

PATIENT COUNSELING

The most important aspect of preoperative patient counseling is the expected postoperative facial function. Patients are told that a facial nerve graft will be needed, although patients with small hemangiomas are informed that it may be possible to preserve the continuity of the facial nerve. Patients should expect a postoperative facial paralysis lasting 6 to 12 months. Ultimate facial function after a facial nerve graft will not be "normal," and the consequences of synkinesis are discussed.

To describe a "good" result after facial nerve grafting, the author tells his patients that the patient will look normal at rest and have active voluntary movement, but it will not be entirely symmetric motion. This asymmetry will be to the extent that family members will notice a difference, but a stranger on the street would not likely turn and stare (Fig. 34–3).

Patients with a preoperative facial nerve palsy are told to expect worse postoperative facial function after nerve grafting. The longer the duration or the greater the severity of the preoperative palsy, the worse the ultimate result. The other potential risks

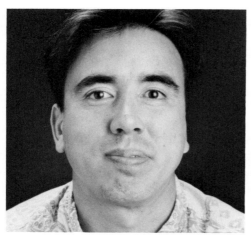

FIGURE 34-3. Patient postoperatively exhibiting a House-Brackmann facial function grade IV one year after facial nerve graft.

internal auditory canal, it can expose the horizontal facial nerve to approximately the midtympanic portion. However, because of the limited access, sewing a graft into the internal auditory canal can be difficult, and posterior fossa access is not provided. For patients with larger tumors or with poor hearing and involvement of the internal auditory canal, posterior fossa, or geniculate ganglion, the translabyrinthine approach can be used. This approach provides wide access for tumor removal and allows placement of a facial nerve graft.

Involvement of the horizontal and vertical facial nerve may also require a transmastoid facial recess approach. Erosion of the external auditory canal may necessitate a canal wall down procedure. The facial nerve can be followed into the parotid should tumor extension require the exposure. A staged procedure may be required in a chronically infected ear that requires an intracranial surgical approach for tumor removal.

Middle Fossa Approach

The initial middle fossa approach is carried out as described for acoustic tumors in Chapter 50. After the craniotomy window is made, the temporal lobe is supported by the House-Urban retractor, and the greater superficial petrosal nerve and the blue line of the superior semicircular canal are identified. The greater superficial petrosal nerve is followed posteriorly to the geniculate ganglion (Fig. 34–4). For patients with tumor involvement in this area, extreme care must be taken during the dissection, as a tumor can distort the anatomy.

The internal auditory canal is skeletonized and the labyrinthine facial nerve identified. The amount of internal auditory canal exposure varies with the degree of tumor extension in that area and the need for access to place a graft (Fig. 34–5). The tegmen bone is also removed to expose the tympanic facial nerve (Fig. 34–6). Care is taken not to touch the ossicular heads with a burr during this removal, as a sensorineural hearing loss will result.

and complications of surgery are also discussed according to the surgical approach needed. For middle fossa and translabyrinthine cases, the risks are similar to those for acoustic tumor patients treated through these approaches (see Chapters 50 and 51).

Patients with tumor involvement of the ossicles may need ossicular reconstruction. In some cases, this procedure is best carried out at a second stage, and the patients are also informed of this possibility.

SURGICAL TECHNIQUES

Preoperative preparation, patient positioning, and instrumentation are described in Chapter 1. For patients needing a facial nerve graft, the upper neck is also prepared for harvesting of the greater auricular nerve.

The surgical approach is selected on the basis of tumor location, tumor size, and level of residual hearing. For small tumors around the geniculate ganglion in patients with good hearing, the middle fossa approach can be used. Besides providing access into the

FIGURE 34-4. Exposure of the geniculate ganglion through the middle fossa approach. A, The greater superficial petrosal nerve and superior semicircular canal are skeletonized. B, Tumor is encountered at the geniculate ganglion.

FIGURE 34-5. The internal auditory canal and labyrinthine facial nerve are exposed medial to the geniculate ganglion.

FIGURE 34-6. After removal of tegmen bone, the facial nerve can be exposed to approximately the midtympanic portion.

FIGURE 34-7. Facial nerve neuroma is seen through a transmastoid approach. The facial recess is opened, and the thin eggshell of bone over the distal facial nerve is removed.

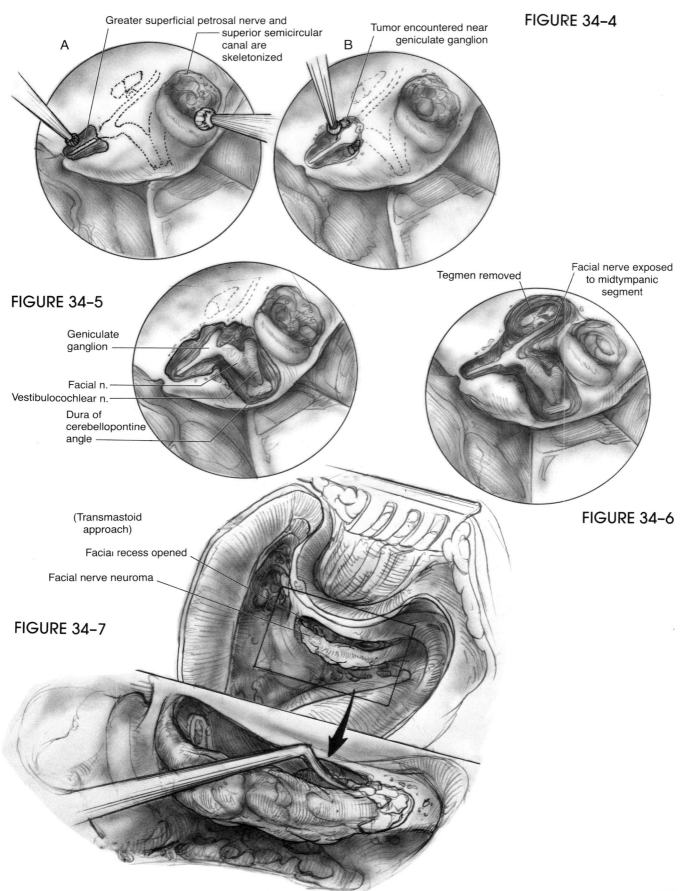

FIGURE 34–4

A Greater superficial petrosal nerve and superior semicircular canal are skeletonized

B Tumor encountered near geniculate ganglion

FIGURE 34–5

Geniculate ganglion

Facial n.

Vestibulocochlear n.

Dura of cerebellopontine angle

Tegmen removed

Facial nerve exposed to midtympanic segment

FIGURE 34–6

(Transmastoid approach)

Facial recess opened

Facial nerve neuroma

FIGURE 34–7

Transmastoid Approach

Should additional distal exposure be needed, a transmastoid approach to the facial nerve can also be performed, as described in Chapter 18. The facial recess is opened and the nerve skeletonized to the stylomastoid foramen. Around the facial nerve, it is best to thin the bone over it with a diamond burr, to use copious irrigation, and then to remove the overlying "eggshell" of bone with an instrument such as a sickle knife or a whirlybird (Fig. 34–7). Because of tumor involvement or the need for additional room, the malleus head and incus can be removed and ossicular reconstruction performed at the end of the procedure.

Translabyrinthine Approach

The translabyrinthine approach is carried out as described in Chapter 51, and the facial nerve is skeletonized. The amount of medial bone removal varies with the tumor extent and the need for access for facial nerve grafting. The bone over the geniculate ganglion can be removed anteriorly to expose the greater superficial petrosal nerve (Fig. 34–8).

Tumor Removal

Tumor removal is accomplished with sharp and blunt dissection. Posterior fossa tumor removal is handled in a way similar to the technique used for acoustic tumors. After the tumor has been removed, frozen sections are taken from the remaining nerve ends to ensure total tumor removal.

In some extraneural tumors (hemangiomas), a plane can be developed between the tumor and nerve, allowing facial nerve preservation. In selected neuroma cases, it may also be possible to remove the tumor while maintaining partial continuity of the facial nerve.

Graft Material

The greater auricular nerve serves as an excellent donor nerve for grafting. The diameter match is good, and the donor deficit is minimal. Adequate length can be obtained to graft from the internal auditory canal to the stylomastoid foramen.

The greater auricular nerve can be found between the angle of the mandible and the tip of the mastoid process on the lateral surface of the sternocleidomastoid muscle,[30] posterosuperior to the external jugular vein (Fig. 34–9). The nerve can be harvested through an oblique skin incision placed in a skin crease. By dissecting the nerve from the posterior aspect of the sternocleidomastoid muscle, ample length is obtained. Another option for a donor graft is the sural nerve (Fig. 34–10), which has a larger diameter and length than the greater auricular nerve.

The ends of the graft are trimmed sharply, and excess fibrous tissue and epineurium are removed from the nerve stumps. Some surgeons advocate reversing the nerve direction to prevent axons from growing out branches of the graft.

Nerve Grafting

Within the temporal bone, if enough of the fallopian canal remains as a trough, placement of the graft in approximation to the nerve end is usually sufficient (Fig. 34–11). The anastomosis can be packed into place with Avitene, which forms a clot over the anastomosis.[31] When sutures are needed, two or three epineurial sutures of 9/0 Deklene II on a T-7 needle (Deknatel) work well (Fig. 34–12). The suture length is trimmed to 6 inches to make it easier to work under the microscope, and a back of a surgical glove is cut, wetted, and placed beneath the anastomosis to give a smooth working surface. The author prefers to cut the graft slightly longer than needed to ensure that no

---

FIGURE 34–8. Translabyrinthine approach with exposure of the geniculate ganglion and greater superficial petrosal nerve. Tumor extends from the internal auditory canal to the tympanic facial nerve.

FIGURE 34–9. The greater auricular nerve is located on the lateral surface of the sternocleidomastoid muscle, posterior to the external jugular vein. It lies between the tip of the mastoid and the angle of the jaw.

FIGURE 34–10. The sural nerve can be found on the lateral surface of the ankle posterior to the lateral malleolus.

FIGURE 34–11. Facial nerve graft is placed in apposition to the proximal facial nerve stump at the labyrinthine segment. Remaining fallopian canal holds graft in place, and sutures are not needed.

FIGURE 34–12. Nerve graft held in approximation to distal mastoid facial nerve stump with two epineurial sutures.

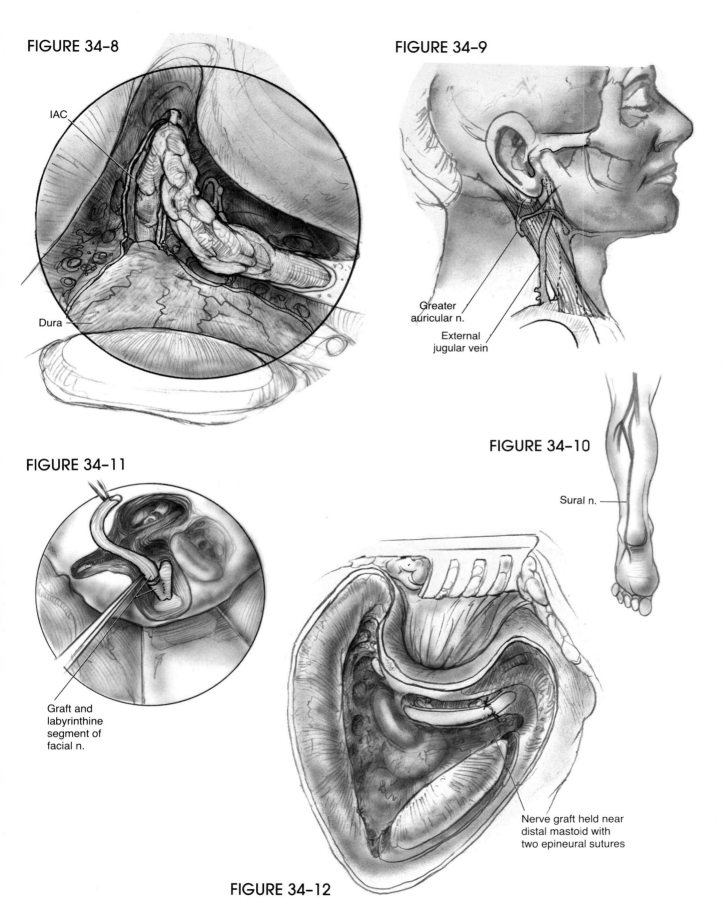

FIGURE 34–8

IAC

Dura

FIGURE 34–9

Greater
auricular n.

External
jugular vein

FIGURE 34–10

Sural n.

FIGURE 34–11

Graft and
labyrinthine
segment of
facial n.

Nerve graft held near
distal mastoid with
two epineural sutures

FIGURE 34–12

tension exists on the anastomosis. If possible, the graft is placed along the normal course of the facial nerve so that if further surgery is required, it can be easily identified. For patients requiring an ossicular reconstruction at a second stage, the graft of the horizontal facial nerve is placed in the epitympanum, superior to the oval window, so that it will not need to be manipulated during later ossicular reconstruction.

The placement of an anastomosis in the internal auditory canal or posterior fossa is much more difficult than that performed within the temporal bone because the intracranial facial nerve has no epineurium (Fig. 34–13). Usually, a single through-and-through suture of 9/0 Deklene is sufficient.[32] The suture is placed on the graft side first. When the suture is placed through the intracranial facial nerve stump, a fenestrated suction is used to support the facial nerve, and the needle is passed into a side hole of the suction (Fig. 34–14).[33]

Rerouting

Depending on the location and length of the facial nerve defect, it may be possible to remove the facial nerve from its canal and reroute it to gain extra length. This maneuver subjects the nerve to a great deal of manipulation and may interfere with its blood supply. However, for a defect in the cerebellopontine angle, rerouting (Fig. 34–15) gains additional nerve length and allows primary anastomosis.

The wounds are closed as described in Chapter 32, and abdominal fat packing is used when indicated. The standard mastoid dressing is used. The postoperative care for tumor removal from the translabyrinthine and middle fossa approaches is similar to that given to patients with acoustic tumors removed through these approaches (see Chapters 50 and 51).

An important aspect of postoperative care is attention to the paralyzed eye. This topic is detailed in Chapter 61. Depending on the anticipated time and quality of facial function recovery, some patients require the placement of an upper eyelid spring.

PITFALLS OF SURGERY

Facial nerve tumors, particularly neuromas, tend to involve the nerve over long distances of its course. Underestimation of tumor extent is an important problem and can be overcome by high-resolution imaging studies. High-resolution computed tomography of the temporal bone can show enlargement and erosion of the fallopian canal and indicate tumor involvement. When needed, gadolinium-enhanced magnetic resonance imaging demonstrates extension of the tumor into the internal auditory canal and posterior fossa.

Many cases in our series were diagnosed elsewhere when a middle ear mass was encountered during tympanotomy to correct a conductive hearing loss. A biopsy must not be done on a middle ear mass in this situation. Of nine tumors for which biopsies were done by the referring surgeons in our series, 88 per cent suffered a postbiopsy facial paralysis (Alavi and Shelton, unpublished data). For a patient going to surgery for a stapedectomy, the development of a postoperative facial paralysis from the biopsy can be extremely disturbing. When a middle ear mass is encountered, the ear should be closed, and a radiologic, not histologic, evaluation should be done. A high-resolution computed tomographic scan showing enlargement of the fallopian canal will yield a diagnosis of facial nerve tumor, and subsequent surgery can be planned based on the extent of the tumor.

The labyrinth is at risk for fistulization by bone erosion caused by tumor growth. Particularly vulnerable are the inferior surface of the lateral semicircular canal at the external genu and the cochlea near the geniculate ganglion. A patient with a facial nerve tumor (particularly one that does not involve the internal auditory canal) who exhibits dizziness or sensorineural hearing loss may have a labyrinthine fistula. Such fistulas can frequently be detected on high-resolution computed tomography. However, the surgeon should always be alert to the possibility of encountering a fistula during surgery and must be prepared to

---

FIGURE 34-13. Facial nerve graft is placed into internal auditory canal through translabyrinthine approach. A single through-and-through suture holds the nerve ends together.

FIGURE 34-14. A fenestrated suction supports the intracranial facial nerve. The suture is passed through the nerve and into a side hole of the suction.

FIGURE 34-15. The facial nerve is rerouted in the translabyrinthine approach to gain approximately 1.5cm of length.

FIGURE 34-13

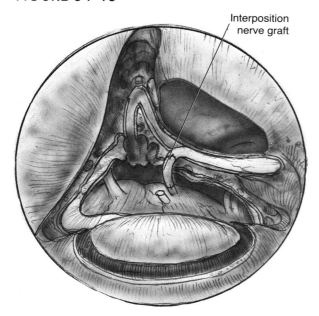

Interposition
nerve graft

FIGURE 34-14

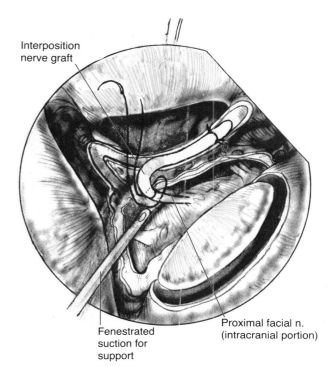

Interposition
nerve graft

Fenestrated
suction for
support

Proximal facial n.
(intracranial portion)

FIGURE 34-15

(Translabyrinthine approach)
Facial nerve rerouted gains
approx. 1.5 cm in length

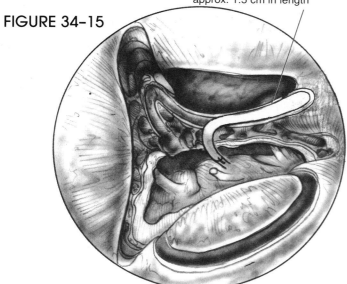

repair it. In patients with a known fistula preoperatively, temporalis fascia can be harvested in anticipation of covering the fistula.

For a nerve graft to function, the anastomosis must be made to viable neural tissue at the nerve stump and not to residual tumor. Frozen section examination of the nerve stump is necessary not only to validate complete tumor removal but also to ensure that no tumor remains at the anastomotic site to impede axonal regrowth.

RESULTS

Facial Nerve Neuromas

A review of 64 facial nerve neuromas removed by members of the House Ear Clinic (Alavi and Shelton, unpublished data) revealed that the facial nerve required repair (graft or primary anastomosis) in 72 per cent of these patients. Of those with 1 year or more of follow-up, 83 per cent of the patients who had undergone repair had facial function graded as a House-Brackmann grade IV or better (Table 34–1). For those with preservation of facial nerve continuity, 70 per cent had postoperative facial function of House-Brackmann grade III or better at 1 year (Table 34–1). Only one patient in long-term follow-up experienced no recovery of postoperative facial function.

Hearing was preserved near the preoperative level (within 10dB pure-tone average and 16 per cent speech discrimination score) in 53 per cent of patients, excluding those undergoing translabyrinthine tumor removal. Sixteen patients had fistulas of the inner ear, 11 involving a lateral semicircular canal, and four involving the cochlea. Hearing was lost in four patients, all fistula cases.

Facial Nerve Hemangiomas

Facial nerve hemangiomas tend to occur at the geniculate ganglion or in the internal auditory canal, with facial nerve repair most often required for tumors at the geniculate ganglion. Of the 34 facial nerve hemangiomas removed by the members of the House Ear Clinic, 47 per cent required facial nerve repair.[18] The vast majority of the repaired nerves achieved a House-Brackmann grade III or IV by 1 year or more after surgery (Table 34–2).

Hearing was maintained near the preoperative level in 64 per cent of patients. One patient had postoperative anacusis from a cochlear fistula caused by the tumor.

COMPLICATIONS AND MANAGEMENT

Postoperative cerebrospinal fluid leaks occurred in 6 per cent of the neuroma series, and postoperative meningitis developed in 3 per cent. Surprisingly, meningitis did not occur in patients who also experienced a cerebrospinal fluid leak. The management of these complications is similar to that after acoustic tumor removal by the translabyrinthine and middle fossa approaches, which are discussed in Chapters 50 and 51, respectively.

TABLE 34–2. Postoperative Facial Nerve Results for 23 Facial Nerve Hemangioma Patients With > 1 Year Follow-up

FACIAL NERVE GRADES*	FACIAL NERVE STATUS	
	Repaired	Intact
I	—	7
II	—	2
III	2	—
IV	8	1
V	1	—
VI	2	—

*House-Brackmann classification.
From Shelton C, Brackmann DE, Lo WW, Carberry JN: Intratemporal facial nerve hemangiomas. Otolaryngol Head Neck Surg 104(1):116–121, 1991.

TABLE 34–1. Postoperative Facial Nerve Function for 34 Facial Nerve Neuroma Patients With > 1 Year Follow-up

FACIAL NERVE* FUNCTION	FACIAL NERVE STATUS		
	Repaired (n = 24)	Intact (n = 10)	Total (n = 34)
I	—	3	3
II	—	1	1
III	9	3	12
IV	11	1	12
V	4	1	5
VI	0	1	1

*House-Brackmann classification.

References

1. Pulec JL: Facial nerve neuroma. Laryngoscope 82(7): 1160–1176, 1972.
2. Rosenblum B, Davis R, Camins M: Middle fossa facial schwannoma removed via the intracranial extradural approach: Case report and review of the literature. Neurosurgery 21(5): 739–741, 1987.
3. Pearman K, Welch AR: Schwannoma of the intratemporal facial nerve. Case report. J Laryngol Otol 94(7): 779–784, 1980.
4. Lilieguist B: Neurinomas of the labyrinthine portion of the facial nerve canal. A report of two cases. Adv Otorhinolaryngol 24: 58–67, 1978.
5. Pulec JL: Facial nerve tumors. Ann Otol Rhinol Laryngol 78: 962–983, 1969.
6. Jackson CG, Glasscock ME III, Hughes G, Sismanis A: Facial paralysis of neoplastic origin: Diagnosis and management. Laryngoscope 90(10Pt1): 1581–1595, 1980.
7. Wiet RJ, Pyle GM, Schramm DR: Middle fossa and intratemporal facial nerve neuromas. Otolaryngol Head Neck Surg 104(1): 141–142, 1991.

8. Lee KS, Britton BH, Kelly DL Jr.: Schwannoma of the facial nerve in the cerebellopontine angle presenting with hearing loss. Surg Neurol 32(3): 231–234, 1989.
9. King TT, Morrison AW: Primary facial nerve tumors within the skull. J Neurosurg 72(1): 1–8, 1990.
10. Dort JC, Fisch U: Facial nerve schwannomas. Skull Base Surg 1: 51–55, 1991.
11. Nelson RA, House WF: Facial nerve neuroma in the posterior fossa: Surgical considerations. In Graham MD, House WF (eds): Disorders of the Facial Nerve. New York, Raven Press, 1982, pp 403–406.
12. Bailey CM, Graham MD: Intratemporal facial nerve neuroma: A discussion of five cases. J Laryngol Otol 97(1): 65–72, 1983.
13. O'Donoghue GM, Brackmann DE, House JW, Jackler RK: Neuromas of the facial nerve. Am J Otol 10(1): 49–54, 1989.
14. Pillsbury HC, Price HC, Gardiner LJ: Primary tumors of the facial nerve: Diagnosis and management. Laryngoscope 93(8): 1045–1048, 1983.
15. Neely JG, Alford BR: Facial nerve neuromas. Arch Otolaryngol Head Neck Surg 100(4): 298–301, 1974.
16. Lipkin AF, Coker NJ, Jenkins HA, Alford BR: Intracranial and intratemporal facial neuroma. Otolaryngol Head Neck Surg 96(1): 71–79, 1987.
17. Wiet RS, Lohan AN, Brackmann DE: Neurilemmoma of the chorda tympani nerve. Otolaryngol Head Neck Surg 93: 119–121, 1985.
18. Shelton C, Brackmann DE, Lo WW, Carberry JN: Intratemporal facial nerve hemangiomas. Otolaryngol Head Neck Surg 104(1): 116–121, 1991.
19. Mangham CA, Carberry JN, Brackmann DE: Management of intratemporal vascular tumors. Laryngoscope 91: 867–876, 1981.
20. Pappas DG, Schneiderman TS, Brackmann DE, et al.: Cavernous hemangiomas of the internal auditory canal. Otolaryngol Head Neck Surg 101: 27–32, 1989.
21. Fisch U, Ruttner J: Pathology of intratemporal tumors involving the facial nerve. In Fisch U (ed): Facial Nerve Surgery. Birmingham, AL, Aesculapius, 1977, pp 448–456.
22. Balkany T, Fradis M, Jafek BW, Rucker NC: Hemangioma of the facial nerve: Role of the geniculate capillary plexus. Skull Base Surg 1: 59–63, 1991.
23. Ylikoski J, Brackmann DE, Savolainen S: Pressure neuropathy of the facial nerve: A case report with light and electron microscopic findings. J Laryngol Otol 98: 909–914, 1984.
24. Glasscock ME, Smith PG, Schwaber MK, Nissen AJ: Clinical aspects of osseous hemangiomas of the skull base. Laryngoscope 94: 869–873, 1984.
25. Tew JM Jr, Yeh HS, Miller GW, Shahbabian S: Intratemporal schwannoma of the facial nerve. Neurosurgery 13(2): 186–188, 1983.
26. Valvassori GE: Neuromas of the facial nerve. Adv Otorhinolaryngol 24: 68–70, 1978.
27. Lo WW, Brackmann DE, Shelton C: Facial nerve hemangioma. Ann Otol Rhinol Laryngol 98(2): 160–161, 1989.
28. Sanna M, Zini C, Gamoletti R, Pasanisi E: Primary intratemporal tumours of the facial nerve: Diagnosis and treatment. J Laryngol Otol 104(10): 765–771, 1990.
29. Murata T, Hakuba A, Okumura T, Mori K: Intrapetrous neurinomas of the facial nerve. Report of three cases. Surg Neurol 23(5): 507–512, 1985.
30. Pulec JL: Facial nerve grafting. Laryngoscope 79: 1562–1583, 1969.
31. House JW: Facial nerve tumors and grafting. In Brackmann DE (ed:) Neurological Surgery of the Ear and Skull Base. New York, Raven Press, 1982, pp 77–80.
32. Barrs DM, Brackmann DE, Hitselberger WE: Facial nerve anastomosis in the cerebellopontine angle: A review of 24 cases. Am J Otol 5: 269–272, 1984.
33. Arriaga MA, Brackmann DE: Facial nerve repair techniques in cerebellopontine angle tumor surgery. Am J Otol 13: 356–359, 1992.

35

Surgery for Cochlear Implantation

WILLIAM M. LUXFORD, M.D.

Although the first attempt to electrically stimulate the auditory system occurred nearly two centuries ago, the development of a cochlear prosthesis to restore hearing to patients with sensorineural hearing loss has happened only over the past three decades. The early pioneering work of Simmons, Michaelson, and House provided the stimulus to encourage others, including Bonfai, Chouard, Clark, Eddington, and the Hochmairs.[1] The initial acceptance of cochlear implants was slow; safety and efficacy were the concerns of the early investigators, and the greatest champions of the implant were the patients themselves. Time and technology increased the benefits gained by most patients from their cochlear implants. As a result, cochlear implants have become more widely accepted with each passing year. Of the more than 5000 patients who have received cochlear implants worldwide, approximately 90 per cent have undergone implantation in only the past 10 years.

Many centers throughout the world have investigated the cochlear implant, and many differences exist in the devices being investigated. In the United States, the Food and Drug Administration (FDA) has monitored these investigations. The FDA has approved the Nucleus 22-channel device manufactured by the Cochlear Corporation for general use in adults and children.[2] Other devices, including the San Francisco device, manufactured by MiniMed,[3] and the Ineraid implant, manufactured by Richards,[4] are undergoing investigational clinical trials controlled by the FDA in adults. Once these devices show safety and efficacy in adults, they will undergo FDA controlled clinical trials in children. The criteria for these groups include age of 18 years or more in adults and age of 2 to 17 years in children, bilateral profound-to-total sensorineural hearing loss, inability to benefit from conventional hearing aids, good physical and mental health, and the motivation and patience to complete a rehabilitation program.[5]

PATIENT SELECTION

Selection criteria of an appropriate implant candidate vary from center to center.

Audiologic Criteria

An audiologic assessment is the primary means of determining implant candidacy. A potential implant candidate has bilateral, profound-to-total sensorineural hearing loss, usually with a three-frequency average (500Hz, 1000Hz, and 2000Hz), pure-tone unaided threshold in the better ear equal to or greater than 95dB. Audiologic testing procedures differ between adults and children.

Adults

The prospective candidate is evaluated with appropriately powerful hearing aids. Factors regarding function with a hearing aid, such as recruitment and discomfort, are considered when the likelihood that the patient might perform better with an implant than with a hearing aid is evaluated.

If the patient cannot obtain an aided speech detection threshold of 70dB sound pressure level or an approximate 53dB hearing level or better, or performs very poorly on discrimination tests with conventional amplification, a cochlear implant is likely to provide greater benefit. Until recently, an implant candidate was commonly thought to be able to achieve no open-set speech discrimination with a hearing aid. However, current data regarding potential performance with an implant indicate that some patients with scores as high as 10 per cent on the W-22 word list may be candidates for a cochlear implant. In addition, an investigational study for the Nucleus 22-channel device is accepting a limited number of adults who may achieve as much as 25 per cent open-set word discrimination in the better ear as long as the poorer ear has less than 10 per cent discrimination, and the binaural score with hearing aids is less than 30 per cent.

A full list of test procedures and criteria for patient selection recommended by the device manufacturers and principal investigators are typically specified in the product labeling or in the training manuals.

Children

Children evaluated for the cochlear implant undergo an extensive audiologic assessment. Tympanometry and otoscopy are performed to rule out middle ear pathology at the time of testing. Acoustic reflexes are measured. In children less than 6 years of age, auditory brainstem response testing is required to confirm a profound hearing loss. Traditional behavioral audiometry or play audiometry with visual, social, or tangible reinforcers is used as needed. If there is no response to sound at maximal levels through the head phones, the child is conditioned to respond to a hand-held bone oscillator to ensure that he or she understands the task.

Discrimination tests are performed with the aid that provides the best warble-tone threshold. With an appropriate hearing aid, the child's performance on the discrimination tests in the ear selected for implantation must be poorer than or equal to the average test results obtained from children using a cochlear implant.

Parent and teacher reports of the child's auditory ability must be consistent with the measured severity of the hearing loss. The child must also have a history of an appropriate hearing aid trial. If recently prescribed hearing aids or ear molds have not yielded optimal results, and if testing reveals that usable hearing may remain, a 3- to 6-month trial with appropriate aids and molds is required before a decision on the implant is made. In these cases, the parents and school are encouraged to provide intense auditory training during the trial period.

Medical Evaluation

The medical evaluation includes a complete history and physical examination to detect problems that might interfere with the patient's ability to complete either the surgical or rehabilitative measures of implantation. Appropriate laboratory studies should be ordered to eliminate any suspected medical disorder.

In adults and children receiving the cochlear implant, the etiology of deafness varies. From the variety of responses to cochlear implantation of patients with the same etiology, the etiology of hearing loss does not seem as important as the onset of loss. For cochlear implant candidates, the onset of profound hearing loss is best described as congenital (hearing loss present at birth) or acquired (hearing loss occurring after birth).

Adults deafened prior to acquisition of verbal language skills (congenital and early acquired) are considered prelingually deaf. Adults deafened after the acquisition of verbal language skills (late acquired) are considered postlingually deaf. Acquired deafness in children can be further defined by age of onset: prelingual ($\leq$1 year), perilingual (1 to 5 years), and postlingual ($\geq$5 years).

For adults, the postlingually deaf individual makes the best implant candidate and comprises the majority of adults receiving implants. A smaller number of adult implant recipients have a congenital or very early onset of hearing loss. Prelingually deaf adults have a long period of auditory deprivation and may have had little experience with sound. Expectations for benefit from a cochlear implant must be adjusted accordingly. Although prelingually and postlingually deaf patients probably receive similar auditory information through a cochlear implant, prelingually deaf adults cannot use the information as effectively and have a higher rate of nonuse of the device.

For children, the later the onset of profound hearing loss the greater the chance that the child will develop an auditory memory and realize the benefit of sound. Unlike adults, children with congenital, prelingual, or perilingual losses are usually able to effectively use the information provided by the implant and have a low rate of nonuse of the device when they receive the implant early.

Another important factor in patient selection is length of profound hearing loss. In a review of adult patients, Dowell et al. found no correlation between age and performance but a highly significant negative correlation between the length of profound deafness and performance.[6] For their patients, the performance was worse if hearing was lost more than 13 years before implantation. They found that patients with prolonged duration of deafness received similar information to that of the other implant patients but were unable to use the information as effectively in the recognition of running speech. Dowell et al. believed that this difference may have been caused by loss of central auditory processing resulting from the long period of sound deprivation.

Duration of profound deafness also seems to be an important factor in selection of an appropriate implant candidate in children, especially in those with onset of hearing loss prior to the acquisition of speech and language.

Even though a shorter duration between onset of hearing loss and implantation is beneficial, the interval must be long enough to be certain of the degree of hearing loss, to determine the full benefits of hearing aids, and to be sure that the profound loss has been accepted by both the patient and the family. The interval is at least 6 months for most adults and may be as long as 1 year for children.

For children, age does seem to be an important issue in patient selection. Teenagers are usually extremely poor candidates for cochlear implants. Although there are many reasons for this, peer pressure and cosmetic issues are the two factors cited most by teenagers who become nonusers. Counseling is an extremely important part of the patient selection with teenagers.

Physical Examination

It is important to identify preoperatively any external or middle ear disease, including perforations of the tympanic membrane, that must be treated prior to cochlear implantation. For young children, the size of the implant in relation to the size of the child's skull must be evaluated, and issues involved with skull maturation must be considered. The distance between the cochlear promontory and the mastoid cortex, the approximate sites of the electrode array, and the receiver-stimulator increases about 1.7cm from birth to adulthood, with one half of the increase occurring during the first 2 years of life.[7] The electrodes must be long enough to tolerate the increase in height and width of the skull that will occur with the child's growth. The accommodation occurs through the gradual straightening of the excess electrode length within the air-containing mastoid cavity.[8]

Radiologic Evaluation

High-resolution computed tomography of the temporal bone is performed in all cases to identify partial or complete ossification of the scala tympani, soft tissue obliteration of the scala, congenital malformation of the inner ear, and surgical landmarks.[9] Complete agenesis of the cochlea and an abnormal acoustic nerve, the result of either congenital malformation, trauma, or surgery, are contraindications for cochlear implant placement.[10]

Cochlear hypoplasia (Mondini's deformity) is not a contraindication for cochlear implantation. Adults and children with incomplete congenital cochlear malformations have received implants successfully.[11]

Ossification or fibrous occlusion of the cochlea or the round window does not exclude a patient from implantation, but it may influence outcome. Occlusion of the cochlea may lead to partial insertion of the electrode carrier. Magnetic resonance imaging has become more useful than computed tomography in the evaluation of the membranous inner ear in detecting cochlear fibrosis.

Promontory Evaluation

Many implant teams perform an electrical stimulation test at either the promontory or the round window membrane.[12] A positive response is a perception of sound on stimulation. Some investigators do not feel that such testing is critical in the selection of candidates because patients with a negative response, particularly at the promontory, may respond to intracochlear stimulation with an implant.

Other Considerations

Although most implant programs no longer require a formal psychological evaluation for implant candidates, numerous other factors are considered important in the final decision to perform the procedure. Counseling is often provided to families who have misconceptions or unrealistic expectations regarding the benefits and limitations of the cochlear implant. Support from family and friends is an important part in the rehabilitative process.

For children, the educational setting can play an important part in the selection process. Children in educational programs in which there is special emphasis on auditory training do better than those in settings with little or no auditory input.[2]

PREOPERATIVE EVALUATION

Once a candidate has been selected, the next decision is which side to place the implant. In the past, we always placed the implant in the worst-hearing ear. With experience, we have learned that the "hearing history" of each ear is important. In the potential candidate with a congenital onset of hearing loss in one ear and an acquired hearing loss in the opposite ear, better implant results would be attained if the acquired ear received the implant. In the potential candidate with different durations of profound hearing impairment in each ear, better results would be attained if the ear that had the shortest duration of deafness received the implant. In the potential candidate who has the same etiology for deafness and a similar duration of deafness in both ears but has used a hearing aid for sound awareness in only one ear with no benefit, as determined by the audiologic test procedures, placing the implant in the ear that used the hearing aid should be discussed with the patient. Potential candidates who have residual hearing in the ear to receive the implant must be told that following implantation with the device's long electrodes, they will likely lose the residual hearing in that ear and be unable to use a hearing aid for sound awareness.

If there is no difference acoustically, then we place the implant in the better surgical ear, based on computed tomographic evaluation. The side with the least ossification or fibrosis within the scala tympani is chosen. Results from vestibular tests should be given the least weight in the selection of the side of cochlear implantation. The ear with the least caloric response should receive the implant.

In children, there are no absolute speech or language selection criteria; however, every child is given a full speech and language assessment, including speech production and expressive and receptive language testing. This information is important in helping the implant staff determine how to most effectively interact with the child. The results of these assessments may also influence the final decision regarding implantation by providing a more complete picture of the child's overall status. Reports from the child's educational setting are extremely helpful in completing the speech and language assessment.

The preimplant audiologic, psychologic, and speech and language evaluations provide baseline information against which improvements with the implant can be judged. These assessments are all repeated at regular follow-up intervals after the procedure.

SURGICAL TECHNIQUE

The details of implantation differ from prosthesis to prosthesis. The cochlear implant should be implanted only by qualified surgeons specifically trained to perform the procedure. Surgeons should avoid allowing any prosthetic material to have contact with the skin of the external ear canal. Therefore, the preferred procedure for placement of an implant in a patient with a normal external ear canal is via the transmastoid facial recess approach to the round window–scala tympani. In patients with mastoid cavities and an absent posterior external ear canal, the preferred procedure is total obliteration of the mastoid and closure of the external ear meatus.

The external ear canal approach to the round window is acceptable in adults. The initial problems of electrode extrusion have been overcome by formation of a deep groove in the external canal and encasement of the electrode in bone. This procedure, however, is not acceptable in children. With the electrode encased in the external ear canal, no accommodation for skull growth occurs. Therefore, the electrode would be displaced from its original intracochlear position over time.

The placement of a cochlear prosthesis in the child is essentially the same as in the adult because the key anatomic structures, including the cochlea, middle ear, ossicles, and tympanic membrane, are in place and in their adult configurations at birth. By age 2 years, the mastoid antrum and facial recess, which provide access to the middle ear for active electrode placement, are adequately developed.

A few modifications are required to accommodate these smaller dimensions of the mastoid process and the thinness of the scalp and temporal squama. The induction coil is firmly anchored to the squamous portion of the temporal bone, and the active electrode is sealed at the round window with connective tissue. Because the same electrode is used in children as in adults, the accommodation for skull growth occurs through gradual straightening of the excess electrode length that is left within the air-containing mastoid cavity. Fortunately, growth-related problems have not been identified in children with implants.

Preoperative Preparation

Implant patients are given the routine instructions that are provided to other patients undergoing mastoid surgery. The use of perioperative antibiotics varies among the implant groups. The author does not routinely use perioperative antibiotics.

Preparation and Draping

As in routine chronic otitis media surgery, the patient is placed in the supine position with the surgeon and surgical nurse at the head of the bed and the anesthesiologist toward the foot. After induction of anesthesia and prior to preparation, the electrodes for monitoring the facial nerve are placed. This monitoring is

used by many physicians. The position of the internal component of the implant is then determined and marked on the external skin surface. This position will vary among devices. Many different incisions have been designed to allow placement of the internal receiver stimulator. The amount of hair to be shaved depends on the design of the incision; the most common preparation technique is to shave approximately four finger breadths above the ear and four finger breadths behind the ear.

Operative Procedure

To prevent receiver-stimulator extrusion through the incision, the incision must be made at least 1cm to 2cm wider than the receiver-stimulator to be used (Fig. 35–1). Good vascular supply to the flap must also be maintained to decrease the chance of the wound not healing.

In adults and older children, the anterior postauricular flap is then elevated in the avascular plane between the scalp and temporalis muscle. Pieces of temporalis muscle are removed at and around the site of the receiver-stimulator. Postoperatively, the scalp heals against the bone around the receiver-stimulator, minimizing the thickness of the scalp over the internal device. As a result, the power required to transfer the stimulus from the external transmitter transcutaneously to the internal receiver is decreased. The decreased distance between the external transmitter and the internal receiver also improves the magnetic attraction between the two devices for those systems. In young children with thin scalps, the postauricular incision is carried down to bone. The temporalis muscle is elevated off the parietal portion of the skull with the skin as a single-layer flap forward to the spine of Henle.

The site for the internal receiver in the skull is created at the position previously determined so that there is a separation of at least 1cm between the incision and the edge of the receiver-stimulator. Suture tunnel holes created on either side of the seat with a guarded burr will be used to help hold the receiver-stimulator in place. The Ineraid implant is the only hard-wired device (i.e., there is a direct connection between the external transmitter and the internal receiver).[13] The percutaneous plug is held in place with bone screws. Percutaneous plugs in children are contraindicated in favor of a totally implanted induction coil.

Almost all implant systems use the transmastoid, facial recess approach to the round window and scala tympani. The mastoidectomy is done using conventional burrs and suction irrigation techniques (Fig. 35–2). Unlike chronic otitis media surgery, the superior and posterior mastoid cortical margins are not saucerized. The margins can be undercut to create a bony overhang that will stabilize the coiled electrode within the mastoid cavity. The bone removal extends back to the sigmoid, but retraction of the sigmoid is not required unless it is far forward. Enough of the bone in the attic is removed so that the top of the incus can be clearly seen. The incus should not be dislocated or removed because this method does not increase surgical exposure. The short process of the incus and its buttress are important landmarks in the development of the facial recess. The posterior bony ear canal wall is thinned without exposing the overlying vascular strip tissue. Thinning of the bony ear canal is necessary because in viewing the round window area, the direction of vision is parallel to the external auditory canal.

The facial recess is then opened (Fig. 35–3). The facial nerve is carefully skeletonized at the mastoid genu to avoid exposure of the nerve sheath. Once the facial recess is opened, the lip of the round window niche is usually visible just inferior to the stapedius tendon and oval window. To get a good look at the round window, one must open the facial recess more inferiorly and posteriorly. Usually, removing the chorda tympani is unnecessary to adequately visualize the round window niche area. If the facial recess is very restricted, the chorda can be removed, but because the chorda enters the middle ear at the level of the annulus, care must be taken not to damage the tympanic membrane.

With a small diamond stone and intermittent suction-irrigation, the lip of the niche is removed, and the round window membrane comes into clear view. To avoid possible damage to the facial nerve, the diamond stone is not rotated when it is passed through the facial recess to the round window area. In cases in which the round window niche is almost hidden under the pyramidal process, one must drill forward and thin the promontory until the scala tympani is entered.

In approximately 50 per cent of cases, the round window niche and membrane are replaced with new bone growth.[14] This condition is more common in patients whose deafness is attributable to meningitis rather than to other diseases.[15] In these cases, the surgeon must drill forward along the basal coil for as much as 4mm to 5mm. Usually, the new bone is white and can be demarcated from the surrounding otic capsule. Following this white plug of bone with the drill will usually lead to the patent scala, allowing placement of the electrode array.[16] If new bone growth completely obliterates the scala tympani, the surgeon can drill superiorly and possibly enter a patent scala vestibuli.[17] In cases with complete ossification of the cochlea, a canal wall down mastoidectomy and closure of the ear canal is performed. A trough around the modiolus is created and the electrode placed in it.[18, 19]

When drilling the round window niche or attempting to create an opening into the scala tympani through new bone growth, the surgeon must direct the burr anteriorly toward the nose (Fig. 35–4). Drilling superiorly may lead to damage to the basilar membrane and osseous spiral lamina, which may result in the loss of ganglion cells. If the surgeon directs the burr inferiorly, a hypotympanic air cell may be accidentally entered, and the active electrode will be placed improperly into this area. Postoperatively, these cases may fail to stimulate. Temporal bone imaging will show that the active electrode is extracochlear. Revision surgery with placement of the electrode array into the scala tympani will remedy this situation. If the surgeon is uncertain of the placement of the electrode, an intraoperative anteroposterior transorbital plane film can be taken to check the electrode position.

FIGURE 35–1. Incision. The shape of the incision may vary from surgeon to surgeon, but it is important to maintain 1cm to 2cm from the edge of the implant to the incision. Good blood supply to the flap must be maintained both superiorly and inferiorly. An alternative incision to the classic wide C-shaped incision is an extension of a postauricular incision near the postauricular crease, extending superiorly over the temporal squama and middle fossa, curving slightly posteriorly at the most superior aspect of the incision. This incision allows a side-to-side closure.

FIGURE 35–2. Cortical mastoidectomy. Superior and posterior margins are not saucerized. Middle fossa plate, sigmoid sinus, antrum, lateral semicircular canal, and short process of the incus are identified.

FIGURE 35–3. Developing a facial recess. The facial nerve in its vertical portion is identified. Care should be taken not to expose the nerve sheath.

FIGURE 35–4. Opening into the scala tympani. The anteroinferior area of the true round window membrane is removed to allow entry into the scala tympani beyond the hook region of the cochlea.

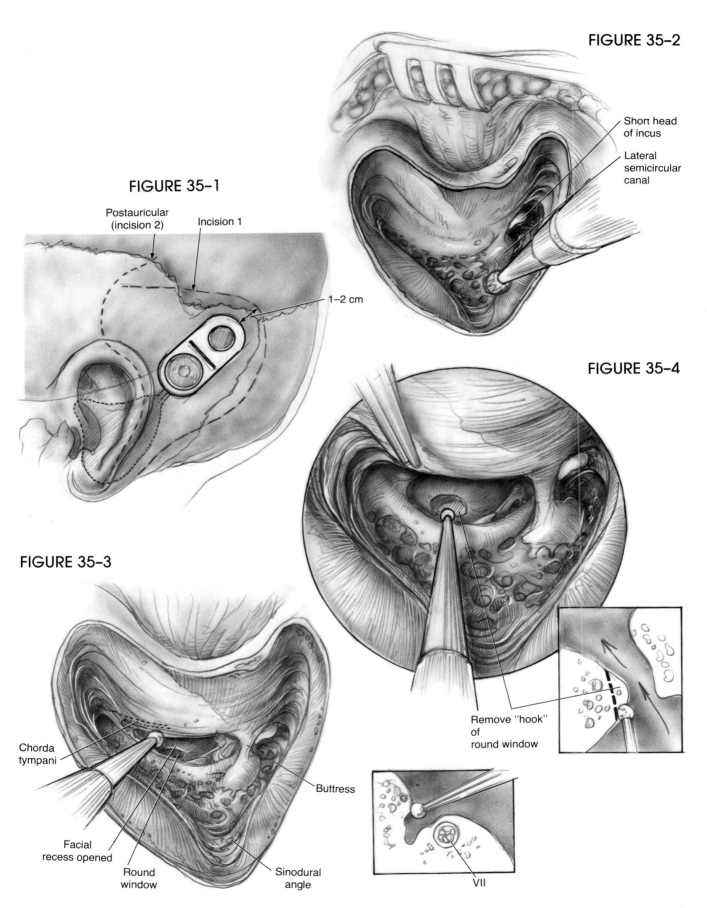

FIGURE 35–1

Postauricular
(incision 2)   Incision 1

1–2 cm

FIGURE 35–2

Short head
of incus

Lateral
semicircular
canal

FIGURE 35–4

Remove "hook"
of
round window

VII

FIGURE 35–3

Chorda
tympani

Buttress

Facial
recess opened

Round
window

Sinodural
angle

Extracochlear electrodes are usually stabilized at the round window. Short and long intracochlear electrodes are advanced carefully into the scala tympani (Fig. 35–5). Either smooth thumb forceps or small two-prong guides are used to direct the electrode tip into the scala tympani. A special electrode insertion tool has been designed to facilitate placement of the MiniMed Clarion electrode. Unlike the straight electrodes of the other implant systems, the MiniMed electrode is precoiled; therefore, there is a right and left cochlear implant electrode.[3]

Most important, force must not be used when any electrode is advanced. Force may lead to insertion trauma to the inner ear structures and may distort the shape of the electrode. Both of these problems can adversely affect the outcome.

If electrocautery is used after placement of the internal receiver, bipolar electrocautery is recommended because it minimizes the possibility of current being passed through the receiver. The postauricular flap is closed in layers, occasionally over a drain. A standard mastoid dressing is placed. If a drain is used, it is usually removed the day following surgery.

Surgery routinely takes 1.5 to 2.5 hours. Patients are usually discharged by the day after surgery, returning for their first postoperative visit about 1 week later. Approximately 4 to 6 weeks later, allowing for resolution of the edema in the postauricular flap, fitting the patient with the signal processor begins.

COMPLICATIONS

The risks of the implant procedure are the same as those for chronic otitis media surgery: infection, facial paralysis, cerebrospinal fluid drainage, meningitis, and the usual risks of anesthesia. All of these risks are remote in chronic otitis media surgery and have proved to be so in implant surgery as well.[20, 21]

Failure of the incision to heal and associated minor infections are the most common problems associated with implant surgery.[22] In a few patients in whom the internal receiver has been placed too close to the wound's edge, or in patients in whom the flap over the internal receiver is too thin, the internal receiver has extruded. As noted earlier, at least 1cm to 2cm must be maintained between the incision and the edge of the internal receiver. The ideal thickness for the flap is 6mm to 7mm. Although too thin a flap may necrose, too thick a flap may diminish device performance by decreasing the transcutaneous transmission of information.

Problems with the facial nerve can occur as the result of both surgery and stimulation.[23] Good surgical landmarks must be maintained when the facial recess is created. Although the facial nerve is identi-

fied, it usually does not have to be uncovered with the facial recess approach. Adequate irrigation at the facial recess must be maintained to help dissipate the heat generated by the turning shaft of the diamond burr used to create the exposure of the round window and entrance into the scala tympani, especially in drill-out cases. To help alleviate the problem of the drill shaft turning against the facial nerve, a drill like the Treace Skeeter could be used. The width of the drill bit shaft is smaller, and a sleeve around most of the length of the shaft protects the surrounding tissues as well. In cases in which the heat from the rotating burr shaft has led to facial nerve problems, the paralysis has been temporary and has resolved over several weeks to several months. Facial nerve paralysis has occurred in patients with congenital malformation of the cochlea and in patients who have undergone radical mastoidectomy many years prior to their implant procedure. In these cases, the facial nerve, either because it is congenitally displaced or exposed by previous surgery, is at greater risk.[24] The use of facial nerve monitoring may decrease the chance of facial nerve trauma.

Cerebrospinal fluid drainage has occurred at both the internal receiver site and the cochlea. In some patients, the temporal squama can be quite thin. In these cases, creating an adequate seat for the internal receiver package requires bony dissection down to the dura. If small dural tears occur, they should be covered with temporalis fascia, and the fascia should be supported with the internal receiver. After insertion of the intracochlear electrode, the cochleastomy is closed with strips of temporalis fascia to prevent perilymphatic fistula development.

A gusher of cerebrospinal fluid is more likely to occur in patients with congenitally malformed inner ears. In these patients, small pieces of Surgicel can be placed through the facial recess opening into the eustachian tube orifice to temporarily occlude the eustachian tube. This procedure should be done prior to opening the scala tympani. Also, closure of the wound should be done in layers, without a drain. I am unaware of any cases that have had persistent cerebrospinal fluid rhinorrhea or leakage of cerebrospinal fluid from the wound site following cochlear implantation.

In adults, the possible effects of the implant on the vestibular system and on tinnitus have been evaluated by clinical monitoring, patient questionnaires, and objective study. No evidence that the implant has significant negative impact in these areas exists.

One concern in extending the cochlear implant program to children was the risk of increased incidence or severity of otitis media, to which children are more prone than adults. Otitis media could have caused the implanted internal coil and the electrode in the mastoid and middle ear to become an infected foreign

FIGURE 35–5

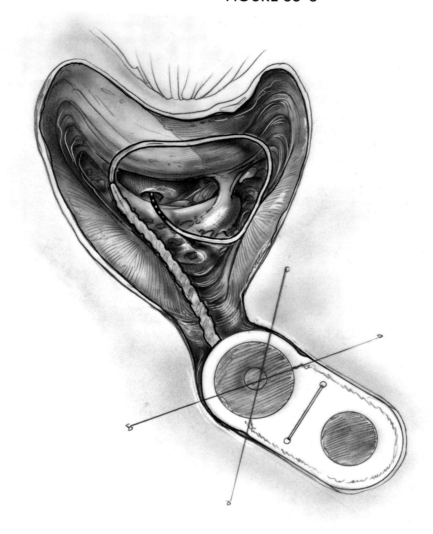

FIGURE 35–5. Electrode insertion and placement of internal receiver package. Electrodes are gently inserted into the scala tympani. After electrode placement, the internal receiver package is fixed in its seat. Soft tissue is placed around the electrode at the round window to create a seal.

body. Further, the infection might extend along the electrode into the inner ear, possibly resulting in meningitis and further degeneration of the auditory system. Information from the clinical trials with 3M/House and Nucleus 22-channel cochlear implants revealed that no increase in incidence or severity of otitis media occurred in children receiving the cochlear implant. In addition, no cases of postoperative meningitis in children have been reported. One case of meningitis in an adult patient with a cochlear implant, however, has been reported.[25]

Chronic otitis media is not a contraindication to cochlear implant surgery. In most cases, because of the prior disease and surgery, the posterior canal wall has been taken down and a radical mastoid cavity created. If no active disease exists, a one-stage surgery can be performed. The mastoid cavity is completely obliterated by everting the external auditory ear canal skin and closing the external auditory canal meatus with a purse-string suture. Although other surgeons have performed a one-stage surgery in the presence of active disease in the middle ear and mastoid cavity, I prefer to perform a two-stage procedure in these cases. The first stage is removal of disease and obliteration of the mastoid cavity, with closure of the external ear canal meatus. Approximately 4 to 6 months later, the second stage can be performed, with placement of the cochlear implant.

REVISION SURGERY

There are two primary reasons for revision surgery: 1) to replace a failed device and 2) to upgrade a system. Revision is possible because human and animal temporal bone studies have shown the following problems either do not occur or are insignificant when the correct surgical technique for implanting electrodes of the different devices is used: degeneration of the remaining viable neural elements due to mechanical trauma to the organ of Corti during insertion or removal of the electrodes, osteogenesis, degeneration of the neural tissue by electrical stimulation, and spread of infection from the middle ear into the inner ear.

For patients undergoing revision surgery of a failed device, either a similar device or an upgrade can be reimplanted in the same ear. Most patients who have undergone revision implant surgery have had a failed device. Experience has shown that it is not difficult to remove and to reinsert a cochlear implant electrode into the scala tympani.[26] However, failure of the cochlear implant sometimes results not from a problem within the internal receiver package but from a migration of the electrode out of the scala tympani and back into the mastoid cavity. In these cases, the scala tympani will fill with fibrosis, and attempting to reinsert an electrode into the tissue-filled scala is very difficult.

The facial nerve is at greater risk in revision cases than in primary cases because the tissue placed around the electrode in the facial recess in the primary case may adhere to a partially exposed facial nerve. Removal of this tissue at revision surgery to allow visualization of the middle ear and promontory must be done carefully.

In patients with functioning devices who are considering revision surgery to upgrade to a new cochlear implant, two options are available: either the ear with or the ear without an implant could be operated on. My preference in most cases with functioning devices is to place the upgrade in the ear without the implant, thus maintaining the patient's only source of hearing. Several years later, if the patient is again interested in an upgrade, I would reimplant in the worst-hearing ear, using the side that provided the least benefit (presumably the side with the oldest implant). I would reimplant an upgrade device in the ear with the presently functioning device if the ear without the implant showed changes on radiographic studies that would hinder the placement of the electrode.

Most patients who have had reimplantation for either a failed device or to upgrade are using their new devices. A few patients who were nonusers of the single-channel systems are also nonusers of the multichannel implants.

Not all of the repairs or upgrades require surgery. The external components (microphone, cables, and speech processors) are repaired or replaced as needed.

REHABILITATION

Surgical implantation of the internal receiver and electrode of the cochlear implant device is only the beginning of the treatment process.[2] Approximately 4 to 6 weeks following surgery, the patient must return to the clinic to be fitted with the external portions of the device. All of the various cochlear implant devices require adjustment of device settings to the individual patient. The more complex the device, the more complex the process for determining appropriate settings. In addition, determining the best fit for a particular patient may involve repeated changes in settings over time as the patient becomes experienced with the sound provided. In addition to setting the device, the patient must be introduced or reintroduced to sound in a manner that provides a realistic idea of the benefit and limitations of the device in relation to the patient's own personal situation. Rehabilitation must also be provided. Most cochlear implant programs include providing information on care and use of the device, simple auditory training, speech reading practice with the added sounds from the cochlear implant, and perhaps training of auditory speech reception skills. Time spent counseling the patient and family members may be considerable.

The amount of rehabilitation and training provided varies from center to center. Further, the amount of time necessary will vary depending on the particular patient and his or her needs. Each cochlear implant manufacturer recommends specific rehabilitation approaches, or provides written materials for implant training, or both. The minimum number of patient hours in the clinic following implantation is usually no less than 40. Regular follow-up visits with objective assessment of performance for the first several years are standard practice.

RESULTS

Cochlear implantation has become a standard rehabilitative approach for profoundly deaf patients who do not benefit significantly from hearing aids. Although many different cochlear implant devices are currently in use, none can provide normal hearing. Most deaf patients who receive a cochlear implant will be able to detect medium-to-loud sounds, including speech, at comfortable listening levels. Many can learn to recognize familiar sounds, such as the doorbell, car horns, telephone ringing, or even the voices of relatives or friends. For many patients, cochlear implants can aid in communication by improving speech reading ability: they are able to combine cues from the sounds and rhythms of speech with what they see. In a smaller number of patients, the implant provides some speech discrimination of words or sentences without the use of speech reading.[2, 4]

The definition of success is different from patient to patient and family to family. Several factors, including age at time of deafness, age at implant surgery, duration of deafness, status of the remaining auditory nerve fibers, training, educational setting, and type of implant, affect the benefit a patient receives from an implant. Memory of previous auditory experience appears to be one of the most important factors. Patients who have had some auditory experience and a short period of deafness may learn to use the sound information provided by the implant more quickly and effectively than those who are born with profound hearing loss or lose their hearing very early in life.

Many professionals are concerned about whether congenitally deaf children can benefit from these devices, whether children in total communication educational programs can benefit, and whether children with cochlear implants are likely to receive the kind of training that will maximize the use of the implant. Experience indicates that, in fact, congenitally deaf children do show significant benefit from the implant, as do children in total communication programs. However, just as with hearing aids, auditory skills are not likely to be maximized without appropriate auditory training.

SUMMARY

Important points about cochlear implant surgery are as follows:

- Cochlear implants are not experimental.
- Cochlear implants are not hearing aids.
- Appropriate candidates have profound bilateral sensorineural hearing loss and do not benefit from conventional amplification.
- Surgical and postoperative complications have been minimal.
- Implants increase auditory abilities and, as a result, improve speech production skills.
- Postlingually deafened adults with a short duration of deafness are excellent candidates for a cochlear implant.
- Although postlingually deafened children in aural programs demonstrate the fastest and greatest development of auditory skills as a group, congenitally and prelingually deafened children show substantial benefit from a cochlear implant.

References

1. Luxford WM, Brackmann DE: The history of cochlear implants. *In* Gray RF (ed): Cochlear Implants. London, Croom Helm, 1985, pp 1–26.
2. Staller SJ, Beiter AL, Brimacombe JA, et al.: Pediatric performance with the Nucleus 22-channel cochlear implant system. Am J Otol 12(Suppl): 126–136, 1991.
3. Schindler RA, Jackler RK, Kessler DK, Merzenich MM: Multichannel cochlear implants: Current status and future directions. *In* Johnson J, et al. (eds): Instructional Courses, Vol I. St. Louis, CV Mosby Company, 1988, pp 195–218.
4. Parkin JL, Randolph LJ: Auditory performance with simultaneous intracochlear multichannel stimulation. Laryngoscope 101: 379–383, 1991.
5. Luxford WM: Cochlear implant indications. Am J Otol 10(2): 95–98, 1989.
6. Dowell RC, Mecklenburg DC, Clark GM: Speech recognition for 40 patients receiving multi-channel cochlear implants. Arch Otolaryngol Head Neck Surg 112: 1054–1059, 1986.
7. O'Donoghue GM, Jackler RK, Jenkins WM, et al.: Cochlear implantation in children: The problem of head growth. Otolaryngol Head Neck Surg 94: 78–81, 1986.
8. Marks DR, Jackler RK, Bates GJ, Greenberg S: Pediatric cochlear implantation: Strategies to accommodate for head growth. Otolaryngol Head Neck Surg 101(1): 38–46, 1989.
9. Gray RF, Evans RA, Freer CEL, et al.: Radiology for cochlear implants. J Laryngol Otol 105: 85–88, 1991.
10. Shelton C, Luxford WM, Tonokawa LL, et al.: The narrow internal auditory canal in children: A contraindication to cochlear implants. Otolaryngol Head Neck Surg 100(313): 227–331, 1989.
11. Silverstein H, Smouha E, Morgan N: Multichannel cochlear im-

plantation in a patient with bilateral Mondini deformities. Am J Otol 9(6): 451–455, 1988.

12. Waltzman SB, Cohen NL, Shapiro WH, Hoffman RA: The prognostic value of round window electrical stimulation in cochlear implant patients. Otolaryngol Head Neck Surg 103(1): 102–106, 1990.

13. Parkin JL: Percutaneous pedestal in cochlear implantation. Ann Otol Rhinol Laryngol 99(10Pt1): 796–800, 1990.

14. Green JD Jr., Marion MS, Hinojosa R: Labyrinthitis ossificans: Histopathologic consideration for cochlear implantation. Otolaryngol Head Neck Surg 104(3): 320–326, 1991.

15. Novak MA, Fifer RC, Barkmeier JC, Firszt JB: Labyrinthine ossification after meningitis: Its implications for cochlear implantation. Otolaryngol Head Neck Surg 103(3): 351–356, 1990.

16. Balkany T, Gantz B, Nadol JB Jr.: Multichannel cochlear implants in partially ossified cochleas. Ann Otol Rhinol Laryngol Suppl 135: 3–7, 1988.

17. Steenerson RL, Gary LB, Wynens MS: Scala vestibuli cochlear implantation for labyrinthine ossification. Am J Otol 11(5): 360–363, 1990.

18. Gantz BJ, McCabe BF, Tyler RS: Use of multichannel implants in obstructed and obliterated cochleas. Otolaryngol Head Neck Surg 98(1): 72–81, 1988.

19. Lambert PR, Ruth RA, Hodges AV: Multichannel cochlear implant and electrically evoked auditory brainstem responses in a child with labyrinthitis ossificans. Laryngoscope 101(1Pt1): 14–19, 1991.

20. Cohen NL, Hoffman RA: Complications of cochlear implant surgery in adults and children. Ann Otol Rhinol Laryngol 100(9Pt1): 708–711, 1991.

21. Webb RL, Lehnhardt E, Clark GM, et al.: Surgical complications with the cochlear multiple-channel intracochlear implant: Experience at Hannover and Melbourne. Ann Otol Rhinol Laryngol 100(2): 131–136, 1991.

22. Haberkamp TJ, Schwaber MK: Management of flap necrosis in cochlear implantation. Ann Otol Rhinol Laryngol 101(1): 38–41, 1992.

23. Niparko JK, Oviatt DL, Coker NJ, et al.: Facial nerve stimulation with cochlear implantation. VA Cooperative Study Group on Cochlear Implantation. Otolaryngol Head Neck Surg 104(6): 826–830, 1991.

24. House JR, Luxford WM: Facial nerve injury in cochlear implantation. Presented at the Southern Section, Triological Society, Boca Raton, FL, January 1993.

25. Daspit CP: Meningitis as a result of a cochlear implant: Case report. Otolaryngol Head Neck Surg 105(1): 115–116, 1991.

26. Parisier SC, Chute PM, Weiss MH, et al.: Results of cochlear implant reinsertion. Laryngoscope 101(9): 1013–1015, 1991.

36

The Audiant Bone Conductor Device

J. V. D. HOUGH, M.D.
MICHAEL McGEE, M.D.

The Audiant is an implantable hearing device that uses the concept of direct bone conduction stimulation by an electromagnetic coil and magnetic implant system.[1] The discovery of the value of implantable rare earth magnets now used in the cochlear implant enabled the development of the Xomed Audiant Bone Conductor. When a rare earth magnet is attached to the skull, magnetic energy not only holds the external device on the head but also provides a means of electromagnetic energy to cause reciprocating bone vibration directly to the inner ear. The microphone of the external device receives sound; its circuitry produces an electromagnetic field, which transcutaneously energizes the magnetic screw attached to the bone. Acoustical energy is thereby transferred by bone conduction directly to the fluids of the inner ear, bypassing both the external and middle ear mechanisms. This device, when properly applied, eliminates almost all the conductive elements of hearing impairment. Its application is clinically predictable, and postoperative complications are rare. At present, it is the only implantable bone conduction device approved by the Food and Drug Administration. However, when compared with alternatives, such as restoration by surgical techniques and the use of modern hearing aids, which can be applied without surgery, the Audiant has limited restrictive applications. Its role, however, is well defined, efficient, and very important for those who cannot reasonably benefit from conventional surgery or from the use of hearing aids.

PATIENT SELECTION

The Audiant is designed for patients with moderate-to-severe bilateral or unilateral conductive hearing loss combined with good sensorineural function in the ear to receive the implant.[2, 3] These patients are either beyond surgery or are unable to benefit from conventional hearing devices for physical or psychologic reasons. Thus, the Audiant may be indicated for patients with conductive hearing impairment who meet the audiometric criteria and have either bilateral or unilateral loss caused by the following:

1. Congenital external or middle ear malformation
2. Open, wet mastoid cavities
3. Inoperable, nonaidable middle ear pathology
4. Chronic external otitis preventing hearing aid use

The candidate should be over 3 years of age, strongly motivated, cognizant of the implications of surgical implantation, free of any generalized disease process that could result in poor wound healing, and unwilling or unable to use conventional air- or bone-conduction hearing aids, as demonstrated by a suitable trial period.

Audiometric Criteria

The patient should have either bilateral or unilateral conductive hearing loss, and the ear to receive the implant should meet the following criteria:[2, 3]

1. Average bone conduction thresholds at speech frequencies (500Hz, 1000Hz, 2000Hz) not worse than 25dB hearing loss, with no single frequency (of 500Hz, 1000Hz, or 2000Hz) worse than 40dB hearing threshold.
2. Average air conduction thresholds at speech frequencies (500Hz, 1000Hz, 2000Hz) not better than 40dB hearing loss.
3. Speech reception threshold not better than 40dB hearing loss.
4. Speech discrimination score not less than 80 per cent.

PATIENT COUNSELING

Patients considering the Audiant implant should be thoroughly counseled in all aspects of the surgical technique and its possible intraoperative and postoperative complications. They should also be instructed in the long-term care of the skin over the implant. The external processor should not be worn until a thorough osseointegration of the implanted screw threads has occurred (12 weeks postoperatively). Likewise, during this time, the overlying skin must have the opportunity to fully heal.

Proper fitting of the external processor is necessary, with adjustments in magnetic strength to allow sufficient strength for holding the device in position on the head, yet not allowing improper compression of the skin, which would cause interference with microcirculation and possible skin necrosis. The external processor, like any other miniature electronic device, requires proper maintenance. Therefore, detailed instruction in its function and physical care should also be given.

The patient should understand approximately what the postoperative hearing perception and threshold will be. Percentage chances of improvement should be clearly defined in understandable terms.

SURGICAL TECHNIQUE[2, 4]

Preparation of the Patient

Shave a large semicircular area behind the pinna. The upper extent of the shaved area should be approximately 3cm above the superior edge of the pinna as it is flattened against the skull. The shaving should extend straight posteriorly and make a curve inferiorly, producing at least 6cm to 8cm posterior to the most posterior edge of the pinna as it is flattened to the skull. This area and the hair, the pinna, the ear canal, the face, and the neck surrounding the area should be scrubbed thoroughly with a povidone-iodine solution or its equivalent.

Anesthetic

A postauricular injection of approximately 5ml of 2 per cent Xylocaine or other brand of lidocaine with 1:100,000 epinephrine should infiltrate the skin over the planned incision site and area of the implantation. For some patients, such as children and uncooperative adults, a general anesthetic may be needed to supplement the above.

Monitoring

Because this procedure is usually done with the patient under sedation but with a local anesthetic, proper monitoring of vital functions, that is, pulse, blood pressure, electrocardiographic reading, and respirations must be done.

Incision

Locating the Implant Site
(Fig. 36–1 and 36–2)

The planned incision and implant site should be marked with the face fully exposed prior to draping.

By palpation, the posterior root of the zygoma may be identified. Its center will be immediately superior to the tragus at the inferior end of the anterior helix. With a ruler, envision a horizontal line aligned from the lower eyelid to the notch above the tragus. Extend this line posteriorly over the temporal bone posterior to the pinna. With a marking pin, mark this line over the mastoid to extend approximately 3cm beyond the posterior margin of the pinna. With the pinna flattened against the skull, measure 2cm from the posterior margin of the pinna on the previously marked horizontal line. Make a mark approximately 1cm above this location. On the normal skull, this point would be the approximate center of the implant site (pilot hole). Mark this site with an X (Fig. 36–2).

The implant must be in the proper position; therefore, to doubly ensure locating this position, the manufacturer has placed in each implant kit a plastic at-the-ear-level template. The use of this marking device is an excellent safety measure to ensure a successful implant location. To use the at-the-ear-level template, place the microphone end over the superior attachment of the pinna, with the hole of the template over the proposed implant site. This area represents the length and width of the Audiant. It should appear on a horizontal plane behind the ear.

Locating the Incision Line

A plastic template incision marker is also provided in the implant kit. This device provides adequate distance between the subsequent scar produced by the incision and the edge of the implant. For skin viability postoperatively, the scar of the incision must not be over the implant (Fig. 36–3).

To use this template, place the hole of the template directly over the previously located X mark for the implant site, as described above. The template may be oriented according to the surgeon's preference, with the incision based accordingly. Mark the skin with an appropriate skin marking pen no more than 180 degrees around the outside circumference of the template to provide the proposed line of incision.

Making the Incision

Make the incision circumferentially on the previously marked incision line through the skin down to subcutaneous tissue.

Preparation of the Flap

After obtaining suitable hemostasis, elevate the skin by sharp dissection in the easily defined subcutaneous plane just below the skin. *Do not* carry the dissection into the deeper layers of muscle and periosteum so as to include this tissue in the skin flap. If the proper subcutaneous tissue plane is maintained during the flap dissection, thinning the flap will probably not be necessary.

If excess subcutaneous tissue exists, remove this tissue with sharp dissection until a thin soft tissue layer remains. At this time, you may choose to use the tissue-measuring Audiant tissue calipers provided in the Hough-Dormer XA-II Instrument Set. Do not thin the skin deeper than the hair follicles.

A total subcutaneous tissue thickness not more than 5mm to 6mm is recommended for adequate magnetic attraction between the implant and the external processor coil. It is not necessary to thin the entire skin flap, only the area over the implant site. It is better to leave the edges of the flap at their original thickness. The steel circular guide cylinder template can be used to determine the approximate size of the area to be thinned. The template can be held on the medial side of the flap to outline this area: roll the skin flap over the forefinger and carefully remove only a thin layer of subcutaneous tissue.

Creating the Implant Pilot Hole

The pilot hole is made in the bone at the implant site marked **X** on the surface of the skin flap. Normally, the hole can be made by fixing vision on the **X** mark while lifting the flap up and placing the burr at that point on the bone. If the location is in doubt, a fine-gauge needle can be inserted through the skin, pointing to that spot on the bone, or perhaps a dot of gentian violet can be put on the area. The pilot hole location is then drilled in the bony cortex with the disposable small collar burr found in the surgical kit. Profuse irrigation should be used during drilling.

Preparation of the Temporal Bone

The guide cylinder template is again used, this time, to remove the soft tissue over the bone around the pilot hole site. Place the center of the circular template at the previously made pilot hole site and incise circumferentially around it down to the cortical bone. Remove the soft tissue plug with its periosteum. With a carbide cutting burr, remove the bone over the area to provide a level implant site. This method prepares a good, even table of bone slightly larger in diameter than the guide cylinder. This flat area will be used to stabilize the guide cylinder during the tapping procedure.

If the area onto which the guide cylinder is to be placed is not relatively flat, the guide cylinder pins may not rest equally on the temporal bone, thereby compromising complete tapping of the implant site. Be cautious not to drill away too much bone over the implant site, which may make the skull too thin to receive the full depth of the implant screw.

Completing the Pilot Hole

Locate the previously made small pilot hole in the bone. This small hole represents the exact point into which the center of the implant will be positioned. Now use the large implant pilot burr to drill a hole into the bone. Irrigate copiously during this procedure. Drill the pilot hole in at least two or three stages, quickly pushing the burr only a short distance into the bone and removing it quickly. With each burr insert, irrigate the pilot hole and allow it to cool. Finally, finish by pushing the burr quickly into the bone to the depth of the "depth-stop" collar of the burr while continuing copious irrigation. The resulting implant pilot hole is now 3.4mm deep with the 4mm implant set and 2.4mm deep with the 3mm pediatric implant set.

Note that using the large implant pilot burr alone *will not result* in a pilot hole deep enough to accommodate the tapping procedure. The diamond finish-ing burr described later must be used to complete the implant pilot hole.

Using the Pilot Diamond Finishing Burr[4]

The pilot diamond finishing burr is used to finish the implant pilot hole. After removing the large implant pilot burr described above, introduce the implant pilot diamond finishing burr into the pilot hole and complete the drilling procedure by penetrating the bone to its depth-stop collar. Again, use quick in-and-out drilling technique and copious irrigation (Fig. 36–4). The implant pilot hole is now 4mm deep for the 4mm (adult) implant and 3mm deep for the 3mm pediatric implant and is ready for the tapping procedure described later.

If a blood vessel is encountered, use bone wax to seal the hole and move the implant pilot hole to a site in a nearby location. Likewise, if cerebrospinal fluid is encountered during the pilot hole preparation, seal the hole with bone wax and proceed to an adjacent location.

It is important to use copious irrigation during the drilling of the implant pilot hole to prevent overheating of the live bone cells. Overheating compromises potential osseointegration of the implant screw.

Using the Guide Cylinder Template[4]

The steel guide cylinder template is a sterile, single-use template with a center "nipple" and three circumferential holes with the same pattern as the guide cylinder pins. The template is used to locate the guide cylinder pin holes on the temporal bone for the tapping procedure described later (Fig. 36–5).

Place the nipple of the guide cylinder template into the newly created implant pilot hole. Holding the template on the bone, rotate it until it is flat on the surface of the implant site. Using the small guide cylinder pin burr, drill the guide cylinder pin holes in each of the three circumferential holes through the template into the underlying bone.

Penetrate the small guide cylinder pin burr through the template holes first to the depth-stop collar for each hole. Then remove the template and finish the holes individually with a second completed thrust with the depth-stop collar burr.

Making the Half-Tap and Full-Tap Threads in the Bone

Assembling the Universal Wrench Handle and Taps

The half-tap and full-tap instruments provided in the Hough-Dormer XA-II Instrument Set are precision-

FIGURE 36-1

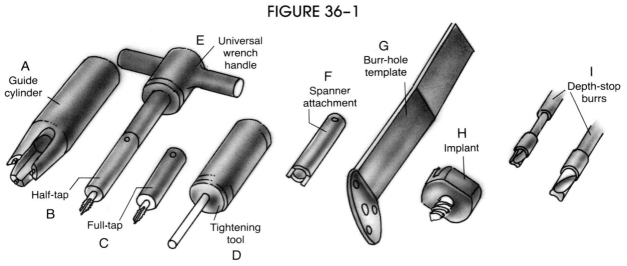

A Guide cylinder

B Half-tap

C Full-tap

D Tightening tool

E Universal wrench handle

F Spanner attachment

G Burr-hole template

H Implant

I Depth-stop burrs

FIGURE 36-2

FIGURE 36-3

FIGURE 36-4

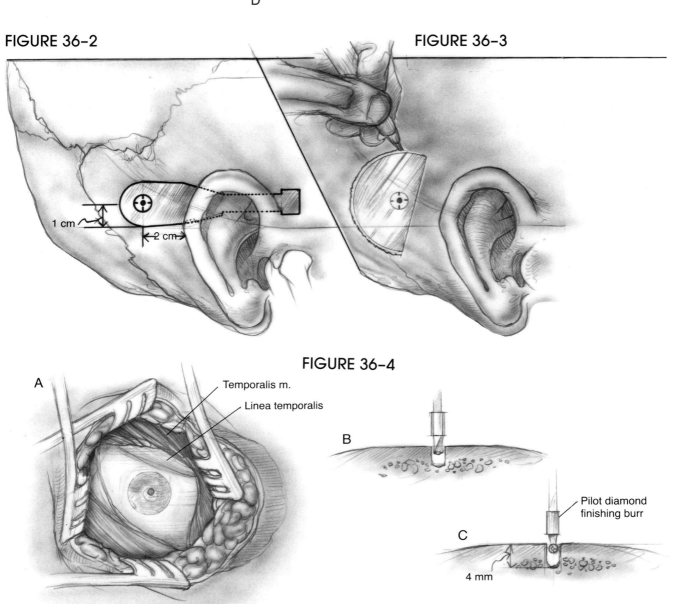

1 cm

2 cm

A Temporalis m.

Linea temporalis

B

C Pilot diamond finishing burr

4 mm

made, very sharp threaded dies designed to precisely make the threads in the bone that receive the implant screw (see Fig. 36–1). It is extremely important that the threaded portions of the taps not be touched by hands or other instruments. Contaminants of foreign materials or damage to the cutting edges may cause injury to the screw threads and compromise implantation.

The half and full taps have a threaded screw on the end opposite the tapping tool that matches a threaded socket at the end of the universal wrench handle opposite the "T." This threaded screw should be introduced into the universal wrench handle and tightened *securely* with the tightening tool (see Fig. 36–1).

If the taps are not securely tightened into the universal wrench handle, they may become loosened or dislodged during the tapping procedure.

When using a 3mm (pediatric) implant, place the plastic ring spacer provided in the 3mm implant set over the universal wrench handle, or use the pediatric-length taps (Fig. 36–6). The purpose of this spacer is to limit the penetration depth of the half and full taps. Place the spacer over the universal wrench handle before starting the tapping procedure. Keep the wrench handle in such a position that the spacer does not slip off while the taps are inserted into the guide cylinder and while the taps are changed. Perform both half- and full-tapping procedures with the spacer in place over the wrench handle. The plastic ring spacer is a sterile, single-use item and should be disposed of after use.

Positioning the Guide Cylinder
(Fig. 36–6)

Keep the guide cylinder upright and perpendicular to the surface of the bone. Engage the three guide cylinder pins into the newly created guide cylinder pin holes. The pins should all penetrate the holes equally, with no separation between the body of the guide cylinder and the bone. If you notice a gap in any of these locations, either redrill the guide cylinder pin holes, as described earlier, or check the flatness of the implant site, also as described earlier.

The guide cylinder should be held in place with the thumb, forefinger, and middle fingers firmly around the guide cylinder and the other fingers resting against the skull with the dorsum of the wrist facing laterally (Fig. 36–7).

Half-Tap Procedure

After assembling the universal wrench handle to the half tap, introduce the assembly into the securely placed and held guide cylinder. It may be necessary to have an assistant hold the patient's head steady at this point. Engage the half tap into the implant pilot hole and rotate the universal wrench handle clockwise while using quite firm, downward pressure with the palm of the hand on top of the universal wrench handle. After securely engaging the tap into the pilot hole with the first complete turn, finish the tap with firm but moderate downward finger pressure. Complete the tapping procedure with 2¾ to 3 total turns of the universal wrench handle. The gap between the universal wrench handle and the head of the guide cylinder will close with 2¾ to 3 turns (Fig. 36–7). This gap is the exact measurement of the depth desired for the finished pilot hole and provides a visible measure of the progress in making this precise penetration.

Do not continue to turn the wrench handle after the gap has been closed between wrench handle and the head of the guide cylinder. This action will cause stripping of the newly made threads in the bone, thus preventing osseointegration of the implant into the temporal bone. Remove the half tap by *gently* and *slowly* turning the universal wrench handle counterclockwise 2¾ turns. It is necessary to *unscrew* the half tap from the newly threaded hole. The tap will not be easily removed by pulling, and such action will damage the threads in the implant pilot hole.

Full-Tap Procedure[2, 4]

After removing the half tap from the guide cylinder, keep the guide cylinder in position while an assistant removes the half tap from the universal wrench handle and replaces it with the full tap. Remember to securely tighten the full tap into the universal wrench handle using the tightening tool.

Introduce the full tap into the guide cylinder, and after it encounters the implant pilot hole, gently turn the universal wrench handle one-half turn counterclockwise, without using any downward pressure. This action allows for the engaging of the full-tap thread in the same location of the already completed half-tap thread.

With a firm, downward pressure (but not as much as used with the half tap) turn the wrench handle clockwise a total of 2¾ turns. The full tap is precisely deepening and finishing the threads already started by the half tap. The gap between the wrench and the guide cylinder will now be closed, and resistance will be encountered (Fig. 36–7).

Remove the full tap by *slowly* turning the wrench handle counterclockwise 2¾ turns. Lift the wrench handle and remove the wrench-tap assembly from the guide cylinder. Remove the guide cylinder at this time and irrigate the pilot hole thoroughly. *Do not use a small lumen section within the threaded hole, as this may damage the threads.*

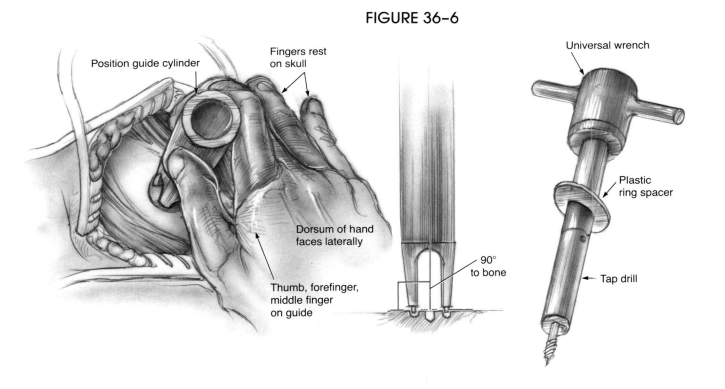

FIGURE 36-5

Burr-hole template

Depth-stop collar

Finish holes without template

FIGURE 36-6

Position guide cylinder

Fingers rest on skull

Dorsum of hand faces laterally

Thumb, forefinger, middle finger on guide

90° to bone

Universal wrench

Plastic ring spacer

Tap drill

Implanting the Magnet Into the Skull[4]

Mounting the Implant on the Insert Tool

Leave the implant in the plastic implant set tray until it is ready to be mounted on the insert tool.

Do not allow the screw threads to come in contact with any foreign material or object (e.g., gloves, instruments, or drapes). Allowing this to occur may compromise the osseointegration of the bone with the screw threads.

Mount the Audiant XA-II implant onto the end of the insert tool by grasping it from the implant set tray by its flat edges with the thumb and forefinger of one hand. Do not touch screw threads. Transfer the implant to the thumb and forefinger of the other hand with the flat surface facing out (Fig. 36–8). Place it onto the end of the insert tool with the screw facing outward.

The magnetic attraction between the magnet of the implant and the end of the insert tool will keep the implant securely in place on the insert tool prior to introducing it into the temporal bone.

Introducing the Implant Using a Two-Handed Technique (Fig. 36–9)

Tilt the insert tool–implant assembly so that you can visualize the insertion of the implant screw into the implant pilot hole. Tip the insert tool–implant assembly upright and hold it by the shaft with the fingers of one hand.

Turn the wings of the insert tool with the thumb and forefinger of the opposite hand counterclockwise one-half turn until the implant thread engages with the thread of the implant pilot hole. You may feel a subtle engaging click of the threads at this time.

Apply downward pressure on the wings of the insert tool with the fingers of one hand. Place the fingers of the opposite hand on the shaft of the insert tool. Now, turn it clockwise 2¾ turns until resistance is felt and the bottom of the implant cap touches the surface of the bone. Gently lift the insert tool off of the implant. Palpate the implant with the thumb and forefinger to check that it is securely seated.

Do not overtighten the implant in the pilot hole, as this action may strip the threads and compromise the osseointegration of the implant. Should this occur, the implant should be removed and a new implant site selected and prepared as described earlier.

Closure of the Incision

Close the wound in two layers, using appropriate sutures and the technique of preference. A small-gauge suction can be used through the incision under the skin to remove blood and serum at the end of the procedure.

DRESSING THE WOUND

Apply a pressure mastoid dressing to the implant site. The dressing may be removed in 48 hours. If excessive swelling occurs, a pressure dressing can remain for 1 week postoperatively, at which time all sutures and dressings may be removed. If a seroma occurs, it may be evacuated, and if excessive swelling still remains, a gentle dressing supported by a tennis sweat band may be necessary for another week.

POSTOPERATIVE PROCESSOR FITTING

After complete tissue healing and total reduction of swelling, the patient may be fitted for an Audiant sound processor, but not before 12 weeks postoperatively. Selection of type of processor (Body, B.T.E., or A.T.E.) is performed at this time. For the A.T.E. processor, selection of magnet strength is also performed, using the Audiant A.T.E. fitting kit (Xomed-Treace produce #50–25255). The processor is ordered as individually needed through the processor certificate included with each implant-certificate package (50–24400 or 50–24300).

The implant should not be regularly stimulated by regular processor use prior to 12 weeks of postoperative healing. This time allows for proper osseointegration of bone tissue to the implant.

The patient's skin in the area of the implant has recently undergone the trauma of surgery. Pay close attention to any changes in the condition of the skin. Fitting a patient with too strong a magnet could cause discomfort and pain. Additionally, pressure from a magnet that is too strong may reduce blood flow to the area, causing irritation. If left unattended, this problem may result in injury to the patient, including tissue necrosis. To allow for safe skin adaptation, a progressive routine of gradually increasing processor use is extremely important. Daily hygiene and observation of the health of the skin is necessary.

RESULTS

In general, the Audiant may be expected to provide hearing to within 5 to 10 dB of the bone conduction threshold.[2, 3, 5, 6] In the analysis of the patient for a possible Audiant implant, the probable result is determined not by the severity of the air-conduction loss, but by the bone-conduction threshold. Regardless of

FIGURE 36-7

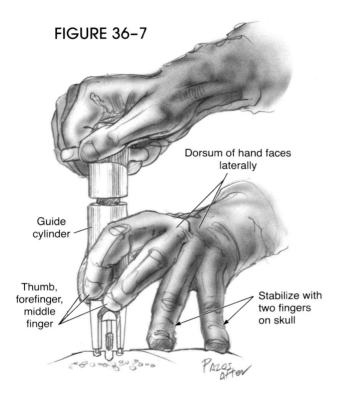

Dorsum of hand faces laterally

Guide cylinder

Thumb, forefinger, middle finger

Stabilize with two fingers on skull

FIGURE 36-8

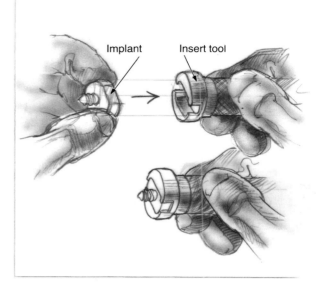

Implant

Insert tool

FIGURE 36-10

Gap

FIGURE 36-9

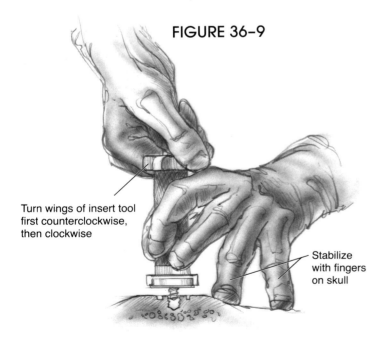

Turn wings of insert tool first counterclockwise, then clockwise

Stabilize with fingers on skull

the extent of the air-bone gap, the Audiant is effective in closure or near closure of that gap (Fig. 36–10).

Recent analysis of all Audiant implants reported in North America indicates that there is a strong tendency for the surgeon to be tempted not to stay within the rigid audiologic criteria prescribed.[6] Nevertheless, when these principles are applied, the results are strongly predictable and beneficial.

Although the number of patients needing the device is small, the Xomed Audiant Bone Conductor is the *only* opportunity for hearing restoration for many patients, that is, those who cannot wear a hearing aid and those for whom surgery is inappropriate. For this reason, it has a vital place in the otologist's armamentarium.[3, 5, 6]

References

1. Hough J, Vernon J, Johnson B, et al.: Experiences with implantable hearing devices and a presentation of a new device. Ann Otol Rhinol Laryngol 95: 60–56, 1986.
2. Hough J, McGee M, Himelick T, Vernon J: The surgical technique for implantation of the temporal bone stimulator (Audiant ABC). Am J Otol 7(5): 315–321, 1986.
3. Hough J, Himelick T, Johnson B: Implantable bone conduction hearing device: Audiant Bone Conductor. Update on our experiences. Ann Otol Rhinol Laryngol 95(5): 498–504, 1986.
4. Audiant Bone Conductor—Implantable Hearing Device XA-II Surgical Technique Manual. Xomed-Treace, a Bristol-Myers Squibb Company.
5. Gates G, Hough J, Gatti W, Bradley W: The safety and effectiveness of an implanted electromagnetic hearing device. Arch Otolaryngol Head Neck Surg 115: 924–930, 1989.
6. Hough JVD, Wilson N, Dormer KJ, Rohrer M: The Audiant Bone Conductor—Update of patient results in North America. [Submitted for publication.]

37

The Bone-Anchored Hearing Aid

ANDERS TJELLSTRÖM, M.D., Ph.D.

In spite of advances in middle ear reconstruction surgery, it is not possible to provide all patients with a dry ear and good hearing. Some patients need amplification. A conventional air-conduction aid is the most common choice, but some patients cannot or should not use such an aid. Bone-conduction transducers are sometimes the hearing aid of choice, but the disadvantages with the conventional type of bone-conduction hearing aids are numerous. The sound quality is generally poor: the sound has to pass through soft tissue, and much of the sound energy is lost there. When the sound waves reach the skull bone they are transmitted with fairly low attenuation and distortion at least to the ipsilateral cochlea. The magnitude of the attenuation of the speech frequencies varies between 7dB and 15dB[1] and the greatest losses are in the important high-frequency range. The attenuation of the sound reaching the contralateral cochlea varies depending on the frequency, but there are also great interindividual differences. Due to the attenuation of the sound energy from the transducer to the inner ear the conventional bone-conduction hearing aid must be driven hard, raising the level of distortion. This problem will be significant in patients with both conduction loss and cochlear dysfunction.

A direct coupling between the transducer and the skull without any soft tissue between is thus of great acoustic advantage. There are, however, other advantages with a direct coupling to the skull, namely, there is no discomfort due to the pressure of the transducer, the position of the hearing aid is stable, and no steel spring over the head, head bands, or heavy frames of glasses are needed.[2–7]

OSSEOINTEGRATION

The possibility of establishing and maintaining a direct anchorage of a hearing aid coupling to the bone of the mastoid process is based on the concept of osseointegration. The term *osseointegration* was coined by professor Per-Ingvar Brånemark of Göteborg, Sweden in 1977 and is defined as "a direct contact between living bone and a loaded implant surface."[8, 9] Implants have been used for many years but primarily to stabilize fractures during healing. Under such circumstances, the choice of implant material is less important. For example, in orthopedic surgery, a plate and screws of different metals and alloys allow healing to take place. However, during healing, the patient is not allowed to load the fracture, which could lead to loss of implant stability and jeopardize fracture healing. When healing has been established, it is not important if the implant material is encapsulated in fibrous tissue. This does become a problem when a whole joint, for example, a hip or a knee, has to be replaced. A zone of fibrous tissue between the implant and the bone will not stand a load in the long run. In the geriatric patient, this problem may be insignificant but in today's sport injuries in young and active patients, this is a larger problem.[10] In oral surgery, implants have been used in the treatment of patients with partial or total edentolousness for many years. The forces used during chewing could be very high (50N to 2000N), and most implants used earlier became loose after loading.

Establishing Osseointegration

To achieve osseointegration the implant material requires careful consideration, as do several other factors, including the surgical technique, which is described in detail later. A combination of hardware and software is necessary for the operation to be successful.[11, 12]

Implant Material

The choice of implant material is very important. The implant material used by the author is commercially pure titanium. This nonalloyed titanium has a purity of 99.75 per cent. The mechanical properties of this implant will change even at very minor changes in its purity. One of the most common titanium implants used in surgery is an alloy called Ti 6Al 4V. This alloy consists of 90 per cent titanium, 6 per cent aluminium, and 4 per cent vanadium. It is possible to establish a direct contact between such an implant and living bone tissue, but the quality and the quantity of this contact are less than that of commercially pure titanium. The reason for these differences is not completely clear but probably involves aluminum ions leaking out from the implant into the tissue and competing with calcium ions at the interface. Local and general reactions of an implant material must be taken into consideration. Aluminum is known to be toxic to the central nervous system, an effect that is especially important to remember when an implant is placed in a young patient who could be expected to have his or her implant in the tissue for 60 to 80 years. Although no neoplastic changes have been reported, this possibility must be remembered when new implant materials are used in the very aggressive environment of the bioliquid. The clinical follow-up with the commercially pure titanium implant material goes back to 1966.[8]

Implant Design

The implants used are screw shaped and have the same type of threads and the same diameter as the implants used by Brånemark intraorally. The implants come in two lengths, 3mm and 4mm, and have a flange that is 5.5mm in diameter (Fig. 37–1). The rationale for having a threaded implant instead of a smooth one is to get a good initial stability. If the implant moves during healing, fibrous tissue instead of bone could result. The flange improves the initial stability but also acts as a protection against too-deep penetration at the time of surgery or later if a direct trauma affects the skin-penetrating coupling.

Implant Surface

The surface of the implant has minor irregularities that will improve the stability of the implant, especially against shear forces. Perhaps an even more important point is to keep the implant surface free from foreign material. Because of the electrophysical properties of the oxide layer that covers the implant when it is machined, the surface is very active and will adhere to foreign material. Such foreign material could jeopardize osseointegration, even if these particles are sterile. Small metal fragments could give rise to electrical currents and induce fibrous tissue instead of bone. The surgeon and nurse must remember this during the different steps of the insertion of the implant.

Loading of the Implant

Originally, a two-stage procedure was used based on the experience from implant surgery in the oral cavity. However, the success rate with permanent implant stability in the mastoid process has been very high, and as the load to the implant is much less than in the oral cavity, a one-stage procedure is today recommended. However, the implant should not be loaded with a hearing aid until 2 to 3 months after surgery. The suggested time span between insertion and loading is based on animal studies performed by Steinemann et al. as well as our clinical experience.[13]

PATIENT SELECTION

The indication for a bone-anchored hearing aid (BAHA) is the need for amplification in a patient who cannot be helped by reconstructive surgery and who cannot use an air-conduction hearing aid. There are two main groups that qualify for a BAHA: patients with chronic ear conditions and patients with external ear atresia. Patients with draining ears or ears that start to drain when the external ear canal is occluded with a hearing aid mold are suitable candidates. Many of these patients will have a combined hearing impairment, and the better the inner ear function the better the chances are for a good result. If the mean

value for the bone conduction from 0.5kHz to 3kHz is better than 45dB and the speech discrimination score is better than 60 per cent, the chances that the patient will have satisfactory hearing are 89 per cent. As many patients have a maximum conductive loss of 60dB, a hearing threshold of 105dB can be helped. Patients with bone conductive hearing loss close to the 45dB level are told that they probably could use the ear level device HC 200 but that a stronger hearing aid, the Superbass HC 220, is available. This hearing aid has a strong transducer fitted to the skin penetration coupling but a conventional body aid. Patients with bone conduction levels as low as 60dB could use this aid.[14, 15]

Patients with bilateral atresia often have normal or near-normal cochlear function and are the ideal patients for the BAHA. Reconstructive atresia surgery is very difficult, and in patients with a Jahrsdoerfer rating of 7 or worse, we often suggest a BAHA instead of reconstructive trials.[16] One advantage of the BAHA is that it will not interfere with atresia surgery later on. This technique could be used in children as young as 3. When these children grow up, an evaluation of their anatomy can be made, as can the final decision about atresia surgery. The BAHA could also be used in patients with special problems, for example, patients with severe otosclerosis in the only-hearing ear, patients with external otitis, and patients who react against all different materials used for ear molds.

Patient selection is of special importance for fitting with a BAHA. The patient must have realistic expectations and be aware that the BAHA has limitations. The patient should also be able to come to regular outpatient follow-up visits and should be able to take care of the skin penetration. Because one of the main reasons for adverse skin reactions is inadequate hygiene, the need to have a high level of personal hygiene must be stressed preoperatively.

Age is not a contraindication per se. The oldest patient operated on was 82, and the youngest, 3 years of age. Psychiatric disease is considered the only contraindication, and when in doubt, a psychiatric consultation is very helpful.

PREOPERATIVE EVALUATION

During the preoperative evaluation, a general ear, nose, and throat examination, audiologic testing with sound thresholds, and speech audiometry are included. In children with congenital malformations, a high resolution computed tomographic scan is done to evaluate the level of the middle cranial fossa, the position of the sigmoid sinus, and whether the facial nerve has an abnormal route. In patients with chronic ear disease, no radiologic examination is made routinely. Even radical surgery will not interfere with the position of the implant for the hearing aid. Because the skin penetration should be in a hairless area, the skin over the mastoid process is examined. If hair follicles are present, the patient is informed that a graft must be taken. A suitable place for the graft is the retroauricular fold. In patients with congenital atresia, skin from the external ear tags could be used, as can skin from the retroauricular fold on the other side.

The patient must be informed about the procedure and what it means to have a skin penetrating implant. The patient is told that he or she must come to regular follow-up visits. The importance of personal hygiene must also be stressed, especially in patients with a greasy skin or seborrhea. However, these conditions and others, like psoriasis and eczema, are not considered as contraindications.[17]

A simple way to give the patient a general idea of how the BAHA will sound is to use the "bite rod," a plastic rod with a hearing aid coupling glued to one end of the rod. The patient is asked to take the rod between the teeth, and the BAHA is attached to the coupling. To avoid acoustic feedback, the patient must close the lips around the rod. If the patient does not have teeth or dentures secured to osseointegrated implants, the rod can be pressed against the skin over the mastoid process. This method, however, is not as good as using the teeth. Another way to evaluate if a BAHA is a good solution for a patient is to provide him or her with a conventional bone-conduction hearing aid for a couple of weeks. The patient is asked to evaluate only the sound quality and to not pay any attention to discomfort or the size of the equipment. If the patient is satisfied with the sound, the chances are very good that he or she will be satisfied with the BAHA.

In patient counseling, it is also stressed that if he or she is sure of the decision and has been provided with a BAHA but for any reason does not like the arrangement, it is very easy to return to the original situation before surgery. Patients may also use the BAHA in combination with other aids if they wish.

SURGICAL TREATMENT

Preoperative Preparation

The surgical procedure is simple and is generally performed under local anesthesia as an outpatient procedure.[11, 18] In children, general anesthesia is used. No antibiotics or steroids are used. The patient is placed on the operating table in the same way as for any type of ear surgery. Before the draping is made, the implant site is marked according to Figure 37–2.

This marking should be made before the external ear is folded anteriorly, as the hearing aid must not touch the pinna because that could cause acoustic feedback. The preoperative preparation is also the same as for any other ear surgery using a postauricular approach. The patient is shaved in the postero superior area behind the ear a radius of 30mm from the implant site. The field is cleaned with 70 per cent alcohol. In patients with congenital malformation, the mastoid process is outlined with surgical ink, and the expected route of the facial nerve is marked. If there is no external ear canal and the patient maybe a future candidate for an auricular prosthesis retained on implants, the site for the hearing aid implant should be about 55mm behind the anticipated external ear meatus. It is often advantageous to place the implant in the linea temporalis because the bone here is normally fairly thick. Above the linea temporalis, the bone over the middle cranial dura may be very thin, especially in malformed children. Below the linea temporalis, air cells are often close to the cortical surface. In the chronic otitis media patient, this is seldom a problem because of the reduced pneumatization of the mastoid process. In patients who have had radical surgery, the cavity is more anterior and will not interfere with the implant site. After the patient and the implant site are cleaned and draped, the area is covered with an adhesive plastic film to prevent even sterile particles from cloth from entering the implant site, which could jeopardize osseointegration. The author prefers using magnifying lenses over the otomicroscope, as this method makes it easier to find the exact axis of direction for the different steps of the procedure.

Special Instruments

The instruments used consist of general surgical instruments and instruments specially designed for this implant surgery, including a drill machine with high- and low-speed functions as well as a feature to reverse the direction of rotation. The torque can also be adjusted. The instruments and the implants and the sound processors are produced by Nobelpharma AB, Göteborg, Sweden.

Standard Instruments

The standard instruments listed are placed by the scrub nurse on a sterile draped Mayo stand and consist of

5 Mosquito clamps
1 Mayo scissors
1 Curved scissors, small
1 Adson forceps
1 Needle holder

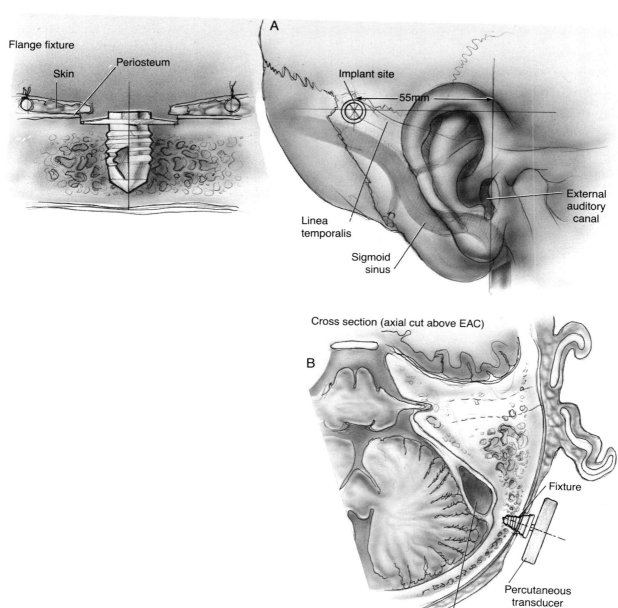

FIGURE 37-1

Flange fixture

Skin

Periosteum

FIGURE 37-2

A

Implant site

55mm

External auditory canal

Linea temporalis

Sigmoid sinus

Cross section (axial cut above EAC)

B

Fixture

Percutaneous transducer

Sigmoid sinus

FIGURE 37-1. The flange fixture.

FIGURE 37-2. Optimal position of the implant to avoid acoustic feedback.

2 Bard-Parker blades
2 Skin hooks, small
2 Self-retaining retractors, small
1 Raspatory
1 Periosteal elevator

Special Instruments

The special instruments are made of either stainless steel or titanium instruments. It is of utmost importance that these instruments are not mixed.

The stainless steel instruments are

Raspatory
Dissector
Open-ended wrench for fixture mount
Open-ended wrench for hearing aid coupling
Cylinder wrench
Screwdriver
Hexagon screwdriver
Screwdriver for hearing aid coupling
Connection to handpiece
Punch
Bowl

The titanium instruments are

Titanium organizer
Cleaning needle
Forceps
Fixture mount
Bowl

The drilling equipment consists of

Control unit with stand and foot control
Motor for high and low speeds
Shank and head

The control unit is draped with a sterile plastic bag and the motor and its cord, with a plastic tube.

The drills and screw taps are sterilely packed and disposable to guarantee maximum sharpness and to avoid the time-consuming cleaning procedure used earlier.

The components used are guide drills with fixed depth to 3mm and 4mm. The *implants* used are flange Fixture, 3mm or 4mm, and hearing aid abutment for the sound processor. The abutment is secured to the flange fixture with an internal screw. During the healing period, a healing cap is used.

Surgical Technique

The different steps of the surgical procedure are illustrated in Figure 37–3.[11, 18] When the implant site has been marked and the surgical field draped with the plastic sheet, 10ml of local anesthesia is injected. The author prefers 1 per cent lidocaine (Xylocaine) with adrenalin. Some of the local anesthesia should be put underneath the periosteum to get perfect anesthesia for the drilling. The 3mm guide drill is attached to the head of the drill, and the switch on the motor is turned to high speed, which is also indicated on the control unit. The drill speed is 1500rpm to 2000rpm. During all drilling, cooling with room-temperature saline is used to avoid unnecessary tissue damage. When the guide drills, which are 1.8mm in diameter, are used, the hole is widened about 2.5mm to 3.0mm. The reasons for this step are that the surgeon gets a better view into the bottom of the hole, the irrigation will reach the site where the cutting takes place, and less bone has to be cut away when the final dimension is established with the countersink. If there is bone at the bottom of the hole when the fixed depth of the 3mm guide drill is all the way down, the short guide drill is changed to the 4mm guide drill. The flange of the guide drill must be down to the bony surface because the countersink is not sharp at its tip. Therefore, if there is soft tissue at the bottom, such as the wall of the sigmoid sinus or the dura of the middle cranial fossa, the hole could still be used for the implant. The next step is to change the drill countersink to the appropriate length. The drill speed is still 1500rpm to 2000rpm, and generous cooling is imperative. The drill should be moved up and down, and the grooves at the side of this spiral drill should be cleaned several times during the drilling. The bone cut away will be collected in these grooves, and when they are filled with bone, the cutting will be reduced and a lot of heat produced. During this phase of the procedure, the final direction of the implant will be established. The implant should be perpendicular to the surface. If it becomes too oblique, there is a risk that the sound processor will touch the skin and cause acoustic feedback.

The hole is now ready for the tapping procedure, which is performed at low speed, 8rpm to 15rpm. The low speed mode will be available by turning the switch on the motor. When the low speed mode is used, the torque can be adjusted on the control unit, as indicated on its window. A torque of 30Ncm is

FIGURE 37–3. The steps of the surgical procedure.

FIGURE 37-3

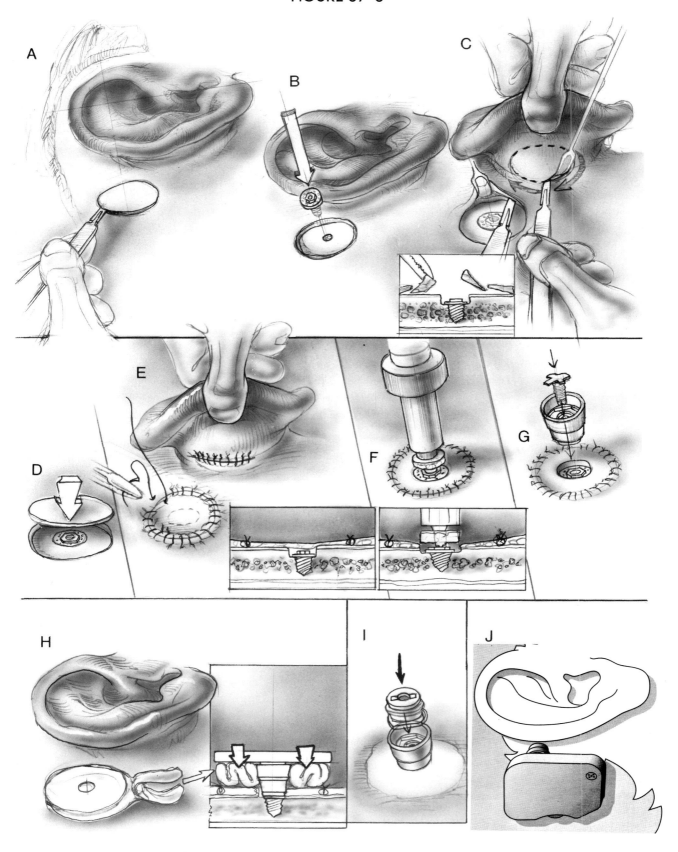

suggested for the standard procedure. In children and in patients with soft and thin bone, 20 Ncm should be used. The exact speed is adjusted by the surgeon through the foot control. The 3mm or 4mm titanium tap is taken from its sterile glass tubing and put into the organizer without being touched with the gloved hand or with any nontitanium instruments. It could be poured into the titanium tray and transferred to its place in the organizer with the titanium forceps. The connection to the hand piece, which is made out of stainless steel and thus could be handled in the normal way, is attached to the hand piece of the motor. The tap is then picked up with the adaptor, which has a spring arrangement that will keep the tap in place. The tap is kept over the implant site, and the motor is started at a low speed. When the correct direction is established, the tap is gently pressed down into the hole. Simultaneous irrigation is essential. When the tap starts to move down, no further pressure is needed because the tap will find its own way. If the tap is stuck before coming to the bottom of the hole, the direction was not correct, and the motor is reversed by use of the knob on the control unit. When the tap is up, the direction is corrected and the tapping is made. If the tap gets stuck several times, a new implant site closeby is prepared. When the tap is removed by reversing the motor, the motor should not be lifted by its shank and head, as the tap could be dislodged.

The implant site is now ready for the implant, the flange fixture, which also comes sterilely packed in a glass cylinder. The fixture is put in the organizer without being contaminated by any nontitanium instrument. The fixture mound is lifted up with the open-ended wrench and secured to the fixture with the internal screw and screwdriver. The hexagon on the top of the fixture must be properly fitted into the hexagonal indentation of the fixture mount. If there is good cortical bone at the implant site, the screw of the fixture mount is tightened more than if the bone is thin and soft. The fixture mount, with the fixture, is picked up with the connection of the hand piece attached to the motor. The implant is kept over the implant site, and the engine is started on low speed. When the correct direction has been established, the fixture will find its way down without any pressure. The implant site should be empty when this part of the procedure is started. Irrigation should not start until the small notches at the tip of the fixture have entered the implant site so that the hole is not filled with saline. As the flange of the implant is coming close to the bone surface, the speed is reduced to get a gentle stop and to avoid damage to the threads in the bone. This step is especially important if the bone is soft. The cylinder wrench is used to manually check that the implant is securely fastened. This has how-

ever to be done with utmost care as very large forces could be produced due to the cantilever effect.

If the fixture is stable, the skin-penetrating abutment is connected directly. If it is not stable, 3 to 4 months are allowed for osseointegration to take place without any load to the implant. In most cases, the implant site is under hair-bearing skin, which is removed. The diameter of the removed skin should be at least 20mm. To establish reaction-free skin penetration, the skin around the implant must not move in relation to the implant. To achieve this, a subcutaneous tissue reduction is made by use of sharp blades and skin hooks. The amount of tissue that should be removed varies among patients, but the aim is to ensure that the edges of the field around the implant site slope gently down. There should be no steps or steep slopes down to the percutaneous coupling of the sound processor. The area closest to the implant is covered with a hairless skin graft taken from the retroauricular fold. The graft is thinned as much as possible and should look almost like a graft taken with a dermatome. The graft is sutured over the fixture with 6.0 nylon monofilament. A hole is punched in the graft for the hearing aid coupling, the abutment. The abutment and its internal screw come sterilely packed. The abutment is held with the open-ended wrench designed for this purpose, and the screw is secured with the four-tipped screwdriver using the wrench to reduce the torque on the fixture. The only reason for grafting is to avoid hair follicles at the implant site; if no follicles are present, only the subcutaneous tissue reduction is made as described. Finally, a healing cap is snapped onto the abutment. This cap will keep an ointment-soaked gauze down to eliminate bleeding and postoperative hematoma. An ordinary mastoid dressing with light pressure is used for 1 day. After that, only a small, light draping is necessary.

POSTOPERATIVE CARE

The day after surgery, the mastoid draping is thus removed and replaced by a light bandage, a "black patch." Five to 7 days after surgery, the patient comes back for the first dressing. The healing cap is tilted off and the gauze is removed. The area is cleaned carefully and left open for about 30 minutes. The healing cap is then put back in place, and a new ointment-soaked gauze is wound under the cap. After another 6 to 7 days, the healing cap is removed and the stitches taken out, including the stitches placed at the graft donor site. The patient is then asked to clean the area very gently with soap and water and also to use some of the same ointment once a day for a couple of weeks. When healing is completed, the patient is informed about the importance of good personal hygiene and are instructed to use soap and water. If a slight irritation occurs, the patient is told to use the ointment prescribed. Having a skin-penetrating abutment will not stop the patient from taking a sauna or from dying or perming the hair. Of course, it is possible to go swimming and diving with the implant. The sound processor must, however, of course be removed! In Figure 37–4 a schematic drawing of the arrangement, including the assembly tool, is presented.[17]

PITFALLS IN SURGERY

The surgical procedure is simple, and since its start in 1977 and after over 1000 implants in the mastoid process, including implants for retention of auricular prostheses, no serious complication has been experienced by the author. In about 10 per cent of cases, the wall of the sigmoid sinus is identified at the bottom of the implant site. In a few cases, the wall has been injured, and slight bleeding has occurred. This condition, however, is very easy to control. If the damage occurs within 2mm, the site is plugged with a piece of periosteum, and another site is identified closeby. If the damage occurs at the final 0.5mm, the hole is widened and threaded, and an implant is put in place. The dura mater of the middle cranial fossa is sometimes seen but seldom damaged. Having the dura at the bottom of the implant site is not considered a contraindication for placing a fixture in that site. In the well-pneumatized mastoid process, air cells are sometimes entered. If the bone is good, contact with an air cell will not call for any special precaution, and the site can often be used. If the amount of bone is very small, another implant site is looked for; good cortical bone for a 4mm fixture may be available within a couple of millimeters. Suction in a site that is in contact with an air cell should be avoided, however, because this situation may lead to a very fast retraction of the drum and could be uncomfortable.

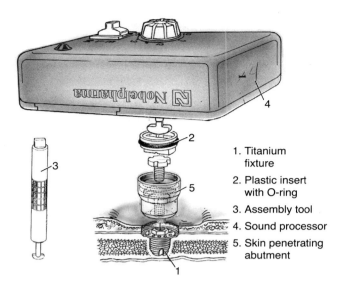

1. Titanium fixture
2. Plastic insert with O-ring
3. Assembly tool
4. Sound processor
5. Skin penetrating abutment

FIGURE 37–4. Schematic drawing of the arrangement with fixture (1), plastic insert with O-ring (2), sound processor (4), and skin-penetrating coupling with coupling screw (5). The assembly tool (3) is also shown.

SOUND PROCESSOR

Six to 8 weeks after surgery, the patient is fitted with the sound processor. Three sound processors are available, but their basic design is the same, and a schematic drawing is seen in Figure 37–5. The main advantage with this direct percutaneous coupling between the bone and the transducer is that the gap between the two components of the transducer could be kept short (50μm). Because of the suspension arrangement, this distance will also be constant. Less power is needed, which means higher output and lower distortion. For a detailed description of the soundprocessor, a paper by Håkansson et al.[2] from 1991 is recommended. The standard sound processor is the HC 200 (Fig. 37–4), which is an ear-level hearing aid that can be used by most patients with a bone-

FIGURE 37–5. The principal design of the transducer. Note the small gap between the two components of the transducer and the suspension arrangement, important for the signal flux.

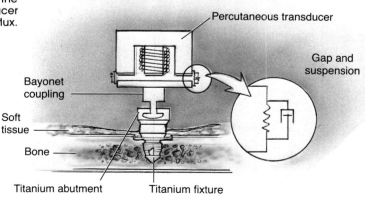

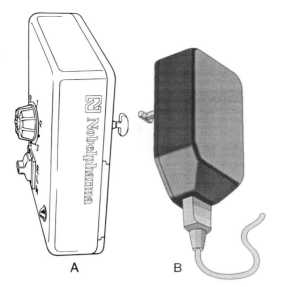

FIGURE 37-6. *A*, Ear level sound processor HC 200. *B*, Superbass sound processor HC 220, which needs a body aid. (From Nobelpharma AB, Göteborg, Sweden.)

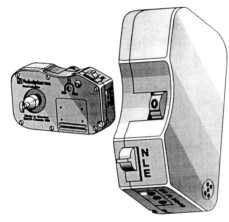

FIGURE 37-7. BAHA Classic 300 (From Nobelpharma AB, Göteborg, Sweden.)

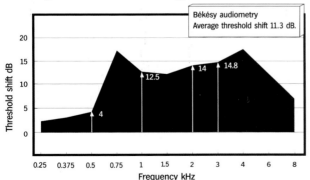

FIGURE 37-8. The threshold shift with and without skin penetration using Békésy audiometry. (From Nobelpharma AB, Göteborg, Sweden.)

conduction threshold of 45dB pure tone average (PTA) for the speech frequencies (0.5kHz to 3kHz) or better. The stronger Superbass HC 220 (Fig. 37–6), is a transducer driven through a body aid. Patients with hearing losses as low as 60dB for bone conduction could use this device. The BAHA Classic 300 (Fig. 37–7), is the smallest of the three and is an ear-level hearing aid. In patients with cochlear function of better than 35dB, this may be a good solution. A BiCROS with a microphone and a telecoil function is also available.

Fitting of the Soundprocessor

When the sound processor is going to be fitted, a plastic insert is fitted into the skin-penetrating coupling. This insert is kept in place with an O-ring illustrated in Figure 37–4. The insertion is made with a small plastic rod that comes with the hearing aid. The insert must be kept absolutely perpendicular to the titanium coupling, and the rectangular ridge of the plastic insert must be in alignment with the rectangular indentation of the coupling. The insert must not be tilted in, as the O-ring will then get cuts that will interfere with its function, will not give the force needed for the retention of the sound processor, and will interfere with the acoustic coupling. This situation can cause distortion and other unwanted sound effects. When the insert is in place, the piston of the sound processor is fitted into the slot of the insert and turned 90°. The placement of the plastic insert is facilitated if the O-ring is moistened in water. The O-ring must be changed every 3 to 6 months, depending on how the patient is handling the hearing aid and the coupling. The plastic insert will also wear and must be exchanged after 1 to 2 years. The coupling arrangement is designed in such a way that if the sound processor is exposed to a strong force, for example, caught by a part of the clothing or by somebody grabbing it, the insert will come out without causing any damage to the implant or to the hearing aid. If this occurs, the insert is replaced in the same way described earlier.

RESULTS

The results in patients equipped with a BAHA were published in detail as a supplement of *Annals of Otology* by Håkansson et al.[14] When direct bone conduction is compared with conventional bone conduction, the improvement for pure tones varies from 5dB to 20dB, depending on the frequency as seen in Figure 37–8. In objective testing, the speech discrimination score measured in noise improves from 50 to 71 per cent in patients who have been using a conventional bone-conduction hearing aid. In patients who had been wearing an air-conduction aid, the improvement was from 50 to 60 per cent. Many patients claimed that there was improved clarity of the sound that is hard to demonstrate in objective tests. In a questionnaire, 89 per cent of the patients with a level of bone conduction better than 45dB and a speech discrimination score better than 60 per cent reported improved hearing.[19] Four per cent reported worse hearing, and 7 per cent, no difference between the old aid and the BAHA. The level of comfort was also high: improved comfort was found in 95 per cent, worse in 3 per cent, and no different in 2 per cent. One of the main advantages expressed by patients with chronic ear conditions was that the drainage from the ear had diminished or disappeared. Another way to evaluate the efficacy of a hearing aid is to determine how many hours per day patients are using the aid. When a group of patients was asked this question, 94 per cent stated that they used it more than 8 hours a day. Another very important advantage reported by patients with chronic ear conditions who had been using air-conduction aids is that the external ear meatus was no longer occluded, and the drainage from the ear canal stopped with the BAHA.

COMPLICATIONS AND MANAGEMENT

Skin

Maintaining reaction-free skin penetration over years is an important consideration with this type of hearing aid. As mentioned earlier, the reduction of subcutaneous tissue is essential and is the responsibility of the surgeon. The patient is responsible for the everyday care. A high level of hygiene is important, and the patient is told to clean the implant area with soap and water regularly. In some patients, this means every day, in others, every second, third, or fourth day. The frequency depends on the general properties of the skin. A patient with greasy skin or seborrhea must be more active than an individual with dry skin free of sebaceous glands. The patient should have mild antibiotic ointment available at home in case of temporary irritation. If irritation occurs, the patient is instructed to intensify the general level of hygiene and use the ointment. The ointment must be applied in small amounts, and the O-ring must be kept free from the ointment. If not, the O-ring will lose some of its physical properties, and the plastic insert could more easily be dislodged. If the irritation persists for a couple of days, the patient should get in touch with the treatment team. One reason for a temporary irritation is that an abutment screw that keeps the coupling secured to the flange fixture has unscrewed itself and needs tightening. These minor movements can be hard to detect without an otomicroscope. The insert must be removed to make such an evaluation possible. Such a loose screw can be tightened with the four-tipped screwdriver and the open-ended wrench as a counterforce without any local anesthesia. If granulation tissue develops, it has to be removed and its cause investigated as described earlier. The removal is often easy with a sterile dental floss or a knife. The plastic insert is temporally exchanged to the healing cap and a gauze with an appropriate antibiotic ointment put in place and kept for several days. In only one of more than 350 patients operated on by the author, the abutment had to be removed because of adverse soft tissue reaction.

In a study based on 1739 observations made at 6-month intervals between 1977 and 1989, no adverse skin reaction occurred in 92.5 per cent of those observations. Seventy-five per cent of the patients never had had an episode of skin reaction around the implant during the same time. A small group (4 per cent) of the patients were responsible for more than 50 per cent of the reactions.

A sensation of pain when the implant is touched is almost always an indication that something is loose. A loose coupling can but will not always cause pain. If the fixture has lost its integration, pain will almost always occur for one or more days before the implant comes out. The risk of losing an implant because of loss of integration is in the range of 2 to 4 per cent over time. Such a loss may occur before the sound processor has been fitted but may also occur as late as 10 years after insertion. Direct trauma is another cause of implant loss. In the author's series of 350 patients, not a single case of osteomyelitis has been diagnosed, and there has been no other serious complication of any kind.

Hearing

A deterioration of function could result from three different causes: the patients hearing may have gone down, the coupling arrangement between the sound processor and the bone may not function as it is supposed to, and a dysfunction of the sound processor may occur.

Patient Hearing

It is a well-known fact that as a patient gets older, the hearing gets worse, especially in the high-frequency range. A draining ear may also influence cochlear function in a negative way. Ototoxic drugs are a third hazard to inner ear function. These are some of the causes the surgeon should remember when a patient is reporting that a BAHA is not working as it used to do. Regular hearing tests are recommended for these patients.

Coupling between Soundprocessor and Bone

One of the most common reasons for dysfunction is that the O-ring has lost its elasticity and will not keep the insert in place with sufficient force. The O-ring may be damaged by rough handling by the patient, for example, if the insert with the O-ring is tilted into the coupling, the O-ring will be damaged. Ointment or other fatty products from the skin may also interfere with the elasticity, or the plastic insert is worn.

The acoustic coupling between the sound processor and the bone is through the piston of the transducer and the coupling screw. After a long time and especially if the patient is using the Superbass HC 220 on maximum output, the piston can cause a groove in the head of the screw, resulting in disturbed acoustic transmission, distortion, and a buzzing sound. The screw should be exchanged. The same type of signal disturbance could result from the coupling screw becoming loose, it should of course be tightened. If the fixture has lost its osseointegration, this condition can result in decreased efficacy, but there is almost always pain associated with touching or shaking the coupling. If the flange fixture has lost its integration, the chance that it will be integrated once again is very small, even if the coupling is removed and the fixture is left without any load. The insertion of a new implant is the solution to this problem.

Defect Sound Processor

The defect sound processor is a third alternative. There is a skull simulator, an artificial mastoid, available to test the sound processor, and a most helpful instrument in determining the reason for a deterioration of function. The longevity for these hearing aids seems to be the same as for conventional hearing aids: ranging from 3 to 5 years.

SUMMARY

Osseointegration has been defined as a direct contact between living bone and a loaded implant surface. Establishment of a lasting anchorage of a titanium implant in the mastoid process has proved to be a safe and simple method for attaching a bone-anchored hearing aid. It is also possible to establish and maintain a reaction-free skin penetration over many years. Of more than 1700 observations of skin reactions around the implant, less than 8% had any irritation and less than 4% needed active treatment. Seventy-five per cent of the patients had never had a single episode of adverse skin reaction. The cochlear function should not be worse than 45 dB for the ear-level device and not worse than 60 dB for the body aid.

The bone-anchored hearing aid is suggested as an alternative in selected hearing-impaired patients in whom reconstructive surgery has been unsuccessful or is contraindicated and in whom a conventional air conduction hearing aid could not or should not be used.

References

1. Brandt A: On sound transmission characteristics of the human skull in vivo. Thesis, Technical report No 61L, Göteborg, Sweden: School of Electrical Engineering, Chalmers University of Technology, 1989.
2. Håkansson B, Tjellström A, Carlsson P: Percutaneous vs transcutaneous transducers for hearing by direct bone conduction. Otolaryngol Head Neck Surg 102(4): 339–344, 1990.
3. Håkansson B, Tjellström A, Rosenhall U: Hearing thresholds with direct bone conduction versus conventional bone conduction. Scand Audiol 13: 3–13, 1984.
4. Håkansson B, Carlsson P, Tjellström A: The mechanical point impedance of the human head, with and without skin penetration. J Acoust Soc Am 80(4): 1065–1075, 1986.
5. Carlsson P, Håkansson B, Rosenhall U, Tjellström A: A speech reception threshold test in noise with the bone-anchored hearing aid. A comparative study. Otolaryngol Head Neck Surg 94(4): 421–426, 1986.
6. Tjellström A: Percutaneous implants in clinical practice. Crit Rev Biocompatibility 1(3): 205–228, 1985.
7. Håkansson B, Tjellström A, Rosenhall U: Acceleration levels and threshold with direct bone conduction versus conventional bone conduction. Acta Otolaryngol (Stockh) 100: 240–252, 1985.
8. Brånemark PI, Hansson B, Adell R: Osseointegration in the treatment of the edentulous jaw. Experience from a 10 year period. Scand J Plast Reconstr Surg 16: 1–132, 1977.
9. Brånemark PI: Introduction to osseointegration. In Brånemark PI, Zarb G, Albrektsson T (eds): Tissue-integrated Prostheses. Chicago, Quintessence Publishing, 1985, pp 11–76.
10. Albrektsson T, Albrektsson B: Osseointegration of bone implants. Acta Orthop Scand 58: 567–577, 1987.
11. Tjellström, A: Osseointegrated systems and their application in the head and neck. Adv Otolaryngol Head Neck Surg 3: 39–70, 1989.
12. Jacobsson M, Tjellström A: Clinical application of percutaneous implants, in high performance biomaterials. In Michael Szycher (ed): A Comprehensive Guide to Medical and Pharmaceutical Applications. Lancaster, Basel, Technomic Publishing Company, 1991, pp 207–229.
13. Steinemann SG, Eulenberger J, Maesuli PA, et al.: Adhesion of bone to titanium. In Christel P, Munier A, Lee AJC (eds): Biological and Biomechanical Performance of Biomaterials. Amsterdam, Elsevier Science Publishers, 1986, pp 409–414.
14. Håkansson B, Lidén G, Tjellström A, et al.: Ten years of experience of the Swedish Bone Anchored Hearing System. Ann Otol Rhinol Laryngol Suppl 99(10Pt2): 1–16, 1990.
15. Abramson M, Fay TH, Kelly JP, et al.: Clinical results with a percutaneous bone-anchored hearing aid. Laryngoscope 99: 707–710, 1989.
16. Jahrsdoerfer RA, Yeakley JW, Aguilar EA, et al.: Grading system for the selection of patients with congenital aural atresia. Am J Otol 13(1): 6–12, 1992.
17. Holgers K-M, Bjursten LM, Thomsen P, et al.: Experience with percutaneous titanium implants in the head and neck—A clinical histological study. Invest Surg 2: 7–16, 1989.
18. Tjellström A: Surgery for the Bone Anchored Hearing Aid. Göteborg Medical Service. Video Library. No. 17/87, 1987.
19. Tjellström A, Jacobsson M, Norvell B, Albrektsson T: Patient attitudes to the bone-anchored hearing aid. Results of a questionnaire study. Scand Audiol 18: 119–123, 1989.

38

Endolymphatic Sac Procedures

MICHAEL M. PAPARELLA, M.D.

Endolymphatic sac surgery for Ménière's disease has been used for more than 65 years. The objective of this operation is to preserve and, if possible, enhance labyrinthine function. Most surgical series demonstrate clinically significant control of vestibular symptoms, including vertigo. The operation has been used successfully to preserve cochlear function and to improve cochlear symptoms. The physiologic role of the endolymphatic sac in normal labyrinthine function has yet to be established, as has the physiologic basis for successful control of symptoms of intractable Ménière's disease by use of endolymphatic sac surgery, although objective and subjective evidence accumulates. Endolymphatic sac surgery offers a patient who has failed medical control of Ménière's disease a nonablative surgical procedure that in most cases results in elimination or control of vertiginous spells, preservation of hearing, and sometimes improvement of hearing along with improvement of other associated labyrinthine symptoms.

Since it was first described in 1927, endolymphatic sac surgery has stood the test of time.[1, 2] This operation, described in all textbooks of otolaryngology, is practiced widely in the United States and throughout the world by leading ear surgeons, some of whom have very large series. It is the only conservative, nondestructive form of surgery that avoids invasion of the labyrinth. Other procedures commonly done today are destructive either to the peripheral labyrinth or to the vestibular nerve. Any procedure that invades the labyrinth is logically going to cause a higher postoperative incidence of labyrinthine dysfunction and deafness. The endolymphatic sac is not part of the labyrinth and exists anterior to Trautmann's triangle within the dura, medial and inferior to the posteroinferior semicircular canal, in a remote location, with communication to the labyrinth via the vestibular aqueduct.

Controversy exists about all methods of treating Ménière's disease, both medical and surgical (including destructive and conservative methods). Indeed, on both philosophic and medical grounds, operations designed to destroy an organ or its parts (irreversible) are more controversial than conservative ones. Opinions regarding diagnosis and treatment of this disease were even stronger in 1861, the year Ménière described this syndrome and, although opinions vary to date, much understanding has developed and more agreement now exists regarding management than existed in those early years.

Endolymphatic sac surgery is now the most commonly done operation for Ménière's disease in the United States and worldwide, with large series having been established by leading otologists. Silverstein[3] sent a questionnaire regarding vestibular nerve section to members of the Otological and Neurotological Society and found that fewer than 3000 nerve sections had been done by all of the members. The majority (approximately two-thirds) consider endolymphatic sac surgery a primary procedure, whereas a smaller number consider vestibular nerve section a primary procedure, even though the questionnaire was directed toward vestibular nerve section. Morrison, in England, has performed more than 2000 endolymphatic sac procedures for Ménière's disease (personal communication, 1992). Huang, a leading otologist in Asia, has performed more than 1700 sac procedures (personal communication, 1992), and Plester and Portmann also have large series (personal communications, 1992 and 1992). Many centers and individuals in the United States, including the author, have series in excess of 1000 cases.

A study by Bretlau et al.[4] has received attention. These authors compared results of sac surgery in 15 patients and with results in patients receiving a "sham" operation. In this small series, numerous questions arise, including criteria for selection of patients, techniques employed, and multiple surgeons.[4a] Their findings were interpreted as being statistically flawed by Pillsbury et al.[5] and four other statisticians of whom the author is aware. The author experienced more than 100 cases before considering publication, and before a sense of comfort and confidence was achieved for favorable short- and long-term results. It is understandable that endolymphatic sac surgery is done more commonly than destructive procedures. One important reason is that Ménière's disease is bilateral in at least one of three cases, more likely closer to one of every two cases, according to Stahle et al.[6] The author has encountered too many patients in whom Ménière's disease has caused deafness in one ear and then later, vertigo and deafness in the second ear. The author has also seen the tragedy of patients who have had surgical treatment resulting in deafness in one ear who would then develop Ménière's disease and deafness in the second ear at a later date.

Perhaps the ultimate trust in, and application of, this procedure is based on its ability to treat a patient who has Ménière's disease in an only-hearing ear that is in the process of developing profound hearing loss, deafness, or both. Studies by the author on the natural history of Ménière's disease suggest that once the progressive form develops, there is an approximate 20 per cent chance that the patient will develop a profound or severe loss or even complete deafness. The author has reluctantly, but successfully, used endolymphatic sac surgery to treat the only-hearing ear in patients with Ménière's disease in approximately 12 patients to date. It was surprising to find that many other leading otologists have a larger experience in this regard. Pulec described endolymphatic sac surgery for an only-hearing ear.[7] To date, Morrison has safely and successfully performed sac surgery in over 100 patients with only-hearing ears.[7a] Huang has performed surgery in 28 cases (personal communication, 1992), Plester, in approximately 15 cases of only-hearing ears (personal communication, 1992).

Certainly, otologists who recommend destructive surgery as a primary modality would never consider such a procedure in an only-hearing ear. An obvious question is, If endolymphatic sac surgery is useful to preserve hearing as a last-step measure why would it not be considered earlier in the disease or preferably on the first ear involved? Because patients are seen in whom Ménière's disease and a severe hearing loss or deafness has developed in the second ear, it is conservative and prudent to do everything possible to preserve hearing in the first ear involved.

The wide application of this conservative procedure is not only for bilateral disease but also for safer treatment for the atypical forms of Ménière's disease (specified later). Endolymphatic sac surgery has had broader acceptance and appeal for otologic surgeons because it provides an opportunity to preserve and, in some instances, enhance function in the vestibular and the cochlear labyrinths. Thus, when patients have predominantly vestibular Ménière's disease with normal or relatively normal hearing, or have cochlear Ménière's disease with relatively little vestibular symptomatology, this conservative procedure can be successfully used in selected cases.

A prudent philosophy and policy for Ménière's disease is that conservative treatment should precede any consideration of surgical treatment. Medical treatment with psychologic support comes first. If cochlear or vestibular symptoms, especially vertigo, become intractable, a conservative surgical procedure, endolymphatic sac enhancement or shunt, can be considered. This procedure can be considered an "extension of conservative treatment" because it has minimal risks and appears to affect pathophysiology beneficially.[8]

The role of endolymphatic sac surgery in treatment of Ménière's disease is in treating patients who develop intractable or progressive Ménière's disease, including vestibular and cochlear symptoms, in spite of adequate and prolonged trials of medical, supportive, empirical management. Because the physiology of the normal labyrinth and the pathophysiology of Ménière's disease are both poorly understood, it is impossible to describe the role of endolymphatic sac surgery with any certainty. Nevertheless, objective and subjective evidence continues to accumulate that suggests strongly that endolymphatic sac surgery enhances the ability of the endolymphatic sac to absorb endolymph. By focusing on what is understood, or reasonably well understood, about Ménière's disease

we are able to diagnose and treat patients conservatively.

Evidence has been reported in previous publications by the author that describes the etiology of Ménière's disease as multifactorially inherited. Occasionally, extrinsic causative factors are known, but a genetic underlying basis most likely leads to the anomalous changes, both physical and chemical, that lead to Ménière's disease. The pathogenesis of Ménière's disease is considered to be based on malabsorption of endolymph. Endolymphatic hydrops was first described by Hallpike and Cairns[9] and also by Yamakawa[10, 11] in 1938. Endolymphatic sac surgery, irrespective of the surgical technique used, likely enhances the absorption of endolymph by 1) decompression, 2) passive diffusion of nanoliters of endolymph along alloplastic material, 3) osmotic changes in pressure that result in an extracellular milieu (pump) around the sac, 4) alteration of blood supply, and 5) most likely, alteration of immune factors in the endolymphatic sac (Fig. 38–1).[8, 12]

PATIENT SELECTION

Generally, indications for surgical procedures on the endolymphatic sac are the development of intractable or progressive Ménière's disease over time and medical empirical management failure (Fig. 38–2). Most patients with Ménière's disease have the nonprogressive form and can be managed medically, indefinitely. Most patients with progressive (intractable) Ménière's disease develop progression over many years, and a minority develop Ménière's disease with destruction of the labyrinth more rapidly, over a brief period of time—a month or a few months, for example. The latter patients therefore need more rapid consideration of intercession. Previous publications by the author indicate that the average duration of disease was approximately 6 years prior to the patient's receiving sac enhancement surgery.[13, 14]

The most common indication for sac procedures is vertigo in classic Ménière's disease, in which patients have characteristic symptoms in all three categories: vestibular symptoms, cochlear symptoms, and aural pressure. Vestibular symptoms include typical episodic attacks of vertigo occurring intermittently at variable intervals; severe disequilibrium or imbalance, which also develops from Ménière's disease; frequent bouts of nausea occurring alone or sometimes with vomiting accompanying the paroxysmal attacks; visually induced vertigo or so-called shopping center nystagmus (these patients will develop dizziness when they look at a computer, read a book, or see movement in a supermarket or shopping center); and positional or motion dizziness, which invariably oc-

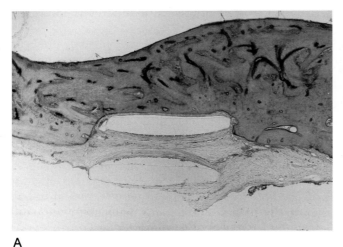

A

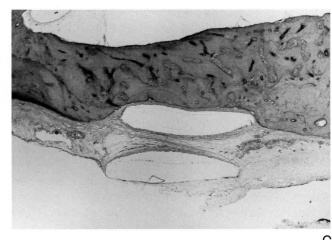

C

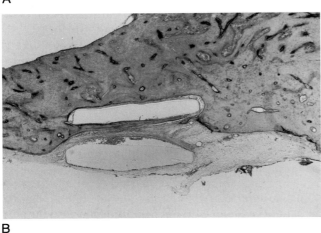

B

FIGURE 38-1. This patient had a sac enhancement operation and died later from unrelated causes. Please note inert silicone sheeting struts within the endolymphatic sac. There is no significant foreign body reaction.

curs during an attack of Ménière's but often between vertiginous episodes as well. Cochlear symptoms include hearing loss, progressive hearing loss, and fluctuating sensorineural hearing loss; tinnitus, which can be disabling, either constant or intermittent, and will often exacerbate during attacks; intolerance of loudness (measured by recruitment studies); and diplacusis or distortion of sound, typically perceived by the patient while listening during a telephone conversation. Aural pressure, a significant component of Ménière's disease, is characteristically perceived as pressure in one (unilateral) or both ears (bilateral) but sometimes as a pressure in the head in general, or a headache or discomfort on the side of the head, or in other regions of the head and neck.

② Another indication for sac surgery is intractable vestibular Ménière's disease. Vestibular Ménière's disease does exist, as clearly evidenced by the study of patients who have classic Ménière's disease because 20 to 50 per cent of them (according to various studies) have vertigo and vestibular symptoms, sometimes occurring over a period of many years (as long as 45 years in one patient). Over time, many of these patients develop cochlear symptoms, allowing the diagnosis of typical Ménière's disease. The role for sac enhancement in the successful treatment of these patients has been described by Miller and Welsh,[15] Paparella and Mancini,[16] Huang,[16a] and Plester (personal communication, 1992).

FIGURE 38-2. This illustration depicts progressive (intractable) Ménière's disease versus nonprogressive Ménière's disease, over time.

③ Cochlear Ménière's disease can occur in the absence of vestibular symptoms.[16b] It can be treated successfully by sac enhancement surgery, especially when there is fluctuating hearing loss. The key is to treat the disease while there are temporary threshold shifts such as can be seen in patients who demonstrate a history of fluctuation. In those who develop a permanent threshold shift due to irrevocable damage from endolymphatic hydrops, surgery may not improve hearing. Nevertheless, many patients have preservation of hearing without progression, as a result of a conservative sac procedure. Pearson[17] has done sac surgery on cochlear Ménière's disease when the diagnosis has been confirmed by positive results on glycerol test and typical electrocorticographic (ECoG) changes. Hearing results have been spectacular in approximately 20 such cases. Morrison has a similar experience (personal communication, 1992).

Although Ménière's disease typically strikes adults, usually occurring during the third and fourth decades, it does occur in children,[18] and the indications for treating children are identical to those for adults:[19] Conservative medical management precedes any consideration of surgery until the disease becomes intractable or progressive. Sac enhancement surgery can also be considered for elderly patients because it is a more conservative procedure, requiring typically one overnight stay in a hospital, in contrast to destructive procedures, which require longer periods of hospitalization, including care in the intensive care unit. Morrison (personal communication, 1992) and Huang (personal communication, 1992) have successfully performed this procedure for elderly patients over 70 years of age. The author has had a similar experience in successfully performing such a procedure in patients who are elderly, including several in their 90s who were otherwise incapacitated.

Ménière's disease can coexist with other diseases, sometimes with a causative or as a coincidental relationship. Multiple otopathologies are not rare.[20] Otosclerosis has been described in association with Ménière's disease. In selected patients, endolymphatic sac enhancement has proved to be useful.[21] Usually, a stapedectomy-sacculotomy is attempted first, particularly if there is a significant conductive component to the hearing loss. The clinical picture of syphilitically induced labyrinthine changes can be identical to Ménière's disease. After exhausting medical management, sac procedures have been used successfully in such patients by Paparella et al.[22] and by Huang and Lin.[23] Ménière's disease has also been found to develop over a period of years following chronic inactive otitis media and mastoiditis. This relationship has been clearly defined in otopathologic studies and clinically in patients.[23a] Endolymphatic sac enhancement has been successful in treating a significant number of these patients, particularly those in a recent study by Huang and Lin.[23b]

④ Bilateral Ménière's disease is another indication for endolymphatic sac surgery. No published author known to this author would consider destructive procedures on the second ear in patients who have bilateral Ménière's disease. The first provocative, or worst, ear is treated first, and if there is intractability in the second ear after months or a period of time that allows for stabilization of the first ear, sac surgery can be considered on the opposite side. Usually, bilateral surgery is unnecessary because once the offending ear with clinical presentation (hearing loss, pressure, and tinnitus) is treated successfully with endolymphatic sac surgery, the patient is comfortable, and the opposite ear often remains stable, and not progressive, especially regarding sensorineural hearing loss. Bilateral sac surgery has been performed in approximately 100 patients by Morrison,[23c] in approximately 80 patients by Huang (personal communication, 1992), and in a similar number of patients by the author.

Earlier congenital anomalies of the inner ear, such as Mondini's deafness, were thought to be treated successfully with endolymphatic sac surgery. A more recent study, however, suggests that the results are not good; therefore, this procedure may not be indicated for patients who have congenital malformations of the inner ear, such as those resulting from Mondini's deafness.[19]

Patients can develop delayed hydrops with onset of vertigo who have developed sudden deafness earlier in their lifetime or childhood deafness from various causes.[24] For example, in children or adults, congenital or acquired forms of deafness, such as meningogenic labyrinthitis, may develop that years later can result in severe vertigo, pressure, and tinnitus in an ear that has a profound hearing loss or that is severely deafened. The author has successfully performed sac surgery in approximately 20 patients in this group, thus requiring same-day discharge or overnight stay without severe disability resulting from destructive labyrinthectomy or nerve section, and without the difficulties with compensation that would ensue from a destructive modality.

Endolymphatic sac revision is another indication for endolymphatic sac surgery. For example, a patient may have had a successful previous endolymphatic sac procedure for a period of 3 or 4 years but subsequently develops characteristic and disabling symptoms of Ménière's disease in the same ear. The patient is told what could be developing, and the patient is advised that often bone tissue (osteoneogenesis) or scar tissue (fibrosis) forms in the region external to the sac to cause reobstruction at that site, and that aditus block can cause formation of tissue and bone in the mastoid. Frequently, scar tissue forms from the undersurface of the inferior wound (skin) contiguous with the adjacent sac.[13, 25] Of course, Ménière's disease can also exacerbate on its own accord. The patient is then advised of the condition and is provided the options of choosing between destructive procedures, such as vestibular nerve section, particularly if there is residual hearing remaining, sac revision, or both. Most patients select a sac revision procedure. Many authors have described sac revision. In the author's experience, the incidence of revision has been approximately 5 per cent, whereas many others have found the incidence of revision to be as high as 10 per cent (Huang, personal communication, 1992; Morrison, personal communication, 1992; Plester, personal communication, 1992).[25–27]

Finally, sac procedures are the only surgical procedures considered in patients who have an only-hearing ear from Ménière's disease. As mentioned, these patients have become deaf in the first ear from the disease or from a destructive procedure, such as labyrinthectomy. Once the second ear becomes intractable and develops severe, progressive, fluctuating deafness, a sac procedure can be considered. Many patients have been successfully treated, as was discussed in the previous section (Huang, personal communication, 1992; Plester personal communication, 1992).[7, 28] The author has performed sac enhancement in 12 such patients, all of whom have preserved hearing; a few have improved hearing, whereas none, thankfully, has developed deafness over a prolonged period of time, in some instances many years.

PREOPERATIVE EVALUATION AND PATIENT COUNSELING

The method of diagnosis for Ménière's disease is documented in detail elsewhere but will be highlighted here.[8] The most important part of the diagnosis is the history, which perhaps contributes 90 per cent or more to the diagnosis. The history starts with the chief complaint, and specifically structured questions are asked in each of three categories (vestibular, cochlear, or aural pressure), depending on the chief complaint. The chief complaint is usually vertigo or vestibular upset; thus, the various specific questions are asked relative to vestibular symptoms of Ménière's disease. If the chief complaint originates in the cochlea, specific symptoms are reviewed regarding hearing loss, fluctuating hearing loss, tinnitus, intolerance of loudness, and diplacusis. The chief complaint may also relate to severe pressure or headache in the region of the ear or head.

Once the history is established, diagnostic studies are performed. The next most important diagnostic study is a routine audiogram consisting of air conduction, bone conduction, speech-reception thresholds, and speech discrimination. Other diagnostic tests follow, depending on indications. Routine diagnostic studies in the author's clinic include mastoid X-rays (especially lateral Law's view) to identify whether the mastoid is pneumatized, sclerotic, diploic, or otherwise pathologic. Studies indicate that hypoplasia exists in the mastoid in patients with Ménière's disease, and that the sigmoid sinus occupies an anterior and deep location. Thus, inexpensive diagnostic information is quickly available in this regard. Plus, if surgery is to take place, X-rays provide a quick guide for rapid drilling in the mastoid; for example, one should be more cautious if the mastoid is sclerotic with a prominent, deep sigmoid sinus, as opposed to a pneumatic sinus.

An audiometric study of brainstem response (ABR) is typically ordered to rule out lesions of the cerebellopontine angle, such as a vestibular schwannoma, although these two diseases result in quite different clinical presentations. ABR has been demonstrated to be 95 per cent accurate. If there may be a space-occupying lesion, magnetic resonance imaging with gadolinium or, less often, a computed tomographic study with enhancement is recommended. An electronystagmogram (ENG) is routinely ordered; ENG results can, however, be normal in up to 52 per cent of patients with Ménière's disease.[29] The patient may have incapacitating classical Ménière's disease and normal ENG results. Posturography and sinusoidal chair testing are used in some centers and have been widely used by the author but have not proved essential or necessary in the diagnosis of Ménière's disease.

Glycerol testing was promoted earlier and continues to be practiced by some, but it is not nearly as commonly employed as it used to be because of lack of persistent relevance. This has been the experience in the author's clinic as well. ECoG can be ordered if it is available; it is not, however, essential. ECoG is typically ordered in the routine battery practiced by the author. After these tests are ordered, the patient continues to be treated medically, if possible, unless the patient has been referred from a specialist, having already had prolonged medical management.

Communication, counseling, and education of the patient is the next important part of management. A patient who understands his or her problem is a far better patient to manage and will have a far better result than a patient who is uninformed about his or her problem. Once a diagnosis is made, it is carefully explained to the patient. An explanation is made concerning the nature of endolymph and the fact that endolymphatic hydrops results form chemical or mechanical obstruction of the vestibular aqueduct and sac. Then, the patient is told how this procedure can reverse pathogenesis, thus allowing for an improved equilibrium of fluid, which provides an excellent opportunity to preserve and sometimes enhance function and ameliorate symptoms.

The patient is advised of the complications, risks, and benefits, both of the disease process and of the procedure. This consideration is important. The risks and complications from progressive Ménière's disease, including deafness, as well as the possibility of deafness from surgery, must be considered. Once the disease has been explained to the patient through diagrams and pictures on the wall, informational reading material is provided the patient. The patient is advised that the goal of surgery is to try to preserve function and, depending on the nature of permanent damage to the labyrinth, to enhance function. The patient is advised that there is no cure for Ménière's disease, but that there is always hope for improvement. Options of treatment, including continued medical conservative treatment, conservative surgical intervention, and destructive surgical intervention, are explained to the patient, reserving destructive procedures for treatment failures (which are uncommon). The patient then chooses from the conservative options.

The following statistics based on the author's published experience are then translated to the patient: the patient is advised that there is an approximate 2 per cent chance that deafness or profound hearing loss might result from the surgery. This loss is not a result of entering the labyrinth but usually relates to the healing process, which will be discussed later. The patient is advised about the cause and pathogenesis of the disease process. The word "recommend" is not used; the problem or disease is described to the patient and the patient is allowed to choose freely among the various options, although destructive surgery is not considered an option at this stage. The incidence of bilaterality or the possibility that the disease may develop in the opposite ear over time is considered by the patient. Patients generally conclude that a conservative approach precedes destructive surgery. In the author's clinic, destructive surgeries, including vestibular nerve section, are not commonly done because conservative approaches have worked for the vast majority of patients over a prolonged period of time.

The patient is advised that there is a 70 per cent chance to stop and ameliorate not only the vertigo but also the associated other vestibular symptoms that accompany Ménière's disease. An additional 20 per cent of patients will continue to have vestibular symptoms, but the attacks will be less severe and less intense, thus allowing continued medical management. They are advised that there is a 90 per cent or better chance that the procedure will help preserve hearing

or that it will not progress so severely over time, and that there is a 30 to 40 per cent chance that the hearing might improve over preoperative threshold levels. The odds of improvement of tinnitus or pressure are slightly better than 50 per cent.[13, 14]

PREOPERATIVE PREPARATION

Antibiotics are not used preoperatively unless there is an associated condition requiring such treatment first. The patient receives general anesthesia and is encouraged to speak with the anesthesiologist ahead of time, if concerns or questions exist.

PREPARATION OF THE SURGICAL SITE, DRAPING, AND POSITIONING

The patient is positioned with the head down at a 45° angle on an operating table that easily moves up or down. The patient is placed in a Juers-Derlacki head holder. One inch of hair is shaved from around the ear. The site is then cleaned with alcohol to remove any oils from the skin. Next, a 2-inch Blenderm tape is used to tape the hair out of the field. A povidone-iodine (Betadine) wash is done with a pat dry, then a povidone-iodine preparation is performed with a pat dry. The site is draped, and the complete site is washed and prepared including the ear canal. The surgeon sits on a comfortable secretarial-type chair and has room to move to the head of the table so that he or she can visualize all aspects within the temporal bone. Sometimes, the patient requires additional Trendelenburg positioning to get the sinodural angle or posterosuperior aspect of the tympanic membrane and canal in a directly vertical position with the position of the binocular microscope.

An air drill is used. Facial nerve monitoring is not used, and in more than 1000 patients, only two have had a temporary nerve palsy; none has had a permanent paralysis. Monitoring by ABR is not used. Steroids and diuretics are not routinely provided.

Monitoring by ECoG is not used by the author. Some individuals have found this to be useful as a monitoring procedure during surgery. ECoG is a method of assessing cochlear function, and because the main indication for surgery in these patients is vertigo or vestibular dysfunction, this test and what it indicates over a brief span of time does not seem likely to provide uniformly accurate information regarding an ultimate postoperative result. Progressive Ménière's disease can be compared to a motion picture that fluctuates over a long period of time. Any test for function, such as ECoG, simulates a "snapshot," or an aspect of labyrinthine function at a given point in time and may not describe the overall course of events. Too many intangibles exist relating to healing and morphologic and physiologic considerations to provide a diagnostic test with predictive relevance. The overall clinical picture, defined primarily by the history and secondarily by audiometric information, the experience and judgment of the surgeon, and the cooperation and understanding by the patient constitute the best prognosis for a favorable result.

SPECIAL INSTRUMENTS

The instruments used by the author have been developed and described elsewhere. Typical and routine instruments are used. An air drill is used and diamond burrs are available; however, the most important burrs are cutting burrs, especially those that can be reversed to provide smooth bony surfaces, stoppage of bleeding, and more cutting action than can be achieved safely with the typical diamond burr. All burrs are available and used. Special instruments are a fenestrometer, to demarcate and measure the solid angle, and a large Hough hoe, used first to enter the sac, followed by whirlybirds. No other special instruments are necessary to perform this operation.

SURGICAL TECHNIQUE

Historical Considerations

The first sac operation, by Portmann in 1927,[1] was simply an exposure of the sac, performed with mallet and gouge without benefit of modern-day magnification.[1] The sac was simply incised with a small knife. Others tried the procedure, but relatively few publications appeared in the literature until an important publication by Yamakawa.[10] In 1954, Yamakawa and Naito published an article that dealt with an interesting modification of Portmann's operation for Ménière's disease. The method involved creating a shunt between the endolymphatic sac and cerebrospinal fluid to avoid postsurgical obliteration of the shunt due to granulation tissue, which was experienced with Portmann's method. This shunt operation also included a surgically induced permanent fistula between the endolymphatic sac and the subarachnoid space.[11, 30]

Credit for popularizing endolymphatic sac surgery deservedly goes to William House, who, because of the availability of the operating microscope and modern otologic techniques, made Portmann's operation much safer. In House's technique, the inner wall of the sac was incised, and a communication was created between the endolymphatic sac and the subarachnoid space; a polytetrafluorethylene (Teflon) tube was placed into this aperture to ensure its patency. Because his early success with this technique showed satisfactory results, House abandoned simple drainage in favor of this shunt surgery in 1962.[31] Gardner continues to favor a modification of the endolymphatic sac to subarachnoid shunt procedure.[32]

After this development, the vast majority of published reports described sac procedures confined to the mastoid. In 1966, Shea reported on a series with promising results, in which a Teflon wick was placed from the sac to the mastoid cavity.[33] Subsequently Shambaugh noted that even when he was unable to identify the sac, simple decompression of the dura around the sac seemed to effect satisfactory results.[34, 34a] Graham and Kemink described a similar observation and experience.[35] Plester's technique included a large incision in the sac, through which a triangular piece of silicone sheeting was inserted; the sac was then covered with a free graft of muscle.[36]

The first inner ear valves were implanted in 1975 and 1976 in Sweden by Stahle et al. and in the United States by Arenberg, who developed a one-way valve placed into the endolymphatic sac with a limb of silicone sheeting extending into the mastoid.[37, 38, 38a] Morrison popularized the capillary endolymphatic shunt in a large series of patients.[39] In this technique, a capillary tube is inserted into the lateral end of the endolymphatic duct, with its distal tip inserted into a silicone sheeting sponge. Paparella and Hanson described their method in 1976[14]; it included a wide exposure of the dura, avoiding the skeletonization of the posterior semicircular canal and draining the sac via a T-strut. Spector and Smith, using a similar method, reported 122 cases over a period of 3 years.[40]

Kitahara et al.'s method of drainage was based on an intramastoid opening of the endolymphatic sac and a folding back of the lateral wall of the sac with an insertion of absorbable gelatin sponge (Gelfoam) into its lumen.[41, 42] Futaki and Nomura used the Kitahara method, in comparison to their modified method of the vein-graft drainage procedure, which showed improved results.[43] Austin also confined his surgery to the mastoid with his method of "capillary endolymph dispersement."[44] Goldenburg and Justus,[45] Brown,[46] Chui et al.[47] Ford,[48] Brackmann and Anderson,[49] and Maddox[50] successfully employed endolymphatic sac procedures confined to the mastoid in sizable series of cases.

In 1987, Brackmann and Nissen reported their results with use of an endolymphatic subarachnoid shunt and an endolymphatic mastoid shunt, showing no statistical differences between the two procedures.[51] Shea et al. through detailed examination and measurements from 40 temporal bones, established reference points by which the conservative surgeon can approach the endolymphatic sac below the level of the posterior semicircular canal. These observations make it unnecessary to risk exposure of the blue line of the posterior canal, thus minimizing risk of labyrinthine injury.[52] Endolymphatic procedures confined to the mastoid are more common than those attempting a communication to the subarachnoid space.

Endolymphatic Sac Enhancement

The method for endolymphatic sac enhancement has been modified during a more than 25-year period. Current surgical principles and steps are summarized in the following paragraphs.

A curvilinear postauricular incision in the skin is placed approximately 1 inch behind the mastoid tip. This method helps avoid postoperative depression of the skin into the mastoid cavity. The posterior tip incision helps reduce scar tissue, which can grow from the subcutaneous wound into the region of the sac postoperatively, especially when accompanied by deficient aeration of the mastoid (Fig. 38–3A).

The mastoid cortex is exposed, a complete simple mastoidectomy is done, and the aditus is widened. The incus is always exposed (the only exception being when there is a lack of mastoid air cells) (Fig. 38–3B and C). The aditus ad antrum is opened widely, including a posterior atticotomy, to expose the head of the malleus. Although usually underdeveloped in patients with Ménière's disease, the facial recess (suprapyramidal recess) can also be opened to encourage postoperative aeration of the mastoid cavity, a very important objective. The tegmen mastoideum and mastoid tip are exposed, the posterior bony wall of the canal is thinned, and the depth of drilling in the mastoid cavity is never extended below the dome of the horizontal semicircular canal or the incus, if a safer depth drilling reference is preferred. The purposes of this procedure are to gain good exposure, especially for later in the procedure; to be able to see the incus and horizontal semicircular canal for orientation; and to make possible later measurements—drilling below the dome of the horizontal canal endangers the posteroinferior semicircular canal. The enlarged aditus helps promote drainage and transfer of air between middle ear and mastoid and helps avoid a postoperative aditus-block syndrome (Fig. 38–3D).

By use of the fenestrometer, measurements are made from the fossa incudis 10mm along the axis of the horizontal semicircular canal and 12mm (approximately 45°) from the linea temporalis. The zone of the solid angle (containing the canals) is demarcated so that further surgery will not enter this zone (Fig. 38–3E). These measurements, based on earlier anatomic dissections, create a demarcated zone to protect the canals and to serve as a landmark for further dissection.

The sigmoid sinus is skeletonized and decompressed throughout its length in the mastoid. Bone over Trautmann's triangle is thinned and removed with mastoid curets or a rongeur (see Figs. 38–3F and G). Because the sigmoid sinus is characteristically prominent in an anterior and medial location in Ménière's disease and is often associated with hypopneumatization of air cells and a small or nonexistent Trautmann's triangle, decompression of the sigmoid sinus enhances subsequent decompression of Trautmann's triangle and the contiguous dura below the solid angle.

Immediately below the demarcated bony zone, an infralabyrinthine cell tract is searched for. Here, a shelf of bone is preserved to contain and hold the silicone sheeting spacers to be placed later for a sustained effect of decompression. Often, infralabyrinthine cells do not exist. In restrictive mastoids (sclerotic or diploic), the anteriorly located facial nerve should be watched for and avoided. The purpose is to expose infralabyrinthine dura because the main body of the sac and its lumen often lie within this area and not posterior to the posteroinferior semicircular canal, as depicted earlier in textbooks. This step also helps dural decompression.

The dura contiguous with the decompressed sigmoid sinus is firmly decompressed (pushed down), especially below the solid angle (Fig. 38–3H). Care must be taken not to traumatize dura above the sac, which is often thin; trauma can lead to drainage of spinal fluid. Sometimes, a prominent bony shelf (operculum) exists below the dura on the side by the posterior cranial fossa and can hamper decompression of the dura. Because of anatomic factors, the dura is often tight in this region, and decompression counteracts this tightness and assists sac enhancement later.

The sac is entered beneath the solid angle. Sac epithelium is visualized by use of a Hough hoe. A whirlybird or other instrument helps bluntly and easily identify the lumen, especially toward the infralabyrinthine region (Figs. 38–3H and I). The entrance to the sac should not be opened to the mastoid cavity so as to prevent fibrous or granulation tissue from invading the sac.

One or two silicone sheeting T-struts are placed within the sac. Depending on the size of the lumen, a selection is made of a preprepared small, medium, or large T-strut. The tail of the strut is placed outside the sac between dura and bone. Small, medium, or large "spacers" or strips of silicone sheeting, as many as possible, are folded above and below the sac between the dura and the bone to decompress the dura and contiguous sigmoid sinus permanently. All silicone is

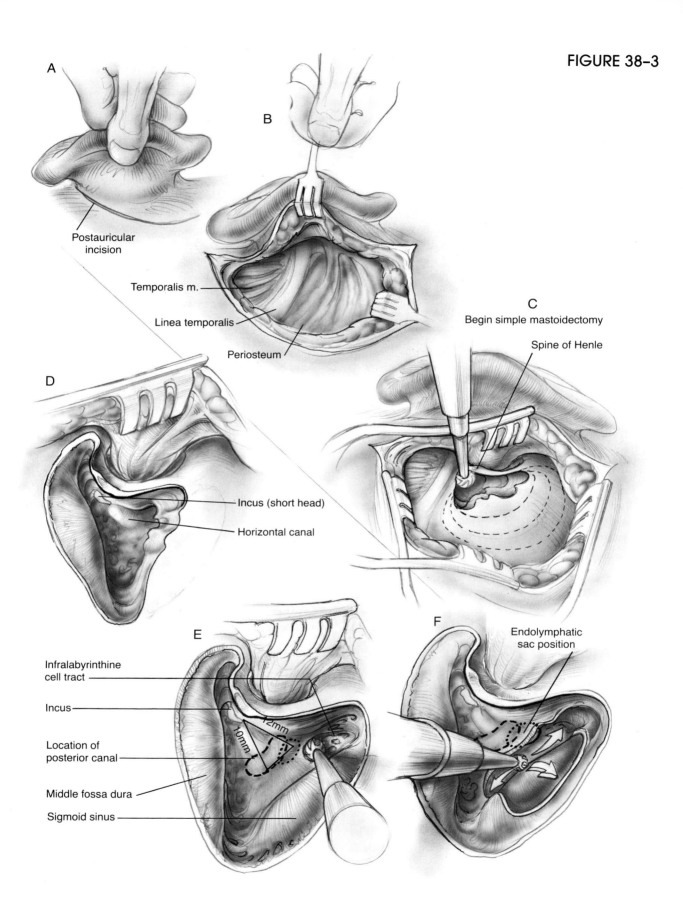

FIGURE 38–3

A

Postauricular
incision

B

Temporalis m.

Linea temporalis

Periosteum

C

Begin simple mastoidectomy

Spine of Henle

D

Incus (short head)

Horizontal canal

E

Infralabyrinthine
cell tract

Incus

Location of
posterior canal

Middle fossa dura

Sigmoid sinus

12mm

10mm

F

Endolymphatic
sac position

FIGURE 38-3 *(continued)*

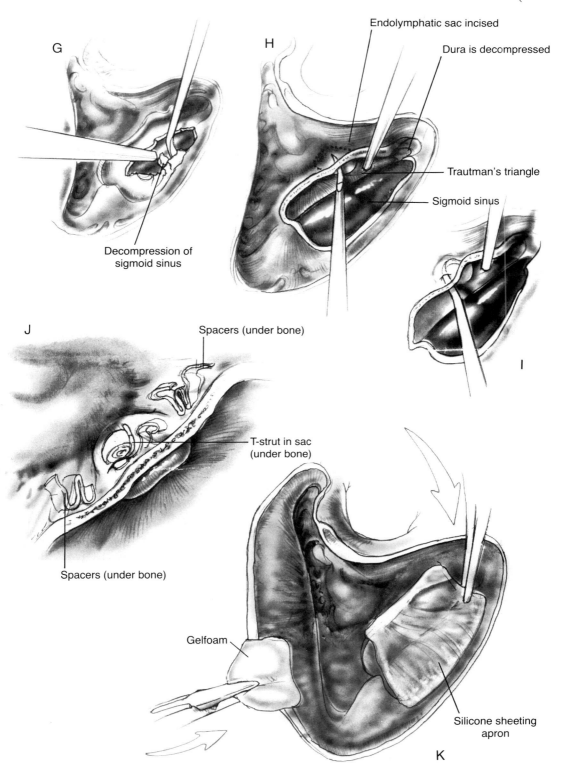

G

Decompression of
sigmoid sinus

H

Endolymphatic sac incised

Dura is decompressed

Trautman's triangle

Sigmoid sinus

I

J

Spacers (under bone)

T-strut in sac
(under bone)

Spacers (under bone)

Gelfoam

Silicone sheeting
apron

K

placed or contained between bone and dura and not in the mastoid. Rubber strips or spacers serve as soft, springlike mechanisms for decompression of dura and sac. T-struts within the lumen enlarge the lumen and help the passive transfer of nanoliters of endolymph. It is important to open and treat the lumen of the sac as well as the surrounding region. This observation is emphasized during revisional sac surgery (Fig. 38–3*J*).

A silicone sheeting apron is placed to cover this region, followed by a large piece or two of absorbable gelatin sponge dipped in a steroid-antibiotic solution and loosely placed to hold the apron in place (Fig. 38–3*K*). The purpose of this step is to help keep fibroblasts from invading the region of the endolymphatic sac. Previous techniques using pedicle grafts, temporalis fascial grafts, and protection by gold foil have been replaced by this original, more effective, and simpler method.

As was done before the lumen of the sac was opened, all bone dust and debris are removed meticulously. Bone dust can enter the middle ear through the aditus and should be irrigated out and removed. All bleeding is stopped, and the wound is closed by use of subcutaneous absorbable sutures followed by skin sutures (vertical or horizontal mattresses) or metal staples. The purpose for this step is to ensure healthy, rapid healing and to avoid infection of the wound.

A ventilation tube is placed in the tympanic membrane, and the middle ear is suctioned through this site. The ventilation tube may not be used if drainage of cerebrospinal fluid occurs. The goal is to promote drainage of operative fluids from the middle ear and mastoid in the immediate postoperative period (2 months). In addition, the tube promotes ventilation to the middle ear and especially the mastoid via the enlarged aditus so as to discourage formation of tissue in the mastoid, both in the short term and long term, and in particular to help avoid aditus block and long-term formation of tissue (granulations, scar, and bone) around the sac, which can lead to subsequent recurrent symptoms and signs of Ménière's disease. The tube has also been helpful in preventing otitis media and barotrauma from flying. The ventilation tube usually extrudes spontaneously in a year or so and is not replaced. The patient's symptoms are not affected when the tube extrudes.

DRESSING THE WOUND AND POSTOPERATIVE CARE

A typical mastoid dressing is applied for the first day, and if the patient has had leakage of cerebrospinal fluid (in fewer than 5 per cent) this dressing may be left on longer. Typically, the dressing is removed and the patient uses no dressing when he or she leaves the hospital the following day.

The patient is hospitalized overnight. Typically, the patient is given empirically amoxicillin or another appropriate broad-spectrum antibiotic to help avoid postoperative inflammation and infection. The patient usually does not require other medication, but if it is required, additional medication is provided. The patient is seen a week later, and the staples or sutures are removed. Although the patient is ambulatory, it takes approximately 2 months for the ear to settle down, at which time an audiogram is usually obtained. Depending on the patient's postoperative status, more frequent visits may be needed. Even after the ear is stabilized and a good result achieved, the patient is advised to have at least an annual or preferably, semiannual, visit to monitor the patient's disease and the status of both labyrinths.

PITFALLS OF SURGERY

In the author's experience, one pitfall of surgery is when a thorough mastoidectomy is not performed. The aditus (often narrow) should be widened to encourage aeration of the mastoid postoperatively. The sigmoid sinus is decompressed routinely; it is almost invariably found in a medial (deep) and anterior position.

Endolymphatic sac surgery can be difficult in many cases because of the pathologic and anatomic characteristics of Trautmann's triangle and surrounding structures. Trautmann's triangle may not exist or be accessible, it may exist in a vertical or horizontal orientation, and it may sometimes exist beneath the sigmoid sinus. Thus, wide decompression of the sigmoid sinus and adjacent dura of Trautmann's triangle can be difficult, depending on these variations.

One should take great care to use a blunt instrument and frequent irrigation when removing bone from the sigmoid sinus because removal of a simple spicule of bone can result in hemorrhage or bleeding from the sinus. Absorbable gelatin sponge is used, followed by adrenalin umbilical tapes gauze, and pressure is applied for a period of time. Then the gelatin sponge can be carefully moved aside, while pressure is still applied, to gain access to the region of the sac underneath the posteroinferior semicircular canal in Trautmann's triangle. The operation is completed.

The subarachnoid space is avoided, but sometimes simple removal of bone above the sac, and especially in elderly patients, will reveal a very thin bluish dura, and cerebrospinal fluid may drain. This is not a serious complication; reverse Trendelenburg's position takes place, pressure is applied, and the operation is completed. If cerebrospinal fluid is draining at the end of the operation, gelatin sponge is packed into this region, followed by adrenalin tapes and gauze packing. The gauze is removed, and once the ear is dry, the wound is closed and the patient advised to keep the head in an upright position and avoid exertion postoperatively. In only one patient has it been necessary to return to the operating room for surgical closure of persistent drainage of cerebrospinal fluid. Cerebrospinal fluid can also flow from trauma to a thin medial wall of the sac. Careful blunt probing of the sac helps avoid this.

One problem can be identification of the sac. The sac is usually easily demarcated and seen, but sometimes it is diffuse without a demarcated border. The sac is typically found beneath and inferior to the posteroinferior canal, and not open in the mastoid. Blunt identification of the lumen helps identify the sac beneath the solid angle. In 97 per cent of patients treated by the author, it has been possible to identify the lumen of the sac. Rarely (in approximately 3 per cent of patients), the sac is so markedly hypoplastic and small that the lumen cannot be found.

Another pitfall is injury to the posteroinferior semicircular canal. This problem has largely been resolved by the measurement, demarcation, and avoidance of the solid angle, as described herein. Key principles include thinning the posterior canal wall and depth drilling above the dome of the horizontal semicircular canal (or incus) in the solid angle. Rarely, the vertical course of the facial nerve can be injured if it is anomalous or, especially, in a tight, sclerotic mastoid. Thinning of the posterior bony canal wall and careful depth drilling, sometimes with a diamond or reverse burr, helps identify the nerve and avoid injury to the nerve.

Hypoplasia of the mastoid air-cell system is commonly seen. A prominent Koerner septum can reduce exposure of the antrum and aditus and must be eliminated. A small number of patients will have no mastoid air cells (sclerotic), and the aditus and landmarks are not seen. The procedure can be accomplished by wide decompression and exposure of the sigmoid sinus. Then, decompression of the sinus and contiguous dura beneath the solid angle permits a narrowed, but usually adequate, exposure of the sac.

A bony shelf sometimes exists as part of the operculum beneath the sac in the posterior cranial fossa. When this happens, it is impossible to decompress the sac, and one has to accept this anatomic anomaly and somehow try to decompress widely around it. An objective is to maintain decompression. Spacers are used for this purpose, below the sac and above the sac, if the dura is not too thin.

Wound healing has been the major problem to date.

This wound is treated with much greater respect than was formerly the case. Many patients have thick subcutaneous tissue, and if that tissue grows into the mastoid postoperatively, it can form a bridge of scar tissue between the postauricular wound (particularly in the region of the tip of the mastoid) and thereby cause reobstruction of the sac. Some patients have smaller mastoids and do not aerate their mastoids well postoperatively, thus encouraging subcutaneous fibrosis to grow into this region and osteoneogenesis to develop subsequently, which can lead to an inadequate result either within a short period of time (if this develops rapidly) or, more typically, over a prolonged period of time. Helpful techniques include meticulous treatment of the wound to stop all bleeding and removal of all bone dust, including bone dust that invariably enters the middle ear and oval window, where it can often result in a small or large conductive hearing loss postoperatively.

Another problem is controlling bleeding from all bony sites. Meticulous care should be taken to stop bony bleeding before the wound is closed. Bony oozing can fill the mastoid with blood, again encouraging fibrosis, and can interfere with aeration of the mastoid, which is essential to getting a good result from this procedure. In instances of revision when we have found the subcutaneous tissue to be thick, we take time to thin it with a plastic scissors to discourage fibrosis from entering the mastoid and region of the sac from the inferior postauricular wound.

RESULTS

The sutures are removed in about a week. The ear is fairly well healed in a week or two, but the patient is advised that it takes about 2 months for the ear finally to settle down from the surgery. In the meantime, the patient is ambulatory and usually functions normally. Many patients are back to work only a few days after surgery. Patients' experience will be individualized because of the vagaries of the disease process and the individual psychological characteristics, attitudes, and ability to heal postoperatively. Medication will be necessary for some patients and not for others.

Patients have also been seen who have had vertigo and other symptoms during the first couple of months postoperatively who have then had a prolonged excellent result over a period of years. Thus, the fact that they have difficulty for the first month or two need not mean that they are going to have a bad result on a long-term basis. Results of this surgery are elimination of vestibular symptoms (in 70 per cent), improvement of them (in 90 per cent), preservation of hearing (in 90 per cent or better), and improvement in hearing (in approximately 30 to 40 per cent). There is a better than 50 per cent chance that the symptoms of pressure and tinnitus will be improved or eliminated as well. A smaller number of patients in the author's series had tinnitus as their chief complaint.

Some patients may require continued medical management but do not require destructive procedures. Clearly one cannot go back and restore function after a destructive procedure, whereas the options for medical, conservative surgical (revision), or destructive procedures are still available to the patient if problems recur.

Silicone sheeting, when placed in the endolymphatic sac, does not cause a severe fibrosis or reaction. During revisional procedures, fibrosis and osteoneogenesis occurred extrinsic to the sac, as a result of wound healing and lack of mastoid aeration in Trautmann's triangle, in the region of the sac and in the mastoid, but not in the lumen of the sac. Typically, at the time of revision, the lumen is intact; there is a yellowish discoloration to the silicone sheeting, suggesting transudation of fluid relating to extracellular ions accumulating in this area, thus substantiating the concept of a change in osmotic potential concomitant with this procedure. In 1984, Belal, in a pathology study of patients who had endolymphatic sac surgery with silicone sheeting, concluded that it did not cause any difficulty.[53] Figure 38–1 shows a temporal bone from the otopathology laboratory at the University of Minnesota from a patient who received sac enhancement surgery; the silicone sheeting was inert, not causing fibrosis or difficulty in the lumen of the endolymphatic sac or around the sac.

COMPLICATIONS

The major complication of endolymphatic sac procedures is 2 per cent deafness or profound hearing loss that usually develops within the first few weeks or within a month or two of surgery. This complication results not so much from entry into the labyrinth as from inflammation in the wound or lack of mastoid aeration postoperatively. Postoperative overt or subclinical and subcutaneous inflammation of the mastoid can invade the endolymphatic sac, causing labyrinthitis and deafness. The wound must be treated meticulously, all bony particles and dust and debris must be cleaned from the wound and its subcutaneous aspects, and all bleeding must be stopped before this wound is closed.

ALTERNATIVE TECHNIQUES

Medical management precedes consideration of conservative surgical management, namely endolymphatic sac enhancement. Vestibular nerve section is reserved for patients who fail conservative management. Destructive labyrinthectomy (rarely necessary) is a last resort. These patients represent a small minority treated in the author's clinic and hospital because the conservative methods of management suffice to control or eliminate symptoms in most patients who have Ménière's disease. Endolymphatic sac revision can be considered for those who have recurrent symptoms (5 to 10 per cent).

During the past 2 years, in selected cases, the author has combined surgery with exposure of the open sac (7 minutes) with absorbable gelatin sponge saturated in streptomycin (or more recently, gentamicin) during endolymphatic sac revision, with successful results. Another useful adjunct to surgery is the extended approach via the facial recess, used in selected cases and in cases of revision in which the mastoid is small and there appears to be aditus block or a potential for aditus block. The facial (suprapyramidal) recess is opened contiguously with the enlarged aditus and posterior attic. This helps the flow of air into the mastoid postoperatively, which helps avoid healing problems and enhances a favorable result.

SUMMARY

A plethora of publications regarding basic science and clinical science aspects of the endolymphatic sac have appeared in the recent literature. Many more studies are needed and can be expected. In the future, the role of the endolymphatic sac in health and disease (e.g., Ménière's disease) will be better understood and its role in treating not only Ménière's disease but also other labyrinthine diseases will unfold.

Acknowledgment

This work was supported in part by NIDCD Grant #8P50 DC-00133 and the International Hearing Foundation.

References

1. Portmann G: The saccus endolymphaticus and an operation for draining the same for the relief of vertigo. Arch Otolaryngol 6: 309, 1927.
2. Portmann M: The Portmann procedure after sixty years. Am J Otol 8(4): 271–274, 1987.
3. Silverstein H: Vestibular neurectomy in the United States—1990. Trans Am Otol Soc 149–156, 1991.
4. Bretlau P, Thomsen J, Tos M, Johnsen NJ: Placebo effect in surgery for Meniere's disease: A three-year follow-up study of patients in a double blind placebo controlled study on endolymphatic sac shunt surgery. Am J Otol 5(6): 558–561, 1984.
4a. Smith WC, Pillsbury HC: Surgical treatment of Meniere's disease since Thomsen. Am J Otol 9: 39–43, 1988.
5. Pillsbury HC, Arenberg IK, Ferraro J, Ackley RS: Endolymphatic sac surgery: The Danish sham surgery study—an alternative analysis. Otolaryngol Clin North Am 92(Pt 1): 113–118, 1983.

6. Stahle J, Stahle C, Med B, Arenberg IK: Incidence of Meniere's disease. Arch Otolaryngol Head Neck Surg 104: 99–102, 1978.
7. Pulec JL: Endolymphatic subarachnoid shunt for Meniere's disease in the only hearing ear. Laryngoscope 91(5): 772–783, 1981.
7a. Morrison AW: Management of Sensorineural Deafness. London, Butterworth's, 1975, pp 109–144.
8. Paparella MM, daCosta SS, Fox R, Yoon TH: Meniere's disease and other labyrinthine diseases. In Paparella MM, Shumrick DA (eds): Otolaryngology: Otology and Neurology. Philadelphia, WB Saunders, 1990.
9. Hallpike CS, Cairns H: Observations on the pathology of Meniere's syndrome. J Laryngol 53: 625–655, 1938.
10. Yamakawa K: Uber die Pathologische Varanderung bei einem Meniere-Kranken. Z Otol 44: 192–193, 1938.
11. Paparella MM, Morizono T, Matsunaga T: Kyoshiro Yamakawa and temporal bone histopathology of Meniere's patients reported in 1938. Arch Otolaryngol Head Neck Surg 118: 660–662, 1992.
12. Paparella MM: Pathogenesis of Meniere's disease and Meniere's syndrome. Acta Otolaryngol (Stockh) 406(Suppl): 10–25, 1984.
13. Liston S, Nissen RL, Paparella MM, daCosta SS: Surgical treatment of vertigo. In Paparella MM, Shumrick DA (eds): Otolaryngology, 3rd ed, Vol II, Otology. Philadelphia, WB Saunders, 1990, pp 1715–1732.
14. Paparella MM, Hanson DG: Endolymphatic sac drainage for intractable vertigo (methods and experience). Laryngoscope 86(5): 697–703, 1976.
15. Miller GW, Welsh RL: Surgical management of vestibular Meniere's disease with endolymphatic mastoid shunt. Laryngoscope 93(Pt 1): 1430–1440, 1983.
16. Paparella MM, Mancini F: Vestibular Meniere's disease. Otolaryngol Head Neck Surg 93(2): 148–151, 1985.
16a. Huang TS, Lin CC: Endolymphatic sac surgery for Meniere's disease: A composite study of 339 cases. Laryngoscope 95 (Pt 1): 1082–1086, 1985.
16b. Williams A, Horton B, Day L: Endolymphatic hydrops without vertigo. Trans Am Otol Soc 35: 116, 1947.
17. Pearson BW, Brackmann DE: Committee on Hearing and Equilibrium: Guidelines for reporting treatment results in Meniere's disease. Otolaryngol Head Neck Surg 93: 579–581, 1985.
18. Meyerhoff WL, Paparella MM, Shea D: Meniere's disease in children. Laryngoscope 88(Pt 1): 1504–1511, 1978.
19. Jackler RK, Luxford WM, Brackmann DE, Monsell EM: Endolymphatic sac surgery in congenital malformations of the inner ear. Laryngoscope 98(7): 698–704, 1988.
20. Paparella MM, Goycoolea MV, Schachern PA: Multiple otological pathologies. Ann Otol Rhinol Laryngol 91: 14–18, 1988.
21. Paparella MM, Mancini F, Liston SL: Otosclerosis and Meniere's syndrome: Diagnosis and treatment. Laryngoscope 94(Pt 1): 623–629, 1984.
22. Paparella MM, Kim CS, Shea DA: Sac decompression for refractory luetic vertigo. Acta Otolaryngol (Stockh) 89(5–6): 541–546, 1980.
23. Huang TS, Lin CC: Endolymphatic sac surgery for refractory luetic vertigo. Am J Otol 12(3): 184–187, 1991.
23a. Paparella MM, deSousa LC, Mancini F: Meniere's syndrome and otitis media. Laryngoscope 93: 1408–1415, 1983.
23b. Huang TS, Lin CC: Surgical treatment of chronic otitis media and Meniere's syndrome. Laryngoscope 101: 900–904, 1991.
23c. Morrison GA, O'Reilly BJ, Chevreton EB, Kenyon GS: Long-term results of revision endolymphatic sac surgery. J Laryngol Otol 104: 612–616, 1990.
24. Nadol JB Jr, Weiss AD, Parker SW: Vertigo of delayed onset after sudden deafness. Ann Otol Rhinol Laryngol 84(6): 841–846, 1975.
25. Paparella MM, Sajjadi H: Endolymphatic sac revision for recurrent Meniere's disease. Am J Otol 9(6): 441–447, 1988.
26. Gya K, Yangihara N: Endolymphatic-mastoid shunt operation: Results of the 24 cases and revision surgery with the Silastic sheet. Auris Nasus Larynx 9(2): 59–66, 1982.
27. House WF, Fraysee B: Revision of the endolymphatic subarachnoid shunt for Meniere's disease. Review of 59 cases. Arch Otolaryngol Head Neck Surg 105(10): 599–600, 1980.
28. Morrison AW: Sac surgery on the only or better hearing ear. Otolaryngol Clin North Am 16: 143–151, 1983.
29. Silverstein H: The effect of the endolymphatic subarachnoid shunt operation on vestibular function. Laryngoscope 88(10): 1603–1611, 1978.
30. Naito T: Notre expérience de l'opération de G Portmann (ouverture du sac endolymphatique dans la maladie de Meniere). Rev Laryngol Otol Rhinol (Bord) 83: 643–645, 1962.
31. House WF: Subarachnoid shunt for drainage of endolymphatic hydrops. Laryngoscope 72: 713–729, 1962.
32. Gardner G: Shunt surgery in Meniere's disease: A follow-up report. South Med J 81(2): 193–198, 1988.
33. Shea JJ: Teflon film drainage of the endolymphatic sac. Arch Otolaryngol Head Neck Surg 83: 316–319, 1966.
34. Shambaugh GE Jr: Surgery of the endolymphatic sac. Arch Otolaryngol Head Neck Surg 83(Suppl): 305–315, 1966.
34a. Shambaugh GE Jr: Effect of endolymphatic sac decompression on fluctuant hearing loss. Otolaryngol Clin North Am 8(2): 537–540, 1975.
35. Graham MD, Kemink JL: Surgical management of Meniere's disease with endolymphatic sac decompression by wide bony decompression of the posterior fossa dura: Technique and results. Laryngoscope 95(Pt 1): 680–683, 1984.
36. Plester D: Surgery of endolymphatic hydrops. J Otolaryngol Soc Aust 3(3): 393–395, 1972.
37. Arenberg IK, Stahle J, Wilbrand H, Newkirk JB: Unidirectional inner ear valve implant for endolymphatic sac surgery. Arch Otolaryngol Head Neck Surg 104(12): 694–704, 1978.
38. Arenberg IK: Results of endolymphatic sac to mastoid shunt surgery for Meniere's disease refractory to medical therapy. Am J Otol 8(4): 335–344, 1987.
38a. Arenberg IK, Balkany TJ: Revision endolymphatic sac and duct surgery for recurrent Meniere's disease and hydrops: Failure analysis and technical aspects. Laryngoscope 92: 1279–1284, 1982.
39. Morrison AW: Cochleostomy or endolymphatic sac surgery for advanced Meniere's disease. Otolaryngol Clin North Am 16(1): 135–142, 1983.
40. Spector GJ, Smith PG: Endolymphatic sac surgery for Meniere's disease. Ann Otol Rhinol Laryngol 92(Pt 1): 113–118, 1983.
41. Kitahara M, Kitano H: Surgical treatment of Meniere's disease. Am J Otol 6(1): 108–109, 1985.
42. Kitahara M, Kitajima K, Yazawa Y, Uchida K: Endolymphatic sac surgery for Meniere's disease: Eighteen years' experience with the Kitahara sac operation. Am J Otol 8(4): 283–286, 1987.
43. Futaki T, Nomura Y: The surgical procedures and evaluation of two modifications of endolymphatic sac surgery: The epidural shunt and vein graft drainage. Acta Otolaryngol (Stockh) 468(Suppl): 117–127, 189.
44. Austin DF: Endolymphatic fistulization. Ann Otol Rhinol Laryngol 93(Pt 1): 534–539, 1984.
45. Goldenburg RA, Justus MA: Endolymphatic mastoid shunt for treatment of Meniere's disease: A five year study. Laryngoscope 93(Pt 1): 1425–1429, 1983.
46. Brown JS: A ten year statistical follow up of 245 consecutive cases of endolymphatic shunt decompression with 328 consecutive cases of labyrinthectomy. Laryngoscope 93(Pt 1): 1419–1424, 1983.
47. Chui RT, McCabe BF, Harker LA: Meniere's disease at the University of Iowa: 1973–1980. Otolaryngol Head Neck Surg 90(4): 482–487, 1982.
48. Ford CN: Results of endolymphatic sac surgery in advanced Meniere's disease. Am J Otol 3(4): 339–342, 1982.
49. Brackmann DE, Anderson RG: Meniere's disease: Results of treatment with the endolymphatic subarachnoid shunt. ORL J Otorhinolaryngol Relat Spec 42(1–2): 101–118, 1980.
50. Maddox HE: Surgery of the endolymphatic sac. Laryngoscope 91(7): 1058–1062, 1981.
51. Brackmann DE, Nissen RL: Meniere's disease: Results of treatment with endolymphatic subarachnoid shunt compared with the endolymphatic mastoid shunt. Am J Otol 8(4): 275–282, 1987.
52. Shea DA, Chole RA, Paparella MM: The endolymphatic sac: Anatomical considerations. Laryngoscope 89: 88–94, 1979.
53. Belal A Jr: Pathology as it relates to ear surgery. IV. Surgery of Meniere's disease. J Laryngol Otol 98(2): 127–138, 1984.

39

Middle Cranial Fossa— Vestibular Neurectomy

UGO FISCH, M.D.
JOSEPH M. CHEN, M.D.

The treatment of Ménière's disease continues to evoke controversy, as evidenced by a multitude of treatment modalities and their claims of efficacy. Medical management in an attempt to alter or stall the course of this condition has proved ineffective, with the exception of symptomatic relief of vertiginous attacks with the use of pharmacologic agents.

In light of the questionable efficacy of endolymphatic sac operation and the undesirable sequelae of a myriad of ablative procedures, vestibular neurectomy has in recent years been accepted as the most effective means to manage recalcitrant and disabling Ménière's disease.

With either the middle fossa or posterior fossa approaches, ablation of vestibular functions and vertigo is reported to be from 85 to 99 per cent,[1-4] greatly exceeding the results of other treatment protocols.

Technical difficulties have been cited by many authors as the major reason for abandoning the middle cranial fossa approach in favor of a predominantly neurosurgical approach from the posterior, especially as collaborative efforts between otoneurology and neurosurgery increase. However, many centers in Europe and South America continue to use the middle fossa approach with great success.[3-6]

The middle cranial fossa vestibular neurectomy performed at the University of Zurich is also known as the transtemporal-supralabyrinthine approach. In contrast to the middle fossa approach of House,[7] which involves significant elevation of the middle fossa dura and retraction of the temporal lobe, the transtemporal-supralabyrinthine access to the internal auditory canal (IAC) is gained through bony reduction, with only minimal retraction of the dura.

PATIENT SELECTION

Patients with unilateral Ménière's disease who suffer incapacitating attacks of vertigo of at least 6 months' duration despite maximal medical therapy are candidates for vestibular neurectomy. These patients usually have residual and fluctuant hearing. Patients with severe-to-profound hearing loss and extremely poor speech discrimination are better managed by a translabyrinthine cochleovestibular neurectomy. The severity of the vertiginous attacks indicative of surgical management is rather subjective and depends more on the patient's functional capacity than on the frequency of attacks.

In bilateral Ménière's disease, surgery could still be contemplated if a dominant side can be identified. Four patients at the University of Zurich underwent bilateral vestibular neurectomies in stages (separated by at least 1 year following good vestibular compen-

sation); surprisingly, postoperative vestibular compensation was shorter and easier after the second operation. These patients have remained symptom-free for 16 to 20 years since surgery. Patients with Ménière's disease suitable for a vestibular neurectomy account for approximately 10 per cent of the whole group.

Unilateral peripheral vertigo without the full spectrum of Ménière's disease may also benefit from vestibular neurectomy.[8] In these patients, it is important to confirm the side of pathology with vestibular function tests if there is no hearing loss to provide a lateralizing sign. Other indications for vestibular neurectomy are rare. Labyrinthine trauma with residual hearing and disabling vertigo after successful stapedectomy with good hearing could be considered.

Contraindications of surgery include the only-hearing ear, signs of central vestibular dysfunction, and poor medical condition. Age over 70 years is a relative contraindication subject to individual assessment.

PREOPERATIVE EVALUATION AND COUNSELING

Prior to surgery, the patient generally undergoes a full auditory-vestibular evaluation that includes full audiometry, electronystagmography, and auditory brain stem response. Electrocochleography and dehydration tests are not part of the test battery performed at the University of Zurich. A high-resolution computed tomographic scan is obtained to rule out a cerebellopontine angle lesion, and it also helps determine perilabyrinthine pneumatization. A Stenver's view is routinely obtained to demonstrate the contours of the floor of the middle cranial fossa as well as the relationship of the meatal plane and superior semicircular canal with respect to the arcuate eminence.

Immunologic evaluation is obtained if autoimmune disorders or significant allergies are suspected. It is not a standard part of the test battery.

Patients are usually referred from other otologists and have been managed conservatively for a prolonged period of time without relief. They are made aware of the efficacy of vestibular neurectomy and its related complications, particularly those pertaining to hearing and facial nerve.

PREOPERATIVE PREPARATION

The patient is premedicated with meperidine (Pethidine, a morphine derivative), 50mg intramuscularly, and atropine, 0.5mg intramuscularly, 30 minutes prior to surgery. A perioperative antibiotic, Chloromycin,

1g intravenously every 8 hours, is started at the time of surgery and continued for the duration of the intravenous infusion, usually for 5 days.

SURGICAL SITE PREPARATION, POSITIONING, AND DRAPING

The night before surgery, the hair over the temporal region is clipped 9cm above and 5cm behind the pinna. This area is shaved and washed with povidone-iodine (Betadine) after the induction of anesthesia.

The patient is secured on the Fisch operating table (Fig. 39–1) in supine position with the head turned to the side. Draping is standard except for a large reservoir plastic bag, which is at the head of the table to catch excess irrigation and blood.

INTRAOPERATIVE MONITORING AND ANESTHETIC CONCERNS

Intraoperative facial nerve monitoring using the Xomed/Treace Nerve Integrity Monitor with percutaneous electromyographic needles is standard. Both unipolar and bipolar stimulating forceps are available. Intracranial pressure is lowered by intraoperative hyperventilation that keeps the P_{CO_2} between 30mm Hg and 40mm Hg. Pharmacologic manipulation with dexamethasone (Decadron, 4mg every 8 hours perioperatively for 4 days) and mannitol (0.5mg/kg intravenously intraoperatively) are also standard. Furosemide is added when necessary. Lumbar cerebrospinal fluid drainage is not routinely performed. Hypotensive anesthesia with sodium nitroprusside is used in most cases to maintain a systolic blood pressure between 80mm Hg and 90mm Hg.

SPECIAL INSTRUMENTS

1. The Fisch operating table (Contraves/Zeiss): motorized table with the center of rotation at the temporal bone, allowing easy remote control for optimal positional changes that can be operated by the scrub nurse or the anesthetist (Fig. 39–1).
2. Articulated middle fossa retractor (Fischer-118200): a self-retaining retractor that allows adjustments in the angle of retraction, tilting, and sideways shifting of the retractor blade (Fig. 39–2).
3. Temporalis muscle retractor (Fischer-118220): a strong, self-retaining retractor with a wide opening span, essential for the exposure of the zygomatic root (Fig. 39–3).

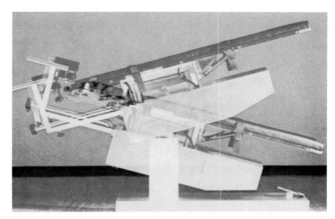

FIGURE 39–1. The Fisch table. (From Fisch U, Mattox DE: Microsurgery of the Skull Base. New York, Thieme, 1988, p 17.)

4. Angled microraspatory (Fischer-118308): specially designed to facilitate dural elevation. Its shoulder retracts the dura away while the tip is used to separate dural attachments to bone (Fig. 39–4).

SURGICAL TECHNIQUE

The objective of the transtemporal supralabyrinthine approach for vestibular neurectomy is to gain access to the IAC through the exenteration of the supralabyrinthine bone, while dural elevation and retraction is limited to no more than 1.5cm. This principle is schematically illustrated in Figure 39–5.

Skin Incision

A preauricular incision is made from approximately the lower edge of the zygomatic root and extended to the temporal area at an angle for about 7cm (Fig. 39–6). The depth of the incision is made to the temporalis fascia, and branches of the superficial temporal artery are divided and clamped. Retraction of the skin edges is provided by securing arterial clamps to the drapes.

Temporal Muscle Flap

After some undermining, the temporalis muscle is well exposed with a self-retaining retractor. Five muscle flaps designed according to Figure 39–7 are developed, elevated from the temporal squama, and retracted away with stay sutures. The temporal squama should be exposed from the root of zygoma to the parietosquamous suture line. A temporalis muscle retractor should be used for the inferior exposure, where the identification of the zygomatic root is essential in the accurate positioning of the craniotomy.

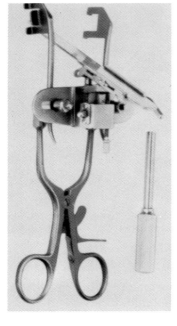

FIGURE 39-2

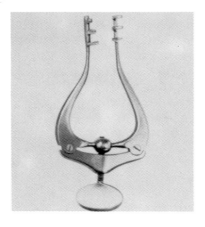

FIGURE 39-3

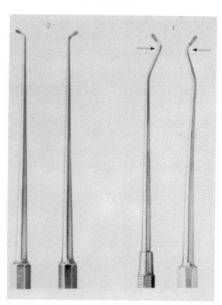

FIGURE 39-4

FIGURE 39-5

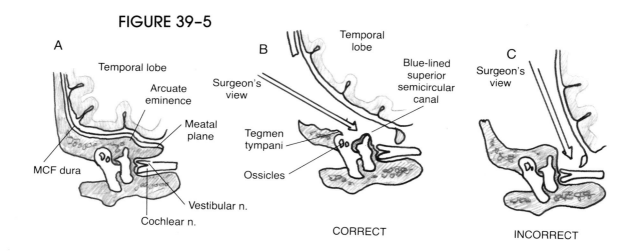

A

Temporal lobe

Arcuate eminence

Meatal plane

MCF dura

Vestibular n.

Cochlear n.

B

Temporal lobe

Surgeon's view

Blue-lined superior semicircular canal

Tegmen tympani

Ossicles

CORRECT

C

Surgeon's view

INCORRECT

FIGURE 39-2. Middle fossa retractor. (From Fisch U, Mattox DE: Microsurgery of the Skull Base. New York, Thieme, 1988, p 426.)

FIGURE 39-3. Temporal muscle retractor. (From Fisch U, Mattox DE: Microsurgery of the Skull Base. New York, Thieme, 1988, p 426.)

FIGURE 39-4. Angled raspatory. (From Fisch U, Mattox DE: Microsurgery of the Skull Base. New York, Thieme, 1988, p 427.)

FIGURE 39-5. A, Middle cranial fossa topography. B and C, Approach. (Redrawn from Fisch U, Mattox DE: Microsurgery of the Skull Base. New York, Thieme, 1988, p 430.)

FIGURE 39-6. Skin incision.

FIGURE 39-7. Muscle flaps.

FIGURE 39-8. Craniotomy.

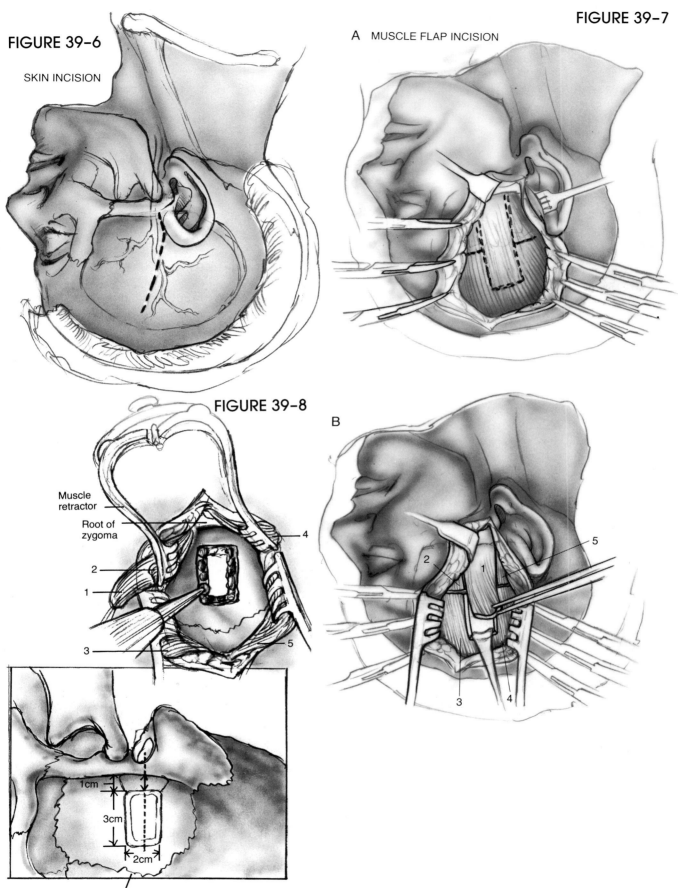

FIGURE 39-6

SKIN INCISION

FIGURE 39-7

A   MUSCLE FLAP INCISION

B

FIGURE 39-8

Muscle
retractor

Root of
zygoma

2

1

3

4

5

5

2

1

3   4

1cm

3cm

2cm

Parietosquamous suture

Craniotomy

A 2cm × 3cm craniotomy (Fig. 39–8) is made perpendicular to, and at least 1cm above, the temporal line, centered over the zygomatic root. This is performed with a 5mm cutting burr on a straight hand piece, and when dura is blue lined, a 4mm diamond burr is used. Care is taken to avoid injuring the dura and branches of the middle meningeal artery, which usually cross the undersurface of the bone flap in its midportion but could be variable.

The bone flap is elevated from the dura with a dura raspatory and is kept in Ringer's solution for later use. The dura is elevated from the edges of the craniotomy to facilitate the placement of the middle fossa retractor. In the region of the middle meningeal arterial branches, this step must be done with care. Sharp edges are removed with a small rongeur to prevent dural laceration.

The craniotomy is extended inferiorly toward the zygomatic arch to the floor of the middle cranial fossa. Lateral extensions of 1cm on each side provide better visibility for the next step (Fig. 39–9).

Dural Elevation

Dural elevation is performed with the microscope. It is perhaps the most delicate part of the operation; if it is not carried out properly, troublesome hemorrhage can occur. It is important to keep the dural elevation to a minimum, and to avoid the region of the middle meningeal artery anteriorly, where significant vascular channels between dura and cranium can be found around the foramen spinosum.

In addition to pharmacologic reduction of the intracranial pressure with mannitol and dexamethasone, cerebrospinal fluid decompression through a small dural incision further facilitates dural elevation. This should be done by first coagulating a small central portion of the dura, and then elevating this area with a hook prior to making an incision (Fig. 39–10).

With the use of a curved suction and angled microraspatory, dural elevation is performed from posteriorly forward. Vascular channels are coagulated and cut close to bone. Persistent bleeding from bone can be controlled by drilling over it with a diamond burr. Oozing from dural vessels at the corners can be con-

trolled with Oxycel packed beneath a cottonoid. Dural attachment to the petrosquamous suture is also coagulated and cut.

Exposure of the Meatal Plane and Arcuate Eminence

Dural elevation is extended to the superior petrosal sulcus and over the arcuate eminence. Moving anteriorly, the meatal plane is reached; this is an area bound by the arcuate eminence, superior petrosal sulcus, and facial hiatus (Fig. 39–11). When the meatal plane is not well defined because of a flat arcuate eminence, it can be identified after blue lining the superior semicircular canal (SCC). If the attachment of the greater superficial petrosal nerve limits the exposure of the meatal plane, it can be separated from dura gently to avoid traction injury of the facial nerve. Meticulous hemostasis in this region is important, and direct coagulation is avoided because of the proximity of the facial nerve.

Introduction of the Middle Cranial Fossa Retractor

The middle cranial fossa retractor can be introduced at this point without the use of a microscope. The self-retaining jaws are firmly attached to the edges of the craniotomy first; the multidirectional stage is slid over the self-retaining portion and loosely placed. The dura is retracted with a suction to reveal the meatal plane to allow the accurate placement of the retractor blade, which is positioned parallel to the superior petrosal sulcus, and its tip just beyond the arcuate eminence (Fig. 39–12). Once the desired position is attained, screws on the multidirectional stage are tightened. Fine adjustments thereafter are done under the microscope.

Bony Exenteration and Blue-lining of the Superior SCC

The operating table is now placed in Trendelenburg's position to better visualize the area over the retractor blade. Bone posterior and lateral to the arcuate eminence is removed with a cutting burr (5 mm), ena-

FIGURE 39-9. Craniotomy extension.

FIGURE 39-10. Cerebrospinal fluid decompression.

FIGURE 39-11. Dural elevation.

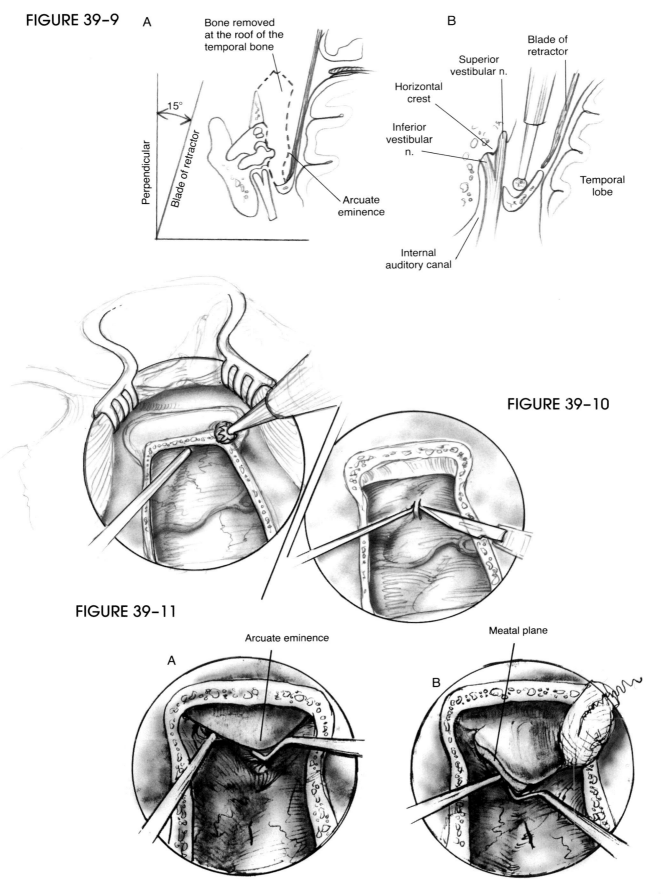

FIGURE 39-9

A

Bone removed at the roof of the temporal bone

15°

Perpendicular

Blade of retractor

Arcuate eminence

B

Superior vestibular n.

Horizontal crest

Inferior vestibular n.

Blade of retractor

Temporal lobe

Internal auditory canal

FIGURE 39-10

FIGURE 39-11

A

Arcuate eminence

B

Meatal plane

bling wider access for the final exposure and the progressive identification of the superior SCC. Because of the variable relationship of the superior SCC to the arcuate eminence, its identification is best accomplished from a posterolateral approach through the pneumatic cells; the yellow compact bone of the SCC can be readily exposed. To blue line the SCC, removal of bone should be done with small diamond burrs (2.3mm, 3.1mm, 4.0mm) in a wide rotatory fashion (Fig. 39–13).

Exposure of the Internal Auditory Canal

Once the blue line of the superior SCC is identified, using a 60° angle centered over the superior canal ampulla, the area of the meatal plane overlying the IAC can be defined. If the surgeon stays within this angle, there is no danger of damaging the facial nerve or the basal turn of the cochlea. The initial drilling is focused over the meatal plane, staying as close as possible to the blue-lined SCC. The axis of the drill is directed medioinferiorly, toward the superior lip of the porus and the medial roof of the IAC. These areas are progressively thinned out, until they are blue lined (Fig. 39–14). The lateral exposure of the IAC involves the removal of bone over the meatal fundus and tegmen tympani (Fig. 39–15). This small triangular area is bordered by the ampulla of the superior SCC, the facial nerve in its labyrinth, and tympanic portions; only 3mm separate the superior ampulla from the genu of the facial nerve. The tegmen is opened if necessary to expose the malleus head and incus for better orientation. Bone over the meatal foramen and the distal superior vestibular nerve (SVN) is removed to clearly identify the vertical crest (Bill's bar), which gives the fundus its inverted W shape. If this is not well defined, the SVN proximal to the ampulla should be exposed. The meatal foramen of the facial nerve should not be unroofed so as to avoid facial nerve injury.

At least one third of the upper circumference of the IAC must be exposed to properly perform a vestibular neurectomy. In particular, the posterior edge of the meatal roof deep in front of the superior SCC must be removed to adequately expose the SVN.

Vestibular Neurectomy

Once the IAC is unroofed from the fundus to the porus, dura over the SVN is opened with a 1.0mm hook. The nerve is identified and cut sharply with a neurectomy knife distal to the vestibular crest (Fig. 39–16). Avulsion of the SVN with a hook is to be discouraged because of the high incidence of deafness associated with this maneuver as a result of either traction or vascular injury to the cochlear nerve.

The meatal dura is incised along the posterior edge toward the porus. The cut end of the SVN is retracted with a microsuction to expose the saccular and singular branches of the inferior vestibular nerve, which are then sectioned with a neurectomy knife. The entire vestibular nerve is stabilized with the suction while the vestibulofacial anastomoses are cut sharply with a neurectomy scissor. The vestibular nerve is now everted with Scarpa's ganglion in full view, which is slightly darker and has a pronounced vascular pattern over it. The vessels are coagulated, and the nerve is then resected proximal to the ganglion (Fig. 39–17). The facial nerve should be only partially exposed, retaining most of its dural cover for protection. The cochlear nerve is hidden beneath the facial nerve and need not be exposed.

Repair of the Floor of the Middle Cranial Fossa

The IAC is covered with a free muscle plug and stabilized with fibrin glue. The tegmen defect is reconstructed with the thinner half of the craniotomy bone flap (wrapped in a gauze and fractured with a rongeur). This bony fragment usually straddles the tegmen defect perfectly and is also fixed in position with fibrin glue (Fig. 39–18). The middle fossa retractor is now removed.

Wound Closure

The dura is elevated with a dural hook and suspended to the adjacent temporalis muscle with 4-0 Vicryl sutures (Fig. 39–19). This action obliterates the dead space between dura and bone and prevents the formation of an epidural hematoma.

FIGURE 39–12. Retractor in position.

FIGURE 39–13. Blue lining the superior SCC.

FIGURE 39–14. Medial internal auditory canal exposure.

FIGURE 39–15. Lateral internal auditory canal exposure.

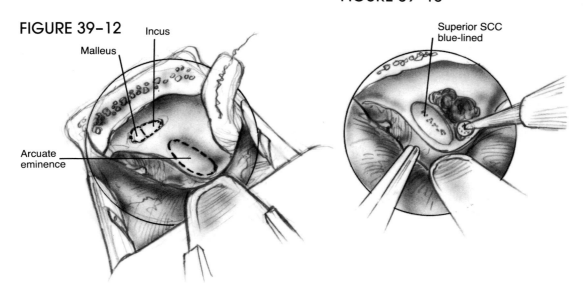

FIGURE 39-12

Malleus

Incus

Arcuate eminence

FIGURE 39-13

Superior SCC blue-lined

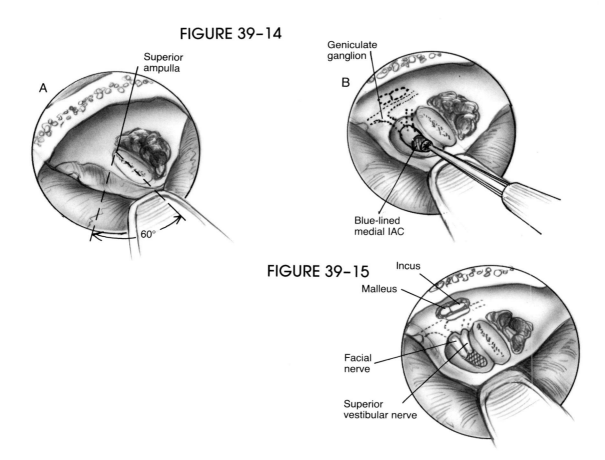

FIGURE 39-14

A

Superior ampulla

60°

B

Geniculate ganglion

Blue-lined medial IAC

FIGURE 39-15

Incus

Malleus

Facial nerve

Superior vestibular nerve

FIGURE 39–16

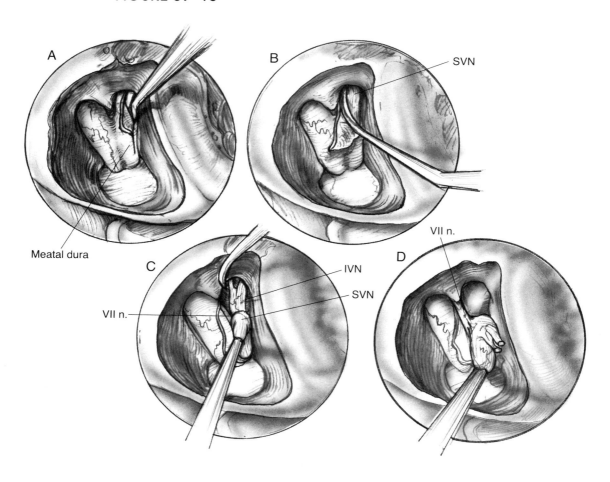

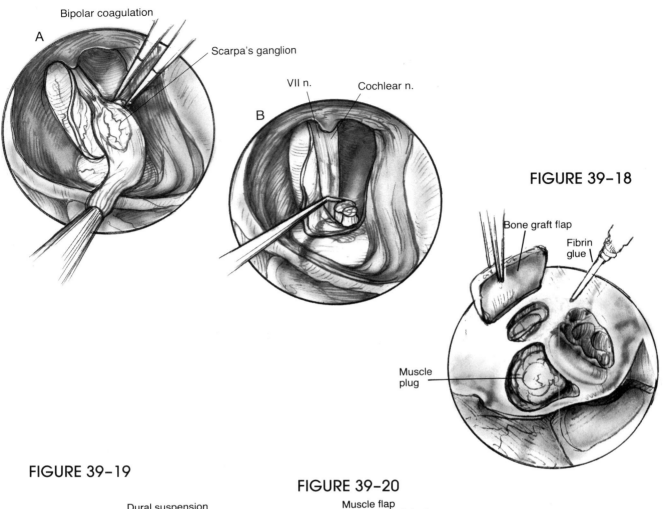

FIGURE 39-17

A

Bipolar coagulation

Scarpa's ganglion

B

VII n.

Cochlear n.

FIGURE 39-18

Bone graft flap

Fibrin glue

Muscle plug

FIGURE 39-19

Dural suspension

4-0 Vicryl

FIGURE 39-20

Muscle flap closure into defect

1

2

3

5

4

The supralabyrinthine cavity is obliterated with the long, anteriorly based muscle flap (#1), which is then sutured to its opposing flap (#5). The craniotomy bone flap is then placed over the upper bony defect, and the remaining muscle flaps are sutured over it (Fig. 39–20).

A single 3.0mm suction drain is placed over the temporalis muscle and brought out through a separate stab incision posteriorly. The skin is closed in two layers with 2-0 catgut and 3-0 nylon sutures.

DRESSING AND POSTOPERATIVE CARE

A compression dressing based over the surgical site is applied following skin closure and is left for 5 days. The patient is kept in the recovery room for at least 24 hours following surgery, with close monitoring of routine and neurologic vital signs every 30 to 60 minutes. Adequate analgesics and antiemetics are ordered to keep the patient comfortably at bed rest. Ambulation and oral intake are started slowly in 2 or 3 days. Subcutaneous heparin is often given in the early convalescent period.

Intravenous antibiotic (Rocephin) is discontinued when the patient no longer requires intravenous infusion. Oral sulfamethoxasole and trimethoprim (Bactrim Forte) is prescribed for at least 5 days. The drain is removed when the daily drainage is less than 10ml, and scalp sutures are removed after 10 days.

TIPS AND PITFALLS

- The root of the zygoma must be well identified to accurately guide the placement of the craniotomy. The craniotomy should be perpendicular to the temporal line, its width not exceeding 2cm, because of the limited opening span of the middle fossa retractor.
- The floor of the middle fossa is usually at the level of the temporal line.
- The elevation of the dura should not exceed 1 cm. The necessary access is gained by removing bone at the floor of the middle fossa.
- If the arcuate eminence is not pronounced (flattened middle fossa), elevate the dura in the area where it is anticipated, that is, in line with the external auditory canal. Remove the pneumatic cells posterior to this region to identify the superior SSC.
- The meatal plane should be identified before the retractor is placed. It is often more medial than expected and may be hidden by a shelf of bone.
- The blue-lined superior SCC is the only essential landmark for the identification of the IAC, but do

not hesitate to open the tegmen tympani to identify the malleus and incus, or the tympanic portion of the facial nerve if more landmarks are needed.
- Adequate exposure of the IAC requires lowering of bone between the superior ampulla and the geniculum of the facial nerve (genicular crest). This procedure must be performed with the utmost care.
- When attempting to identify the blue line of the IAC, work medially toward the porus rather than laterally to avoid injuring the labyrinthine segment of the facial nerve.
- Clearly identify the vertical crest (Bill's bar) by thinning the bone over the meatal foramen. Do not open the meatal dura before the completing bone removal, because the pressure of the cerebrospinal fluid suspends the facial and vestibular nerves against the dura and thus facilitates identification.
- The intrameatal facial nerve often appears to impinge on and partially cover the SVN. The posterior roof of the IAC close to the superior SCC must be removed to adequately expose and identify the cleavage plane between the nerves for the subsequent neurectomy.
- Always cut the vestibular nerve with a neurectomy knife rather than avulse the nerves with a hook. This will prevent inadvertent traction on the cochlear nerve and its vascular supply, resulting in deafness.
- Look for a loop of the anteroinferior cerebellar artery before cutting the nerve close to the porus.
- Lateral suspension of the dura decreases the dead space and will prevent epidural hematoma formation.
- To avoid perforation, overzealous blue lining of the superior SCC and its ampulla is discouraged. If it does occur, however, the area of opening should be immediately covered with a piece of fascia, with bone dust pate or wax applied over it, and stabilized with fibrin glue.
- The basal turn of the cochlea should not be encountered if the 60° rule is followed. However, one must be cautious when a change of color is observed in the bone while working anteriorly. Avoid working deep in the bone without an adequate view around the tip of the burr. Perforation of the basal turn of the cochlea should also be managed as described above.

RESULTS

Follow-up of 3 to 15 years was available in 281 vestibular neurectomy patients operated on at the University of Zurich from 1967 to 1988.[8] Of these, 218 of the operations were for Ménière's disease, including four patients who underwent staged operations for bilateral disease, whereas 63 were for other forms of peripheral vestibular disorder. The success rate of transtemporal vestibular neurectomy to alleviate intractable vertigo was 98.2 per cent for the Ménière's group, and 96.8 per cent for the peripheral vestibular disorder group.

In 61 per cent of the Ménière's group, evidence suggests a stabilizing effect of the surgery on residual hearing. An initial hearing improvement of more than 15dB was seen in 12 per cent of patients, with some improvement lasting for as long as 7 years, but invariably hearing deterioration ensued. Although difficult to explain, this hearing improvement could be due to 1) the division of cochlear efferents traveling with the vestibular nerve, 2) the reduction in the rate of endolymph production resulting from the devascularization and destruction of the dark cell areas, or 3) a change in the parasympathetic innervation of the inner ear subsequent to the sectioning of the olivocochlear bundle in the vestibulofacial anastomosis.[9]

COMPLICATIONS

Vestibular compensation usually takes a few weeks, and most patients are back to work in a few months. Twenty per cent of the patients complain of a mild, transient dizziness after rapid head movements in the first postoperative year. Two per cent suffer from incomplete vestibular compensation and continue to experience disabling vertigo.

Complications specifically associated with this approach include a 2 per cent sensorineural hearing loss. This complication is most likely a result of traction injury of the cochlear nerve and unrecognized perforation of the semicircular canal. Transient facial paresis is seen in 3.2 per cent of cases and occurs 5 to 7 days following surgery. Recovery is expected within 1 to 3 months.

Transient cerebrospinal fluid rhinorrhea during the first 5 to 7 days occurs in 6 per cent of patients, all successfully treated with conservative measures. One case of epidural hematoma was noted and required evacuation with no sequela. No meningitis, temporal lobe epilepsy, and atrophy were associated with this technique.

ALTERNATIVE TECHNIQUES

The indication for endolymphatic sac surgery appears to be hearing preservation only in patients with early-stage disease. The long-term results at the University of Zurich have been equally disappointing as those reported by others.[10-12]

Endolymph-perilymph shunting procedures and peripheral labyrinthine ablation by either medical or surgical means continue to find support in many centers.[13-17] Many are of historical interest only, whereas others, such as intratympanic injection of vestibulotoxic medications, show some promise; however, the results both in the control of vertigo and in preventing hearing loss make them less than desirable alternatives. Vestibular neurectomy and neurotomy (nerve section) appear to offer the best control of intractable vertigo refractory to medical therapy.

Retrolabyrinthine and retrosigmoid vestibular nerve sections[1, 2, 11] have been recently proposed as alternatives to the middle fossa (transtemporal-supralabyrinthine) vestibular neurectomy. It is, however, more logical to divide the vestibular nerve fibers in the distal IAC where fibers are distinct to achieve a complete section, while preserving the cochlear nerve. Also, the resection of the vestibular nerve, including Scarpa's ganglion, ensures that regeneration does not occur. Furthermore, one is less likely to encounter large vessels in the distal portion of the IAC. These three important anatomic considerations are not adequately addressed with the posterior fossa approaches and must be kept in mind when comparing long-term results of the various surgical options.

Although the surgical access to the IAC in the transtemporal-supralabyrinthine approach is narrower compared with that of the standard middle fossa approach, the dangers associated with temporal lobe retraction are practically eliminated. The posterior fossa approach entails more risks of severe cerebrospinal fluid leaks, meningitis, deafness, permanent facial paralysis, and intracranial hemorrhage, not to mention a very common sequela of permanent headache[2] that is often downplayed.

We concur that the transtemporal-supralabyrinthine approach is challenging and demands a thorough knowledge of the temporal bone; however, these challenges are similar to those of other neurotologic procedures.

References

1. House JW, Hitselberger WE, et al.: Retrolabyrinthine section of the vestibular nerve. Otolaryngol Head Neck Surg 92: 212–215, 1984.
2. Silverstein H, Norrell H, et al.: Microsurgical posterior fossa vestibular neurectomy: An evolution in technique. Skull Base Surg 1: 16–25, 1991.
3. Fisch U, Mattox D: Microsurgery of the Skull Base. Thieme Medical Publishers, New York, 1988.
4. Garcia-Ibanez E, Garcia-Ibanez JL: Middle fossa vestibular neurectomy: A report of 373 cases. Otolaryngol Head and Neck Surg 88: 486–490, 1980.
5. Castro D: Transtemporal supralabyrinthine vestibular neurectomy for Ménière's disease. In Fisch U, Yasargil MG (eds): Neurological Surgery of the Ear and Skull Base. Berkeley, Kugler & Ghedini Publications, 1989.
6. Portmann M, Sterkers JM, Charachon R, Chouard CH: Le conduit auditif interne-anatomie, pathologie, chirurgie. Paris, Librairie Arnette, 1973, pp 102–117.

7. House WF: Surgical exposure of the internal auditory canal and its contents through the middle cranial fossa. Laryngoscope 71: 1363–1365, 1961.
8. Kronenberg J, Fisch U, Dillier N: Long-term evaluation of hearing after transtemporal supralabyrinthine vestibular neurectomy. *In* Nadol JB (ed): The Second International Symposium on Ménière's Disease. Amsterdam, Kugler & Ghedini Publications, 1989, pp 481–488.
9. Chouard CH: Acousticofacial anastomosis in Ménière's disorder. Arch Otolaryngol Head Neck Surg 101: 296–300, 1975.
10. Bretlau P, Thomsen J, Tos M, Johnsen NJ: Placebo effect in surgery for Ménière's disease: Nine-year follow-up. Am J Otol 10: 259–261, 1989.
11. Glasscock ME, Jackson CG, Poe DS, Johnson GD: What I think of sac surgery. Am J Otol 10: 230–233, 1989.
12. Brown JS: A ten year statistical follow-up of 245 consecutive cases of endolymphatic shunt and decompression with 328 consecutive cases of labyrinthectomy. Laryngoscope 93: 1419–1424, 1983.
13. Schuknecht HF: Cochleosacculotomy for Ménière's disease: Theory, technique, and results. Laryngoscope 92: 853–854, 1982.
14. Pennington CL, Stevens EL, Griffin WL: The use of ultrasound in the treatment of Ménière's disease. Laryngoscope 80: 578–581, 1980.
15. Wolfson RJ: Labyrinthine cryosurgery for Ménière's disease—Present status. Otolaryngol Head Neck Surg 92: 221–227, 1984.
16. Shea J: Perfusion of the inner ear with streptomycin. Am J Otol 10: 150–155, 1989.
17. Moller C, Odkvist LM, Thell J, et al.: Vestibular and audiologic functions in gentamycin-treated Ménière's disease. Am J Otol 9: 383–391, 1989.

40

Retrolabyrinthine/ Retrosigmoid Vestibular Neurectomy

HERBERT SILVERSTEIN, M.D.

SETH I. ROSENBERG, M.D.

Today, vestibular neurectomy is an accepted procedure to preserve hearing and relieve vertigo associated with unilateral vestibular disorders refractory to medical management. A survey of the American Otological Society and the American Neurotologic Society in 1990 indicated that almost 3000 vestibular neurectomies had been performed in the United States.[1] Ninety-five per cent of these were posterior fossa vestibular neurectomies, either retrolabyrinthine, retrosigmoid, or combined approaches. In this series, representing the experience of 58 surgeons, the cure rate was greater than 90 per cent, as was the reported patient satisfaction. The goals of vestibular neurectomy are to cure vertigo by completely denervating the vestibular system while preserving patients' hearing at the preoperative level. Classical Ménière's disease is the most common inner ear disorder treated by vestibular neurectomy; however, the procedure is also useful in treating selected cases of recurrent vestibular neuronitis, traumatic labyrinthitis, and vestibular Ménière's disease.

From 1978 to 1985, the retrolabyrinthine vestibular neurectomy (RVN) approach (anterior to sigmoid sinus) was used to transect the vestibular nerve in the posterior fossa. From 1985 to 1987, the retrosigmoid-internal auditory canal (RSG-IAC) approach (posterior to sigmoid sinus) was used, and from 1987 to the present, the combined retrolabyrinthine-retrosigmoid (combined R-R) approach (posterior to the sigmoid sinus) was used.[2–5] In this chapter, 171 consecutive vestibular neurectomies performed for the treatment of Ménière's disease using the RVN (78 cases), RSG-IAC (14 cases), and the combined R-R (79 cases) approaches are presented.

PATIENT SELECTION

Patient's choice is the strongest consideration in the decision of when to perform vestibular neurectomy. Some patients may have one or two severe Ménière's attacks a month, and their lifestyles may not be sufficiently affected to warrant a surgical procedure to correct their problem. Other patients with only two or three attacks a year can be so severely affected that they live in constant dread of the next recurrence. In some patients, the loss of a warning signal (e.g., change in hearing, tinnitus, or aural fullness) prior to their attack of vertigo is what motivates them to have surgery.

Contraindications to vestibular neurectomy include bilateral vestibular disease, poor medical condition, ataxia or other indications of a possible significant central nervous system involvement, and vertigo arising from an only-hearing ear. Unless a patient is experiencing an acute Ménière's attack, he or she should

be able to perform a tandem gait test reasonably well. Vertigo from an ear with very poor hearing (i.e., greater than 80dB speech reception threshold or less than a 20 per cent discrimination score) is usually more appropriately treated with a transcochlear eighth-nerve section.[6, 7]

A previous endolymphatic sac operation or mastoidectomy is not a contraindication for posterior fossa vestibular neurectomy. When the patient is healthy and has good balance function, old age is also not a concern. Vestibular neurectomy has been done successfully in patients over 70 years old with excellent results and little additional morbidity. However, elderly persons usually take longer to regain good balance function postoperatively than do younger individuals.

PREOPERATIVE EVALUATION AND PATIENT COUNSELING

Before surgery can be considered, objective evidence of unilateral inner ear disease should be provided by audiogram, electronystagmography, or electrocochleography. An auditory evoked brainstem response helps rule out a central disorder and provides a baseline for intraoperative eighth-nerve monitoring. A high-resolution computerized tomographic scan is obtained before surgery primarily to identify the singular canal in the internal auditory canal (IAC) and to measure the overall length of the IAC. These dimensions are significant if the posterior rim of the IAC is drilled to expose the eighth nerve within the canal. A magnetic resonance imaging study is generally not required.

Patients are told that the goals of vestibular neurectomy are to relieve their episodic vertigo and preserve their hearing. They should expect to have vertigo immediately after surgery that usually lasts 3 to 5 days. Imbalance may last for several weeks or months, but most patients resume their normal activities within 3 weeks. All patients are encouraged to increase their activity as soon as possible after surgery.

SURGICAL ANATOMY

The surgical anatomy of the right ear is described as if the patient were supine and the head were turned away from the surgeon (Fig. 40–1). At the labyrinthine end of the IAC, six separate branches of the seventh and eighth cranial nerves enter the temporal bone: the facial nerve, nervus intermedius, superior vestibular, saccular, singular (posterior ampullary), and cochlear nerves. The transverse (falciform) crest,

FIGURE 40-1

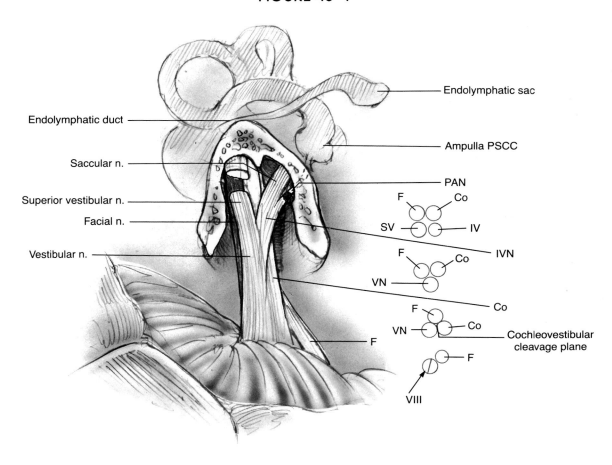

FIGURE 40-1. Anatomy of the seventh and eighth cranial nerves as seen from otologic surgical position. Note 90° rotation of cochlear and vestibular nerves. PSCC: posterior semicircular canal; PAN: posterior ampullary nerve; SV: superior vestibular nerve; IVN: inferior vestibular nerve; VN: vestibular nerve; Co: cochlear nerve; VIII: eighth cranial nerve; F: facial nerve.

which lies in a perpendicular plane, divides the lateral IAC into superior and inferior compartments. A vertical crest of bone (Bill's bar) separates the superior half of the IAC into an anterosuperior quadrant containing the facial nerve and nervus intermedius, and a posterosuperior quadrant containing the superior vestibular nerve. Anteriorly and inferior to the transverse crest lies the cochlear nerve, hidden from the surgeon by the inferior vestibular nerve. The singular nerve lies in a separate canal (singular canal) that enters the IAC in the posteroinferior quadrant, approximately 2mm medial to the transverse crest. This reliable landmark is the point at which drilling stops when the posterior wall of the internal auditory canal is being surgically removed. The inferior vestibular nerve is formed when the saccular nerve joins the singular nerve just medial to the transverse crest.

The superior vestibular nerve innervates the superior semicircular canal, horizontal semicircular canal, utricle, and part of the saccule. The inferior vestibular nerve innervates the saccule (saccular nerve) and the posterior semicircular canal (singular nerve).

The separation between the cochlear and vestibular nerves, the cochleovestibular cleavage plane at the labyrinthine end of the IAC, lies in the superoinferior plane, with the vestibular nerves occupying the posterior half of the IAC. Between the transverse crest and the porus acusticus, the superior and inferior vestibular nerves fuse. Laterally, within the IAC is a constant, well-delineated cleavage between these two nerves.[8]

At the distal end of the IAC, the cochlear nerve lies anterior to the inferior vestibular nerve. The cochlear and inferior vestibular nerves fuse within the IAC, just medial to the transverse crest. The cochlear and vestibular nerves then rotate 90° so that the cochlear nerve, which at first lies anterior to the inferior vestibular nerve, rotates to lie caudal and inferior to the vestibular nerve as it enters the porus acusticus.[9] Most of the rotation occurs within the IAC; only slight rotation occurs in the cerebellopontine angle (Fig. 40–1). The cochlear nerve leaves the brainstem caudal and slightly dorsal to the vestibular nerve. The flocculus of the cerebellum covers 5mm of the eighth cranial nerve at the brainstem.

After the vestibular and cochlear nerves fuse within the IAC, the cochleovestibular cleavage plane usually persists grossly and histologically.[8] The vestibular fibers remain segregated and are cephalad or superior; the cochlear fibers are caudal or inferior. Occasionally, inferior vestibular fibers will run with the cochlear nerve, whereas the efferent cochlear fibers run in the inferior vestibular nerve. Near the labyrinth, the cochleovestibular cleavage plane runs in a superoinferior direction and, because of rotation, in an anteroposterior direction in the cerebellopontine angle. In the cer-

ebellopontine angle, the cochleovestibular cleavage plane appears grossly as a fine septum along the eighth cranial nerve in 75 per cent of patients.[8]

In the lateral IAC, the facial nerve is positioned in the anterosuperior quadrant, anterior to the superior vestibular nerve, running to a ventral-caudal position as it exits the brainstem. The facial nerve remains ventrally positioned and hidden by the eighth cranial nerve along much of its entire course. In the IAC, the facial nerve is connected to the superior vestibular nerve by the Rasmussen facial-vestibular anastomosing fibers, and in the cerebellopontine angle, the facial nerve lies adjacent to, but distinct from, the eighth nerve. Although it remains hidden from the surgeon's view by the eighth cranial nerve, the facial nerve can easily be seen by gentle retraction of the superior vestibular nerve in the IAC or the eighth nerve in the cerebellopontine angle. The facial nerve exits the brainstem 3mm ventral and usually caudal to the eighth nerve root entry zone. In the IAC, the seventh nerve appears whiter than the eighth nerve; in the cerebellopontine angle it appears more gray.

The nervus intermedius, which may consist of a single nerve or multiple bundles, runs between the seventh and eighth nerves through their entire course. The nervus intermedius enters the brainstem closest to the eighth nerve and usually delineates the cochleovestibular cleavage plane on the anterior surface of the eighth nerve.

PREOPERATIVE PREPARATION

The shave preparation that has been done at the patient's bedside is examined for adequacy. Any excess hair is removed in the operating room. Perioperative intravenous antibiotics are given, usually nafcillin (2gm) in three doses: the first preoperatively, the second during surgery, and the third 8 hours later. Intravenous mannitol (1.5gm/kg to a maximum of 100gm) is administered when the drilling begins, causing contraction of the cerebellum and allowing a wider exposure of the cerebellopontine angle.

SURGICAL SITE PREPARATION, DRAPING, AND POSITIONING

Injections are made with 1 per cent lidocaine (Xylocaine) and epinephrine 1:100,000 into the postauricular area. A plastic Steri-Drape (#1010, 3M, Minneapolis, MN) is cut into thirds and used to border the surgical area. Benzoin is used to secure the drape. The skin preparation is done using gel prep, a thick gelatin-like povidone-iodine. The area is blotted dry, and a Steri-Drape II (#20–45) is placed over the surgical site. The sterile area is covered with a split-contoured sheet. A hole is cut in the drape for placement of the Silverstein wrist rest (Diversatronics, Norristown, PA) bar; the horseshoe and bar are inserted and adjusted to the proper height, and a sterile drape tape is used to seal the opening. The wrist rest allows the surgeon to comfortably support his or her wrists on the horseshoe during surgical manipulations.[10] An abdominal preparation is done on the left lower quadrant. Abdominal adipose tissue is obtained at the onset of the procedure; a suction drain is used to prevent hematoma formation. This tissue is used to obliterate the surgical defect in the RVN and the combined R-R vestibular neurectomy procedures.

A magnetic mat to hold instruments is placed on the drapes across the patient's chest. A Ziess OPMI 6 (Zeiss, Thornwood, NY) on a Neuro Contravus I base (Zeiss) microscope with a $250\times$ magnification lens is used. The Super Lux Light source (Dyonics, Andover, MA) provides brilliant illumination during the surgical procedure. The 35mm Contax camera and the Sony 3CCD camera DXC 750 MD are attached to the microscope beam splitter to document parts of the procedure. One of the two television monitors in the room can be viewed by the surgeon, and the other can be seen by the scrub technician.

To reduce tangling of suction tubing and electrical cords, a polyvinyl chloride (PVC) cord holster attaches by Velcro straps to the undersurface of the Mayo stand. The drill cords, the monitor cords, and the suction and irrigation tubes are placed through PVC tubes, which keeps them from getting tangled on the surgical field. Five-inch-long PVC tubes, glued to a flat, plastic plate and attached to the end of the Mayo stand, are used to hold drills, suction tips, and cautery tips. Two suction irrigator setups with silicone tubing are used with Essar suction tips (Xomed-Treace, Jacksonville, FL). A 1000ml saline irrigation bag is placed inside a pneumatic blood pressure cuff applying constant pressure of 150psi to deliver a constant stream of irrigation fluid. The Essar irrigation suction tips contain a pressure-sensitive valve controlled by the thumb and forefinger that allows the fluid to pass through the irrigation tip; the index finger applied to the regulator hole controls the suction.

The facial nerve is monitored by both mechanical pressure sensor (WR-S8 monitor, WR Medical Electronics, Stillwater, MN) and electromyography (Brackmann monitor, WR Medical Electronics, Stillwater, MN) connected to the Wiegand Computer (WR Medical Electronics, Stillwater, MN) and NIM-2 (Xomed-Treace, Jacksonville, FL).[11] The hook wires and needle electrodes for the Brackmann electromyographic monitor are placed in the orbicularis oris and the frontalis muscles. The strain gauge sensor for the Silver-stein WR-S8 facial nerve monitor-stimulator is placed in the patient's mouth, and the set screw is tightened. The sensor is tested by tapping on the face, which activates the alarm. The cable from the sensor is secured with a strip of Micropore tape to the patient's neck. This helps eliminate artifact created by motion of the drapes pulling the sensor wires during surgery. A molded surgical mask (3M, Minneapolis, MN) is placed over the sensor and taped into place to prevent the surgical drapes from putting pressure on the mouth piece and setting off the alarm. A slit is made in the mask to allow for the endotracheal tube.

To help preserve serviceable hearing during vestibular neurectomy, eighth nerve action potentials in combination with brainstem auditory evoked responses and electrocochleography have been used. Electrodes are placed on the forehead (ground) and ear lobe for intraoperative monitoring of brainstem and direct eighth nerve potentials using the Nicolet Pathfinder (Nicolet, Madison, WI). Intraoperative eighth nerve monitoring enhances the surgeon's ability to preserve hearing and allows the surgeon to inform the family immediately after surgery that hearing will probably be unchanged, if appropriate.[12, 13]

A major difficulty encountered during vestibular neurectomy in the posterior fossa is that in approximately 25 per cent of cases, the cochleovestibular cleavage plane is not readily identifiable.[8] Recently, a flushed-tipped, bipolar electrode recording probe was used to directly record responses to monaural click stimuli from the cochlear nerve, but not from surrounding tissue. This technique has been used to help identify the cochleovestibular cleavage plane.[14]

SPECIAL INSTRUMENTS

Several unique instruments have been developed for vestibular neurectomy (Fig. 40–2).[15] A modified Penfield elevator is used to elevate bone of the endolymphatic sac or dura, so that a small rongeur can be used to remove this bone quickly. The Silverstein lateral venous sinus retractor (Storz)[16] is used to compress and retract the lateral venous sinus posteriorly to provide greater exposure of the posterior fossa during retrolabyrinthine vestibular neurectomy. The arachnoid dissector allows the surgeon to incise arachnoid and release cerebrospinal fluid from the cerebellopontine angle cistern. A long sickle knife is used to start the separation between the cochlear and vestibular nerves. The nerve separator is a blunt, slightly curved instrument used to complete the separation developed in the cochleovestibular cleavage plane. A 3mm mirror is used to view the eighth-nerve complex from the anterior side. The malleable nerve hook is used when it is necessary to develop a cleav-

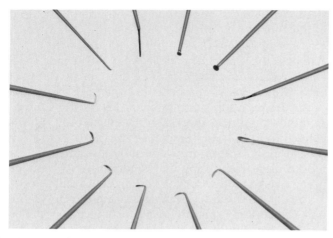

FIGURE 40-2. The series of microsurgical instruments for vestibular neurectomy in the posterior fossa.

age plane from the anterior aspect of the nerve. Leutje microscissors are used to transect the vestibular nerve. Round knives (1mm, 2mm, and 3mm) are used to separate the eighth nerve from the flocculus and the facial nerve if they are intimately related. All these instruments are manufactured by Storz Instrument Company, St. Louis, MO.

These instruments are also available with insulated handles, which can be attached via the "SACS" (adapter for continuous stimulation) to the Silverstein WR-S8 facial nerve monitor or Brackmann monitor (WR Medical Electronics, Stillwater, MN). The instruments can then become electrical probe tips as well as dissectors.

SURGICAL TECHNIQUE

Middle Fossa Vestibular Neurectomy

From 1963 to 1978, the middle fossa (subtemporal) approach was exclusively used by the senior author to section the vestibular nerve. Results for vertigo relief were good, but the procedure was formidable, anatomic landmarks were difficult, and complications, such as facial nerve weakness or deafness, occurred.[17, 18] Patients over 60 years of age were generally not candidates. The procedure was technically difficult and carried a high risk of complications; thus many patients who had significant disability were not enthusiastically offered a middle fossa vestibular neurectomy. This procedure is discussed in greater detail in Chapter 39.

Posterior Fossa Vestibular Neurectomy

Retrolabyrinthine Approach

In 1978, the senior author developed the RVN approach to the posterior cranial fossa for vestibular neurectomy.[19, 20] Although the approach was previously used for trigeminal nerve section, its application for selective vestibular nerve section had not been described.[21]

A 4cm × 5cm anteriorly based U-shaped postauricular incision is made (Fig. 40–3). The flap is elevated with the periosteum and postauricular muscles as one layer. A simple mastoidectomy is performed, and the sigmoid sinus and posterior fossa dura just behind the sinus and in front of it are exposed. The endolymphatic sac is widely exposed and the bone overlying the posterior semicircular canal identified. The sigmoid sinus is collapsed with a retractor, and the dura incised in a C shape anterior to the sigmoid sinus based on the labyrinth (Fig. 40–4). A Penrose drain is placed over the cerebellum, which is gently retracted until the arachnoid is opened with a blunt instrument (arachnoid knife) to allow cerebrospinal fluid to escape. The cerebellum will fall away from the temporal bone allowing exposure of cranial nerves 5, 7, 8, 9, 10, and 11. After the cleavage plane is visualized under high-power magnification, a longitudinal incision is made in the cleavage plane, the cochlear and vestibular fibers are separated, and the vestibular nerve is transected.

Several landmarks are helpful in finding the cleavage plane. The vestibular nerve often appears grayer, and the cochlear nerve whiter; the cochlear fibers are more numerous, averaging 31,000, whereas the vestibular fibers average 18,000. A fine blood vessel frequently courses on the surface between the cochlear and vestibular fibers. A mirror can be used to view the anterior surface of the eighth nerve because the cleavage plane is sometimes more visible from this surface. The nervus intermedius, which usually lies in the cleavage plane, can also be seen anteriorly. A bipolar electrode recording probe has been recently developed to identify a physiologic cleavage plane.[14] The superior half of the eighth cranial nerve is transected when a cleavage plane cannot be readily identified. Most vestibular fibers will be cut, and most cochlear fibers will be spared through this technique. The dura is closed with three or four interrupted 4-0 silk sutures, and the mastoid cavity is filled with abdominal adipose tissue. Unfortunately, this approach results in a 10 per cent incidence of cerebrospinal fluid leak.[3]

FIGURE 40–3. A 4cm × 5cm U-shaped postauricular incision used for all approaches.

FIGURE 40–4. The posterior fossa as seen through the retrolabyrinthine approach.

FIGURE 40-3   FIGURE 40-4

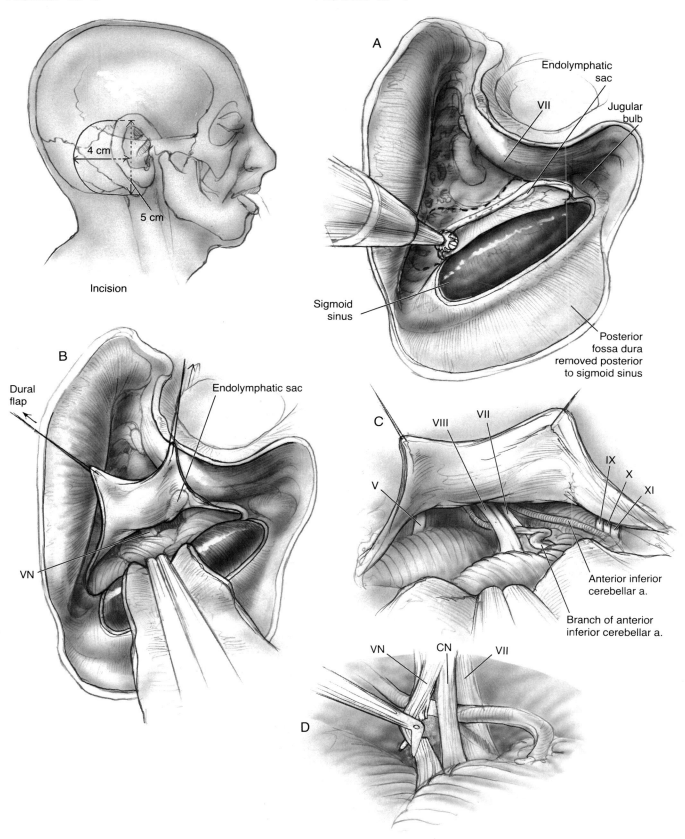

Incision

Retrosigmoid–Internal Auditory Canal Approach

In 1985, in an attempt to perform a more complete vestibular neurectomy nearer to the labyrinth, to improve vertigo relief and hearing preservation, and to decrease the incidence of cerebrospinal fluid leak, the RSG-IAC approach was developed.[22] Because the cleavage plane between cochlear and vestibular fibers is more completely developed within the IAC, a more complete and selective vestibular neurectomy can be performed by cutting the nerve within the IAC.

In this procedure, a posterior fossa craniotomy is performed immediately behind the lateral sinus, and the cerebellum is retracted to give exposure to the seventh and eighth cranial nerves and the IAC. The first major landmark seen in the posterior fossa above the jugular foramen is the white linear fold of dura, the jugular dural fold (Herb's fold). The jugular dural fold extends approximately 2cm from the anterior aspect of the foramen magnum overlying the junction of the lateral sinus and jugular bulb and attaching to the temporal bone 7mm medial to the endolymphatic duct. The jugular dural fold lies 7mm to 9mm lateral to the exit of the ninth nerve. The anterior aspect of the fold usually points to the eighth cranial nerve, which is 7mm to 10mm medial. The posterior wall of the IAC is removed to the singular canal, thereby exposing the branches of the eighth cranial nerve (Fig. 40–5). The superior vestibular nerve and the singular nerve are sectioned. The inferior vestibular fibers that innervate the saccule are not divided because of their close association with cochlear fibers. The saccule has no known vestibular function in humans, so sparing these fibers does not result in postoperative vertigo attacks.

This procedure offers several advantages over the RVN. No abdominal fat is needed to fill the defect; thus, the procedure can be performed on thin patients. Because the exposure does not enter the mastoid, patients who have had chronic mastoiditis, a sclerotic mastoid, or an anterior-lying sigmoid sinus can be candidates for the RSG-IAC approach.

Combined Retrolabyrinthine-Retrosigmoid Approach

A further evolution of the vestibular neurectomy procedure, the combined R-R approach, was developed in 1987.[23] The combined R-R approach incorporates the advantages of the RVN and RSG-IAC approaches and also allows the surgeon to assess the cochleovestibular cleavage plane in the posterior fossa and decide where the neurectomy should be performed. If a good cochleovestibular cleavage plane exists, the vestibular nerve section will be done in the cerebellopontine angle. If not, the IAC can be opened and the superior vestibular and posterior ampullary nerves sectioned within the IAC. In this approach, a limited mastoidectomy is done. The sigmoid sinus is exposed from the transverse sinus inferiorly 3cm, and the posterior fossa dura is exposed for 1.5cm posterior to the sigmoid sinus. The dural incision is made 3mm behind and parallel to the sigmoid sinus for 2.5cm (Fig. 40–6). The sigmoid sinus is retracted anteriorly using stay sutures placed in the dural cuff. This provides an improved wide exposure of the posterior wall of the temporal bone and posterior fossa without retraction of the cerebellum. After the cerebellopontine angle cistern is opened, the eighth nerve is examined, and, if a cleavage plane is present, the vestibular nerve section is performed in the cerebellopontine angle, as in the retrolabyrinthine approach (Fig. 40–7). If no cleavage plane is identified, the dura is reflected off the temporal bone, the IAC is opened with a diamond burr, and the superior vestibular and singular nerves are divided, as in the retrosigmoid approach (see Fig. 40–5). The mastoid air cells are sealed with bone wax, the dura is closed with 4-0 braided nylon in a watertight fashion, and the surgical defect is filled with abdominal adipose tissue.

DRESSING AND POSTOPERATIVE CARE

A mastoid dressing is applied in the operating room at the end of the procedure. The dressing is left in

---

FIGURE 40–5. The retrosigmoid internal auditory canal vestibular neurectomy. Note the 90° rotation of the eighth nerve from the ear to the brain. Most of the rotation occurs in the internal auditory canal (IAC). Note the superior vestibular nerve and posterior ampullary nerves that are transected, whereas the saccular nerve is spared. This allows for complete denervation of the vestibular labyrinth without damaging the cochlear nerve.

FIGURE 40–6. Combined retrolabyrinthine-retrosigmoid vestibular neurectomy. Dura is transected behind sigmoid sinus (right ear).

FIGURE 40–7. Combined retrolabyrinthine-retrosigmoid vestibular neurectomy in the cerebellopontine angle. There is a good cochleovestibular cleavage in the cerebellopontine angle, and the neurectomy is done in the posterior fossa (right ear). The vestibular nerve has been transected.

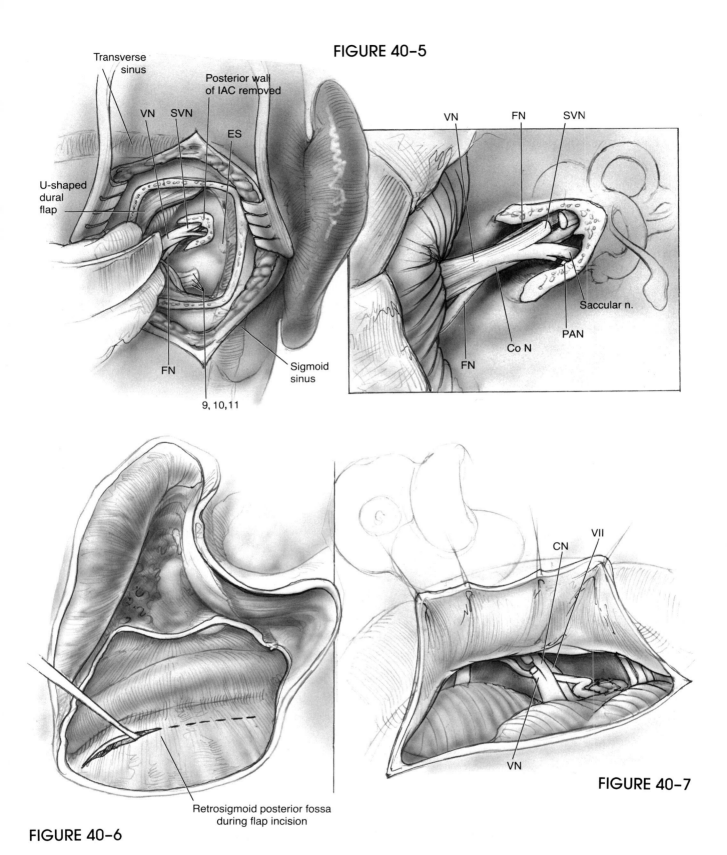

FIGURE 40-5

Transverse
sinus

VN SVN

Posterior wall
of IAC removed

ES

U-shaped
dural
flap

FN

9, 10, 11

Sigmoid
sinus

VN   FN   SVN

Saccular n.

PAN

Co N

FN

Retrosigmoid posterior fossa
during flap incision

FIGURE 40-6

CN   VII

VN

FIGURE 40-7

place for 48 to 72 hours unless it soaks with blood or cerebrospinal fluid.

For the first 24 hours postoperatively, the patient is observed in a neurosurgical intensive care unit. On the first postoperative day, the Foley catheter and arterial lines are removed. The abdominal dressing and suction drain are left in place for 24 to 48 hours. Early activity is encouraged; the patients usually sit up, stand, and ambulate on the first postoperative day. Patients are usually discharged on the fourth to sixth postoperative day.

Patients are seen 1 week postoperatively for suture removal and audiogram. One month postoperatively, a repeat audiogram and electronystagmography with iced caloric testing is obtained. The electronystagmography is obtained to document the percentage of reduced vestibular response. All patients are encouraged to resume an active lifestyle and are given a program of vestibular rehabilitation by a therapist. Most patients not only maintain their preoperative lifestyle but also return to activities they had given up because of their Ménière's disease, including golf, tennis, bicycling, and running. More than 90 per cent of patients consider themselves to be more active following recovery than before surgery.

PITFALLS OF SURGERY

Bleeding from injury to the sigmoid sinus or jugular bulb is usually managed by placing an Avitene (Alcon, Humacao, Puerto Rico) surgical pack over the bleeding site and holding it in place with a cottonoid neurosurgical sponge. Bleeding from a large mastoid emissary vein is controlled with a microfibrillar collagen (Avitene) pack; however, this can be prevented if a stump of vein, which can be cauterized, is left on the sigmoid sinus. If the emissary vein can be seen before bleeding occurs, dissection should proceed with a diamond burr. When the dura is opened small vessels can be cut inadvertently. Bleeding is controlled with microbipolar cautery set at 20 watts. Lifting the dura and cutting with scissors helps avoid cutting these vessels.

After the dura is opened there is a slight chance that brain swelling may occur. This effect is prevented by lowering the PCO_2 during surgery by hyperventilating the patient and by giving the patient mannitol (1.5gm/kg) intravenously when the bone work begins. Damage to the cerebellum is prevented by using a Penrose drain placed against the cortex while retracting the cerebellum to gain exposure of the cerebellopontine angle and by releasing cerebrospinal fluid. In younger patients, the cerebellum may be tense and protrude slightly through the dural incision. Gentle pressure against the Penrose drain lying

on the cerebellum will allow cerebrospinal fluid to escape. The Penrose drain is slid along the cerebellum at the inferior margin of the wound toward the ninth cranial nerve. After cerebrospinal fluid is released from the cerebellopontine angle by opening the arachnoid layer with a blunt instrument, the cerebellum will fall away from the temporal bone and allow good exposure of the cerebellopontine angle without cerebellar retraction. If brain swelling occurs from trauma to the cerebellum and the posterior fossa cannot be easily exposed, it is best to back out and close the wound. We have not had to do this in any case. Care must be taken not to traumatize the petrosal veins located above the fifth cranial nerve and near the tentorium. Because of the brain shrinkage from mannitol, these veins are stretched and can easily rupture. Bleeding is controlled with Avitene or electrocautery.

When the thin arachnoid layer is dissected away from the seventh and eighth cranial nerves, bleeding from small vessels may occur. This bleeding is prevented by cauterizing the vessel with an irrigating microbipolar cautery and transecting with a microscissors. Sometimes, the flocculus of the cerebellum is adherent and hides much of the eighth cranial nerve. By use of a round knife, the flocculus must be dissected away from the eighth cranial nerve. Locating cranial nerves 5, 9, and 10 helps orient the surgeon to the vestibular portion of the eighth cranial nerve (the superior half is closest to the fifth cranial nerve). To prevent injury to the facial nerve, a small mirror is used to look on the anterior aspect of the eighth cranial nerve. Occasionally, the facial nerve is attached to the vestibular nerve and must also be separated with a round knife. The surgeon can avoid facial nerve injury by seeing the nerve before the vestibular neurectomy is performed. The cleavage between the cochlear and vestibular nerve is first made with a sharp sickle knife, then completed with an electrified nerve separator. This instrument, electrified at 0.05mA with the Silverstein adapter for continuous stimulation, alerts the surgeon if the facial nerve is in proximity on the anterior side of the cleavage plane.

Unless the nerve separator can be seen emerging from the anterior aspect of the eighth cranial nerve and the facial nerve is not near the vestibular nerve, only about 80 per cent of the vestibular nerve is transected with the Luetje microscissors. The transection is then completed with a sharp sickle knife that is also electrified, thereby avoiding injury to the facial nerve and the internal auditory artery. Total hearing loss can occur if the internal auditory artery is interrupted during the vestibular neurectomy. Such a loss is more likely to occur if a 3mm to 4mm section of nerve is removed for histologic study; this is not recommended as a routine procedure. If the facial nerve is inappropriately transected, it must be repaired at the time of surgery with a greater auricular nerve graft, which would be a technically demanding procedure. Fortunately, none of our patients has suffered a facial nerve injury. Because this procedure is done in the posterior fossa, a neurosurgeon should be available in the event of an unusual complication with which the otologist is unfamiliar. Most intraoperative complications are prevented by using careful, gentle microsurgical techniques.

RESULTS

Retrolabyrinthine Vestibular Neurectomy

Results of RVN have been good. In 78 patients, 88 per cent were completely cured of their vertigo, and 7 per cent were substantially improved; only 5 per cent noted no change postoperatively. Overall patient satisfaction with the procedure was 93 per cent, and sensorineural hearing has been maintained to within 20dB of the preoperative level in 70 per cent. Some patients experienced a mild conductive loss in the low frequencies, probably secondary to bone dust fixing the stapes or adipose tissue impeding the ossicular chain.

Retrosigmoid–Internal Auditory Canal Vestibular Neurectomy

RSG-IAC produced a 90 per cent cure rate in 14 patients, and hearing results are similar to those of the retrolabyrinthine vestibular neurectomy. This procedure was originally thought to have several advantages over the RVN. Because no abdominal fat is needed to fill the defect, the procedure can be performed on thin patients. Because the exposure does not enter the mastoid, patients who have had chronic mastoiditis or a sclerotic mastoid or those with an anteriorly lying sigmoid sinus are good candidates. Complications have been infrequent, except for severe postoperative headache in 75 per cent of the patients. Fifty per cent of the patients have had significant headaches that are difficult to control with nonnarcotic analgesics and last for many months. Two years after undergoing the procedure, 25 per cent still experience severe headaches requiring continuous medication. The cause for this problem is unknown. This problem is perplexing, particularly because this approach has been used successfully for vascular decompression or section of the fifth cranial nerve. Drilling the bone from the IAC or bone dust may have produced an arachnoiditis with resultant headache. Postoperative headaches remain a major concern and have tempered our enthusiasm for the classic RSG-IAC vestibular neurectomy.

Combined Retrolabyrinthine-Retrosigmoid Vestibular Neurectomy

The combined R-R procedure is a significant improvement over the two previous procedures. Because much less bone removal is needed than in the retrolabyrinthine approach, the surgical time is shortened. In addition, the surgeon has the option of opening the IAC and cutting the vestibular nerve more laterally where the cochleovestibular cleavage plane is better defined. The incidence of cerebrospinal fluid leak (2.5 per cent) is also markedly reduced. The advantage that this procedure has over the retrosigmoid approach is that cerebellar retraction is not necessary and the bony defect is smaller. In 79 patients, vertigo was cured in 90 per cent. Hearing was preserved within 20dB of preoperative levels in 86 per cent of patients, and discrimination maintained to within 20 per cent of the preoperative level in 77 per cent of patients. Drilling the posterior lip of the IAC for vestibular neurectomy apparently results in headache complaints in 50 per cent of patients. Using the R-R approach, fewer than 10 per cent of patients had the IAC drilled for better exposure of the vestibular nerve. In the last 50 cases, the IAC was not drilled. With the use of the bipolar recording probe, few if any patients will need to have the IAC drilled for better exposure of the vestibular nerve.

COMPLICATIONS: INCIDENCE AND MANAGEMENT

Postoperative Complications

Early postoperative bleeding in the posterior fossa requires assessment by a neurosurgeon. The wound may have to be opened immediately. This complication has not occurred in our series. Meningismus with mild temperature elevation occurring soon after surgery usually represents a chemical meningitis caused by small amounts of blood in the cerebrospinal fluid and requires no treatment.

Wound infection secondary to serum collected beneath the flap in the postauricular crease is treated by incision and drainage, culture of the pus, and appropriate antibiotic treatment. This complication is prevented by keeping the skin flap and muscle layer together when elevating the skin flap, and by using perioperative antibiotics such as nafcillin. No wound infection has been seen in the past 75 cases, and, fortunately, none has ever progressed to meningitis. Several days postoperatively, if a spiking temperature elevation with nuchal rigidity and headache occurs, a spinal tap for culture and sensitivity should be done, and the patient should be treated for meningitis. We have not yet had to treat this complication.

Following RVN, the most common early complication is cerebrospinal fluid leak (10 per cent) from the wound edge or through the eustachian tube. Initially, these were treated by immediate re-exploration of the wound and repacking with adipose tissue. Now, a cerebrospinal fluid leak is treated with continuous lumbar drainage for 3 or 4 days. In this series, after lumbar drainage, all acute cerebrospinal fluid leaks stopped without re-operation. Because the dura cannot be closed watertight with the retrolabyrinthine exposure, no way has been found to prevent the high incidence of cerebrospinal fluid leaks. When the dural incision can be closed watertight, as in the combined R-R approach, the incidence of cerebrospinal fluid leak is greatly reduced. In this series, no cases of facial paralysis, meningitis, or death have occurred.

Late Complications

The cause for postoperative headache (75 per cent) after RSG-IAC vestibular neurectomy remains a mystery. Twenty-five per cent of patients continue to have headaches for years after surgery, but they eventually improve over several years. Using the combined R-R approach and drilling the IAC only in cases in which a cleavage plane cannot be determined helps minimize this side effect of surgery. When IAC drilling is required, in the combined R-R procedure, which is less extensive than the retrosigmoid approach and does not require cerebellar retraction, it appears to reduce the severity of the headache.

About 5 per cent of patients will continue to have some vertigo. Usually, the vertigo is mild, and the patients' quality of life is greatly improved from prior to vestibular neurectomy. There are several explanations for this. Some patients (1 per cent) will develop bilateral Ménière's disease. These patients are offered subtotal streptomycin ablation if their symptoms warrant further treatment. Patients with vertigo secondary to some cause other than Ménière's disease have a higher failure rate than those with classical Ménière's disease. In some patients, all vestibular fibers may not have been transected.[24] It is important to obtain an electronystagmography with iced caloric testing 6 months postoperatively to document complete vestibular ablation. If some vestibular function remains and the patient continues to have severe episodic vertigo, imbalance, or tinnitus, a transcochlear eighth-nerve section is recommended. This has been performed eight times (4 per cent) in our series.

References

1. Silverstein H, Wanamaker H, Flanzer J, Rosenberg S: Vestibular neurectomy in the USA 1990. Am J Otol 13: 23–30, 1992.
2. Silverstein H, Norrell H, Rosenberg S: An evolution of approach in vestibular neurectomy. Otolaryngol Head Neck Surg 102: 374–381, 1990.
3. Silverstein H, Norrell H, Rosenberg S: The resurection of vestibular neurectomy: A 10-year experience with 115 cases. J Neurosurg 72: 533–539, 1990.
4. Silverstein H, Norrell H, Smouha E, Jones R: Combined retrolab-retrosigmoid vestibular neurectomy: An evolution in approach. Am J Otol 10: 166–169, 1989.
5. Silverstein H, Rosenberg S: Vestibular neurectomy via the posterior fossa. In Silverstein H, Rosenberg S (eds): Surgical Techniques of the Temporal Bone and Skull Base. Philadelphia, Lea & Febiger, 1992, pp 175–194.
6. Silverstein H: Transmeatal labyrinthectomy with and without cochleovestibular neurectomy. Laryngoscope 86: 1777–1791, 1976.
7. Jones R, Silverstein H, Smouha E: Long-term results of transmeatal cochleovestibular neurectomy: An analysis of 100 cases. Otolaryngol Head Neck Surg 100: 22–29, 1989.
8. Silverstein H: Cochlear and vestibular gross and histologic anatomy (as seen from the postauricular approach). Otolaryngol Head Neck Surg 92: 207–211, 1984.
9. Silverstein H, Norrell H, Haberkamp T, McDaniel A: The unrecognized rotation of the vestibular and cochlear nerves from the labyrinth to the brainstem: Its implications in surgery of the eighth cranial nerve. Otolaryngol Head Neck Surg 95: 543–549, 1986.
10. Silverstein H: Silverstein wrist rest. Otolaryngol Head Neck Surg 89: 305–306, 1981.
11. Silverstein H, Rosenberg S: Intraoperative facial nerve monitoring. Otolaryngol Clin North Am 24: 709–725, 1991.
12. Silverstein H, Wazen J, Norrell H, Hyman S: Retrolabyrinthine vestibular neurectomy with simultaneous monitoring of eighth nerve action potentials and electrocochleography. Am J Otol 5: 552–555, 1984.
13. McDaniel A, Silverstein H, Norrell H: Retrolabyrinthine vestibular neurectomy with and without monitoring of 8th nerve potentials. Am J Otol (Supp) 23–6, 1985.
14. Rosenberg S, Martin W, Pratt H, et al.: A bipolar electrode recording technique. Am J Otol [In press].
15. Silverstein H: Microsurgical instruments and nerve stimulator-monitor for retrolabyrinthine vestibular neurectomy. Otolaryngol Head Neck Surg 94: 409–411, 1986.
16. Silverstein H: Silverstein lateral venous sinus retractor. Otolaryngol Head Neck Surg 89: 303–304, 1981.
17. Glasscock M, Kveton J, Christiansen S: Middle fossa vestibular neurectomy: An update. Otolaryngol Head Neck Surg 92: 216–220, 1984.
18. Silverstein H, Norrell H, Haberkamp T: A comparison of retrosigmoid IAC, retrolabyrinthine, and middle fossa vestibular neurectomy for treatment of vertigo. Laryngoscope 97(2): 165–173, 1987.
19. Silverstein H, Norrell H: Retrolabyrinthine surgery: A direct approach to the cerebellopontine angle. In Silverstein H, Norrell H (eds): Neurological Surgery of the Ear, Vol II, Birmingham, AL, Aesculapius, 1979, p. 318.
20. Silverstein H, Norrell H: Retrolabyrinthine surgery: A direct approach to the cerebellopontine angle. Otolaryngol Head Neck Surg 88: 462–469, 1980.
21. Hitselberger WE, Pulec JL: Trigeminal nerve (posterior root) retrolabyrinthine selective section. Arch Otolaryngol Head Neck Surg 96: 412–415, 1972.
22. Silverstein H, Norrell H, Smouha E: Retrosigmoid-Internal auditory canal approach vs. retrolabyrinthine approach for vestibular neurectomy. Otolaryngol Head Neck Surg 97: 300–307, 1987.
23. Silverstein H, Norrell H, Smouha E, Jones R: Retrolabyrinthine or retrosigmoid vestibular neurectomy: Indications. Am J Otol 8: 414–418, 1987.
24. Rosenberg S, Silverstein H, Norrell H, White D: Audio and vestibular function after vestibular neurectomy. Otolaryngol Head Neck Surg 104: 139–140, 1991.

41

Cochleosacculotomy

HAROLD F. SCHUKNECHT, M.D.
MICHAEL J. McKENNA, M.D.

The surgical treatment for Ménière's disease can be classified into two groups, according to mode of action: 1) procedures that have the objective of total or partial ablation of vestibular function and 2) procedures that are intended to enhance the drainage of endolymph by fistulization of the membranous labyrinth and decompression of the endolymphatic sac. Endolymphatic drainage procedures can be further divided into 1) external shunts that attempt to drain excessive endolymph from the endolymphatic sac into the mastoid or subarachnoid space and 2) internal shunts that attempt to drain excessive endolymph into the perilymphatic space. The cochleosacculotomy operation falls into the latter group, that is, an internal shunt procedure.

PHYSIOLOGIC, ANATOMIC, AND PATHOLOGIC RATIONALE

Ménière's disease is characterized pathologically by progressive endolymphatic hydrops that is probably related to a disturbance in endolymphatic sac function. This condition must be differentiated from non-progressive endolymphatic hydrops in which the hydrops is the result of a single traumatic or inflammatory insult to the labyrinth, causing a permanent but not progressive endolymphatic hydrops.[1]

The symptoms of progressive endolymphatic hydrops can be correlated with two principal types of pathologic change: 1) distentions and ruptures of the endolymphatic system[2, 3] and 2) alterations in the cytoarchitecture of the auditory and vestibular sense organs, sometimes accompanied by atrophic changes. Coincident with rupture, there is sudden contamination of the perilymphatic fluid with neurotoxic endolymph (140mEq per liter of potassium) that causes paralysis of the sensory and neural structures and is expressed clinically as episodic vertigo, fluctuating hearing loss, or both. The American Academy of Otolaryngology—Head and Neck Surgery (AAO-HNS)[4] recommended that these episodes be designated the "definitive" symptoms of Ménière's disease. As the disease progresses, there are changes in the cytoarchitecture of the sense organs that consist of distortion and atrophy of the sensory cells and supporting cells as well as disruption and deformation of their gelatinous aprons. These alterations impair the motion mechanics of the sense organs resulting in permanent functional deficits. The symptoms for the auditory system are hearing loss and tinnitus, and for the vestibular system are constant or recurring sensations of unsteadiness, described as being off-balance, floating, tilting, falling, or spinning, and are often aggravated by head movement. The AAO-HNS recommended that they be known as "adjunctive" symptoms. To be successful, surgical procedures based on facilitating drainage of endolymph should alleviate definitive symptoms and arrest the progression of adjunctive symptoms.

Among the internal shunt procedures are the sacculotomy of Fick,[5, 6] the tack operation of Cody,[7, 8] the otic-perotic shunt of Pulec and House,[9] and the cochleosacculotomy.[10] In the sacculotomy and tack procedures, picks are introduced through the footplate of the stapes to puncture the saccule with the hope of producing a permanent fistula in the saccular wall by which excessive endolymph can drain into the perilymphatic space. This approach, however, fails to consider the histopathologic observation that in Ménière's disease, the distended saccule often fills the vestibule; its distended wall is adherent to the footplate and could not be fistulized into the perilymphatic space by these maneuvers.[11] The otic-perotic shunt, as conceived by House and Pulec, involves the placement of a platinum tube through the basilar membrane to connect the scala media and scala tympani; however, the procedure is not surgically feasible because of the small size of the cochlear duct.

The cochleosacculotomy operation consists of creating a fracture-disruption by impaling the osseous spiral lamina and cochlear duct with a pick introduced through the round window. The rationale is supported by two histopathologic observations and muted by a third.

1. Histologic study of the temporal bones from patients with Ménière's disease shows that the distended membranous labyrinth may fistulize permanently in any area. Such spontaneous fistulization may account for the long remissions and even permanent arrest of symptoms of episodic vertigo and fluctuating hearing loss in some patients.

2. Animal experiments have shown that surgical disruption of Reissner's membrane[12] or the walls of the utricle, saccule, or semicircular canals[13] results in prompt healing of the fistulas. However, it has been shown in experimental studies on cats[14–16] and guinea pigs[17] that fracture-disruption of the osseous spiral lamina and cochlear duct can sometimes result in a permanent communication between the endolymphatic and perilymphatic spaces. Furthermore, those experiments clearly demonstrate that such fistulas exist without impairing the hearing for frequencies other than those tonotopically located immediately adjacent to the fistulas.

3. Histopathologic findings in human temporal bones of persons with Ménière's disease that militate against the success of internal shunts is that the distended membranes in some cases block the flow of endolymph toward such a fistula.[18] For this rea-

son, a successful cochleosacculotomy fistula will not relieve symptoms in all instances.

PATIENT SELECTION

Some otolaryngologists believe that surgery is never indicated for the relief of symptoms of Ménière's disease because in the normal course of the disease, the vertigo eventually subsides. This approach has merit if the patient is not unduly handicapped. In many cases, however, the disequilibrium erodes occupational efficiency as well as recreational and family lifestyle to the extent that invasive therapy is justified. This approach applies to patients having frequent and severe vertiginous episodes unrelieved by medication and those having falling attacks (Tumarkin's otolithic catastrophy).[19]

Some general considerations need to be addressed before cochleosacculotomy is recommended. The diagnosis of Ménière's disease must be unequivocal. Other disorders that cause fluctuating hearing loss and episodic vertigo, such as otosyphilis, inner ear autoimmune disease, perilymph fistula, demyelinating diseases, and intracranial neoplasms must be ruled out. The operation is not recommended for patients who present audiovestibular symptoms that are atypical for progressive endolymphatic hydrops. There should be no evidence of involvement of Ménière's disease or other disorders that might be progressive in the opposite ear. It is prudent to require a duration of symptoms of at least 1 year. The opposite ear becomes involved in almost 50 per cent of cases, sometimes many years after the onset of symptoms in the first ear.

Cochleosacculotomy is the procedure of choice for patients who for health reasons are at risk for the stress of postoperative vertigo and who should not have general anesthesia, as well as for elderly patients who often compensate poorly to procedures that ablate vestibular function. It has the advantage of being technically simple to perform, is almost totally free of morbidity, and carries little or no risk of mortality. Labyrinthectomy is more certain than cochleosacculotomy to relieve disabling episodic vertigo; however, it has the disadvantage of producing severe postoperative vertigo, permanent hearing loss, and in some cases, prolonged disequilibrium. For these reasons, some patients may choose to have a cochleosacculotomy as a first attempt to resolve their vertigo problem.

SURGICAL TECHNIQUE

The ear is prepared and draped similarly to any transcanal procedure. The operation is performed under local anesthesia. With the aid of a nasal speculum, the fibrocartilaginous external auditory canal is infiltrated circumferentially in four positions with 1% lidocaine (Xylocaine) containing 1:100,000 epinephrine, using a 27-gauge 1.5-inch needle. The ear canal is dilated with the nasal speculum, which also serves to diffuse the anesthetic solution uniformly into the tissues. An ear speculum of the surgeon's preference is introduced into the ear canal and locked in an adjustable speculum holder, thus freeing both of the surgeon's hands. The posterior aspect of the bony canal is exposed, and the skin of the bony canal is infiltrated at two sites with 1% lidocaine containing 1:1000 epinephrine, using a 30-gauge 1.5-inch needle. The beveled opening of the needle must be introduced flush against the bone at an obtuse angle, and the blanching area of infiltration should extend to the tympanic annulus from the 6 to 12 o'clock position. Adjustments of the speculum and speculum holder are made as often as necessary to achieve optimum exposure of the surgical field.

Incisions are made, and a triangular skin flap is elevated to the tympanic annulus (Fig. 41–1A). Bleeding must be meticulously controlled at all times. The tympanomeatal flap is elevated by lifting the tympanic annulus from its sulcus and folding the flap into the anterior tympanomeatal angle of the ear canal (Fig. 41–1B). The chorda tympani nerve and the ossicles are not disturbed. The ear speculum is locked into a position that exposes the round window niche and posterior aspect of the hypotympanum. In rare cases, the round window niche is partly hidden behind the posteroinferior part of the bony tympanic annulus, in which case a small burr is used to remove sufficient bony annulus to allow access to the round window niche.

Usually, the round window niche will accommodate a 3mm right-angled pick without removal of bone. The pick is advanced through the round window membrane, which may or may not be visible. The pick is guided in the direction of the oval window while hugging the lateral wall of the inner ear to ensure that the cochlear duct is traversed (Fig. 41–1C). When the pick has been introduced to its full 3mm length, the end of the pick will be located beneath the footplate of the stapes. Occasionally, the subiculum, which is a ridge of bone lying in the boundary between the round window niche and sinus tympani, interferes with introduction of the pick. It can readily be shaved down with a 2mm burr. Occasionally, the overhanging bony lip of the round window niche must be removed to accommodate the pick (Fig. 41–1D). In this case, a 2mm (rather than a 3mm) pick is used to avoid excessively deep penetration into the vestibule and possible injury to the utricular macula (Fig. 41–2). Rarely, a high jugular bulb blocks access to the round window niche, in which case it may be necessary to abort the operation (Fig. 41–3).

Occasionally, a slight loss of resistance is felt as the pick passes through the cochlear partition and causes the planned fracture-disruption of the osseous spiral lamina and cochlear duct (Fig. 41–4). Usually, the patients experience no sensation as the pick is advanced, but a few have noted momentary vertigo, and several have reported hearing a "click." The maneuver does not produce vertigo, presumably because the vestibular sense organs are not mechanically disturbed, and the endolymph from the fistulized area drains into the scala tympani rather than into the perilymphatic space of the vestibule. The pick is withdrawn, and the perforation in the round window membrane is sealed by a tissue graft of perichondrium or adipose tissue. The operation is terminated by returning the tympanomeatal flap to its original position. Strips of silk cloth are laid over the incisions, and a round synthetic rubber sponge of appropriate size is placed in the canal to maintain slight pressure on the skin flap. Cotton is placed in the ear canal. A few patients note slight unsteadiness for a day or two; however, all feel well enough to be discharged from the hospital on the following day. The packing is removed 1 week later, at which time the tympanic membrane and canal wall skin should be well healed.

Serial hearing tests at weekly intervals show a sensorineural hearing loss for 2 to 3 weeks, followed by recovery in most cases (Irwin Ginsberg, Personal communication). The authors first test hearing 6 weeks after surgery, when the hearing has stabilized. The complications of cochleosacculotomy are about the same as those for stapedectomy and include perforation of the tympanic membrane, tears of the jugular bulb, postoperative otitis media, sensorineural hearing loss, facial nerve injury, and perilymph fistula. The only significant complication in cochleosacculotomies performed by the authors, other than sensorineural hearing loss, was one case of otitis media that resulted in profound sensorineural hearing loss in the infected ear.

RESULTS

The authors' experience consists of 120 cochleosacculotomies performed since April 1979. The first assessment of results was made in 1982,[10] when it was reported that with a mean follow-up time of 4.32 months, 88 per cent of 51 patients were relieved of disabling vertigo, and hearing losses of greater than 20dB occurred in 23 per cent. The second assessment was in 1984,[20] when it was reported that 76 per cent of 83 patients were relieved of disabling vertigo, and hearing was worse in 49 per cent (15dB threshold loss [average for 500Hz, 1000Hz, 2000Hz] or 15 per cent discrimination loss). The third assessment was made in 1985[21] on 90 cases with a mean follow-up time of 22.3 months: relief of disabling vertigo occurred in 72.6 per cent and hearing losses in 45 per cent (same criteria), including 12.2 per cent who experienced profound hearing loss. The last assessment of results was done in 1991[22] on 120 patients with a mean follow-up time of 6.9 years: 70 per cent experienced relief of disabling vertigo, and in 35 per cent, the hearing loss was aggravated (same criteria), including 10 per cent who experienced profound hearing loss as a result of the operation.

The success rates reported for either internal or external endolymphatic shunt procedures should be viewed with some caution. For example, in a review of 834 articles published on Ménière's disease between 1952 and 1975, Torok[23] found that almost without exception, advocates of either medical or surgical treatment reported success rates in the range of 60 to 80 per cent. Not only is there a strong placebo effect, but sudden prolonged remission of symptoms are characteristic of Ménière's disease. However, some patients who had vertiginous attacks on a weekly basis (or more often) had a total cessation of attacks following cochleosacculotomy. In the management of disabling Ménière's disease, the discerning otologist will find cochleosacculotomy to be a useful alternative to vestibular nerve section and labyrinthectomy in selected cases.

FIGURE 41–1. *A*, Skin incisions are made in the posterior wall of the bony external auditory canal. *B*, The tympanomeatal flap is elevated and reflected into the anterior tympanomeatal angle. *C*, A 3mm right-angled pick is advanced through the round window membrane in the direction of the oval window. *D*, If the niche will not accommodate a 3mm right-angled pick, the bony lip of the round window is removed, and a 2mm right-angled pick is used to accomplish the cochleosacculotomy.

FIGURE 41-1

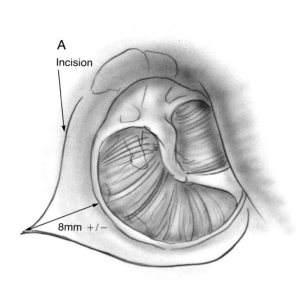

A

Incision

8mm +/−

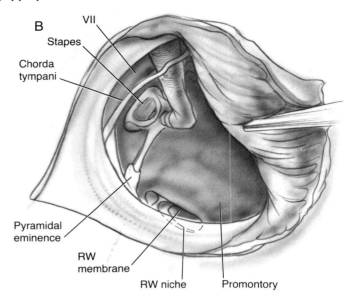

B

VII

Stapes

Chorda
tympani

Pyramidal
eminence

RW
membrane

RW niche

Promontory

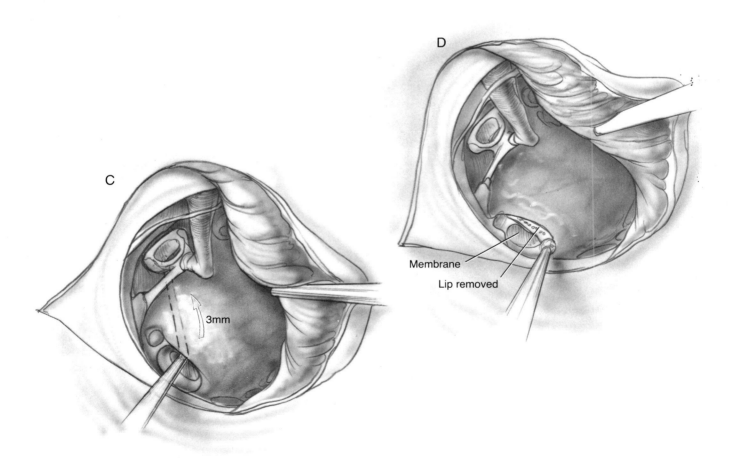

C

3mm

D

Membrane

Lip removed

FIGURE 41-2

FIGURE 41-3

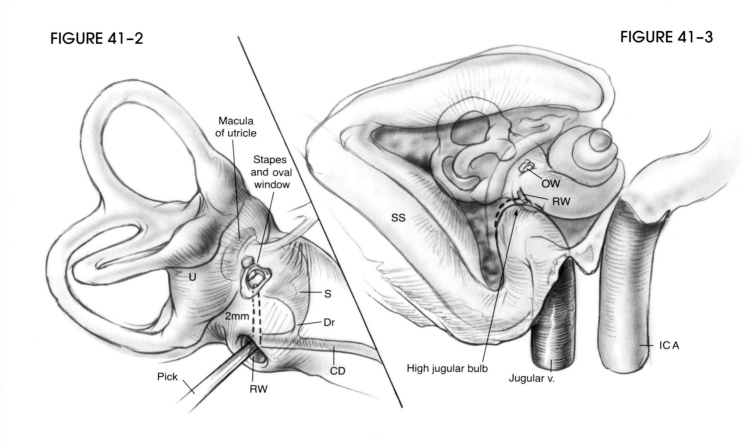

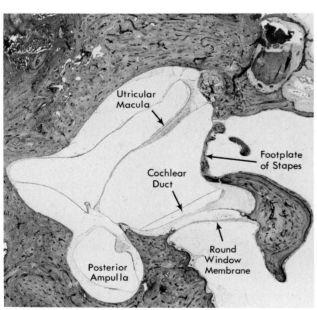

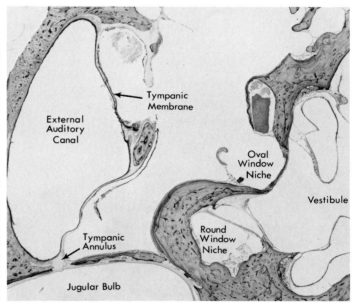

Key to abbreviations

S	Saccule	RW	Round window	OW	Oval window
Dr	Ductus reuniens	SV	Scala vestibuli	OSL	Osseous spiral lamina
CD	Cochlear duct	ST	Scala tympani	M	Macula
U	Utricle	SS	Sigmoid sinus		

FIGURE 41-4

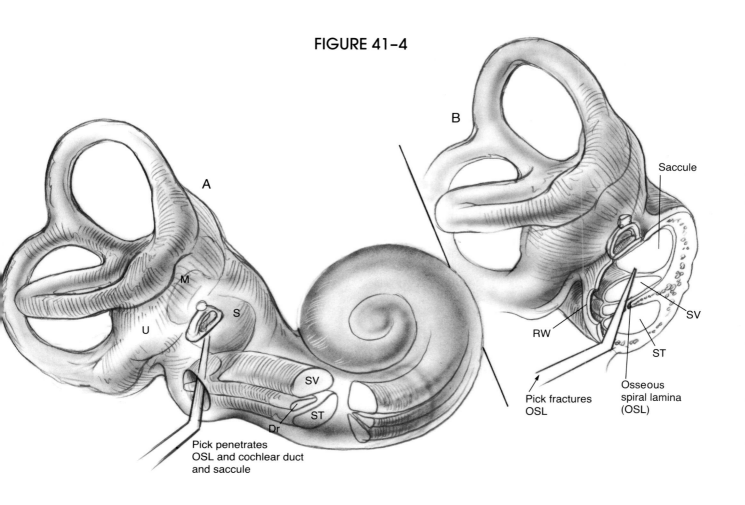

FIGURE 41-2. This vertical section of a normal ear demonstrates the anatomic features of the middle and inner ears that are relevant to cochleosacculotomy.

FIGURE 41-3. This vertical section of a normal ear shows a high jugular bulb abutting the tympanic annulus and encroaching on the round window niche. Other sections show a reduced orifice leading to a small niche. It is not feasible to attempt cochleosacculotomy in such cases.

FIGURE 41-4. The 3mm right-angled pick is shown penetrating the dilated cochlear duct and dilated saccule.

References

1. Schuknecht HF, Gulya AJ: Endolymphatic hydrops: An overview and classification. Ann Otol Rhinol Laryngol 92: (Suppl 106) 1–20, 1983.
2. Schuknecht HF: Ménière's disease: A correlation of symptomatology and pathology. Laryngoscope 73: 651–665, 1963.
3. Dohlman GF: On the mechanism of the Ménière attack. Arch Otorhinolaryngol 212: 301–307, 1976.
4. Committee on Hearing and Equilibrium: Report of Subcommittee on Equilibrium and its Measurement. Ménière's disease: Criteria for diagnosis and evaluation of therapy for reporting. Trans Am Acad Ophthalmol Otolaryngol 76: 1462–1464, 1972.
5. Fick IA van N: Decompression of the labyrinth. A new surgical procedure for Ménière's disease. Arch Otolaryngol 79: 447–458, 1964.
6. Fick IA van N: Ménière's disease: Aetiology and a new surgical approach: Sacculotomy. J Laryngol Otol 80: 288–306, 1966.
7. Cody DTR, Simonton KM, Hallberg OE: Automatic repetitive decompression of the saccule in endolymphatic hydrops (tack operation). Preliminary report. Laryngoscope 77: 1480–1501, 1967.
8. Cody DTR: The tack operation for endolymphatic hydrops. Laryngoscope 79: 1737–1744, 1969.
9. Pulec JL: Ménière's disease. The otic-perotic shunt. Otolaryngol Clin North Am 1: 643–648, 1968.
10. Schuknecht HF: Cochleosacculotomy for Ménière's disease: Theory, technique and results. Laryngoscope 92: 853–858, 1982.
11. Schuknecht HF: Pathology of Ménière's disease as it relates to the sac and tack procedures. Ann Otol Rhinol Laryngol 86: 677–682, 1977.
12. Duval AJ III, Rhodes VT: Ultrastructure of the organ of Corti following intermixing of cochlear fluids. Ann Otol Rhinol Laryngol 76: 688–708, 1967.
13. Kimura RS, Schuknecht HF: Effect of fistulae on endolymphatic hydrops. Ann Otol Rhinol Laryngol 84: 271–286, 1975.
14. Schuknecht HF, Neff WD: Hearing losses after apical lesions in the cochlea. Acta Otolaryngol (Stockh) 42: 263–274, 1952.
15. Schuknecht HF, Sutton S: Hearing losses after experimental lesions in basal coil of cochlea. Arch Otolaryngol 57: 129–142, 1953.
16. Schuknecht HF, Seifi A El: Experimental observations on the fluid physiology of the inner ear. Ann Otol Rhinol Laryngol 72: 687–721, 1963.
17. Kimura RS, Schuknecht HF, Ota CY, Jones DD: Experimental study of sacculotomy in endolymphatic hydrops. Arch Otorhinolaryngol 217: 123–137, 1977.
18. Schuknecht HF, Rüther A: Blockage of longitudinal flow in endolymphatic hydrops. Eur Arch Otorhinolaryngol 248: 209–217, 1991.
19. Tumarkin A: Otolithic catastrophe. A new syndrome. BMJ 2: 175–177, 1936.
20. Schuknecht HF: Cochlear endolymphatic shunt. Am J Otol 5: 546–548, 1984.
21. Schuknecht HF, Bartley M: Cochlear endolymphatic shunt for Ménière's disease. Am J Otol (Suppl): 20–22, 1985.
22. Schuknecht HF: Cochleosacculotomy for Ménière's disease: Internal endolymphatic shunt. Op Tech Otolaryngol Head Neck Surg 2: 35–37, 1991.
23. Torok N: Old and new in Ménière's disease. Laryngoscope 87: 1870–1877, 1977.

42

Chemical Labyrinthectomy: Methods and Results

EDWIN M. MONSELL, M.D., Ph.D.
STEPHEN P. CASS, M.D.
LEONARD P. RYBAK, M.D., Ph.D.

In 1944, streptomycin was isolated from cultures of a soil organism, *Streptomyces griseus*.[1] This drug displayed broad-spectrum antibacterial activity and was the first found to be effective against tuberculosis. Because effective treatment of tuberculosis with streptomycin required prolonged therapy, ototoxicity became evident soon after introduction of the drug. As early as 1948, streptomycin was used to treat patients with unilateral Ménière's disease specifically on the basis of its vestibulotoxic effects.[2]

Aminoglycosides exert their toxic effects on the hair cells of the inner ear by two general mechanisms. First, aminoglycosides bind to the plasma membrane and displace calcium and magnesium. This event results in acute but reversible interference with calcium-dependent mechanical-electrical transduction channels.[3] Second, aminoglycosides are transported into the cell by an energy-dependent process. Within the cell, the drug binds to phosphatidylinositol. This event is associated with progressive disruption of the plasma membrane and inhibition of the second messenger inositol triphosphate. With progressive disruption of the second messenger system and the plasma membrane, cell death occurs.[4–6]

Aminoglycosides do not seem to be concentrated in cochlear fluids, but the elimination half-life increases with chronic administration, suggesting sequestration of the drug by hair cells.[7] Amikacin, dihydrostreptomycin, and kanamycin are primarily cochleotoxic, whereas gentamicin and streptomycin are primarily vestibulotoxic. At high doses, streptomycin is also cochleotoxic. For example, streptomycin, 25 mg per kg per day, administered systemically to cats resulted in loss of vestibular hair cells only, but at 100 mg per kg per day, both vestibular and cochlear hair cells were lost.[8]

The hair cells of the cristae, the ampullae, and the cochlea degenerate to different degrees following the administration of aminoglycosides. The primary vestibular neurons, the cochlear nuclei, and the vestibular nuclei are not directly affected, even at high doses.[8, 9] The basal turn of the cochlea is the region most susceptible to permanent loss of hair cells, resulting in an initial loss of high-frequency hearing. Although the mechanisms of this differential toxicity are incompletely understood, several contributing factors have been identified, including the route of administration, dose variables, and the specific aminoglycoside used.

Damage to vestibular dark cells, which are thought to play a role in the production of endolymph, has been reported following administration of doses of aminoglycoside below the threshold for damage to hair cells. Impaired function of dark cells may be beneficial in Ménière's disease.[10, 11]

INTRANEOUS APPLICATION OF STREPTOMYCIN

INTRAMUSCULAR APPLICATION OF STREPTOMYCIN

Clinical Studies

Between 1948 and 1980, eight investigators reported on a total of 49 patients treated with intramuscular streptomycin for unilateral or bilateral Ménière's disease.[12] In the first extensive studies of intramuscular streptomycin, Schuknecht[13, 14] administered 0.75g to 1.75g intramuscularly every 12 hours. Treatment continued until there were no ice water caloric responses in the diseased ear or ears. The total doses ranged from 13.5g to 89g; mean, 39g. Schuknecht's experience with intramuscular streptomycin therapy in 20 patients is notable for its long-term (1 to 19 yrs) follow-up.[15] All patients became severely ataxic and most suffered oscillopsia early in the course of treatment, but none experienced hearing loss. Ninety-five per cent of patients had no posttreatment vertigo. Thirty-five per cent had persistent ataxia, and 15 per cent had persistent oscillopsia. Hearing was stabilized in 90 per cent of patients. Thus, when a totally ablative dose of intramuscular streptomycin was administered, vertigo was controlled and hearing preserved. Unfortunately, patients who undergo total vestibular ablation may still be disabled by chronic dysequilibrium, ataxia, and oscillopsia.[16]

To limit the chronic oscillopsia and ataxia that follows total bilateral vestibular ablation, subtotal or titration treatment protocols with streptomycin were developed.[17–20] Gradually accreting cumulative doses of streptomycin were administered until episodic vertigo was controlled, but some vestibular function was preserved to prevent oscillopsia.

Treatment Method for Subtotal Vestibulectomy

The authors' suggestions have been adapted from established protocols and modified by our own experience.[17–20] From the standpoint of the clinical skills required by the practitioner and the potential morbidity to patients, the administration of aminoglycosides for vertigo by any route of administration should be considered as great an undertaking as surgical treatment. Because not all the problems and pitfalls of any technique can be conveyed in a printed article, we advise that streptomycin treatment be learned under the guidance of a practitioner experienced in its use.

Indications

Intramuscular streptomycin may be considered for patients with disabling episodic vertigo caused by

Ménière's disease in the following three situations: 1) simultaneously active Ménière's disease in both ears, especially when it is unclear from which ear the attacks of vertigo are arising, 2) Ménière's disease in an only-hearing ear, or 3) in the second ear following an ablative procedure on the opposite side, such as selective vestibular neurectomy. It is essential to determine to what extent a patient may be disabled by the definitive episodic vertigo of Ménière's disease as defined by the American Academy of Otolaryngology and Head and Neck Surgery (AAO-HNS).[21, 22] Patients disabled primarily by continuous dysequilibrium, ataxia, oscillopsia, or motion intolerance are generally not good candidates for vestibular destructive procedures of any type, because their symptoms result from a failure of central compensation, from the perception of dysequilibrium in the presence of normal balance performance, or from both.[23, 24]

It is important to identify patients with Cogan's syndrome, luetic hydrops, and autoimmune disease of the ear because these patients may respond to nondestructive medical treatment, such as corticosteroids. Patients with markedly reduced caloric function prior to treatment with streptomycin should be managed with additional caution because they may develop permanent dysequilibrium or oscillopsia and the loss of additional vestibular function. Consideration should be given to treating such patients with lower doses of streptomycin over a longer period of time.

Pretreatment Evaluation and Patient Counseling

The pretreatment evaluation requires a complete history and physical examination, including a neurologic examination, observation of eye movements, and vestibulospinal examination. The vestibulospinal examination consists of observation of gait, tandem gait, Romberg's, and tandem Romberg's maneuvers. A simple, effective assessment of postural stability can be performed in the examination room or at bedside by having a patient stand on four to six inches of dense foam with eyes closed. The foam produces unreliable proprioceptive input to postural control mechanisms so that subjects must depend on vestibular input when eyes are closed. Normal persons have no difficulty standing on the foam, but patients with bilateral loss of vestibular function or an acute vestibular loss will fall when forced to rely solely on vestibular cues to maintain posture. Baseline audiometric and laboratory vestibular function tests are performed, including electronystagmography, rotational testing, and posturography. Renal function tests are performed as indicated.

It is essential to distinguish clearly between two phenomena in patients with Ménière's disease who are undergoing intramuscular treatment with aminoglycosides: 1) vertigo due to the disease and 2) the syndrome of acute bilateral vestibular loss caused by vestibulotoxicity. Vertigo is the hallucination of motion, that is, the perception of motion when none is occurring. The vertigo of Ménière's disease occurs without provocation, consists of a spinning or rotating sensation always with spontaneous nystagmus, lasts 20 minutes to several hours, and is accompanied by dysequilibrium and nausea that may last for hours.

The syndrome of acute bilateral vestibular loss may include rotational vertigo, but the vertigo is related to treatment rather than being spontaneous. Commonly, patients experience discomfort associated with rapid head movements, a sense of disorientation in space, and ataxia. Patients may also manifest oscillopsia, a disturbing sensation of the visual field bobbling as the patient walks about or rides in a car. This phenomenon results from impairment or loss of the vestibulo-ocular reflex, which helps maintain a stable image on the retina during head movement. Oscillopsia may be temporary or permanent following a bilateral loss of vestibular function.[15, 16, 25]

These distinctions are important because symptoms due to Ménière's disease are indications to resume treatment, whereas symptoms due to vestibulotoxicity are indications to halt treatment. Occasionally, the clinician may find it difficult to make this distinction from a patient's history. In such cases, caution would dictate that treatment be discontinued until the situation is clarified by repeated observations over time.

Patient counseling is extremely important. Patients are counseled that the purpose of the titration streptomycin therapy is to control the recurrent episodes of vertigo typical of Ménière's disease, and that disability due to dysequilibrium may replace disability due to episodic vertigo. Patients need to understand that treatment may be protracted and that additional courses of streptomycin may be needed in the future. Other risks and complications include hearing loss, tenderness from the deep intramuscular injections, nausea, perioral or peripheral numbness or tingling, rash, and fever. Renal, visual, and hematologic effects have also been reported with prolonged treatment with aminoglycosides.

Special discussion is required for patients with abnormal renal function because renal toxicity is a potential complication of aminoglycosides. Careful monitoring of renal function and consultation with a nephrologist is recommended to ensure safe treatment of a patient with impaired renal function. Occasionally, a patient will report allergy to aminoglycosides. In this case, the nature of the allergy is explored, and an intradermal test dose is considered.

Treatment Technique

Therapy may start with streptomycin sulfate injected intramuscularly, 1g twice a day for 5 days, that is, 10g total cumulative dose. After this initial course, clinical reassessment is performed by interview, vestibulospinal physical examination, audiometry, and vestibular function tests. If studies remain unchanged, there is no clinical indication of decreased vestibular function, and the patient continues to suffer vertigo, additional streptomycin may be given. For example, a second course could consist of additional streptomycin sulfate injected intramuscularly, 1g twice a day for 5 days, that is, 10g in the second course and a total cumulative dose of 20g. After administration of the first 20g of total cumulative dose, we recommend that additional doses be smaller, for example, streptomycin sulfate injected intramuscularly, 1g once a day for 5 days, that is, 5g per increment.

Streptomycin injections should be stopped when any of the following occurs: 1) episodic vertigo ceases or seems to abate; 2) the syndrome of acute vestibular loss appears or worsens; 3) balance performance worsens on the vestibulospinal examination; 4) laboratory tests of vestibular function demonstrate loss of vestibular function, such as reduction of caloric responses, increase in phase or decrease in gain of the vestibulo-ocular reflex on rotational testing, or a fall on posturography when forced to rely solely on vestibular cues; or 5) hearing declines. It is important to proceed with treatment slowly and cautiously. The effects of streptomycin can be delayed, and if the reduction of vestibular function continues to complete ablation, ataxia and oscillopsia may persist chronically. If episodic vertigo recurs, additional courses of streptomycin can be given as indicated.

Results

The long-term results of intramuscular subtotal streptomycin therapy for bilateral Ménière's disease are known from only one report.[25] Nineteen patients were reviewed, with follow-up from 2 to 9 years. Recurrent vertigo was controlled in 95 per cent of patients within the first 6 to 18 months following treatment. At last follow-up, 63 per cent of patients reported having had no recurrence of vertigo. Persistent mild dysequilibrium occurred in 60 per cent of patients without recurrent vertigo, and oscillopsia persisted in 16 per cent of patients.[25]

APPLICATION OF STREPTOMYCIN TO THE LATERAL SEMICIRCULAR CANAL

Experimental Studies

Kimura et al.[26] reported that the application of gentamicin to the lateral semicircular canal of normal guinea pigs produced a selective vestibular lesion. Sensory cell degeneration occurred in the utricular maculae and in all but one of the cristae of the superior, lateral, and posterior canals of 27 ears. The saccular maculae were less affected. All cochleas were normal except one, which had a small lesion of outer hair cells at the basal turn. Fenestrated control ears were normal throughout. Kimura et al.[27] repeated some of their experiments with streptomycin after producing experimental endolymphatic hydrops by occlusion of the endolymphatic duct. Hydropic ears sustained substantial cochlear lesions, as well as vestibular lesions, when streptomycin was applied to the lateral semicircular canal. Fenestration of the lateral canal without drug application produced a significant cochlear lesion, but not a vestibular lesion.

Clinical Studies

The application of streptomycin to the labyrinth through the lateral semicircular canal (labyrinthotomy with streptomycin infusion, LSI) was introduced by Shea and Norris[28] and by Shea.[29] The rationale of this procedure was that application to the vestibular labyrinth might cause more drug to reach the vestibular hair cells than cochlear hair cells and produce a more selective lesion with a single treatment. Accomplishment of this route of administration requires the performance of a mastoidectomy and an opening of the bony otic capsule.

Surgical Method

The technique of LSI was described by Shea and Norris.[28] The technique of one of the authors (EMM) is reviewed to describe the method of administration of a drug to the lateral semicircular canal. A simple mastoidectomy is performed, and the lateral semicircular canal is identified. The bone of the dome of the semicircular canal is gradually thinned with a diamond burr. A double blue-line technique is used to create a fenestration of the lateral semicircular canal. This opening is located as close to the ampullated end of the lateral semicircular canal as possible while trauma to the short process of the incus is avoided. The technique involves thinning the bone at the edges of the bony canal so that an island of thicker bone remains between two parallel areas of thinner bone. The island is then removed gently with a fine pick. The double blue-line technique dates from the era of fenestration surgery for otosclerosis and may be less traumatic to the inner ear than drilling an opening into the lateral semicircular canal directly. The ovoid opening need be only 0.5mm to 1.0mm in diameter.

The tip of a fine-bore needle mounted on a tuberculin syringe is inserted just inside the bony lip of the fenestration. A small amount of fluid containing streptomycin is slowly infused into the perilymphatic space of the lateral semicircular canal. Slow, gentle infusion over several minutes may help avoid hydrodynamic trauma to the inner ear. As the streptomycin solution is slowly infused, some perilymph is displaced and flows out of the labyrinth with some of the infusate. Opening the lateral semicircular canal in Ménière's disease results in enhancement of the ratio of the summating potential to the action potential of the electrocochleographic recording, primarily by reduction in the amplitude of the action potential. The ratio is not changed during infusion of streptomycin but may decline slightly after the fenestration is closed.[30]

The volume of fluid, the composition of the diluent (lactated Ringer's solution or other physiologic solution), the amount of streptomycin in the solution delivered, the amount of time over which the fluid is introduced, and whether the streptomycin solution is followed by a rinse of a physiologic solution without streptomycin are important technical variables that affect the amount of streptomycin administered and the amount of trauma to the inner ear. After the drug is infused, the fenestration is closed with a thick piece of temporalis muscle and fascia. The postauricular wound is closed in the usual manner.

On the basis of animal experiments, Shea initially recommended puncturing the lateral membranous canal in hydropic ears to release endolymph, possibly decompressing endolymphatic hydrops acutely[28, 29, 31] but has subsequently withdrawn this recommendation.

Results

In 1989, a multicenter study was initiated to produce an independent study of LSI results for hearing preservation and control of vertigo. Preliminary data from this and other studies have been reported.[12, 30] The results for control of vertigo and disability are not available because of the short follow-up (less than 2 years); however, early hearing results have been reported.

Preoperative pure-tone averages ranged from 14dB to 76dB hearing loss, with a mean of 54dB (SD = 14). Postoperative pure-tone averages ranged from 25dB to 110dB hearing loss, with a mean of 76dB. Four patients (9 per cent) had an early postoperative hearing result that was better than the preoperative hearing level.[22] In 11 patients (23 per cent), the hearing was unchanged, and in 32 (68 per cent) it was worse. In 27 patients (57 per cent), the postoperative pure-tone level was 71dB or worse (severe-to-profound hearing loss). Hearing outcome (change in pure-tone average or word recognition) did not seem to be a function of patient age, sex, side of surgery, duration of hearing loss prior to surgery, whether the patient

had had a surgical procedure on the ear prior to the LSI, or which surgeon performed the procedure. A trend was identified that suggested that patients with milder preoperative losses may sustain less hearing damage from LSI. Opening the endolymphatic space of the lateral membranous canal resulted in more loss of hearing than when the membranous canal was not opened ($P = 0.05$).

The postoperative follow-up time ranged from 1 to 18 months, with a mean of 10 months. Eight patients (17 per cent) had secondary procedures for control of vertigo during the first few postoperative months.

Discussion

Silverstein reported that patients with good hearing seemed to be more resistant to hearing loss from streptomycin applied intratympanically.[19, 20] There appeared to be less postoperative hearing loss from LSI when the preoperative pure tone average was 40dB or better.

Findings in patients with vestibular disorders appear to corroborate findings in the guinea pig model, that is, that the hydropic ear shows more sensitivity to aminoglycoside ototoxicity than the normal ear, and that there is less selectivity of lesions between vestibular and cochlear hair cells in hydropic ears.[27]

The long-term results (2 or more years) for hearing preservation and control of vertigo by LSI are not known. Consequently, this procedure should not be considered an established treatment.

INTRATYMPANIC GENTAMICIN THERAPY

Experimental Studies

Intratympanic injection of aminoglycosides allows treatment of unilateral Ménière's disease without producing systemic toxicity or effects on the opposite ear. Tracer studies have demonstrated that the primary route of entry into the inner ear is through the round window membrane.[32–36] A secondary route of entry into the inner ear may be through the annular ligament of the stapes.[26, 37]

Following the application of intratympanic streptomycin in guinea-pigs, Lindeman[38] found that the cristae of the semicircular canals are most sensitive to degeneration, followed by the utricle, then the saccule and the cochlea. The preferential vestibular toxicity after intratympanic injection is also dependent on dose. For example, application of 8mg of streptomycin to the round window membrane of the cat produced only vestibular toxicity, whereas 20mg to 40mg produced both cochlear and vestibular toxicity.[39] These experimental results emphasize the potential for cochlear toxicity due to the primary route of entry

TABLE 42–1. Review of Literature on Intratympanic Aminoglycoside Therapy

AUTHOR AND REFERENCE	NUMBER OF PATIENTS TREATED	AMINO-GLYCOSIDE	DOSAGE	TREATMENT END POINT	CONTROL OF VERTIGO (%)	LOSS OF CALORIC RESPONSE (%)	HEARING PRESERVED (%)	TINNITUS DISAPPEARED OR IMPROVED (%)	AURAL FULLNESS IMPROVED (%)
Schuknecht[14]	8	Streptomycin	50–300mg/dose 350–600mg total dose	Vestibular ablation	63	63	37	NR	NR
Beck and Schmidt[43]	43	Gentamicin	30mg/day	Vestibular ablation	91	NR	42	86	95
	40	Gentamicin, 40mg/ml	"6 doses planned"	First ototoxic reaction	92	0	85	95	100
	Total 83								
Lange[42]	92	Streptomycin Tobramycin, Gentamicin, 40mg/ml	60mg/day, "typically several days"	First ototoxic reaction	90	NR	76	35	43
Moller et al.[46]	15	Gentamicin 30mg/ml	15–30mg/dose 1–11 doses, mean = 5	First ototoxic reaction	93	100	66	82	78
Sala[47]	62	Gentamicin 30mg/ml	Up to 30mg/day 1–8 doses, mean = 3.5	First ototoxic reaction	86	51	70	76	78
Blessing and Schlenter[48]	82	Gentamicin 40mg/ml	1 or 2/day 5–40mg/dose × 7 days	Ablative nystagmus or hearing loss	89	28	67	NR	NR
Laitakari[49]	20	Gentamicin 40mg/ml	0.2ml/day × 3 days, then 0.2ml qod 3–12 doses, mean = 5.3	Ablative nystagmus	90	70	55	NR	NR
Nedzelski et al.[45]	20	Gentamicin 26.7mg/ml pH 6.4	0.65ml tid × 4 days 52mg/dose × 4 = 208 mg	12 doses or first ototoxic reaction	90	85	80	NR	NR
Magnusson and Padoan[44]	5	Gentamicin 30mg/ml pH 6.4	30mg/ml bid 2 doses for 1 day	2 doses	100	100	100	0	NR

bid = twice a day; NR = not reported; qod = every other day; tid = three times a day.

into the inner ear through the round window membrane. This situation necessitates careful control of the dose of intratympanic aminoglycosides if preferential vestibular toxicity is to be achieved.

Clinical Studies

The use of intratympanic aminoglycosides to induce a chemical labyrinthectomy for the treatment of unilateral Ménière's disease was introduced by Schuknecht.[13, 14] He reported on the results of eight patients given large daily doses of streptomycin (150 to 600 mg per day) for 1 to 7 days. The treatment end point was the onset of signs and symptoms of vestibular ablation. The treatment was successful in controlling vertigo in five of eight patients, all of whom lost substantial hearing in the treated ear. Although hearing was preserved in the remaining three of eight patients, persistent vertigo necessitated surgical labyrinthectomy. Schuknecht found that complete control of vertigo with intratympanic streptomycin required abolition of ice water caloric responses, which resulted in loss of hearing.

Lange[40, 41, 42] reported on an extensive experience in which various aminoglycosides were used to treat Ménière's disease. In his group of 92 patients, Lange reported that 90 per cent had no further episodes of severe vertigo, and hearing remained unchanged in 76 per cent of patients.

To reduce the incidence of hearing loss, Beck and Schmidt[43] used a modified protocol. Gentamicin was administered at 30mg per day and stopped after 6 days or at the slightest indication of ototoxicity. In 40 patients treated with the modified regimen, control of vertigo occurred in 92.5 per cent of patients. Eighty-five per cent of patients maintained hearing. The studies by several authors showed remarkably similar results, 86 to 93 per cent control of vertigo and 55 to 70 per cent hearing preservation in a total of 123 patients (Table 42–1).

In contrast to the administration protocols discussed earlier, there are two reports on a predetermined number of gentamicin doses without reliance on a clinical endpoint.[44, 45] Nedzelski et al. formulated a well-defined intratympanic gentamicin treatment protocol consisting of gentamicin injections three times per day for 4 days (gentamicin solution, 26.7mg per ml, pH 6.4, total dose approximately 208mg). Treatment was stopped after 12 doses or if signs or symptoms of inner ear toxicity appeared. In a series of 20 patients with at least 2 years' follow-up (AAO-HNS criteria), vertigo was controlled in 90 per cent, and disability was absent in 85 per cent. Hearing was maintained in 85 per cent and improved in 25 per cent.[45]

In a study to characterize the delayed effects of intratympanic gentamicin, Magnusson and Padoan[44] treated 5 patients with 2 doses of gentamicin (30mg per ml, pH 6.4), given 12 hours apart. The first symptom of an ototoxic reaction noted by the patients was a sensation of unsteadiness occurring 2 to 5 days (mean, 3.2 days) after the injections. Vertigo and nystagmus were noted 3 to 8 days (mean, 5.1 days) after the injections. At 1 year follow-up, vertigo was controlled (with a loss of caloric responsiveness in the treated ear) and hearing preserved in all five patients.[44]

This preliminary study raises the question of whether very low intratympanic doses of gentamicin may be effective in controlling vertigo and preserving hearing. Because this technique may not totally ablate vestibular function, vertigo may recur, but hearing is usually preserved. Additional gentamicin can be used if vertigo recurs.

Combining results from several studies shows that vertigo was controlled in about 90 per cent of 387 patients. Some patients required additional gentamicin injections or surgery.

Preservation of hearing varied from 55 to 85 per cent, with up to 25 per cent of patients showing improved hearing. The preliminary results suggest that the dose schedule and total dose may be significant factors in hearing preservation. A beneficial effect of intratympanic gentamicin treatment on tinnitus and aural fullness was also reported by some authors (Table 42–1).

Treatment Techniques

Indications

Intratympanic aminoglycoside therapy may be considered in any patient with disabling vertigo, sensorineural hearing loss (fluctuating or fixed), tinnitus, and aural fullness consistent with unilateral Ménière's disease that is persistent and refractory to previous medical or surgical management. Because intratympanic aminoglycoside therapy is a nonsurgical outpatient treatment, elderly patients and those with significant surgical or anesthetic risks may be treated safely and thus are primary candidates. Intratympanic aminoglycoside therapy can also be used to avoid additional surgery in patients with recurrent vertigo and a return of caloric function following previous ablative vestibular surgery. Patients with profound hearing loss are excellent candidates for intensified treatment.

The data on efficacy of intratympanic aminoglycoside therapy to control vertigo and its safety in preservation of hearing are almost exclusively from patients with Ménière's disease. Most patients with non-Ménière's vestibulopathy have normal hearing. For these reasons we do not currently recommend intratympanic aminoglycoside therapy in the primary treatment of vertigo caused by disorders other than Ménière's disease.

Pretreatment Evaluation and Counseling

A full diagnostic assessment is made, including a complete history, physical examination, neurologic examination, observation of eye movements, vestibulospinal examination, vestibular function testing (electronystagmography, posturography, and rotational chair stimulations) and an audiometric evaluation.

Retrocochlear disorders are excluded. Metabolic disorders are screened with blood tests as indicated. Given the low total dose of gentamicin used, the need to withhold treatment based on abnormal renal function is rare.

Patients are counseled that the purpose of the intratympanic gentamicin injections is to control the recurrent episodes of vertigo typical of Ménière's disease. The expectation and time course of posttreatment unsteadiness or dysequilibrium typical of unilateral vestibular ablation are explained. Moreover, the possibility that additional courses of gentamicin may be needed in the future or that surgical ablation may be required to control vertigo is reviewed. The possibility of increased hearing loss, including a profound loss of hearing that would be unaidable, is reviewed. Hearing preservation results from the literature and personal series are discussed. Potential positive and negative effects on aural fullness and tinnitus are explained.

Preparation of Gentamicin Solution

Gentamicin solution may be used either as a stock solution of 40mg per ml with a pH of about 5.4, or the gentamicin solution may be buffered to a pH of 6.4 to reduce the sting associated with intratympanic injection. One method to prepare the buffered solution is as follows: 1.5ml of gentamicin solution (40mg per ml) is injected into a sterile 5ml vial. An 0.6M sodium bicarbonate per liter solution is prepared by combining 2ml of 8.4 per cent sodium bicarbonate and 1.36ml of sterile water in a 5ml sterile vial. Add 0.5ml of the 0.6M sodium bicarbonate solution to the sterile vial containing 1.5ml of gentamicin to form 2ml of a solution of gentamicin (30mg per ml, pH 6.4) ready for injection.

Injection Technique

The patient should be comfortably positioned supine with the head turned away from the ear to be treated (Fig. 42–1). This position is maintained for 30 minutes following the injection, and the patient is instructed

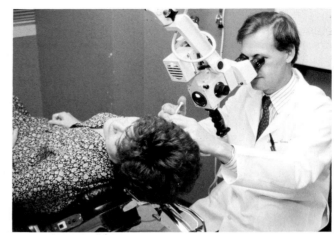

FIGURE 42–1. Patient positioning for intratympanic injection of gentamicin.

not to swallow or clear the middle ear during this period. A small injection site on the surface of the tympanic membrane is anesthetized with a small drop of phenol, and the gentamicin is injected into the middle ear using a tuberculin syringe and a 27-gauge needle (Fig. 42–2). Typically, about 0.5ml of solution fills the middle ear.

Administration Protocols

Numerous administration protocols have been described. Nedzelski et al.[45] applied gentamicin intratympanically three times a day for 4 days. Patients were hospitalized during this period or treated as outpatients. The placement of an infusion catheter into the middle ear facilitated the frequent injection of gentamicin.

The protocol introduced by Beck and Schmidt[43] has been used by multiple investigators. Gentamicin was applied intratympanically once a day until the earliest sign of ototoxicity was observed. One to 12 doses were given (mean, four to six doses).

An alternative outpatient technique is under development and investigation by one of the authors (SPC). The rationale is to reduce the risk of hearing loss while maintaining control of vertigo by giving less medication per dose and extending the time of treatment with repeated applications as necessary. One intratympanic injection of approximately 0.5ml of gentamicin, 30mg per ml, pH 6.4, is given each week. If weekly audiometric results are unchanged, weekly injections are continued to reach a total of four doses (40mg to 60mg total dose). Treatment is stopped early if auditory toxicity is noted. Additional doses may be given if vertigo is not controlled or recurs. Although experience with this protocol is preliminary ($n = 25$), vertigo has been consistently controlled, caloric function has been ablated, and hearing preserved.

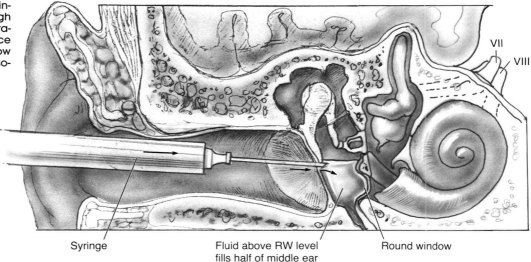

FIGURE 42–2. Intratympanic injection of gentamicin through a pinhole perforation. Gentamicin fills a middle ear space and bathes a round window membrane with antibiotic solution.

VII

VIII

Syringe   Fluid above RW level fills half of middle ear   Round window

SUMMARY

Subtotal bilateral chemical labyrinthectomy by intramuscular streptomycin administration is an accepted treatment for disabling vertigo due to bilaterally active Ménière's disease or Ménière's disease in an only-hearing ear. Long-term results show preservation of hearing and control of vertigo in most cases, although chronic dysequilibrium and oscillopsia remain as problems for some patients. Consequently, this treatment should be reserved for patients who are disabled and meet criteria for treatment.

Application of streptomycin to the lateral semicircular canal appears to cause a higher rate of hearing loss than does intramuscular or transtympanic application. Long-term results for hearing preservation and efficacy of control of vertigo with standard reporting methods are not known for application to the lateral semicircular canal. Reports of early postoperative results indicate a high rate of hearing loss. This approach is not accepted treatment at the present time.

Intratympanic application of gentamicin results in some cases of early posttreatment hearing loss, although vertigo is usually well controlled. Patients with posttreatment vertigo can be retreated easily. A current trend in transtympanic application is to use a fixed number of doses rather than treating until ototoxicity is clinically evident. Also, smaller doses are given over longer periods of time. Intratympanic gentamicin is a promising treatment that should be reserved for patients with classic Ménière's disease who meet appropriate treatment criteria.

References

1. Sande MA, Mandell GL: Antimicrobial agents. *In* Gilman AG, Rall TW, Nies AS, Taylor P (eds): Goodman and Gilman's The Pharmacological Basis of Therapeutics, 8th ed. New York, Pergamon Press, 1990, pp 1098–1116.
2. Fowler EP: Streptomycin treatment of vertigo. Trans Am Acad Ophthalmol Otolaryngol 52:239–301, 1948.
3. Ohmori H: Mechano-electrical transduction currents in isolated vestibular hair cells of the chick. J Physiol 359:189–217, 1985.
4. Rybak LP:Ototoxic mechanisms. *In* Altschuler RA, Hoffman DW, Bobbin RP (eds): Neurobiology of Hearing. New York, Raven Press, 1986, pp 441–454.
5. Williams SE, Smith DC, Schacht J: Characteristics of gentamicin uptake in the isolated crista ampullaris of the inner ear of the guinea pig. Biochem Pharmacol 36:89–95, 1987.
6. Williams SE, Zenner H, Schacht J: Three molecular steps of aminoglycoside ototoxicity demonstrated in outer hair cells. Hear Res 30:11–18, 1987.
7. Henley CM III, Schacht J: Pharmacokinetics of aminoglycoside antibiotics in inner ear fluids and their relationship to ototoxicity. Audiology 27:137–147, 1988.
8. McGee T, Olszewski J: Streptomycin sulfate and dihydrostreptomycin toxicity. Arch Otolaryngol Head Neck Surg 75:295–311, 1962.
9. Berg K: The toxic effect of streptomycin on the vestibular and cochlear apparatus. Acta Otolaryngol (Stockh) (Suppl 157):1–77, 1951.
10. Park J, Cohen G: Vestibular ototoxicity in the chick: Effects of streptomycin on equilibrium and on ampullary dark cells. Am J Otolaryngol 6:117–127, 1982.
11. Pender D: Gentamicin tympanoclysis: Effects on the vestibular secretory cells. Am J Otolaryngol 6:358–367, 1985.
12. Monsell EM, Shelton C, et al: Labyrinthotomy with streptomycin infusion: Early results of a multicenter study. Am J Otol [In press].
13. Schuknecht HF: Ablation therapy for the relief of Ménière's disease. Laryngoscope 66:859–870, 1956.
14. Schuknecht HF: Ablation therapy in the management of Ménière's disease. Acta Otolaryngol (Stockh) (Suppl 1132): 1–42, 1957.
15. Wilson W, Schuknecht S: Update on the use of streptomycin therapy for Ménière's disease. Am J Otol 2: 108–111, 1980.
16. "J. C.": Living without a balance mechanism. N Engl J Med 246:458–460, 1952.
17. Graham MD, Kemink JL: Titration streptomycin therapy for bilateral Ménière's disease: A progress report. Am J Otol 5: 534–535, 1984.
18. Graham MD, Sataloff RT, Kemink JL: Titration streptomycin therapy for bilateral Ménière's disease: A preliminary report. Otolaryngol Head Neck Surg 92: 440–447, 1984.
19. Silverstein H: Streptomycin treatment for Ménière's disease. Ann Otol Rhinol Laryngol 93 (Suppl 112): 44–88, 1984.
20. Silverstein H, Hyman SM, Feldbaum J, Silverstein D: Use of streptomycin sulfate in the treatment of Ménière's disease. Otolaryngol Head Neck Surg 92: 229–232, 1984.

21. Alford BR: Ménière's disease: Criteria for diagnosis and evaluation of therapy for reporting. Trans Am Acad Ophthalmol Otolaryngol 76: 1462–1464, 1972.
22. Subcommittee on Equilibrium: Ménière's disease: Criteria for diagnosis and evaluation of therapy for reporting. AAO-HNS Bulletin, July 1985: 6–7.
23. Konrad HR: Intractable vertigo—when not to operate. Otolaryngol Head Neck Surg 95:482–484, 1986.
24. Monsell EM, Brackmann DE, Linthicum FH: Why do vestibular destructive procedures sometimes fail? Otolaryngol Head Neck Surg 99: 472–479, 1988.
25. Langman AW, Kemink JL, Graham MD: Titration therapy for bilateral Ménière's disease: Follow-up report. Ann Otol Rhinol Laryngol 99:923–926, 1990.
26. Kimura RS, Iverson NA, Southard RE: Selective lesions of the vestibular labyrinth. Ann Otol Rhinol Laryngol 97:577–584, 1988.
27. Kimura RS, Lee K-S, Nye CL, Trehey JA: Effects of systemic and lateral semicircular canal administration of aminoglycosides on normal and hydropic inner ears. Acta Otolaryngol (Stockh) 111: 1021–1030, 1991.
28. Shea JJ, Norris CH: Streptomycin perfusion of the labyrinth. In Nadol JB (ed): Second International Symposium on Ménière's Disease. Amsterdam, Kugler & Ghedini, 1989.
29. Shea JJ: Perfusion of the inner ear with streptomycin. Am J Otol 10: 150–155, 1989.
30. Monsell EM: Electrocochleographic recording in patients undergoing labyrinthotomy with streptomycin infusion. In Arenberg IK (ed): Surgery of the Inner Ear. Amsterdam, Kugler & Ghedini, 1991.
31. Konishi S, Shea JJ: Experimental endolymphatic hydrops and its relief by interrupting the lateral semicircular duct in guinea pigs. J Laryngol Otol 89:577–592, 1975.
32. Smith B, Myers M: The penetration of gentamicin and neomycin into the perilymph across the round window membrane. Otolaryngol Head Neck Surg 87:888–891, 1978.
33. Saijo S, Kimura R: Distribution of HRP in the inner ear after injection into the middle ear cavity. Acta Otolaryngol 97:593–610, 1984.
34. Goycoolea M, Carpenter A, Muchow D: Ultrastructural studies of the round-window membrane of the cat. Arch Otolaryngol 113:617–624, 1987.
35. Kawauchi H, DeMaria T, Lim D: Endotoxin permeability through the round window. Acta Otolaryngol (Suppl 457): 100–115, 1988.
36. Lundman L, Bagger-Sjoback D, Holmquist L, Juhn S: Round window membrane permeability. Acta Otolaryngol (Suppl 457): 73–77, 1988.
37. Jahnke K: Transtympanic application of gentamicin with cochlea protection. In Nadol JB (ed): Second International Symposium on Ménière's Disease. Amsterdam, Kugler & Ghedini, 1989.
38. Lindeman H: Regional differences in sensitivity of the vestibular sensory epithelia to ototoxic antibiotics. Acta Otolaryngol 67: 177–189, 1969.
39. Cass S, Bouchard K, Graham M: Controlled application of streptomycin to the round window membrane of the cat. Otolaryngol Head Neck Surg 103: 223, 1990.
40. Lange G: Isolierte Medikamentose Ausschaltungeines Gleichgewichtsorganes beim Morbus Meniere mit Streptomycin-Ozothin. Arch Klin Exp 191: 545–549, 1968.
41. Lange G: Transtympanic treatment for Ménière's disease with gentamicin sulfate. In Vosteen K-H, Schuknecht HF, Pfaltz CR, et al. (eds): Ménière's Disease, Pathogenesis, Diagnosis and Treatment. Stuttgart, Georg Thieme Verlag, 1981.
42. Lange G: Gentamicin and other ototoxic antibiotics for the transtympanic treatment of Ménière's disease. Arch Otorhinolaryngol 246: 269–270, 1989.
43. Beck C, Schmidt CL: Ten years of experience with intratympanically applied streptomycin (gentamicin) in the therapy of morbus Ménière. Arch Otorhinolaryngol 221: 149–152, 1978.
44. Magnusson M, Padoan S: Delayed onset of ototoxic effects of gentamicin in treatment of Ménière's disease. Acta Otolaryngol 111: 671–676, 1991.
45. Nedzelski J, Schessel D, Bryce G, Pfleiderer A: Chemical labyrinthectomy: Local application for the treatment of unilateral Ménière's disease. Am J Otol 13: 18–22, 1992.
46. Moller C, Odkvist L, Thell J, et al: Vestibular and audiologic functions in gentamicin-treated Ménière's disease. Am J Otolaryngol 9: 383–391, 1988.
47. Sala T: Transtympanic administration of aminoglycosides in patients with Ménière's disease. Arch Otorhinolaryngol 245: 293–296, 1988.
48. Blessing R, Schlenter W: Langzeitergebnisse der Gentamicin-Therapie des Morbus Meniere. Laryngorhinootologie 68: 657–660, 1989.
49. Laitakari K: Intratympanic gentamicin in severe Ménière's disease. Clin Otolaryngol 15:545–548, 1990.
50. Monsell EM, Cass SP, Rybak LP: Aminoglycoside treatment for vertigo: Development and current status. Adv Otolaryngol Head Neck Surg 7: 174–188, 1993.

43

Transcanal Labyrinthectomy

JOSEPH B. NADOL, Jr., M.D.

MICHAEL J. McKENNA, M.D.

Labyrinthectomy is an effective surgical procedure for the management of unremitting or poorly compensated unilateral peripheral vestibular dysfunction in the presence of ipsilateral, profound, or severe sensorineural hearing loss. The physiologic rationale is that central vestibular compensation is more rapid and complete for unilateral absence of peripheral vestibular function than for unilateral abnormal function, either episodic or chronic.[1]

Unilateral vestibular ablation has been advocated for over six decades. Selective or total eighth nerve transection by the suboccipital approach was introduced by Dandy in 1928.[2] Destruction of the peripheral end organs of the vestibular labyrinth was introduced by Jansen in 1895 for complications of suppurative labyrinthitis.[3] This technique was applied to unilateral peripheral vestibular disturbance by Milligan[4] and by Lake[5] in 1904 and was reintroduced by Cawthorne[6] in 1943 as a canal wall up technique. In his original description, Cawthorne apparently ablated only the lateral semicircular canal. However, in its current form, complete vestibular ablation is accomplished by exenteration of all three of the semicircular canals and both maculae.

The earliest report of a transcanal procedure for vertigo is credited to Crockett, who in 1903 described removal of the stapes as an effective treatment for vertigo.[7] Lempert described an endaural transmeatal approach to the oval and round windows for Ménière's disease.[8] In this procedure, the stapes was removed and the round window punctured to "decompress" the membranous labyrinth. However, there was no mention of the importance of destruction of the vestibular end organs. The modern transcanal labyrinthectomy for unilateral peripheral vestibular dysfunction was introduced by Schuknecht in 1956[9] and by Cawthorne in 1957.[10] In a series of papers, Schuknecht's technique evolved to emphasize the importance of destruction of all five vestibular end organs.[11-13] The importance of total ablation of peripheral vestibular function was also emphasized by Armstrong[14] and Ariagno.[15]

PATIENT SELECTION

The modern complete transcanal labyrinthectomy is an extremely effective treatment option for unilateral peripheral vestibular dysfunction. Rates of control of vertigo in the range of 95 to 99 per cent have been achieved by several authors. The modified Cawthorne transmastoid labyrinthectomy and the translabyrinthine vestibular or eighth nerve section are equally effective options for ablation of peripheral vestibular dysfunction. However, the transcanal labyrinthectomy has the obvious advantages of a more direct approach to the vestibular end organs, a shorter operating time, and a lower morbidity, particularly for postoperative facial nerve dysfunction and cerebrospinal fluid leak.

Medical management appropriate to the unilateral vestibular disorder, including vestibular supressants and diuretics for Ménière's disease, should be attempted prior to consideration of labyrinthectomy. These forms of medical management are less successful for poorly compensated peripheral vestibular dysfunction, such as the sequelae of vestibular neuronitis, labyrinthitis, or trauma. In these cases, rehabilitative vestibular physical therapy should be attempted prior to labyrinthectomy. Labyrinthectomy should be performed only when it has been clearly demonstrated that the vestibular dysfunction is unilateral and when the ipsilateral hearing loss is severe or profound. Although the published indications for labyrinthectomy have included hearing levels poorer than a 50dB speech reception threshold and a 50 per cent discrimination score, in view of the incidence of bilateral Ménière's disease of 10 to 40 per cent, as reported by Greven et al.[16] and Paparella and Griebie,[17] labyrinthectomy should be reserved for cases in which the hearing loss is severe to profound, generally with a speech reception threshold of 75dB or worse and a speech discrimination score of less or equal to 20 per cent. This threshold for labyrinthectomy should be increased if hearing in the contralateral ear is not in the normal or near-normal range. Given the acute and often protracted vestibular disturbance following labyrinthectomy, this procedure should be done only for debilitating peripheral vestibular dysfunction. That is, the patient with only mild or infrequent attacks may be best treated nonoperatively. Obviously, the definition of handicapping vertigo also depends on many other clinical factors, such as age, intercurrent disease, and occupation of the patient.

A successful labyrinthectomy depends not only on total ablation of peripheral vestibular dysfunction but also on compensation for this unilateral vestibular loss. In general, negative indicators for successful vestibular compensation include increased age, visual disturbances, obesity, sedentary lifestyle, arthritis or other lower limb dysfunction, dependent personality, or clear indication of secondary gain.

PREOPERATIVE EVALUATION

A complete history and otolaryngologic and head and neck examination should be performed. Bilateral behavioral audiometry, including pure-tone thresholds for air and bone conduction and speech discrimination, are necessary. Vestibular testing should include at least bilateral caloric function, best done by electronystagmography. This assessment is necessary to evaluate the possibility of bilateral vestibular dysfunction and also to confirm vestibular dysfunction in the affected ear based on audiometry and history. Hallpike positional testing and evaluation for the presence of the fistula and Hennebert's signs should be done.[18] A neurologic exam should be done to rule out concurrent cranial nerve, cerebellar, or other neurologic dysfunction that would belie the working diagnosis of a peripheral unilateral vestibular dysfunction. Radiographic assessment with computed tomography and magnetic resonance imaging is not essential in every case. However, the symptoms and findings of long-standing unilateral Ménière's disease may be similar to those caused by lesions of the posterior fossa. In general, magnetic resonance imaging with gadolinium enhancement is useful to rule out cerebellopontine angle or other tumors and demyelinating lesions. In summary, the ideal candidate for labyrinthectomy is an individual with unremitting or uncompensated peripheral vestibular dysfunction with severe-to-profound unilateral sensorineural hearing loss, unilateral vestibular dysfunction on electronystagmography, and lack of neurologic and radiographic evidence of central neurologic disease.

In general, the functional outcome is better in patients with unilateral Ménière's disease than in those with other peripheral vestibular dysfunction. In some patients with Ménière's disease, the electronystagmogram will be normal. In such cases, labyrinthectomy is justified if the symptoms and signs are sufficiently localizing to be convincing of unilateral peripheral dysfunction. Thus, the presence of fluctuating or severe-to-profound sensorineural loss, ipsilateral tinnitus, and aural symptoms concurrent with Ménière's attack is sufficient to warrant labyrinthectomy, even in the presence of normal caloric function if other selection criteria are met. The patient should be aware that postoperative vertigo will be more severe when preoperative function is normal or nearly so in the affected ear.

PREOPERATIVE PATIENT COUNSELING AND INFORMED CONSENT

Preoperative counseling should include a discussion of the natural history of Ménière's disease, including both the spontaneous rate of remission of approximately 70 per cent within 8 years as well as the 10 to 40 per cent incidence of involvement of the second ear.[19] In addition, the patient should be aware that all hearing will be lost in the ear receiving surgery and that the effect on tinnitus is unpredictable. The patient must be aware that immediately postoperatively there

will be a period of vertigo much like a typical attack and that this episode will continue for several days. In addition, a period of protracted disequilibrium may occur, and in those with negative indicators for compensation, there may be some degree of permanent disability that requires a rehabilitative program. A discussion of alternative treatments for the vestibular symptomatology of Ménière's disease should be well understood by the patient. The discussion should include medical regimens, alternative ablative techniques, including transmastoid or translabyrinthine approaches, and selective ablative techniques through the middle or posterior fossa to save residual hearing. Particularly in the aged or in patients with other negative indicators for compensation, a round window labyrinthotomy should be considered and discussed with the patient as a possible alternative to labyrinthectomy. This procedure has the advantage of not resulting in a protracted period of disequilibrium and does not preclude a labyrinthectomy, if necessary. In addition, the usual risks of ear surgery should be discussed, including paresis or paralysis of the facial nerve, perforation of the tympanic membrane, dysgeusia, failure of the procedure to achieve the desired result, the possible need for revision or secondary procedures, spinal fluid leakage or meningitis, and the fact that harvesting of a fat graft may be necessary.

SURGICAL TECHNIQUE

General anesthesia is required because of the violent vestibular response during removal of the vestibular end organs. One exception may be in a revision labyrinthectomy in an ear with minimal residual vestibular function. In such cases, local anesthesia may allow intraoperative confirmation that the site of residual vestibular function has been located. The patient is placed in a supine position in a head holder with the head positioned similar to any transcanal procedure. Hair is shaved one-half inch around the auricle and prepared with an antiseptic solution. Generally, systemic antibiotics and steroids are not required.

Facial nerve monitoring is usually not done in primary labyrinthectomy but may be useful in a revision case if there is considerable scarring in the oval window area. No special instruments are necessary, but an instrument to remove the utricle from the recesses of the vestibule and a probe to mechanically destroy the cristae of the three semicircular canals should both be available. For these purposes, a 4mm right-angled hook or a whirlybird from the Austin middle ear instrument set are useful. A microdrill is necessary to widen the oval window or to connect the oval and round windows for exposure.

Incision and Exposure

The procedure is done by the transcanal approach in most cases. Occasionally, with a very narrow meatus, an endaural incision or postauricular transcanal approach may be useful. An anteriorly based tympanomeatal flap, somewhat longer than that used for stapedectomy, is elevated to allow wide curettage in the oval and round window areas (Fig. 43–1). The horizontal segment of the facial nerve, the entire stapes footplate, and the entire round window niche should all be easily visible after elevation of the flap and curettage of the posterior aspect of the bony tympanic annulus.

Preparation for Opening the Vestibule

The incus is removed. The stapedial tendon is then sectioned and the stapes removed in a rocking motion in an anteroposterior direction to allow removal of the stapes without fracture. Every effort should be made to avoid aspiration of the vestibule at this time to avoid displacement of the utricle. To obtain access to the vestibular end organs, the oval window may simply be enlarged at its anterior and inferior aspects (Fig. 43–2), or the oval and round windows may be connected to remove a segment of the promontory (Fig. 43–3). At this juncture, an attempt may be made to expose the posterior ampullary nerve. It may be exposed near the posterior aspect of the round window niche (Figs. 43–2 and 43–3), which affords the surgeon an opportunity to practice identification and section of the posterior ampullary nerve and also helps guarantee a more complete labyrinthectomy. In a study of labyrinthectomy in the cat, Schuknecht[23] reported that subtotal destruction of the vestibular end organs occurred in ten of 24 ears and that the crista of the posterior semicircular canal was the end organ most commonly missed.

Removal of Vestibular End Organs

Total mechanical destruction of the five vestibular end organs is the goal of this surgery. The normal position of the vestibular end organs and their relationship to the oval and round windows is shown in Figure 43–4. However, endolymphatic hydrops or intraoperative loss of perilymph may cause displacement of these end organs. For example, during aspiration or loss of perilymphatic fluid, the utricle usually retracts superiorly to lie medial to the horizontal segment of the facial nerve. Before aspiration of the vestibule, the utricle should be removed with a 4mm hook, whirlybird, or utricular hook in the superior aspect of the vestibule (Fig. 43–5). The utricle is substantial and can easily be seen under low power of the operating microscope. Avulsion of the utricle from the vestibule will usually result in avulsion of the cristae of both lateral and superior semicircular canals as well, but not that of the posterior semicircular canal. The saccule is destroyed mechanically by aspiration of the medial aspect of the vestibule in the area of the spherical recess. Manipulation of the medial aspect of the vestibule must be done with care to avoid fracture of the cribrose area, which would result in profuse leakage of cerebrospinal fluid from the internal auditory canal. Any residual neuroepithelium of the cristae of the three semicircular canals is then destroyed by mechanical probing. The surgeon can feel the 4mm hook drop into the ampullary ends of the bony canals (Fig. 43–6). This entire technique should be practiced in the temporal bone laboratory to gain both familiarity with the anatomy and proficiency in this procedure.

After destruction of the vestibular end organs, the vestibule is usually packed with absorbable gelatin sponge (Gelfoam) or, preferably, a small fat graft from the ear lobe (Fig. 43–7). Some surgeons recommend the use of streptomycin-soaked gelatin sponge in the medial aspect of the vestibule to guarantee destruc-

---

FIGURE 43–1. Incisions for transcanal labyrinthectomy. The anteriorly based tympanomeatal flap should be slightly wider and longer than that used for stapedectomy to allow wide curettage of the bony tympanic annulus. Curettage should allow visualization of the horizontal segment of the facial nerve and the entire oval and round window niches.

FIGURE 43–2. Access to the vestibule may be achieved by widening the oval window niche by removing a segment of promontory. At this time the posterior ampullary nerve (PAN) may be located in the floor of the round window niche. This step is facilitated by removal of the round window overhang.

FIGURE 43–3. As an alternative way of exposure of the vestibule, the round and oval windows may be connected to remove the lateral aspect of the promontory.

FIGURE 43–4. The normal anatomic positions of the five vestibular end-organs are superimposed on the surgical exposure.

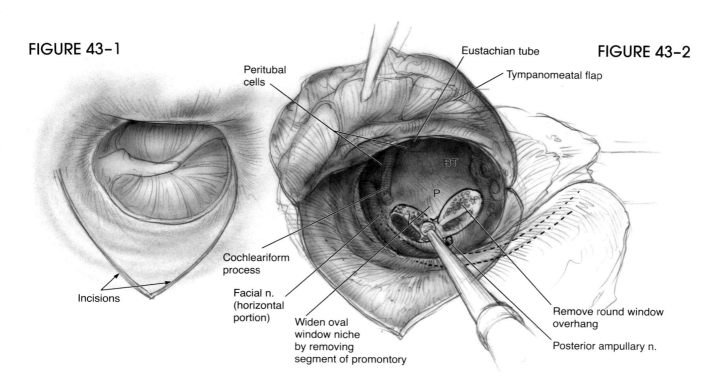

FIGURE 43–1

Incisions

FIGURE 43–2

Peritubal cells

Eustachian tube

Tympanomeatal flap

Cochleariform process

Facial n. (horizontal portion)

Widen oval window niche by removing segment of promontory

Remove round window overhang

Posterior ampullary n.

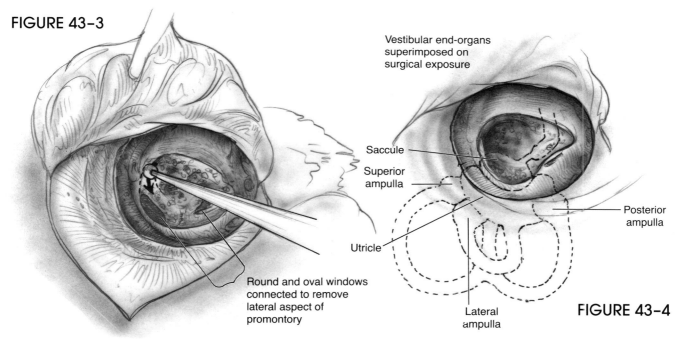

FIGURE 43–3

Round and oval windows connected to remove lateral aspect of promontory

Vestibular end-organs superimposed on surgical exposure

Saccule

Superior ampulla

Utricle

Lateral ampulla

Posterior ampulla

FIGURE 43–4

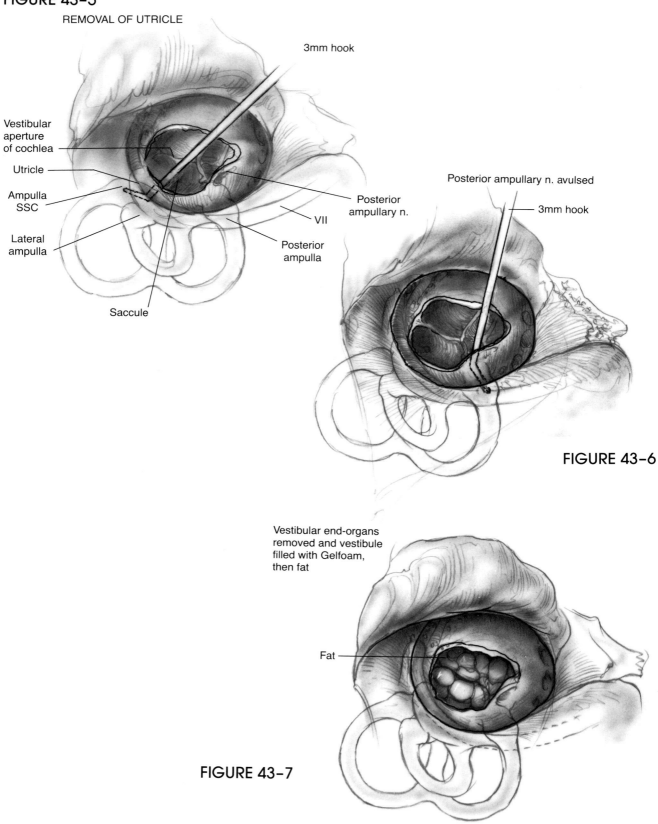

FIGURE 43-5

REMOVAL OF UTRICLE

3mm hook

Vestibular
aperture
of cochlea

Utricle

Ampulla
SSC

Lateral
ampulla

Saccule

Posterior
ampullary n.

VII

Posterior
ampulla

Posterior ampullary n. avulsed

3mm hook

FIGURE 43-6

Vestibular end-organs
removed and vestibule
filled with Gelfoam,
then fat

Fat

FIGURE 43-7

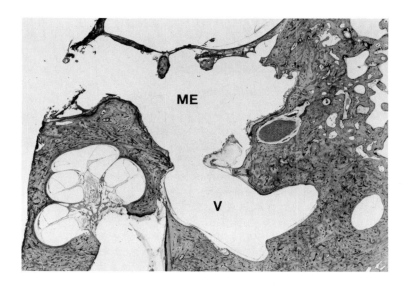

FIGURE 43-8. The vestibule (V) remains in communication with the middle ear (ME) 14 years following a transcanal labyrinthectomy.

tion of residual neuroepithelium. As seen in Figure 43–8, the absence of a tissue graft of the open oval window results in a pneumolabyrinth postoperatively. Generally, this result does not cause a problem, but a tissue seal with fat or fascia provides a better barrier between the middle ear and spinal fluid spaces. Leakage of spinal fluid after aspiration of the vestibule should be repaired with a tissue seal. In such cases, the tympanomeatal flap is then returned to the posterior canal wall and held in place with packing, and the procedure is terminated.

POSTOPERATIVE CARE

The degree of postoperative vestibular disturbance is positively correlated with preoperative residual vestibular function. That is, individuals with normal or near-normal caloric response preoperatively have a more severe reaction than those with minimal or no vestibular response. Third-degree nystagmus, nausea, and vomiting can be expected. Control of the vestibular symptomotology may be achieved with promethazine or droperidol. Vestibular suppressants should be tapered as quickly as possible, given the evidence that they may impair or slow central compensation for unilateral vestibular ablation. Rapid advancement of physical activity should be encouraged, including sitting and ambulation with assistance in the first few days. The patient may be discharged when he or she is relatively self-sufficient and ambulating without assistance. This improvement may take from 3 to 7 days.

At the first postoperative visit at 1 week, the packing is removed, and progressive activity is encouraged. The patient is seen 1 month postoperatively to evaluate residual symptoms, progress, and compensation and to ascertain healing of the tympanic membrane and ear canal. At this time, there is usually no residual spontaneous nystagmus, and a caloric test of the ear that had surgery, using 20ml of ice water and Frenzel's lenses, is used to ascertain the completeness of unilateral vestibular ablation. Further follow-up is dependent on the patient's progress.

FIGURE 43-5. Removal of the utricle can be accomplished with a 4mm hook (as shown), a utricular hook or a whirly bird. Removal of the utricle often results in simultaneous avulsion of the ampullary ends of the lateral and superior canals, but not that of the posterior canal.

FIGURE 43-6. After removal of the utricle and aspiration of the saccule, any residual neuroepithelium of the three semicircular canals is destroyed by mechanical disruption using a 3mm to 4mm angled hook.

FIGURE 43-7. After avulsion and destruction of the vestibular end organs, the vestibule is filled with absorbable gelatin sponge soaked in gentamicin or streptomycin solution and a tissue graft, such as fat.

SURGICAL COMPLICATIONS AND MANAGEMENT

Intraoperative Complications

Cerebrospinal Fluid Leakage

Fracture of the cribrose bone on the medial aspect of the vestibule results in profuse spinal fluid leakage from the internal auditory canal. The leakage can be controlled by a tissue graft using fascia, or subcutaneous fat, or both, to seal the vestibule.

Failure to Find Utricle

Identification and removal of the utricle is essential to a complete labyrinthectomy. When perilymph has been aspirated from the vestibule, the utricle may retract superiorly under the horizontal segment of the facial nerve. The use of a modified right-angled hook (utricular hook) (Fig. 43–5) or a right-angled 20F suction may aid in retrieval. Alternately, the utricle will remain fixed to the lateral and superior semicircular canals, which may be palpated in the depths of the vestibule. A wide exposure achieved by removing the bone from the inferior aspects of the oval window or by connecting the round and oval windows improves access to the vestibule and its contents.

Facial Nerve Injury

The facial nerve may be damaged in its horizontal segment. Care must be taken, particularly in retrieval of the utricle, to avoid trauma to the medial aspect of the horizontal segment of the nerve. Treatment of injury to the facial nerve should follow the usual principles of management of iatrogenic injury. A delayed facial paresis occurs infrequently and may be managed expectantly.

Postoperative Complications

Incomplete Labyrinthectomy

The incidence of incomplete labyrinthectomy in many series is under 5 per cent. However, persistent postoperative vestibular symptoms or failure to compensate following labyrinthectomy may signal residual neuroepithelium and vestibular function in the operated ear. A postoperative ice water caloric test is valuable, if the results are positive, to confirm the presence of functional neuroepithelium. However, absence of induced symptoms or nystagmus on postoperative ice water caloric test does not necessarily indicate total destruction of the vestibular end organs. In the presence of persistent symptoms or poor compensation following surgery in the absence of contralateral disease, the possibility of an incomplete labyrinthec-

tomy should be considered despite the absence of caloric response.

Management of suspected incomplete labyrinthectomy should include revision surgery. One option is revision transcanal labyrinthectomy with the patient under local anesthesia using the patient's response during manipulation of the vestibule as a means of localizing residual neuroepithelium. However, this is frequently a difficult procedure with fibrous tissue and, occasionally, new bone formation within the vestibule. A more certain means of ablating vestibular function in such cases is a transmastoid labyrinthectomy and translabyrinthine vestibular nerve section.

HISTOPATHOLOGY OF LABYRINTHECTOMY

Postmortem histopathology of temporal bones from patients who, in life, underwent labyrinthectomy have been reported by Belal et al.,[20] Linthicum et al.,[21] Pulec,[22] and Schuknecht,[23] and all have reported examples of incomplete mechanical disruption of the vestibular end organ after transcanal labyrinthectomy. These results underscore the importance of proper exposure, removal of the utricle, and thorough probing of the ampullae. In an animal study of labyrinthectomy, Schuknecht reported that the neuroepithelium of the posterior semicircular canal persisted in 10 of 24 ears. This fact argues for wider exposure of the vestibule by connecting the oval and round windows and for selective destruction of the posterior ampullary nerve, as recommended by Gacek, as an additional step to guarantee complete labyrinthectomy.[24] Both Linthicum et al.[21] and Belal et al.[20] reported traumatic neuroma within the vestibule following labyrinthectomy (Fig. 43–9). Both groups interpret this finding as an indication of the superiority of the translabyrinthine vestibular neurectomy. However, in one case, a traumatic neuroma was also described after transmastoid labyrinthectomy and section of the superior vestibular nerve. In an experimental study in the cat, Schuknecht reported no evidence of regeneration of vestibular nerve fibers or formation of traumatic neuroma following labyrinthectomy.[23] In temporal bone specimens from human subjects who had undergone transcanal labyrinthectomy during life, degeneration of the vestibular nerve was seen in one, and a proliferation of nerve fibers was identified in another (Fig. 43–10). However, no evidence exists to suggest that nerve fibers, whether residual or regenerative, can contribute to afferent vestibular input if the vestibular neuroepithelium distal to it has been destroyed.

Two patients are cited by Linthicum et al.[21] as examples of failure of labyrinthectomy because of trau-

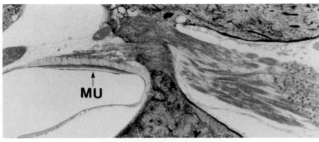

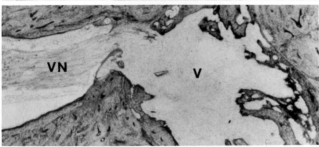

FIGURE 43-9. Histopathology of the superior vestibular nerve 36 months after transcanal labyrinthectomy in the cat. The unoperated control ear (A) at the level of the normal macular utriculi (MU). In the ear that had undergone labyrinthectomy (B), there was moderate degeneration of the vestibular nerve (VN), new bone and fibrous tissue within the vestibule (V), and no evidence of proliferation of the remaining vestibular nerves.

matic neuroma. In the first case, reported by Hilding and House,[25] the neuroma was uncovered at revision labyrinthectomy, but there was no evidence that the persistent symptoms resulted from the neuroma rather than from residual neuroepithelium.

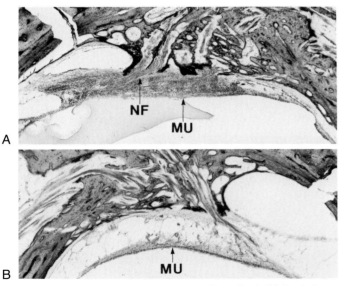

FIGURE 43-10. Histopathology 4 months after left labyrinthectomy. The macular utriculi (MU) of the ear that had surgery (A) shows atrophy. However, the stroma of the macula is intact, and there has been proliferation of nerve fibers (NF) within it. The superior vestibular nerve and macular utriculi (MU) of the unoperated side (B) appear normal.

In the second case, reported by Pulec,[22] a traumatic neuroma was identified by postmortem temporal bone histopathology in a patient with persistent vestibular symptoms for 10 years after labyrinthotomy, not labyrinthectomy. In addition, despite no response on the premortem caloric testing, the ampulla of the posterior semicircular canal was normal. In this case, the persistent vestibular symptoms probably resulted from residual vestibular neuroepithelium rather than from the traumatic neuroma.

RESULTS OF SURGERY

The reported results as measured by ablation of caloric function or cure of the patient have varied considerably. For example, Linthicum et al.[21] reported that only 17 of 25 patients (60 per cent) who underwent labyrinthectomy were cured or improved by this approach, and therefore they advocated translabyrinthine nerve section as a more reliable method of ablating vestibular function. However, Ariagno found a 98 per cent success rate in controlling peripheral vestibular disorders through transcanal labyrinthectomy, emphasizing the need for total destruction of the vestibular end organs by joining the oval and round windows.[15] Hammerschlag and Schuknecht reported a cure of episodic vertigo in 120 of 124 patients (96.8 per cent) by transcanal labyrinthectomy.[26] The remaining four patients had continuing disequilibrium, and three with persistent vestibular response by postoperative ice water caloric tests were cured by revision transcanal labyrinthectomy, resulting in an overall cure rate of 99 per cent.

SPECIAL CONSIDERATIONS

The advent of cochlear implantation as a possibility for rehabilitation of the profoundly deaf and the fact that 10 to 40 per cent of patients with Ménière's disease have bilateral involvement require consideration of the implications for eventual implantation after any surgical procedure for management of vestibular disturbance. Chen et al.[27] reported on three temporal bone cases from patients who in life had undergone labyrinthectomy, two by the transcanal route and one by the transmastoid approach. Based on the patency of the cochlear duct, remaining spiral ganglion and neural elements, and maintenance of the organ of Corti as evaluated by histopathologic study, these authors predicted that labyrinthectomy would not preclude subsequent cochlear implantation. In six patients who had undergone previous unilateral transmastoid labyrinthectomy, Lambert et al.[28] reported that round window electrical stimulation resulted in a psychophysical response to stimulus in all patients and electrically evoked middle latency response in five of six patients. Kveton et al.[29] reported an ear deafened by transmastoid labyrinthectomy with subsequent successful cochlear implantation resulting in speech comprehension comparable to that of patients deafened by other causes.

References

1. Stockwell CW, Graham MD: Vestibular compensation following labyrinthectomy and vestibular neurectomy. *In* Nadol JB Jr (ed): Second International Symposium for Ménière's disease. Amsterdam, Kugler & Ghedini Publishers, 1989, pp 489–498.
2. Dandy WE: Ménière's disease: Its diagnosis and a method of treatment. Arch Surg 16: 1127–1152,1928.
3. Jansen A.: Referat uber die operationsmethoden bei den verschiedenen otitischen gehirukoneplikationen. Verh Dtsch Otol Gesell (Jena), 1895, p 96.
4. Milligan W: Ménière's disease: A clinical and experimental inquiry. Br Med J 2: 1228,1904.
5. Lake R: Removal of the semicircular canals in a case of unilateral aural vertigo. Lancet i: 1567–1568,1904.
6. Cawthorne TE: The treatment of Ménière's disease. J Laryngol Otol 58: 63–71,1943.
7. Crockett EA: The removal of the stapes for the relief of auditory vertigo. Ann Otol Rhinol Laryngol 12: 67–72,1903.
8. Lempert J: Lempert decompression operation for hydrops of the endolymphatic labyrinth in Ménière's disease. Arch Otolaryngol Head Neck Surg 47: 551–570,1948.
9. Schuknecht HF: Ablation therapy for the relief of Ménière's disease. Laryngoscope 66: 859–870,1956.
10. Cawthorne T: Membranous labyrinthectomy via the oval window for Ménière's disease. J Laryngol Otol 71: 524–527,1957.
11. Schuknecht HF: Ablation therapy in the management of Ménière's disease. Acta Otolaryngol Suppl (Stockh) 132: 1–42,1957.
12. Schuknecht HF: Destructive therapy for Ménière's disease. Arch Otolaryngol Head Neck Surg 71: 562–572,1960.
13. Schuknecht HF: Destructive labyrinthine surgery. Arch Otolaryngol Head Neck Surg 97: 150–151,1973.
14. Armstrong BW: Transtympanic vestibulotomy for Ménière's disease. Laryngoscope 69: 1071–1074,1959.
15. Ariagno RP: Transtympanic labyrinthectomy. Arch Otolaryngol Head Neck Surg 80: 282–286,1964.
16. Greven AJ, Oosterveld WJ: The contralateral ear in Ménière's disease. Arch Otolaryngol Head Neck Surg 101: 608–612,1978.
17. Paparella MM, Griebie MS: Bilaterality of Ménière's disease. Acta Otolaryngol (Stockh) 97: 233–237,1984.
18. Nadol JB Jr: Positive "fistula sign" with an intact tympanic membrane. Arch Otolaryngol Head Neck Surg 100: 273–278,1974.
19. Silverstein H, Smouha E, Jones R: Natural history versus surgery for Ménière's disease. *In* Nadol JB Jr (ed): Second International Symposium for Ménière's disease. Amsterdam, Kugler & Ghedini Publishers, 1989, pp 543–544.
20. Belal A, Ylikoski J: Pathology as it relates to ear surgery. II. Labyrinthectomy. J Laryngol Otol 97: 1–10,1983.
21. Linthicum FH, Alonso A, Denia A: Traumatic neuroma. Arch Otolaryngol Head Neck Surg 105: 654–655,1979.
22. Pulec JL: Labyrinthectomy: Indications, technique and results. Laryngoscope 84: 1552–1573,1974.
23. Schuknecht HF: Behavior of the vestibular nerve following labyrinthectomy. Ann Otol Rhinol Laryngol 91 (5 Suppl 97): 16–32,1982.
24. Gacek RR: Transection of the posterior ampullary nerve for the relief of benign paroxysmal positional vertigo. Ann Otol Rhinol Laryngol 83: 596–605,1974.
25. Hilding DA, House WF: "Acoustic neuroma": Comparison of traumatic and neoplastic. J Ultrastruct Res 12: 611–623, 1965.
26. Hammerschlag PE, Schuknecht HF: Transcanal labyrinthectomy for intractable vertigo. Arch Otolaryngol Head Neck Surg 107: 152–156, 1981.
27. Chen DA, Linthicum, RH, Rizer FM: Cochlear histopathology in the labyrinthectomized ear: Implications for cochlear implantation. Laryngoscope 98: 1170–1172,1988.
28. Lambert PR, Ruth RA, Halpin CF: Promontory electrical stimulation in labyrinthectomized ears. Arch Otolaryngol Head Neck Surg 116: 197–201,1990.
29. Kveton JF, Abbott C, April M, et al.: Cochlear implantation after transmastoid labyrinthectomy. Laryngoscope 99: 610–613,1989.

44

Translabyrinthine Vestibular Neurectomy

RALPH A. NELSON, M.D., M.S.

Successful surgery for vertigo is predicated on three ① conditions, the first of which is altering or denervating the peripheral end-organ. If the symptoms do not originate in the end-organ, surgery is unlikely to be ② of value. Second, surgery is warranted only when dysequilibrium is significantly disabling or handicapping. Because major surgery for vertigo will often produce minor but noticeable sequelae, such as poor postdenervation central compensation, we must ensure that the cure is not worse than the disease. Third, ③ the patient must have shown a failure to respond to medicinal or noninvasive measures. If all these criteria are met, surgery may be considered.

The type of surgical intervention considered depends on several criteria, including ① surgical expertise and experience, ② residual hearing in the ear to be operated on, ③ condition of the opposite ear, ④ auditory needs of the patient, and ⑤ site of lesion. If the surgeon does not have the knowledge, training, and facilities to perform certain procedures, choices become limited. The levels of residual hearing also will dictate which procedures are best suited because a destructive labyrinthectomy may be quite appropriate when no residual hearing exists, but a hearing-conservation procedure will be used in most other circumstances. Last, the specific site of a peripheral lesion may have some influence on the procedure selected. As an example, a labyrinthectomy may not help patients with dizziness originating from a vestibular nerve tumor located medial to the end organ.

The translabyrinthine vestibular nerve section is the gold standard for denervation procedures. It is both a ① postganglionic nerve section, because of the labyrinthectomy used to access the internal auditory canal ② (IAC), and a preganglionic procedure, because of the vestibular nerve section. Some controversy surrounds the significance or even existence of traumatic neuromas in postganglionic procedures. Numerous traumatic neuromas have been documented in the House Ear Institute temporal bone collection,[1] and persisting balance problems in some patients have been attributed to these neuromas. Because of these histologic findings and the symptoms accompanying them, we prefer preganglionic surgeries whenever feasible.

The single largest drawback to the translabyrinthine vestibular nerve section is the sacrifice of residual hearing. In the past, a hearing level of 50 per cent speech discrimination and 50dB loss was felt to be the dividing line between serviceable and nonserviceable hearing; however, with the advent of better hearing aids and greater understanding of the role of binaural hearing in central processing, the parameters of serviceability have been expanded. This is especially true in situations in which the remaining ear is marginal or could become diseased, such as in Ménière's syndrome.[2]

Preoperative radiologic, auditory, vestibular and metabolic testing is not specific for translabyrinthine vestibular nerve section. Such testing is performed as a part of the dizziness evaluation done to determine the origin of symptoms. Surgery is not scheduled until these problems have been addressed.[3] These studies ensure that unrecognized pathology has not been missed, and in the case of vestibular function tests, that the proper end organ is operated on. It is necessary to point out, however, that in a large series of translabyrinthine eighth nerve sections, there was no direct correlation between success or failure of surgery and the degree of reduced vestibular response, as seen on electronystagmography.[4] This finding undoubtedly results from the inability of standard electronystagmography to test the function of the inferior vestibular nerve.

SURGICAL TECHNIQUE

Surgery is performed with the patient under general anesthesia and placed on the table in reverse to allow for table manipulations and to allow the seated surgeon to sit comfortably with knees under the table. The patient is supine, and the head is turned to the side facing away from the surgeon. The anesthesia machine is at the foot of the table and is connected to the endotracheal tube by extended tubing (Fig. 44–1). A sterile, hairless area is prepared 2cm above and 5cm behind the ear, and the field is draped off. The high-speed drill with various cutting burrs and suction irrigation with sterile saline are on the field. Monopolar and bipolar electrocautery are available. If it is to be used, seventh cranial nerve monitoring equipment is set up and the electrodes inserted.

An incision is made approximately 1cm above and behind the postauricular crease and follows the contour of the auricle (Fig. 44–2). A plane is established in the galea-aponeurotic layer lateral to the temporalis muscle, and the auricle is turned forward. A thick periosteal flap is created by incising this tissue along the linear temporalis just anterior to the incision line, and then inferiorly to the mastoid tip. This flap is elevated off the mastoid cortex and retracted forward with a large self-retaining retractor. The staggered two-layer incision provides better closure to prevent cerebrospinal fluid leaks.

The high-speed drill with a large cutting burr and constant suction irrigation is used to perform a cortical mastoidectomy. The posterior external bony canal wall is thinned, the bone over the tegmen is thinned, and the sigmoid sinus is skeletonized (Fig. 44–3). We frequently eggshell the bone over the sinus and decompress it by collapsing it with thumb pressure, leaving tiny, fragmented pieces of bone, similar to the

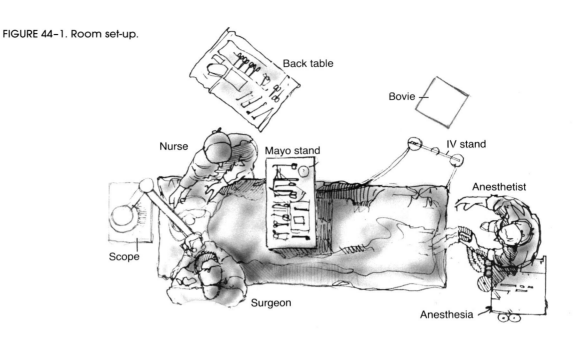

FIGURE 44-1. Room set-up.

Back table

Bovie

Nurse

Mayo stand

IV stand

Anesthetist

Scope

Surgeon

Anesthesia

armor of medieval chain mail, over the highly vulnerable sigmoid sinus to protect it from damage from instruments entering and exiting the wound (Fig. 44-4). The sinus is easily collapsed and gives needed exposure medially. The sinodural angle is opened as far back on the cortex as possible. Because the vestibule lies under the facial nerve anteriorly, an angulated view via the sinodural angle is necessary to visualize the contents of the vestibule and eventually identify landmarks used to excise the superior vestibular nerve.

Bone over the posterior fossa dura is thinned out but not removed. The labyrinth is skeletonized and the cells of the mastoid tip opened. The labyrinthectomy is performed by opening the crown of the lateral (horizontal) semicircular canal on its posterior border and following the half-opened canal posteriorly to the posterior canal. The lateral canal is only half opened to protect the external genu of the facial nerve until careful trimming can be done. The posterior canal, having been opened, can be traced to its confluence with the superior semicircular canal, where the two canals combine to become the common crus (Fig. 44-5). The common crus may then be followed directly forward to the vestibule (Fig. 44-6).

The posterior surface of the facial nerve over the external genu is now thinned carefully, and the anterior limb of the posterior canal is followed to its ampulla at the inferior pole of the elliptical recess. The lateral canal is opened anteriorly and medially to its ampullated end, and the ampulla of the superior canal identified next to that of the lateral is opened. The superior canal is opened along the tegmen throughout its course, which curves back to the common crus.

With all the canals and the vestibule opened, all soft tissue elements of the membranous labyrinth should be removed. This step would be the normal end point of the postauricular, postganglionic labyrinthectomy but only sets the stage to skeletonize the IAC in a translabyrinthine vestibular nerve section and preganglionic denervation (Fig. 44-7).

A key factor in successful exploration of the IAC is clear identification of the IAC contents. Identification is possible only if the soft tissue contents are not violated in the removal of bone during IAC skeletoniza-

Postauricular incision

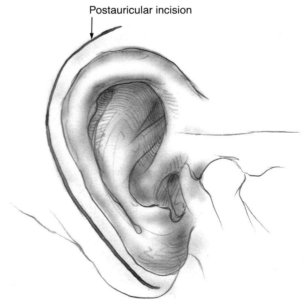

FIGURE 44-2. Postauricular incision.

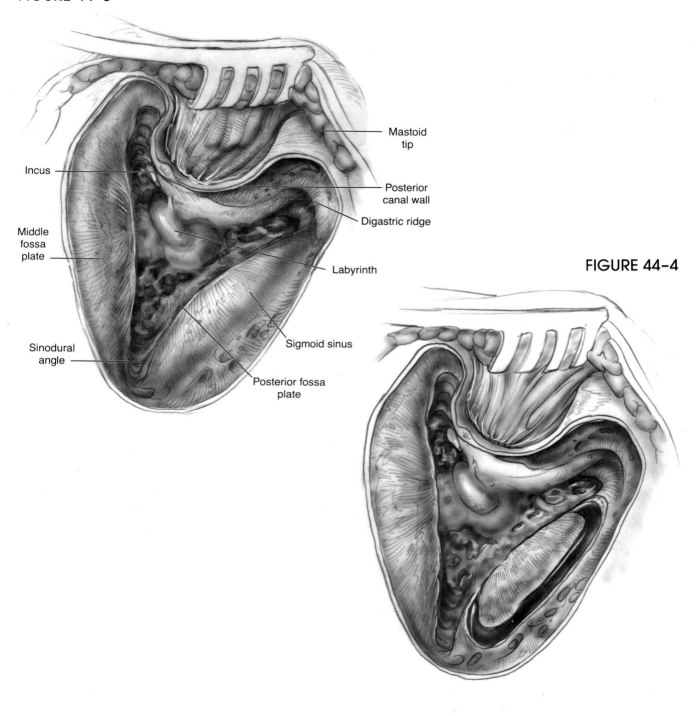

FIGURE 44-3

Incus

Middle
fossa
plate

Sinodural
angle

Mastoid
tip

Posterior
canal wall

Digastric ridge

Labyrinth

Sigmoid sinus

Posterior fossa
plate

FIGURE 44-4

FIGURE 44-3. Cortical mastoidectomy.

FIGURE 44-4. Sigmoid sinus decompression—"Bill's island."

FIGURE 44-5. Opening the semicircular canals.

FIGURE 44-6. Opening the vestibule.

FIGURE 44-7. Cleaning the vestibule.

FIGURE 44-8. Skeletonizing the internal auditory canal.

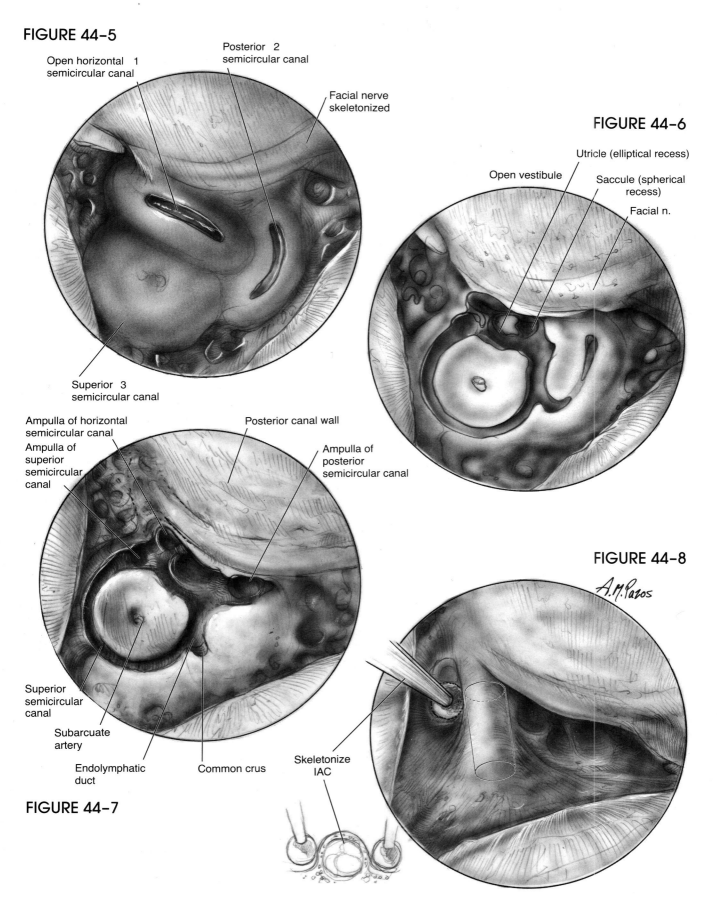

FIGURE 44-5

Open horizontal 1
semicircular canal

Posterior 2
semicircular canal

Facial nerve
skeletonized

Superior 3
semicircular canal

FIGURE 44-6

Open vestibule

Utricle (elliptical recess)

Saccule (spherical recess)

Facial n.

Ampulla of horizontal
semicircular canal

Ampulla of
superior
semicircular
canal

Posterior canal wall

Ampulla of
posterior
semicircular canal

Superior
semicircular
canal

Subarcuate
artery

Endolymphatic
duct

Common crus

Skeletonize
IAC

FIGURE 44-8

A. M. Pazos

FIGURE 44-7

tion. Loss of part or all of any of the soft tissue landmarks places all of the other contents at great risk because of the difficulty in differentiating the nerves from one another. The purpose in using the facial nerve–vestibular nerve tissue plane when dissecting the IAC is to enable identification of the facial nerve in its normal position and extend the dissection into the diseased area, where those relationships are sometimes more difficult to ascertain.

A useful technique for IAC skeletonization is blue lining the IAC throughout the area to be opened. The thin bony cover protects the soft tissue structures within the IAC. Blue lining actually starts at the vestibule because this is where the bone is thinnest. The nerves of the IAC exit into the bony labyrinth through perforations in the thin bone separating the fundus of the internal auditory canal from the vestibule. This naturally blue-lined area can be used as a starting point for skeletonization of the remainder of the canal. Removal of bone should extend to the porus acusticus and should cover 180° of the lateral side of the canal. The general orientation of the IAC is that the fundus is lateral just medial to the vestibule. The superior border is along a line drawn between the superior semicircular canal ampulla and the sinodural angle, and the inferior border is along the line starting at the posterior semicircular canal ampulla drawn posteriorly parallel to the superior border. The IAC angles away from the surgeon in an anterolateral to a posteromedial direction very deep to the sigmoid sinus (Fig. 44–8).

Once the IAC is adequately skeletonized, the irrigation fluid is changed to a solution of 0.25% bacitracin in saline, and the wound thoroughly rinsed. The thin bone over the canal is lifted away with a small, right-angled pick. The perforated area where the superior vestibular nerve enters both the lateral and the superior ampullae is thinned very carefully, and a 1mm hook is used to avulse the superior vestibular nerve from the vestibular nerve recess that it makes in the labyrinthine bone lateral to the fallopian canal. As the superior vestibular nerve is reflected, the facial nerve comes into view deep to the plane of dissection (Fig. 44–9). If the facial nerve is not immediately visible, the hook can be used to palpate the bone of the vestibular nerve recess ("Bill's bar," or the lateral wall of the fallopian canal) until the edge of the fallopian canal is found and the hook easily (and gently!) inserted into this labyrinthine segment of the canal.

With the superior vestibular nerve separated from the facial nerve (vestibulofacial fibers will have to be lysed), the inferior vestibular nerve is also avulsed with the singular nerve to the posterior semicircular canal. Because the singular nerve frequently leaves the inferior nerve midway out of the IAC, the surgeon must be careful to check for it. Failure to include the singular nerve may spell failure for the entire operation.

Scarpa's ganglion lies midway out of the IAC. The avulsed ends of the two vestibular nerves are reflected and the fused nerves sectioned medial to the ganglion. The specimen is sent to a pathologist for examination (Fig. 44–10).

Although the cochlear nerve may also be sectioned, this action would preclude its use in a cochlear implant if that opportunity arises. Generally, implantation is not a strong consideration, but sometimes a cochlear nerve section may be entertained as a possible solution to overwhelming tinnitus symptoms. Because elimination of tinnitus is not guaranteed, this approach is rarely encouraged.

Hemostasis is achieved through bipolar cautery and the application of bovine collagen (Avitene). Control of cerebrospinal fluid leak is achieved through dural closure with 4-0 silk sutures when possible, but primarily through packing. The IAC and labyrinthine defects are sealed with strips of adipose tissue obtained from the abdominal wall, and the mastoid incision is closed with interrupted, slow-absorbing sutures in a two-layer fashion, first, the thick periosteal flap, and then, a subcuticular closure of the skin. Steri-Strips are placed over the incision, and a bulky mastoid dressing is applied. The abdominal wall incision is usually drained. The patient is watched in intensive care for a day with hourly neurologic checks and then is moved to a step-down room when neurologic stability is assured. The abdominal drain is removed in 1 day, and the Steri-Strips in 1 week.

Cx: Complications seen with translabyrinthine neurectomy in order of frequency include cerebrospinal fluid leak, meningitis, and facial nerve paralysis. Facial paralysis can be considered the consequence of working in an area in which the nerve is anatomically at risk. Avoidance is the best medicine for this problem: the surgeon should be certain of the nerve's location and treat it with respect. Postoperative steroids or limited decompression of the nerve, particularly in the labyrinthine segment, may be useful in preventing seque-

---

FIGURE 44–9. Establishing the plane between the seventh and eighth nerves.

FIGURE 44–10. Section of the vestibular nerves medial to Scarpa's ganglion.

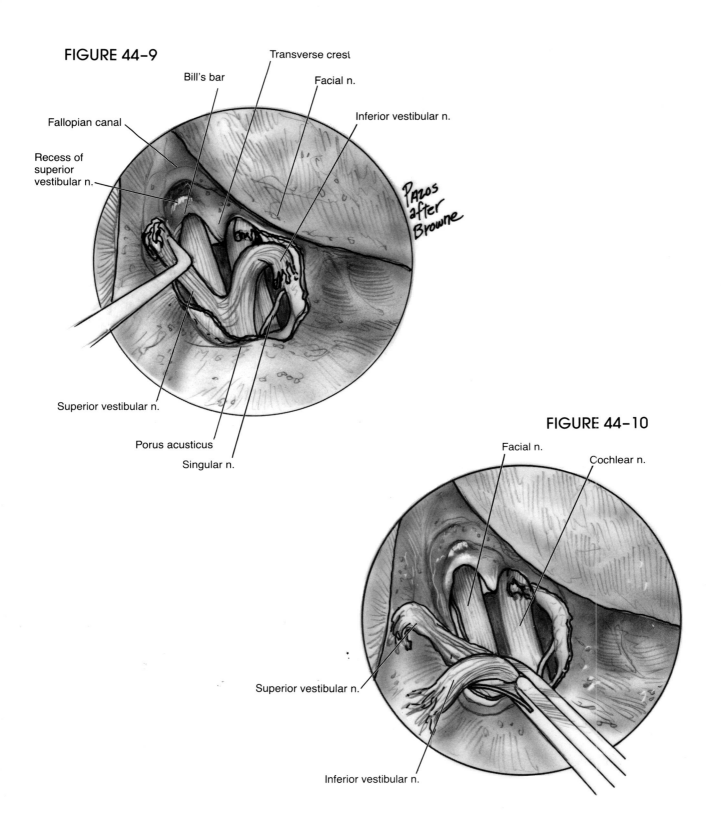

FIGURE 44-9

Fallopian canal

Recess of
superior
vestibular n.

Bill's bar

Transverse crest

Facial n.

Inferior vestibular n.

*Pazos
after
Browne*

Superior vestibular n.

Porus acusticus

Singular n.

FIGURE 44-10

Facial n.

Cochlear n.

Superior vestibular n.

Inferior vestibular n.

lae when the nerve is known to have been abused. We do not routinely employ perioperative antibiotics other than the bacitracin irrigation because of the fear of encouraging subclinical infections, which might become apparent only after release from the hospital. When fever and meningismus occur, a spinal tap is performed and appropriate antibiotic coverage instituted.

Cerebrospinal fluid leaks are aggressively pursued within 2 to 3 days to prevent retrograde contamination and meningitis. Initially, a tight head dressing is applied, and the patient is placed on carbonic anhydrase inhibitors, such as acetazolamide (Diamox). The patient is placed at bed rest in a semi-Fowler position. If resolution of the leak is not seen within 2 days, the wound is explored, usually with the patient under local anesthesia, and the adipose plug readjusted.

Patients are encouraged to sit up and dangle their legs on the first or second postoperative day, and to begin ambulation with help as soon as possible thereafter. Discharge from hospitalization occurs between the fifth and eighth days. Patients are checked in the office within the next 7 days to be certain that the postoperative progress is satisfactory.

Results of translabyrinthine vestibular nerve section indicate that our ability to properly diagnose the etiology of vertigo is imperfect. If complete denervation of the end organ is accomplished (and translabyrinthine neurectomy is the most complete denervation theoretically possible), vertigo should be absent postoperatively. However, we find that with the exception of Ménière's syndrome, which has a 93 per cent cure, our ability to control vertigo is 80 per cent or higher. Inability to properly diagnose the origin of the vertigo or inability of the central nervous system to compensate for the denervation are logical explanations for these statistics.[4]

References

1. Linthicum FH, Alongso A, Denia A: Traumatic neuroma: A complication of transcanal labyrinthectomy. Arch Otolaryngol Head Neck Surg 105: 654–655, 1979.
2. Shelton C, Hitselberger WE, House WF, Brackmann DE: Hearing preservation after acoustic tumor removal: Long-term results. Laryngoscope 100: 115–119, 1990.
3. Nelson RA, Brackmann DE: Clinical problems in Diagnosis and Documentation of Ménière's Disease. Immunobiology, Histophysiology and Tumor Immunology in Otolaryngology. Proceedings of 2nd International Academic Conference, Utrecht, The Netherlands. Berkeley, CA, Kugler, 1987, pp 3–8.
4. Nelson RA: Labyrinthectomy and translabyrinthine nerve section. *In* Brackmann DE (ed): Neurological Surgery of the Ear and Skull Base. New York, Raven Press, 1982.

45

Posterior Ampullary Nerve Section for Benign Paroxysmal Positional Vertigo

RICHARD R. GACEK, M.D.

Benign paroxysmal positional vertigo (cupulolithiasis, or BPPV) is a disorder of the semicircular canal system, usually the posterior semicircular canal.[1] This balance symptom is produced by a cupula of the sense organ that has been transformed into a gravity-sensitive structure because of deposits probably derived from degenerated otoconia of the utricular macula.[2] Dislodgement of utricular otoconia may result from head injury, viral labyrinthitis, aging, or traumatic inner ear surgery. Patients with this disorder complain of a rotatory experience when the head is placed in either the head-back or the to-the-side positions.[3] The vertiginous experience typically has a duration of less than 1 minute and reappears briefly when the original position is resumed. In severe cases, nausea and vomiting may accompany the vertiginous experience. Repeat positioning results in decreased vestibular signs and symptoms.

The Hallpike maneuver[4] is used diagnostically to reproduce the patient's symptoms and nystagmus (Fig. 45–1). The direction of nystagmus is typically a rotatory one that occurs in a counterclockwise direction when the right ear is nearest the floor and clockwise when the left ear is downmost. The type and direction of nystagmus are determined by the anatomic projections of the posterior canal sense organ.[1] These projections are diagrammed in Figure 45–2 and summarize the input of the posterior semicircular canal to the inferior rectus and the superior oblique muscles, which on excitation produce the rotatory type of nystagmus described with Hallpike positioning maneuver. Because many patients with this disorder have normal hearing, a selective denervation of the posterior canal sense organ without invading the labyrinthine capsule is desirable to preserve hearing. The nerve to the ampullary posterior canal crista travels in a separate canal (singular canal) and can be approached from a middle ear direction.

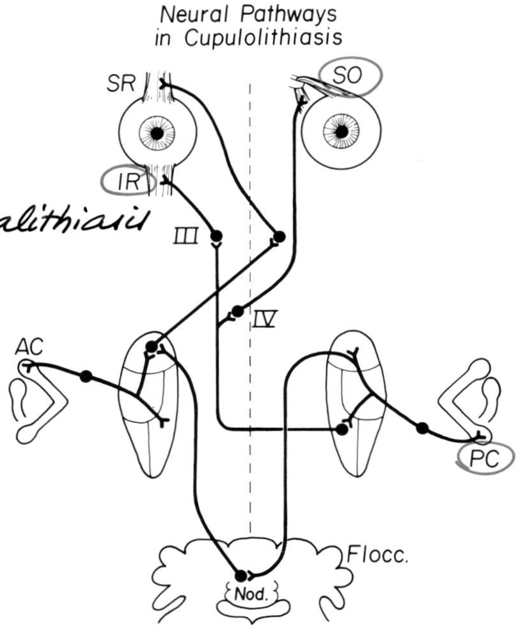

There is another group of patients with balance symptoms, not typically paroxysmal positional vertigo, resulting from incomplete ablation of labyrinthine function, attempted either by labyrinthectomy or vestibular nerve transection. Because the posterior canal sense organ and its nerve supply are anatomically inaccessible in these procedures, they may escape ablation. This residual function of the posterior canal sense organ may be responsible for persistent symptoms following vestibular ablation procedures. In these patients, transection of the singular nerve can be performed to provide relief of their symptoms.

FIGURE 45–2. Diagram of the neural pathways responsible for nystagmus response during provocative test and following singular neurectomy. AC = anterior canal; PC = posterior canal; SR = superior rectus; IR = inferior rectus; SO = superior oblique; III = oculomotor nucleus; IV = trochlear nucleus; Nod. = nodulus; Flocc. = flocculus. (Modified from Baloh RW, Spooner JW: Downbeat nystagmus: A type of central vestibular nystagmus. Neurology 31: 304–310, 1981, as in Gacek RR: Pathophysiology and management of cupulolithiasis. Am J Otolaryngol 6: 66–74, 1985.)

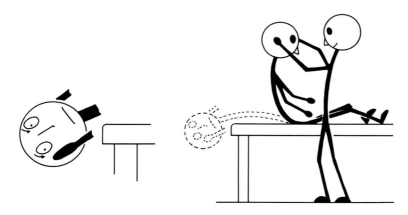

FIGURE 45–1. Diagram of the maneuver used to demonstrate nystagmus in positional vertigo. (From Carmichael EA, Dix MR, Hallpike CS: Pathology, symptomatology and diagnosis of the organic affections of the eighth nerve system. Br Med Bull 12: 146–152, 1956.)

PATIENT SELECTION

Because the vast majority of patients with BPPV undergo spontaneous resolution within a 6- to 12-month period, or may be only mildly disabled by their symptoms, surgical treatment is not frequently employed.[5] Exercise programs that use the head and neck and upper trunk muscles may be helpful in reducing the severity of symptomatology and promoting spontaneous resolution.[6] However, for a small **dx:** group of patients who demonstrate chronic positional vertigo for more than 1 year and are sufficiently disabled from their normal activities, singular neurectomy (SN) has provided a very effective means of relief from the disabling symptoms.[1, 7] Some patients with chronic BPPV continue to live with their symptoms by avoiding the provocative position and changing their lifestyle. Surgical relief is offered only to those who request it and are willing to accept a 4 per cent risk of hearing loss.

PREOPERATIVE EXAMINATION

The evaluation and diagnosis of BPPV consists of an accurately obtained history documenting labyrinthine trauma, such as head injury, viral labyrinthitis, inner ear surgery, or aging, as well as tests of auditory and vestibular function. Most patients with this syndrome are middle aged (mean age is in the sixth decade). There is a 2:1 female predominance. The vast majority of patients have a normal ear examination, although an occasional patient with chronic middle ear inflammatory disease experiences BPPV. The patients with chronic inflammatory disease should undergo surgical eradication of the inflammatory disease to control vestibular symptoms. The functional evaluation consists of pure-tone and speech audiometry as well as electronystagmographic assessment of the vestibular sensitivity by the caloric method. Auditory brain stem response and electrocochleographic examinations are not necessary in the evaluation of a patient with this disorder.

Dx: The most important diagnostic test is the Hallpike maneuver properly performed with or without Frenzel's glasses with the patient on an examining room table (see Fig. 45–1). The test has been well described in the literature[4] and consists of the examiner taking the patient's head down to a head-hanging position, first right and then left, from the sitting position and observing the patient's ocular response along with his or her subjective vestibular experience. Posterior canal BPPV typically produces a rotatory nystagmus either clockwise or counterclockwise after a latency of a few seconds. The nystagmus builds to a crescendo and then disappears over a period of 25 to 30 seconds but reappears when the sitting position is again assumed. Repeat testing produces less nystagmus and subjective symptoms, supporting the peripheral location of the pathology. It is important to test both right and left head-down positions because approximately 15 to 18 per cent of patients with BPPV have bilateral disease[8] that is usually worse in one ear than the other. In patients with unilateral cupulolithiasis, a nystagmus response is not seen when the contralateral (non-involved) ear is placed geotropically because the gravity-sensitive cupula is deflected utriculopetally (opposite to hair cell polarization). When the involved ear is geotropic, cupular deflection is utriculifugal and in the direction of hair cell polarization, thereby causing depolarization (Fig. 45–3). Occasionally, the Hallpike test may reveal a horizontal nystagmus with the same time characteristics and fatigability observed with the rotatory nystagmus.[9] These patients are not candidates for singular neurectomy, as their symptoms may be caused by pathology in other labyrinthine sense organs, such as the lateral canal crista.

MRI: Because a central nervous system lesion has been identified rarely in patients with similar findings, an imaging study, such as enhanced magnetic resonance imaging or computed tomographic scan, of the posterior fossa is recommended to rule out the slim chance of a central lesion being responsible for the positional vertigo.

Once a patient has been identified as having BPPV of the peripheral type, the degree of disability from the positional vertigo must be determined from an evaluation of the patient's work and lifestyle. If the

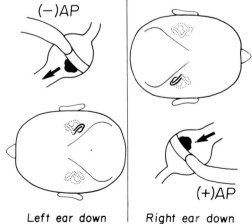

FIGURE 45–3. Explanation for different responses of right posterior semicircular canal in right ear down and left ear down position tests. AP = action potentials. (From Gacek RR: Pathophysiology and management of cupulolithiasis. Am J Otolaryngol 6: 66–74, 1985.)

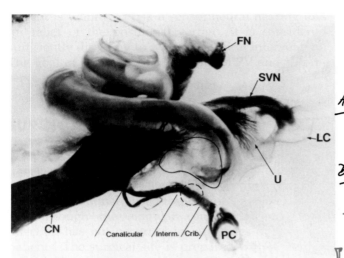

FIGURE 45-5. Dissection of human labyrinth and its nerve supply shows the relationship of the singular nerve to the round window membrane *(solid line)*. Dashed circular line indicates the point for transection of the nerve. The three divisions of the singular canal are explained in the text. (From Gacek RR: Transection of the posterior ampullary nerve for the relief of benign paroxysmal positional vertigo. Am Otol Rhinol Laryngol 83: 596–605, 1974.)

a small piece of adipose tissue will satisfactorily control the leak. On a few occasions, the SN was exposed at its entrance into the recess for the posterior canal ampulla (Fig. 45–6). After the tympanic membrane and flap are returned to their original position, a small pack is used to hold them in position for approximately 1 week while healing occurs. A small cotton ball in the external auditory meatus and a small outer ear dressing is applied for the first 24 hours. Beyond that, a sterile cotton ball is placed in the external au-

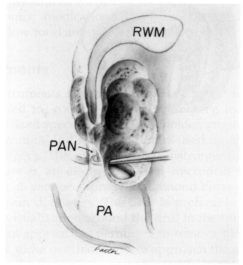

FIGURE 45-6. Diagram of the surgical exposure and probing of singular canal aperture into the recess for posterior canal ampulla. RWM: Round window membrane; PAN: Posterior ampullary nerve; PA: Posterior canal ampulla. (From Gacek RR: Pathophysiology and management of cupulolithiasis. Am J Otolaryngol 6: 66–74, 1985.)

ditory meatus and the pack is removed in 1 week's time at an outpatient visit.

POSTOPERATIVE CARE

Oral antibiotics are used routinely for 1 week. Postoperatively, patients have varying degrees of ataxia and dizziness; some patients are able to leave the hospital 1 day after surgery; others require from 2 to 4 days. The Hallpike maneuver, when carried out on the first postoperative day, does not demonstrate a rotatory nystagmus as in the preoperative positional test but instead will demonstrate a downbeat vertical nystagmus reflecting the imbalance between eye muscles supplied by the complementary vertical canals. There is an unopposed pull of the superior rectus from the contralateral anterior canal following denervation of its coplaner posterior canal. This nonfatiguing positional downbeat nystagmus will be observed for 1 to 3 days and usually parallels the patient's ability to leave the hospital. Vestibular exercises are not necessary but may help allow some patients to complete the compensatory process necessary to overcome the vestibular deficit created by singular neurectomy.

PITFALLS OF SURGERY

The primary risk of this surgery is injury to the cochlea through the round window membrane. This injury can be avoided by carefully identifying the round window membrane and avoiding injury to it with instrumentation, particularly the drill. Maintaining a ridge of bone between the attachment of the round window membrane and the site created for exposing the singular canal is helpful in avoiding this undesirable result. Another significant complication of the procedure is not finding the singular canal and the nerve. Because of variability in the anatomic position of the canal, this may occur when the singular canal is located superiorly under the round window membrane attachment. The use of local anesthesia to permit the patient's response when the canal is exposed and probed is crucial in avoiding this pitfall of surgery.

RESULTS

To date, 125 patients have undergone singular neurectomy in a series dating back to 1972.[7] All but four of these patients have had complete relief of the positional vertigo, and only four have experienced a sensorineural hearing loss as a result of the surgery.

PATIENT SELECTION

Because the vast majority of patients with BPPV undergo spontaneous resolution within a 6- to 12-month period, or may be only mildly disabled by their symptoms, surgical treatment is not frequently employed.[5] Exercise programs that use the head and neck and upper trunk muscles may be helpful in reducing the severity of symptomatology and promoting spontaneous resolution.[6] However, for a small group of patients who demonstrate chronic positional vertigo for more than 1 year and are sufficiently disabled from their normal activities, singular neurectomy (SN) has provided a very effective means of relief from the disabling symptoms.[1, 7] Some patients with chronic BPPV continue to live with their symptoms by avoiding the provocative position and changing their lifestyle. Surgical relief is offered only to those who request it and are willing to accept a 4 per cent risk of hearing loss.

dx:

PREOPERATIVE EXAMINATION

The evaluation and diagnosis of BPPV consists of an accurately obtained history documenting labyrinthine trauma, such as head injury, viral labyrinthitis, inner ear surgery, or aging, as well as tests of auditory and vestibular function. Most patients with this syndrome are middle aged (mean age is in the sixth decade). There is a 2:1 female predominance. The vast majority of patients have a normal ear examination, although an occasional patient with chronic middle ear inflammatory disease experiences BPPV. The patients with chronic inflammatory disease should undergo surgical eradication of the inflammatory disease to control vestibular symptoms. The functional evaluation consists of pure-tone and speech audiometry as well as electronystagmographic assessment of the vestibular sensitivity by the caloric method. Auditory brain stem response and electrocochleographic examinations are not necessary in the evaluation of a patient with this disorder.

dx: The most important diagnostic test is the Hallpike maneuver properly performed with or without Frenzel's glasses with the patient on an examining room table (see Fig. 45–1). The test has been well described in the literature[4] and consists of the examiner taking the patient's head down to a head-hanging position, first right and then left, from the sitting position and observing the patient's ocular response along with his or her subjective vestibular experience. Posterior canal BPPV typically produces a rotatory nystagmus either clockwise or counterclockwise after a latency of a few seconds. The nystagmus builds to a crescendo and then disappears over a period of 25 to 30 seconds but

reappears when the sitting position is again assumed. Repeat testing produces less nystagmus and subjective symptoms, supporting the peripheral location of the pathology. It is important to test both right and left head-down positions because approximately 15 to 18 per cent of patients with BPPV have bilateral disease[8] that is usually worse in one ear than the other. In patients with unilateral cupulolithiasis, a nystagmus response is not seen when the contralateral (non-involved) ear is placed geotropically because the gravity-sensitive cupula is deflected utriculopetally (opposite to hair cell polarization). When the involved ear is geotropic, cupular deflection is utriculifugal and in the direction of hair cell polarization, thereby causing depolarization (Fig. 45–3). Occasionally, the Hallpike test may reveal a horizontal nystagmus with the same time characteristics and fatigability observed with the rotatory nystagmus.[9] These patients are not candidates for singular neurectomy, as their symptoms may be caused by pathology in other labyrinthine sense organs, such as the lateral canal crista.

MRI: Because a central nervous system lesion has been identified rarely in patients with similar findings, an imaging study, such as enhanced magnetic resonance imaging or computed tomographic scan, of the posterior fossa is recommended to rule out the slim chance of a central lesion being responsible for the positional vertigo.

Once a patient has been identified as having BPPV of the peripheral type, the degree of disability from the positional vertigo must be determined from an evaluation of the patient's work and lifestyle. If the

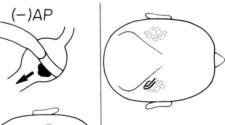
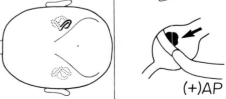

Cupulolithiasis
Right Posterior Semicircular Canal

(−)AP

Left ear down | Right ear down

(+)AP

FIGURE 45–3. Explanation for different responses of right posterior semicircular canal in right ear down and left ear down position tests. AP = action potentials. (From Gacek RR: Pathophysiology and management of cupulolithiasis. Am J Otolaryngol 6: 66–74, 1985.)

patient is willing to risk a sensorineural hearing loss for relief of the positional vertigo, it is considered sufficiently disabling to warrant surgical intervention. The goal of SN is to eliminate the BPPV and to preserve hearing.

SURGICAL TECHNIQUE

The preoperative preparation is similar to that for any transcanal middle ear surgery; preoperative or intraoperative antibiotics are not used. Postoperative antibiotics are routinely used to prevent ascending infection through the singular canal. However, such infection has not occurred in our series of over 125 patients. The surgical site is prepared with a sterilizing solution, such as povidone-iodine (Betadine), and draped for transcanal surgery. A bifenestrated drape with an opening for the patient's face and one that fits around the auricle is available commercially. The patient is in a prone position with the head turned so that the operated ear is facing up toward the surgeon and the head is in a somewhat dependent position, the ear canal is then on a straight line with the surgeons's view. A small amount of hair is shaved around the postauricular area so that the drape can adhere to the skin surface. The surgical procedure is carried out with the patient under local anesthesia with 1 per cent lidocaine (Xylocaine) with 1:100,000 dilution of adrenaline injected into the external auditory meatus and the posterior and inferior canal wall skin. A 27-gauge needle is helpful to successfully place the local anesthetic in the subperiosteal layer of the ear canal and dissect down to the level of the tympanic annulus. Medically assisted anesthesia with intravenous medication from an anesthesiologist helps allow local anesthesia to be effective.

Instruments

The instruments for this procedure are the same as those used for routine middle ear surgery, including various sized speculae, speculum holder, angled canal wall elevators, and hooks and picks used in oval window surgery. The most essential instrument for this procedure is an electric-powered microdrill for use through an ear speculum with diamond burrs of 1mm and 0.5mm diameters. The drill is preferably angled so that visualization around the drill in the transcanal speculum approach is permitted to remove the round window niche overhang and to approach the singular canal in the floor of the round window niche. Monitoring of hearing or facial nerve is not included in our experience, although monitoring of auditory function may be useful in determining any untoward event in auditory function from the surgical procedure. With

the patient under local anesthesia, the surgeon can monitor the patient's subjective symptoms of vertigo and pain when the singular nerve is transected and can observe a vertical or rotatory nystagmus at this transection.

Surgery

After elevation of the tympanomeatal flap, the drill is used to remove the overhang of the round window niche so that the entire round window membrane can be visualized from anteriorly to posteriorly (Fig. 45–4). Often, a mucous membrane fold will cover the aperture of the round window niche and should not be confused with the round window membrane. This membrane fold is dissected free with small hooks and picks so that the round window membrane can be clearly identified by its dark gray appearance and by its displacement when the ossicular chain is depressed. After the round window membrane has been satisfactorily exposed, the drill is used to create a depression in the floor of the round window niche just inferior to the bony attachment of the posterior segment of the round window membrane. This bony depression is deepened to a level of 2mm, at which point the singular canal is usually encountered and is recognized by the white myelinated nerve bundle that runs slightly at an angle to the alignment of the round window membrane (Fig. 45–5). If the singular canal is not identified at the level of 2mm or more, the singular canal may be superiorly located under the attachment of the round window membrane. The drill can then be used to enlarge the base of the bony depression in the floor of the niche to reach the singular canal from the inferior direction by undercutting the attachment of the round window membrane. In these cases, identification of the nerve in the singular canal is highlighted by the patient's abrupt response of vertigo or pain.

The canal is then probed with a small, right-angled hook, probing only the proximal end of the singular canal. Probing the distal end of the canal is not advised because of the proximity to the posterior canal ampulla. After repeated probing of the canal with destruction of the nerve tissue, the bony defect is drilled lightly to place bone dust into the canal lumen. This dust should form a bony barrier to regeneration of nerve fibers. Absorbable gelatin sponge (Gelfoam) may then be used to fill the bony defect. Because the segment of singular canal exposed is either the intermediate or the cribrose segment, cerebrospinal leak is not usually encountered. The nerve is surrounded by cerebrospinal fluid in the proximal canalicular segment, which lies inferior to the floor of the vestibule. Rarely, a leak of spinal fluid may be seen if the singular canal is probed too far proximally. In these cases,

FIGURE 45-4

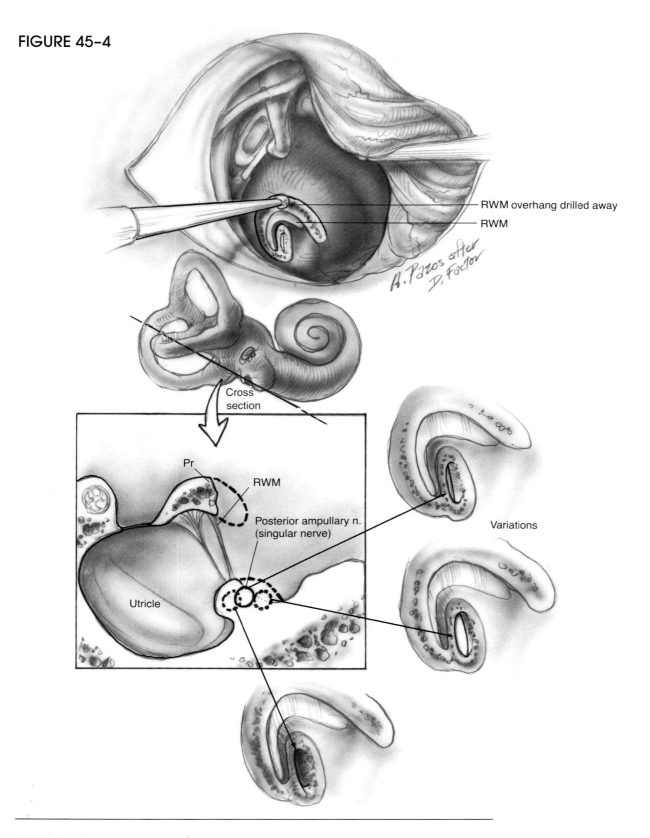

FIGURE 45-4. Surgical view of the right middle ear with a corresponding vertical section taken through the round window niche. The three most common variations in the anatomy of the singular canal are shown. RWM = round window membrane; Pr = promontory. (Redrawn from Gacek RR: Pathophysiology and management of cupulolithiasis. Am J Otolaryngol 6: 66-74, 1985.)

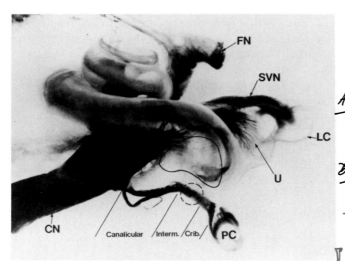

FIGURE 45-5. Dissection of human labyrinth and its nerve supply shows the relationship of the singular nerve to the round window membrane *(solid line)*. Dashed circular line indicates the point for transection of the nerve. The three divisions of the singular canal are explained in the text. (From Gacek RR: Transection of the posterior ampullary nerve for the relief of benign paroxysmal positional vertigo. Am Otol Rhinol Laryngol 83: 596-605, 1974.)

a small piece of adipose tissue will satisfactorily control the leak. On a few occasions, the SN was exposed at its entrance into the recess for the posterior canal ampulla (Fig. 45–6). After the tympanic membrane and flap are returned to their original position, a small pack is used to hold them in position for approximately 1 week while healing occurs. A small cotton ball in the external auditory meatus and a small outer ear dressing is applied for the first 24 hours. Beyond that, a sterile cotton ball is placed in the external au-

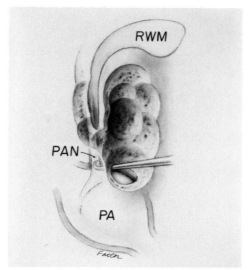

FIGURE 45-6. Diagram of the surgical exposure and probing of singular canal aperture into the recess for posterior canal ampulla. RWM: Round window membrane; PAN: Posterior ampullary nerve; PA: Posterior canal ampulla. (From Gacek RR: Pathophysiology and management of cupulolithiasis. Am J Otolaryngol 6: 66–74, 1985.)

ditory meatus and the pack is removed in 1 week's time at an outpatient visit.

POSTOPERATIVE CARE

Oral antibiotics are used routinely for 1 week. Postoperatively, patients have varying degrees of ataxia and dizziness; some patients are able to leave the hospital 1 day after surgery; others require from 2 to 4 days. The Hallpike maneuver, when carried out on the first postoperative day, does not demonstrate a rotatory nystagmus as in the preoperative positional test but instead will demonstrate a downbeat vertical nystagmus reflecting the imbalance between eye muscles supplied by the complementary vertical canals. There is an unopposed pull of the superior rectus from the contralateral anterior canal following denervation of its coplaner posterior canal. This nonfatiguing positional downbeat nystagmus will be observed for 1 to 3 days and usually parallels the patient's ability to leave the hospital. Vestibular exercises are not necessary but may help allow some patients to complete the compensatory process necessary to overcome the vestibular deficit created by singular neurectomy.

PITFALLS OF SURGERY

The primary risk of this surgery is injury to the cochlea through the round window membrane. This injury can be avoided by carefully identifying the round window membrane and avoiding injury to it with instrumentation, particularly the drill. Maintaining a ridge of bone between the attachment of the round window membrane and the site created for exposing the singular canal is helpful in avoiding this undesirable result. Another significant complication of the procedure is not finding the singular canal and the nerve. Because of variability in the anatomic position of the canal, this may occur when the singular canal is located superiorly under the round window membrane attachment. The use of local anesthesia to permit the patient's response when the canal is exposed and probed is crucial in avoiding this pitfall of surgery.

RESULTS

To date, 125 patients have undergone singular neurectomy in a series dating back to 1972.[7] All but four of these patients have had complete relief of the positional vertigo, and only four have experienced a sensorineural hearing loss as a result of the surgery.

COMPLICATIONS

Infection and delayed healing of the tympanic membrane should not occur in the hands of a trained otologic surgeon. The primary problem following this surgery is a recurrence of symptoms.

Recurrence of vertigo following singular neurectomy may be caused by incomplete transection of the singular nerve in the operated ear or by BPPV or cupulolithiasis involving the contralateral ear. Carefully performed Hallpike maneuvers with documentation of the nystagmus response are necessary to determine the presence of positional vertigo in either ear. Approximately 15 to 18 per cent of patients may exhibit bilateral cupulolithiasis. Other forms of dysequilibrium may be experienced by patients following singular neurectomy and are related to inadequate vestibular compensation to the ablation procedure.

ALTERNATIVE TECHNIQUES

Patients with chronic disabling BPPV that is not responsive to conservative methods of management may be considered for other methods of surgical ablation. The procedure of posterior canal occlusion through a mastoidectomy approach has been recently described by Parnes and McClure,[10] who cited a high percentage of effective relief from positional vertigo and no apparent significant incidence of sensorineural hearing loss. Although the procedure is based on the theory that compression of the membranous canal will immobilize the endolymph fluid compartment, preventing the cupular displacement, a more plausible explanation for the relief of positional symptoms by the surgical procedure is degenerative effect on the posterior canal sense organ sensitivity as a result of a surgical labyrinthitis. The delay (up to 8 weeks) in the disappearance of the positive Hallpike response following surgery as well as the reversible sensorineural hearing loss that usually occurs following the procedure are clinical signs that suggest labyrinthitis. Careful observation over time and reporting of results will be necessary to decide on the usefulness of this procedure. Furthermore, this procedure requires a mastoidectomy performed under general anesthesia and poses some risk of injury to the facial nerve.

Total ablation of the vestibular input from the labyrinth by selective vestibular nerve section is another approach to ablating the posterior canal activity. Unfortunately, this procedure also ablates remaining vestibular labyrinth function, thus unnecessarily denervating the input from important sense organs, such as the utricular macula, the saccule, and the two cristae supplied by the superior vestibular division. In addition, the morbidity associated with vestibular nerve section is significantly higher than with singular neurectomy.

Finally, in the rare patient who may have cupulolithiasis involving the posterior canal in an only hearing ear, a possible treatment would be the parenteral administration of streptomycin sulfate to ablate vestibular function by a titrated method.

References

1. Gacek RR: Pathophysiology and management of cupulolithiasis. Am J Otolaryngol 6: 66–74, 1985.
2. Schuknecht HF: Cupulolithiasis. Arch Otolaryngol Head Neck Surg 90: 113–126, 1969.
3. Barany R: Diagnose von Krankheitserscheinungen im Bereiche des Otolithenapparates. Acta Otolaryngol (Stockh) 2: 434–437, 1921.
4. Carmichael EA, Dix MR, Hallpike CS: Pathology, symptomatology and diagnosis of the organic affections of the eighth nerve system. Br Med Bull 12: 146–152, 1956.
5. Barber HO: Positional nystagmus, especially after head injury. Laryngoscope 74: 891–944, 1964.
6. Brandt T, Daroff RB: Physical therapy for benign paroxysmal positional vertigo. Arch Otolaryngol Head Neck Surg 106: 484–485, 1980.
7. Gacek RR: Singular neurectomy update. II. Review of 102 cases. Laryngoscope 101: 855–862, 1991.
8. Longridge NS, Barber HO: Bilateral paroxysmal positioning nystagmus. J Otolaryngol 7: 395–400, 1978.
9. McClure JA: Horizontal canal BPV. J Otolaryngol 14: 30–35, 1985.
10. Parnes LS, McClure JA: Posterior semicircular canal occlusion for intractable benign paroxysmal positional vertigo. Ann Otol Rhinol Laryngol 99: 330–334, 1990.

46

Posterior Semicircular Canal Occlusion for Benign Paroxysmal Positional Vertigo

LORNE PARNES, M.D.

Benign paroxysmal positional vertigo (BPPV) is the commonest vestibular end-organ disorder: in one busy vestibular clinic, BPPV accounted for 17 per cent of diagnoses.[1] Patients complain of brief vertigo spells, often accompanied by nausea but rarely vomiting. The actual duration of the spells (5 to 15 seconds) is usually much shorter than what the patient describes (10 seconds to 5 minutes). Spells are induced by characteristic head movements, such as rolling to the affected side while supine or extending the neck while upright. Less common precipitating movements include bending forward, arising from a supine position, and rotating the head. When the disease is very active, in addition to the brief positional vertigo episodes, patients may complain of protracted, nonspecific imbalance and dizziness accompanied by mild lassitude.

BPPV is most often an idiopathic disorder. The commonest identifiable cause is head or temporal bone trauma.[2] Other less common causes include viral labyrinthitis, vestibular neuronitis, stapedectomy, perilymph fistula, Ménière's disease, and chronic otitis media.[3–8]

Three factors provide conclusive evidence that BPPV is a disorder of the posterior semicircular canal of the undermost ear during the provocative Hallpike maneuver, the diagnostic test for BPPV. First, various combinations of rotatory, vertical, and oblique nystagmus may be seen in response to the Hallpike maneuver, depending on the position of the globe within the orbit during the nystagmus. However, the nystagmus profile correlates with the known neuromuscular pathways arising from the crista of the undermost posterior canal.[9–12] Second, in a postmortem temporal bone study, Schuknecht and Ruby[13] identified large basophilic deposits attached to the posterior canal cupula in three specimens. These three patients had premortem documentation of BPPV affecting the same ear. They coined the term *cupulolithiasis* to describe this finding. Third, when successful, selective denervation of the undermost posterior canal (singular neurectomy) cures this condition.[14]

The Hallpike maneuver begins by quickly rotating the patient back from a sitting to a head-hanging position with the head turned 45° and the affected ear facing down toward the floor. This maneuver serves to rotate the undermost posterior semicircular canal in the earth vertical plane, thereby inducing a characteristic oculomotor response of rotatory nystagmus, which from the examiner's viewpoint has its fast phase beating clockwise with the left ear down and counterclockwise with the right ear down. There is a brief latent period (usually 2 to 5 seconds but as long as 10 to 20 seconds) between the patient's assuming the head-hanging position and the onset of the nystagmus. The patient complains of accompanying vertigo and often nausea. The vertigo and nystagmus briefly crescendo, plateau, and then gradually decrescendo with a typical limited total duration of 10 to 30 seconds. Once the nystagmus stops, the patient is returned to the sitting position, where after a short latent period, a milder reverse-direction nystagmus occurs with a less intense sensation of vertigo. Fatigability occurs whereby the nystagmus and vertigo responses decrease in intensity and duration with each repeated maneuver at the same sitting. Because standard electronystagmography does not record rotational eye movements, normal electronystagmographic positional testing should not preclude the diagnosis of BPPV. The necessity for direct visualization of the eyes during the Hallpike maneuver cannot be overstated.

BPPV must be differentiated from other causes of vertigo and nystagmus. The history is usually quite typical, and a positive response to the Hallpike maneuver is virtually diagnostic, assuming that all features are present. To my knowledge, no cases of other lesions perfectly replicating all of the classic features of a positive Hallpike maneuver have been reported.

BPPV has three types of clinical courses. Most common is the self-limited variety that subsides spontaneously over weeks to months. A second group of patients experience remissions and recurrences ranging from weeks to years. A still smaller group seem to have the more permanent form of this disorder. In one busy vestibular clinic, about 30 per cent of untreated patients had symptoms lasting longer than 1 year.[8]

PATHOPHYSIOLOGY

Under normal physiologic conditions, the cupula has the same density as the surrounding endolymph. Therefore, the semicircular canals are normally not sensitive to gravity (linear acceleration). However a fixed cupular deposit would render the posterior canal crista gravity sensitive.[15] Rotation of the canal in the earth vertical plane during the Hallpike maneuver produces cupular displacement through the gravitation pull on the deposit, resulting in nystagmus and vertigo. This condition, so-called cupulolithiasis, likely represents the more permanent form of this disorder.

The more common self-limited form and the form with remissions and recurrences likely has a different pathophysiologic mechanism. Free-floating endolymph particles within the posterior canal produce a Hallpike response identical to that of a fixed cupular deposit.[16] Because the posterior canal is the most dependent part of the vestibular labyrinth, free-floating endolymph particles have a predilection for settling in the posterior canal endolymph. With the head upright, the most dependent part of the canal is the area just posterior and inferior to the ampulla on the side of the cupula opposite the utricle. As the posterior canal rotates during the Hallpike maneuver, the particles initially rotate upward because of their inertia. After a short latent period, gravity pulls them down and away from the cupula (utriculofugal) to a more dependant position. Their hydrodynamic drag creates an endolymph current in the same direction, thereby displacing the cupula away from the utricle. Utriculofugal displacement of the posterior canal cupula increases the resting discharge rate of the first-order neurons. As known from previous animal studies, this action produces excitation of the ipsilateral superior oblique and contralateral inferior rectus muscles,[9] which causes counterclockwise eye rotation with stimulation of the left posterior crista and clockwise rotation with right-sided stimulation. However, the fast component of the induced nystagmus will be in the opposite direction, corresponding with the clinical features of typical BPPV. These free-floating posterior canal particles have in fact been identified in vivo in patients undergoing surgery for BPPV.[17] This theory of free-floating particles is an important concept as it relates to the treatment of this condition.

PREOPERATIVE PATIENT COUNSELING AND CONSERVATIVE MANAGEMENT

First and foremost, the patient must be reassured that this inner ear disorder is relatively benign and most often self-limited. To date, effective medical management for BPPV remains unproven experimentally.[18] The most efficacious means of vertigo control is avoidance of the specific provocative head movements that induce the attacks. Most patients already use this approach by not lying on the affected side and by not extending the neck to look upward. Patients who stringently avoid these movements may have more prolonged courses because the absence of provocative movements prevents dispersement of the particles from the canal.

Most cases of BPPV resolve spontaneously over weeks to months without any treatment. Brandt and Daroff[19] recommended a rigorous course of physiotherapy under heavy sedation during several days of hospitalization. They felt that the exercises shook free the otolithic debris from the cupula. Unfortunately, other clinicians could not reproduce their excellent results (Personal communication). Semont et al.[20] reported excellent results using a technique called the "liberatory maneuver." They theorized that this technique liberated deposits from the cupula and reported a 92 per cent success rate following two maneuvers.

Epley: My limited experience with the liberatory maneuver was not quite as favorable. Furthermore, the maneuver was difficult to perform in elderly, frail patients; therefore, a modified technique, coined the "particle-repositioning maneuver," was recently adapted.[21] This new technique, similar to the canalith repositioning procedure described by Dr. John Epley at various instruction courses, is based on the free-floating particle pathophysiologic theory of BPPV. For the purpose of this discussion, it is important to remember that the cupula forms a complete barrier across the ampullated end of the canal that is impermeable to endolymph and free-floating particles. Therefore, free-floating posterior canal endolymph particles can exit the canal only through the common crus.

The current particle repositioning technique (Fig. 46–1) begins with the patient seated lengthwise on the examining table. The Hallpike maneuver is then performed by rotation of the posterior semicircular canal of the undermost (affected) ear in the earth vertical axis. The examiner should observe the classic nystagmus response, which confirms the diagnosis, and then reassure the patient as the vertigo subsides. The patient maintains this position for 2 to 3 minutes after resolution of the nystagmus, thereby allowing the particles to settle in their new dependant position closer to the common crus. In the second stage, the patient rolls laterally onto the opposite side with the head turned 45° downward. This stage is performed in a smooth, continuous motion, and the neck is kept extended until it reaches the final position, at which time the neck is flexed. This method serves to rotate the posterior canal 180° in the plane of gravity, allowing the free-floating particles to follow the natural curve of the canal and continue their relative course through the common crus into the utricle.

While the examiner supports the patient's head, a secondary nystagmus response is usually noted, once again following a short latent period. A nystagmus response that replicates the initial nystagmus (positive response) during the Hallpike maneuver can result only from further passage of the particles in the same ampullofugal direction. Such passage would lead them through the common crus into the utricle, where they would no longer induce a pathologic response. Conversely, a secondary nystagmus that reverses direction from that of the Hallpike maneuver may occur through two possible mechanisms. In one, the particles reverse their direction of movement because of an improperly performed maneuver, resulting in a utriculopetal endolymph current. Cupulolithiasis is the other possible mechanism underlying reversal nystagmus. The gravitational effect on a fixed cupular deposit results in utriculofugal cupular deflection during the Hallpike maneuver (Fig. 46–1B), as would be

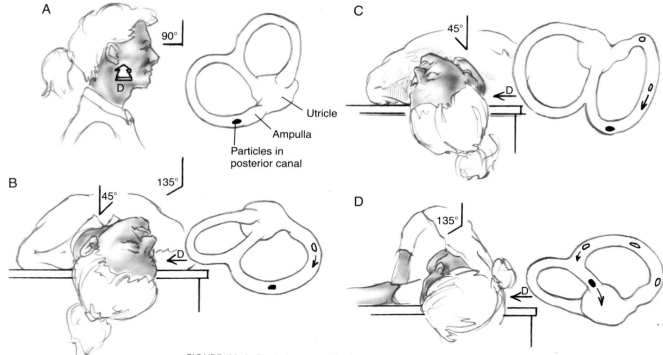

FIGURE 46-1. Particle repositioning maneuver—4 positions, right ear. Schematic representation of patient and concurrent movement of labyrinth, specifically the posterior and superior semicircular canals. In each position, dark oval represents new position of particle conglomerate in most dependant part of posterior canal, and open oval represents previous position. A, Patient seated. B, Patient in Hallpike head position. Particles gravitate in amupullofugal direction, causing counterclockwise rotatory nystagmus (right ear). Position is maintained for 2 to 3 minutes. C, Mid position and D, final position of second stage of maneuver performed in one steady continuous motion. Particles continue gravitating in ampullofugal direction through common crus into utricle. Eyes are observed for nystagmus response. Position is maintained for 1 to 2 minutes; then patient sits up. D = direction of view of labyrinth.

seen with free-floating particles. The position assumed during the second stage of the particle-repositioning maneuver effectively rotates the posterior canal 180° in the earth vertical plane (Fig. 46–1D). This action reverses the gravitational pull on the cupula, resulting in utriculopetal cupular displacement and a reversal of the nystagmus response.

Outcome: After another 1 to 2 minutes, the patient sits back up and is observed for nystagmus. With a successful maneuver, no nystagmus occurs when the patient returns to the upright position because the particles have been removed from the canal. This result is in contrast to that of the conventional Hallpike maneuver, in which one notes a reversal nystagmus. Patients are then instructed to maintain an upright position for 48 hours, theoretically to prevent particle reentry into the posterior canal. Patients are then reassessed 1 month later, and if necessary, the maneuver is repeated.

Several other clinical findings help support the free-floating particle theory as the mechanism underlying most cases of BPPV. In some patients with classic his-

> *90% response. ~50% recurrence.*

tories of BPPV, an initial Hallpike maneuver often fails to induce a positive response. I have noted that in many of these patients, a vigorous headshake may often elicit a latent response. In these cases, the head shake may overcome the particle conglomerate's inertia or its minor adherence to the membranous canal wall, allowing for its mobilization.

Free-floating particles may also explain the fatigability of a conventional Hallpike maneuver. Each maneuver likely causes increased endolymph dispersion of the particle conglomerate, resulting in a smaller mass effect with each subsequent maneuver and reducing the degree of hydrodynamic drag and endolymph current. In several patients, a repeat Hallpike maneuver 30 to 60 minutes after a fatigued response often elicits the same maximal response seen during the initial Hallpike maneuver. Theoretically, the particles have had time to reassemble into the large conglomerate mass within the endolymph of the posterior canal.

Parnes and Price-Jones demonstrated very favorable results in 38 patients treated with the particle-repositioning maneuver.[21] More than half of the patients had the more chronic form of this disorder and had had constant symptoms for more than 1 year. Despite this history, 88 per cent remain cured, with minimum follow-up times of 6 months. Three of the four patients who did not respond demonstrated a reversal secondary-stage nystagmus response during the particle-repositioning maneuver. Apparently, reversal nystagmus predicts a poor outcome. This supports the theory that a fixed cupular deposit (cupulolithiasis) underlies the "permanent" cases of BPPV. However, the vast majority of patients had "positive" responses to the maneuver; therefore, free-floating *PSCO.* particles appear to be the most common cause of BPPV. The exact etiology of these particles remains unknown.

PATIENT SELECTION

Rx / Sx:

Operative intervention is offered for intractable cases ① in which symptoms are severe enough to significantly affect the patient's occupation or lifestyle. The current criteria include failure to respond to the particle-re② positioning maneuver and the observation of reversal ③ nystagmus. Since I started using the particle-repositioning maneuver, the number of surgical cases has *SN:* decreased dramatically. Until recently, singular neu*cons* rectomy was the gold standard of operative treatment.[14, 22–24] However, the procedure is technically dif① ficult, is performed by very few surgeons, and yields ② ③ variable rates of failure and sensorineural hearing ④ loss.[25, 26] Furthermore, Ohmichi et al.[27] showed that the ⑤ singular nerve is inaccessible through a tympanotomy approach in 14 per cent of human temporal bones.

The newer procedure of posterior semicircular canal occlusion evolved to circumvent the shortcomings of singular neurectomy. Money and Scott[28] initially used this technique in feline vestibular physiology experiments. Plugging individual semicircular canals blocked their receptivity to angular acceleration without influencing the responses of the other ipsilateral vestibular receptors. Although posterior canal occlusion was at first a theoretical remedy for BPPV, the main concern in applying this technique to humans was its possible detrimental effect on hearing. This problem was not addressed in the original cat studies. Therefore, Parnes and McClure[29] carried out a study in guinea pigs to measure the effect of canal occlusion on hearing using brain stem auditory evoked responses. The hearing responses remained relatively unchanged during follow-up times as long as 6 months.

To test the hypothesis that canal occlusion would indeed abolish BPPV, two patients fortuitously pre-

sented with intractable BPPV in ears with coexisting profound sensorineural hearing losses. With no hearing to lose, both agreed to undergo what at that time was an experimental procedure. Both patients were relieved of their BPPV and have remained symptom-free for 4 years.[30, 31] In addition, both maintained postoperative lateral semicircular canal function as measured by caloric responses. This important finding supports the postulate that the procedure's success results from its isolated direct effect on the posterior canal and not from a generalized destructive process of the vestibular labyrinth.

The theoretical intent of the procedure is to compress the membranous labyrinth closed against the opposite bony wall, thereby creating a closed, fluid-filled (endolymph) space between the plug and cupula, both of which are impermeable to endolymph. Because fluid cannot expand or compress without a change in temperature, this action eliminates all endolymph movement within the posterior canal, effectively fixing the cupula. The canal no longer responds to the gravitational effect on a fixed cupular deposit, eliminating the BPPV. In addition, the canal no longer responds to physiologic angular acceleration. However, because the deficit is constant and permanent, gradual compensation occurs through central adaptation.

Singular neurectomy eliminates the resting discharge from the posterior semicircular canal crista, creating a static vestibular asymmetry[32] between the two posterior canals. This effect results in immediate postoperative vertigo at rest and spontaneous rotatory nystagmus. However, posterior canal occlusion does not disturb the resting neuronal discharge from the occluded canal, and therefore, most patients do not have spontaneous postoperative vertigo or nystagmus at rest unless their conditions are complicated by other factors. Both singular neurectomy and posterior canal occlusion result in a dynamic vestibular asymmetry,[32] itself resulting in motion sensitivity. The dynamic asymmetry gradually resolves because of central adaptation, as does the static vestibular asymmetry.

PREOPERATIVE EVALUATION

contraindx:

Preoperative evaluation includes a routine audio① gram. The procedure is not recommended in an only- or significantly better–hearing ear. Preoperative electronystagmography and evoked response audiometry are not necessary. A high-resolution computed tomographic scan of the temporal bone defines the anatomy and ensures that the posterior canal is indeed accessible through a transmastoid approach. To date, all posterior canals have proven to be accessible.

② *acute/chronic OM*

SURGICAL TECHNIQUE

 Abx:

Perioperative broad-spectrum antibiotic coverage is necessary only for ears with a past history of otitis media. Obviously, the procedure is contraindicated during acute or subacute episodes of otitis media. The patient is placed in the supine position with the head turned 45° toward the opposite side. The surgical site, preparation, and draping are performed in a routine fashion. Intraoperative auditory and facial nerve monitoring are not necessary.

With the patient under general anesthesia, a limited mastoidectomy is performed through a postauricular incision (Fig. 46–2*A*). The antrum is opened, providing exposure of the lateral canal. Identification of the tegmen and digastric ridge is not necessary. The sigmoid sinus is identified, from which bone removal proceeds anteriorly along the cerebellar plate toward the posterior canal. Once the posterior canal otic capsule is identified, the bone is blue lined with progressively smaller diamond burrs and copious suction irrigation. The target zone for the occlusion is the area at, or just inferior to, a line extending posteriorly from the lateral posterior canal. Because this part of the posterior semicircular canal is furthest from the ampulla and vestibule, manipulation in this region is theoretically least likely to induce other vestibular or cochlear damage.

Using an 0.8mm diamond burr, a 3mm segment of canal is skeletonized 180° around the outer circumference down to endosteum, creating a 1mm by 3mm endosteal island (Fig. 46–2*B*). Bone removal should proceed evenly along the circumference so that once the endosteum is violated and perilymph is exposed, all drilling can cease. The endosteal island is removed with a fine, 90° pick to expose the perilymph (Fig. 46–3). Great care must be taken to not suction directly on the perilymph and especially the membranous labyrinth. At this stage, the exact outline and limits of the membranous labyrinth are usually not clearly discernable. However, at this stage, particles were first iden-tified within the posterior canal in two previously reported patients[17] and in two subsequent patients. Although not essential, perilymph may be gently "wicked" away with a cottonoid to expose the membranous labyrinth, at which time the membranous duct collapses. In canals with particles, perilymph removal allows for confirmation that these are indeed free-floating particles within the endolymph.

Dry bone chips previously gathered from the mastoidectomy are mixed with one drop of a two-component fast-acting human fibrinogen glue (Tisseel, Immuno, Vienna, Austria). Once set (about 30 seconds), it forms an easily workable but malleable plug with a firm consistency (Fig. 46–4). The plug is gently but firmly inserted through the fenestra with the intention of completely filling the canal lumen and thereby compressing the membranous labyrinth closed (Fig. 46–5). The membranous labyrinth is surprisingly quite resistant to tearing, providing that no shearing forces are applied. The bone chips within the plug will cause intracanal ossification that leads to complete permanent occlusion of the canal.

If commercially prepared fibrinogen glue is not available, autologous glue may be fashioned from the patient's own serum. Alternatively, some surgeons have successfully used plugs made from periosteum or fascia.

After completing the plug insertion, the fenestra and surrounding bone are covered with a piece of temporalis fascia, which is maintained in place by several more drops of fibrinogen glue (Fig. 46–6). A good tissue seal is necessary to prevent a postoperative perilymph fistula.

The incision is closed in two layers, and a standard mastoid dressing is applied. A drain is not necessary. The dressing is maintained for 1 or 2 days.

In a variation of this technique, Anthony[33] successfully treated BPPV by applying an HGM Argon laser to the blue-lined posterior canal. The laser burns are purported to create fibrous bands within the canal, leading to obstruction of the membranous duct.

FIGURE 46–2. *A*, Exposing the right posterior semicircular canal otic capsule. *B*, Creating the 1mm by 3mm endosteal island with a small diamond burr. *C*, Cross-sectional view.

FIGURE 46–3. *A*, Lifting out the endosteal island with a fine, 90° pick. *B*, Magnified lateral view.

FIGURE 46–4. Creating the plug with two-component fibrinogen glue and mastoid cortex bone chips.

FIGURE 46–5. *A*, Tamping plug through fenestra into the canal. *B*, Cross-section schematic of canal shows intact but occluded membranous canal.

FIGURE 46–6. Covering fenestra and surrounding bone with fascia and glue.

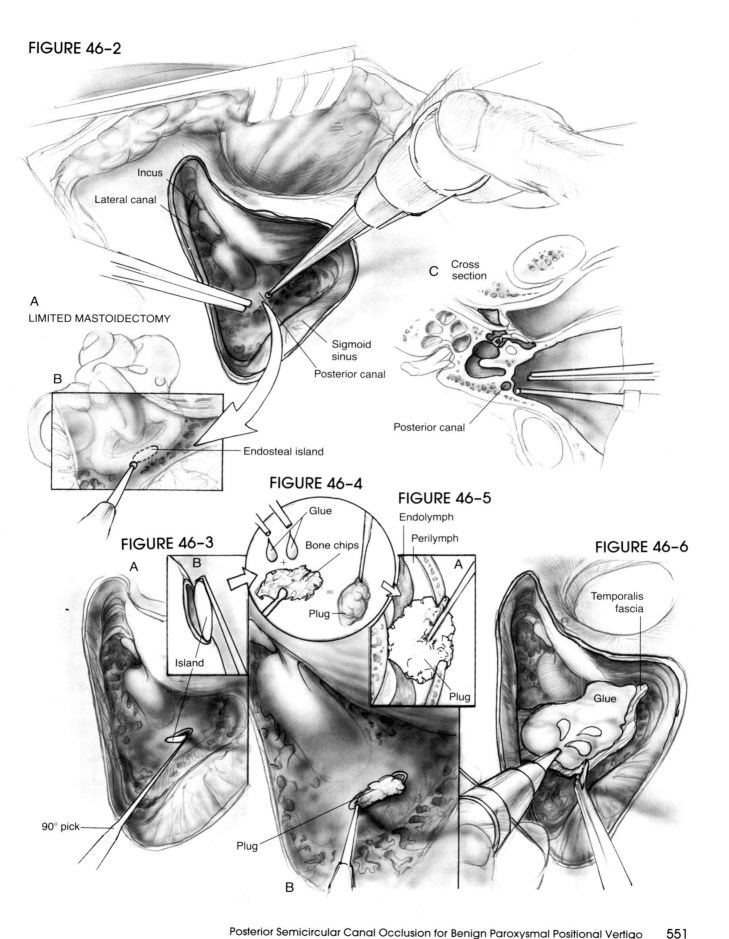

FIGURE 46-2

Incus

Lateral canal

A
LIMITED MASTOIDECTOMY

Sigmoid sinus

Posterior canal

B

Endosteal island

C Cross section

Posterior canal

FIGURE 46-4

Glue

Bone chips

+

=

Plug

FIGURE 46-5

Endolymph

Perilymph

A

Plug

FIGURE 46-3

A

B

Island

90° pick

Plug

B

FIGURE 46-6

Temporalis fascia

Glue

Posterior Semicircular Canal Occlusion for Benign Paroxysmal Positional Vertigo   551

48

Drainage Procedures for Petrous Apex Lesions

DERALD E. BRACKMANN, M.D.
NEIL A. GIDDINGS, M.D.

With the help of cranial computed tomography (CT) and magnetic resonance imaging (MRI), petrous apex lesions can be correctly diagnosed preoperatively. Consequently, cystic lesions requiring drainage should be approached with procedures designed for drainage, not total en bloc removal. Although the transmastoid infralabyrinthine procedure has been the usual approach for these lesions, transcanal infracochlear drainage offers a more dependent drainage site. The eventual role of the various approaches for petrous apex drainage will depend on the long-term follow-up of these patients.

Advances in radiologic imaging during the past decade have made it possible to reliably differentiate lesions of the petrous apex preoperatively. The development of CT scanning was the first major step in imaging the temporal bone since the development of polytomography. CT scanning gives the surgeon the ability to visualize the size of the lesion and its relationship to vital structures, including the internal auditory canal, cochlea, vestibular labyrinth, carotid artery, and jugular bulb. It also helps characterize the border of the lesion as expansile or invasive, which may differentiate between benign lesions and malignant neoplasms. MRI of the temporal bone added the capability of characterizing the substance of the lesion rather than its effect on bony interfaces, allowing the surgeon to distinguish between mucus, fat, cholesterol granuloma, cholesteatoma, and neoplasm. The combination of CT, with its superior bone imaging algorithms, and MRI, with its enhanced tissue imaging capabilities, allows the surgeon to differentiate accurately and reliably between benign cystic lesions, normal anatomic variants, and neoplastic lesions of the petrous apex.

Patients with petrous apex lesions present with various symptoms and physical findings. The most widely recognized finding is Gradenigo's syndrome, consisting of retro-orbital pain, otorrhea, and ipsilateral sixth cranial nerve paresis. The signs and symptoms of noninflammatory or neoplastic lesions may be more subtle. Hearing loss and vestibular abnormalities are frequently associated with lesions of the petrous apex as they enlarge and compress the internal auditory canal. The facial nerve is relatively resistant to paresis from slowly expansile lesions but may be involved early with neoplastic lesions of the petrous apex or non-neoplastic lesions compressing the internal auditory canal.

Pain may be present with benign or cystic lesions but is commoner in neoplastic lesions. Its distribution is dependent on the region involved. The mastoid cavity is innervated by cranial nerve IX and may radiate pain into the neck. Middle fossa and superior petrosal regions are innervated by cranial nerve V and may be perceived as retro-orbital or facial pain. Le-

sions extending into the posterior fossa may cause pain along the routes of distribution of cranial nerves IX, X, and the first three cervical nerves.[1] Although 80 per cent of adult mastoid bones are aerated, only 30 per cent of petrous bones have air cells extending to the apex, and up to 7 per cent may have asymmetric pneumatization of the petrous apex.[2, 3] The increasing use of MRI of the head and neck makes it imperative that the clinician can differentiate pathology from normal variant in the temporal bone. Common lesions of the petrous apex and their associated radiologic findings are summarized in Table 48–1.

Asymmetric pneumatization is clearly seen on CT scanning, but supplementary MRI may be needed to rule out pathologic lesions in a symptomatic ear. Normal bony architecture can be seen on CT scanning, with hyperintensity on MRI T1 scans and hypointensity on T2 because of the large fat content in marrow. Retained mucus in the air cells also presents with normal bony architecture on CT scan but is hypointense on T1- and hyperintense on T2-weighted MRI scans. Cholesteatoma is usually associated with chronic otitis media but may arise from congenital rest cells in the petrous apex. Because of its high water content, cholesteatoma is isointense with cerebrospinal fluid on CT and displays a hypointense T1 and hyperintense T2 image on MRI. Cholesterol granuloma is isointense with brain on CT scanning and presents a classic image on MRI with hyperintensity on T1 and T2. Radiologic descriptions of other, less common lesions are also summarized in Table 48–1. Differentiating between chordoma, chondroma, and chondrosarcoma of the temporal bone remains difficult, even with the scanning techniques currently available. The area of origin and the age of the patient must be considered when the pathology of destructive lesions of the petrous apex is determined.[4–6]

PATIENT SELECTION

Most surgical approaches to the petrous apex were developed in the preantibiotic era for drainage of petrous apex abscesses and cure of Gradenigo's syndrome. With the arrival of modern antibiotics, infectious processes of the petrous apex have severely declined in frequency, but these same approaches may be equally effective in draining cystic lesions of the petrous apex.

Air cell tracts extend above, below, and anterior to the otic capsule, allowing the potential of safe passage to the petrous apex. Approaches that follow superior air cell tracts include middle fossa,[7] through the superior semicircular canal,[8] the attic, and the root of the zygomatic arch.[9] Approaches below the inner ear include the infralabyrinthine and the infracochlear.[10–13]

TABLE 48–1. Radiologic Appearance of Common Petrous Apex Lesions

LESION	COMPUTED TOMOGRAPHY	MAGNETIC RESONANCE IMAGING		
		T1	T2	Enhancement
Retained mucus	Normal bony architecture, nonenhancing	Hypointense	Hyperintense	No
Mucocele	Hypodense, expansile smooth border, nonenhancing	Hypointense	Hyperintense	No
Asymmetric pneumatization	Normal bony architecture, nonenhancing	Hyperintense	Hypointense	No
Cholesteatoma	Loss of normal air cells, nonenhancing, isointense with CSF	Hypointense	Hyperintense	No
Cholesterol granuloma	Expansile smooth border, occasional rim enhancement, isointense with brain	Hyperintense	Hyperintense	No
Metastatic lesion	Destructive, indistinct border	Isointense	Hyperintense	Yes
Chordoma	Aggressive bone destruction, calcification	Isointense: 75% Hypointense: 25%	Hyperintense	Yes
Chondroma	Aggressive bone destruction, calcification	Hypointense to isointense	Hyperintense	Yes
Chondrosarcoma	Aggressive bone destruction, calcification	Hypointense to isointense	Hyperintense	Yes

CSF = cerebrospinal fluid.

Anterior approaches have been described by Ramadier, Eagleton, and Lempert, who used the triangle between the anterior border of the cochlea, the carotid artery, and the middle fossa dura.[14–16] All these approaches are used for drainage of inflammatory disease processes that are not responsive to antibiotic therapy or simpler operations for chronic ear disease (Fig. 48–1).

Infralabyrinthine, infracochlear, and trans-sphenoidal approaches are most commonly chosen for drainage of cystic lesions of the petrous apex in an ear with serviceable hearing. These lesions are frequently detected at an asymptomatic stage with today's imaging techniques. Because the natural history of small benign cystic lesions is not well documented, surgical drainage should be reserved for patients with larger lesions or with symptoms, including pain, visual changes, diplopia, hearing loss, vertigo, or facial nerve weakness. For patients without serviceable hearing, these lesions should be drained through a translabyrinthine approach. Because other vital structures may be affected by enlargement of the cyst, delaying surgery in symptomatic patients provides no advantage.

Cholesterol granuloma is the most common cystic lesion of the petrous apex, occurring 30 times less frequently than acoustic neuroma.[17] It may develop in any aerated portion of the temporal bone but most commonly occurs in the mastoid air cells distant to a lesion that prevents normal aeration. Cholesterol granuloma of the petrous apex probably develops when a pathologic process or trauma obstructs the air cell tracts to a well-pneumatized petrous apex.

The treatment for cholesterol granuloma of the temporal bone is drainage and re-establishment of adequate aeration to the involved area. The cyst wall is composed of a fibrous connective tissue. It is free of keratinizing squamous epithelium that characterizes cholesteatoma, and complete removal of the cyst is not necessary.

Solid tumors of the temporal bone and cholesteatoma are removed when first identified rather than after further symptoms develop because these symptoms frequently reveal further involvement of other vital structures. Drainage procedures are obviously inadequate treatment for these lesions, and all reasonable efforts should be made to remove them entirely. Total removal may require the sacrifice of cranial nerves and major vascular structures.

PREOPERATIVE EVALUATION AND PATIENT COUNSELING

Preoperative evaluation of these patients is based upon their symptoms. Patients presenting with hearing loss are evaluated initially with audiometric testing, including air, bone, and speech reception thresholds and speech discrimination scores. Electronystagmography is performed in patients who complain of imbalance or vertigo. In patients with otherwise normal results on physical examination, asymmetric hearing is next evaluated with auditory brainstem response testing. If these results are abnormal, an MRI scan is indicated. In patients with cranial nerve involvement other than the eighth nerve, with asymmetric hearing, auditory brainstem response testing is not performed, and the physician proceeds directly to an MRI scan.

Patients who have normal hearing but have other cranial nerve deficits that may be referable to the petrous apex may be screened with either a high-resolution, thin-section CT of the temporal bone or an MRI with gadolinium. If an abnormality is found, all patients undergo air, bone, and speech reception thresholds and speech discrimination audiometric testing before surgery to document hearing levels before a procedure that jeopardizes hearing.

Preoperatively, patients are counseled to expect resolution of pain, if present, and the possibility of improvement in cranial nerve function if it is decreased preoperatively. Cranial nerves that have been affected for shorter periods of time seem to have a better prognosis and fewer long-standing deficits than those affected longer. Patients are reminded this is a drainage procedure whose goal is to decompress the lesion and provide an aerated cavity, if possible. The goal is not the removal of the lesion, and close follow-up may be necessary. Recurrence of the lesion secondary to inadequate drainage is usually heralded by the return of preoperative symptoms. Follow-up MRI frequently reveals a cholesterol granuloma cyst that remains full of fluid, but the T1-weighted image is hypointense, compared with the preoperative hyperintense image on T1 views. A return of hyperintensity on the T1 image suggests inadequate drainage in a symptomatic lesion.[18]

SURGICAL TECHNIQUES

Infralabyrinthine Drainage of the Petrous Apex

The patient is prohibited from eating and drinking for at least 8 hours preoperatively. Unless an infectious process is suspected, no preoperative antibiotics are used.

The surgical ear is prepared similarly to any other chronic otitis media case operated on through a postauricular approach. Hair is shaved to one fingerbreadth above the auricle and two fingerbreadths behind the postauricular crease. Surgical preparation is an antibacterial scrub followed by painting with antibacterial solution. Sterile Mastisol is applied around the auricle and allowed to dry. An adhesive aperture drape is placed over the ear, and sterile sheets cover the patient. Routine chronic otitis media instruments and drill are the only equipment required.

1. The patient is placed in a supine position with the involved ear facing up. The surgeon sits at the side of the patient with the patient's head turned away.
2. A postauricular incision is made 1cm behind the postauricular crease down to the temporalis fascia superiorly, and through the periosteum below the temporal line. A second incision is made through the temporalis muscle and fascia at the temporal line, beginning above the external auditory canal and ending posteriorly at the postauricular incision, allowing the periosteum to be raised and the ear reflected anteriorly. Temporalis muscle is reflected superiorly.
3. A simple mastoidectomy is performed, removing all air cells from Trautmann's triangle (bordered by the middle fossa dural plate superiorly, the semicircular canals anteriorly, and the sigmoid sinus posteriorly) (Fig. 48–2A).
4. The facial nerve should be identified in its vertical portion but need not be exposed.
5. Mastoid air cells are removed from the mastoid tip, and the sigmoid sinus is followed until the jugular bulb is identified. The superior aspect of the jugular bulb forms the most inferior portion of the opening into the petrous apex.
6. The posterior half of the horizontal and the inferior portion of the posterior bony semicircular canal are skeletonized, and care is taken not to expose the membranous portions of the canals.
7. Once the semicircular canals and the jugular bulb are clearly defined, the infralabyrinthine air cell tract is followed toward the petrous apex with a diamond burr or curette until the cystic lesion is encountered and opened.
8. Once the lesion is entered, it is evacuated with suction and copious irrigation. All fluid and loose debris are removed. Removal of tissue lining the cavity is neither necessary nor possible with this approach.
9. The largest silicone sheeting catheter that fits into the newly created opening is placed and retained by friction to prevent stenosis of the drainage site (Fig. 48–2B).
10. The periosteum is reapproximated with absorba-

FIGURE 48–1. Surgical approaches for drainage of the petrous apex.

FIGURE 48–2. *A,* Exposure of the cyst in the infralabyrinthine cell tract. An island of bone protects the retracted sigmoid sinus (Bill's bar). *B,* A silicone tube placed into the interior of the cavity drains into the inferior mastoid cavity.

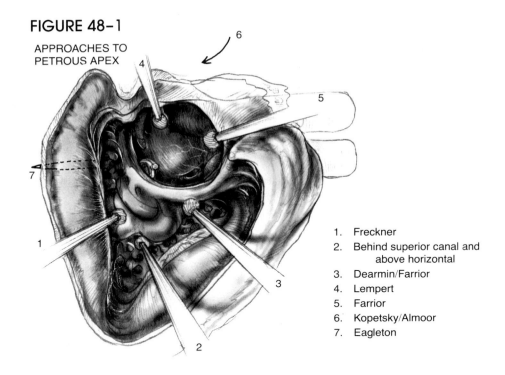

FIGURE 48-1

APPROACHES TO
PETROUS APEX

1. Freckner
2. Behind superior canal and
   above horizontal
3. Dearmin/Farrior
4. Lempert
5. Farrior
6. Kopetsky/Almoor
7. Eagleton

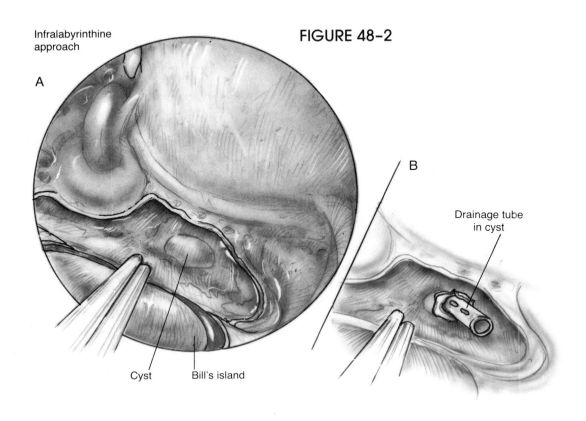

FIGURE 48-2

Infralabyrinthine
approach

A

B

Drainage tube
in cyst

Cyst   Bill's island

ble suture, and the subcutaneous tissue and skin are closed in layers, followed by the placement of a mastoid pressure dressing.

The mastoid pressure dressing is formed by placing Telfa over the postauricular incision. One half a cotton ball is placed in the concha and two 4 × 4 gauze pads are folded in half and placed in the postauricular crease. A soft, absorbant bolster is then placed over the auricle and the mastoid region. A four-inch Kling bandage is then wrapped anteriorly to posteriorly and secured by cinching down with a tracheotomy tie one inch posterior to the lateral orbital rim.

Most patients are admitted to the hospital for one night after this surgery. The dressing is removed the following day, and the incision is cleaned, if necessary. If skin sutures were used, they are removed 1 week later. The patient is allowed to get the postauricular incision wet at this time and should be instructed to clean the incision once per day for the next 2 weeks with hydrogen peroxide to reduce crusting on the incision.

Pitfalls

Infralabyrinthine drainage has been the most commonly employed procedure in the United States for drainage of these cystic lesions. However, it is not without risk to the facial nerve, jugular bulb, and otic capsule. Surgeons attempting this procedure should be intimately familiar with the neural and major vascular anatomy of the petrous bone. When a large cystic lesion expands along the infralabyrinthine cell tracts, this approach may be the simplest. With a small lesion, following this cell tract to the area of pathology may be difficult. Probably the greatest limitation to this approach is its extreme difficulty when used in patients with a high jugular bulb. The drainage opening may be narrowed significantly, even if it is possible to decompress the jugular bulb and retract it inferiorly during the surgical procedure. Consequently, this approach should not be chosen when the jugular bulb is high or narrows the surgical approach to the apex. Injury to the jugular bulb can be temporarily controlled with external packing and light pressure. At this time, the surgeon should arm himself or herself with adequate suction and large sheets of Surgicel. The Surgicel is removed, and the damaged jugular bulb inspected as well as possible. For small lacerations, a small sheet of Surgicel is placed over the bulb and packed in place with absorbable gelatin sponge (Gelfoam). A large defect in the jugular bulb requires that a large piece of Surgicel be placed through the defect into the lumen of the vein. Small pieces should not be placed near the defect or into the lumen because of the possibility of embolization to the lung.

Absorbable gelatin sponge is packed over the Surgicel, usually controlling the bleeding with light pressure.

Injury to the posterior or horizontal semicircular canal requires early recognition of the surgical misadventure. Little or no suction should be used to inspect the fenestration. A small piece of temporalis fascia is placed over the defect, and bone wax is used to secure the fascia and provide a watertight seal. If recognized early, hearing may be preserved, although vertigo will be present for several weeks in the postoperative period.

Transcanal Infracochlear Approach to the Petrous Apex[12]

In 1984, Farrior described a transcanal approach to small glomus jugulare tumors of the hypotympanum.[11] The infracochlear approach to the petrous apex is a combination of this technique and the subcochlear approach described by Ghorayeb and Jahrsdoerfer.[13]

1. A postauricular incision is made, and the auricle is reflected anteriorly.
2. The membranous external auditory canal is completely transected laterally (Fig. 48–3A).
3. A tympanomeatal flap is elevated from 2 o'clock to 10 o'clock, leaving the tympanic membrane attached at the umbo and the superior canal wall.
4. The external auditory canal is enlarged anteriorly and inferiorly to expose the hypotympanum. The chorda tympani is followed inferoposteriorly to laterally to define the extent of posterior dissection possible without injury to the facial nerve (Fig. 48–3B).
5. Air cells are removed below the cochlea in the hypotympanum to expose the course of the carotid artery and the jugular bulb. The round window provides the superior line of dissection, and Jacobson's nerve leads to the "crutch" of the carotid and jugular bulb (Fig. 48–3C).
6. Removal of air cells continues medially. If the plane of dissection remains below the round window, the internal auditory canal structures will not be at risk (Fig. 48–3D).
7. The cholesterol granuloma cyst is entered and drained. The newly created "window" is enlarged as far anteriorly as possible to the carotid artery, as far inferiorly as the jugular bulb, and superiorly to the inferior aspect of the basal turn of the cochlea (Fig. 48–3E).
8. A silicone catheter of appropriate size is introduced, if necessary, to stent the opening (Fig. 48–3F).
9. The soft tissue of the external auditory canal is

returned to its normal position, gelatin sponge is packed within the membranous external auditory canal, and bone paté (previously obtained during initial drilling) is placed between the canal wall and the newly enlarged bony canal (Fig. 48–3*G*).
10. The postauricular incision is closed, and a mastoid dressing is applied (Fig. 48–3*H*).

Postoperative dressings, care, and length of hospitalization are similar to those used for the infralabyrinthine approach, except in the care of the external auditory canal. The patient is seen 1 week postoperatively to check the postauricular incision and to ensure that excessive drainage is not occurring from the external auditory canal. The packing should be moist without evidence of active drainage. If excessive drainage or evidence of infection is present, the patient is prescribed antibiotic ear drops (Cortisporin otic suspension) three times a day. If the packing is dry, the patient begins using the ear drops 2 weeks after surgery, two drops three times a day, until the packing is removed 1 month postoperatively. At this point, the tympanic membrane should be intact and the canal skin healing well. Small areas of exposed bony external auditory canal will epithelialize within 1 to 2 months.

This procedure is similar to the infralabyrinthine approach, in that both involve an area of the temporal bone to which most otolaryngologists have little exposure. The surgery need not be difficult, but surgeons must spend time in the temporal bone laboratory familiarizing themselves with the relative positions of the basal turn of the cochlea, the jugular bulb, and the carotid artery. After the soft tissue of the canal is reflected superiorly, a large amount of the bone lateral to the annulus can be removed with a cutting burr. Once the hypotympanum is entered, the surgeon should switch to successively smaller diamond burrs until the cyst is entered.

Injury to the jugular bulb is treated as was described for the infralabyrinthine approach. Injury to the basal turn of the cochlea is more serious than opening into a semicircular canal. It should be approached with minimal suction, and the placement of temporalis fascia should be secured by bone wax. Despite early recognition, the prognosis for hearing is much poorer when the cochlea is violated than when the semicircular canals are violated.

This approach may cause injury to the infratemporal portion of the carotid artery. The carotid arterial wall may be thinner in the temporal bone than in the neck. Every effort should be made to leave a thin wall of bone over the carotid artery. If the artery is violated, immediate control can usually be achieved with packing and pressure to the middle ear and external auditory canal. This injury is potentially life-threatening and requires the expertise of a vascular surgeon. Distal control may be achieved with an intra-arterial catheter threaded past the point of injury, and proximal control is achieved in the neck. Once proximal and distal control are achieved, the injury can be directly repaired. Obviously, occlusion of the carotid artery runs the risk of cerebral infarct.

RESULTS

No large series documenting the superior effectiveness of any one procedure exists. All procedures would be expected to relieve pain, if it was present preoperatively, and may allow the recovery of some cranial nerve dysfunction. Gherini et al.[17] reported that hearing was preserved in 83 per cent of patients who had useful preoperative hearing, but no improvement occurred in those with preoperative hearing impairment. Vertigo, if present preoperatively, usually resolves with adequate decompression.[19] Several patients displayed recovery of cranial nerve function other than the cochlear nerve, but this return of function is not universal, even after adequate decompression.[17, 19, 20]

COMPLICATIONS AND MANAGEMENT

All procedures that approach the petrous apex may cause injury to major vessels and cranial nerves. Each approach has its own set of risks. Table 48–2 compares the common procedures used for drainage of petrous apex lesions. The experience of the surgeon, the position of the lesion, and the needs of the patient all need to be addressed.

The infralabyrinthine approach is the most familiar to otolaryngologists and head and neck surgeons. It is a direct extension of the simple mastoidectomy that may be accomplished with minimal morbidity in patients with a large cyst that has expanded between the labyrinth and the jugular bulb. Smaller cysts that are more medially based become more challenging, and a high jugular bulb may preclude this approach entirely. Care must be taken not to disturb the endolymphatic sac or damage the endolymphatic duct during this dissection. Damage to these areas may lead to endolymphatic hydrops. This technique drains the cyst farther from the eustachian tube than any other otologic technique and, consequently, may be more prone to failure. Because of the debris that is never completely removed from these cysts, the mastoid itself may become poorly aerated, leading to the potential for long-term failure.

The transcanal infracochlear approach has the advantage of a direct approach to the petrous apex and

FIGURE 48–3

Infracochlear approach to petrous apex

A

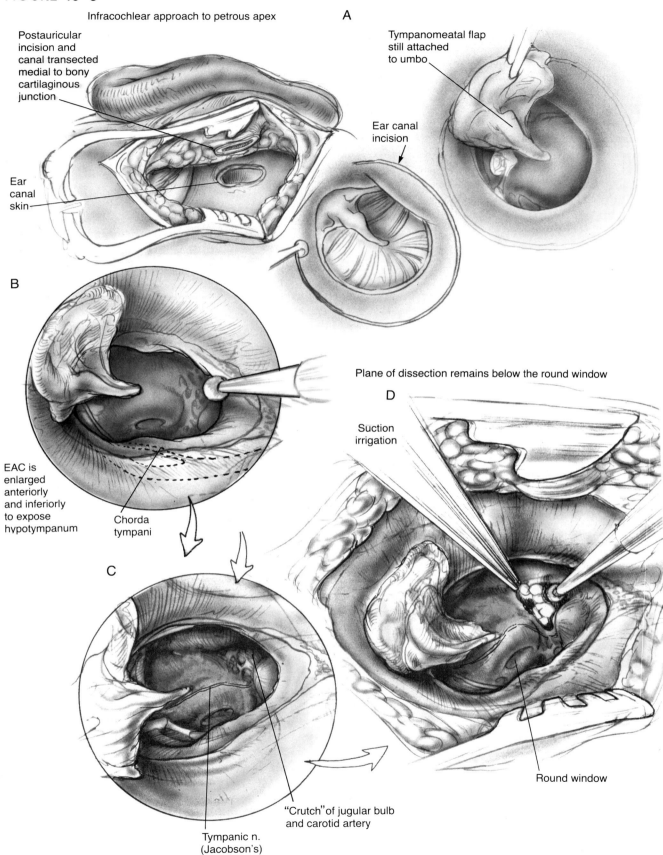

Postauricular incision and canal transected medial to bony cartilaginous junction

Ear canal skin

Tympanomeatal flap still attached to umbo

Ear canal incision

B

EAC is enlarged anteriorly and inferiorly to expose hypotympanum

Chorda tympani

Plane of dissection remains below the round window

D

Suction irrigation

C

Tympanic n. (Jacobson's)

"Crutch" of jugular bulb and carotid artery

Round window

FIGURE 48-3 *(continued)*

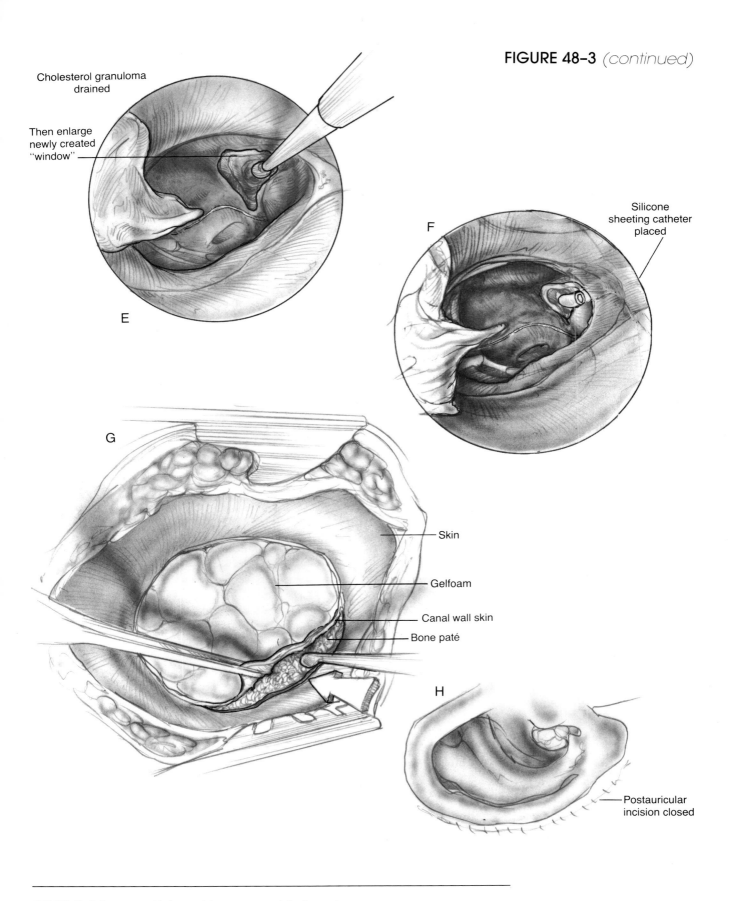

Cholesterol granuloma drained

Then enlarge newly created "window"

E

F

Silicone sheeting catheter placed

G

Skin

Gelfoam

Canal wall skin

Bone paté

H

Postauricular incision closed

FIGURE 48-3. Transcanal infracochlear approach to the petrous apex.

TABLE 48–2. Common Drainage Approaches to the Petrous Apex

PROCEDURE	STRUCTURES AT RISK	ADVANTAGES	DISADVANTAGES
Infralabyrinthine	Jugular bulb, bony labyrinth, facial nerve	Direct approach that is more familiar to most otolaryngologists	Difficult with high jugular bulb Drainage into mastoid cavity far from eustachian tube
Transcanal infracochlear	Jugular bulb, carotid artery, cochlea	Direct drainage near the mouth of the eustachian tube Can be revised with transtympanic procedure	Anatomy may be challenging to those not familiar with hypotympanum and major vessels of temporal bone
Trans-sphenoidal	Carotid artery, optic nerve, cavernous sinus, maxillary nerve, pituitary gland	Direct approach to large cysts that are in contact with posterior wall of sphenoid sinus Opening into cyst may be directly observed in clinic with endoscope	Sphenoid anatomy is highly variable Can only be used for "giant" cysts in contact with sphenoid High rate of failure
Translabyrinthine or subtotal petrosectomy	Labyrinth, jugular bulb, internal auditory canal	Cyst and wall can be removed if desired	Profound postoperative sensorineural hearing loss
Middle fossa	Temporal lobe, cochlea, labyrinth, internal auditory canal, greater superficial petrosal nerve	Drains cyst directly into bony eustachian tube	Middle fossa craniotomy poorly tolerated in elderly Drainage is not dependent Temporal lobe may obstruct drainage path

the maintenance of normal ear anatomy. It requires familiarity with the surgical anatomy of the hypotympanum, but the surgical landmarks are easily identified. The round window is easily seen, and careful removal of bone with a diamond burr reveals the location of the jugular bulb and carotid artery. If major vessel damage occurs, it is easily temporized with direct pressure until the situation can be controlled with direct vessel repair or permanent packing. It also drains the cyst close to the opening of the eustachian tube into the middle ear space, which makes obstruction less likely. Complete transection of the soft tissue external auditory canal may lead to mild stenosis in the postoperative period. If this occurs, it is easily managed and corrected with the placement of a foam ear insert used by audiologists for routine audiometric testing. The insert maintains gentle pressure on the area of stenosis while allowing passage of sound down the central lumen.

ALTERNATIVE TECHNIQUES

Several other techniques are available for exposure of the petrous apex.

Trans-sphenoidal Approach to Petrous Apex Lesions

Trans-sphenoidal drainage of petrous apex cysts may be the most simple and straightforward approach to large cysts that have a large surface area against the posterior wall of the sphenoid sinus. This technique is obviously not useful when the cyst does not impinge upon the sphenoid sinus. The risk of damage to the cochlea and labyrinth is decreased with this technique, but the risk to the carotid artery increases, and an added risk of damage to the optic nerve exists (a frequently reported complication of endoscopic sinus surgery). This technique also has a high failure rate when compared with otologic drainage procedures for cholesterol granuloma of the petrous apex. Thedinger et al.[19] reported that 80 per cent of patients who had a trans-sphenoidal initial approach for drainage eventually required one or more procedures to effectively drain the lesion. In their series, the only patient who required revision surgery after an otologic procedure had had a middle fossa attempt that did not provide dependent drainage.

1. An external ethmoidectomy sphenoidotomy, intranasal sphenoethmoidectomy, intranasal sphenoidotomy, trans-septal sphenoidotomy, or transpalatal approach may be used to expose the posterior and lateral walls of the sphenoid sinus.[19, 21]
2. Indentations in the lateral and superior walls may reveal the location of vital nervous and vascular structures, including the pituitary gland, optic nerve, maxillary nerve, carotid artery, and cavernous sinus.
3. A cruciate incision is made in the posterior sphenoid sinus mucosa, and flaps are elevated from the bony posterior wall.
4. Based on preoperative CT scanning, a diamond burr or sharp chisel is used to remove a small portion of the posterior bony wall of the sphenoid sinus. Pituitary rongeurs are used to enlarge the

bony orifice as much as possible without violating vital structures, exposing the cystic lesion.

5. The cyst wall is opened, and the contents are drained. The cyst is irrigated, and all debris is removed. The mucosal flaps previously raised are laid into the cavity, and no synthetic drain is used.
6. A large sphenoidotomy is performed for postoperative inspection and cleaning.
7. If an intranasal approach was used, the sphenoid sinus should remain unpacked, but the nasal cavity may be lightly packed. If an external approach was chosen, the wound is closed in layers.

With the increased interest in endoscopic sinus surgery, the trans-sphenoidal approach to the petrous apex is gaining in popularity. Unfortunately, this approach does not work in smaller lesions that do not directly abut the posterior wall of the sphenoid sinus. Many endoscopists have gained a great deal of expertise with the surface anatomy of the sphenoid and other paranasal sinuses. This procedure should not be confused with routine sinusotomy or removal of infected mucosa from the sinus walls. This approach to draining the petrous apex requires bone removal from the posterior wall of the sphenoid sinus, placing the carotid artery and optic nerve at risk. Skilled endoscopists perform this procedure with a low complication rate, but those with less experience would do well to note that the sphenoid sinus is the most variable in form of any bilateral cavity or organ in the human body. The sphenoid sinus may vary in length from four to 44mm, in width from 2.5 to 34mm, and in height from 5 to 33mm.[23]

Subtotal Petrosectomy

Fisch and Mattox[24] describe a subtotal petrosectomy in combination with removal of the otic capsule to gain full exposure of the petrous apex. This technique offers the advantage of direct exposure from the carotid artery to the sigmoid sinus in an anteroposterior direction and exposure from the hypotympanum to the middle fossa dura in an inferosuperior direction. The contents of the internal auditory canal are left undisturbed, and the facial nerve does not require transposition, making complete removal of benign lesions of the petrous apex, including cystic structures with their lining matrix, possible. Unfortunately, this increased exposure results in total sensorineural hearing loss with the removal of the otic capsule.

1. A postauricular incision is made down to the temporalis fascia superiorly and through the periosteum posteriorly and inferiorly. A second incision is made along the temporal line through the tem-

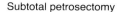

Subtotal petrosectomy

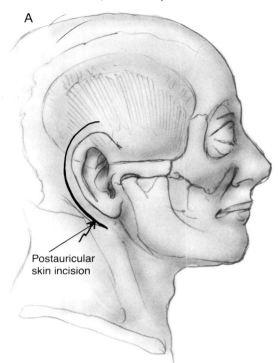

FIGURE 48–4. *See legend on page 577.*

poralis muscle, the auricle is reflected anteriorly, and the cartilaginous canal is transected. External auditory canal epithelium is everted, and the canal is sutured closed with a layer of periosteum sutured medially to form a two-layer closure (Fig. 48–4A).
2. A canal wall down tympanomastoidectomy is performed, and the posterior canal wall is lowered to the level of the facial nerve (Fig. 48–4B).
3. The mastoid tip cells are removed to the level of the digastric muscle (Fig. 48–4C).
4. The remaining external auditory canal skin, tympanic membrane, and annulus are removed after section of the incudostapedial joint and tensor tympani muscle (Fig. 48–4D).
5. Retrolabyrinthine, supralabyrinthine, supratubal, infralabyrinthine, and retrofacial air cells are then removed under direct vision. The bony labyrinth and cochlea are also removed without transposition of the facial nerve (Fig. 48–4E).
6. The lesion and its matrix or capsule are then removed under direct vision (Fig. 48–4F).
7. The remaining mucosa is gently curetted from the middle ear space. The introitus from the middle ear to the eustachian tube is drilled with a diamond burr, and the remaining mucosa is cauterized. The tube is obliterated with bone wax, muscle, and then fibrin glue (Fig. 48–4G).

The therapy for glomus tumors of the temporal bone continues to be controversial. Because the clinical characteristics and growth rates of these tumors are variable, the full gamut of management has been recommended from observation alone through radiation therapy and surgical management. Although there are isolated case reports of prolonged survival without treatment, these lesions can be quite deadly. The studies of Brown, Spector et al., Rosenwasser, and others have documented mortality rates from five per cent to 13 per cent for glomus jugulare tumors.[1-5] This chapter outlines the diagnostic and preoperative evaluation, surgical techniques, and results and complications in the management of glomus tumors of the temporal bone.

PATIENT SELECTION

Temporal bone glomus tumors are neoplasms of the normal paraganglioma in the temporal bone that principally occur in the adventitia of the dome of the jugular bulb but are also found in the submucosa of the cochlear promontory within the tympanic plexus. Numerous classification schemes have been proposed for these lesions, primarily by their origin (tympanic plexus versus jugular bulb) and the anatomic extent of lesion. The clinical surgical classification proposed by Antonio De la Cruz is particularly useful in planning the clinical management of patients with glomus tumors. The extent of the tumor is described by the involvement of structures of the temporal bone and skull base. A series of operations that correspond to the extent of the tumor is used (Table 49–1).

TYMPANIC TUMOR. This lesion arises from the glomus body of the promontory along Jacobson's nerve. The tumor is confined entirely to the mesotympanum, and all of its borders can be seen with routine otoscopy. This small tumor could not arise from the jugular bulb or it would extend beyond the inferior margins of the tympanic annulus. Although no additional studies are necessary to define the extent of the tumor, any vascular tumor of the middle ear must be differentiated from an aberrant carotid artery or a dehiscent jugular bulb. The aberrant carotid artery lies more anteriorly and is paler than the glomus tumor. The jugular bulb lies more posteriorly and is darker blue. If there is any question about the existence of either of these lesions, cranial computed tomography (CT) must be done to exclude them.

TYMPANOMASTOID TUMOR. Like the tympanic tumor, this lesion arises from the glomus body on the promontory. However, it extends beyond the tym-

TABLE 49–1. Glomus Tumor Classification and Surgical Approach

CLASSIFICATION	SURGICAL APPROACH
Tympanic	Transcanal
Tympanomastoid	Mastoid-extended facial recess
Jugular bulb	Mastoid-neck (possible limited facial nerve rerouting)
Carotid artery	Infratemporal fossa
Transdural	Infratemporal fossa/intracranial

panic annulus inferiorly or posteriorly. Because there is no way clinically to delineate the tumor's extent, any patient with a tumor that extends beyond the tympanic annulus must have a thorough radiographic evaluation. The key feature of this tumor category is that studies will show that the lesion does not involve the jugular bulb itself. However, tympanomastoid tumors may extend into the mastoid and into the retrofacial air cells.

JUGULAR BULB TUMOR. This lesion arises from the glomus body of the dome of the jugular bulb. It may extend into the middle ear and also into the bulb itself. This lesion is limited to involvement of the middle ear, mastoid, and the jugular bulb. By definition, it does not extend onto the carotid artery or medially into the skull base or intracranially.

CAROTID ARTERY GLOMUS TUMOR. This lesion arises from the jugular bulb but extends beyond the confines of the jugular bulb and vein and contacts the carotid artery. Small tumors of this category may involve only the carotid artery at the skull base, whereas larger tumors may extend far medially and may also involve the horizontal portion of the internal carotid artery and the petrous apex.

TRANSDURAL TUMOR. These lesions arise from the jugular bulb and extend not only to the internal carotid artery but also through the jugular foramen intracranially.

GLOMUS VAGALE TUMOR. These lesions arise from the glomus body along the vagus nerve at the base of the skull. Because glomus vagale tumors do not begin within the temporal bone, they are often larger than glomus tumors of the temporal bone itself because they later produce symptoms of pulsatile tinnitus and hearing loss. Clinically, these lesions produce vocal cord paralysis prior to the onset of hearing loss or tinnitus or the appearance of a vascular middle ear mass. In contrast, glomus tumors of the temporal bone produce otologic symptoms prior to the onset of vocal cord paralysis.[6]

PREOPERATIVE EVALUATION

Thorough preoperative evaluation permits surgical planning for complete and safe tumor removal. Advances in imaging technology now permit accurate preoperative assessment of tumor involvement within the temporal bone. The following tests are routinely used in the evaluation of patients with glomus tumors of the temporal bone.

ROUTINE HEARING TESTS. Air, bone, and speech audiometry are performed to assess the degree of conductive and sensorineural hearing impairments.

CRANIAL COMPUTED TOMOGRAPHY. The mainstay of assessment of glomus tumors of the temporal bone is thin-section (1.5mm thick) cranial CT using the bone algorithm. Tumors confined to the middle ear and mastoid are distinguished from tumors that involve the jugular bulb. Extensive lesions that extend onto or medial to the internal carotid artery and those that extend transdurally are also defined by this technique. In many cases, cranial CT is the only examination necessary for planning treatment. Because the jugular bulb is the major consideration in preoperative planning, cranial CT has supplanted retrograde jugular venography in assessing involvement of the jugular bulb.

MAGNETIC RESONANCE IMAGING. Because bone involvement by tumor is not clearly demonstrated on magnetic resonance imaging (MRI), this technique provides only adjunctive information regarding the extent of tumor involvement. If the diagnosis is at all in question, MRI combined with CT provides exquisite preoperative guidance in the differential diagnosis of petrous apex lesions.[7] MRI can indicate occlusion of the jugular bulb and vein because the normal flow signals will be altered. In intradural tumors, MRI can more clearly delineate the tumor-brain interface and the relationship of the lesion to the intradural structures. MRI must be interpreted cautiously because T1 images of glomus tumors may overestimate the degree of tumor involvement. Marrow-containing bone of the petrous apex is hyperintense and indistinguishable from enhancing tumor in the petrous apex. Magnetic resonance angiography and magnetic resonance venography offer another diagnostic tool in evaluating glomus tumors. In their present form, however, magnetic resonance angiographic techniques cannot provide adequate imaging resolution to define feeding vessels to the tumor. The role of these techniques in the preoperative assessment of glomus tumors has not been fully clarified.[8, 9]

ARTERIOGRAPHY. Four-vessel angiography is necessary when cranial CT demonstrates a glomus tumor involving the jugular bulb, carotid artery, or intradural structures. The principle indication for angiography is to assess the involvement of the internal carotid artery by tumor. Additionally, this technique assures preoperative identification of additional glomus lesions, if present. Although estimates vary, paragangliomas are multicentric in approximately 10 per cent of nonfamilial cases and 33 per cent in familial cases.

BRAIN PERFUSION AND FLOW STUDIES. For tumors that abut the internal carotid artery, it is necessary to assess the adequacy of the cerebral cross-perfusion from the contralateral internal carotid artery. Cross-compression angiography, stump pressure measurements, and clinical evaluation during test occlusion of the involved carotid are basic guides to the risk of stroke in the event that the affected carotid artery must be sacrificed. Xenon blood flow and radioisotope studies offer much more precise quantification of the risk of stroke and the possible need for surgical replacement of the internal carotid artery.[10] In certain cases with extensive invasion of the carotid artery and acceptable results on the perfusion studies of the contralateral artery, the involved carotid artery may be permanently occluded with a detachable balloon. If the preoperative studies indicate that the patient cannot withstand permanent occlusion of the artery, then graft replacement of the carotid is necessary if the carotid is injured during tumor removal.

Preoperative flow studies provide only risk information in the event of carotid injury. The decision to proceed with surgery or permanent occlusion in the face of poor results on the flow studies must be individualized based on factors such as the patient's age, health status, extent of disease, and previous treatment.

EMBOLIZATION. Large glomus tumors may result in significant intraoperative blood loss. We have found that preoperative embolization of feeding vessels can significantly reduce such loss.[11] The embolization is usually performed with Ivalon and is performed at the time of angiography 1 or 2 days before surgery.

BIOPSY. Biopsy of vascular middle ear masses is not recommended. The clinical and radiographic appearance of glomus tumors is characteristic enough to permit definitive management without a tissue diagnosis. Efforts at obtaining a tissue diagnosis prior to completion of the radiologic evaluation can result in injury to an aberrant carotid artery or a high jugular bulb as well as significant bleeding from the tumor itself.

PATIENT COUNSELING

Patients with tympanic and tympanomastoid glomus tumors are advised of the routine risks of exploratory tympanotomy and tympanomastoidectomy surgery. However, as will be discussed in the *Results* section of this chapter, the prognosis for these patients is excellent if total tumor removal is accomplished.

Patients with jugular bulb, carotid artery, or transdural tumors should be aware of the additional risks inherent in complete removal of their tumors. Specifically, facial nerve transposition is generally necessary and carries the attendant risk of facial paresis. Furthermore, these patients should be aware of the risk of lower cranial nerve injury and possible vascular complications as well. Any patient with intradural tumor extension must be aware of the risks of craniotomy, including postoperative hemorrhage, cerebrospinal fluid leakage, meningitis, and stroke.

SURGICAL APPROACHES

The following surgical techniques are used for removal of glomus tumors of the temporal bone. Notice that the specific approaches described correspond to the tumor classification system described earlier.

Transcanal Approach

The transcanal approach is used for small glomus tympanicum tumors that are limited to the mesotympanum. Because the entire circumference of the tumor is visible within the middle ear, preoperative imaging studies are not necessary. However, if there is any doubt of the possibility of an aberrant internal carotid artery, preoperative CT scanning should be obtained to exclude this possibility. The tympanomeatal flap is modified with the inferior incision extending more anteriorly so that the inferior aspect of the tympanic membrane can be elevated. The tumor is identified on the promontory (Fig. 49–1).

The inferior tympanic branch of the ascending pharyngeal artery supplies the glomus tympanicum tumor. The vessel may be controlled with bipolar cautery or a small piece of oxidized cellulose (Surgicel) to occlude the bony canaliculus from which the vessel arises. It is critical to avoid unipolar cautery on the tympanic promontory, as this may severely injure the cochlea.

The tumor is then removed with cup forceps. The brisk bleeding from the distal end of the artery anterior to the stapes (near the cochleariform process) is difficult to control directly; however, it usually clots readily. Small pledgets of oxidized cellulose assist in hemostasis, and the tympanomeatal flap is replaced

and the ear canal packed. No specific dressing is necessary, and the patient is ready for hospital discharge the following day. Accurate preoperative assessment is critical for success with the transcanal approach for glomus tympanicum tumors. If the entire circumference of the lesion is not visible through the meatus, the hypotympanotomy or mastoid-extended facial recess approach should be considered.

Tumors with limited hypotympanic extension without posterior involvement on CT scan may be removed by a modified transcanal (hypotympanic) approach.[12] After a postauricular incision is performed with transection of the ear canal, a superiorly based tympanomeatal flap is elevated to permit access to the inferior aspect of the tympanic ring. This bone is progressively drilled until the inferior limit of the tumor is identified. The drilling involved with this exposure is usually much less than the drilling required for the transcanal infracochlear drainage procedures for the petrous apex described in Chapter 48.

Mastoid-Extended Facial Recess Approach

The mastoid-extended facial recess approach is used for tympanomastoid glomus tumors. The tumor may extensively involve the middle ear and mastoid but has arisen from the glomus tympanicum body and does not involve the jugular bulb. Preoperative CT evaluation is critical before this approach is undertaken. Because the limits of the tumor are not visible through the tympanic membrane, CT provides an assessment of the extent of tumor involvement. Patient preparation and draping are performed as for a routine tympanomastoidectomy. A wide shave is performed, and the incision is made 1.5cm posterior to the postauricular sulcus. After a complete mastoidectomy, the facial recess is opened. The extended facial recess exposure is performed by further bone removal inferiorly accomplished by severing the corda tympani nerve and following the fibrous annulus of the tympanic membrane as a landmark. Such an approach allows complete exposure of the middle ear and the hypotympanum. After the tumor is exposed, bipolar cautery is helpful in shrinking the tumor and in controlling the blood supply. Oxidized cellulose packs are used to further tamponade the main arterial supply in the hypotympanum, and the tumor is removed with cup forceps. The tumor can be stripped from the ossicles if necessary.

Extension of glomus tympanicum tumors into the retrofacial air cells is managed by direct exposure. A cutting burr is used to remove the air cells inferior to the labyrinth and beneath the facial nerve, thereby leaving the facial nerve suspended with a thin layer of bone to allow the surgeon access to the entire hypotympanum (Fig. 49–2). A small curette is used to remove bits of tumor from crevices in the hypotympanum. The dome of the jugular bulb can be inspected to be certain that it is free of tumor.

Extensive tumor involvement may necessitate removal of the ossicles and tympanic membrane. In such circumstances, a tympanoplasty and ossicular reconstruction may be accomplished in the routine manner. Similarly, if the tumor has produced extensive destruction of the posterior canal wall, such cases may be managed with a canal wall down technique combined with tympanoplasty and mastoid obliteration after complete tumor removal. At the conclusion of the procedure, a mastoid dressing is applied, and the patient is usually ready for discharge by the first postoperative morning.

Mastoid and Neck Approach

The mastoid and neck approach is used for small glomus jugulare tumors. These tumors involve the jugular bulb but do not extend onto the internal carotid artery or into the neck or posterior fossa. The preoperative evaluation of these patients may include angiography because involvement of the jugular bulb raises the question of possible carotid artery involvement. Continuous intraoperative facial nerve monitoring is used. Additionally, electromyographic electrodes in the sternocleidomastoid muscle are useful for monitoring cranial nerve XI, electrodes in the lateral pharyngeal wall can monitor cranial nerve IX, and electrodes in the vocalis muscle can monitor cranial nerve X. The procedure is performed by initially completing the same exposure as that described in the mastoid-extended facial recess approach (Fig. 49–2), then amputating the mastoid tip. The periosteum of the digastric groove is followed anteriorly until it turns abruptly laterally at the stylomastoid foramen. Drilling laterally along the digastric ridge both anteriorly and posteriorly frees the entire mastoid tip. The incision is then carried into the neck along the anterior border of the sternocleidomastoid muscle. This muscle is freed from the mastoid tip and retracted posteriorly. The mastoid tip can then be removed by grasping it with a Kocher clamp and cutting with a curved Mayo scissors along the bone. The posterior belly of the digastric muscle is identified and freed from the digastric groove and retracted anteriorly to allow exposure of the major neurovascular structures of the neck. Once the internal jugular vein is identified and dissected free from surrounding tissues, it is occluded with multiple 2-0 silk sutures. The jugular vein is followed over the transverse process of the first cervical vertebra into the base of the skull. In this fashion, the eleventh cranial nerve is identified (usually lateral to the vein) and preserved.

In limited tumors that do not extend into the neck or skull base, it is usually possible to preserve the ninth, tenth, and eleventh cranial nerves. The neck exposure is necessary to permit ligation of the jugular vein.

Exposure of the sigmoid sinus and jugular bulb is then completed with diamond burrs. Although limited tumors do not involve the medial wall of the jugular foramen, the tumor arises from the dome of the jugular bulb, and the bulb must be resected in continuity with the tumor. The proximal sigmoid sinus is controlled with extraluminal packing of oxidized cellulose. Preservation of the bone over the midportion of the sigmoid sinus permits extraluminal packing of this portion of the sigmoid sinus. Because the jugular vein has been tied in the neck, the sigmoid sinus may be opened just distal to the proximal packing. Bleeding occurs at this point from the patent inferior petrosal sinus and condylar vein. Oxidized cellulose is advanced into the jugular bulb to control this bleeding. This packing must not be placed too firmly, as a weakness of cranial nerves IX, X, and XI may result.

The tumor is now ready for resection in continuity with the dome of the jugular bulb. Bipolar cautery helps in hemostasis and shrinkage of the tumor bulk. Once the tumor and dome of the jugular bulb are excised, hemostasis is completed with oxidized cellulose packing (Fig. 49–3). Complete tumor resection is accomplished, and if the tympanic membrane or ossicles are involved, reconstruction may be performed as described earlier. It is usually possible to preserve the ninth, tenth, and eleventh cranial nerves with these limited tumors unless there is preoperative involvement of these structures. Postoperatively, these patients are cared for in the intensive care unit because the possibility of an acute lower cranial neuropathy or major postoperative hemorrhage exists. Usually, minimal morbidity is associated with this approach, and patients are stable and may be discharged from the hospital within a few days. The major pitfall associated with this approach is related to inaccurate preoperative assessment of tumor extent. The mastoid-neck approach is too limited if the tumor extensively involves the carotid artery.

Mastoid and Neck with Limited Facial Nerve Rerouting

A useful modification of the mastoid-neck approach adds a limited facial nerve rerouting to the procedure. Additional exposure in the mastoid-neck approach may be achieved by totally decompressing the facial nerve from the second genu throughout the entire vertical segment. The periosteum of the facial nerve at the stylomastoid foramen is preserved, but the fi-

FIGURE 49-1

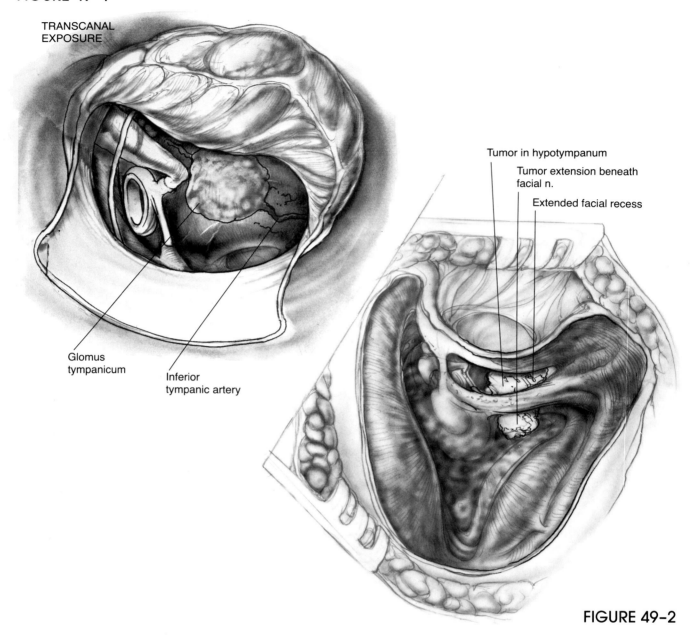

TRANSCANAL
EXPOSURE

Glomus
tympanicum

Inferior
tympanic artery

Tumor in hypotympanum

Tumor extension beneath
facial n.

Extended facial recess

FIGURE 49-2

FIGURE 49-1. Transcanal exposure of glomus tympanicum tumor limited to the promontory.

FIGURE 49-2. The facial recess has been opened widely and extended inferiorly to expose tumor in the hypotympanum. Tumor extension beneath the facial nerve is exposed by removing the retrofacial air cells and skeletonizing the facial nerve.

FIGURE 49-3. Completed procedure using mastoid-neck approach. The jugular bulb is resected along with the tumor after proximal and distal vessels are controlled.

FIGURE 49-4. Mastoid-neck approach with limited facial nerve rerouting. Displacement of the facial nerve exposes larger tumors of the jugular bulb.

FIGURE 49-3

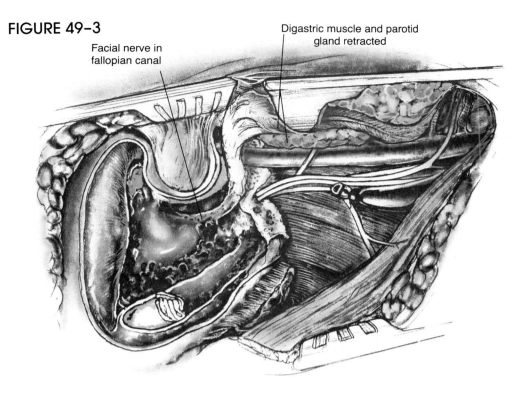

Facial nerve in
fallopian canal

Digastric muscle and parotid
gland retracted

FIGURE 49-4

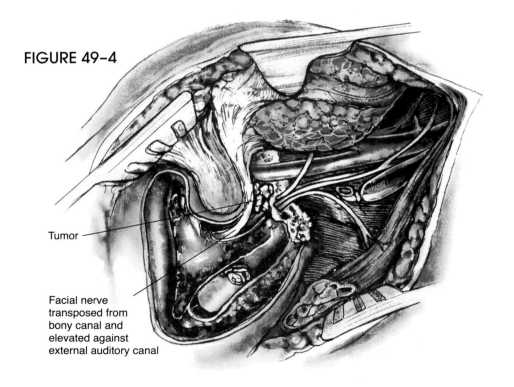

Tumor

Facial nerve
transposed from
bony canal and
elevated against
external auditory
canal

brous attachments to the nerve in its vertical portion are sharply transected. The mobilized nerve can be transposed laterally along with the periosteum at the stylomastoid foramen and the attached posterior belly of the digastric muscle. A suture through the stylomastoid periosteum can be used to hold the nerve laterally and prevent traction on this structure. Such transposition of the facial nerve will permit further bone removal in the area of the vertical facial canal and retrofacial air cells along the infralabyrinthine air cell tract (Fig. 49–4). This modification of the mastoid and neck approach with limited facial nerve rerouting is ideal for neuromas of the jugular foramen because they are not as intimately involved with the carotid artery as are glomus tumors. The surgeon should be cautious about applying this approach for glomus tumors that involve the carotid artery. The annulus and posterior canal wall still limit the surgeon's view of the vertical portion of the carotid artery if extensive manipulation is necessary in this area.

Infratemporal Fossa Approach

The development of the infratemporal fossa approach by Fisch has been a significant advance in our ability to totally remove large glomus jugulare tumors.[13] Previous approaches that did not remove the external auditory canal or reroute the facial nerve did not allow adequate exposure of the tumor or internal carotid artery (Fig. 49–5). There are eight distinct steps in the infratemporal fossa exposure: 1) patient preparation, 2) management of the ear canal and tympanic ring, 3) mastoidectomy, 4) initial preparation of the jugular vein and neck exposure, 5) transposition of the facial nerve, 6) completion of the neck exposure and identification of the lower cranial nerves and skull base carotid artery, 7) tumor removal and intracranial extension, and 8) wound closure. Continuous facial nerve monitoring and electromyographic monitoring of the lower cranial nerves are employed as previously described.

A wide shave is performed, and a large postauricular incision is made in a C-shaped fashion. The incision is carried anteriorly, and the ear canal is tran-

sected slightly medially to the bone-cartilage junction of the ear canal. Cartilage is removed from the ear canal to permit fashioning of the ear canal as a cuff that can be everted. The skin of the meatus is closed with 5-0 nylon sutures. The periosteum of the postauricular area is elevated as a flap and sutured behind the opening in the meatus to further reinforce the closure (see Chapter 60, Figs. 60–4 and 60–5). Next, a mastoidectomy is completed, and the facial recess is opened to allow separation of the incudostapedial joint. The posterior wall of the ear canal can then be removed with rongeurs and cutting burrs. The remaining skin of the ear canal as well as the tympanic membrane, malleus, and incus are removed. Next, the facial nerve is decompressed from the geniculate to the stylomastoid foramen. An eggshell-thin layer of bone is left over the nerve itself. By use of cutting and diamond burrs, the bone of the tympanic ring is progressively removed, the level of the jugular bulb is identified, and the bone over the temporomandibular joint and vertical segment of the petrous carotid artery is removed anteriorly (Fig. 49–6).

Attention is then focused on the neck. The incision is continued vertically along the anterior border of the sternocleidomastoid muscle, the mastoid tip is removed as previously described, the jugular vein is identified, and ligatures are placed around the vein but are not yet tied at this point. The carotid artery is identified and marked with a ligature. The posterior belly of the digastric muscle is transected.

Next, the facial nerve is transposed. The transposition technique originally described by Fisch has been modified because of temporary and sometimes permanent residual facial weakness.[14] Rather than exposing the facial nerve in the parotid, the surgeon transposes the nerve with periosteum of the stylomastoid foramen and elevates the entire tail of the parotid.[15] After decompressing the nerve, the remaining eggshell-thin bone over the facial nerve is removed with a blunt instrument. The multiple fibrous connections along the descending portion of the nerve are sharply transected. The tympanic portion of the nerve does not have such adhesions, and this section elevates readily. The posterior belly of the digastric muscle is

---

FIGURE 49–5. The overlying facial nerve prevents exposure of the internal carotid artery for tumor removal.

FIGURE 49–6. Temporal bone dissection completed. The facial nerve is skeletonized and the tympanic ring removed. The carotid artery and jugular bulb with tumor are exposed.

FIGURE 49–7. Facial nerve transposed anteriorly. A large suture tacks the periosteum of the stylomastoid foramen and facial nerve superiorly to avoid tension on the transposed nerve.

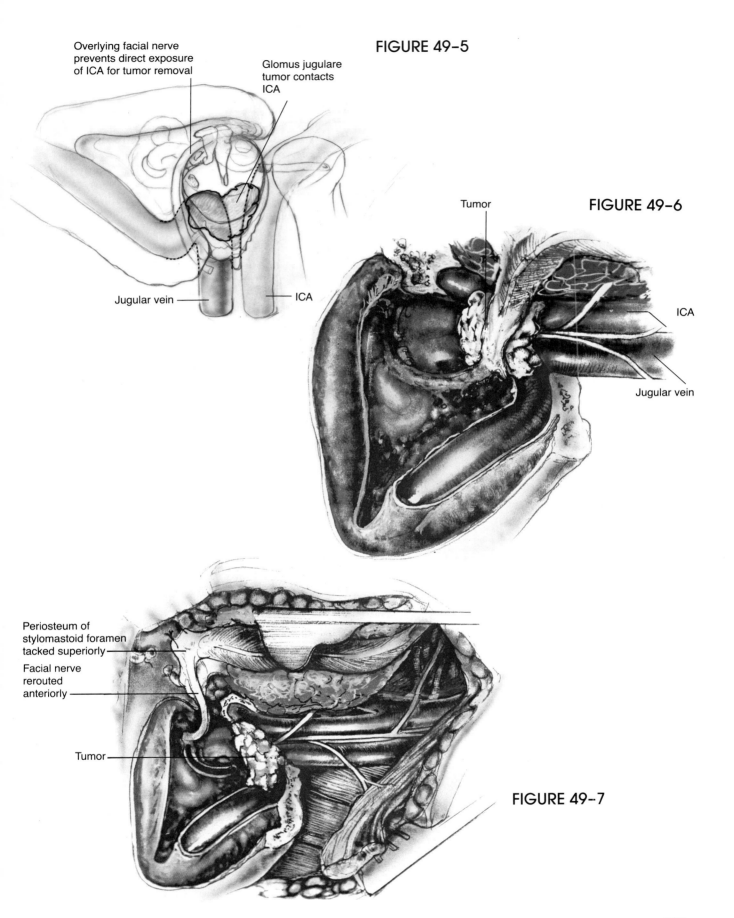

FIGURE 49-5

Overlying facial nerve prevents direct exposure of ICA for tumor removal

Glomus jugulare tumor contacts ICA

Jugular vein

ICA

FIGURE 49-6

Tumor

ICA

Jugular vein

Periosteum of stylomastoid foramen tacked superiorly

Facial nerve rerouted anteriorly

Tumor

FIGURE 49-7

moved anteriorly because the fascia of this muscle contributes to the stylomastoid foramen periosteum. The nerve can then be transposed anteriorly along with the tail of the parotid. A large suture is placed through the periosteum of the stylomastoid foramen and attached to the soft tissues in the area of the root of the zygoma (Fig. 49–7), thereby elevating the facial nerve and preventing it from being stretched when retractors are placed. The use of continuous facial nerve monitoring during this maneuver has significantly improved postoperative facial nerve function.[16]

After the facial nerve is decompressed and elevated, a large Perkins retractor is placed beneath the angle of the mandible, and the entire mandible is retracted forward. This exposure avoids the need to resect the mandibular condyle, even in large tumors that extend into the infratemporal fossa extensively. The remaining bone over the distal sigmoid sinus, jugular bulb, and vertical portion of the petrous carotid artery can be removed with diamond burrs. Attention is once again focused in the neck, where the internal carotid artery is followed through the skull base into its intratemporal course. The lower cranial nerves (IX, X, and XI) are followed into the jugular foramen as well. The twelfth cranial nerve is also identified and followed to its foramen.

The jugular vein is doubly ligated and transected between ligatures, and the external carotid artery is ligated. If the tumor extends intradurally, the proximal sigmoid sinus is doubly ligated with silk sutures passed through openings in the dura with an aneurysm suture passer (Fig. 49–8). If the tumor is not intradural, then the sigmoid can be packed with Surgicel without violating the dura. The jugular vein is then elevated, and the tumor in the area of the jugular bulb is freed inferiorly to superiorly following the jugular vein into the jugular bulb. The tumor is freed from the carotid artery anteriorly, and bleeding from the caroticotympanic vessels is controlled with bipolar cautery. If the tumor is adherent to the internal carotid artery, it is best to leave a portion of it on the artery and remove the bulk of the tumor. Tumor hemostasis is continued with bipolar cautery and oxidized cellulose packing of the inferior petrosal sinus; the tumor can be removed in continuity with the dome of the jugular bulb. If the last bit of the tumor from the carotid artery is not removed until the conclusion of

the procedure, a small entry into the carotid artery that may occur at the location of the caroticotympanic artery can be repaired directly (Fig. 49–9).

Small intracranial tumor extensions are usually removed at the time of removal of the jugular bulb because this is the usual location of dural penetration. If there is extensive intracranial extension, however, a decision must be made about whether to attempt total removal of the tumor. The decision is largely based on the amount of blood lost to this point. If blood loss has been limited to less than 3000ml, as is almost always the case, removal of the intracranial extension of the tumor may proceed. However, if the amount of blood loss has been greater, problems with bleeding may occur despite the replenishment of the known clotting factors with fresh frozen plasma and platelet packs. In such cases, a two-stage procedure with removal of the intracranial portion of the tumor at a later date is planned.

The removal of the intracranial portion of the tumor is often easier than the removal of tumor within the temporal bone. By the time one is ready for the removal of the intracranial extension, the blood supply has often been controlled. The blood supply to the intracranial portion of the tumor is often discrete and can be controlled with bipolar cautery as with other cerebellopontine angle tumors (Fig. 49–10). If tumor has been left along the internal carotid artery, it is now removed. Closure is accomplished by closing the eustachian tube with oxidized cellulose, muscle, and strips of abdominal fat (Fig. 49–11). If cerebrospinal fluid has been encountered, continuous lumbar drainage is used for approximately 5 days until the wound is sealed (see Chapter 60). A drain is left in the neck wound and removed on the first postoperative morning. A pressure dressing is placed for 4 postoperative days.

One technique with encouraging results in cases with large blood loss has been the use of a Cell Saver (Hemonics, Braintree, MA) (which is commonly used in cardiovascular surgery). By use of a special irrigating suction device with a heparinized reservoir, intraoperative blood loss can be salvaged and prepared for replacement to the patient during the same procedure. Additionally, we routinely counsel patients on preoperative autologous donation of blood to minimize the need for banked blood replacement.

FIGURE 49–8. The jugular vein and sigmoid sinus are doubly ligated. If the tumor does not extend intradurally, the sigmoid is occluded with extraluminal packing.

FIGURE 49–9. Final piece of tumor removed from carotid artery. The artery may be repaired with vascular suture if injury occurs with total tumor removal.

FIGURE 49-8

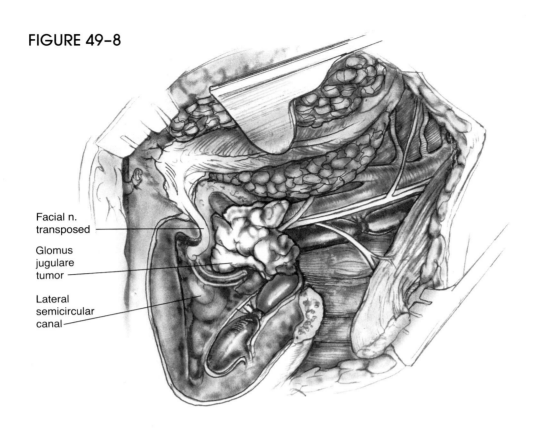

Facial n. transposed

Glomus jugulare tumor

Lateral semicircular canal

FIGURE 49-9

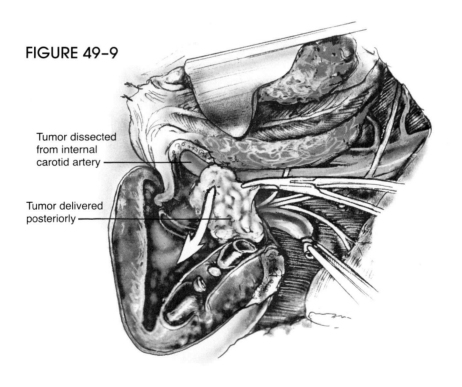

Tumor dissected from internal carotid artery

Tumor delivered posteriorly

FIGURE 49-10

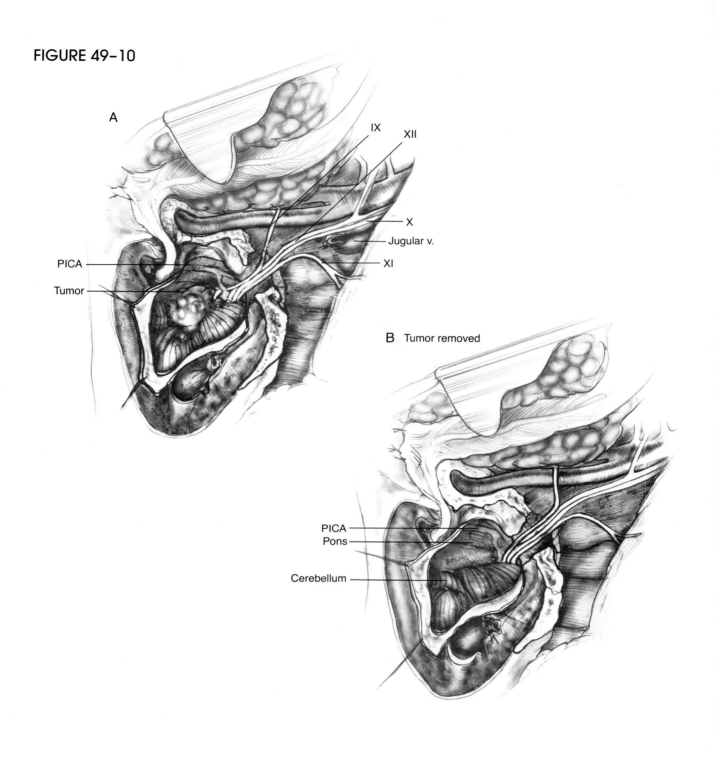

A

IX XII

X

Jugular v.

XI

PICA

Tumor

B Tumor removed

PICA

Pons

Cerebellum

FIGURE 49-10. Removal of the intracranial extension of tumor. Intracranial feeding vessels are controlled by bipolar cautery.

FIGURE 49-11. The eustachian tube is closed with oxidized cellulose and muscle. For intracranial tumors, the dura is sutured to the extent possible. Strips of abdominal fat obliterate the middle ear and mastoid.

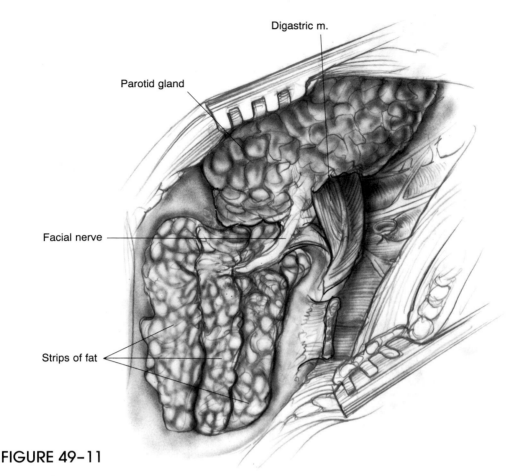

Parotid gland

Facial nerve

Strips of fat

Digastric m.

FIGURE 49–11

RESULTS

GLOMUS TYMPANICUM TUMORS. O'Leary et al. recently reviewed the results of glomus tympanicum surgery at the House Ear Clinic.[17] Seventy-three glomus tympanicum tumors (tympanic tumor or tympanomastoid tumor) were managed at the House Ear Clinic between 1957 and 1990. Eighty per cent of these required a mastoid-facial recess approach, and in twenty per cent, a transcanal removal was possible. Although significant intraoperative blood loss occurred (average, over 500ml), the morbidity was minimal. Hearing levels remained stable: the mean speech reception threshold increased 1dB postoperatively. Of the five complications, three were residual tympanic membrane perforations requiring a secondary tympanoplasty. One patient developed a cholesteatoma postoperatively. One patient developed a facial nerve weakness requiring re-exploration and facial nerve decompression with an ultimately good outcome (II/VI on the House-Brackmann scale). This series demonstrated that the critical feature of glomus tympanicum management is total tumor resection. The three cases in which an incomplete resection was performed resulted in tumor recurrence. Overall, the recurrence rate in this series was less than 5 per cent.

GLOMUS JUGULARE TUMORS. Green et al. recently reviewed the House Ear Clinic experience with glomus jugulare tumors (jugular bulb, carotid artery involvement tumors, and intradural tumors) between 1980 and 1991.[18] During this interval, 52 patients were surgically treated for glomus jugulare tumors who had undergone no prior radiotherapy or surgery. The techniques involved were the infratemporal fossa approach in 83 per cent, the mastoid-neck approach in 7 per cent, and the mastoid-neck with limited facial nerve mobilization in 10 per cent. Complete surgical removal was possible in 85 per cent of the patients. Eight patients required transection of the facial nerve for complete tumor removal. These patients underwent segmental grafting or greater auricular nerve reconstruction. The mean intraoperative blood loss was 1500ml. Long-term facial function was good: 95 per cent of patients had grade I/VI or II/VI facial function at 1-year follow-up or greater. Nearly 20 per cent of patients required a vocal cord augmentation procedure. However, no patient required a tracheotomy in the immediate postoperative period. Four patients required prolonged nasogastric tube feeding, and two ultimately requiring gastrostomy. Eighty-five per cent of the patients were able to resume the same activity level as before surgery.

COMPLICATIONS

GLOMUS TYMPANICUM TUMORS. Glomus tympanicum surgery risks the same morbidity as that involved in tympanomastoid surgery. The management of associated facial nerve, tympanic membrane, sigmoid sinus, and healing complications is identical to that in tympanomastoid surgery for chronic otitis media.

GLOMUS JUGULARE TUMORS. As illustrated in the *Results* section, the categories of morbidity in glomus jugulare surgery include facial nerve injury, lower cranial nerve dysfunction, carotid artery injury, bleeding problems, and intracranial complications. Direct tumor infiltration of the facial nerve necessitates transection of the involved segment and replacement of that segment with a nerve graft using standard techniques. The advent of continuous intraoperative facial nerve monitoring has significantly improved postoperative facial nerve function in infratemporal fossa surgery.[16] In our experience, the need for tracheotomy or gastrostomy has been infrequent (<4 per cent). We recommend early vocal cord augmentation for vagal paralysis.[18, 19]

The possibility of carotid artery injury must be anticipated. Careful preoperative imaging, including CT scans and angiography, are helpful in defining the anatomic relationships of the tumor to the internal carotid artery. Preoperative flow studies (i.e., balloon occlusion or xenon or technetium blood flow studies) are helpful in predicting how well a patient will tolerate total occlusion of the internal carotid artery. The indications for replacement versus permanent occlusion have been summarized elsewhere.[20] The possibility of significant intraoperative blood loss must be anticipated. Autologous blood donation has been helpful in avoiding transfusions of banked blood. In the weeks preceding surgery, the patient donates his or her own blood for possible autologous transfusion perioperatively. Similarly, the cell saver, which recycles the patient's intraoperative blood loss, may reduce the requirement for banked blood transfusions. The limiting factor, however, is that the use of the cell saver cannot be combined with absorbable hemostatic packing (i.e., oxidized cellulose, Avitene, or gelatin sponge), so the value of this technology has not been fully assessed for glomus jugulare surgery. Finally, the surgeon must be cognizant of the extent of blood replacement and be certain that the appropriate ratio of platelets and fresh frozen plasma are replaced in addition to the red cell products themselves.

Intracranial glomus tumor extension should be managed cooperatively with a neurosurgeon. The techniques for tumor removal are similar to those employed for other posterior fossa neoplasms. Specifically, the possibility of intracranial hemorrhage, wound infection, and cerebrospinal fluid leakage may require neurosurgical expertise. In our experience, patients with cerebrospinal fluid fistulae respond to conservative management with pressure dressing and lumbar drainage.

ALTERNATIVE TECHNIQUES

The role of radiation therapy in the management of glomus jugulare tumors is still controversial. Histologic studies have proved that the effects of irradiation appear to be on the blood vessels and fibrous elements of the tumor rather than on the tumor cells themselves.[21] These tumors often begin growing after a 10- to 15-year period of control. Accordingly, we favor radiation therapy in elderly patients with symptomatic glomus tumors or in patients who otherwise could not withstand a surgical removal. We recommend surgery as definitive therapy for patients who are medically stable enough to undergo an operative procedure.

SUMMARY

Modern imaging studies accurately delineate the extent of glomus tumors of the temporal bone. Microsurgical techniques allow total removal of even the largest tumors with acceptable morbidity and virtually no mortality. We favor surgical management of glomus tumors except in the elderly or infirm, in whom radiation therapy is a reasonable alternative.

References

1. Rosenwasser H: Carotid body-like tumor of the middle ear and mastoid bone. Arch Otolaryngol 41: 64–67, 1945.
2. Bickerstaff ER, Howell JS: The neurological importance of tumors of the glomus jugulare. Brain 76: 576–593, 1953.
3. Steinberg N, Holz WG: Glomus jugulare tumors. Arch Otolaryngol Head Neck Surg 82: 387–394, 1965.
4. Brown JS: Glomus jugulare tumors revisited: A ten-year statistical follow-up of 231 cases. Laryngoscope 95: 284–285, 1985.
5. Spector GJ, Fierstein J, Ogura JH: A comparison of therapeutic modalities of glomus tumors in the temporal bone. Laryngoscope 86: 690–696, 1976.
6. Leonetti JP, Brackmann DE: Glomus vagale tumors: The significance of early vocal cord paralysis. Otolaryngol Head Neck Surg 100: 533–537, 1989.
7. Arriaga MA, Brackmann DE: Differential diagnosis of primary petrous apex lesions. Am J Otol 12(6): 470–474, 1991.
8. Arriaga MA, Lo WWM, Brackmann DE: Imaging case study of the month. Magnetic resonance angiography of synchronous bilateral carotid body paragangliomas and bilateral vagal paragangliomas. Ann Otol Rhinol Laryngol 101: 955–957, 1992.
9. Rogers GP, Brackmann DE, Lo WWM: Magnetic resonance angiography, a technique for evaluation of skull base lesions. Am J Otol 14 (1): 56–62, 1993.
10. Janecka IP, Sekhar LN, Horton JA: General blood flow evalua-

tion. *In* Cummings CW, et al. (eds): Otolaryngology Head and Neck Surgery Update II. St. Louis, Mosby Year Book, 1990, pp 54–63.

11. Murphy TP, Brackmann DE: Effects of preopererative embolization on glomus jugulare tumors. Laryngoscope 99: 1244–1247, 1989.

12. Farrior JB: Glomus tumors—Postauricular hypotympanotomy. Arch Otolaryngol Head Neck Surg 86: 367–373, 1967.

13. Fisch U: Infratemporal fossa approach for glomus tumors of the temporal bone. Ann Otol Rhinol Laryngol 91: 474–479, 1982.

14. Fisch U, Fagan P, Valvanis A: The infratemporal fossa approach for the lateral skull base. Otolaryngol Clin North Am 17(3): 513–552, 1984.

15. Brackmann DE: The facial nerve in the infratemporal approach. Otolaryngol Head Neck Surg 97: 15–17, 1987.

16. Leonetti JP, Brackmann DE, Prass RC: Improved preservation of facial function in the infratemporal fossa approach to the skull base. Otolaryngol Head Neck Surg 101: 74–78, 1989.

17. O'Leary MJ, Shelton C, Giddings N, et al.: Glomus tympanicum tumors: A clinical perspective. Laryngsocope 101: 74–78, 1989.

18. Green JD, Nguyen CD, Arriaga MA, et al.: Technical modifications in the surgical management of glomus jugulare tumors. Laryngoscope [In press].

19. Neterrville JD: Primary Thyroplasty in Glomus Jugulare Surgery. Oral presentation, American Neurotology Society Fall Meeting, Washington DC, September 13, 1992.

20. deVries EJ: A new method to predict safe resection of the internal carotid artery. Laryngoscope 100: 85–89, 1990.

21. Brackmann DE, House WF, Terry R, et al.: Glomus jugulare tumors: Effect of irradiation. Trans Am Acad Ophthalmol Otolaryngol 76: 1423–1431, 1972.

50

The Middle Fossa Approach

WILLIAM F. HOUSE, M.D.
CLOUGH SHELTON, M.D.

The middle fossa approach for vestibular nerve section was reported as early as 1904; however, hammer and chisel were used at that time, which put the facial nerve at risk.[1] The middle fossa approach did not have widespread application until refined by the senior author (WFH) in 1961.[2] The approach was used initially for decompression of the internal auditory canal in cases of extensive otosclerosis. That therapy was later abandoned, but it became evident that this approach was suitable for removal of acoustic tumors. Initially, the middle fossa approach was used for tumors of all sizes. However, further experience demonstrated that it was most suitable for small tumors,[3–5] and that preservation of hearing and facial nerve function was possible in a significant proportion of operated patients.[6] The middle fossa approach was used infrequently until the recent development of gadolinium-enhanced magnetic resonance imaging. With this development, a larger number of acoustic tumors are diagnosed when they are small and before hearing has been significantly affected, making an attempt at hearing preservation desirable.

The middle fossa approach provides complete exposure of the contents of the internal auditory canal, allowing removal of laterally placed tumors without the need for blind dissection.[7] This exposure ensures total removal and is well suited for the removal of very small acoustic tumors.[8] The facial nerve can be located in its bony canal, allowing positive identification in a location not involved by tumor.

The middle fossa approach is technically difficult because of the lack of robust landmarks and the limited exposure. Bleeding in the posterior fossa can be difficult to control because of the limited access. Because of its location in the superior aspect of the internal auditory canal, the facial nerve is subjected to more manipulation in this approach than in other approaches.[9, 10] In the past, facial nerve results in middle fossa cases have not been as good as those from the translabyrinthine approach for similar-sized tumors.[11] However, the routine use of the facial nerve monitor has helped improve these results.

Several authors use an extended middle fossa approach for large tumors.[12–14] The tentorium is divided to give wider access to the posterior fossa. Some also perform a labyrinthectomy to enlarge the exposure when hearing preservation is not attempted.[15–17]

INDICATIONS

The primary indications for the middle fossa approach are a small acoustic tumor, with less than 5mm *1am* extension into the cerebellopontine angle, and good preoperative hearing. For hearing conservation surgery, we use the arbitrary audiometric criteria of

OR 60/50 rule

speech reception threshold of better than 30dB and speech discrimination score of better than 70 per cent, although these indications must be individualized to the needs of the patient.[18] Some advocate attempting hearing preservation in the removal of small acoustic tumors if any measurable preoperative hearing exists.[19] Patients older than 60 years do not tolerate the middle fossa approach as well as younger patients because of the fragility of the dura and retraction of the temporal lobe.

PREOPERATIVE EVALUATION

Several preoperative factors may predict postoperative hearing preservation. The most obvious is tumor size. Intuitively, the smaller the tumor, the easier it is to remove and the more likely one is to save hearing. This trend has been substantiated by several authors.[11, 20, 21] Some have also found that the better the preoperative hearing, the more likely it will be preserved,[22, 23] whereas others have failed to identify such a relationship.[11, 21, 24] Also, an intact preoperative stapedial reflex has been associated with successful postoperative hearing preservation.[22]

Several authors have reported a relationship between preoperative auditory brain stem response audiometry (ABR) and hearing preservation.[16, 21] In one report, hearing was preserved in 78 per cent of patients with an intra-aural wave V latency difference of 0.4 milliseconds or less.[11] For latency differences of 0.5 to 2.0 milliseconds, the hearing preservation rate dropped to 58 per cent. In patients with no response on the ABR, postoperative measurable hearing remained in only 50 per cent. Thus, patients with a more normal preoperative ABR result apparently have a greater success rate for postoperative hearing preservation. This result may reflect less tumor involvement of the cochlear nerve. However, one report did not find preoperative ABR to be predictive of hearing outcome.[25]

Tumors arising from the superior vestibular nerve have a higher rate of hearing preservation than those arising from the inferior vestibular nerve. Acoustic tumors developing in the inferior portion of the internal auditory canal may involve the cochlear nerve earlier and more severely.[26] In a series of middle fossa acoustic tumor removals, 68 per cent of patients whose tumors were found intraoperatively to arise from the superior vestibular nerve had measurable hearing preservation, whereas only 43 per cent of patients whose tumors originated from the inferior vestibular nerve had measurable postoperative hearing.[11] This difference was statistically significant. Preoperative electronystagmography (ENG) may predict tumor origin and, thus, hearing preservation. The caloric response reflects superior vestibular nerve function. In the presence of a small acoustic neuroma, a normal caloric response indicates an inferior vestibular nerve tumor, whereas a decreased response suggests a tumor arising from the superior vestibular nerve. Of a group of 54 patients who had preoperative ENG, hearing was preserved in 64 per cent with hypoactive caloric responses, whereas postoperative hearing remained in only 45 per cent of those with normal caloric responses.[11] The association of normal caloric tests with nonpreservation of hearing has also been reported by others.[10, 16]

For intracanalicular tumors, the x-ray appearance may predict success at hearing preservation. Small tumors that enlarge the internal auditory canal have a poorer prognosis for hearing preservation (Jackler, Personal communication, 1990). In the junior author's experience, these small tumors that expand the canal are very adherent to the cochlear nerve, which adversely affects the hearing outcome.

PATIENT COUNSELING

After a thorough discussion of the relevant anatomy and the necessity to treat acoustic tumors, the options regarding surgical approaches to remove acoustic tumors are described to the patient. For those with small tumors and relatively good preoperative hearing, the issues of hearing preservation are discussed. We tell such patients that there is an approximate 50 per cent chance of saving some measurable hearing and a 30 per cent chance of saving the hearing to near the preoperative level. Should the preoperative ENG and ABR be favorable (see earlier), they are informed that the prognosis for hearing preservation is above average.

The patient is told that there is an approximate 90 per cent chance that normal or nearly normal facial nerve function will be obtained in the long term, but that there is a 50 per cent chance of having temporary facial paralysis in the early postoperative period. Although the facial nerve results for either the middle fossa or retrosigmoid approach are excellent, our best and most consistent facial nerve results occur with the translabyrinthine approach. We feel that the patient should be informed that there is a small but definite risk for attempted hearing preservation.

Patients with preoperative tinnitus are counseled that the problem will likely get better but probably will not disappear. Patients with no preoperative tinnitus have an approximate 25 per cent chance of developing it postoperatively.[27] Other important possible complications are discussed, including cerebrospinal fluid leak, meningitis, serious brain complications, death, and blood transfusion options. The patient usu-

ally donates one unit of autologous blood prior to surgery.

Recuperation can take weeks to months, and most patients are back at work within 6 weeks. The patient should expect to be dizzy postoperatively, and the rapidity of the central compensation greatly influences the time course of the recuperation.

SURGERY

Preoperative Preparation

We do not usually use preoperative or postoperative antibiotics, but despite this, the incidence of postoperative meningitis is very low. Because of the long-distance referral nature of our practices, we prefer that the patient stay in the institution's geographic area in case he or she develops postoperative meningitis.

Intraoperative furosemide and mannitol are given to allow easier temporal lobe retraction. The junior author (CS) also routinely uses a single dose of dexamethasone (Decadron) intravenously at the beginning of surgery. His clinical impression is that the incidence of delayed facial paralysis is reduced by this measure. This single dose of steroid does not seem to adversely affect wound healing. Long-acting muscle relaxants are avoided during surgery so as not to interfere with facial nerve monitoring.

Please see Chapter 1 for details of surgical site preparation and draping. Also described in this chapter are the instruments used, including the House-Urban middle fossa retractor.

Surgical Anatomy

The surgical anatomy of the temporal bone from the middle fossa approach is compact but complex (Fig. 50–1). Landmarks are not as apparent as with other approaches through the temporal bone, so laboratory dissection is very useful for the surgeon to become familiar with the anatomy from above.

Anteriorly, the limit of the dissection is the middle meningeal artery, which is lateral to the greater superficial petrosal nerve. The arcuate eminence marks the position of the superior semicircular canal and may be readily apparent in some patients but obscure in others. Kartush et al. cautioned that the relationship between the arcuate eminence and the superior semicircular canal may be variable in some patients, but the superior canal tends to be perpendicular to the petrous ridge.[28] Medially, the superior petrosal sinus runs along the petrous ridge.

Surgical tolerances are very tight in the area of the lateral internal auditory canal. The labyrinthine portion of the facial nerve lies immediately posterior to the basal turn of the cochlea. Bill's bar separates the facial and superior vestibular nerves. Slightly posterior and lateral to this area is the vestibule and ampullated end of the superior semicircular canal.

Identification of the geniculate ganglion can be accomplished by tracing the greater superficial petrosal nerve posteriorly to it. If the tegmen is unroofed, the geniculate is found to be slightly anterior to the head of the malleus.

The internal auditory canal lies approximately on the same axis as the external auditory canal; this relationship is useful in orienting the surgical field.[12] The more medial one progresses along the internal auditory canal, the more space exists around it,[29] allowing for safe dissection in this area.

Several methods can be used to locate the internal auditory canal and are reviewed in detail elsewhere.[12, 28] We prefer to follow the facial nerve in a retrograde fashion to the internal auditory canal (see later). In some cases, after the geniculate ganglion has been identified, the junior author (CS) employs the technique of Garcia-Ibanez and Garcia-Ibanez,[30] which involves drilling on the bisection of the angle formed by the blue line of the superior semicircular canal and greater superficial petrosal nerve. The internal auditory canal can be initially located in the "safe" medial area of the temporal bone and followed laterally.

Surgical Technique

The patient is placed in the supine position with the head turned to the side. The surgeon is seated at the head of the table and the anesthesiologist at the foot. An incision is made in the pretragal area and extended superiorly in a gently curving fashion (Fig. 50–2). An inferiorly based U-shaped flap is fashioned of the temporalis muscle and fascia and is reflected inferiorly.

By use of a cutting burr, a craniotomy opening is made in the squamous portion of the temporal bone (Fig. 50–3). It is located approximately two thirds anterior and one third posterior to the external auditory canal and is approximately 2.5cm². This bone flap is based on the root of the zygoma as close to the floor of the middle fossa as possible. During creation of this flap, care is taken to avoid laceration of the underlying dura. The bone flap is set aside for later replacement.

The dura is elevated from the floor of the middle fossa. The initial landmark is the middle meningeal artery, which marks the anterior extent of the dissection. Frequently, venous bleeding will be encountered from this area and can be controlled with oxidized cellulose (Surgicel). Dissection of the dura proceeds in a posterior to anterior fashion. In approximately 5 per cent of cases, the geniculate ganglion of the facial nerve will be dehiscent, but injury can be avoided with dural elevation. The petrous ridge is identified, and care is taken not to injure the superior petrosal sinus. The arcuate eminence and greater superficial petrosal nerve are identified. These are the major landmarks to the subsequent intratemporal dissection. Once the dura has been elevated, typically with a suction irrigator and a blunt dural elevator, the House-Urban retractor is placed to support the temporal lobe. To maintain a secure position, the teeth of the retaining retractor should be locked against the bony margins of the craniotomy window (Fig. 50–4). By use of a large diamond burr and continuous suction irrigation, the blue line of the semicircular canal is identified at the arcuate eminence. This structure makes an approximately 45° to 60° angle with the internal auditory canal.

The greater superficial petrosal nerve is located medial to the middle meningeal artery (Fig. 50–5) then followed posteriorly to the geniculate ganglion (Fig. 50–6). The labyrinthine portion of the facial nerve is identified medial to the ganglion. Care must be taken to avoid the cochlea, which lies only a few millimeters anterior to the labyrinthine portion of the facial nerve.

Bone is removed from the superior surface of the internal auditory canal down to the porus acusticus. The lateral end of the internal auditory canal is dissected, Bill's bar and the superior vestibular nerve are identified (Fig. 50–7). Medially, 180° of bone can be removed from its circumference (Fig. 50–8). This exposure must narrow laterally because of the location of the inner ear.

FIGURE 50-1. Surgical anatomy of the temporal bone as viewed from the middle fossa approach.

FIGURE 50-2. Incision begins in the pretragal area and extends 7cm to 8cm superiorly in a gently curving fashion.

FIGURE 50-3. Two thirds of the craniotomy window is located anterior to the external auditory canal.

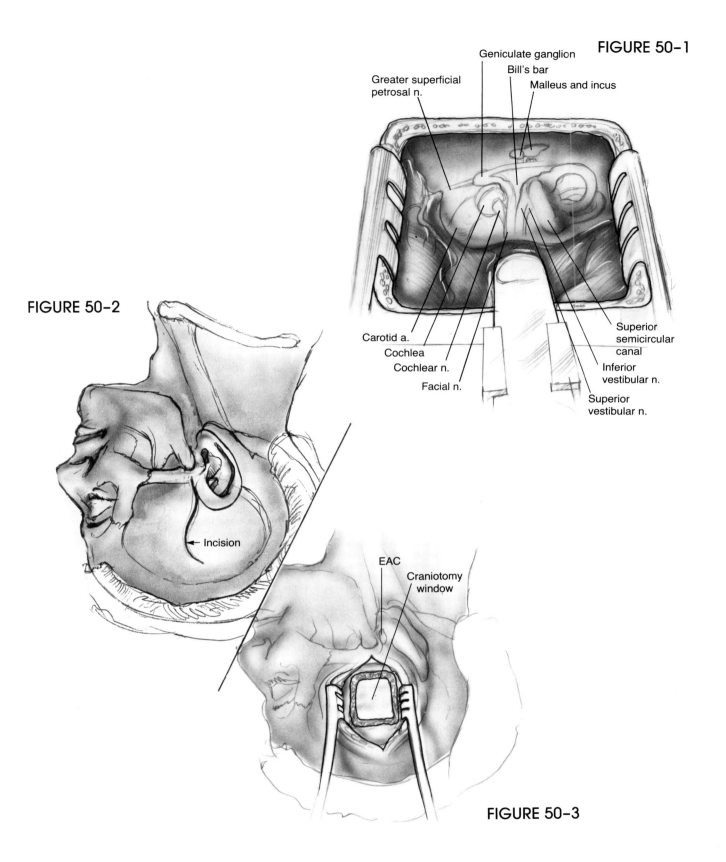

FIGURE 50-1

Greater superficial
petrosal n.

Geniculate ganglion

Bill's bar

Malleus and incus

Carotid a.

Cochlea

Cochlear n.

Facial n.

Superior
semicircular
canal

Inferior
vestibular n.

Superior
vestibular n.

FIGURE 50-2

Incision

EAC

Craniotomy
window

FIGURE 50-3

Since William F. House first began removing acoustic tumors through the translabyrinthine approach in 1960,[1, 2] we at the House Ear Clinic have been using this approach for most of our acoustic tumor removals. To date, we have removed about 2750 acoustic neuromas with this approach. The translabyrinthine procedure allows excellent access to the cerebellopontine angle (CPA) and exposure of the entire facial nerve from the brainstem to the stylomastoid foramen. The approach is extradural through most of the surgery. The primary disadvantage is sacrifice of hearing.

In patients with poor or no hearing, the translabyrinthine approach is ideal for acoustic neuromas; facial nerve lesions, such as neuromas; trauma due to operative injury; or head trauma. The approach has many advantages. It is the most direct route to the structures of the CPA (Figs. 51–1 and 51–2).[3] The lateral end of the internal auditory canal (IAC) can be dissected to ensure complete tumor removal from this area and allow consistent anatomic identification of the facial nerve.[4] The approach also offers exposure of the mastoid, tympanic, and labyrinthine portions of the facial nerve. Identification of the facial nerve in the mastoid is possible after removal of the semicircular canals (Fig. 51–3). Because the labyrinth has been removed, the labyrinthine segment of the nerve is readily followed into the IAC. The IAC and CPA can be exposed widely if the lesion involves the facial nerve in the posterior fossa. The facial nerve is readily accessible from the brainstem to the stylomastoid foramen and beyond into the parotid gland. Many procedures other than acoustic tumor removal can be performed through this approach, including excision of other tumors (e.g., meningiomas, cholesteatomas involving the petrous bone and posterior fossa, cholesterol granulomas, glomus tumors, and adenomas), decompression of the facial nerve, and repair of the nerve either by direct end-to-end anastomoses or by nerve grafting (Fig. 51–4). For tumors involving the area anterior to the internal auditory nerve at the clivus, the standard translabyrinthine approach is modified to allow anterior exposure (Fig. 51–5). The facial nerve is removed from the fallopian canal in the tympanic and mastoid segments and is reflected anteriorly. The cochlea is then removed to provide excellent exposure anterior to the IAC (see Chapter 54 on the transcochlear approach).

A major advantage of the translabyrinthine approach is that the patient is in the supine position with the head turned away from the surgeon (Figs. 51–6 and 51–7). This position eliminates some of the possible complications of the classic suboccipital approach to the CPA in which the sitting position is used, including risks of air embolism and injury to the cerebellum from retraction. In addition, quadraplegia has been reported in association with the sitting position.[5] The translabyrinthine approach poses no danger of air embolism and does not require retraction of the cerebellum. The brain and surrounding structures are less likely to be injured because much of the surgery is extradural.

PATIENT SELECTION

Tumor size and residual hearing are the principal factors influencing the choice of the translabyrinthine approach. We use the translabyrinthine approach in most cases if the tumor extends into the CPA more than 1cm and in all cases of nonserviceable hearing in the tumor ear. When tumors are confined to the IAC in an ear with serviceable hearing, we use the middle cranial fossa approach in an attempt to save hearing. In some patients with good hearing, the retrosigmoid approach is chosen, primarily for tumors in the CPA with minimal extension into the IAC.

Our definition of serviceable hearing is a pure-tone average threshold better than 50dB, a speech discrimination score of greater than 50 per cent, or both. This definition is referred to as the 50/50 rule. Of course, exceptions exist if the hearing in the contralateral ear is poor, or if bilateral tumors are present. In such cases, we may attempt tumor removal through the

---

FIGURE 51–1. Magnetic resonance image of large acoustic neuroma, illustrating the direct route to the cerebellopontine angle through the mastoid and labyrinth.

FIGURE 51–2. Postoperative computed tomographic scan of patient shown in Figure 51–1. Note the extent of removal of bone from the mastoid and labyrinth.

FIGURE 51–3. Facial nerve identified in mastoid portion after removal of semicircular canals. Note the island of bone over the sigmoid sinus.

FIGURE 51–4. Facial nerve graft through the translabyrinthine approach. A greater auricular nerve graft has been placed from the internal auditory canal to the proximal mastoid facial nerve.

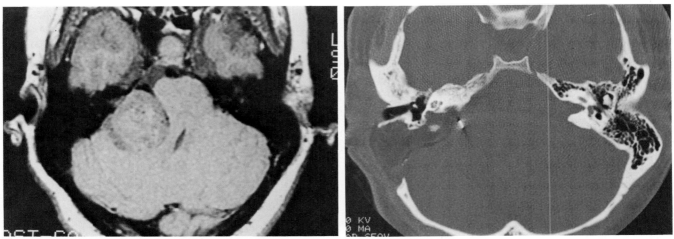

FIGURE 51-1

FIGURE 51-2

FIGURE 51-3

FIGURE 51-4

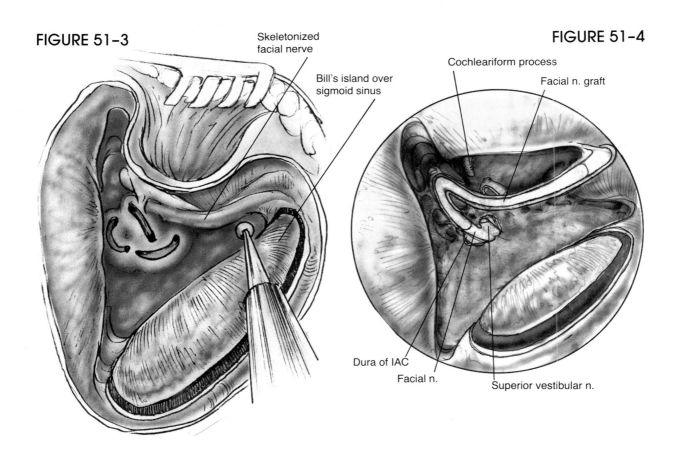

Skeletonized facial nerve

Bill's island over sigmoid sinus

Cochleariform process

Facial n. graft

Dura of IAC

Facial n.

Superior vestibular n.

middle fossa approach, even if the tumor extends up to 1cm into the CPA. We may use the retrosigmoid approach in an attempt to save hearing if the tumor is smaller than 1.5 or 2cm and does not extend into the lateral half of the IAC.

SURGICAL PROCEDURE

The procedure is performed with the patient under general endotracheal anesthesia with inhalation agents. Muscle relaxants are used only for the induction because they may interfere with facial nerve monitoring, which is used in all cases. A nasogastric tube and Foley catheter are placed. A generous amount of hair is shaved from the postauricular and temporal areas. The skin is cleaned with povidone-iodine (Betadine), and a plastic Vi-Drape is placed to cover the entire area. Because facial nerve monitoring is routine during all of our translabyrinthine procedures, needle electrodes are inserted into the orbicularis oris muscles before the drape is applied. The lower abdomen is also prepared and draped to allow for the harvesting of fat.

One per cent lidocaine (Xylocaine) with epinephrine 1:100,000 is injected into the postauricular region. The epinephrine assists with homeostasis. The incision is performed about 2 to 4cm posterior to the auricular sulcus and is curved anteriorly to allow anterior retraction of the pinna. The posterior curve of the incision allows exposure of the area posterior to the sigmoid sinus. This exposure is important to allow access to the CPA. The Lempert elevator is used to elevate the periosteum off the bone of the mastoid. Soft tissue must be removed from the posterior edge of the external auditory canal to an area far posterior to the sigmoid sinus, and care must be taken not to tear the skin off the external auditory canal. We use a self-retaining retractor with rings to hold a small suction catheter, which helps to remove blood and irrigation fluid from the wound.

A complete mastoidectomy is performed with a high-speed drill, using various sizes of cutting and diamond burrs. Removing bone posterior to the sigmoid sinus is crucial to expose the dura over the posterior cranial fossa. A small island of bone ("Bill's island," named for William F. House, MD, who first suggested it) is left over the otherwise exposed sigmoid sinus (Fig. 51–8). This bony cover protects the sigmoid sinus from the shaft of the burr as the drilling proceeds medially to remove the labyrinth. The dissection continues with the removal of all bone covering the posterior fossa dura medial to the sigmoid sinus and down to the labyrinth. All bone over the sinal dural angle and a small amount of bone over the middle fossa dura adjacent to the angle must be removed. I prefer to perform all of the lateral bone work before beginning the labyrinthectomy to obtain better exposure of the deep structures.

After the complete mastoidectomy is performed and the bone is removed from posterior fossa dura, sigmoid sinus, and some of the middle fossa dura, the deepest point of dissection shifts to the sinal dural angle. The labyrinthectomy begins with the removal of the lateral semicircular canal and extends posterior to the posterior canal. The bone removal is continued inferior and anterior toward the ampullated end of this canal (Fig. 51–9). The posterior semicircular canal is opened inferiorly to the vestibule and superiorly to the common crus and the vestibule. The facial nerve is identified in its descending portion in the mastoid and skeletonized to just proximal to the stylomastoid foramen. We prefer to identify the facial nerve after the posterior semicircular canal has been removed so that the side of the diamond burr, rather than the end of the burr, can be used. This method helps reduce the possibility of injury to the nerve. With this portion of the facial nerve identified, the remainder of the bone of the inferior IAC is removed to the vestibule. After opening the vestibule widely, the removal of the superior portion (nonampullated end) of the posterior canal is carried to the common crus, which is composed of the nonampullated ends of the posterior and superior semicircular canal.

The common crus is opened to the vestibule. The superior canal is now opened and removed to its ampullated end in the vestibule. This portion of the su-

FIGURE 51–5. Meningioma involving the internal auditory canal and extending anterior to the clivus can be removed through the translabyrinthine-transcochlear approach.

FIGURE 51–6. Patient placed in the supine position with head turned away from surgeon. Anesthesiologist is at foot of table.

FIGURE 51–7. The surgeon is seated with the operating microscope. The nurse is across the table. Note the facial nerve monitor at lower left.

FIGURE 51–5

Meningioma

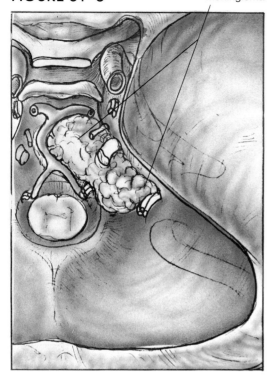

FIGURE 51–6

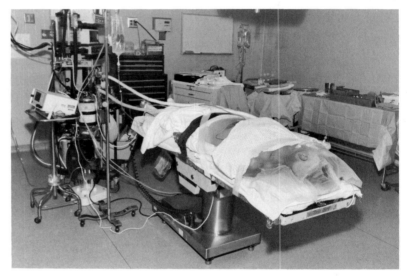

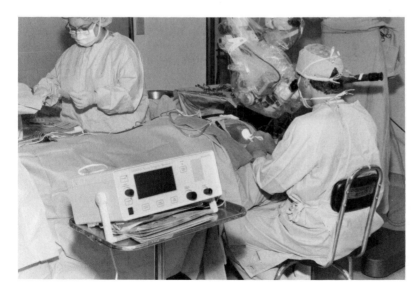

FIGURE 51–7

perior canal identifies the area where the superior vestibular nerve exits the lateral end of the IAC. Similarly, the singular nerve exits the IAC at the posterior semicircular canal ampulla, and the inferior vestibular nerve exits the canal at the saccule and the spherical recess. Identification of these structures delineates the superior and inferior extents of the IAC. As the bone posterior to the IAC is removed, the vestibular aqueduct and the beginning of the endolymphatic sac are removed. An eggshell thickness of bone is left over the dura of the IAC and posterior fossa to avoid injury to the underlying structures until all of the bony dissection is completed (Fig. 51–10).

The IAC is not entered at this time because bone must be removed medially to the porus acusticus. The canal runs deep from the vestibule and away from the surgeon. A great deal of bone must be removed to properly expose the contents of the canal and the CPA. Bone is removed around the canal superiorly and inferiorly to expose at least 210 degrees of the circumference of the canal. The dura of the canal and the posterior fossa is not opened until all bone removal has been accomplished. The inferior limit of bone removal is the cochlear aqueduct and the jugular bulb. The cochlear aqueduct enters the posterior fossa directly inferior to the midportion of the IAC, superior to the jugular bulb (Fig. 51–11).[6] The cochlear aqueduct is an important landmark to identify because it is one of the limits of dissection in the area inferior to the IAC. It identifies the location of the neural compartment of the jugular foramen anterior to the jugular bulb. By not removing bone from anterior and deep to the cochlear aqueduct, injury to cranial nerves IX, X, and XI is avoided. Bone is removed from the inferior portion of the IAC and particularly the inferior lip, thereby affording access to the inferior poll of the tumor in the CPA.

The bone is removed from the superior, lateral IAC last because of its close proximity to the facial nerve. Bone should be removed from the superior lip of the IAC. This dissection is tedious because the facial nerve often underlies the dura along the anterosupe-

rior aspect of the IAC. The surgeon must be very careful not to allow the burr to drop into the canal and possibly injure the nerve. As with the inferior lip, all of the bone must be removed from the superior lip to allow access to the superior poll of the tumor. With the superior lip, the facial nerve may be close to the surface, making this part of the removal laborious.

The facial nerve is identified as it exits the lateral end of the IAC at the vertical crest of bone ("Bill's bar," named after William F. House, M.D.) by use of a sharp 3mm hook. The hook is passed carefully along the inside of the superior distal IAC until Bill's bar is palpated (Fig. 51–12). The facial nerve monitor frequently sounds a warning as the hook passes along the nerve at the proximal portion of the fallopian canal.

All of the dissection thus far has been extradural, and morbidity should be minimal. Once the facial nerve canal has been identified, the dura of the posterior fossa over the midportion of the IAC is opened with sharp scissors. The length of the incision depends on the size of the tumor. For smaller tumors and nerve sections, the incision is made close to the IAC. For larger tumors, it is started closer to the sigmoid sinus. The incision extends to the IAC, then curves superiorly and inferiorly around the porus acusticus. The surgeon must take care to avoid vessels on the surface of the tumor and adjacent to the dura. Posteriorly, the petrosal vein lies close to the dura. The IAC is opened over the inferior vestibular nerve and reflected superiorly to avoid injury to the facial nerve. Cottonoids are placed posteriorly between the tumor and the cerebellum. This plane must be developed accurately to separate the major vessels of the CPA from the tumor.

With larger tumors, the size of the tumor is reduced by the use of the House-Urban dissector (Fig. 51–13). The surface of the tumor is carefully inspected first to identify nerves. Occasionally, the facial nerve is deflected posteriorly. The tumor capsule is incised, and the dissector is inserted to begin the intracapsular removal of the bulk of the tumor. Excessive manipula-

FIGURE 51–8. Mastoidectomy with exposure of the sigmoid sinus. Note that a small bony island is left over the sinus to protect it from the shaft of the burr.

FIGURE 51–9. Completed labyrinthectomy with ampullated ends of posterior and superior semicircular canals.

FIGURE 51–10. All bone has been removed, exposing the dura of the posterior fossa and the internal auditory canal.

FIGURE 51–11. Bone has been removed from the internal auditory canal (IAC) and the posterior fossa. The cochlear aqueduct can be seen inferior to the IAC and superior to the jugular bulb.

FIGURE 51-8

MASTOIDECTOMY

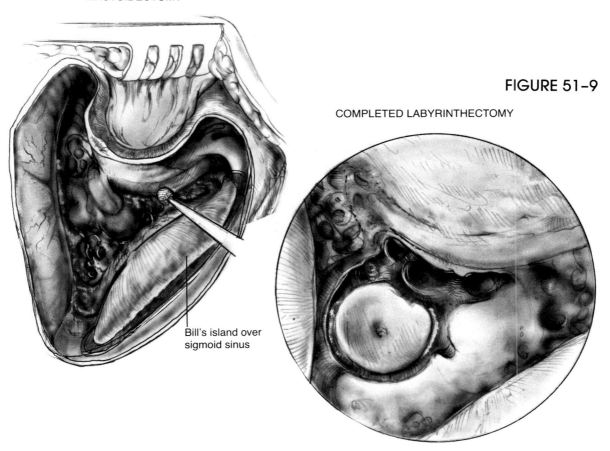

Bill's island over
sigmoid sinus

FIGURE 51-9

COMPLETED LABYRINTHECTOMY

FIGURE 51-10

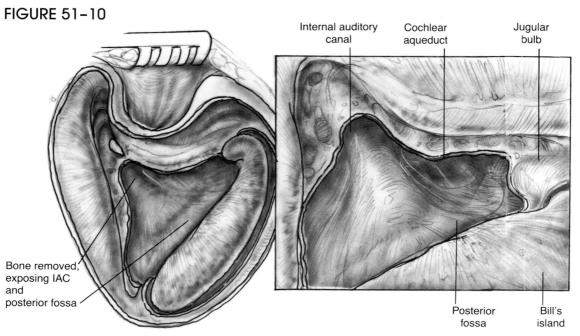

Bone removed,
exposing IAC
and
posterior fossa

Internal auditory
canal

Cochlear
aqueduct

Jugular
bulb

Posterior
fossa

Bill's
island

FIGURE 51-11

tion of the tumor must be avoided because it can cause traction on the facial nerve. The capsule of the tumor is then collapsed into the interior of the tumor, greatly facilitating the dissection of the tumor from the CPA. The tumor is then followed to the brainstem. The plane between the tumor and the brainstem is developed with sharp and blunt dissection. Cottonoids are placed between the brainstem and the tumor. At this point, attempts are made to identify the facial nerve superiorly. It is usually anterior to the tumor but may be draped over the top of the tumor. The ninth cranial nerve is identified inferiorly. In cases of large tumors, the ninth nerve may be stretched over the surface of the tumor. The physician should take care in this stage because excessive manipulation may cause a change in the pulse rate. During this phase of the tumor removal, avoidance of injury to surrounding structures is greatly facilitated by the use of the fenestrated neurotologic suction tip.[7]

Bill's bar is again palpated with a long hook. The hook is passed slightly anteriorly and medially until it falls over Bill's bar into the facial canal, thereby positively identifying the facial nerve. The hook is then withdrawn from the facial canal and placed under the superior vestibular nerve, which is avulsed and separated from the facial nerve. The vestibular nerve and tumor are separated from the facial nerve in the IAC and carefully dissected medially to the porus acusticus and into the CPA (Fig. 51–14). Some tumors involve the lateral end of the IAC, complicating identification of the facial nerve in the canal. In these cases, bone is removed from the proximal fallopian canal to allow positive identification of the facial nerve where it is not involved with tumor. This maneuver greatly reduces injury to the facial nerve.

It may be necessary to identify the facial nerve at the brainstem, and to begin to separate the tumor from the facial nerve, medially to laterally. Careful and patient dissection is usually successful in separating the facial nerve from the tumor as the tumor is dissected out of the posterior fossa. Continuous intraoperative facial nerve monitoring has greatly facilitated this process. The use of scissors to carefully free

the nerve from the tumor causes less trauma than the use of blunt dissection to establish this plane.

As the tumor is dissected free, bleeding is controlled with bipolar cautery and, in rare instances, clips. Only the vessels that enter the tumor capsule are coagulated. The other vessels are freed from the tumor capsule. A small blood vessel may accompany the eighth nerve. As the nerve is cut, control of bleeding with bipolar cautery or a clip may be necessary. Careful control of bleeding produces minimal blood loss. With an average blood loss of about 250cm^2, our patients rarely need transfusions. As a precaution, we offer patients the opportunity to withdraw one or two units of their own blood up to 1 month before the scheduled surgery.

During the drilling, the wound is periodically irrigated with a solution containing bacitracin to reduce the chance of infection. After the drilling has been completed, the bacitracin irrigant is attached to the suction irrigator used during the dissection of the tumor. This solution cannot be used during drilling because it tends to produce foam. Using this technique, we have reduced the rate of meningitis in our patients.

Closure involves the use of abdominal fat, and if the opening is large, a partial closure of the dura. Fat is obtained from the lower abdomen through a small transverse incision. The wound is closed with subcuticular sutures, and a Penrose drain is inserted. The fat is cut into strips and soaked in the bacitracin irrigant. The dura is closed with 4-0 silk along the posterior fossa incision. The strips of fat are inserted through the opening into the dura and IAC openings, extending about 2cm into the angle. These strips are tightly packed into the defect and expand on both sides of the dura to prevent leakage. Additional fat is packed into the attic. The incus may be removed so that the eustachian tube and the middle ear can be packed with muscle. The mastoid is also filled with fat. The wound is closed in layers with 0-chromic and 3-0 Vicryl sutures. Steri-Strips are applied to both wounds, and a head dressing and abdominal pressure dressings are applied.

surgicel → ET
temporalis m → ME. attic

FIGURE 51-12. The internal auditory canal (IAC) is skeletonized, and bone is removed to expose 180 to 240 degrees of the canal. The facial nerve is identified as it exits the IAC at Bill's bar.

FIGURE 51-13. The House-Urban dissector is used for intracapsular removal of tumor bulk.

FIGURE 51-14. The vestibular nerve and tumor are separated from the facial nerve in the internal auditory canal and dissected to the porus acusticus and the cerebellopontine angle.

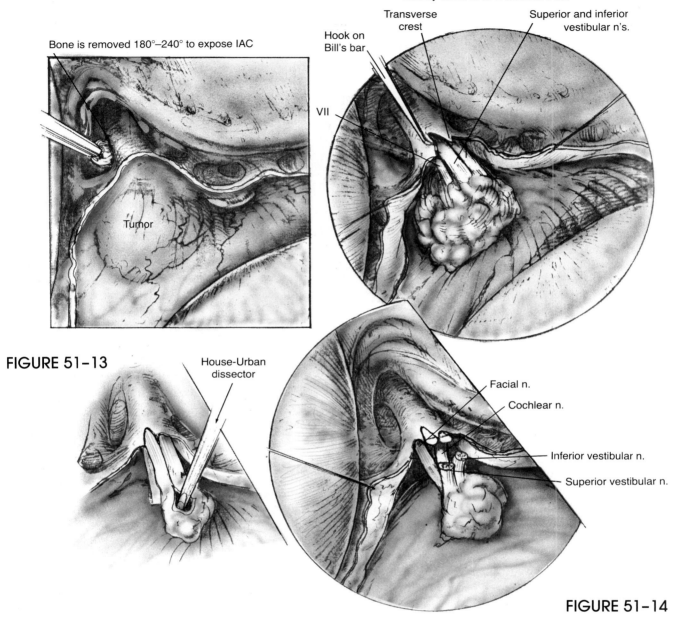

FIGURE 51-12

Identify facial n. as it exits Bill's bar

Transverse crest

Superior and inferior vestibular n's.

Hook on Bill's bar

VII

Bone is removed 180°–240° to expose IAC

Tumor

FIGURE 51-13

House-Urban dissector

Facial n.

Cochlear n.

Inferior vestibular n.

Superior vestibular n.

FIGURE 51-14

POSTOPERATIVE CARE

The abdominal drain is removed the following day. To prevent vomiting and aspiration, a nasogastric tube is inserted at anesthesia induction in the operating room and is attached to suction. This tube is also removed the following day. In addition, the urinary catheter inserted at the beginning of the procedure is removed on postoperative day one or two. The head dressing remains for 3 days, and the Steri-Strips remain for 1 week.

The patient stays in the intensive care unit for 1 or 2 days after surgery and then is transferred to a standard room. Progressive ambulation starts the day after surgery. The patient sits on the side of the bed, stands by the bed, and is encouraged to sit in a chair. We believe that early ambulation helps reduce complications and speed recovery.

Vital signs and temperature are monitored frequently during the first 2 or 3 days after surgery. In addition, the nurses are instructed to observe the patient for possible cerebrospinal fluid leak and neurologic changes. If the patient has drainage from the nose, the nurses test it for glucose and alert the physician.

COMPLICATIONS

Facial Nerve

Facial nerve weakness or paralysis is not a complication but a risk that cannot be entirely eliminated. The primary concern of most patients undergoing tumor removal is the ultimate facial nerve result. Continuous intraoperative facial nerve monitoring and meticulous dissection of the tumor from the facial nerve usually yield good facial nerve results. Eighty per cent of the results of surgery on all tumor patients are House-Brackmann grade I or II. Only about 5 per cent of patients have a grade VI outcome. If the facial nerve is intimately involved with the tumor or if the tumor is a facial neuroma, preservation of the anatomic continuity of the facial nerve may not be possible. We feel that repairing the nerve during the initial surgery is important. With the translabyrinthine approach, the nerve can be identified in the labyrinthine segment, exposed in the tympanic and mastoid portions, and either rerouted or an interposed graft sutured to the proximal and distal portions of the nerve. Suturing the nerve in the CPA is difficult; if this is possible, usually only one suture can be placed. The result allows for normal facial tone and good emotional and voluntary motion. Mass action or synkinesis is always present. Grade III is the best result that can be expected.

When a primary anastomosis or nerve graft is not possible, or if facial nerve function does not return after 1 year, we perform a facial-hypoglossal (VII-XII) anastomosis. It gives good resting tone, fair voluntary motion with synkinesis, and usually a grade IV recovery. If the nerve has been paralyzed for several years and the patient has poor tone, we combine the VII-XII anastomosis with a temporalis muscle transposition to the orbicularis oris. This procedure gives an immediate cosmetic improvement to the face at rest and gradual return of voluntary motion over 6 to 12 months.

Bleeding

The most dramatic and potentially fatal complication is an early postoperative hematoma in the CPA. This complication is manifested by signs of increased central nervous system pressure, such as loss of consciousness and nonreactive pupils. If is managed by immediate opening of the wound and removal of the fat while the patient is in the intensive care unit. This is an advantage of the translabyrinthine approach, in that the angle may be rapidly decompressed for this uncommon complication. The patient is taken back to surgery, and the bleeder is identified and controlled. Bleeding is part of the procedure. The most dramatic bleeding occurs if the sigmoid sinus is entered. Opening of the sinus produces profuse bleeding, and because the bleeding is venous, it is easy to stop with light pressure over the sinus. Bleeding is controlled with extraluminal packing with Surgicel, and great care is taken to prevent the packing from entering the lumen of the sinus. If this occurs, the packing will enter the pulmonary circulation, resulting in a pulmonary embolism. If the lumen of the jugular bulb is opened, the jugular vein is ligated in the neck, and the bulb is packed to control bleeding. This complication is very rare. Arterial bleeding is seldom a problem. Great care is taken to identify and avoid the anterior cerebellar artery because thrombosis or injury to this artery can be fatal. Fortunately, this is extremely rare with modern microsurgical techniques.

Cerebrospinal Fluid Leak

Before 1974, we used temporalis muscle to close the dura, and our incidence of cerebrospinal fluid leak was as high as 20 per cent.[2] Since we began using abdominal fat instead, this incidence has been reduced to less than 7 per cent in translabyrinthine acoustic tumor removals.[8]

Most leaks can be stopped with a pressure head dressing and bed rest with the patient's head elevated. Typically, we leave the dressing in place for 3 or 4 days. If the leak continues with the dressing in place, or if it recurs when the dressing is removed, a lumbar spinal drain is inserted, and the patient is placed at bed rest for 3 to 4 days. If the leak still persists, the patient is taken back to surgery, the wound is reopened, the leak is located, and additional fat is placed. Usually, we harvest additional fat. If excess fat is harvested at the original surgery, it can be frozen and used in case of a later leak. Spinal fluid leaks usually occur in the first 5 days, if at all.

Meningitis *3%*

The incidence of meningitis has been falling with the use of bacitracin irrigation and reduced surgical time. In the past few years, only about 3 per cent of postoperative patients have had meningitis,[8] for which a causative agent is rarely identified. A spinal tap is performed when the patient has a fever, elevated white blood cell count, and a stiff neck. If the cerebrospinal fluid white blood cell count is greater than 100, we use high doses of intravenous antibiotics. In addition to the cell count, the spinal fluid is cultured for both anaerobic and aerobic bacteria, and total protein and glucose levels are measured. In typical meningitis patients, the cerebrospinal fluid protein level is elevated, and the glucose level is reduced. Antibiotics are altered if the cultures so indicate. The usual response to treatment is reduction in fever, drop in white blood cell count, and reduction in headache. The spinal tap is repeated on the fourth or fifth treatment day. Treatment is continued until the cerebrospinal fluid cell count is below 100 and the cerebrospinal fluid is composed mostly of monocytes.

RESULTS

The total number of acoustic neuromas removed· at the House Ear Clinic now approaches 3000. With experience and refinements of technique, the results have progressively improved.

A recent review from our database of acoustic tumor cases provides data from 1302 patients who underwent a translabyrinthine acoustic tumor removal between 1982 and 1993. Their mean age was 50.0 years, and 46 per cent were male and 54 per cent were female. Tumor size varied from 0.5 to 6.5cm,

with a mean size of 2.4cm. Operating time averaged 3.3 hours. Three (0.2 per cent) deaths occurred in this series.

Data on long-term (≥ 6 months) facial nerve function as determined by the House-Brackmann scale were available on 889 cases, with a mean follow-up time of 2.1 years. Of these, 58.2 per cent had a grade I function; 12.6 per cent, grade II; 13.2 per cent, grade III; 7.8 per cent, grade IV; 3.3 per cent, grade V; and 5.1 per cent, grade VI. For cases undergoing surgery since the advent of facial nerve monitoring in 1988 and with at least 1 year follow-up, 59 per cent of the 312 patients had grade I facial nerve function; 15.4 per cent had grade II; 9.3 per cent, grade III; 7.7 per cent, grade IV; 4.2 per cent, grade V; and 4.5 per cent, grade VI.

SUMMARY

The translabyrinthine approach to tumors involving the temporal bone and CPA offers excellent and safe exposure. We have used this approach for more than 30 years to remove more than 2700 tumors. Our experience has yielded many refinements of the original procedure, and we continue to seek improvements to lower the morbidity. Mortality now approaches zero. We continue to feel that the translabyrinthine approach is the approach of choice for most acoustic neuromas.

References

1. House WF: Acoustic neuroma (Monograph). Arch Otolaryngol Head Neck Surg 80: 598–757, 1964.
2. House WF: Translabryinthine approach. *In* House WF, Luetje CM (eds): Acoustic Tumors, Vol 2: Management. Baltimore, University Park Press, 1979, pp 43–87.
3. Brackmann DE: Translabyrinthine removal of acoustic neurinomas. *In* Brackmann DE (ed): Neurological Surgery of the Ear and Skull Base. New York, Raven Press, 1982, pp 235–241.
4. House WF, Leutje CM (eds): Acoustic Tumors, Vol 1. Baltimore, University Park Press, 1979.
5. Hitselberger WE, House WF: A warning regarding the sitting position for acoustic tumor surgery (Editorial). Arch Otolaryngol Head Neck Surg 106: 69, 1980.
6. Brackmann DE, Green D: Translabyrinthine approach for acoustic tumor removal. Otolaryngol Clin North Am 25: 311–329, 1992.
7. Brackmann DE: Fenestrated suction for neuro-otologic surgery. Trans Am Acad Ophthalmol Otolaryngol 84: 975, 1977.
8. Rodgers GK, Luxford WM: Factors affecting the development of cerebrospinal fluid leak and meningitis after translabyrinthine acoustic tumor surgery. Laryngoscope 103:959–962, 1993.

Editorial Comment

Neurotologic approaches to cranial base tumors are a team endeavor in which the neurotologist and the neurosurgeon must be fully familiar with the other members' techniques. A frequent comment by former clinical fellows after completing training at the House Ear Clinic is that differences exist in the removal of acoustic tumors, especially larger tumors, between neurosurgeons familiar with the translabyrinthine approach and those who are adjusting to this anterior exposure.

The editors have invited William E. Hitselberger, M.D. to provide the neurosurgical prospective on tumor removal through the translabyrinthine approach. With a personal experience of over 3000 acoustic tumors removed with this technique, Dr. Hitselberger's insights are particularly relevant for neurotologic teams in the early phases of collaboration.

Neurosurgical Techniques in Acoustic Tumor Surgery

WILLIAM E. HITSELBERGER, M.D.

The strategy for the removal of an acoustic neuroma depends on whether the tumor is large or small. The techniques used in each of these situations, although similar, vary enough in important details that differences are described and emphasized here. The slight variation in technique is necessary because of the variation in the difficulty in preserving neurologic structures in each of these situations. Although variations exist in the technique used, the size of an acoustic neuroma is not a limiting factor in the choice of the translabyrinthine approach. In 30 years and more than 3000 acoustic neuromas, I have never found a tumor that was too large to take out through this approach.

REMOVAL OF THE SMALL ACOUSTIC TUMOR

In the removal of both the small and the large acoustic neuroma through the translabyrinthine approach, the importance of exposure can not be overemphasized. Adequate exposure of the tumor is the sine qua non of the procedure. Bone removal should include the bone over the middle fossa dura, the sigmoid sinus should be skeletonized so that it can be easily compressed, and bone removal should extend down to the jugular bulb. The posterior fossa dura should be cleared and easily retractable. The internal auditory canal should be skeletonized for at least 180 degrees from the posterior presentation. The labyrinthine portion of the facial nerve should be identified and uncovered.

During the drill-out of the internal auditory canal, the rotation of the drill is very important because the facial nerve is near the surface of the canal and exposed to a greater degree when the tumor is small than when it is larger. In a larger tumor, the tumor usually acts as a buffer between the facial nerve and the drill. If the drill is rotating into the internal auditory canal, the bit can catch on the bony edge, and the fast-moving burr may injure the nerve.

The dura should be opened over the end of the internal auditory canal, and the facial nerve should be positively identified both visually and with the facial nerve stimulator. The nerve at the end of the canal is anterior and superior to the superior vestibular nerve. The plane between these nerves can be readily developed if the bony dissection of the internal auditory

canal has been completed at its lateral extent. After division of the facial-vestibular anastomosis, the plane between the superior vestibular nerve and the facial nerve leads the surgeon into the plane between the facial nerve and the tumor. This latter plane is then carried medially down to the porus acusticus.

At this point, the nerve may be bound down in adhesions and tumor. High magnification (40×) may be necessary to keep the facial nerve plane delineated from the adhesions and tumor. Facial nerve dissection may be facilitated if the nerve is identified at the brainstem. The facial nerve arises anterior and medial to the cochleovestibular nerve. The anteroinferior cerebellar artery usually crosses between the seventh and eighth nerves near the brainstem. The facial nerve is generally quite distinct and has a whiter color than the eighth nerve because of a heavier concentration of myelin.

Developing the facial nerve plane from medial to lateral leads to the medial extent of the tumor. Sometimes, the tumor will then "shell out" from the bed of the eighth nerve. More importantly, the continuing plane of the facial nerve can be developed back to the porus. Thus, the facial nerve plane is developed from both the medial brainstem side and the lateral internal auditory canal side. Usually, once the facial nerve has been cleared from the surface, the tumor can be easily delivered. Thus, the importance of facial nerve dissection lies both in the preservation of the facial nerve and in the delineation and ultimate removal of the tumor.

Blood vessels lying on the surface of the tumor should be dissected free without coagulation, if possible. This method preserves the blood supply to the adjacent brainstem as well as the facial nerve. A very fine bayonet forceps and scissors can be used to free the vessels from the surface of the tumor without coagulation.

After the tumor has been removed, the tumor bed is carefully evaluated for any small bleeders. Bipolar coagulation set at a low level and oxidized cellulose are generally sufficient to treat such bleeding.

REMOVAL OF THE LARGE ACOUSTIC NEUROMA

The bony removal for a large acoustic neuroma, although similar to that for a small neuroma, varies enough that important variations should be mentioned. Wide, adequate exposure is the key and is accomplished by thorough removal of bone over the middle fossa, posterior fossa, and internal auditory canal. Additionally, bone should be removed for at least 1cm posterior to the sigmoid sinus over the subocciput. Even with a contracted mastoid, adequate exposure can be obtained for removal of any-sized neuroma if the bone removal has been exploited to the maximum. Another key for removal of a large acoustic neuroma from the cerebellopontine angle is extradural retraction. If the bone removal is inadequate, this retraction against the residual bone is impossible. Bony overhangs at the external genu of the facial nerve and the overhang of the posterior external auditory canal should also be removed.

The facial nerve is identified at the end of the internal auditory canal as in a smaller tumor. This dissection can be more difficult if the end of the canal is distorted by an impacted tumor, which is occasionally invasive into the otic capsule. After identification of the facial nerve at the end of the internal auditory canal, the dura is opened over the posterior fossa anterior to the sigmoid sinus. The tumor may bulge into the dural opening. A rapid decompression of the interior of the tumor can be carried out with the House-Urban rotary dissector, starting from the posterosuperior compartment of the tumor adjacent to the tentorium. At this point, I am not concerned with moderate venous bleeding; rather, the goal is rapid debulking of the tumor. Coagulating small bleeding vessels is unnecessary—these stop bleeding when the tumor is removed.

Once the tumor has been decompressed, the cisterna lateralis is emptied of spinal fluid. This step further adds to the available space and allows even greater room for retraction. The position of the facial nerve should be ascertained with the facial nerve monitor before radical resection of the tumor is undertaken. Usually, the facial nerve is anterior to the tumor, but it may be superiorly placed. Rarely, it can even be in a posterior position, which is an especially dangerous position for the facial nerve because the surgeon must operate past the facial nerve to remove the tumor, subjecting it to increased risk.

After decompression of the tumor, the facial nerve dissection can be started. High magnification (40×) and sharp dissection are best suited for this process. The nerve is usually stretched and attenuated by the tumor. The facial nerve monitor is invaluable in delineating the nerve when it has been thinned out over the surface of the tumor. The facial nerve dissection proceeds from both the medial and lateral ends of the tumor.

Vascular radicles are removed from the surface of the tumor, avoiding coagulation whenever possible. A large branch of the petrosal vein is usually positioned on the posterior medial surface of the tumor and should be sought after, identified, and dealt with, either with preservation, if easily accomplished, or with bipolar coagulation.

After tumor removal, all bleeding points in the tumor bed should be controlled with bipolar coagulation. The smallest bipolar coagulating tips possible should be used to avoid excessive heat and facial nerve injury.

52

Retrosigmoid Approach to Tumors of the Cerebellopontine Angle

ROBERT K. JACKLER, M.D.
DAVID W. SIM, F.R.C.S.Ed.(ORL)

exposure may be further compromised by a low transverse sinus course, particularly if the patient also has a short neck and a prominent shoulder. This problem of restricted exposure may be overcome by combining the retrosigmoid approach with an anterosigmoid, retrolabyrinthine decompression to allow anterior retraction of the sigmoid sinus.[6] A highly placed jugular bulb restricts access to the internal auditory canal (IAC) and can make the dissection of the inferior bony trough between the canal and the bulb difficult. Occasionally, the bulb may even extend superiorly to overlap the IAC, partially obscuring access to the medial aspect of the canal.[7]

PREOPERATIVE EVALUATION AND PATIENT COUNSELING

Clinical history, physical examination, pure-tone and speech audiometry, and an imaging study (preferably, gadolinium-enhanced magnetic resonance imaging [MRI]) constitute the minimal preoperative evaluation for a patient with a CPA tumor. In nonacoustic tumors, computed tomographic scanning for evaluation of the osseous characteristics of the cranial base and angiography to address vascular anatomy and possibly to perform embolization are occasionally indicated. Neither vestibular diagnostic testing nor auditory evoked responses are routinely obtained in patients already diagnosed with an acoustic neuroma.[8]

Numerous factors affect the selection of posterior fossa craniotomy for tumors of the CPA.[7, 9, 10] As advocates of selective management of these lesions according to the unique attributes of each tumor and the potential surgical options, we involve the patient in the discussion of the relative advantages and disadvantages of each technique. In most cases, an obvious choice can be made, whereas in others, patient preference is important. Our customary preoperative counseling includes the anticipated and potential risks to hearing, balance, and facial motor function. Less common complications discussed include CSF leak, meningitis, cerebrovascular accident, and death.[11] Although blood transfusion is seldom required, we encourage the patient to donate a unit of autologous blood.

PATIENT SELECTION

Common Indications in Neurotology

Hearing Preservation

The primary aim of acoustic neuroma management is removing the threat of progressive tumor growth while avoiding injury to the central nervous system. Preservation of cranial nerve function (facial movement, facial sensation, and hearing), which has become the primary focus of acoustic neuroma surgery in recent years, is a secondary goal. Acoustic tumors lie in three groups in terms of potential for hearing preservation. Those for whom hearing preservation is highly improbable generally undergo translabyrinthine removal. Criteria that place an individual into this group include poor hearing (< 30 per cent speech discrimination, > 70dB speech reception threshold); large CPA component (> 3cm), and deep penetration of the IAC. Conversely, individuals with good hearing (> 70 per cent speech discrimination, < 30dB speech reception threshold), small CPA component (< 1cm), and shallow IAC involvement are considered excellent candidates for a hearing conservation approach.[7] It is difficult to codify a set of rules concerning selection of a hearing conservation approach for the substantial group of patients who lie between these parameters. Each surgical team must rely on their own criteria, based on experience, together with the patient's wishes in coming to a selection of surgical approach. Undoubtedly, neurotologists would always favor undertaking a hearing conservation approach, even when the chances of success were remote, were there not potential adverse consequences from the endeavor. The lower morbidity of the translabyrinthine approach, especially in terms of persistent headache and CSF leak, leads the clinician away from the retrosigmoid hearing conservation approach when the chances of success are limited.

The concept of useful hearing is context dependent. In a patient with a normal contralateral ear, imperfect residual hearing in the tumor ear is often of little practical benefit. When hearing in the contralateral ear is impaired or threatened, such as in cases of bilateral acoustic neuromas associated with neurofibromatosis type 2, a conservative approach to hearing conservation is prudent, occasionally even at the expense of complete tumor excision.[12]

Hearing preservation is seldom achieved when tumors with a CPA component exceeding 2 cm in diameter are removed.[13] However, this rule should not be applied in nonacoustic CPA tumors (e.g., meningiomas), because hearing preservation is frequently achieved even with large tumors.[14]

The retrosigmoid approach is able to expose a variable amount of the IAC without violating the inner ear while the canal is being drilled open. Two factors should be considered in the decision of whether hearing conservation via the retrosigmoid approach is feasible: the depth to which the tumor penetrates the IAC and the degree of IAC exposable in that patient. The relationship between the inner ear and the lateral-most extension of the tumor into the IAC may be predicated by preoperative gadolinium-enhanced MRI.[15]

Acoustic Neuroma in a Patient With Chronic Otitis Media

Although patients with acoustic neuromas rarely have concomitant chronic middle ear infection, in those who do the translabyrinthine approach for acoustic neuroma resection is contraindicated. However, the retrosigmoid approach may also open into potentially contaminated mastoid air cells lying behind the sigmoid sinus as well as into air cells that may surround the IAC. To avoid potential intracranial infection, chronic middle ear infection should be controlled with tympanoplasty, antibiotics, or both, before tumor surgery whenever possible.[7]

Tumors Extending Into Inferior Portion of the Cerebellopontine Angle

The retrosigmoid approach provides the best access to the lower portion of the CPA and is readily extendible to expose the foramen magnum when required. Transtemporal approaches to the CPA are limited in their inferior exposure by the sigmoid sinus and the jugular bulb. Acoustic neuromas seldom extend into the inferior reaches of the CPA. Even when they do, the capsular peel is readily mobilized superiorly after tumor debulking. However, meningiomas and other extra-axial tumors usually do not mobilize easily and are often entwined with the lower cranial nerves (IX through XII) and vital vascular structures (e.g., posteroinferior cerebellar and vertebral arteries). In such cases, the retrosigmoid approach is chosen for its superior ability to expose this region. In neurofibromatosis type 2 patients, concurrent schwannomas on the lower cranial nerves are a common finding at the time of acoustic neuroma surgery. The retrosigmoid approach permits a thorough inspection of the jugular foramen contents as well as the dural lining of the posterior cranial base for possible early meningioma formation. Small, asymptomatic schwannomas on the lower cranial nerves are typically left alone, whereas early meningiomas are excised.

Revision Surgery

The retrosigmoid approach is favored in cases of recurrence following a previous translabyrinthine removal of an acoustic neuroma to avoid the dural scar from the prior procedure and to allow identification of the facial nerve as it emerges for the fat graft located in the surgical defect.

Relative Contraindications

Deep Extension Into the Internal Auditory Canal

Generally, tumors extending into the lateral one third of the IAC are not resectable by the retrosigmoid approach without destroying hearing. In such cases, the translabyrinthine approach ensures complete resection and reduces operative morbidity.[7]

Extension Into the Cranial Base

Tumor penetration into the posterolateral cranial base is a relative contraindication to the retrosigmoid approach. CPA tumors that invade the temporal bone (other than the medial two thirds of the IAC), the jugular foramen, or the hypoglossal canal are generally best addressed via a lateral, transbasal craniotomy.

Large Tumors

Although large CPA tumors (> 3cm) may be approached through either the retrosigmoid or translabyrinthine technique, we prefer to use the latter because it provides ample exposure and minimizes the need for cerebellar retraction. In addition, when the pons and the cerebellar peduncle are substantially displaced medially and posteriorly, the translabyrinthine approach, by virtue of its more anterior placement, provides a more favorable angle of view posteriorly toward the brainstem interface. In cases of facial nerve disruption, which is commoner in large tumors, the translabyrinthine approach affords more reconstructive options through mastoid meatal rerouting.[7]

PATIENT PREPARATION AND POSITIONING

At University of California, San Francisco (UCSF), the operation is carried out by a multidisciplinary team consisting of a neurotologist, neurosurgeon, neuro-anesthesiologist, neurophysiologist, and specialized operating room nurses. The operation is carried out with the patient under general anesthesia. A short-duration muscle relaxant is used to facilitate endotracheal intubation. Thereafter, anesthesia is maintained with inhalational agents alone, avoiding the use of muscle relaxants, which would prevent effective intraoperative cranial nerve electrophysiologic monitoring. In addition to the routine neuroanesthesia monitoring equipment, antithrombotic stockings and a urinary catheter are used. The retrosigmoid approach may be carried out in one of three surgical positions: supine, lateral supine ("park bench position"), and sitting.[10] Supine is the favored position because it affords excellent exposure and carries the lowest risk of complication, as is discussed later.

The patient is secured in the optimal operating position by means of a headholder attached to the bed frame (e.g., Mayfield). This apparatus facilitates exposure of the suboccipital region while the patient is in the supine position. Optimal surgical field exposure is obtained by a combination of head rotation, neck flexion, and ipsilateral shoulder elevation. Excessive neck torsion should be avoided to prevent cervical injury as well as to reduce the risk of cerebellar swelling secondary to compromised flow through the vertebral venous system. The cranial nerve–monitoring electromyographic electrodes are placed into the muscles supplied by cranial nerves V, VII, and XI. When intraoperative auditory brainstem monitoring is indicated, scalp electrodes are placed, and an earphone is inserted into the ipsilateral external auditory canal.[16]

We favor using an operating room table with enhanced lateral rotation capability (up to 30 degrees), which permits optimal visualization of the lateral end of the IAC at a comfortable working angle. When the surgeon works at relatively extreme rotations, the patient must be securely supported on the operating table by a lumbar support and placed on the contralateral side to the operative exposure, with both chest and thigh safety straps. The bed is reversed, with the patient's head on the foot section to allow the surgeon to sit during the microsurgical portion of the procedure.

A perioperative prophylactic antibiotic with good CSF penetration (e.g., ceftizoxime, 2g administered intravenously) is administered. Mannitol (1gm/kg) is administered intravenously when the scalp incision is made so that its effectiveness in reducing brain swelling coincides with dural entry. We do not routinely give corticosteroids, except in patients with larger tumors (> 3cm) or in those with peritumoral brain edema, when dexamethasone (10mg) is administered intravenously. To reduce the risk of CSF fistulization, an indwelling lumbar CSF drain is used when extensive peri-IAC pneumatization is encountered.

SURGICAL SITE PREPARATION

We ask the patient to wash his or her hair thoroughly either the morning of surgery or on the evening before with an antiseptic shampoo. In the operating room, after induction of anesthesia, the hair over the suboccipital area is removed with electric clippers. The upper neck is included in the operative site, thereby allowing potential access to the great auricular nerve

in case a graft is required for facial nerve reconstruction. The scalp is washed with povidone-iodine soap, and the clipped area is shaved. To improve attachment of adhesive drapes, the surgical site is defatted with alcohol and dried. Sterile drapes are placed 1cm from the hair edge around the prepared scalp and held in place with surgical adhesive (e.g., Mastisol). The field is then prepared with povidone-iodine solution and dried. Sterile towels are placed around the operative field and held into position by an adhesive plastic sheet.

SPECIAL INSTRUMENTS

Various instruments are used for the retrosigmoid approach to the CPA, including craniectomy instruments, retractors, a high-speed surgical drill with a selection of cutting and diamond burrs, suction and suction-irrigation tips of both the fenestrated and nonfenestrated types, bipolar cautery, microdissection instruments, and a binocular operating microscope.

We perform the craniectomy with an Acra-Cut disposable cranial perforator burr-hole maker in a Hudson brace, a system that allows rapid bone removal while minimizing the chance of dural or venous sinus injury. The craniectomy is completed with rongeurs. To retract the thick suboccipital musculature, a deep-bladed Weitlaner-type retractor is used. For brain retraction, several sizes of malleable blades are used that may be held in position in several ways. We prefer to use the Apfelbaum base, which combines a Weitlaner-type retractor with a moveable arm to affix the retractor. Other options for basing the brain retractors during retrosigmoid craniotomy include a C-clamp placed on the headholder frame or a table-based system (e.g., Greenberg).

Either an electric or air-powered drill is suitable to use for this approach. When the exposure is narrow, an angled handpiece is advantageous because it is less obstructing to the surgeon's point of view. An operating microscope with an inclinable optical pathway is desirable to accommodate the variety of exposure angles required during the procedure while maintaining a comfortable operating position. Insulated bipolar cautery forceps are essential for obtaining hemostasis during CPA tumor surgery. Both large tips for handling substantial vessels and slender, fine tips for use when the coagulation must be confined to a narrow region are needed. We have found that a self-irrigating system (e.g., Malis bipolar irrigating system) is valuable because it discourages tissue adhesion to the forcep tips.

We use a microsurgical instrument set that includes sharp and blunt dissectors in various shapes and sizes, needles, and small bone curettes (e.g., Rhoton microneurosurgical instruments). A set of sharp scissors of different sizes and angles is also important. Many special tools are available to facilitate rapid intracapsular debulking of the tumor. We prefer to use an ultrasonic surgical aspirator (Cavitron, CUSA), which allows debulking without traction or torsion, minimizes hemorrhage, and respects tumor capsular planes, thereby avoiding inadvertent neural or vascular injury. Other options include the surgical laser and a rotatory surgical aspirator (House-Urban).

Operating room electrical circuitry and neuroanesthesia electrical monitoring equipment should be grounded and electronically quiet, to minimize 60 Hz noise production, which interferes with the cranial nerve electrophysiologic monitoring setup. The specialized equipment for intraoperative cranial nerve monitoring used in our institution has been described elsewhere in detail.[16]

SURGICAL TECHNIQUE

Acoustic neuroma excision by the retrosigmoid approach to the CPA can be subdivided into seven stages: (1) craniectomy, (2) exposure of the CPA, (3) exposure of the IAC, (4) tumor resection, (5) hemostasis, (6) IAC closure, and (7) craniotomy closure.

Craniectomy

A curvilinear paramedian incision 3cm behind the postauricular sulcus is made down to bone. The cervical muscles are detached anteriorly and posteriorly, exposing the mastoid and suboccipital areas. Emissary venous bleeding is controlled with bone wax. The mastoid tip is exposed, and the posterior belly of digastric muscle is elevated from its groove. Dissection directly on the bone preserves the occipital nerves and vessels. A posterior fossa craniotomy window of approximately 3 × 3cm is made in the retrosigmoid approach. Anteriorly, it is bounded by the sigmoid sinus, superiorly, by the transverse sinus. The craniectomy begins with two to three closely approximated burr holes. The burr holes are joined up with ronguers, thus creating a craniotomy window. The bone fragments are collected and stored in sterile antibiotic-saline solution for replacement in the cranial defect at the end of the procedure. Development of the craniectomy anteriorly usually opens the mastoid air cell system to a variable degree. Once the bony craniectomy is complete, the opened mastoid air cells are sealed with bone wax. Wax is also used to control bleeding from diploic bone at the craniotomy margins. Many styles of dural opening are described in the literature. We use a posteriorly based dural flap to enter the posterior fossa. The posterior fossa dura is opened 2 to 3mm from its junction with the sigmoid and transverse sinus dura and at a similar distance from the inferior bony margin. The dural flap is then reflected posteriorly. Small, relaxing incisions are made superiorly and inferiorly in the marginal dura to create small anterior and superior dural flaps, which are then retracted with stay sutures, thereby completing the dural opening.

Exposure of the Cerebellopontine Angle

Once the dural flap has been reflected posteriorly, it and the craniotomy margins are covered with moist Telfa strips. To drain CSF from the cisterna magna, the cerebellum is gently retracted superiorly with a polytetrafluoroethylene (Teflon)–coated malleable retractor. The arachnoid of the cistern is then lanced with a bayoneted suction tip, which decompresses the posterior fossa, relaxes the cerebellum, and allows it to fall away medially. Premature medially directed cerebellar retraction, before draining the cisterna magna, risks inducing massive cerebellar swelling. After this maneuver, the retractor is withdrawn and repositioned anteriorly to develop posteromedial cerebellar retraction. Retraction in this manner, accompanied by division of arachnoid bands and bridging veins, opens the CPA. The degree of CPA exposure required varies with the size and location of the tumor being addressed. Superiorly, the petrosal veins (or Dandy's veins), which lie just below the tentorium cerebelli and run parallel to the course of the trigeminal nerve, may hinder exposure or appear to be in jeopardy of tearing with retraction. When necessary, these may be coagulated and divided. After their division, the superior pole of the cerebellar hemisphere falls posteromedially away from the tentorium, thereby providing access to the superior aspect of the CPA.

The cerebellar flocculus often overlies the brainstem root entry zones of cranial nerves VII and VIII and must be gently mobilized from the cerebellar peduncle and lateral pontine surfaces. A tuft of choroid plexus, emanating from the lateral recess of the fourth ventricle, is also frequently encountered in this area. Mobilizing these structures from the root entry zone need not necessarily be performed during hearing conservation procedures when the proximal portion of the nerves are not involved with tumor, because this maneuver places the internal auditory artery at risk. The cranial nerve electrophysiologic monitoring circuitry is then tested by stimulating cranial nerve XI, which is usually readily accessible at the inferior pole of the exposure. Particular attention is paid to the location of the anteroinferior cerebellar artery (AICA) and its branches. Inferiorly, the posteroinferior cerebellar artery may be seen in relation to the lower cranial nerves, and superiorly the superior cerebellar artery may be identified coursing through the region of the tentorial notch. In acoustic neuroma surgery, we prefer to begin the drill excavation of the internal auditory canal at a relatively early stage, before extensive opening of the arachnoid planes above and below the CPA component. This method helps reduce bone debris contamination of the subarachnoid space.

Exposure of the Internal Auditory Canal (Figs. 52–3 through 52–6)

Exposure of the IAC and its contents involves removal of the bone surrounding the posterior, superior, and inferior aspects. Optimal canal visualization may be obtained through a combination of rotation of the operating table away from the side of the surgeon and microscope positioning. These maneuvers bring the posterior petrous face into view centered over the region of the IAC. To locate the canal, the opening of the meatus is gently probed with a blunt, right-angled hook. Before IAC opening begins, the operative field is set up to contain as much bone debris as possible and to prevent its dissemination into the subarachnoid space. Absorbable gelatin sponge (Gelfoam) pledgets are placed into the superior and inferior portions of the CPA. A rectangular-shaped rubber dam is fashioned from a surgical glove, placed over the occluding pledgets, and held in place with the cerebellar retractor. An H-shaped dural incision, centered on the long axis of the IAC, is outlined on the posterior petrous face by use of a bipolar cautery. Once the dura has been incised with the tip of a No. 11 blade, superior and inferior dural flaps are elevated with a small Lempert's mastoid elevator. The surgeon should exercise caution when incising inferiorly because the jugular bulb is occasionally dehiscent on the posterior petrous face. Similarly, the incision should not be carried too far laterally because laceration of the sigmoid sinus can occur. Care is taken to identify and preserve the endolymphatic sac and duct, which are located posterolaterally. The dura can usually be elevated off the endolymphatic sac. The entry point of the vestibular aqueduct into bone is a useful anatomic landmark. When the bony dissection of the IAC does not extend lateral to the operculum of the aqueduct, the labyrinth is unlikely to be breached.

The posterior IAC wall is then rapidly removed by the drilling of a trough over the posterior petrous face. Drilling from medial to lateral in the line of the IAC reduces the risk of the burr slipping into the CPA. The canal should be opened only as much as required to expose the lateral-most aspect of the tumor. Excessive bony opening does not further enhance exposure but may increase the risk of CSF leak through the opening of additional petrous air cells. Initially, the bone is removed with a cutting burr until the IAC dura is identified through a thin bony plate. To expose the dura of the posterior aspect of the IAC, the dural cuff of the meatus is first elevated from the thin resid-

FIGURE 52–3. Step 1 of exposure of the internal auditory canal during the retrosigmoid approach. After localization of the porus acusticus through palpation with a ball hook, an H-shaped dural incision is created over the long axis of the internal auditory canal. Dural flaps are then reflected anteriorly and posteriorly to expose the posterior aspect of the petrous pyramid. The dura can usually be dissected from the posterior surface of the endolymphatic sac. To maximize the possibility of hearing preservation, care must be exercised to avoid avulsion of the sac from its aqueduct. Prior to the commencement of drilling, Gelfoam pledgets are positioned above and below the 7 to 8 neurovascular bundle in the posterior fossa in an effort to minimize the spread of bone dust onto arachnoidal surfaces.

FIGURE 52–4. Step 2 of exposure of the internal auditory canal during the retrosigmoid approach. A cutting burr is used to rapidly excavate the bone overlying the internal auditory canal. Once the canal dura is encountered, a diamond burr is used. Drilling is carried out from medial to lateral (from porus to fundus), in part to minimize the possibility that the drill could accidentally run into the posterior fossa.

FIGURE 52–5. Step 3 of exposure of the internal auditory canal during the retrosigmoid approach. A diamond burr is used to create deep troughs around the internal auditory canal that should extend well deep to the canal plane to provide adequate room for microdissection with the angled instruments needed to safely remove the facial nerve from the tumor. Particular care should be exercised while the superior trough is developed because the facial nerve may lie immediately beneath the dura in this location.

FIGURE 52–6. Step 4 of exposure of the internal auditory canal during the retrosigmoid approach. In preparation for tumor removal, the dura of the internal auditory canal is incised. After an incision along the length of the canal is created with upbiting scissors, two small relaxing incisions are created at both the porus and the fundus to develop dural flaps. These are then reflected anteriorly and posteriorly to expose the canal contents.

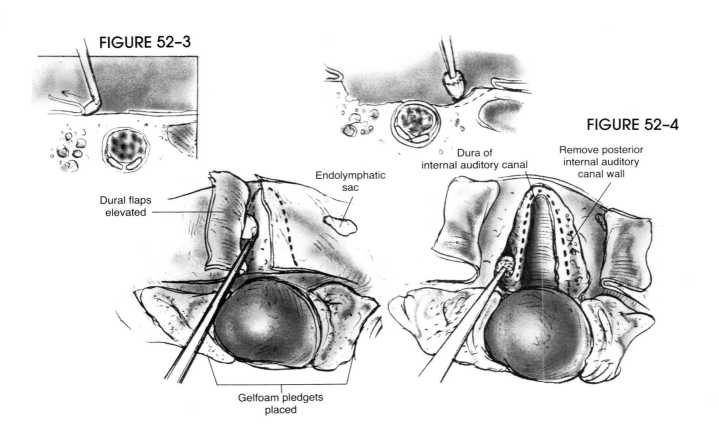

FIGURE 52-3

FIGURE 52-4

Dural flaps elevated

Endolymphatic sac

Dura of internal auditory canal

Remove posterior internal auditory canal wall

Gelfoam pledgets placed

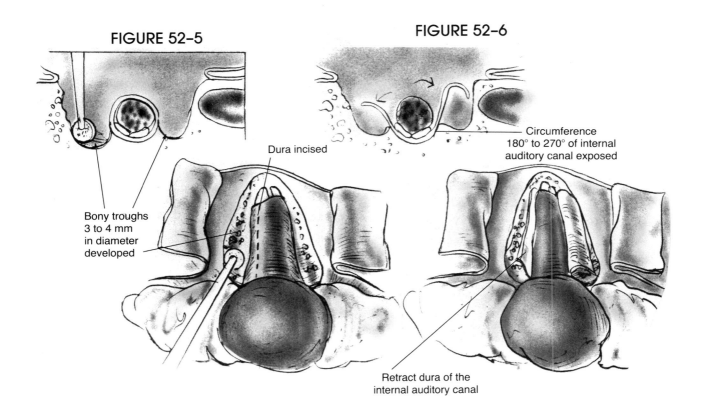

FIGURE 52-5

FIGURE 52-6

Dura incised

Circumference 180° to 270° of internal auditory canal exposed

Bony troughs 3 to 4 mm in diameter developed

Retract dura of the internal auditory canal

ual plate. Then, the remaining bony shell over the posterior aspect of the IAC is drilled away. To reduce the risk of traumatizing the IAC dural lining or its neural structures, removal of the last eggshell of bone is accomplished with diamond burrs. Diamond burrs are more controllable by virtue of their reduced tendency to run and are less likely to cause injury if they come into contact with soft tissue structures.

Bony troughs, 3 to 4mm in diameter, are then developed above and below the canal. These troughs are important for three reasons: (1) to provide working space for the insertion of angled instruments needed to establish a plane of dissection between the tumor and the facial and cochlear nerves, (2) to permit visualization of the facial nerve when it is acutely angled superiorly or inferiorly as a result of tumor displacement, and (3) to enhance exposure of the anterior aspect of the CPA. In preparation for the drilling of bony troughs around the canal, the IAC dura is elevated from the upper and lower canal walls with a blunt dissector. The troughs, which should be widest at the level of the porus, are then excavated with a cutting burr. As the troughs are developed, a thin shell of bone is left over the dura of the superior and inferior walls of the IAC. Once the troughs are fully developed, the remaining bony shells are progressively thinned with the side of the diamond burr until the dura is exposed. Copious irrigation is used to prevent thermal injury to neural structures. Often, the IAC dura can be gently retracted with a fenestrated suction, permitting completely atraumatic removal of the remaining bony eggshell fragments, which can then be elevated from the exposed IAC dura. This technique exposes between 180 to 270 degrees of the IAC circumference. Caution must be exercised in development of the superior and inferior troughs because of the proximity of the facial nerve and the jugular bulb, respectively. The width of the inferior trough varies with the location of the jugular bulb. When the jugular bulb is unusually high, creating an inferior bony trough at the level of the meatus may be impossible, although exposure of the fundus is typically unhindered. Compensating for the limited inferior access associated with a high jugular bulb is usually possible through creation of an unusually wide and deep superior trough. Additional exposure of the IAC from above may also be gained through retraction of the tentorium.

In hearing conservation attempts, the lateral extent of the IAC opening should be restricted to approximately the medial two thirds of the IAC because opening of the lateral one third to expose the fundus may result in a breach of the vestibule or crus commune, militating against hearing conservation. The decision as to how far laterally the IAC is opened depends on the lateral intracanalicular extent of the

tumor, which may be predicted with considerable accuracy from the preoperative gadolinium-enhanced MRI.[15, 17] Alternatively, the lateral opening can be limited on the premise that an indirect inspection and clearance of the tumor from the lateral IAC can be satisfactorily achieved. However, this method has the attendant risk of leaving residual tumor in the lateral IAC. To avoid this problem, some have advocated blind curettage using special right-angled curettes followed by inspection of the fundus with a small mirror or endoscope to validate the extent of tumor resection. We have found that with these methods, distinguishing residual tumor from the transected vestibular nerves and traumatized dura is sometimes difficult. Dissection of tumor from the fundus without direct visualization risks leaving well-vascularized residual tumor with the potential for clinically significant recurrence.[18, 19] We advocate exposure of the IAC laterally to a point beyond the tumor interface, where the naked seventh and residual eighth nerves may be visualized. At times, this process may require opening the canal to the fundus, with resultant entry into labyrinthine structures and sacrifice of residual hearing.

After completion of the IAC exposure, the rubber dam and gelatin sponge pledgets are removed. The dura of the IAC is opened along the long axis of the canal with sharp, upturned, right-angled microscissors working from a medial to lateral direction. This incision is placed slightly eccentrically and is biased to the superior side to avoid the creation of a long flap over the facial nerve course. The dural flaps are then reflected superiorly and inferiorly, exposing the IAC contents.

Acoustic Neuroma Resection
(Figs. 52–7 through 52–9)

Attention is now turned to planning the actual resection of the tumor, the size of the tumor largely dictating the actual sequence and pattern of removal. We prefer to initially dissect the IAC because this step helps to ascertain the probable course of the facial nerve outside of the porus into the CPA and allows early identification of the facial nerve. Then, a test run of the neural monitoring system can be performed in which positive identification of the nerve by its anatomic relationships is possible. In many cases, ascertaining whether the tumor has arisen from the superior or inferior vestibular nerve is possible. When only one of these nerves is visible on the posterior surface of the tumor, it may be assumed that the other was the nerve of origin. Dissection is commenced laterally by identification of the plane between the facial nerve and the tumor. A fine-tipped dissector is insinuated between the superior dural leaf of the canal and the tumor while gentle downward pressure and a rotating motion are applied. Gradually, this process brings into view the interface between the facial nerve and the lateral end of the tumor. Once this plane has become established, a sharp, right-angled instrument is used to dissect the tumor from the posterior surface of the facial and cochlear nerves. All tissue superficial to this plane, including the tumor and both vestibular nerves, is then transected either with curved microscissors or through an upward motion with the sharp edge of the dissector. When the intracanalicular tumor component is bulky, it may require debulking to a variable degree to permit microdissection of the capsular peel from the facial and cochlear nerves. This initial dissection of the intracanalicular portion should proceed only to the lip of the porus acusticus or just beyond it, to avoid dissection of the typically most adherent section at this stage. It is important to avoid inducing neuropraxic injury, which might impair later electrical identification of the facial nerve medially at its brainstem exit.

After removal of the intracanalicular portion of the tumor, the CPA component is addressed. The posterior capsule is swept with the neural monitoring probe to assure that the facial nerve is not on this surface (a rarity in acoustic neuroma). A rectangular incision is made in the posterior capsule with the point of a No. 11 blade, and the peel is then resected with scissors. Intracapsular debulking may be carried out with cupped forceps, sharp dissection with scissors, an ultrasonic aspirator (e.g., Cavitron), a rotatory aspiration device (e.g., House-Urban), or the surgical laser. We favor using the CUSA because it efficiently removes the tumor core while respecting its capsule, thus avoiding potential injury of adherent nerves and vessels. Tumor resection then proceeds with alternate intracapsular debulking, followed by microdissection of the thin capsule from the brain surface and cranial nerves, and ultimately, resection of the liberated capsular segment.

The most crucial aspect of CPA tumor removal is identification and preservation of the cranial nerves and blood vessels that lie draped on the capsular surface. In larger tumors, the medial tumor brain dissection plane commences posteriorly along the middle cerebellar peduncle. Once this arachnoid plane has become established, it is gradually developed onto the lateral surface of the pons. Attention is turned inferiorly to the probable root entry zone of the seventh and eighth nerve complexes. As an aid to facial nerve identification, electrical stimulation is periodically performed along the meniscus of dissection. The course and appearance of the nerve varies depending on its displacement by the tumor. It may be thinned and fanned to a variable degree, making it difficult to delineate from surrounding thickened arachnoid tissue without the use of the microneural stimulator.

The brainstem entry of the eighth nerve is usually encountered lateral to and immediately above the seventh nerve entry zone. A small branch of AICA typically passes between the two nerves and may be a useful guide in orienting the surgeon. In hearing conservation approaches, the vestibular fibers must be separated from the cochlear fibers and divided proximally to establish a tumor dissection plane. When no effort is being made at hearing preservation, the eighth nerve may simply be transected, a maneuver that simplifies identification of the proximal seventh nerve. Once the proximal plane over these two nerves is established, an arachnoid plane can be developed between them and the tumor capsule. While the tumor capsule is dissected, both large and small arteries, potential AICA branches, are meticulously preserved. Vessels directly entering the tumor capsule can generally be safely coagulated and divided at the capsular surface without adverse consequences.

While the tumor neural plane is dissected, use of the microneural stimulator (e.g., Xomed Treace-Yingling) with a curved, pliable wire allows blind stimulation of the yet undissected anterior capsule. By localizing the facial nerve course before dissecting the tumor nerve interface, the surgeon may rapidly resect uninvolved capsule and direct meticulous efforts along the actual course of the nerve. Although the course of the facial nerve varies, it characteristically lies anterior to the tumor, occasionally with a somewhat anterosuperior or anteroinferior bias. In small tumors, the entire dissection may be accomplished from a medial to lateral direction. In larger tumors, however, medial-to-lateral dissection becomes difficult when the nerve is anteriorly angulated toward the porus acusticus. When this occurs, we return to the lateral tumor nerve interface at the end of the IAC and work medially. Alternatively, the anterior tumor capsule with attached nerve may be lifted and rotated to bring the facial nerve course into the surgeon's view. However, this action is quite traumatic to the facial nerve and risks disruption of its attenuated fibers. We prefer to dissect the tumor from the facial nerve in situ without mobilizing it from its bed, where it lies supported by an arachnoidal mesh. When the facial nerve is both splayed and tightly adherent to the tumor capsule, removing the last remnant of capsule may not be possible without disruption of the nerve.[20] In such cases, we prefer to perform a near-total removal, leaving a thin velum of capsule, only 1 to 2mm thick, attached to the nerve. We believe that this minuscule residual capsule, hanging free in the CPA, is unlikely to generate a recurrent tumor.[18] By contrast, tumor left in the distal IAC or in contact with brainstem possesses a vascular supply and is at higher risk of regrowth.

Several modifications in the strategy of tumor removal are used during hearing conservation approaches. The direction of dissection should be from medial to lateral, whenever possible, to reduce the risk of traumatic avulsion of the delicate cochlear nerve fibers from their entry into modiolus. Throughout the cochlear nerve dissection, changes in auditory brainstem responses relative to the previously recorded baseline waveforms obtained at the start of the procedure are reported. Continuity of the cochlear nerve is maintained if possible; however, tumor adherence to it may necessitate its resection. Even when the cochlear nerve is well preserved during dissection, hearing is often lost because of interruption of the cochlear blood supply. This may occur either in the CPA, where the labyrinthine artery branches from a loop of AICA, or in the IAC, where it courses between the inferior vestibular and cochlear nerves.

After tumor resection, anatomic and electrical continuity of the cochlear and facial nerves is checked. The facial nerve stimulation threshold voltage at the root entry zone and the intraoperative auditory brainstem response waveform pattern and latencies are recorded. We believe that electrophysiologic monitoring of the auditory nerve is not clearly beneficial, other than in the prognostic sense, in the maintenance of hearing. However, monitoring of the facial nerve is indispensable if an optimal outcome is to be obtained.

Hemostasis

After the tumor resection is completed, the wound is irrigated with bacitracin-saline solution, the blood clot is removed, and all bleeding points are identified and controlled with bipolar cautery or by application of thrombin-soaked gelatin sponge. As a means of detecting subtle or intermittent bleeding, the anesthesiologist gives the patient a Valsalva maneuver for 20 seconds. Because postoperative hemorrhage into the CPA is a potentially devastating complication, hemostatic efforts should be diligent.

Internal Auditory Canal Closure
(Fig. 52–10)

The bony troughs developed for the IAC exposure are inspected for opened air cells by palpation with a ball hook. Inspection of the cut bony edge may also be carried out through use of a 90 degree angled rigid endoscope. Bone wax is applied to a small cottonoid and smeared over the exposed bony trough surfaces to seal overtly and covertly opened air cells to prevent CSF leakage. A small muscle graft is harvested from the exposed cervical muscles and is used to seal the IAC. A 7.0 monofilament nylon suture is placed through the dural flaps of the posterior petrous face. The muscle plug is then positioned in the IAC and the

FIGURE 52–7. Step 1 of removal of an acoustic neuroma via the retrosigmoid approach. After the intracanalicular portion of the tumor is debulked, the lateral-most extension of the tumor is reflected medially, and a plane between the tumor capsule and the facial nerve is developed. This maneuver ensures complete removal of the tumor from the fundus. It also affords an early opportunity to confirm the function of the cranial nerve monitoring system by stimulation of the distal facial nerve under direct vision in a region where it is characteristically not especially adherent to the tumor surface.

FIGURE 52–8. Step 2 of removal of an acoustic neuroma via the retrosigmoid approach. The main portion of the tumor in the cerebellopontine angle is rapidly debulked. To facilitate rapid and safe tumor removal, we use a Cavitron ultrasonic aspirator. The tumor capsule is first liberated from the cerebellum and middle cerebellar peduncle. The pontine surface, including the root entry zones of cranial nerve VII and VIII can then be exposed. In larger tumors, the lesion must also be microdissected from the trigeminal and lower cranial nerves (IX and X) as well.

FIGURE 52–9. Step 3 of removal of an acoustic neuroma via the retrosigmoid approach. Characteristically, the facial nerve is most adherent to the tumor capsule between the brainstem surface and the anterior lip of the porus acusticus. Liberation of the nerve from the tumor surface in this location often requires particularly delicate microdissection techniques.

FIGURE 52–10. Closure of the internal auditory canal defect at the completion of a retrosigmoid craniotomy. After waxing of the cut bony walls to seal any transected air cells, a muscle graft harvested from the nuchal area is mortised into the bony defect. The graft is retained in position by sutures, which are anchored in the dural flaps previously developed from the posterior petrous surface.

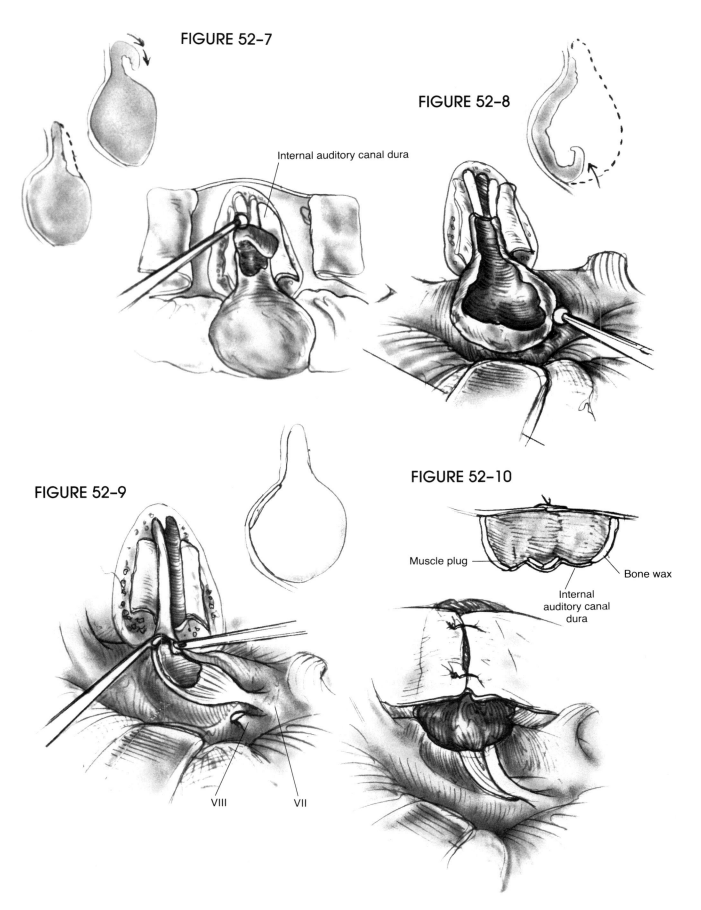

FIGURE 52-7

Internal auditory canal dura

FIGURE 52-8

FIGURE 52-9

FIGURE 52-10

Muscle plug

Bone wax

Internal
auditory canal
dura

VIII   VII

suture tied. Auditory and facial nerve monitoring is maintained until the muscle plug is secured in place so that any possible neural irritation induced by its placement can be identified.

Craniotomy Closure

After removal of all the cottonoids and Telfa strips, the dural flap is sutured back into place with multiple, closely positioned, interrupted 4.0 braided nylon (Surgilon) sutures. At closure of the dura, bacitracin-saline solution is instilled into the subarachnoid space. The margins of the craniectomy are then reinspected for opened air cells and smeared with bone wax as indicated. When the transected air cells are large, rather than merely impacting the wax into the exposed cavities, a thin sheet of wax is applied. A gelatin sponge pad cut in the shape of the craniectomy defect is placed over the dura, and the previously preserved bone chips are replaced. In our experience, the bone regenerates over several months into a strong, bony plate that restores the cranial contour. After removal of the remaining retractors, the soft tissues of the neck are closed in a series of layers with interrupted 2.0 braided nylon (Surgilon) sutures, closing any potential dead space, after the wound is irrigated with antibiotic solution. The skin is sutured with interrupted 4.0 nylon sutures. Electromyographic electrodes, ground pads, and the external auditory canal earphone are removed after completion of wound closure and dressing.

DRESSING

After closure of the wound, the wound is cleaned, dried, and covered with a Telfa strip over, which a sterile adhesive, Op-Site or similar dressing, is applied. To discourage subcutaneous accumulation of CSF, a mastoid-type padded pressure bandage is applied. The dressing is removed 48 hours after surgery, and the wound is inspected and left open to the air. The skin sutures are removed 7 to 10 days after surgery.

POSTOPERATIVE CARE

The anesthesiologist awakens the patient, ideally with a smooth extubation that avoids straining and coughing. Antiemetics are given prophylactically to prevent vomiting, which could cause aspiration and associated pneumonitis during recovery from anesthesia. Postoperative monitoring is carried out initially in the postanesthetic care unit and then in the neurosurgical intensive care unit for 24 hours after surgery. After the initial 24-hour period, patients spend an average of 5 to 6 days on a hospital ward staffed by nurses experienced in postcraniotomy care. In addition to the monitoring of temperature, cardiorespiratory status, consciousness level, and fluid balance, both the nursing staff and patients are instructed to identify and report any CSF wound leakage or rhinorrhea.

Should a postoperative facial palsy be present, its grade is recorded according to the House-Brackmann scale, and preventative eye care is instituted. When eye closure is incomplete, artificial tears are applied hourly, or more often as needed, while the patient is awake. During sleep, a plastic eye shield is placed to prevent drying and development of corneal abrasion. Special attention needs to be directed toward patients with dysfunction of both the facial and trigeminal nerves. When the cornea is dry, exposed, and insensitive, early gold weight placement is performed even when facial nerve recovery is expected.

Moderate-to-severe headache for several days is typical and may require narcotic analgesia for a variable period. Global headache that is delayed in onset by several days may signify the evolution of meningitis, either aseptic or bacterial, and is discussed later. We try to wean the patients from narcotics quickly and try to get their headaches under control with simple nonsteroidal anti-inflammatory preparations. In those relatively few cases in which corticosteroids have been used, they are tapered over a 7- to 10-day period. Vertigo can be controlled with parenterally administered antivertiginous agents if the condition is severe and with oral agents, if it is mild. In general, we prefer avoiding vestibular suppressants in the postoperative period because they may retard vestibular compensation.

Both diet and increasingly independent mobilization are encouraged under the guidance of a dietitian and physical therapist. We usually restrict the fluid intake for 3 days to a total of 1.5 L/24-hour period. Most patients are able to start a light diet 24 to 48 hours after surgery. Constipation and straining are avoided by the administration of stool softeners to prevent aggravation of headache and possible development of CSF leakage. Most patients begin to mobilize around 48 hours after surgery, although they have been encouraged to actively exercise their legs while they are recumbent in bed to reduce the risk of deep venous thrombosis. Antiembolism stockings are maintained until the patient is mobile. Mobilization usually takes the form of initially sitting at the bedside chair, followed by accompanied walks to the bathroom and then farther afield to the hospital corridors, and then onto a trial of practice on the stairs. Walking aids are provided by the physical therapist as required by the patient, depending on his or her progress. We usually discourage hair washing until 1 week after surgery to prevent the wound from getting wet and macerated. Patients may use a dry shampoo if desired.

Most patients are usually ready for discharge 5 to 7 days after surgery. Even when all other functions have recovered fully, easy fatigability often persists for 1 to 3 months postoperatively. The convalescent period required before returning to full-time employment and all the previous activities of daily living varies but is usually 2 to 3 months.

RESULTS

Historically, the primary issue in acoustic neuroma surgery was the survival of the patient. Fortunately, with the evolution of microsurgical techniques, mortality from acoustic neuroma surgery has become very low: less than 2 per cent in most recent series. Contemporary emphasis includes tumor control and, particularly, functional preservation. However, before the data from our own experience and the data published in the literature are addressed it is important to appreciate that limited international standardization exists in the criteria used for reporting results on degree of resection,[21] facial nerve function,[22] and hearing preservation.[23]

In our opinion, the goal of acoustic neuroma resection should be tumor control, and not necessarily complete resection in every case. Nevertheless, we perform a complete removal in most cases. Incomplete removal can be considered in two categories: subtotal and near-total excision. Subtotal removal, in which a substantial bulk of tumor remains, is seldom performed except in elderly or infirm individuals of short anticipated lifespan in whom shortening of the operative procedure is felt to be in the patient's interest. We have encountered several symptomatic recurrences in this group of patients, especially in individuals with cystic tumors. As previously discussed, near-total excision, in which a thin peel of capsule is left on the most adherent portion of the facial nerve, is occasionally used. Although few data are published on the recurrence risk for this group of patients, we have observed many individuals with serial gadolinium-enhanced MRI and have yet to encounter a recurrence. The decision to undertake a near-total resection depends on the patient's age (i.e., less desirable in a younger individual) and preference as to whether the slightly higher risk of recurrence is justified by the improved facial nerve outcome.

Numerous papers appear in the literature on the subject of facial nerve preservation in acoustic neuroma surgery citing varying degrees of success. Because these are difficult to compare and draw conclusions from, we confine our commentary to our own series at UCSF. In our experience, facial nerve outcome from the retrosigmoid approach is similar to that from the other methods of removing acoustic neuromas for tumors of similar size.[24] In UCSF acoustic neuroma, patients, anatomic continuity of the facial nerve was maintained in 99.2 per cent of cases. Of course, anatomic continuity does not necessarily imply functional integrity. The probability of a grade 1 or 2 facial function at 1 year after surgery in the context of tumor size was 100 per cent for tumors less than 1cm; 90 per cent for those 1 to 3cm; and 82 per cent for those greater than 3cm.

With regard to hearing preservation, most published series address residual "measurable" hearing in contrast to the much more relevant concept of "useful" hearing.[25] For a patient with a unilateral acoustic neuroma, it could be argued that unless the conserved hearing maintains an interaural difference of less than 30dB hearing loss with good speech discrimination (> 50 per cent), then it would be unlikely to be of benefit. Preservation of useful hearing has been reported to be achieved in 25 to 58 per cent of hearing conservation candidates.[13] Very little information is available on the long-term follow-up of patients with preserved hearing. In two published series, significant late decline occurred in 22 to 56 per cent of ears with successful hearing conservation.[26, 27] Factors relevant to success in hearing conservation approaches to acoustic neuroma include tumor size in the CPA, the depth to which the tumor penetrates the IAC, pure-tone hearing level, and auditory brainstem response results. A full discussion of these criteria is beyond the scope of this chapter. It is not yet well established whether intraoperative auditory monitoring materially improves hearing conservation results. In one study using auditory brainstem response monitoring, it was found to be of marginal benefit overall, with the possible exception of tumors less than 1 cm in diameter.[28] Results with either the middle fossa or the retrosigmoid approach are similar for intracanalicular tumors.[13, 23, 25, 29, 30] Incomplete resection also has a potential role in hearing preservation, particularly in patients with neurofibromatosis type 2 or in those with a tumor in an only-hearing ear.[12, 31]

COMPLICATIONS

The common complications of the retrosigmoid approach to the CPA are persistent headache and CSF leakage.[11, 32, 33] Less common complications include (aseptic or bacterial) meningitis, hydrocephalus, cerebellar dysfunction, vascular compromise (thrombosis and hemorrhage), and problems associated with patient malpositioning during surgery. Of course, medical complications, such as pulmonary thromboembolism and pneumonia, may also occur but are not specific to surgery of this region. Although the potential complications of acoustic neuroma surgery are similar among the various operative approaches, their relative incidence varies considerably. In the retrosigmoid approach, both persistent headache and CSF leakage occur more frequently than with the other techniques used in approaching CPA tumors.

Vascular Complications

Hemorrhage

Vascular complications may be extra-axial or intra-axial. The main extra-axial problem is bleeding into the CPA. CPA hematomas may cause brainstem compression and acute obstructive hydrocephalus. The incidence of acute CPA hematomas has been reported from 0.5 to 2 per cent; however, with modern hemostatic techniques, the incidence is probably considerably less frequent.[11] This diagnosis should be suspected when a patient does not promptly awake after surgery or has a delayed deterioration in the level of consciousness. The diagnosis may be made by non-contrast computed tomographic scan in which fresh blood appears as a hyperdense mass in the CPA and extrinsic pontine compression is noted. If serious neurologic sequelae or even death are to be avoided, prompt surgical evacuation of the hemorrhage is essential. Intra-axial pontine hemorrhage may occur, particularly after removal of very large tumors that have greatly deflected the brainstem. Although major parenchymal hemorrhage is rare, minor amounts of intrinsic pontine bleeding are quite often evident radiographically after extirpation of giant tumors. Presumably, these result form the sudden re-expansion of the deeply compressed parenchyma. Supratentorial intra-axial hemorrhages have been reported after retrosigmoid approaches performed with the patient in the sitting position. These hemorrhages were associated with hypertension and may have resulted from subcortical venous tearing resulting from mechanical stress induced by the sitting position.[34-36] Extradural hematoma formation, a concern in the middle fossa approach, is uncommon after the retrosigmoid approach.

Anteroinferior Cerebellar Artery Syndrome

Brainstem infarction may occur after damage to the AICA, the vascular supply to the pons and cerebellar peduncle. Mechanisms of injury include disruption, cauterization, and arteriospasm with thrombosis. A full-fledged AICA syndrome is very serious and is often fatal because it results in the loss of respiratory center control.[37] Partial interruption of flow in the AICA system, avulsion of one or more of its branches, or obstruction of a nondominant AICA may result in an incomplete AICA syndrome. We have recently recognized several patients operated on for acoustic neuromas greater than 3cm in diameter in whom gadolinium-enhanced MRI detected an infarction in the region of the middle cerebellar peduncle. These patients had unilaterally impaired cerebellar function and required prolonged physical therapy rehabilitation.[38]

Nonvascular Complications

Complications From Patient Positioning

As with any craniotomy, air embolism through breach of the major venous sinuses is a potential hazard. However, this risk is minimal when a supine or lateral patient position is used.[39] Air embolism is the main complication of the sitting position and has been reported in up to 30 per cent of cases. When the sitting position is used, intraoperative monitoring with precordial Doppler ultrasonography alerts the anesthesiologist to venous air entry. The initial maneuvers to perform when air embolism has been detected are to flood the field with fluid and lower the head of the bed.

Quadriplegia (in four cases) and paraplegia have also been reported after acoustic neuroma resection in the sitting position. The degree of cervical flexion in the absence of protective spinal reflexes during anesthesia was thought to have caused spinal cord compression and infarction.[40, 41] In both the supine and lateral supine positions, the unconscious patient must be handled carefully, especially when the headholder is positioned. Excessive head rotation risks cervical injury and may obstruct vertebral venous drainage and contribute to cerebellar swelling. Excessive downward displacement of the shoulder risks traction injury on the brachial plexus.

As with any prolonged surgical procedure, adequate padding under pressure points is important to avoid pressure ulceration. Despite the best of precautions, patients frequently complain of discomfort over the ischium or other bony prominences for a few weeks postoperatively.

Cerebrospinal Fluid Leakage

CSF leakage is the commonest postoperative complication, occurring in approximately 15 per cent of patients who undergo retrosigmoid approaches for acoustic neuroma. The patient must be counseled to recognize and report CSF leakage so that steps can be taken to rapidly control it to prevent infectious meningitis. CSF leak occurs either directly through the wound or indirectly through the ear and auditory tube to the nasopharynx, where it presents as a watery rhinorrhea or salty postnasal discharge. CSF escape into the ear may occur through opened and unsealed mastoid air cells in the region of the craniectomy or through air cells opened and unsealed in the bony IAC dissection.[42] CSF drainage often stops spontaneously with simple fluid restriction and avoidance of straining. The use of acetazolamide, a carbonic anhydrase–inhibiting diuretic, may also be of benefit. Alternatively, the early use of a lumbar CSF drain for 48 to 72 hours may halt the drainage. Some have advocated (1) wound re-exploration with rewaxing of the bone to close covert open air cells, (2) replacement of the muscle graft plug to close CSF leakage, and (3) continued lumbar drainage.[39] We prefer to address persistent, intractable CSF otorhinorrhea transtemporally. When useful residual hearing is present, a canal wall up mastoidectomy is performed, perilabyrinthine cells are copiously waxed, the fossa incudis is occluded with a fascia graft, and fat is used to obliterate the cavity. When the operated ear is deaf, a canal wall down mastoidectomy is performed. The external auditory canal is sutured closed, and the auditory tube is sealed under direct vision with bone wax and muscle. The mastoid air cells are also waxed, and the cavity is obliterated with fat. Lumbar CSF drainage is maintained for approximately 72 hours after surgery.

Aseptic and Bacterial Meningitis

Entry of blood and bone dust into the subarachnoid space can result in aseptic meningitis. Care is taken during the drilling of the posterior petrous face during the IAC exposure to prevent contamination of the subarachnoid space with bone dust. Gelatin sponge is placed in the CPA superior and inferior to the tumor and seventh-eighth nerve complex, and a rubber dam is placed over the cerebellum. After completion of the bone work, the wound is thoroughly irrigated and the bone debris removed. Similarly, throughout the tumor dissection and at its completion, a combination of suction and irrigation is used to prevent the buildup of blood and clots because both blood and bone debris produce an irritative or chemical, aseptic, meningitis.[11]

To reduce the risk of bacterial meningitis, intravenous prophylactic antibiotics are administered at the start of surgery and bacitracin is added to the irrigant solution used to flush the CPA at the end of the procedure. This complication should be suspected if the patient develops headache, fever, and malaise in the first postoperative week. Nuchal rigidity, usually considered a sign of meningeal irritation, is of limited information following RS craniotomy, as the neck muscles may be in spasm owing to direct surgical trauma. Bacterial meningitis may also occur in the late postoperative period, particularly when a CSF leak is present. The clinician is wise to maintain a high degree of suspicion about bacterial meningitis and, when in doubt, obtain a sample of CSF via lumbar puncture for analysis. In patients in whom the clinical picture is suggestive, intravenous antibiotics should be instituted pending results of culture and sensitivity testing.

Hydrocephalus

Hydrocephalus can occur as a result of blood and bone debris contamination of the posterior fossa subarachnoid space. Particulate and proteinaceous debris becomes ingested by arachnoid granulations, impairing their absorptive capabilities, which results in raised intracranial pressure. Cerebellar retraction with subsequent swelling at release may also result in the development of hydrocephalus.[11]

Cerebellar Dysfunction

Prolonged cerebellar retraction may result in edema and swelling and possibly contusion, with resultant dysmetria and impaired balance in the postoperative period.

Persistent Headache

Headache is encountered more frequently after the retrosigmoid approach than after other types of posterior fossa craniotomy.[43, 44] In our experience, nearly all retrosigmoid patients have substantial headache during the first postoperative month. By 3 months after surgery, approximately one third continue to complain of this symptom. By one year, around 15 per cent of patients continue to have chronic moderate-to-severe headaches, compared with very few headaches for those who underwent the translabyrinthine procedure. Some individuals are unable to return to work or resume other life activities because of this symptom. Of interest, the highest incidence of persistent headache in our series has been in patients with small tumors who underwent the retrosigmoid approach in an effort to preserve hearing. Although the headache may have myriad presentations, it is most commonly either frontal or referred to the area of surgery and is often triggered by cough. Numerous potential underlying causes exist for chronic headache after retrosigmoid craniotomy including aseptic meningitis, coupling of the suboccipital dura to the nuchal musculature, occipital neuralgia, and even exacerbation of an underlying headache tendency, such as migraine. Although numerous mechanisms are possible, we believe that most are a result of chronic arachnoiditis incited by contamination with bone dust and blood at the time of surgery.

Residual or Recurrent Tumor

We prefer to revise recurrent tumors after retrosigmoid craniotomy using a translabyrinthine approach. This method avoids the previously scarred dural areas and tends to present more favorable arachnoid dissection planes during the early portion of the procedure.[45]

Acknowledgment

Figures 52–1 to 52–10 were adapted from artwork produced by the authors for a work in preparation, *Atlas of Surgical Neurotology*, which is to be published by CV Mosby. The original drawings in this chapter were produced by Christine Gralapp, MA.

References

1. Krause F: Zur Freilegung der hinteren Felsenbeinflache und des Kleinhirns. Beitr Klin Chir 37: 728–764, 1903.
2. Rhoton AL Jr, Tedeschi H: Microsurgical anatomy of acoustic neuroma. Otolaryngol Clin North Am 25: 257–294, 1992.
3. Lang J: Clinical Anatomy of the Posterior Cranial Fossa and its Foramina. New York, Thieme, 1991.
4. Lang J Jr, Samii A: Retrosigmoidal approach to the posterior cranial fossa. An anatomical study. Acta Neurochir (Wien) 111: 147–153, 1991.
5. Camins MB, Oppenheim JS: Anatomy and surgical techniques in the suboccipital transmeatal approach to acoustic neuromas. Clin Neurosurg 38: 567–588, 1992.
6. Silverstein H, Morrell H, Smouha E, Jones R: Combined retrolab-retrosigmoid vestibular neurectomy. An evolution in approach. Am J Otol 10: 166–169, 1989.
7. Jackler RK, Pitts LH: Selection of surgical approach to acoustic neuroma. Otolaryngol Clin North Am 25: 361–387, 1992.
8. Selesnick SH, Jackler RK: Clinical manifestations and audiologic diagnosis of acoustic neuromas. Otolaryngol Clin North Am 25: 521–551, 1992.
9. Cohen NL, Hammerschlag P, Berg H, Ransohoff J: Acoustic neuroma surgery: An eclectic approach with an emphasis on hearing preservation. Ann Otol Rhinol Laryngol 95: 21–27, 1986.
10. Cohen NL: Retrosigmoid approach for acoustic tumor removal. Otolaryngol Clin North Am 25: 295–310, 1992.
11. Wiet RJ, Teixido M, Liang JG: Complications in acoustic neuroma surgery. Otolaryngol Clin North Am 25: 389–412, 1992.
12. Glasscock ME III, Hart MJ, Vrabec JT: Management of bilateral acoustic neuroma. Otolaryngol Clin North Am 5: 449–469, 1992.
13. Shelton C: Hearing preservation in acoustic tumor surgery. Otolaryngol Clin North Am 25:609–621, 1992.
14. Nassif PS, Shelton C, Arriaga MM: Hearing preservation following surgical removal of meningiomas affecting the temporal bone. Laryngoscope 102: 1357–1362, 1992.
15. Blevins N, Jackler RK, Pitts LH: The retrosigmoid approach to the IAC: A radioanatomic study. Otolaryngol Head Neck Surg 1994 [in press].
16. Yingling CD, Gardi JN: Intraoperative monitoring of facial and cochlear nerves during acoustic neuroma surgery. Otolaryngol Clin North Am 25: 413–448, 1992.
17. MacDonald CB, Hirsch BE, Kamerer DB, Sekhar L: Acoustic neuroma surgery: Predictive criteria for hearing preservation. Otolaryngol Head Neck Surg 104: 128, 1991.
18. Lye RH, Pace-Balzan A, Ramsden RT, et al: The fate of tumour rests following removal of acoustic neuromas: An MRI Gd-DTPA study. Br J Neurosurg 6: 195–201, 1992.
19. Thedinger BS, Whittaker CK, Luetje CM: Recurrent acoustic tumor after a suboccipital removal. Neurosurgery 29: 681–687, 1991.
20. Kemink JL, Langman AW, Niparko JK, Graham MD: Operative management of acoustic neuromas: The priority of neurologic function over complete resection. Otolaryngol Head Neck Surg 104: 96–99, 1991.
21. Moffat DA: Synopsis on near-total, subtotal or partial removal. Acoustic Neuroma. *In* Tos M, Thomsen J (eds): Proceedings of the First International Conference on Acoustic Neuroma. Copenhagen, August 25–29, 1991. New York, Kugler Publications, 1992, pp 983–984.
22. Baer S, Tos M, Thomsen J, Hughes G: Synopsis on: Grading of facial nerve function after acoustic neuroma treatment. Acoustic Neuroma. *In* Tos M, Thomsen J (eds): Proceedings of the First International Conference on Acoustic Neuroma. Copenhagen, August 25–29, 1991. New York, Kugler Publications, 1992, pp 993–995.
23. Sanna M, Gamoletti J, Tos M, Thomsen J: Synopsis on: Hearing preservation following acoustic neuroma surgery. Acoustic Neuroma. *In* Tos M, Thomsen J (eds): Proceedings of the First International Conference on Acoustic Neuroma. Copenhagen, August 25–29, 1991. New York, Kugler Publications, 1992, pp 985–987.
24. Lalwani A, Jackler RK, Pitts LP: Facial nerve function following acoustic tumor surgery. Otolaryngol Head Neck Surg 1994 [in press].
25. Hinton AE, Ramsden RT, Lye RH, Dutton JE: Criteria for hearing preservation in acoustic schwannoma surgery: The concept of useful hearing. J Laryngol Otol 106: 500–503, 1992.
26. Shelton C, Hitselberger WE, House WF, Brackmann DE: Long-term results of hearing after acoustic tumor removal. Acoustic Neuroma. *In* Tos M, Thomsen J (eds): Proceedings of the First International Conference on Acoustic Neuroma, Copenhagen, August 25–29, 1991. New York, Kugler Publications, 1992, pp 661–664.
27. McKenna MJ, Halpin C, Ojemann RG, et al: Long-term hearing results in patients after surgical removal of acoustic tumors with hearing preservation. Am J Otol 13: 134–136, 1992.
28. Slavit DH, Harner SG, Harper CM Jr, Beatty CW: Auditory monitoring during acoustic neuroma removal. Arch Otolaryngol Head Neck Surg 17: 1153–1157, 1991.
29. Atlas MD, Harvey C, Fagan PA: Hearing preservation in acoustic neuroma surgery: A continuing study. Laryngoscope 102: 779–783, 1992.
30. Samii M, Matthies C, Tatagiba M: Intracanalicular acoustic neurinomas. Neurosurgery 29: 189–198; Discussion 198–199, 1991.
31. Wigand ME, Haid T, Goertzen W, Wolf S: Preservation of hearing in bilateral acoustic neurinomas by deliberate partial resection. Acta Otolaryngol (Stockh) 112: 237–241, 1992.
32. Mangham CA: Complications of translabyrinthine vs suboccipital approach for acoustic tumor surgery. Otolaryngol Head Neck Surg 99: 396–400, 1988.
33. Ebersold MJ, Harner SG, Beatty CW, et al: Current results of the retrosigmoid approach to acoustic neurinoma. J Neurosurg 76: 901–909, 1991.
34. Haines JH, Maroon JC, Janetta PJ: Supratentorial intracerebral hemorrhage following posterior fossa surgery. J Neurosurg 49: 881, 1978.
35. Harders A, Gilbach J, Weigel K: Supratentorial space occupying lesions following infratentorial surgery: Early diagnosis and treatment. Acta Neurochir (Wien) 74: 57, 1985.
36. Seiler RW, Zurbrugg HR: Supratentorial intracerebral hemorrhage after posterior fossa operation. Neurosurgery 18: 472, 1986.
37. Atkinson J: The anterior cerebellar artery. Its variations, pontine distribution, and significance in the surgery of cerebello-pontine angle tumours. J Neurol Neurosurg Psychiatry 12: 137–151, 1949.
38. Sim DW, Jackler RK, Pitts LH: Cerebellar peduncle infarction after acoustic neuroma surgery. 1994 [in press].
39. Harner SG, Beatty CW, Ebersold MJ: Retrosigmoid removal of acoustic neuroma: Experience 1978–1988. Otolaryngol Head Neck Surg 103: 40–45, 1990.
40. Hitselberger WE, House WF: A warning regarding the sitting position for acoustic tumor surgery. [Editorial] Arch Otolaryngol Head Neck Surg 106: 69, 1980.
41. Samii M, Turel KE, Penker G: Management of seventh and eighth nerve involvement by cerebellopontine angle tumors. Clin Neurosurg 32: 242, 1985.
42. Smith PG, Leonetti JP, Grubb RL: Management of cerebrospinal fluid otorhinorrhea complicating the retrosigmoid approach to the cerebellopontine angle. Am J Otol 11: 178–180, 1990.
43. Schessel DA, Nedzelski JM, Rowed Feghali JG: Headache and local discomfort following surgery of the cerebellopontine angle. Acoustic Neuroma. *In* Tos M, Thomsen J: Proceedings of the First International Conference on Acoustic Neuroma. Copenhagen, August 25–29, 1991. New York, Kugler Publications, 1992, pp 899–904.
44. Broberg T, Sim DW, Jackler RK, Pitts LH: Headache after acoustic neuroma surgery: Comparison of the retrosigmoid and translabyrinthine approaches. 1994 [In Press].
45. Beatty CW, Ebersold MJ, Harner SG: Residual and recurrent acoustic neuromas. Laryngoscope 97: 1168–1171, 1987.

53

The Transotic Approach

JOSEPH M. CHEN, M.D.
UGO FISCH, M.D.

The transotic approach to the cerebellopontine angle (CPA) was first introduced in 1979 in response to the limitations of the translabyrinthine technique. The objective of this approach is to obtain a direct lateral exposure and the widest possible access to the CPA through the medial wall of the temporal bone, from the superior petrosal sinus to the jugular bulb, and from the internal carotid artery to the sigmoid sinus. The tympanic and mastoid portions of the fallopian canal are left in situ. This transtemporal access is achieved at the expense of bony exenteration rather than cerebellar retraction.

In spite of well-documented technical details,[1] there is a general misconception equating the transotic approach with the transcochlear approach[2] of House and Hitzelberger. Significant differences exist between the two approaches in the extent of exposure, the management of the facial nerve, and the obliteration of the surgical cavity.

As a natural extension of subtotal petrosectomy, which forms the basis of lateral and posterior skull base surgery at the University of Zurich,[1] the transotic approach was initially designed for acoustic neuromas and has since expanded to include other pathology. Several modifications were also made over the years to optimize its use.[3-5]

INDICATIONS

ACOUSTIC NEUROMA. Although the transotic approach, like the translabyrinthine approach, can be used for tumors of all sizes, it is ideal for tumors of 2.5cm or less in their medial-lateral extent, in patients with *no* serviceable hearing. In this clinical setting, the transotic approach offers the best possible exposure for tumor extirpation and the preservation of facial nerve and with minimal morbidity.

Tumors larger than 2.5cm that cause significant brain stem compression are managed by the neurosurgery department as a matter of departmental policy at the University of Zurich. Small intracanalicular tumors in patients with good hearing (using the 50/50 rule of at least 50dBHL and 50 per cent discrimination score) are managed through a middle cranial fossa (transtemporal-supralabyrinthine) approach (see Chapter 39).

OTHER LESIONS. Other lesions involving the CPA or the temporal bone with invasion of the internal auditory canal (IAC) or the otic capsule could also be approached via the transotic technique. They include

- Epithelial cysts (congenital cholesteatoma)
- Arachnoid cysts
- Hemangiomas
- Giant cholesterol and mucosal cysts
- Jugular foramen schwannomas
- Temporal paragangliomas (glomus tumors)

These lesions can be quite extensive and may require a combined infratemporal fossa type A or B approach for added exposure.

PREOPERATIVE EVALUATION

The evaluation for retrocochlear lesions, such as acoustic neuromas, is fairly standard at the University of Zurich and includes routine audiometry, auditory brainstem response, electronystagmography, and magnetic resonance imaging with gadolinium enhancement. High-resolution computed tomography is still performed for bony assessment of lesions within or invading the temporal bone.

Facial nerve status is recorded clinically using the Fisch grading system[6] and quantified by electroneuronography prior to surgery.

In addition to a candid discussion of surgical and postoperative complications, patients are made aware *Adv.* of the advantages of the transotic approach specifically ① with regard to the preservation of the facial ② nerve and the complete obliteration of the surgical cavity, with blind sac closure of the external auditory canal to minimize cerebrospinal fluid leak. The option of conservative management by close monitoring with serial magnetic resonance imaging to follow tumor growth is presented to all patients and is recommended for patients with nonprogressive longstanding symptoms, especially the elderly; patients with small tumors and normal hearing; patients with significant medical illnesses; or those who refuse to undergo surgery. These patients are made aware that rapid tumor growth will ultimately require surgical attention, and that facial nerve function and hearing preservation may be compromised as a result of the delay in surgery.

SURGICAL TECHNIQUES

Preoperative Preparation

The patient is premedicated with meperidene (Pethidine, a morphine derivative), 50 mg, and atropine, 0.5 mg intramuscularly, 30 minutes before surgery. Perioperative antibiotic, Chloromycetin (1g intravenously every 8 hours), is given at the time of surgery until the removal of intravenous infusion, usually by the third day after surgery.

Surgical Site Preparation, Positioning, and Draping

The night before surgery, hair over the temporoparietal region (10cm) is clipped. This area is shaved and washed with povidone-iodine (Betadine) after the induction of anesthesia. The abdomen and the contralateral leg are also shaved and prepared for fat harvesting and the possible need of a sural nerve graft.

The positioning and draping for this procedure are similar to those described in Chapter 1, with some minor differences. The patient is secured in supine position on the Fisch operating table (see Chapter 39), with the head turned away from the surgeon. A large plastic bag is incorporated into the draping to catch excess irrigation and blood.

Intraoperative Monitoring and Concerns

Intraoperative facial nerve monitoring using the Xomed nerve integrity monitor (NIM-II) and percutaneous electromyographic needles is standard with this approach. Intracranial pressure is lowered by intraoperative hyperventilation that keeps the P_{CO_2} between 30mmHg and 40mmHg. Pharmacologic manipulation with dexamethasone (Decadron, 4 mg every 8 hours perioperatively and 4 days postoperatively) and mannitol (0.5mg per kg intravenously intraoperatively) are also standard. Furosemide is added when necessary. Lumbar cerebrospinal fluid drainage is not routinely performed. Hypotensive anesthesia with sodium nitroprusside is used in most cases to maintain a systolic blood pressure between 80mmHg and 100mmHg.

Techniques of Surgery

Skin Incision

A postauricular incision is placed along the hairline to keep it behind the operative cavity (Fig. 53–1). The incision is made from the mastoid tip to the temporal region for the surgical approach; its superior extension *(dotted lines)* is made at the time of wound closure for the exposure of the temporalis muscle flap.

Blind Sac Closure of the External Auditory Canal

A mastoid periosteal flap is developed while the postauricular skin flap is elevated. The external auditory canal is transected and its skin elevated, everted externally, and closed as a blind sac. A second layer of closure using the mastoid periosteal flap ensures a complete seal (Fig. 53–2).

Subtotal Petrosectomy: Exposure of Jugular Bulb and Petrous Carotid

A complete mastoidectomy is performed, and the remaining external auditory canal skin, tympanic membrane, and ossicles are removed in a stepwise fashion. The tympanic bone is progressively thinned out, and a complete exenteration of the pneumatic spaces (retrofacial, retrolabyrinthine, supralabyrinthine, hypotympanic, infralabyrinthine, and pericarotid) is carried out. Figure 53–3 shows the surgical cavity at the completion of this step. The middle fossa dura, sigmoid sinus, and jugular bulb are blue lined; the fallopian canal and the vertical portion of the petrous carotid artery are skeletonized. The mastoid tip is removed to reduce the depth of the surgical cavity.

Obliteration of the Eustachian Tube

The mucosa of the membranous eustachian tube orifice is coagulated and the bony canal obliterated with bone wax at the isthmus. An additional muscle plug will be used prior to closure.

Exenteration of the Otic Capsule

With the completion of subtotal petrosectomy, the surgical cavity is divided into two compartments by the fallopian canal (Fig. 53–4). Because the enlarged IAC lies mostly deep within the anterior compartment, the advantage of the transotic approach to fully access this region is clear.

To begin this step, the semicircular canals are removed and the vestibule opened as in the translabyrinthine approach. The posterior aspect of the IAC is exposed from the fundus to the porus, leaving a thin layer of bone over the meatal dura. The posterior fossa dura of the posterior compartment is exposed caudal to the superior petrosal sinus and anterior to the sigmoid sinus. Retrofacial cells are subsequently removed to gain access over the inferior aspect of the IAC.

Attention is now focused on the anterior compartment. The cochlea is drilled away to expose the enlarged IAC, which lies predominantly within this compartment, and as the dissection is carried forward, the dura anterior to the porus is also exposed. Bony reduction between the jugular bulb and the inferior aspect of the IAC requires working beneath and over the fallopian canal, which is left in its anatomic position across the surgical field. Sufficient bone is left surrounding the canal to prevent accidental fracture.

The cochlear aqueduct is identified between the jugular bulb and the IAC. The arachnoid of the aqueduct is opened to allow the outflow of cerebrospinal fluid,

FIGURE 53-1

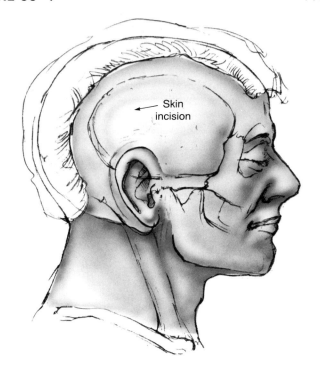

Skin incision

FIGURE 53-2

Blind sac closure of the external auditory canal after eversion of the canal skin

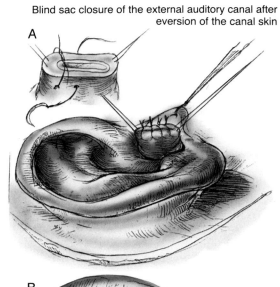

A

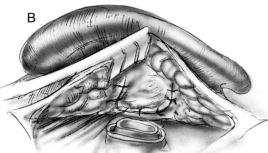

B

FIGURE 53-3

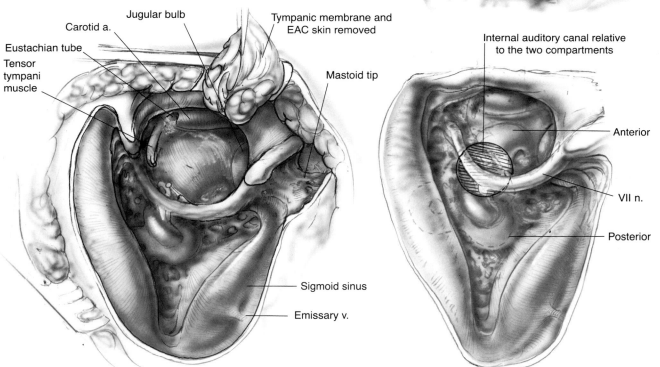

Jugular bulb

Carotid a.

Eustachian tube

Tensor tympani muscle

Tympanic membrane and EAC skin removed

Mastoid tip

Sigmoid sinus

Emissary v.

Internal auditory canal relative to the two compartments

Anterior

VII n.

Posterior

FIGURE 53-4

FIGURE 53-5

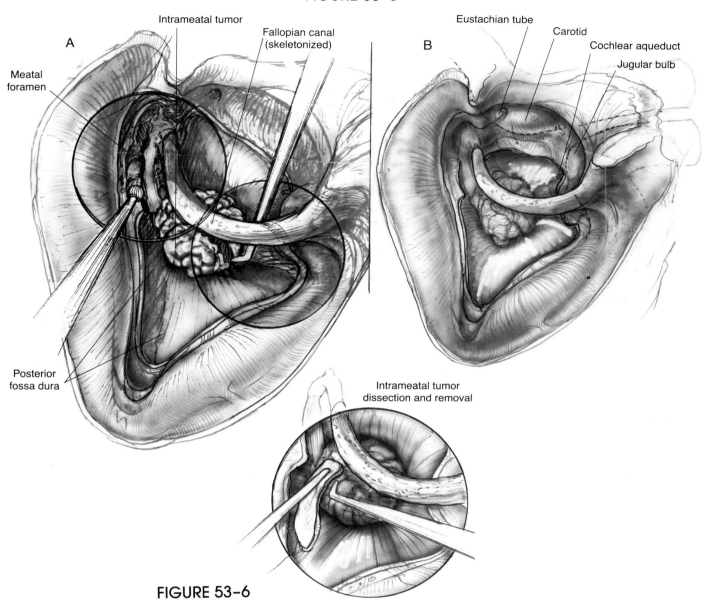

A — Meatal foramen · Intrameatal tumor · Fallopian canal (skeletonized) · Posterior fossa dura

B — Eustachian tube · Carotid · Cochlear aqueduct · Jugular bulb

Intrameatal tumor dissection and removal

FIGURE 53-6

FIGURE 53-1. Skin incision.

FIGURE 53-2. Blind sac closure of the external auditory canal.

FIGURE 53-3. Subtotal petrosectomy.

FIGURE 53-4. Position of the internal auditory canal.

FIGURE 53-5. Exposure of the internal auditory canal and posterior fossa dura.

FIGURE 53-6. Intrameatal tumor dissection.

thereby decompressing the lateral cistern before the posterior fossa dura is opened.

The tensor tympani muscle and bone medial to it are removed to gain more anterior access; likewise, bone medial to the carotid artery is removed as much as possible.

Unroofing of the Labyrinthine Portion of the Facial Nerve

Since 1988, the unroofing of the labyrinthine segment of the facial nerve from the meatal foramen to the geniculate ganglion has been incorporated as a standard step in the transotic approach. The meatal foramen can be found approximately 2mm anterior and superior to the meatal fundus. This exposure will provide additional room for that portion of the facial nerve most likely to suffer traction injury and edema subsequent to tumor manipulation. Also, the labyrinthine portion of the facial nerve serves as an important landmark while further access over the porus is gained along the superior petrosal sinus.

The completed exposure is shown in Figure 53–5. The posterior fossa dura surrounding the porus is circumferentially exposed from the carotid artery to the sigmoid sinus, and from the jugular bulb to the level of the superior petrosal sinus.

Tumor Removal

A few instruments are required for tumor removal. Bayonet and angled bipolar forceps, cup forceps, microraspatories, and a long suction with finger control are the most essential.

The intrameatal portion of the tumor is approached first and is separated from the facial nerve until the level of the porus. Figure 53–6 illustrates the advantage of the additional space obtained with the transotic exenteration, whereby the intrameatal portion of the tumor can be easily displaced and mobilized during its removal.

The posterior fossa dura is incised between the sinodural angle and the posterior edge of the porus. The incision is extended superiorly and inferiorly along the porus (Fig. 53–7). It is important to elevate the dura with a hook prior to making an incision to prevent the inadvertent injury of vessels over the cerebellum. The dural edges must be cauterized before extending the incision to facilitate hemostasis. One must also be acutely aware of the variations of the course of the anterior inferior cerebellar artery (AICA) and its branches.

The superior and inferior dural flaps are retracted with 4-0 Vicryl sutures, which are clipped to the wound edges (Fig. 53–8). The full extent of the tumor can usually be demonstrated: the posterior pole of the tumor abuts against the cerebellum, the petrosal vein, and the AICA courses anteroinferior to the tumor.

Intracapsular reduction of the tumor can now commence and is continued until tumor margins can be seen without tension being placed on the facial nerve. During this step, the meatal dura at the superior pole of the porus is not detached, so as to render some stability to the tumor. It is of utmost importance to handle the tumor meticulously; manipulations should be carried out with suction over a cottonoid, and the displaced facial nerve should always be in view to avoid undue traction (Fig. 53–9).

Bleeding is diminished by coagulation of all visible vessels over the tumor capsule. The main blood supply to the tumor generally runs along the eighth nerve, and some may come from branches of the AICA: they should be coagulated, cut on the tumor, and gently pulled away.

With sufficient reduction, separation of the facial nerve can now be attempted. The advantage of the transotic approach is now easily appreciated, as the displaced facial nerve can be followed in its entirety. The dural attachments of the tumor at the porus are cut, and the nerve can be gently grasped with bipolar forceps and teased away from the tumor (Fig. 53–10). Likewise, the AICA can be separated from the nerve by using the tips of the forceps or by pulling on the coagulated branches.

At the inferior pole of the tumor, the origin of the eighth nerve and the course of the AICA looping around it are identified. In many instances, the root exit zone of the facial nerve, always anterior to the eighth nerve, is identified only after the eighth nerve is cut.

FIGURE 53–7. Dural incision.

FIGURE 53–8. Initial cerebellopontine angle exposure.

FIGURE 53–9. Intracapsular tumor reduction.

FIGURE 53–10. Intracranial facial nerve dissection.

FIGURE 53–11. View of cerebellopontine angle after tumor removal.

FIGURE 53-7

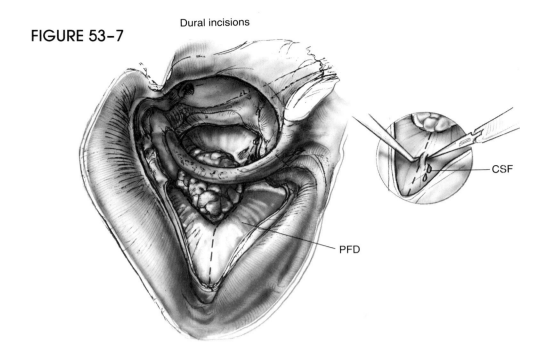

Dural incisions

CSF

PFD

FIGURE 53-8

Initial CPA exposure

AICA

Petrosal v.

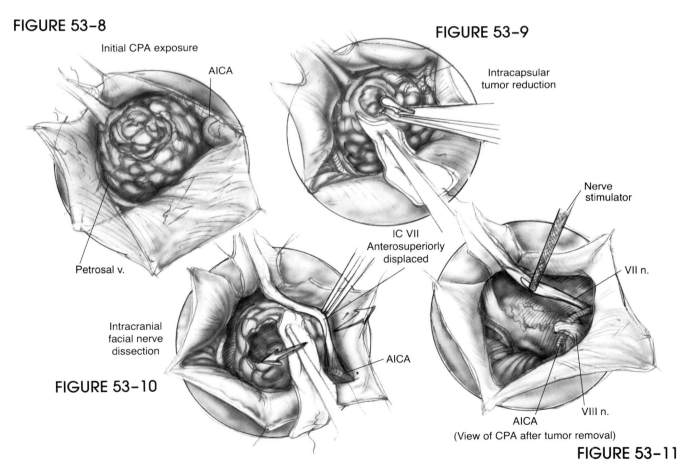

FIGURE 53-9

Intracapsular
tumor reduction

Intracranial
facial nerve
dissection

IC VII
Anterosuperiorly
displaced

AICA

FIGURE 53-10

Nerve
stimulator

VII n.

VIII n.

AICA
(View of CPA after tumor removal)

FIGURE 53-11

The anterior access of the transotic approach offers an unparalleled view to an area that is usually partially hidden from the surgeon during suboccipital or translabyrinthine surgery.[7, 8] In this exact region, the facial nerve is most tenuous and frequently appears as a thin, transparent band. Any manipulation not under direct vision can easily rupture the nerve.

Once it is completely detached from all vital structures, the tumor can now be removed. The complete exposure of the CPA and all of its structures are illustrated in Figure 53–11.

The facial nerve is stimulated electrically to obtain a threshold response. Despite a normal response intraoperatively, the patient may still demonstrate an immediate or delayed facial paralysis due to impaired vascular supply and the inevitable trauma to the nerve during dissection. If stimulation fails to produce a response or facial contraction, and if the anatomic integrity of the nerve is precarious, it is best to proceed with nerve grafting immediately. Failure to do so while waiting for the improbable return of facial function may delay reinnervation for up to 2 years. The details of intracranial-intratemporal and hypoglossal-facial crossover grafting techniques are beyond the scope of this chapter and are documented elsewhere.[1, 9]

Wound Closure

A musculofascial graft that is slightly larger than the dural defect is taken from the temporalis muscle. It is placed under the dura and fixed in place with the two 4-0 Vicryl sutures used previously as stay sutures (Fig. 53–12). These sutures are passed through the edges of the graft and secured to the dura. A small muscle graft is also used as a plug to supplement the prior wax obliteration of the eustachian tube. Both grafts are stabilized with fibrin glue.

A second layer of closure with abdominal fat grafts is to follow. A large piece of fat is first passed under the fallopian canal and firmly anchored (Fig. 53–13). Several small pieces of fat are used to fill out the surgical cavity and are also stabilized with fibrin glue.

The temporalis muscle is now transposed and sutured in place with 2-0 Vicryl sutures. Additional fat is placed under the muscle flap to create a slight compressive tension (Fig. 53–14). This type of closure has consistently minimized the incidence of postoperative cerebrospinal fluid leaks and demonstrates another advantage of the transotic approach. A small plastic suction drain is inserted over the muscle flap while the skin incision is closed in two layers with 2-0 Dexon and 3-0 nylon sutures.

Dressing and Postoperative Care

The suction drain is removed as soon as a compression dressing is applied. Dressing is left in place for 5 days, and if there is any evidence of cerebrospinal fluid leak or subcutaneous cerebrospinal fluid accumulation, the compression dressing is reapplied.

The patient is transferred to the recovery room extubated and fully awake. Routine and neurologic vital signs are closely monitored every 30 to 60 minutes. Adequate analgesics and antiemetics are ordered to keep the patient comfortably at bed rest, usually for 72 hours after surgery. Ambulation and oral intake are started slowly thereafter. Subcutaneous heparin is often given during the early convalescent period. An oral antibiotic (Bactrin Forte) is prescribed for at least 5 days after intravenous fluid and Chloromycetin therapy are discontinued.

Head and abdominal wound sutures are removed on day 12, and leg sutures after 2 weeks. The patient is discharged from hospital at this time, barring any complication.

Tips and Pitfalls

The transotic approach is more than a combination of the translabyrinthine and transcochlear approaches. It uses the complete infralabyrinthine compartment of the temporal bone, from the carotid artery to the sigmoid sinus, and from the jugular bulb to the superior petrosal sinus. It provides the largest possible transtemporal access to the CPA, which can be best appreciated by comparing the cross-sectional surgical exposure of the transotic approach with the translabyrinthine approach shown in Figure 53–15.

The preservation of the facial nerve in its anatomic position within the fallopian canal does not limit the visibility or illumination. Enough bone must be kept surrounding the canal initially during subtotal petro-

FIGURE 53–12. Dural closure.

FIGURE 53–13. Fat obliteration of the surgical cavity.

FIGURE 53–14. Temporalis muscle flap.

FIGURE 53–15. Cross-sectional views of the transotic approach versus the translabyrinthine approach.

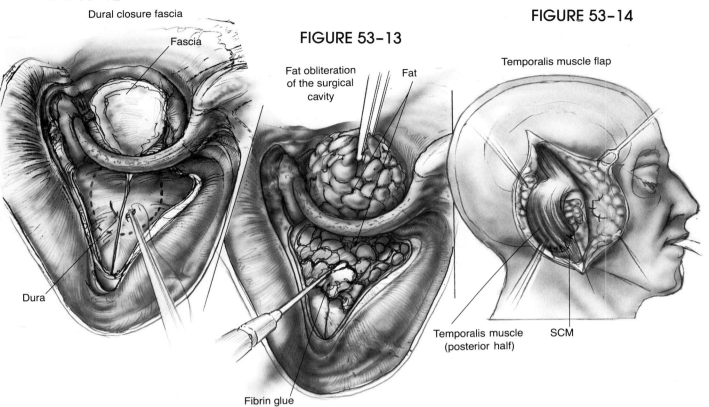

FIGURE 53-12

Dural closure fascia

Fascia

Dura

FIGURE 53-13

Fat obliteration of the surgical cavity

Fat

Fibrin glue

FIGURE 53-14

Temporalis muscle flap

Temporalis muscle (posterior half)

SCM

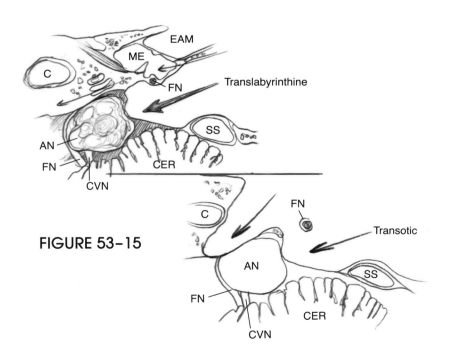

FIGURE 53-15

EAM

ME

C

FN

Translabyrinthine

SS

AN

FN

CVN

CER

C

FN

Transotic

AN

FN

SS

CVN

CER

sectomy and subsequently while the otic capsule is exenterated. Skeletonization of the fallopian canal must be done progressively as the surgical cavity enlarges, and with only diamond burrs. Bone surrounding the proximal tympanic segment of the facial nerve and of the superior aspect of the IAC should be left intact to support the facial nerve.

If the fallopian canal is inadvertently fractured during dissection, it will most likely remain undisplaced and will not impede surgery. If no significant torsion or traction has occured, no major adverse effects should result, provided that no further manipulation occurs. The fractured edges can be supported with fibrin glue, and at the time of closure, abdominal fat will adequately render support from beneath. If the fracture is displaced and unstable, a small, malleable aluminum strip can be used as a retractor and can maintain the fallopian canal in position. If this is not possible, the nerve may have to be fully unroofed and transposed anteriorly as in infratemporal fossa type A approach. This situation, however, has not occurred in our hands.

The three fundamental principles for the removal of acoustic neuromas are

1. Perform intracapsular reduction of the tumor to progressively gain better visibility around the circumference of the tumor.
2. Expose tumor from lateral to medial. Coagulate all visible vessels over the tumor capsule and remove the devascularized portion in a piecemeal fashion.
3. Separate the facial nerve from the tumor and not vice versa.

Cerebrospinal fluid outflow following the opening of the cochlear aqueduct will decompress the lateral cistern before the dural incision is made. It also indicates that the pars nervosa of the jugular foramen and the lower cranial nerves have not yet been reached by the tumor.

Even in the presence of a high jugular bulb, a few millimeters of exposure can be obtained between it and the IAC to allow adequate access to the inferior pole of the tumor. Unroofing and compressing the jugular bulb to gain more exposure is unnecessary and dangerous. If access to the CPA is severely limited by the jugular bulb, the facial nerve can be unroofed and transposed anteriorly, as in the infratemporal fossa type A approach.

Bony exenteration to expose the posterior fossa dura should be done in a stepwise fashion, gaining as much exposure of the posterior fossa dura around the porus as possible. The time spent in the initial bony exenteration may be tedious at first, but it is well rewarded by much-expanded access and improved illumination, which facilitate tumor removal dramatically.

Do not open the dura until all bony work has been completed and hemostasis perfectly controlled. While incising the dura, beware of the AICA, which may loop underneath. Make the initial cut in the center of the exposure to avoid this artery, which usually lies in the inferior half of the CPA.

Perform intracapsular reduction of the tumor while it is still attached to the meatal dura at the superior pole of the porus to prevent excessive traction on the facial nerve. It also stabilizes the tumor during reduction.

The major blood supply of acoustic tumors runs along the eighth nerve. Always check for vessels on the undersurface of the tumor prior to removal.

The most delicate portion of the facial nerve is just proximal to the acoustic porus, where the nerve can be flattened to a thin transparent band. It is most frequently pushed anteriorly and superiorly. Keep an eye on this area while working deeper in the CPA.

If the facial nerve appears to be significantly traumatized and cannot be stimulated at the end of surgery, proceed directly to an intracranial-intratemporal grafting or XII–VII cross-innervation procedure, depending on the clinical setting. Spontaneous return of function with conservative treatment is not likely to occur.

Do not resect posterior fossa dura to gain exposure. Retract the dural edges with stay sutures.

Do not forget to obliterate the eustachian tube with both bone wax and a muscle plug to prevent cerebrospinal fluid rhinorrhea.

Fat graft anchored under the fallopian canal will support the musculofascial repair and prevent lateralization of these autogenous tissues.

RESULTS

Between 1979 and 1990, 147 consecutive transotic approaches were performed for the removal of unilateral acoustic neuromas by the senior author (UF). Tumors in this series were limited in size from 1.0cm to 2.5cm in their medial-lateral extension. Tumors may fill the lateral cistern, abutting but without significantly compressing the brainstem.

Complete tumor removal was achieved in all cases. Optimal visualization of the facial nerve was obtained, and the anatomic preservation of the nerve was possible in 139 cases (94.6 per cent). In eight cases in which facial nerve integrity could not be preserved, intracranial-intratemporal nerve grafting resulted in an average of 66 per cent return of facial function by the Fisch facial nerve grading system (or House-Brackmann grade III), during a mean follow up of 4 years.

Sixty-six patients in this series were available for

TABLE 53–1. 2-Year Postoperative Facial Function

TUMOR SIZE (cm)	n	PER CENT RECOVERY				
		100	80–99	60–79	40–59	0–39
1.0–1.4	14	100	—	—	—	—
1.5–2.5*	52	61	19	12	4	4
Total	66	70	15	9	3	3

*No difference in facial function following removal of tumors of 1.5cm to 1.9cm versus 2.0cm to 2.5cm.

follow-up of at least 2 years. Tumors of 1.0cm to 1.4cm were removed with no incidence of permanent facial injury, and 80 per cent of patients with tumors of 1.5cm to 2.5cm had normal or near-normal facial function (Table 53–1). Since 1988, the unroofing of the labyrinthine portion of the facial nerve has been a standard step in the transotic approach, which is felt to be a major contributing factor in the diminished incidence of delayed facial palsy in acoustic neuroma surgery.

COMPLICATIONS AND MANAGEMENT

The obliteration of the surgical cavity and eustachian tube, along with the blind sac closure of the external auditory canal, has significantly lowered the incidence of cerebrospinal fluid leak. In the series mentioned earlier, 4 per cent of patients developed a subcutaneous cerebrospinal fluid collection without leakage, and the collections usually resolved within 3 to 4 weeks with conservative management, including bed rest and prolonged compressive dressing over the surgical site.

Three patients (4 per cent) developed either immediate or delayed cerebrospinal fluid leaks and were treated with lumbar drainage and bed rest; only one required surgical revision. One patient had meningitis and responded to antibiotic treatment without sequelae. Most notably is the lack of any other central nervous system complication in this series. One unfortunate death occurred as a result of postoperative pulmonary embolism and cardiorespiratory failure. Wound infection with necrosis of the abdominal fat graft or temporalis muscle flap was a rare complication and was thought to be the inciting cause in the case of meningitis.

ALTERNATIVE TECHNIQUES

When and how acoustic neuromas should be operated are issues of ongoing and often emotional debates. If surgery is contemplated, the aim is obviously to try to obtain the safest and best possible exposure that will allow complete tumor extirpation and the preservation of facial nerve. Hearing preservation is of secondary concern if the opposite ear is functional.

Translabyrinthine and suboccipital approaches are perhaps the most established and popular techniques, whereas the middle fossa approach has traditionally been reserved for small tumors in patients with serviceable hearing; an extended version of the middle fossa approach has gained popularity in some centers to remove tumors up to 4.5cm,[10, 11] despite a seemingly high morbidity.[12] The relative efficacy of each of these approaches is difficult to quantify without a randomized multi-institutional study.

Our own experience with the translabyrinthine removal of acoustic neuromas prior to 1979 was unsatisfactory in many respects, and those problems were subsequently rectified with the transotic approach.[1] There are three advantages of the transotic approach over the translabyrinthine approach:

1. A wider surgical access with a near circumferential exposure of the IAC and the porus acusticus. This added exposure is particularly important in the presence of a high-riding jugular bulb and an anteriorly positioned sigmoid sinus.
2. The direct visualization and access to the anterior CPA where the facial nerve is most tenuous and vulnerable.
3. A much reduced rate of cerebrospinal fluid leakage as a result of permanent closure of the ear canal and eustachian tube and complete obliteration of the surgical cavity.

References

1. Fisch U, Mattox D: Microsurgery of the Skull Base. New York, Thieme Medical Publishers, 1988.
2. House WF, Hitzelberger WE: The transcochlear approach to the skull base. Arch Otolaryngol Head Neck Surg 102: 334–342, 1976.
3. Jenkins HA, Fisch U: The transotic approach to resection of difficult acoustic tumors of the cerebellopontine angle. Am J Otol 2: 70–76, 1980.
4. Gantz BJ, Fisch U: Modified transotic approach to the cerebellopontine angle. Arch Otolaryngol Head Neck Surg 109: 252–256, 1983.
5. Chen JM, Fisch U: The transotic approach in acoustic neuroma surgery. J Otolaryngol 22:331–336, 1993.
6. Burres S, Fisch U: The comparison of facial grading systems. Arch Otolaryngol Head Neck Surg 112: 755–758, 1986.
7. Whittaker CK, Leutje CM: Translabyrinthine removal of large acoustic neuromas. Am J Otol 7 (Suppl): 155–160, 1985.
8. Gardner G, Robertson JH, et al.: Transtemporal approaches to the cranial cavity. Am J Otol 7 (Suppl): 114–120, 1985.
9. Fisch U, Lanser MJ: Facial nerve grafting. Otolaryngol Clin North Am 24: 691–708, 1991.
10. Wigand ME, Haid T, et al.: Extended middle cranial fossa approach for acoustic neuroma surgery. Skull Base Surg 1: 183–187, 1991.
11. Kanzaki J, Ogawa K, et al.: Results of acoustic neuroma surgery by the extended middle cranial fossa approach. Acta Otolaryngol Suppl (Stockh) 487: 17–21, 1991.
12. Kanzaki J, Ogawa K, et al.: Postoperative complications in acoustic neuroma surgery by the extended middle cranial fossa approach. Acta Otolaryngol Suppl (Stockh) 487: 75–79, 1991.

54

Transcochlear Approach to Cerebellopontine Angle Lesions

ANTONIO DE LA CRUZ, M.D.
SUJANA S. CHANDRASEKHAR, M.D.

The transcochlear approach is the most direct surgical route to midline intracranial lesions arising from the clivus and cerebellopontine angle masses arising anterior to the internal auditory canal. These lesions often extend around the basilovertebral artery and, because traditional surgical approaches were limited by the cerebellum and the brainstem, have been considered inoperable by many surgeons. The transcochlear approach is not thus limited and is designed primarily for meningiomas arising from the petroclinoid ridge, intradural clivus lesions, congenital petrous apex epidermoids, and primary intradural epidermoids anterior to the internal auditory canal.

Adv of other approaches

Evolution of the transcochlear approach resulted from an inability to excise the base of implantation and control the blood supply of these near-midline and midline tumors. Total removal of these lesions through a suboccipital approach is often not possible because of the interposition of the cerebellum and the brainstem.[1, 2] The transpalatal-transclival approach was tried for these intradural midline lesions, with little or no success.[3] The exposure is inadequate, the field is at quite a distance from the surgeon, the blood supply is lateral, away from the surgeon's view, and intracranial problems with oral contamination occur. The retrolabyrinthine approach is limited in its forward extension by the posterior semicircular canal. Tumor access with the translabyrinthine approach is limited anteriorly by the facial nerve, which impedes removal of the tumor's base of implantation, which is anterior to the internal auditory canal, around the intrapetrous carotid artery, or anterior to the brainstem. The recent development of the anterior extended middle fossa approach enables complete removal of petroclinoid meningiomas and is used in patients with useful hearing.[4] The primary limitation with this approach is that it cannot access tumors with inferior extension below the level of the inner ear.[5, 6]

The transcochlear approach was developed by House and Hitselberger in the late 1960s and early 1970s[2, 3] as an anterior extension of the translabyrinthine approach. It involves complete rerouting of the facial nerve posteriorly and allows removal of the petrous bone, which exposes the intrapetrous internal carotid artery. This approach affords wide exposure of the anterior cerebellopontine angle, cranial nerves V, VII, VIII, IX, X, and XI, both sixth cranial nerves, the clivus, and the basilar and vertebral arteries. The contralateral cranial nerves and the opposite cerebellopontine angle are also visible. It is the only approach during which the tumor base and its arterial blood supply from the internal carotid artery are removed.[2] The addition of excision and closure of the external auditory canal, recently advocated by Brackmann (Personal communication, 1993), further increases the anterior exposure.

ADVANTAGES OF THE TRANSCOCHLEAR APPROACH. This approach requires no cerebellar or temporal lobe retractors. Exposure and dissection of the petrous apex and clivus ensure complete removal of both the tumor and its blood supply. This is of particular importance in meningiomas. Careful handling and constant monitoring of the facial nerve during rerouting prevent injury to the intratemporal portion of the nerve. However, meningiomas often invade the nerve, and cholesteatomas tend to wrap themselves around it. If the facial nerve is lost during tumor removal, we recommend immediate repair by end-to-end anastamosis or nerve graft interposition.

DISADVANTAGES OF THE TRANSCOCHLEAR APPROACH. The main disadvantages of this approach are sacrifice of residual hearing in the operated ear and risk of temporary facial palsy. This technique is used when no serviceable hearing exists in the involved ear, or when the tumor is too far inferior for the extended middle fossa craniotomy approach. With the use of continuous facial nerve monitoring, the incidence of permanent facial nerve palsy is low.

PATIENT EVALUATION AND PREOPERATIVE COUNSELING

Individuals with tumors that require transcochlear surgery may have minimal symptomatology, and the tumors are quite large at the time of diagnosis.[1, 7] Unilateral hearing loss and tinnitus are the presenting complaints in 80 per cent of petrous apex epidermoids. Imbalance, ataxia, and parietal or vertex headache may be the only complaints in 20 per cent.[8] With petrous apex cholesteatomas, persistent otorrhea and facial twitch are common. Patients with meningiomas and intradural epidermoids may be nearly symptom-free until they present with fifth cranial nerve findings and signs of increased intracranial pressure.[9, 10] There is a relatively high rate of jugular foramen syndrome in patients with meningiomas.[1] Seizures, dysarthria, and late signs of dementia from hydrocephalus were common presenting symptoms in the past.[8]

Evaluation proceeds with examination of the cranial nerves and audiometry. Hearing and vestibular function are frequently normal, and acoustic reflex decay or abnormal auditory brainstem response audiometric results may be the only anomalies.[2] Radiographic evaluation using high-resolution computed tomography (CT) with contrast enhancement magnetic resonance imaging (MRI), or both, is essential for diagnosis and surgical planning (Fig. 54–1).[11] Petrous apex and intradural epidermoids are expansile, spherical, or oval lesions, with scalloping of a bony

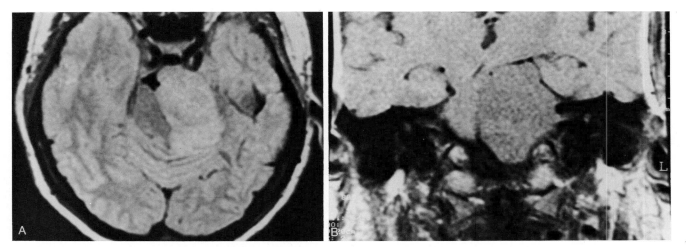

FIGURE 54-1. Axial (*A*) and coronal (*B*) gadolinium-enhanced magnetic resonance image of a large, left-sided ependymoma. Note extension of the tumor superiorly, displacing the tentorium, and medially, across the midline. Inferiorly, the tumor approaches the foramen magnum, and anteriorly, it extends into the middle cranial fossa via the porus trigeminus and abuts the internal carotid artery at the cavernous sinus. This tumor was removed in its entirety via the transcochlear approach.

edge on CT. They are isodense to brain on CT, with capsular enhancement. On MRI, they are hypointense on T1- and hyperintense on T2-weighted images. Meningiomas enhance on CT and MRI. Localization of the tumor may also require angiography. In tumors surrounding or invading the intratemporal carotid artery, preoperative balloon occlusion, embolization, or both, are indicated. Both balloon occlusion of the carotid artery and selective embolization are performed at least 1 day before the neurotologic surgery, and the patient is sedated but awake. This state ensures early identification of negative neurologic sequelae. If necessary, the balloon can be deflated immediately to restore cerebral perfusion. Radioisotope or xenon studies are used to assess cerebral perfusion during occlusion studies. Positron-emission tomography is another useful adjunctive diagnostic modality in this situation.

Patients are counseled regarding the serious nature of their tumor. The natural history of petrous apex epidermoids is that they grow and may become superinfected. Treatment is difficult when such infection occurs, and meningitis, sepsis, and death may result. Intracranial epidermoid tumors spread through the cisterns and subarachnoid planes to neighboring regions; petrous ridge meningiomas grow and are space-occupying lesions that increase intracranial pressure. Thus, surgical intervention is advised. After surgery, intracranial pressure is reduced, and cranial nerve symptoms improve. Risks and complications in the immediate postoperative period include transient vertigo, complete hearing loss, and temporary facial nerve paresis, as well as infection, bleeding, cerebrovascular accidents, and death.

SURGICAL TECHNIQUE

Overview

A wide mastoidectomy and labyrinthectomy are performed, exposing the internal auditory canal. The external auditory canal may be removed, and the meatus may be closed. The facial nerve is completely skeletonized, with transection of the greater superficial petrosal and chorda tympani nerves, and is rerouted posteriorly out of the fallopian canal. The cochlea is completely drilled out, and the internal carotid artery is identified. A large triangular window is created into the skull base. Its superior boundary is the superior petrosal sinus; inferiorly, it extends below and medial to the inferior petrosal sinus into the clivus. Anteriorly is the internal carotid artery, and the apex of the triangle is just beneath Meckel's cave. After tumor removal, the dura is reapproximated, and abdominal fat is used to fill the mastoidectomy defect and to cushion the facial nerve.

Setup

General endotracheal anesthesia with arterial blood pressure monitoring is used, and a urinary catheter and a nasogastric tube are inserted. Long-acting muscle relaxants are avoided because they may produce false-negative responses from the intraoperative facial nerve monitor, which is used in all cases. Anesthesia is kept light so that changes in blood pressure and pulse brought about by tumor manipulation are not masked. Prophylactic third-generation cephalosporin antibiotics and steroids are used routinely before the skin incision is made. Venous antiembolism compression boots are placed on the patient's legs before the procedure begins.

The patient is placed supine on the operating table, with the head turned to the opposite side, and is maintained in a natural position without fixation. The surgeon sits at the side of the patient's head. This position avoids air embolization, minimizes surgeon fatigue, and allows stabilization of the surgeon's hands during the microsurgical procedure.

Incision

A retroauricular incision is made 3cm behind the postauricular fold, starting 1cm above the ear and ending below the mastoid tip. If the intracranial carotid artery and/or the lower cranial nerves are involved, the incision may be extended inferiorly into the neck to provide control of the great vessels and to obtain exposure of the lower cranial nerves. The superior limb of the incision extends to the level of the fascia temporalis. Inferiorly, the periosteum is incised above the linea temporalis from the level of the zygomatic root anteriorly to a point 1cm posterior to the sigmoid sinus. The periosteal incision is carried inferiorly to the mastoid tip. The periosteal elevator is used to free the periosteum from the underlying cortex, to the sinodural angle posteriorly, and forward to the level of the external auditory canal. The external auditory canal skin is either not elevated, avoiding a possible route for infection, or is completely excised, including canal skin and tympanic membrane, and the meatus is closed in two layers.

Mastoidectomy (Fig. 54–2)

A complete simple mastoidectomy is carried out with cutting and diamond burrs and continuous suction-irrigation. Bone removal is started along two lines, one along the linea temporalis, and another tangential to the external canal. The mastoid antrum is opened, and the lateral semicircular canal is identified. This canal is the most reliable landmark in the temporal bone and allows the dissection to proceed toward delineating the fallopian canal and the osseous labyrinth.

The external opening of the mastoid cavity must be as large as possible and is extended posterior to the sigmoid sinus, exposing 1 to 2cm of suboccipital (posterior fossa) dura. The larger the size of the tumor, the further back the posterior fossa dura is exposed, to a maximum of 2 to 3cm. Removal of bone over the sigmoid sinus is performed with diamond burrs, leaving an island of bone (Bill's island) over the dome of the sinus. This process avoids injury to the sinus from burr shafts. If bleeding occurs that cannot be con-

trolled with preservation of the sigmoid sinus, it is reduced with bipolar cautery, and the sinus is packed with oxidized bovine cellulose (Surgicel), or it is ligated. The mastoid emissary vein is dissected, and bleeding is controlled with bipolar cautery, a mixture of Surgicel and bone wax, or plain Surgicel packing.

Bone is removed from the sinodural angle along the superior petrosal sinus. The mastoid air cells are exenterated from the sinodural angle, thereby skeletonizing the dura of the posterior fossa and the posterior 1cm of middle fossa dura.

Labyrinthectomy and Exposure of the Internal Auditory Canal
(Fig. 54–3)

The operating microscope is brought into place, and dissection of the perilabyrinthine cells down to the lateral semicircular canal is completed. The facial nerve is identified between the nonampullated end of the lateral semicircular canal and the stylomastoid foramen. At this time, exposing the perineurium of the nerve is not necessary, but it should be clearly and unmistakeably identified in its vertical lie.

The lateral semicircular canal is fenestrated, and the membranous portion is identified and followed anteriorly to its ampullated end and posteriorly to the posterior semicircular canal. All three membranous and bony semicircular canals are removed, as well as the saccule and utricle in the vestibule.

The dissection proceeds along the sinodural angle, and the dura of the posterior fossa is exposed anteriorly. The cells over the jugular bulb are removed, skeletonizing it. The internal auditory canal is identified, beginning inferiorly and then around to the porus acusticus, using the faciform (transverse) crest and vertical crest (Bill's bar) as identifying landmarks. The dissection and removal of the roof of the internal auditory canal is performed with diamond burr.

Facial Nerve Dissection

After removal of the incus, the facial nerve is completely skeletonized from the internal auditory canal to the stylomastoid foramen, including the geniculate ganglion, with diamond burrs. An extended facial recess opening is created (Fig. 54–3), and an area comprising 180 degrees of the bony fallopian canal is uncovered (Fig. 54–4). The greater superficial petrosal nerve is cut at its origin from the geniculate ganglion with the incudostapedial joint knife. The nerve is then reflected posteriorly out of the bony fallopian canal by use of dental excavators, and care is taken to avoid traction on the nerve, especially near the second genu, which is the site of several branches to the stapedius muscle (Fig. 54–5).

Closure of the External Auditory Canal

When further anterior exposure is required, removal and closure of the external auditory canal is included (see Chapter 60 on management of cerebrospinal fluid leaks). The canal skin is transected at the bony-cartilaginous junction and is undermined laterally. Extra cartilage is removed, and the skin is closed with interrupted nylon sutures in a dimple-like fashion at the external auditory meatus. A periosteal flap is used to oversew the undersurface of the canal skin. After removal of all of the canal skin, the tympanic membrane, and the malleus, the bony external auditory canal is drilled out and excised circumferentially. Care is taken to avoid entering the glenoid fossa (see Chapter 60 on the infratemporal approach for illustrations).

Transcochlear Drill-Out

The fallopian canal has been removed, the promontory and ossicles have now been exposed, and the stapes has been removed. Starting with the basal coil, the cochlea is completely drilled out (Fig. 54–6). Bone removal is carried forward to the internal carotid artery, and the inferior extent of bone removal extends to the inferior petrosal sinus and jugular bulb. Superiorly, the superior petrosal sinus is exposed to Meckel's cave. Medially, bone removal extends to the clivus. At this stage, a large window, covered by dura, has been created into the skull base (Fig. 54–7). Its boundaries are superiorly, the superior petrosal sinus; inferiorly, below and medial to the inferior petrosal sinus into the clivus; anteriorly, the internal carotid artery; and medially, the lateral clivus. The apex of the triangle is just beneath Meckel's cave. In certain cases, the internal carotid artery must be sacrificed for complete tumor removal. Carotid resection affords greater anterior exposure, and the risks attendant to this procedure are minimized if the patient has tolerated preoperative balloon occlusion of the artery.

Tumor Removal (Fig. 54–8)

With petrous ridge meningiomas, arterial feeder vessels from the internal carotid artery are encountered and eliminated at this stage. The diamond burr is used to excise these vessels and the base of implantation at the petrous tip. Using this approach, the surgeon removes the root of the tumor. The dura is now opened posterior to the internal auditory canal, and the opening is extended as far forward as is necessary for complete tumor exposure.

The facial nerve is seen on the posterior surface of tumors. The junction of the intracranial portion of the facial nerve and the skeletonized intratemporal portion is now identified, and the entire nerve is reflected posteriorly. The nerve is protected with a moist absorbable gelatin sponge (Gelfoam) pledget.

The tumor capsule is opened, and the main mass of the tumor is removed. As the dissection proceeds forward and medially, the basilar artery and sixth cranial nerves are identified anterosuperiorly. The vertebral arteries appear posteroinferiorly. The tumor capsule is removed from these vessels and their major tributaries under direct vision. In tumors extending across the midline, the basilar artery and its major branches can be dissected posteriorly off the tumor capsule. When the lesion is removed in this fashion, the cranial nerves and the internal auditory canal in the opposite cerebellopontine angle come into view.

Closure

After the tumor has been removed, hemostasis is secured. The dura is reapproximated, and the facial nerve is freed and reflected forward. The eustachian tube orifice is plugged with Surgicel, bone wax, and bone paté. Abdominal fat is used to fill the mastoid and skull base defect, as well as to form a bed for the facial nerve. The postauricular incision is closed in three layers, and a compressive dressing is placed securely about the head. Lumbar drainage may be instituted and continued for 5 days.

POSTOPERATIVE CARE

The patient is observed in the intensive care unit for 48 hours after surgery and remains in the hospital for 7 days. Steroids are continued for 48 hours, but antibiotics are not routinely continued after the perioperative period. Early mobilization and ambulation allow for speedy return of balance.

RESULTS

In 1982, De La Cruz[1] reviewed the results of 16 patients in whom the transcochlear approach was used. A combination transcochlear–middle fossa approach was used in the three cases involving dumbbell-shaped tumors in both the posterior and middle cranial fossae. Total tumor removal was possible in 13 of the 16 patients. Each of the other three patients had had surgery elsewhere and presented with large recurrent meningiomas and extensive neurologic deficits preoperatively. During the transcochlear approach, scraps of tumor were left behind on the vertebral artery in two of these cases. None of these patients has had tumor recurrence.

Four patients had facial paresis or twitch preoperatively; of the other 12, four had permanent facial pa-

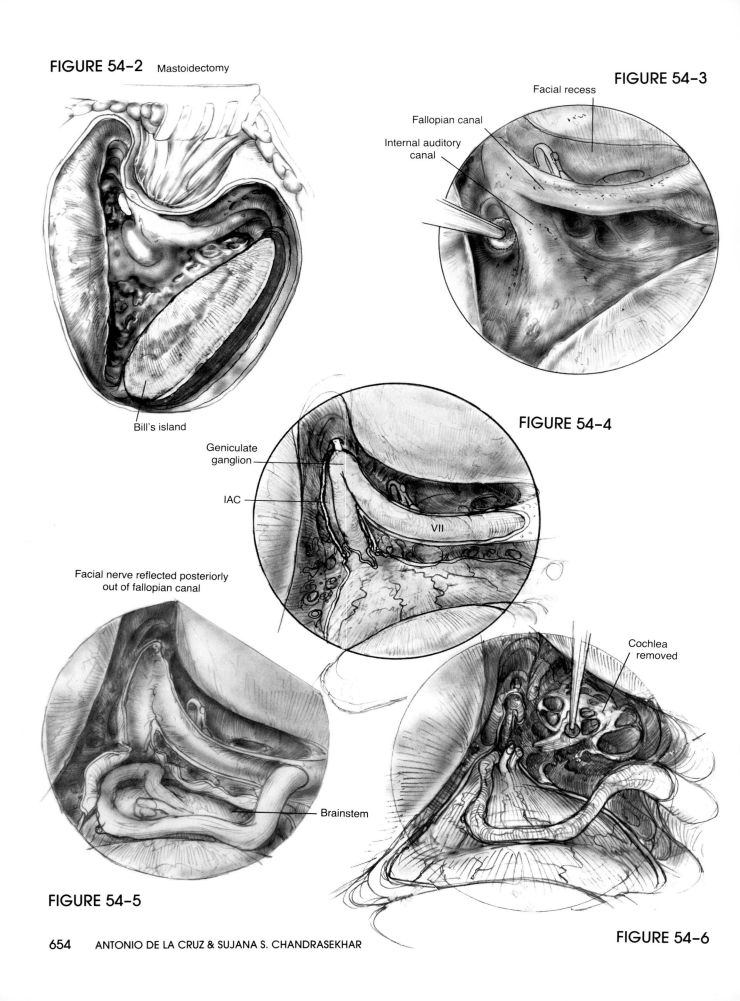

FIGURE 54-2 Mastoidectomy

Bill's island

FIGURE 54-3

Facial recess

Fallopian canal

Internal auditory
canal

Facial recess

FIGURE 54-4

Geniculate
ganglion

IAC

VII

Facial nerve reflected posteriorly
out of fallopian canal

Brainstem

Cochlea
removed

FIGURE 54-5

FIGURE 54-6

FIGURE 54-7

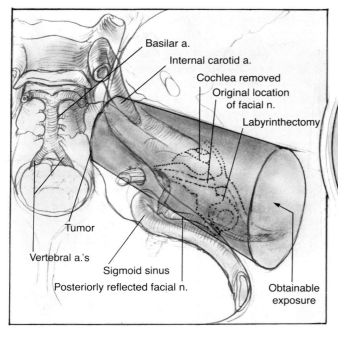

Basilar a.

Internal carotid a.

Cochlea removed

Original location of facial n.

Labyrinthectomy

Tumor

Vertebral a.'s

Sigmoid sinus

Posteriorly reflected facial n.

Obtainable exposure

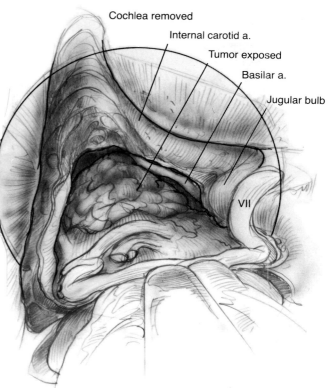

Cochlea removed

Internal carotid a.

Tumor exposed

Basilar a.

Jugular bulb

VII

FIGURE 54-8

FIGURE 54-2. Transcochlear approach: mastoidectomy. There is wide exposure of the posterior and middle fossa dura, with identification of the bony labyrinth and skeletonization of the sigmoid sinus, preserving Bill's island over the dome.

FIGURE 54-3. Transcochlear approach: exposure of the internal auditory canal (IAC), skeletonization of the facial nerve from the IAC to the stylomastoid foramen, and extended facial recess. The labyrinthectomy has been completed.

FIGURE 54-4. Transcochlear approach: the bone over the facial nerve is removed. At this point, the greater superficial petrosal nerve (GSPN) will be sectioned.

FIGURE 54-5. Transcochlear approach: location of the facial nerve after it is completely reflected posteriorly out of the bony fallopian canal.

FIGURE 54-6. Transcochlear approach: cochlear drill-out.

FIGURE 54-7. Transcochlear approach: exposure obtained at the skull base at the completion of the approach.

FIGURE 54-8. Transcochlear approach: tumor removal.

ralysis due to tumor involvement of the nerve, and seven had temporary paresis with good-to-excellent recovery of facial function. This paresis was attributed primarily to the excessive manipulation necessary for total tumor removal, and these patients were operated on before facial nerve monitoring was available.

Two deaths occurred in this series. One individual had bleeding from the vertebral artery 1 week postoperatively, requiring clipping of the vessel, with subsequent infarction of the brainstem; the other was diabetic and succumbed 1 month postoperatively to gram-negative shock from pyelonephritis. He was one of the patients reported as having a "permanent" facial paralysis. Autopsy revealed no evidence of residual tumor on the facial nerve or elsewhere.

A comparison to the report by Yamakawa et al.[10] of results with the suboccipital approach reveals subtotal tumor removal in 17 of 29 patients with intracranial epidermoids and tumor recurrence in seven patients. One of 14 patients with cerebellopontine angle tumors had postoperative seventh nerve paralysis, six had abducens palsy, four had dysphagia, and two had deafness.

The report by Yasargil et al.[12] published in the same year analyzed results in 43 patients, 35 with epidermoid tumors and the rest with intracranial dermoid tumors. No recurrences were seen. Aseptic meningitis and transient cranial nerve palsies were the most common complications. Two deaths were reported.

COMPLICATIONS AND THEIR MANAGEMENT

Temporary facial nerve paresis is the most common complication. If facial paresis occurs, prompt eye care is essential: adequate lubrication with drops, nighttime ointments, and a moisture shield prevents ocular complications. Unless the facial nerve has been severed, surgical intervention for facial reanimation is not indicated. The best approach in individuals with even complete facial paralysis after transcochlear surgery, if the facial nerve is anatomically intact, is eye care and "watchful waiting" because the great majority of these patients recover to an acceptable grade of facial function within the first year after surgery.

Other cranial nerve palsies may occur and should be addressed individually. The neurotologist must attain a good working relationship not only with a neurosurgeon but also with an ophthalmologist and a laryngologist, to help in the management of these cranial nerve deficits.

Intracranial bleeding is controlled at the time of surgery. Close observation of the patient in the intensive care unit for the initial 48 hours postoperatively allows early recognition of a delayed postoperative intracranial hemorrhage. In these cases, treatment consists of immediate reopening of the surgical wound and removal of the fat in the intensive care unit while the operating room is being prepared, and then operative evacuation of the hematoma and control of the bleeding site or sites.

Meningitis is not unusual after complete excision of intracranial epidermoids,[12, 13] and the incidence increases when the tumor capsule is left in place.[14] Meningitis may be fatal if it is infectious and requires aggressive antibiotic therapy. More commonly, however, it is a chemical meningitis, and the patient is treated with dexamethasone. Normal-pressure hydrocephalus can occur and is treated with acetazolamide (Diamox). Postoperative pain is not as severe as that seen with the suboccipital approach and is managed adequately with oral analgesics.

With this approach, tumor recurrence is rare when all of the visible tumor has been removed. Patients with recurrences do not present typically and may have vague complaints of unsteadiness or trigeminal neuropathy several years after the initial resection.[1] Biannual follow-up with gadolinium-enhanced MRI is necessary. In cases of suspected tumor regrowth or recurrence, complete re-evaluation is performed, and removal of the recurrent tumor is advised.

SUMMARY

Access to midline intracranial lesions, intradural clival tumors, and cerebellopontine angle tumors arising anterior to the internal auditory canal has been difficult. The transcochlear approach mobilizes the facial nerve, removes the cochlea, and dissects the internal carotid artery, allowing direct exposure of these lesions and of midline and contralateral structures. Total removal of the tumor and its base and blood supply is accomplished with this approach. The transcochlear approach is recommended for these lesions in patients with poor or no hearing. Its safety and efficacy encourage its use.

References

1. De La Cruz A: The transcochlear approach to meningiomas and cholesteatomas of the cerebellopontine angle. *In* Brackmann DE (ed): Neurological Surgery of the Ear and Skull Base. New York, Raven Press, 1982, pp 353–360.
2. House WF, De La Cruz A: Transcochlear approach to the petrous apex and clivus. Trans Am Acad Ophthalmol Otolaryngol 84: 927–931, 1977.
3. House WF, Hitselberger WE: The transcochlear approach to the skull base. Arch Otolaryngol Head Neck Surg 102: 334–342, 1976.
4. Hitselberger WE, Horn KL, Hankinson H, et al: The middle fossa transpetrous approach for petroclival meningiomas. Skull Base Surg 3(3): 130–135, 1993.

5. Shiobara R, Ohira T, Kanzaki J, Toya S: A modified extended middle cranial fossa approach for acoustic nerve tumors: Results of 125 operations. J Neurosurg 68: 358–365, 1988.
6. Wigand ME, Haid T, Berg M: The enlarged middle cranial fossa approach for surgery of the temporal bone and of the cerebellopontine angle. Arch Otol Rhinol Laryngol 246: 299, 1989.
7. Brackmann DE, Anderson RG: Cholesteatomas of the cerebellopontine angle. In Silverstein H, Norrell H (eds): Neurological Surgery of the Ear. 1979, pp 340–344.
8. De La Cruz A, Doyle KJ: Congenital epidermoids of the petrous apex. In Jackler RA, Brackmann DE (eds): Neurotology. York, PA, Spectrum [In press].
9. Nager GT: Epidermoids involving the temporal bone: Clinical, radiological, and pathological aspects. Laryngoscope 2(Suppl): 1–22, 1975.
10. Yamakawa K, Shitara N, Genka S, et al: Clinical course and surgical prognosis of 33 cases of intracranial epidermoid tumors. Neurosurgery 24(4): 568–573, 1989.
11. Mafee MF: MRI and CT in the evaluation of acquired and congenital cholesteatomas of the temporal bone. J Otolaryngol 22(4): 239–248, 1993.
12. Yasargil MG, Abernathy CD, Sarioglu AC: Microneurosurgical treatment of intracranial dermoid and epidermoid tumors. Neurosurgery 24(4): 561–567, 1989.
13. Cantu RC, Ojemann RG: Glucosteroid treatment of keratin meningitis following removal of a fourth ventricle epidermoid tumor. J Neurol Neurosurg Psychiatry 31: 75, 1968.
14. Guidetti B, Gagliardi FM: Epidermoid and dermoid cysts. J Neurosurg 47: 12–18, 1977.
15. De La Cruz A: Transcochlear approach to lesions of the cerebellopontine angle and clivus. Rev Laryngol Otol Rhinol (Bord) 102(1–2): 33–36, 1981.

55

The Middle Fossa Transpetrous Approach for Access to the Petroclival Region (Extended Middle Fossa Approach)

KARL L. HORN, M.D.

HAL HANKINSON, M.D.

WILLIAM E. HITSELBERGER, M.D.

Removal of petroclival neoplasms remains one of the most formidable challenges to skull base surgeons for numerous reasons. Lesions of the petrous apex and clivus are uncommon, and this region is not commonly frequented by either neurotologists or neurosurgeons. The nuances of surgical anatomy are therefore less familiar to most surgeons than other regions of the skull base that are more commonly involved with pathologic processes. Access to lesions of the petroclival region through any surgical approach is difficult because of interposed vital structures, including the cerebellum, brainstem, cranial nerves, vascular structures, and temporal bone. Surgical approaches to this area require the surgeon to make difficult decisions about working around these structures or removing vital structures to improve exposure. These difficulties have led to the use of numerous surgical approaches to the petroclival region.

SURGICAL APPROACHES TO THE PETROCLIVAL REGION

For many years, the petroclival area has been approached through the conventional suboccipital craniotomy. In this procedure, the surgeon's view of the petrous tip and clivus is obscured by the brain stem, branches of the anteroinferior cerebellar artery, and cranial nerves 5 through 9. Overhanging cerebellum requires at least minimal retraction, and the surgeon must work at an uncomfortable distance from the lesion.

Although midline transclival approaches have proved helpful for extradural tumors, these procedures have limitations for intradural lesions.[1] The surgeon must work at a considerable distance from the operative field once the tumor is exposed. Tumor manipulation is difficult because of the restricted surgical field. Hemostasis and cerebrospinal fluid leakage are difficult to manage, and the potential for postoperative meningitis is significant.

The infratemporal approach offers excellent exposure of structures inferior to the otic capsule, but exposure of the clivus requires removal of the otic capsule, displacement of the internal carotid artery, or both. This procedure always requires rerouting of the facial nerve and obliteration of the middle ear.[2]

The widest exposure of the petroclival area is provided by the transcochlear approach, which is an anterior extension of the translabyrinthine approach. In this exposure, bone removal is carried anterior to the internal auditory canal after rerouting of the facial nerve posteriorly and removing the cochlea. In its modified form, the complete petrous apex is removed, and dissection may be continued into the clivus.[3] The major advantage of this approach is wide exposure of

the cerebellopontine angle and the petroclival area. The major disadvantages to this technique are unilateral deafness and transient facial weakness.

The disadvantages of hearing loss and transient facial weakness have led several authors to avoid removal of the otic capsule. The petrosal approach extends the retrolabyrinthine or presigmoid approach by transection of the superior petrosal sinus and the tentorium.[4] This approach provides wide exposure of the petroclival region but often obviates removal of bone that may be involved with tumor. The subtemporal-preauricular infratemporal approach provides removal of bone of the petrous apex and clivus; however, it entails removal of the carotid artery from its bony canal, transection of the eustachian tube, and often, removal of the mandibular condyle.[5] Spetzler et al. recently organized many of these concepts into three supratentorial and infratentorial approaches in which the superior petrosal sinus and tentorium are always cut.[6] The amount of bone removed varies and may include retrolabyrinthine, translabyrinthine, or transcochlear techniques. Ligation and section of the sigmoid sinus may be done when deemed necessary and safe.

Although all of these techniques may be used to approach petroclival lesions, they are formidible procedures that may not be required for lesions anterior to the internal auditory canal. The middle fossa transpetrous approach, which is more anteriorly centered than most other techniques, provides access to the petroclival region anterior to the internal auditory canal and requires removal of few if any vital structures. This technique is a modification of the middle fossa approach that has been used for many years in acoustic tumor surgery. Most of the anatomy and technique are therefore familiar to skull base surgeons.

In 1931, Eagleton was the first to approach the petroclival region through a middle fossa transpetrous approach.[7] However, interest in this approach has been renewed only recently by Kawase et al. and House et al.[8, 9] In the middle fossa transpetrous approach, the anterior cerebellopontine angle is entered through a middle fossa or subtemporal craniotomy by removal of bone medial to the petrous carotid artery and cochlea. Kawase et al. used this approach for access to lower basilar aneurysms in two patients, whereas House et al. used the approach for removal of a fifth-nerve schwannoma in one patient and petroclival meningioma in a second patient. The roughly triangular area of bone removed medial to the carotid artery has become known as Kawase's triangle.

SURGICAL ANATOMY

The underlying principle of the operation described in this chapter is to provide access to the posterior fossa through a middle fossa approach. This concept is not new and has been used in acoustic tumor surgery for many years. This technique differs from the traditional and more recently discussed widened middle fossa techniques for acoustic tumor surgery by virtue of its anterior dissection.[10–12] In the middle fossa transpetrous technique, the petrous apex anterior to the internal auditory canal and medial to the carotid artery is removed (Fig. 55–1). The opening into the anterior portion of the posterior fossa may be significantly enlarged by transection of the tentorium over the area of petrous bone removal. A sound understanding of the anatomy of the petrous apex and the tentorium attached to the petrous apex is necessary to safely perform this procedure.

PETROUS APEX

As noted by Paullus et al. and others, the petrous apex has both superior (middle fossa) and posterior (posterior fossa) surfaces.[13–15] The tentorium is attached to the temporal bone at the angle of intersection of these two surfaces. The superior petrosal sinus runs in a sulcus along the edge of the petrous bone roughly at the angle of intersection of the superior and posterior surfaces in the area of dural attachment.

The superior surface of the petrous apex forms the posterior medial floor of the middle fossa. The petrosquamous suture separates the petrous and squamous portions of the temporal bone and is often a site of dural attachment to the middle fossa floor. The most important clinical significance of the petrosquamous suture line is its relationship to the greater superficial petrosal nerve. The greater superficial petrosal nerve is always medial to the petrosquamosal suture and runs in a groove on the superior surface of the petrous apex from the facial hiatus toward the foramen lacerum.

The arcuate eminence lies posterior to the facial hiatus, and the bone between these two structures overlies the internal auditory canal. Fisch and Mattox have termed this surface of bone the *meatal plane*.[16] Anterior and lateral to the greater superficial petrosal nerve is the foramen spinosum and the middle meningial artery. Anterior and medial to the foramen spinosum is the foramen of ovale for the third division of the trigeminal nerve. The foramen ovale represents the most anterior portion of surgical dissection for the middle fossa transpetrous approach. A line connecting the foramen spinosum and the foramen ovale is parallel to the horizontal petrous carotid artery.

The posterior surface of the petrous bone is roughly triangular in shape. Anterior to the internal auditory canal, this surface is bounded above by the superior petrosal sinus and the tentorium. Inferiorly, this triangle is bounded by the inferior petrosal sinus and

the petro-occipital synchondrosis. Anterior to the internal auditory canal, no structures pass through the dura on the posterior surface of the petrous apex.

Within the petrous apex anterior to the internal auditory canal are two important structures: the cochlea and the internal carotid artery. The basal turn of the cochlea lies beneath the geniculate ganglion and the labyrinthine segment of the facial nerve. The posterior loop of the petrous carotid artery is anterior to the cochlea, and the basal turn is usually separated from the artery by 1mm to 2mm of bone. The course of the greater superficial petrosal nerve on the floor of the middle cranial fossa is roughly parallel to the course of the horizontal petrous carotid artery within the petrous apex.

TENTORIUM

The tentorium is attached to the petrous ridge, posterior clinoid process, and anterior clinoid process. Transection and retraction of the tentorium above the area of petrous bone removal greatly improves the exposure of the middle fossa transpetrous approach. Several structures are in close relationship to the tentorium in this area. The most significant structure is the petrosal vein (Dandy's vein), which usually enters the superior petrosal sinus just posterior to Meckel's cave. However, the site of entry of the petrosal vein into the superior petrosal sinus is variable, and it may be inadvertently injured as the tentorium and superior petrosal sinus are sectioned.[17] In addition, the tentorium may be laced with a plexus of otherwise unnamed veins that may complicate section of the structure.

The tentorium receives arterial supply from several sources. In approximately one quarter of cases, the superior cerebellar artery sends a branch to the undersurface of the free edge of the tentorium.[18] Such a vessel may be encountered as the tentorium is divided above the anterior petrous ridge.

The trochlear nerve enters the free edge of the tentorium in the posterior portion the oculomotor trigone. Although the nerve is not in the tentorium that is sectioned above the petrous apex, this nerve may be injured as the anterior dural leaf is retracted for exposure. The extended course and delicate nature of the trochlear nerve make it particularly susceptible to injury. The trigeminal nerve is less vulnerable but may be injured by injudicious trauma caused by such procedures as cautery.

SURGICAL TECHNIQUE

The patient is placed in the supine position and given general anesthesia. Electrodes for monitoring the sixth and seventh cranial nerves are inserted. The hemicranium is shaved, the skin is cleaned with povidone-iodine (Betadine), and self-adhering plastic drapes are applied. The incision begins at the tragal notch and extends 7cm to 8cm anterosuperiorly (Fig. 55–2). The plane between the skin and temporalis fascia is developed with blunt dissection. The temporalis fascia is opened, and the exposed temporalis muscle is reflected inferiorly over the zygomatic arch. We have not found it necessary to transect the zygomatic arch to improve exposure or to displace the temporalis muscle out of the field. A self-retaining retractor is placed beneath the remaining temporalis muscle, exposing the squamous temporal bone. A 3cm × 5cm bone flap is removed, thereby exposing the temporal dura (Fig. 55–3). The craniotomy is located two thirds anterior and one third posterior to the external auditory canal. Bone is removed to the floor of the middle cranial fossa with rongeurs and drill. Hyperventilation, osmotics, and spinal drainage are used when appropriate.

The dura is elevated from the floor of the middle cranial fossa by posterior-to-anterior dissection. This direction of dissection is used to avoid injury to an exposed geniculate ganglion or inadvertent elevation of the greater superficial petrosal nerve with resultant traction of the facial nerve. The dura is firmly adherent to the petrosquamosal suture and may require cauterization and sharp dissection. The greater petrosal nerve is medial to this structure. The temporal lobe is elevated with a self-retaining retractor.

The middle meningeal artery, the greater superficial nerve, and the arcuate eminence are identified (Fig. 55–4). A diamond burr is used to expose the geniculate ganglion and to blue line the superior semicircular canal. The labyrinthine segment of the facial nerve is followed into the fundus of the internal auditory canal (Fig. 55–5). The internal auditory canal is skeletonized but not opened. The middle meningeal artery is clipped or cauterized at the foramen spinosum and transected. The third division of the trigeminal nerve (V3) is identified at the foramen ovale, which lies anteromedial to the foramen spinosum.

Bone within Glasscock's triangle is removed (Fig. 55–6). This triangle is bordered laterally by a line from the arcuate eminence to the foramen spinosum, anteriorly by the third division of the fifth nerve, and medially by the groove for the greater superficial petrosal nerve. The greater superficial petrosal nerve lies over the horizontal petrous carotid artery. The nerve is sacrificed to prevent traction of the geniculate ganglion and to allow wide exposure of the carotid artery. The horizontal petrous carotid artery is skeletonized from the posterior loop to V3. Dissection should not be extended behind the posterior loop of the internal carotid artery, because of close proximity of the cochlea. Dissection may be extended medial to V3 by transection of the nerve or by bone removal from the anterolateral foramen ovale and mobilization of V3 anterolaterally.

Removal of bone medial to the horizontal carotid canal and cochlea is continued inferiorly to the level of the inferior petrosal sinus (Kawase's triangle). The posterior fossa dura has thus been exposed from the internal auditory canal to Meckel's cave and from the superior petrosal sinus above to the inferior petrosal sinus below. The dura is opened through an inferiorly based flap.

The dissection may be extended medially into the clivus by transection of the inferior petrosal sinus in the petro-occipital synchondrosis. Dissection above the level of the tentorium may be accomplished by transection of the superior petrosal sinus and tentorium. This is performed by an incision in the middle fossa dura just lateral to the superior petrosal sinus from the internal auditory canal to the third root of the trigeminal nerve. The superior petrosal sinus is clipped or coagulated, and the tentorium is transected in the midportion of this incision (Fig. 55–7). Special care is taken to avoid injury to the petrosal vein or trochlear nerve. The tumor is debulked with mechanical techniques or the fiberoptic argon laser. After tumor removal, the defect is obliterated with abdominal adipose tissue, and the bone flap is wired in place. The wound is closed in layers.

FIGURE 55–1. Skull base from above showing area of petroclival bone removal.

FIGURE 55–2. Skin incision extending from tragus 7cm to 8cm superiorly.

FIGURE 55–3. Reflection of temporalis muscle flap and 3cm × 5cm craniotomy.

FIGURE 55–4. Elevation of dura from middle fossa floor with identification of the middle meningeal artery, greater petrosal nerve, and arcuate eminence.

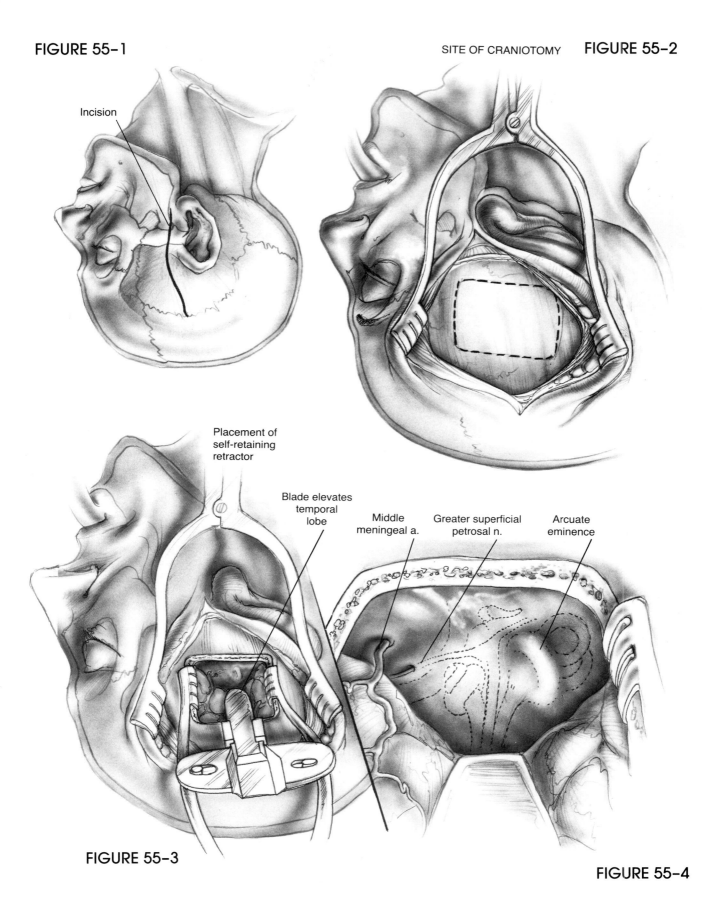

FIGURE 55-1

Incision

Placement of
self-retaining
retractor

Blade elevates
temporal
lobe

Middle
meningeal a.

Greater superficial
petrosal n.

Arcuate
eminence

FIGURE 55-3

FIGURE 55-4

FIGURE 55-5

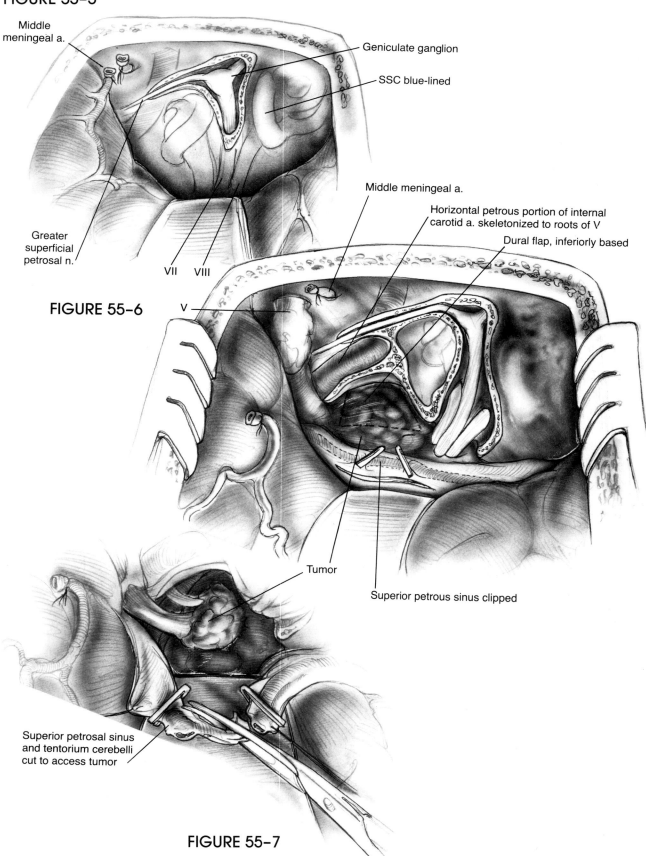

Middle meningeal a.

Geniculate ganglion

SSC blue-lined

Greater superficial petrosal n.

VII VIII

FIGURE 55-6

Middle meningeal a.

Horizontal petrous portion of internal carotid a. skeletonized to roots of V

Dural flap, inferiorly based

V

Tumor

Superior petrous sinus clipped

Superior petrosal sinus and tentorium cerebelli cut to access tumor

FIGURE 55-7

MIDDLE FOSSA TRANSPETROUS APPROACH

The middle fossa transpetrous approach has been used for removal of petroclival neoplasms and for access to basilar artery aneurysms.[19, 20] Large meningiomas have been removed through this approach by us and others.[19, 20] The technically limiting factor of this procedure is not tumor size alone. Indeed, tumors extending well across the midline and above the anterior tentorial incisura have been removed through this approach. However, because hearing preservation is a primary objective of the procedure, dissection is limited anatomically by the internal auditory canal. Lesions that extend posterior to the internal auditory canal require use of different technique, such as the transcochlear approach, or the addition of second technique, such as the suboccipital or extended retrolabyrinthine approaches. The addition of other surgical approaches to the middle fossa transpetrous approach may result in removal of considerable bone anterior, inferior, and posterior to the otic capsule and middle ear without loss of hearing or facial nerve function.

The most significant disadvantage of the middle fossa transpetrous approach is the frequent necessity of transecting the third division of the fifth nerve for bone removal at the petrous tip. Except for numbness of the chin, transection of this nerve has caused little functional disability. Another disadvantage to this technique is temporal lobe retraction. Although not reported by other authors, we have seen one patient with temporary expressive aphasia that was attributed to temporal lobe retraction.

References

1. Miller E, Crockard HA: Transoral transclival removal of anteriorly placed meningiomas at the foramen magnum. Neurosurgery 20: 966–968, 1987.
2. Fisch U, Pillsbury HC: Infratemporal fossa approach to lesions in the temporal bone and base of the skull. Arch Otolaryngol Head Neck Surg 105: 99–107, 1979.
3. Horn KL, Hankinson HL, Erasmus MD, et al.: The modified transcochlear approach to the cerebellopontine angle. Otolaryngol Head Neck Surg 104: 37–41, 1991.
4. Al-Mefty O, Fox JL, Smith RR: Petrosal approach for petroclival meningiomas. Neurosurgery 22: 510–517, 1988.
5. Sekhar LN, Schramm VL, Jones NF: Subtemporal-preauricular infratemporal fossa approach to large lateral and posterior cranial base neoplasms. J Neurosurg 67: 488–499, 1987.
6. Spetzler RF, Daspit CP, Pappas CTE: Combined approach for lesions involving the cerebellopontine angle and skull base: Experience with 30 cases. Skull Base Surg 1: 226–234, 1991.
7. Eagleton WP: Unlocking the petrous pyramid for localized bulbar (pontile) meningitis secondary to suppuration of the petrous apex. Arch Otolaryngol Head Neck Surg 13: 386–422, 1931.
8. Kawase T, Toya S, Shiobara R, et al.: Transpetrosal approach for aneurysms of the lower basilar artery. J Neurosurg 63: 857–861, 1985.
9. House WF, Hitselberger WE, Horn KL: The middle fossa transpetrous approach to the anterior-superior cerebellopontine angle. Am J Otol 7: 1–4, 1986.
10. House WF: Surgical exposure of the internal auditory canal and its contents through the middle cranial fossa. Laryngoscope 71: 1363–1385, 1961.
11. House WF: Middle cranial fossa approach to the petrous pyramid: A report of 50 cases. Arch Otolaryngol Head Neck Surg 78: 406–469, 1963.
12. Wigand ME, Haid T, Berg M, et al.: Extended middle cranial fossa approach for acoustic neuroma surgery. Skull Base Surg 1: 183–187, 1991.
13. Paullus WS, Pait TG, Rhoton AL: Microsurgical exposure of the petrous portion of the carotid artery. J Neurosurg 47: 713–726, 1977.
14. Leonitti JP, Smith PG, Linthicum FH: The petrous carotid artery: Anatomic relationships in skull base surgery. Otolaryngol Head Neck Surg 102: 3–12, 1990.
15. Andrews JC, Martin NA, Black K, et al.: Middle cranial fossa transtemporal approach to the intrapetrous internal carotid artery. Skull Base Surg 1: 142–146, 1991.
16. Fisch U, Mattox D: Microsurgery of the Skull Base. New York, Thieme Medical Publishers, 1988.
17. Lang J: Clinical Anatomy of the Posterior Cranial Fossa and Its Foramina. New York, Thieme Medical Publishers, 1988.
18. Ono M, Ono M, Rhoton AL, et al.: Microsurgical anatomy of the region of the tentorial incisura. J Neurosurg 60: 365–399, 1984.
19. Pensak ML, Lovern HV, Keith RW: Subtemporal transpetrosal approach to the petrous apex. Presented at the American Otological Society, 125th Meeting. Marriott Desert Springs Resort, Palm Desert, CA, April 12 and 13, 1992.
20. Velut S, Jan M: Anterior petrosectomy during approach to the petroclival area. In Schmidek HH (ed): Meningiomas and Their Surgical Management. Philadelphia, WB Saunders, 1991, pp 435–450.
21. Hitselberger WE, Horn KL, Hankinson HL, et al.: The middle fossa transpetrous approach for petroclival meningiomas. Skull Base Surg 3:130–135, 1993.

FIGURE 55-5. Identification of the geniculate ganglion and facial nerve.

FIGURE 55-6. Removal of bone anterior to the internal auditory canal and medial to the internal carotid artery.

FIGURE 55-7. Transection of the tentorium.

56

The Lateral Infratemporal Fossa Approaches

DOUGLAS E. MATTOX, M.D.

If it were not for the facial nerve passing through the temporal bone and arborizing in the face, lateral approaches to the skull base would have been devised decades ago. Several recent surgical technical advances have led to rapid proliferation of approaches to the lateral skull base. The realization that the facial nerve could be mobilized out of the fallopian canal without significant postoperative facial morbidity was seminal in the development of lateral approaches.[1] Second, techniques were developed to reflect the upper branches of the facial nerve with the attached muscles, which allows access to the skull base without paralysis of the upper part of the face.[2] Third, the concept that large segments of facial bone can be removed and replaced has simplified access and reconstruction. Last, the advent of reliable microvascular free flaps has been invaluable in the safe reconstruction of defects that risk confluence or contamination of the intracranial cavity with the paranasal sinuses or nasopharynx.[3]

Approaching skull base tumors laterally has several advantages, including wide exposure of the infratemporal fossa and identification of the carotid artery proximal to the lesion, allowing it to be traced as it passes into the tumor and controlled if hemorrhage occurs.

The objective of this chapter is to present a graded series of progressively more radical approaches to the lateral skull base with illustrative examples.

PATIENT SELECTION

Patients with tumors of the infratemporal fossa extending to the parasellar region, cavernous sinus, clivus, and lateral nasopharynx are candidates for lateral approaches. Small midline lesions are best handled with anterior midfacial approaches. Generally accepted signs that a malignant tumor is unresectable include multiple cranial nerve palsies or cavernous sinus invasion.

PREOPERATIVE PREPARATION

Preoperative consultation should be obtained from all potential members of the skull base team, including the neurosurgeon, neurophthalmologist, otolaryngology and head and neck surgery specialist, plastic and reconstructive surgeon, general surgeon, radiation oncologist, and anesthesiologist. Preoperative pulmonary, cardiac, and nutritional status should also be evaluated and problems corrected well in advance of the surgery.

Preoperative evaluation almost always includes imaging with both computed tomography (for bone margins and destruction) and magnetic resonance (for soft tissue margins). Arteriography, with embolization when appropriate, is necessary to define the blood supply of the tumor and occlude its major feeding vessels. In cases in which occlusion, injury, or resection of the internal carotid artery are likely, preoperative carotid occlusion with neurologic evaluation, electroencephalography, or cerebral blood flow studies are imperative to assess the patient's ability to tolerate carotid sacrifice.[4, 5] When carotid sacrifice is certain, preoperative permanent balloon occlusion of the carotid is preferred to intraoperative resection because the patient can be kept in better hemodynamic balance, monitored, and evaluated without postsurgical neurologic deficits and other confounding variables introduced by the surgery.

The patient should be fully informed of the objectives, benefits, and potential risks of these massive surgical undertakings. It should be made clear to the patient if there is a real chance for "cure" of the lesion or if the procedure is palliative for the relief of pain or mass effect or is prophylactic, for instance, to prevent compression of a remaining optic nerve. The potential risks of this kind of surgery are so overwhelming that one can question if any individual outside the field can truly give informed consent, but the neurologic, functional, and cosmetic risks must be carefully explained to the patient, and all questions must be answered.

INFRATEMPORAL FOSSA TYPE A APPROACH

The infratemporal fossa type A approach was the first lateral approach to the skull base (Fig. 56–1). It was designed primarily for resection of lesions in the inferior portion of the temporal bone, primarily the jugular bulb.[1] The major impediment to surgery of the jugular bulb is the facial nerve, which crosses the center of the bulb just a few millimeters lateral to it. In the type A approach, the facial nerve is elevated from the fallopian canal from the geniculate ganglion to the stylomastoid foramen. The nerve is permanently transposed anteriorly, giving unobstructed access to the sigmoid sinus, jugular bulb, and carotid artery (Fig. 56–2). A drawback of this approach is that the middle ear is sacrificed and the external auditory canal is permanently closed, resulting in a permanent conductive hearing loss.

The type A approach is most commonly used for glomus jugulare tumors. It can also be used for cholesteatomas and cholesterol cysts of the petrous apex and for neuromas of cranial nerves 9, 10, 11, and 12 in the jugular foramen. It is described in detail in Chapter 49.

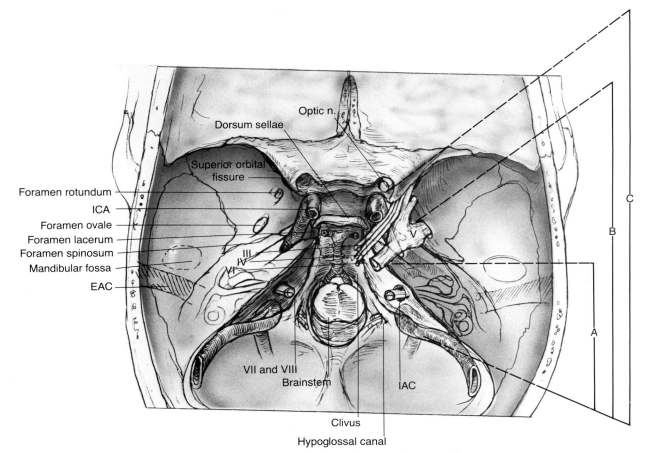

FIGURE 56-1. The different exposures obtained with the Fisch types A, B, and C approaches to the infratemporal fossa.

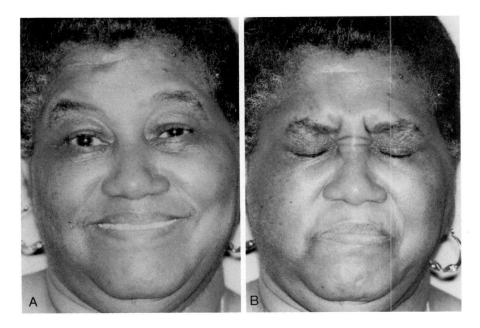

FIGURE 56-2. *A-B*, A 62-year-old patient 1 month after a Fisch infratemporal type A approach. Note the facial symmetry and function. Her immediate postoperative facial function was the same as shown here.

INFRATEMPORAL FOSSA TYPES B AND C APPROACHES

Type B

The Fisch type B approach is applicable to lesions of the petrous apex (apical cholesteatoma and cholesterol cyst) and for lesions of the clivus (chordomas). It differs from the type A approach in that the facial nerve is left in situ in its fallopian canal and is *not* transposed. Exposure is obtained by reflecting the zygomatic arch and temporalis muscle inferiorly and removing bone of the lateral skull base to provide access to the infratemporal fossa (Fig. 56–3). In rare instances in which a lesion also involves the jugular foramen area or the cervical spine, a combined type A and type B approach can be performed. In this situation, the facial nerve must be transposed forward and backward during the procedure, depending on the surgical area being exposed.[6]

A wide postauricular incision is used, and the superior limb can extend all the way to the eyebrow if needed for anterior exposure. The inferior limb is extended into the neck for the control of the great vessels. The external auditory canal is permanently closed as a blind sac. The ear is reflected forward, and the soft tissues are dissected from the anterior surface of the remaining cartilaginous external auditory canal, tympanic bone, and stylomastoid suture line. The main trunk of the facial nerve is identified and followed to its bifurcation. The portion of the facial nerve in greatest jeopardy in the type B approach is the frontal branch; therefore, to protect it, the upper branches of the facial nerve are followed from the bifurcation over the zygomatic arch until they disappear into the facial musculature. Because the nerve is kept in direct vision, it can be protected when the temporalis muscle and zygomatic arch are reflected inferiorly.

The frontal branch of the facial nerve is gently pulled below the body of the zygomatic arch, and the periosteum is divided and retracted until the bone is fully exposed from its origin over the external auditory canal to the orbital process. The arch is divided as far anteriorly and posteriorly as possible. Drill holes may be made in the anterior arch for rewiring at the end of the procedure. The attachments of the masseter muscle along the inferior border of the zygomatic arch are left undisturbed to provide a secure vascular supply for the bone. The zygomatic arch is reflected inferiorly over the frontal branch of the facial nerve. Temporalis muscle is elevated from its attachments to the parietal skull and reflected inferiorly based on its attachment to the mandible.

The tympanic and mastoid air cell system is completely exenterated (subtotal petrosectomy). This procedure includes removal of the external auditory canal skin, tympanic membrane, malleus, and incus, and total exenteration of all pneumatic cell tracks within the tympanomastoid space. The facial nerve is identified within its fallopian canal, but a thin layer of protective bone is left over the nerve. The vertical segment of the internal carotid artery identified in the anterior middle ear space is followed as it passes medial to the eustachian tube.

The entire anterior and inferior tympanic ring is removed down to the level of the eustachian tube. The ligamentous attachments of the condyle to the glenoid fossa are incised. For additional room, the articular disk of the temporal mandibular joint can be removed. Once these attachments are fully removed, the infratemporal fossa retractor can be inserted over the mandibular condyle and temporalis muscle. Opening the retractor will push the condyle inferiorly and provide access to the infratemporal fossa. Care must be taken that the infratemporal fossa retractor does not slip behind the condyle and exert force on the main trunk of the facial nerve.

The bone of the skull base is removed, starting at the glenoid fossa and continuing to the infratemporal fossa. This bone is quite thick, and skeletonization down to the dura will provide a significant amount of room and exposure anterior and medial to the glenoid fossa. The spinous process, middle meningeal artery, and third division of the trigeminal nerve can be identified. If exposure deep in the infratemporal fossa is needed, the artery and nerve can be coagulated with bipolar forceps and then divided. The bony and cartilaginous eustachian tube are completely removed, exposing the horizontal portion of the carotid canal as it passes through the foramen lacerum. The tensor tympani muscle can be totally removed for complete exposure.

The carotid artery can be mobilized from the ca-

FIGURE 56–3. The exposure obtained in the type B approach.

FIGURE 56–4. The area of bone removal for the infratemporal fossa approach type A. The area of bone removal in the preauricular infratemporal approaches.

FIGURE 56–3

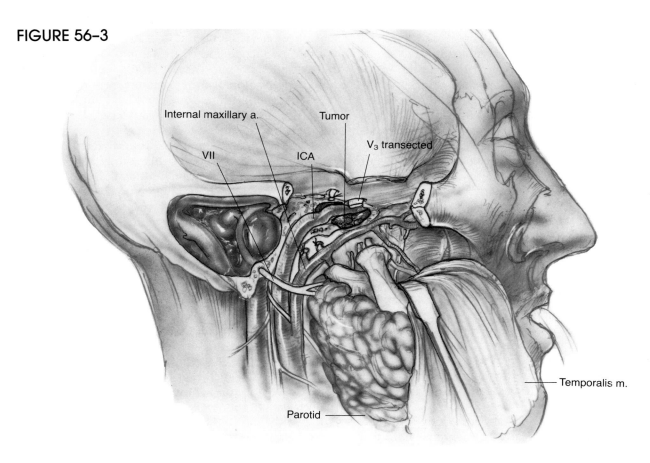

Internal maxillary a.   Tumor

VII   ICA   V₃ transected

Temporalis m.

Parotid

FIGURE 56–4

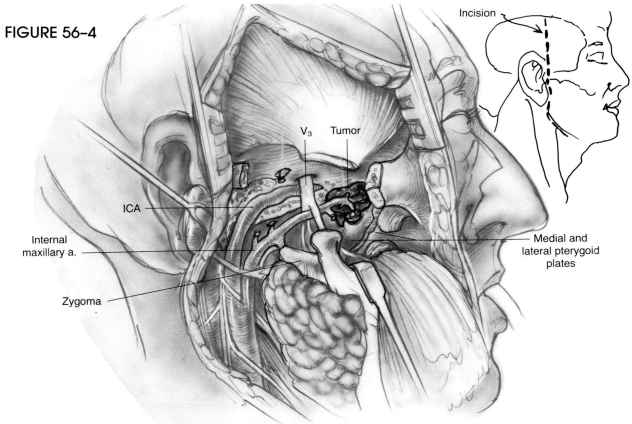

Incision

V₃   Tumor

ICA

Internal
maxillary a.

Medial and
lateral pterygoid
plates

Zygoma

rotid foramen to the foramen lacerum and reflected inferiorly and anteriorly. The combination of rerouting the facial nerve and elevating the carotid artery will expose the entire petrous apex.

The wound is closed by obliterating the cartilaginous eustachian tube with sutures and lining the cavity with a free revascularized flap or pedicled temporalis muscle graft. If additional soft tissue obliteration is required, abdominal fat can be harvested and placed in the wound. The wound is closed in layers, as previously described.

Type C

The type C approach is a logical anterior extension of the type B approach. It is used for lesions of the anterior infratemporal fossa, sella, and nasopharynx. The major modifications distinguishing the types B and C approaches are resection of the pterygoid plates, and skeletonization and possible transection of the second division of the trigeminal nerve. The lateral wall of the nasopharynx, eustachian tube orifice, posterior maxillary sinus, and posterior nasopharyngeal wall past the midline can all be resected through the type C approach.

The initial exposure is performed exactly the same as the type B approach. The facial nerve is again left in its normal anatomic position. The carotid artery is skeletonized from the carotid foramen to the foramen lacerum. The mandibular branch of the trigeminal and the middle meningeal artery are transected. The mandible, zygomatic arch, and temporalis muscle are reflected inferiorly. The lateral surface of the pterygoid process is identified, and the soft tissues are elevated from it. The base of both the medial and lateral plates of the pterygoid process are drilled away, exposing the lateral wall of the nasopharynx. The external pterygoid muscle is separated from the condylar process and removed with the residual pterygoid process. The nasal cavity can then be entered, depending on the site of the lesion. Usually, the nasopharynx is entered anteriorly just behind the maxillary sinus. The mucosa is opened and the incision continued superiorly around the eustachian tube. The entire peritubal area can then be outlined and resected en bloc. Inferiorly, the excision can be extended as far inferiorly as the upper surface of the palate. Superiorly, the dissection can be carried medially to the carotid artery to the cavernous sinus and parasellar region. The entire lateral wall of the sphenoid sinus can easily be removed in this approach. Dissection of the perasellar region can be exposed extradurally through this approach.

Closure is more difficult than in the type A or B approach because there is a wide connection between the nasopharynx and the operative site that requires closure with viable tissue. This step is performed by widely mobilizing the entire temporalis muscle and reflecting it into the wound. Partial separation from the lateral portion of the coronoid process may facilitate this mobilization; however, blood supply to the muscles must be preserved. The muscles should be sutured around the nasopharyngeal defect. If additional soft tissue obliteration is required, a vascularized free flap, ideally, the rectus abdominis, provides good soft tissue obliteration and negligible donor defect. Abdominal fat should not be used because of the risk of contamination of the wound with nasopharyngeal secretions.

DIRECT PREAURICULAR APPROACHES

In many instances, the lesion is well anterior to the middle ear, and, therefore, exenteration of the tympanomastoid space is unnecessary. Such lesions can be approached with a direct preauricular approach (Fig. 56–4).[7–9] The incision is similar to those described above, except that it is brought through the preauricular crease far enough to identify and protect the facial nerve at the stylomastoid foramen. To protect the frontal branches of the facial nerve, the soft tissue elevation of the forehead should be carried beneath the temporalis fascia. The edge of the periosteum over the zygomatic arch is divided sharply to allow elevation of the periosteum in continuity with the fascia (Figs. 56–5 and 56–6). This elevation is extended anteriorly until the entire lateral orbital rim is exposed. The zygomatic arch and lateral orbital rim can be reflected inferiorly as described earlier or can be removed en bloc and reinserted as a free graft at the end of the surgery.

Once the temporalis muscle is reflected out of the way, the attachments around the glenoid fossa can be divided and the condyle mobilized inferiorly. Deep to the mandibular condyle, the tympanic ring can be followed medially and its anterior edge drilled away to reveal the anterior portion of the carotid canal. Once identified, the carotid is followed as it turns anteriorly in the foramen lacerum. The same landmarks in the infratemporal fossa (middle meningeal, foramen ovale, eustachian tube, pterygoid plates, clivus) can be found through this approach as was described for the type B and C approaches.

LATERAL FACIAL DISASSEMBLY

More aggressive approaches to the skull base require sacrifice of some branches of the facial nerve. Although transection and reanastomosis of the main

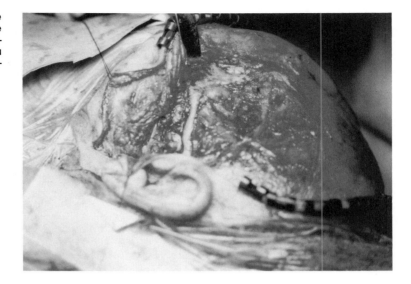

FIGURE 56-5. Intraoperative photograph showing the reflection of a bicoronal flap and exposure of the temporalis muscle and zygomatic arch. The dissection has been carried beneath the temporalis fascia to avoid trauma to the facial nerve and facial musculature.

trunk can be performed, the long-term functional results are better when the nerve branches are transected as far peripherally as possible. Arriaga and Janecka[10] described a lateral facial disassembly procedure that fits these requirements (Figs. 56–7 and 56–8). A Weber-Fergusson incision is combined with a cervical-preauricular incision to form a large, inferiorly based facial flap. The frontal branches of the facial nerve are sacrificed as the incision follows the upper margin of the zygomatic arch. These branches can be reanastomosed at the end of the procedure. Development of the skin flaps exposes the entire facial skeleton from the midline to the external auditory canal. Depending on the exposure needed, the lateral maxilla with the attached lateral orbital wall and zygomatic arch can be removed en bloc for exposure of the maxilla, infratemporal fossa, nasopharynx, and parasellar area. The bony skeleton is replaced at the end of the case. Resection of a tumor requiring this much exposure almost certainly requires obliteration of the dead space with a vascularized free muscle flap.[11, 12]

ADJUNCTIVE MEASURES

When the tumor has substantial intradural and extradural extensions, the decision must be made whether

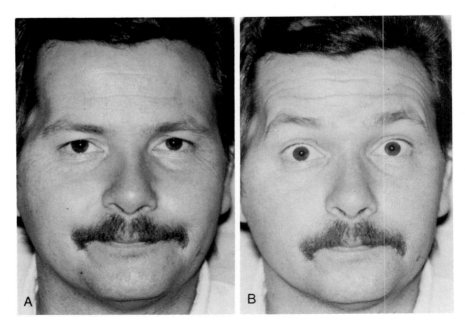

FIGURE 56-6. A-B, Postoperative photographs of patient showing full preservation of movement of the upper face.

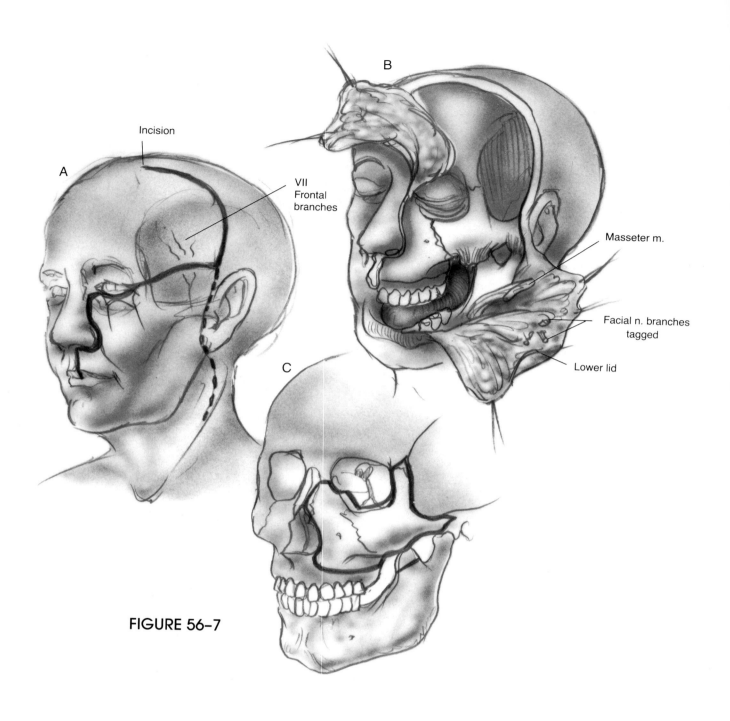

Incision

A

VII
Frontal
branches

B

Masseter m.

Facial n. branches
tagged

Lower lid

C

FIGURE 56-7

FIGURE 56-7. The lateral facial disassembly showing skin incisions and extent of possible bony removal. (Modified from Arriaga MA, Janecka IP: Facial translocation approach to the cranial base: The anatomic basis. Skull Base Surg 1:26, 1991.)

FIGURE 56-8. *A*, Preoperative photograph of a patient with a large recurrent meningioma. Note that in this case, the upper branch of the facial nerve will be sacrificed for safe exposure of the tumor. *B*, Preoperative magnetic resonance imaging. *C*, Intraoperative photograph showing the exposure of the tumor. *D*, Postoperative CT scan. The dead space left by the tumor has been filled with a rectus abdominis free flap.

FIGURE 56-8

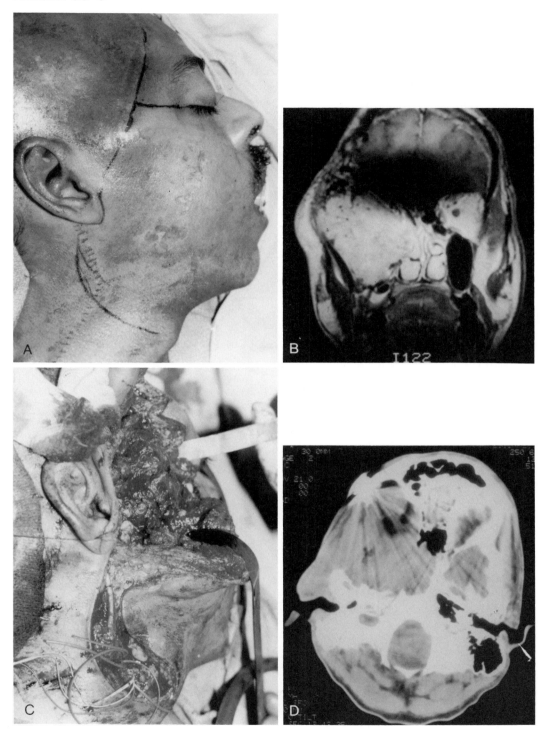

to attempt a one-stage intracranial-extracranial resection or to perform a two-stage resection. Although single-stage resections have been reported by several authors, many others prefer a two-stage resection. Fisch described a two-stage approach for removing large glomus tumors.[13] The first stage was a lateral approach that involved removing all accessible tumor and sealing the wound, including the eustachian tube, against cerebrospinal fluid leak. A second-stage neurosurgical intervention can be performed without risk of cerebrospinal fluid leak through a contaminated wound.

Alternatively, the order of the resections can be reversed.[7] The first stage entails a craniotomy and placement of fascia lata (neodura) between the brain and the tumor. After a short period of healing, a second-stage lateral approach is performed with the knowledge that the brain and subarachnoid space are secured from the surgical field.

RESULTS AND COMPLICATIONS

The results of radical approaches to the skull base are largely dependent on the location and biology of the lesion.[14] Jackson et al.[15] observed a 40 to 50 per cent long-term survival after craniofacial resection of malignant tumors. Donald[16] found an overall 47 per cent 2-year survival without recurrence among 262 patients with malignant disease pooled from nine centers.

Complications, especially cranial nerve deficits, are also dependent on the location of the lesion. Extensive resections of the skull base often lead to large dead spaces that communicate with both the subarachnoid space and the aerodigestive tract. Providing an adequate seal for the cerebrospinal fluid and obliterating this space is vital to the successful healing of the patient. Although temporalis muscle flaps have been used for this purpose, the temporalis muscle is often too small and has been devascularized during the resection. In this instance, obliteration of the dead space with a vascularized free flap is the technique of choice.

SUMMARY

The art and science of lateral approaches to the skull base is advancing rapidly. Radical techniques for approach and resection of tumors have been developed. Future efforts must focus on the long-term results and morbidity from these heroic measures as well as the development of adjuvant techniques.

References

1. Kumar A, Fisch U: The infratemporal fossa approach for lesions of the skull base. Adv Neurosurg 10: 187, 1983.
2. Jackson IT, Marsh WR, Bite U, Hide TA: Craniofacial osteotomies to facilitate skull base tumor resection. Br J Plast Surg 39: 153–160, 1986.
3. Hardesty RA, Jones NF, Swartz WM, et al.: Microsurgery for macrodefects: Microvascular free-tissue transfer for massive defects of the head and neck. Am J Surg 154: 399–405, 1987.
4. Andrews JC, Valavanis A, Fisch U: Management of the internal carotid artery in skull base surgery. Laryngoscope 99: 1224–1229, 1989.
5. de Vries EJ, Sekhar LN, Horton JA, et al.: A new method to predict safe resection of the internal carotid artery. Laryngoscope 100: 85–88, 1990.
6. Fisch U, Mattox DE. Microsurgery of the Skull Base. New York, Georg Thieme, 1988.
7. Holliday MJ, Nachlas N, Kennedy DW: Uses and modifications of the infratemporal fossa approach to skull base tumors. Ear Nose Throat J 65: 101–106, 1986.
8. Sekhar LN, Schramm VL Jr, Jones NF: Subtemporal-preauricular infratemporal fossa approach to large lateral and posterior cranial base neoplasms. J Neurosurg 67: 488–499, 1987.
9. Gates GA: The lateral facial approach to the nasopharynx and infratemporal fossa. Otolaryngol Head Neck Surg 99: 321–325, 1988.
10. Arriaga MA, Janecka IP: Facial translocation approach to the cranial base: The anatomic basis. Skull Base Surg 1: 26–33, 1991.
11. Jones NF, Sekhar LN, Schramm VL: Free rectus abdominis flap reconstruction of the middle and posterior cranial base. Plast Reconstr Surg 78: 471–479, 1986.
12. Jones NF, Schramm VL, Sekhar LN: Reconstruction of the cranial base following tumor resection. Br J Plast Surg 40: 155–162, 1987.
13. Fisch U: Infratemporal fossa approach for extensive tumors of the temporal bones and skull base. In Silverstein H, Norrell H (eds): Neurological Surgery of the Ear. Birmingham, Aesculapius, 1977, pp 35–53.
14. Jackson IT: Advances in craniofacial tumor surgery. World J Surg 13: 440–453, 1989.
15. Jackson IT, Bailey MH, Marsh WR, Juhasz P: Results and prognosis following surgery for malignant tumors of the skull base. Head Neck 13: 89–96, 1991.
16. Donald PJ: Skull base surgery: Combined results of treatment of malignant disease. Skull Base Surg 2: 76–79, 1992.

57

The Petrosal Approach

C. PHILLIP DASPIT, M.D.
ROBERT F. SPETZLER, M.D.

This chapter describes our surgical management of patients with extensive posterior fossa lesions via the petrosal approach as well as its variations and indications for use. Malis[1] first popularized the combination of the subtemporal and posterior fossa approaches, which improves exposure of lesions in the clivus or medial petrous region. We have divided this approach into three variations[1a]: 1) the *retrolabyrinthine*, (petrous bone resection with preservation of hearing), 2) the *translabyrinthine* (greater petrous bone resection and sacrifice of hearing), and 3) the *transcochlear* (maximum petrous drilling, sacrifice of hearing, and transposition of the facial nerve).

These three variations maximize temporal bone drilling and therefore provide exquisite exposure of the clivus and petrous region with minimal or no brain retraction. The superior petrosal sinus is always sacrificed, and the tentorium is completely cut. The sigmoid sinus can be transected or kept intact, depending on the venous drainage and the degree of exposure required. The combined skills of a neurosurgeon and a neuro-otologist maximize the operative exposure of the clivus and medial petrous region.

PATIENT SELECTION

Patients with extremely large lesions that extend above and below the tentorial incisura can be treated successfully via the petrosal approach. The petrosal approach can be used whenever exposure is needed from the sphenoid ridge and cavernous sinus to the foramen magnum and anterior cervical spinal cord. We have used this procedure successfully to treat 83 patients with tumors, aneurysms, cavernous malformations, and arteriovenous malformations, 46 of whom have been reviewed in detail elsewhere.[1]

PREOPERATIVE EVALUATION AND PATIENT COUNSELING

Magnetic resonance imaging in the axial, coronal, and sagittal planes and, recently, three-dimensional reconstructions using computed tomographic parallel processing are invaluable in the preoperative localization of the lesion and in the selection of the most advantageous surgical route. The location, size, and relationship of the lesion to important structures of the brain must be mapped accurately.

Each patient's evaluation must then be individualized to determine three important factors: 1) if the lesion can be accessed through noneloquent brain, 2) if the potential resulting neurologic deficits are acceptable, and 3) if the risks preclude operative intervention. Pre-existing neurologic deficits, coexisting lesions, or bony defects from previous procedures must also be considered when the appropriate avenue of surgical attack is chosen.

If high-resolution vascular imaging is needed, angiography can be used to evaluate the carotid artery. If the blood supply to a lesion needs to be decreased preoperatively, it can be embolized at that time.

The team describes the planned surgical procedure and its potential risks and complications to the patient and family members. In particular, risks involving all cranial nerves are discussed, as are procedures for repair and rehabilitation. The need for long-term imaging follow-up, especially in cases of meningiomas, is emphasized.

PREOPERATIVE PREPARATION

All patients are given steroid-antibiotics before surgery. Methylprednisolone sodium succinate (Solu-Medrol, 8mg to 12mg) is given at induction and repeated every 8 hours for 2 to 3 days. Patients who are not allergic to penicillin receive a third-generation cephalosporin (50mg per kg). Patients who are allergic to penicillin receive an intravenous aminoglycoside (80mg) and intravenous vancomycin (1gm).

Arterial and venous (peripheral and central) access is obtained by the neuroanesthesiologist. Compressed spectral electroencephalographic readings and somatosensory evoked potentials, as well as facial nerve and other cranial nerve function, are monitored on all patients. The auditory brain stem response is monitored bilaterally or only in the contralateral ear if ipsilateral hearing is sacrificed. Barbiturates are administered intravenously when the dura is opened (thiopental, 1 to 3mg per kg loading dose) and titrated to the point of electroencephalographic burst suppression. Besides improving the patient's tolerance to focal ischemia, the marked decrease in cerebral blood flow slackens the brain, allowing easier and safer retraction. Pressure is also controlled by the use of diuretics or by drainage of spinal fluid in patients who already have a ventriculostomy.

SURGICAL SITE PREPARATION

The surgical team consists of a neurosurgeon versed in skull base and vascular surgery and a neuro-otologist versed in all transmastoid-transcochlear procedures. The patient is positioned supine on the operating table. The head is turned parallel to the floor, slightly inclined downward, and fixed to the operating table with the Mayfield head holder. Appropriate shoulder support is provided.

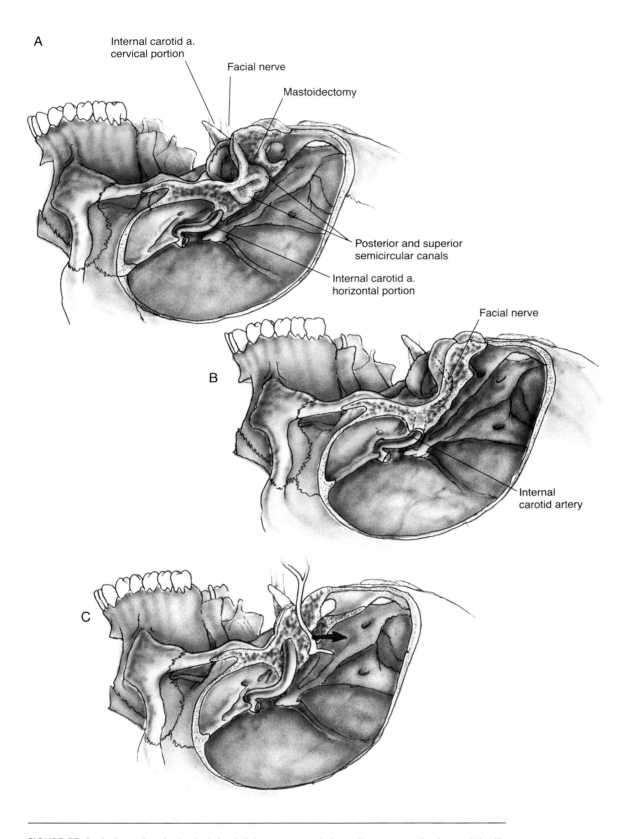

A, An extended retrolabyrinthine approach from the surgeon's viewpoint with skeletonized posterior and superior semicircular canal and mastoidectomy. B, Translabyrinthine approach from the surgeon's view. All three semicircular canals have been removed. C, Transcochlear approach from the surgeon's view with posteriorly transposed facial nerve for maximum exposure. (Reprinted with permission of the Barrow Neurological Institute.)

FIGURE 57–1.

The incision begins at the level of the zygoma 1cm anterior to the ear and continues in a gentle, curving fashion around the ear to just below the mastoid tip. If greater exposure is needed, the posterior limb of the incision can be extended further posteriorly. For maximum inferior lateral exposure of the foramen magnum, it can even be combined with the far lateral suboccipital approach.[2-4]

SPECIAL INSTRUMENTS

The Midas Rex (Midas Rex, Fort Worth, TX) high-speed drill system is used for the mastoidectomy portion of the procedure, and the Osteone system (Hall Surgical, Santa Barbara, CA) is used with the Zeiss operating microscope (variable 200mm to 400mm focal length) for more detailed bone removal. Suction irrigation is used continuously. An ultrasonic aspirator, with fine-tip unipolar attachments for cutting and coagulation, is used if a tumor must be debulked.

DETAILS OF SURGICAL TECHNIQUE[1]

The lateral side of the skull is exposed by retracting the scalp inferiorly with fish hooks attached to a Leyla bar.[5] This maneuver exposes the zygoma, lateral temporal bone, external auditory meatus, and mastoid region. A craniotomy that allows exposure of the sigmoid sinus is performed. The neuro-otologist performs this approach through the temporal bone.

If hearing is to be preserved, an extended retrolabyrinthine approach is performed (Fig. 57–1A). The posterior and superior semicircular canals are skeletonized by drilling as far anteriorly as possible, both above and below the otic capsule, to expose as much

dura as possible. The bone is removed over the superior petrosal sinus and the sigmoid sinus. An intraoperative view shows the exposed superior petrosal sinus, sigmoid sinus, and jugular bulb with the dura intact. The endolymphatic sac and duct are preserved. The neurosurgeon turns a bone flap from the temporal and occipital craniotomy across the transverse sinus.

If greater exposure is required, the translabyrinthine approach, which sacrifices hearing, is used (Fig. 57–1B). The approach is performed as described earlier, but all three semicircular canals are completely removed, and the posterior half of the internal auditory canal is completely skeletonized. More bone can therefore be removed from the face of the petrous pyramid. By removing all the bone overlying the sigmoid sinus and, if necessary, over the jugular bulb, the surgeon gains more working room and a greater exposure of the clivus inferiorly. The posterior external auditory canal and the bone overlying the mastoid segment of the facial nerve should also be thinned. The distal end of the superior vestibular nerve in the vestibule is referenced for easier identification of the facial nerve as it exits the internal auditory canal. The labyrinthine segment of the facial nerve can usually be seen through the thinned bone after cautious drilling in this region with a diamond bit. The subtemporal-suboccipital craniotomy is then performed.

The transcochlear approach is used for lesions that require maximum exposure and a very flat angle of approach to the clivus (Fig. 57–1C). The external auditory canal is transected and oversewn in two layers. Following the translabyrinthine exposure, the facial nerve is removed from its bony canal within the temporal bone. After the greater superficial petrosal nerve has been sectioned, the facial nerve is transposed posteriorly. The dura of the internal auditory canal is

FIGURE 57–2. Postsurgical three-dimensional computed tomographic scan of bone reconstruction compares petrous bone resection by the retrolabyrinthine approach on the left with total petrous bone resection by the transcochlear approach on the right. (From Spetzler RF, Daspit CP, Pappas CTE: The combined supra- and infratentorial approach for lesions of the petrous and clival regions: Experience with 46 cases. J Neurosurg 76: 588–599, 1992.)

FIGURE 57–3. Craniotomy. A dotted line indicates dural incision with preservation of sigmoid sinus and clips across superior petrosal sinus. Alternative dural incision (inset) crosses both superior petrosal and sigmoid sinuses. (Reprinted with permission of the Barrow Neurological Institute.)

FIGURE 57–4. If the sigmoid sinus is sacrificed, the ipsilateral vein of Labbé will drain contralaterally as it reliably enters the lateral sinus above the junction of the superior petrosal and sigmoid sinuses. (Reprinted with permission of the Barrow Neurological Institute.)

FIGURE 57–5. The temporal lobe and the cut tentorium are protected by retractors. The base of the temporal lobe along with the cut tentorium is elevated without stretching the vein of Labbé. The ipsilateral petrous region, the entire clivus, and the cranial nerves are exposed. (Reprinted with permission of the Barrow Neurological Institute.)

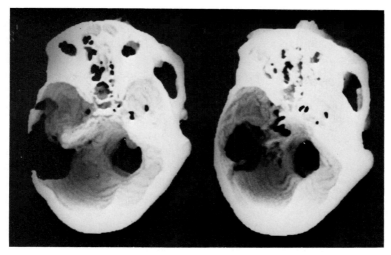

FIGURE 57-2

FIGURE 57-3

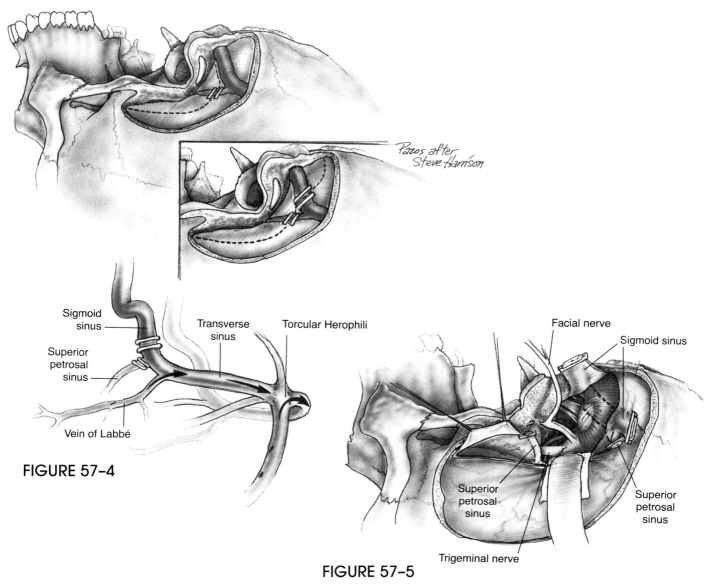

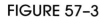

Pazos after
Steve Harrison

Sigmoid
sinus

Superior
petrosal
sinus

Transverse
sinus

Torcular Herophili

Vein of Labbé

FIGURE 57-4

Facial nerve

Sigmoid sinus

Superior
petrosal
sinus

Superior
petrosal
sinus

Trigeminal nerve

FIGURE 57-5

used to protect the facial nerve. The entire tympanic portion of the temporal bone is removed, and the periosteum of the temporal mandibular joint is exposed. The internal auditory canal and cochlea are removed. The jugular bulb is exposed by removing the bone that separates it from the internal carotid artery at the skull base. Care should be taken to avoid injuring the ninth, tenth, or eleventh cranial nerves. The bony wall of the carotid is removed to the siphon. Sufficient carotid artery can be exposed to allow a direct petrous-portion internal carotid artery to subarachnoid internal carotid artery saphenous vein bypass, if necessary.[6, 7] All bone medial to the carotid is removed, thereby exposing dura to the petrous tip. If direct exposure of the internal carotid artery is unnecessary, a thin rim of bone may be left surrounding the vessel. Bone is also removed from the floor of the middle fossa plate down to the horizontal segment of the internal carotid artery. The difference of the amount of petrous ridge resection between the retrolabyrinthine and transcochlear approaches can best be appreciated with postoperative computed tomographic reconstruction (Fig. 57–2).

Elevating the craniotomy flap exposes a large dural surface. Standard methods of brain shrinkage and monitoring as described earlier are implemented as required. The dura is incised over the temporal lobe at the anterior limit of the craniotomy (Fig. 57–3). The incision is extended posteriorly to at least 1cm below where the superior petrosal sinus enters the sigmoid sinus. Care should be exercised to avoid injuring a low-lying vein of Labbé that is attached to the temporal dura or tentorium. If the sigmoid sinus is not to be sacrificed, the dural incision crosses the superior petrosal sinus to join with a dural incision in front of the sigmoid sinus (Fig. 57–3). If necessary, another incision behind the sigmoid allows access in front and back of the sinus.[8]

The sigmoid sinus can be sacrificed if it can be angiographically verified that the sagittal sinus is the major drainage to the contralateral sigmoid sinus and that the confluence of this sinus is patent (Fig. 57–4). For further assurance that the sigmoid sinus can be sacrificed safely, a 25-gauge needle is inserted into the sinus, and the pressure is recorded before and after occlusion of the sinus below the clip. In our experience, intravascular pressure has not increased more than 7mm Hg with sigmoid sinus occlusion when patency was demonstrated angiographically. If pressure in the sigmoid sinus rises more than 10mm Hg with temporary occlusion, the sinus is kept intact. We have kept the sigmoid sinus intact in one third of the cases, based on preoperative angiography or because the additional exposure provided by sectioning the sigmoid sinus became unnecessary. If the sigmoid sinus is sacrificed, the ipsilateral vein of Labbé will drain contralaterally because it reliably enters the lateral sinus above the junction of the superior petrosal and sigmoid sinus (Fig. 57–4). If the sigmoid sinus is preserved and the posterior temporal lobe must be elevated because a tumor extends superiorly, the vein of Labbé, which is indirectly tethered to the skull base via the sigmoid sinus, must be protected.[9]

Once the dural incisions have been completed, the temporal lobe and the cut tentorium are protected by retractors that allow the base of the temporal lobe to be elevated without stretching the vein of Labbé (Fig. 57–5). This maneuver exposes the ipsilateral petrous region, the entire clivus, and the cranial nerves. Tumors and vascular lesions can be resected or clipped between any adjacent pair of cranial nerves by microsurgical techniques (Figs. 57–6 to 57–13). These approaches provide the maximum angle of exposure along the skull base and require minimal or no brain retraction.

At closure, the temporal and occipital dura are reapproximated. Abdominal adipose tissue, temporalis muscle, and fibrin glue are used to obliterate the temporal bone resection of the exposure. Temporary 3- to 5-day lumbar spinal drainage is used to control leakage of cerebrospinal fluid (CSF).

DRESSING AND POSTOPERATIVE CARE

A routine mastoid head dressing is applied for 2 days. Antibiotics are continued for 2 days unless patients have an intrathecal catheter. Steroids are tapered im-

FIGURE 57–6. After the translabyrinthine petrous bone resection. The sigmoid sinus has been transected, and the dura of the temporal and posterior fossae has been opened. Between the clips on the superior petrosal sinus, the tentorium will be cut along its entire length. (From Spetzler RF, Daspit CP, Pappas CTE: The combined supra- and infratentorial approach for lesions of the petrous and clival regions: Experience with 46 cases. J Neurosurg 76: 588–599, 1992.)

FIGURE 57–7. Schematic drawing showing the exposure of the basilar artery and neck of the aneurysm among cranial nerves V, VII, and VIII. The sixth cranial nerve is draped over the aneurysm dome. (From Spetzler RF, Daspit CP, Pappas CTE: The combined supra- and infratentorial approach for lesions of the petrous and clival regions: Experience with 46 cases. J Neurosurg 76: 588–599, 1992.)

FIGURE 57-6

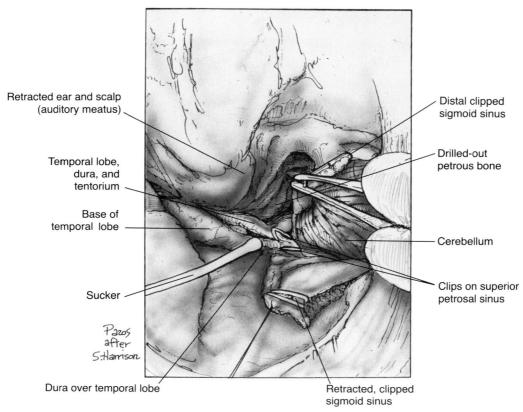

Retracted ear and scalp (auditory meatus)

Temporal lobe, dura, and tentorium

Base of temporal lobe

Sucker

Pazos after S. Harrison

Dura over temporal lobe

Distal clipped sigmoid sinus

Drilled-out petrous bone

Cerebellum

Clips on superior petrosal sinus

Retracted, clipped sigmoid sinus

FIGURE 57-7

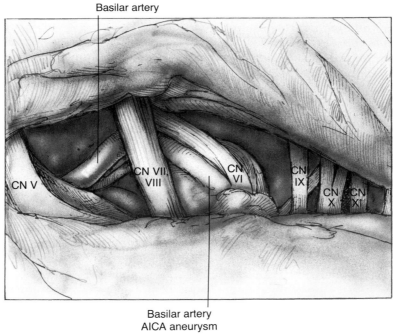

Basilar artery

CN V

CN VII, VIII

CN VI

CN IX

CN X

CN XI

Basilar artery AICA aneurysm

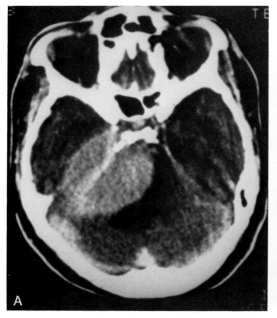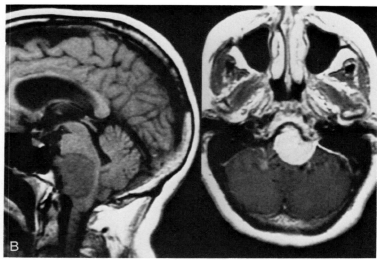

FIGURE 57-8. *A,* Computed tomographic scan demonstrating a classic medium-sized meningioma suitable for the petrosal approach. It is located in both the middle and the posterior fossae, straddling the petrous ridge. *B,* A magnetic resonance image demonstrates the extent of the tumor along the length of the clivus. The brainstem, along with the basilar artery, is markedly elevated. (From Spetzler RF, Daspit CP, Pappas CTE: The combined supra- and infratentorial approach for lesions of the petrous and clival regions: Experience with 46 cases. J Neurosurg 76: 588–599, 1992.)

mediately after surgery and withdrawn within 2 to 3 days. Ambulation is encouraged as soon as possible but may have to be delayed if the patient has a lumbar drain. Lumbar drains are typically maintained for 3 days after surgery to decrease the incidence of CSF leaks. The patient's diet is advanced as soon as possible.

RISKS OF SURGERY

Whether the petrosal approach proceeds anteriorly to the horizontal portion of the internal carotid artery and the siphon depends on the type of lesion, the location of the mass, and the patient's hearing function. The three variations of the petrosal approach maintain the advantages of minimal cerebellar retraction and positive facial nerve identification in the lateral internal auditory canal and offer better visualization of the dissection plane between brainstem and tumor.

The sigmoid sinus can be preserved through use of a dural opening similar to the one described by Samii et al.[8] and Al-Mefty et al.[9] The base of the temporal lobe can be elevated safely without risking injury to the vein of Labbé when the cut sigmoid sinus and the cut tentorium are elevated along with the temporal

lobe. These variations of the petrosal approach can give exposure anterior to the brainstem, toward the middle fossa, and inferior to the foramen magnum. The major arterial vessels of the brainstem are also accessed more readily for clipping aneurysms, removing arteriovenous malformations, or obtaining hemostasis during tumor removal.

The indications for a particular variation of the petrosal approach depend on the function of the seventh and eighth cranial nerves, the amount of temporal bone that must be removed for adequate exposure, and the amount of brainstem compression present. If function of the seventh and eighth cranial nerve is to be preserved and an anterior exposure to the brainstem is not needed, the retrolabyrinthine variation is adequate: it allows entry into the cerebellopontine angle anterior to the sigmoid sinus but requires more retraction than the other variations.

If more anterior visualization of the brainstem is needed or if the patient has little or no hearing, the translabyrinthine variation is appropriate. This variation gives a more direct anterolateral approach to the cerebellopontine angle and provides greater exposure because more of the petrous bone is resected. The function of the facial nerve is preserved, but the risk of a CSF leak is increased. The transcochlear variation gives additional exposure anterior to the brainstem

FIGURE 57-9

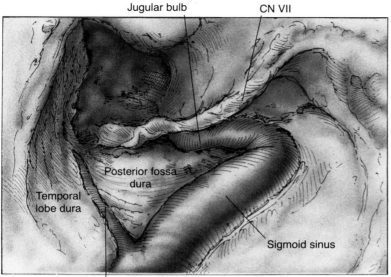

Jugular bulb   CN VII

Posterior fossa dura

Temporal lobe dura

Sigmoid sinus

Superior petrosal sinus

FIGURE 57-10

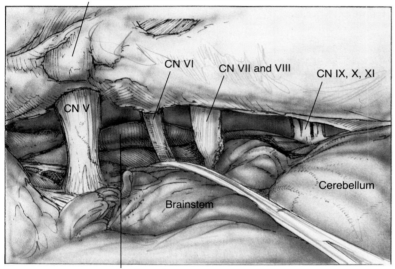

CN in Meckel's cave after tumor removal

CN VI   CN VII and VIII   CN IX, X, XI

CN V

Cerebellum

Brainstem

Basilar artery

FIGURE 57-9. After the petrous bone drilling by the transcochlear approach. The sigmoid sinus and the jugular bulb have been exposed, and the superior petrosal sinus can be seen entering the sigmoid sinus. The drilled-out seventh cranial nerve lies over the jugular bulb. The greater superficial petrosal branch has been cut to allow mobilization of the seventh cranial nerve. Compare the additional bone resection achieved using this transcochlear approach with that of the translabyrinthine approach shown in Figure 57-6B. (From Spetzler RF, Daspit CP, Pappas CTE: The combined supra- and infratentorial approach for lesions of the petrous and clival regions: Experience with 46 cases. J Neurosurg 76: 588-599, 1992.)

FIGURE 57-10. The meningioma after removal. Cranial nerves V through XI, along with the basilar artery, have been exposed. This very flat approach to the clivus can be achieved only through the transcochlear approach. (From Spetzler RF, Daspit CP, Pappas CTE: The combined supra- and infratentorial approach for lesions of the petrous and clival regions: Experience with 46 cases. J Neurosurg 76: 588-599, 1992.)

and is indicated when maximum exposure is needed. It provides a very flat angle of approach to the clivus. However, it not only has the disadvantages associated with the translabyrinthine approach, it also increases the risk of facial nerve paresis or paralysis.

Of course, the routine anterior subtemporal approach or posterior fossa approach should be used when appropriate. The anterior subtemporal approach provides exposure for tumors in the upper third of the clivus without significant lateral petrous extension, just as the suboccipital approach is adequate for tumors of the posterior fossa that do not extend into the middle fossa or that do not extend too far contralaterally. However, the petrosal approach offers maximum exposure with minimal retraction for tumors in the middle portion of the clivus or for tumors that cross the medial petrous ridge and extend into the posterior and middle fossa and into Meckel's cave and the cavernous sinus.

Although the sacrifice of the sigmoid sinus is optional, it permits more elevation of the temporal lobe than is otherwise possible without stretching the vein of Labbé. As long as appropriate venous drainage can be verified, no risk appears to be associated with sacrificing the sigmoid sinus.

The facial nerve can be transposed in several ways. For an anterior transposition, the nerve can be completely removed from its canal, and the parotid gland can be dissected. Brackmann[10] moves the nerve anteriorly along with the surrounding soft tissue of the stylomastoid foramen. The nerve, which is not completely transposed, is thereby left with better postoperative function. Although most patients experience postoperative facial paresis, function returns completely or almost completely after several months. Proper use of intraoperative monitoring techniques can help preserve facial nerve function. Facial paralysis from interruption of the nerve may be restored by facial anastomosis or interposition nerve grafting or by an anastomosis of the hypoglossal-facial nerves.

RESULTS

We reported on a series of 46 patients who underwent the petrosal approach[1] but have now used this approach to treat a total of 83 patients. Of the 46 patients, 42 did well after surgery and returned to their premorbid occupations. Two patients needed home nursing care. One patient who recently underwent surgery is home recuperating. The remaining patient underwent surgery in April 1991 and developed hydrocephalus from his previous subarachnoid hemorrhage. The patient received a ventriculoperitoneal shunt. In 42 of the 46 cases, the patients' lesions were grossly extirpated, as could be ascertained through the operating microscope and postoperative magnetic resonance imaging studies. Four meningiomas were incompletely removed. In these patients, a clear arachnoid plane between the tumor and the brainstem–perforating arteries and basilar artery could not be established. Therefore, no attempt was made to remove all the tumor from these structures.

The outcome of the last 37 patients is similar to that of the patients already reported, except that one patient had a severe postoperative hemorrhage that required re-exploration and removal of a hematoma from the brainstem. This patient now has significant hemiparesis.

We obtained gross total removal in most of our patients. Because most of the lesions were meningiomas, we emphasize that the patients are not cured and must be followed long term to check for recurrences. Facial nerve recovery after the transcochlear approach has been variable, but most patients recover to a House grade III. Most patients have been discharged after 1 or 2 weeks of hospitalization.

Complications

Facial nerve injury was the highest postoperative complication, as would be expected from surgical ma-

---

FIGURE 57–11. A more anterior view exposing cranial nerves III through VIII. Notice the opened Meckel's cave, where the residual tumor can now be easily removed. (From Spetzler RF, Daspit CP, Pappas CTE: The combined supra- and infratentorial approach for lesions of the petrous and clival regions: Experience with 46 cases. J Neurosurg 76: 588–599, 1992.)

FIGURE 57–12. After removal of a large clivus meningioma. Posteriorly to anteriorly, this view allows excellent visualization of the hypophyseal stalk. Notice the preserved fine vascular network on the brainstem. Maintaining the arachnoid over the brainstem to protect the vascularity is a primary goal, when possible. (From Spetzler RF, Daspit CP, Pappas CTE: The combined supra- and infratentorial approach for lesions of the petrous and clival regions: Experience with 46 cases. J Neurosurg 76: 588–599, 1992.)

FIGURE 57–13. An anterior-to-posterior view after resection of a large meningioma provides a dramatic demonstration of the cranial nerves and vascular structure of this region. (From Spetzler RF, Daspit CP, Pappas CTE: The combined supra- and infratentorial approach for lesions of the petrous and clival regions: Experience with 46 cases. J Neurosurg 76: 588–599, 1992.)

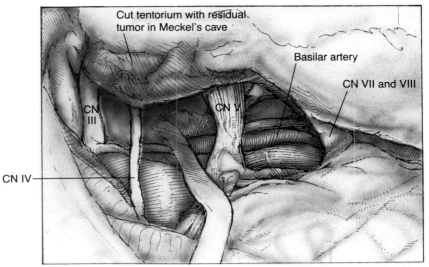

FIGURE 57–11

Cut tentorium with residual tumor in Meckel's cave

Basilar artery

CN VII and VIII

CN III

CN V

CN IV

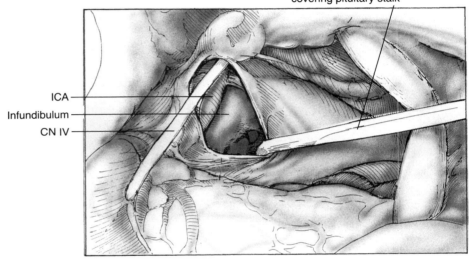

Dissector holding back arachnoid covering pituitary stalk

FIGURE 57–12

ICA

Infundibulum

CN IV

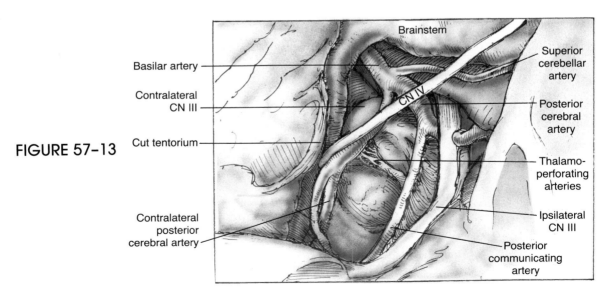

FIGURE 57–13

Brainstem

Superior cerebellar artery

Basilar artery

Contralateral CN III

Cut tentorium

CN IV

Posterior cerebral artery

Thalamo-perforating arteries

Ipsilateral CN III

Contralateral posterior cerebral artery

Posterior communicating artery

nipulation.[1] Wound healing was not a major problem. The second most common complication associated with the petrosal approach was CSF leakage, especially in patients who were not drained expectantly. Few wounds required re-exploration to stop a CSF leak—almost all stopped leaking after lumbar drainage. The rates of occurrence for decreased gag reflex, abducens nerve paresis, numbness, aphasia, sepsis, hemiparesis, pneumonia, and hematoma are low.[1] No operative deaths occurred.

Our rates of morbidity and mortality[1] after surgery compare favorably with those of previously published reports. Before the use of the operative microscope, operative mortality was more than 50 per cent for clival and petrous meningiomas.[11] With the use of the microscope, mortality has dropped to 11 per cent in Mayberg's and Symon's[11] series and to 9 per cent in Al-Mefty's et al.[9] series. As would be expected, the incidence of cranial nerve deficits from surgical manipulation is high after these procedures. Both Mayberg and Symon[11] and Al-Mefty et al.[9] reported that cranial nerve deficits occurred in more than 50 per cent of their patients.

ALTERNATIVE TECHNIQUES

Both neurosurgeons and neuro-otologists have modified the combined approach. House and Hitselberger[12] described a combined suboccipital-petrosal approach to remove large cerebellopontine angle tumors. Their translabyrinthine approach extends beyond the sigmoid sinus into the suboccipital area to achieve a wider view of the cerebellopontine angle than afforded by either the translabyrinthine or suboccipital approach alone. The sigmoid sinus can be mobilized anteriorly or posteriorly or even divided if the contralateral transverse sinus is patent. This combined translabyrinthine-suboccipital exposure is useful for very large tumors. This exposure permits good visualization of the brainstem medially and the facial nerve laterally while minimizing brain retraction. Hemostasis is better controlled because the dissection plane between the brainstem and tumor can be well visualized, and the major arterial vessels are therefore more readily accessed.

Malis[13] has used a combined suboccipital-subtemporal approach for clival, clivotemporal, and basilar tumors. The vein of Labbé is preserved by ligating the lateral sinus between the entrance of the vein of Labbé posteriorly and the sigmoid sinus and superior petrosal sinus anteriorly. After the sinus is divided, the tentorium may be divided along the petrosal apex, sparing the superior petrosal sinus. The tentorium, lateral sinus, temporal lobe, and vein of Labbé are

retracted upward, exposing the clivus down toward the foramen magnum.

House[14] modified this approach by including the transcochlear approach, which extends the translabyrinthine exposure of the petrous bone forward into the cerebellopontine angle and provides excellent exposure of tumors and the arterial system anteriorly and anterolaterally to the brainstem. Excellent exposure is also obtained by rerouting the facial nerve.

Morrison and King[15] described a translabyrinthine-transtemporal approach for exposing the cerebellopontine angle upward into the middle fossa by drilling the petrous temporal bone. The superior petrosal sinus and tentorium cerebelli are then divided. Patients with tumors reaching down into the foramen magnum are not candidates for this approach, because visualization is inadequate. Using a similar approach with an incomplete labyrinthectomy, Bochenek and Kukwa[16] drilled out the lateral aspect of the petrous bone posteriorly to the level of the compact plate of the sigmoid sinus and medially to the lateral semicircular canal. The tentorium cerebelli was divided, and the superior petrosal sinus was kept patent. The goal of this approach was to gain a better exposure of the cerebellopontine angle than could be obtained through the labyrinth.

In 1977, Fisch[17] first described the infratemporal approach, which combines a partial posterior and inferior petrosectomy with a cervicofacial approach. The jugular foramen is exposed well by the infratemporal approach. Combining the transcochlear approach of House and Hitselberger and the infratemporal approach of Fisch, Pellet et al.[18] created the widened transcochlear approach. Their approach involves a petrosectomy that connects the posterior fossa to the superior carotid region. Saddlebag-shaped tumors extending into the posterior fossa and the infratemporal region can be removed in one stage.

SUMMARY

The indications for a variation of the petrosal approach depend on the function of the eighth cranial nerve, the amount of temporal bone that must be removed for adequate exposure, and the amount of brainstem compression. The amount of exposure needed to remove the lesion safely must be weighed against the permanent sacrifice of hearing or the temporary loss of facial nerve function. Of course, the routine anterior subtemporal approach or posterior fossa approach should be used when appropriate. The former provides exposure for tumors in the upper third of the clivus without significant lateral petrous extension. The latter is adequate for tumors of the posterior fossa that do not extend into the middle fossa or that do not extend too far contralaterally.

We recommend the petrosal approach and its appropriate variations for large lesions of the posterior fossa. These approaches permit exquisite exposure for tumor removal, arteriovenous malformation resection, and aneurysm clipping in the petroclival region and yield an acceptable rate of morbidity and mortality. The technique illustrates the evolution of neuro-otologic skull base approaches that allow access to transtentorial pathology.

References

1. Decker RE, Malis LI: Surgical approach to midline lesions at base of skull. J Mt Sinai Hosp 37: 84–102, 1970.
1a. Spetzler RF, Daspit CP, Pappas CTE: The combined supra- and infratentorial approach for lesions of the petrous and clival regions: Experience with 46 cases. J Neurosurg 76: 588–599, 1992.
2. Heros RC: Lateral suboccipital approach for vertebral and vertebrobasilar artery lesions. J Neurosurg 64: 559–562, 1986.
3. Sen CN, Sekhar LN: An extreme lateral approach to intradural lesions of the cervical spine and foramen magnum. Neurosurgery 27: 197–204, 1990.
4. Spetzler RF, Grahm TW: The far-lateral approach to the inferior clivus and the upper cervical region: Technical note. Barrow Neurol Inst Q 6(4): 35–38, 1990.
5. Spetzler RF: Two technical notes for microsurgery. Barrow Neurol Inst Q 4(2): 38–39, 1988.
6. Sekhar LN, Sen CN, Jho HD: Saphenous vein graft bypass of the cavernous internal carotid artery. J Neurosurg 72: 35–41, 1990.
7. Spetzler RF, Fukishima T, Martin N, et al.: Petrous carotid-to-intradural carotid saphenous vein graft for intracavernous giant aneurysm, tumor, and occlusive cerebrovascular disease. J Neurosurg 73: 496–501, 1990.
8. Samii M, Ammirati M, Mahran A, et al.: Surgery of petroclival meningiomas: Report of 24 cases. Neurosurgery 24: 12–17, 1989.
9. Al-Mefty O, Fox JL, Smith RR: Petrosal approach for petroclival meningiomas. Neurosurgery 22: 510–517, 1988.
10. Brackmann DE: The facial nerve in the infratemporal approach. Otolaryngol Head Neck Surg 97: 15–17, 1987.
11. Mayberg MR, Symon L: Meningiomas of the clivus and apical petrous bone. Report of 35 cases. J Neurosurg 65: 160–167, 1986.
12. House WF, Hitselberger WE: The transcochlear approach to the skull base. Arch Otolaryngol Head Neck Surg 102: 334–342, 1976.
13. Malis LI: Surgical resection of tumors of the skull base. In Wilkins RH, Rengachary SS (eds): Neurosurgery. New York, McGraw-Hill, 1985, pp 1011–1021.
14. House WF: Translabyrinthine approach. In House WF, Luetje CM (eds): Acoustic Tumors, Vol 2, Management. Baltimore, University Park Press, 1979, pp 43–87.
15. Morrison AW, King TT: Experiences with a translabyrinthine-transtentorial approach to the cerebellopontine angle. Technical note. J Neurosurg 38: 382–390, 1973.
16. Bochenek Z, Kukwa A: An extended approach through the middle cranial fossa to the internal auditory meatus and the cerebello-pontine angle. Acta Otolaryngol (Stockh) 80: 410–414, 1975.
17. Fisch U: Infratemporal fossa approach for extensive tumors of the temporal bone and base of the skull. In Silverstein H, Norell H (eds): Neurological Surgery of the Ear. Birmingham, AL, Aesculapius, 1977, pp 34–53.
18. Pellet WT, Cannoni M, Pech A: The widened transcochlear approach to jugular foramen tumors. J Neurosurg 69: 887–894, 1988.

58

Treatment of Bilateral Acoustic Neuromas

RICHARD T. MIYAMOTO, M.D.

KAREN L. ROOS, M.D.

ROBERT L. CAMPBELL, M.D.

The presence of bilateral acoustic neuromas is the hallmark of neurofibromatosis type 2 (NF-2) (Fig. 58–1). However, despite this unique hallmark, NF-2 has only recently been recognized as a distinct clinical entity. Prior to 1987, all patients with phenotypic manifestations of neurofibromatosis, that is, cafe au lait macules or subcutaneous neurofibromas, were considered to be at risk for developing bilateral acoustic neuromas, but extensive screening programs infrequently identified these tumors. The National Institutes of Health Consensus Development Conference on Neurofibromatosis in 1987[1] clarified this inconsistency by identifying two clinically and genetically distinct forms of neurofibromatosis. Clinical criteria differentiating these forms of neurofibromatosis have greatly assisted clinicians in determining which patients are at risk of developing bilateral acoustic neuromas and which are not.

When acoustic neuromas occur bilaterally, initial treatment planning is directed toward the prevention of life-threatening sequelae. Although the preservation of auditory function is of paramount concern, this goal has been documented infrequently. With the advent of auditory brainstem response testing, advanced imaging techniques, and new genetic information, bilateral acoustic neuromas can be identified at an early stage when hearing preservation is feasible. Successful surgical intervention that eliminates the inevitable total, bilateral deafness can now be attained in selected patients.[2–11] When surgical removal of the tumors and hearing preservation cannot be accomplished, new technology incorporating electrical stimulation of the auditory system provides a therapeutic option in the aural rehabilitation of these patients.

CLASSIFICATION OF NEUROFIBROMATOSIS (Table 58–1)

Neurofibromatoses primarily affect cell growth of neural tissues and can cause tumors to grow on nerves at any time and at any location. A wide range of expressivity may be seen, even within a family, and variant forms may exist that confound classification in some patients. Resultant manifestations may be innocuous or may be progressive and result in significant morbidity or even mortality.

Neurofibromatosis Type 1

The most common type of neurofibromatosis, neurofibromatosis type 1 (NF-1), affects approximately one in 4000 individuals. This disorder was previously labeled von Recklinghausen's disease or peripheral neurofibromatosis. Individuals with NF-1 typically have multiple café au lait macules, Lisch's nodules, optic nerve gliomas, and dermal, subcutaneous, and plexiform neurofibromas. A diagnosis of NF-1 is made in an individual in whom at least two of the following seven features are found:

1. Six or more café au lait spots larger than 5mm in children and 15mm in teenagers and adults
2. Two or more neurofibromas or one plexiform neurofibroma
3. Freckling in the axilla or groin areas
4. Optic nerve glioma
5. Two or more iris hamartomas (Lisch nodules)
6. A distinctive bony lesion, such as sphenoid wing dysplasia or thinning of the long bone cortex, with or without pseudoarthrosis
7. A first-degree relative with NF-1 according to the above criteria

Neurofibromatosis Type 2

NF-2 affects approximately one in 40,000 individuals. NF-2 is characterized by bilateral acoustic neuromas; presenile lens opacities; dermal, subcutaneous, and plexiform neurofibromas; and brain and spinal cord tumors. NF-2 has also been referred to as "hereditary bilateral vestibular schwannoma syndrome" to emphasize that the origin of the eighth cranial nerve tumors is the vestibular nerve, not the acoustic nerve, and that the tumors are schwannomas and not true neuromas. The previously applied term "central neurofibromatosis" is no longer used. A diagnosis of NF-2 is made in an individual who has bilateral eighth cranial nerve tumors or a first-degree relative (parent, sibling, or child) with NF-2 and either a unilateral eighth cranial nerve tumor or two of the following:

1. Dermal or subcutaneous neurofibromas
2. Plexiform neurofibroma
3. Schwannoma
4. Glioma
5. Juvenile posterior subcapsular cataract

Although NF-1 and NF-2 are distinctly different disorders, they share many clinical characteristics. Both NF-1 and NF-2 are autosomal dominant disorders; therefore, 50 per cent of the offspring of individuals with NF-1 and NF-2 will be affected. Both disorders demonstrate high penetrance but with great variability of expression and severity from one individual to another. Approximately 50 per cent of the cases of NF-1 and NF-2 are the result of sporadic mutations; this mutation rate is the highest for any human genetic disorder described to date. Eighty per cent of the mutations of the NF-1 gene are of paternal origin.

TABLE 58–1. Features of Neurofibromatosis (NF) Types 1 and 2

PARAMETER	NF-1	NF-2
Synonyms	Peripheral NF	Central NF
	von Recklinghausen's	Bilateral acoustic NF
Incidence	30/100,000	3/100,000
Age of onset	First decade	Second or third decade
Skin manifestations		
Cutaneous neurofibromas	95% have more than two	Over 30% have more than one
Over 5 café au lait spots	Found in most	Rare
Intertriginous freckles	Usually present	Rare
Eye manifestations		
Lisch's nodules	Present in over 90%	Rare
Lens abnormalities	Not reported	Posterior capsular cataract in over 50%
Bony abnormalities	Common	Not reported
Central nervous system tumors		
Acoustic neuromas	None documented in familial cases	Bilateral in 96%
Other brain tumors	Optic glioma, 2%–15%	9%–100% depending on type of NF-2
Spinal cord tumors	Occasional	Common in several types of NF-2

Modified from Ferris NJ, Siu KH: Neurofibromatosis 2: Report of an affected kindred, with a discussion on imaging strategy. Australas Radiol 34(3): 229–233, 1990.

In spite of the similarities, clear distinguishing differences exist between NF-1 and NF-2. The age of onset of signs and symptoms is earlier in NF-1. In fact, the diagnosis may be made at birth or during infancy by examination of the skin. The typical hyperpigmented macules or café au lait spots are found predominantly on the trunk and appear within the first year of life in most individuals with NF-1 and are present by age 4 years in most affected children. Neurofibromas appear just before puberty and increase in number and size throughout adulthood. The clinical manifestations of NF-2 are more subtle. Signs of NF-2 may not become apparent until puberty or early

adulthood but may appear as late as the seventh decade of life. Therefore, individuals at risk of inheriting the NF-2 gene must be followed up closely for many years for signs of the development of an acoustic neuroma. Although individuals with either disorder may have café au lait spots and neurofibromas, those with NF-2 tend to have a smaller number of café au lait spots and neurofibromas than those with NF-1. Axillary freckling is unique to those with NF-1. An individual who clearly has NF-1 is not at risk for developing an acoustic neuroma.

All individuals with bilateral acoustic neuromas have NF-2 by definition and are at risk for developing other tumors, such as meningiomas, schwannomas, gliomas, ependymomas, and plexiform neurofibromas. Recently, Eldridge and Parry[12] suggested a further subclassification of NF-2. Three broad groupings emerged from a study of families with multiple members affected and individuals representing sporadic cases when age at onset, rate of progression of hearing loss, and presence or absence of associated brain and spinal cord tumors were correlated.

The first type of NF-2, described by Feiling in 1920 and Gardner in 1930, is characterized by onset of hearing loss in the third and fourth decade and few, if any, associated brain and spinal cord tumors. Hearing may be preserved until late in life, especially in males. The second type of NF-2 was described by Wishart in 1822. It is characterized by earlier onset of hearing loss, more rapid progression to spontaneous deafness, and multiple brain and spinal cord tumors. Brain tumors include other cranial nerve schwannomas and meningiomas, which may develop on the optic nerve sheath and may be bilateral in the posterior fossa. Spinal tumors include extramedullary and paraspinal schwannomas and meningiomas, as well as intramedullary low-grade astrocytomas and epen-

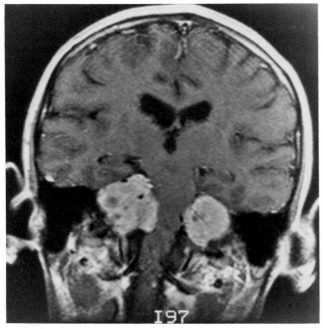

FIGURE 58–1.

dymomas. Because the clinical course may be rapid, reproduction is often impaired, and cases tend to be sporadic. The third type of NF-2 was described by Lee and Abbott. This form displays variable age at initial hearing loss and at spontaneous deafness. A distinguishing feature is the early morbidity due to associated tumors, which tend to be numerous, especially when they involve the spinal cord. Cerebellopontine angle meningiomas, meningiomatosis en plaque of the falx, and schwannomatosis of spinal nerve roots are common.

The ophthalmologic examination may help distinguish between NF-1 and NF-2 in an individual with café au lait macules and neurofibromas. Both forms of neurofibromatosis may be accompanied by distinct eye changes that can be definitive in diagnosis. Lisch nodules of the iris occur in more than 85 per cent of postpubertal patients with NF-1 but have been reported in only one patient with NF-2.[13] They are melanocytic hamartomas that appear as yellow or brown, raised, dome-shaped lesions on the surface of the iris. Posterior subcapsular opacities of the lens are seen in approximately 40 to 50 per cent of individuals with NF-2 but have not been described in patients with NF-1.[14] This association is of interest because the gene for NF-2 and one of the genes controlling beta-B2 lens crystallin are in the same region on the long arm of chromosome 22. Optic gliomas, although seen in NF-1, are not seen in NF-2.

MOLECULAR GENETICS

Neurofibromatosis Type 1

The gene for NF-1 was identified by genetic linkage analysis and found to be on chromosome 17.[15] Subsequently, two unrelated patients with NF-1 were identified who had translocations disrupting chromosome 17 at band 17q11.2. This finding helped localize the NF-1 gene to band 17q on the long arm of chromosome 17 near the centromere.[16]

Neurofibromatosis Type 2

The gene for NF-2 has been localized to the middle of the long arm of chromosome 22. The initial clue for the location of the NF-2 gene was uncovered by the application of a primary mechanism of tumorigenesis in humans that was discovered in embryonal tumors to the formation of tumors associated with NF-2. By this mechanism, tumor growth occurs in a two-step process. The initial event is a primary mutation that results in the formation of an allele, a change in a DNA sequence at a point on a chromosome, that is recessive at the cellular level to the normal allele. The growth of a tumor occurs only after an additional

change, such a loss of a chromosome, allows for expression of the altered allele.[17]

Individuals with NF-2 frequently develop meningiomas as well as acoustic neuromas. The development of a menigioma is associated with a loss of one copy of chromosome 22. As demonstrated by Seizinger et al.,[17] the formation of an acoustic neuroma is also specifically associated with loss of genes on chromosome 22, suggesting that chromosome 22 might contain a locus for a tumor-suppressor gene or antioncogene. Loss of this gene allows for malignant transformation of certain cells. These same investigators subsequently demonstrated specific loss of alleles from chromosome 22 in two acoustic neuromas, two neurofibromas, and one meningioma from individuals with NF-2.[18] Only a portion of the long arm of chromosome 22 was deleted in the two acoustic neuromas, narrowing the chromosomal location of the gene causing NF-2 to the region near the center of the long arm of chromosome 22. By linkage analysis of a large kindred with NF-2, Rouleau et al.[19] and Wertelecki et al.[20] were able to pinpoint the locus for this disorder at the center of the long arm of chromosome 22 (22q11.1–22q13.1).

Clinical Manifestations

The initial symptoms of an acoustic neuroma are loss of hearing, tinnitus, or dysequilibrium. The hearing loss is a progressive sensorineural hearing loss, usually with poor discrimination. Although the tumors arise from the vestibular nerves, acute vertigo is uncommon because the slow growth pattern allows the ear to compensate as the tumor enlarges. These tumors may become symptomatic for the first time over a wide age range, from age 10 to age 60, although most become symptomatic between ages 20 to 40 years. The rate of growth of acoustic neuromas in patients with NF-2 is unpredictable. NF-2 should be ruled out in any patient who develops an acoustic neuroma before the age of 40.

The initial evaluation of an individual whose condition is highly suggestive of NF-2 should include pure-tone audiometry and a T1-weighted magnetic resonance (MR) scan with gadolinium. The gadolinium-enhanced MR scan is the best neuroimaging procedure for detecting small intracanalicular neuromas and can detect these tumors in children before they are symptomatic. Brainstem auditory evoked response and acoustic reflex studies are helpful screening procedures.

Individuals with NF-2 should have annual ophthalmologic evaluations. A posterior subcapsular opacity of the lens is present in 40 to 50 per cent of individuals with NF-2 by age 30 and may produce progressive visual loss.[21]

Patients with NF-2 are at risk for developing central nervous system tumors, particularly Schwann cell tumors. These tumors develop on spinal nerve roots, within the spinal cord, particularly in the cervical cord area, and on the cranial nerves. The tumors can grow very rapidly. An MR scan of the entire neural axis in patients with NF-2 is useful in detecting asymptomatic schwannomas along the spinal cord. Individuals with NF-2 are also at risk for menigiomas, spinal ependymomas, and astrocytomas.

All individuals younger than age 40 with a sporadic, unilateral acoustic neuroma should be examined carefully for neurofibromas, café au lait spots, posterior subcapsular cataracts, and abnormalities on neurologic examination that suggest the presence of other central nervous system tumors. Follow-up evaluation with gadolinium-enhanced MR scan and pure-tone audiometry enables early detection of an acoustic neuroma on the contralateral side, if this develops.

MANAGEMENT

When acoustic neuromas occur bilaterally (NF-2), initial treatment planning is influenced by tumor size at the time of diagnosis and their anticipated growth pattern and the patient's age and hearing status. The growth pattern of acoustic neuromas is unpredictable: some tumors grow slowly over many years, whereas others may enlarge rapidly, resulting in deafness, cerebellar dysfunction, or brainstem compression.

Initial treatment planning must be directed toward the prevention of life-threatening sequelae resulting from brainstem compression or increased intracranial pressure. After this concern has been addressed, the preservation of auditory function in at least one ear is of great concern. However, hearing preservation has been an elusive goal in NF-2 patients because bilateral acoustic neuromas have a tendency to invade rather than compress adjacent nerves.[22] This renders difficult the definitive treatment of bilateral acoustic tumors while preserving hearing.

Surgical intervention is currently the only definitive treatment for enlarging acoustic tumors. As a general rule, acoustic tumors of any size should be removed when aidable hearing is not present and the patient is suitable for an elective operation. When serviceable or aidable hearing is present and the tumor does not appear to adhere to the brainstem on preoperative imaging studies, hearing preservation surgery may be appropriate. Because most acoustic neuromas arise from the superior or inferior vestibular nerves, preservation of the cochlear nerve and its blood supply is feasible in some cases through the use of microsurgical techniques. Two surgical approaches have been applied. The middle fossa approach described by William House is appropriate for small intracanalicular tumors or tumors that extend slightly medial to the porus acusticus.[22a] The retrosigmoid or suboccipital approach may be applied for intracanalicular tumors or for some slightly larger tumors that extend into the cerebellopontine angle. The intracranial course of the cochlear nerve can be traced from its origin at the pontomedullary junction to the lateral end of the internal auditory canal just proximal to its entrance into the cochlea. Intraoperative monitoring of facial and cochlear nerve function have augmented the current surgical technique.

Although size is only one tumor characteristic influencing hearing preservation, the likelihood of tumor invasion into the cochlear nerve is less if the tumor can be detected early in its course. Current imaging techniques using MR with gadolinium have greatly enhanced our ability to detect tumors. However, the invasive tendencies of acoustic neuromas cannot be assessed by preoperative imaging. Only by surgical exploration can these properties be determined. If the tumor is invading the cochlear nerve, subtotal removal and decompression of the internal auditory canal may delay progression of hearing loss.[23]

Clinical Approaches

There are six basic management strategies for patients with bilateral acoustic neuromas. Each has specific indications and disadvantages. Individualization of management is a prerequisite.

HEARING PRESERVATION SURGERY—TOTAL TUMOR REMOVAL. The two surgical approaches applicable are the middle fossa and retrosigmoid approaches. The indications and limitations discussed in previous chapters for these approaches also apply to bilateral tumors. The difficult decision often involves which side lesion to attempt (larger versus smaller tumor and better versus worse-hearing ear). Usually the larger tumor and poorer hearing ear are operated first. If hearing is successfully preserved on one side, the other side may be considered for surgery 6 months following the initial procedure.

OBSERVATION WITHOUT SURGICAL INTERVENTION. A small tumor in an only-hearing ear or bilateral tumors too large for hearing preservation are usually managed by observation. Close clinical and MRI follow-up (initially at 6 months and then annually) allows adequate assessment of brainstem compression or hydrocephalus. The patients must understand the importance of notifying the otologist of any symptoms that may signify tumor growth or brainstem compression. Surgery is considered when further hearing loss develops, clinical symptoms increase, or the tumor reaches sufficient size for brainstem compression (usually 3cm). The observation time is an important opportunity for educational rehabilitation, counseling, signing and lip-reading classes, and family screening.

MIDDLE FOSSA CRANIOTOMY—INTERNAL AUDITORY CANAL DECOMPRESSION WITHOUT TUMOR REMOVAL.

This technique is an option for patients undergoing observation who experience fluctuation or progression of hearing loss. The goal of this strategy is to relieve the constriction on the cochlear nerve and blood supply without subjecting the patient to the increased risk of hearing loss if tumor debulking is initiated. The basic principles of middle fossa tumor surgery apply. The dura of the IAC and porus acusticus is incised; however, the tumor is not removed or debulked. This technique has been successfully employed to stabilize and even improve hearing in patients with bilateral tumors.[23]

RETROSIGMOID PARTIAL TUMOR REMOVAL.

The theory for partial tumor removal is preservation of the seventh and eighth nerves by removing only those portions of the tumor farthest from the nerves. Although this approach is advocated in some centers,[23a] its success has been limited. Debulking the tumor may affect the blood supply along the cochlear nerve, and rapid regrowth of tumor from the well-vascularized capsule is common.

NONHEARING PRESERVATION—TOTAL REMOVAL.

When hearing preservation is not an issue, the goal of management is total tumor removal and facial nerve preservation. Translabyrinthine or retrosigmoid techniques are suitable, although distal IAC exposure of the seventh nerve is often more direct with the translabyrinthine approach. Hearing rehabilitation can be accomplished with a cochlear implant if the cochlear nerve is preserved, or the auditory brainstem implant (see Chapter 59) if the cochlear nerve is transected.

STEREOTACTIC RADIOSURGERY (RADIATION THERAPY).

Stereotactic surgery is closed-skull destruction of a precisely definable intracranial tissue through use of ionizing radiation. This technique, which combines a stereotactic delivery device with ionizing radiation, was initially described by Leksell[29] in 1951. In 1968, Larsson et al.[30] designed and applied the first gamma knife stereotactic radiosurgical unit. The dose of radiation in stereotactic radiosurgery is delivered by means of several evenly distributed and precisely collimated beams of ionizing radiation. The radiation dose gradient is extremely sharp at the target tissue, resulting in a radiation lesion that is sharply circumscribed. Tissue adjacent to the target structures sustain little damage.

Stereotactic radiosurgery is a treatment alternative for some NF-2 patients. However, this approach is not without morbidity. Progressive hearing deterioration or deafness has been reported in 64 per cent, transient facial paralysis in 12 per cent, facial hypesthesia in four per cent, and progressive tumor growth in 34 per cent. Hydrocephalus has also been reported as a complication of stereotactic radiosurgery.[31]

Additionally, disadvantages of this technique include radiation-induced fibrosis, which complicates tumor removal when surgery becomes necessary owing to continued tumor growth. Similarly, this fibrosis may produce anatomic distortion that prevents successful placement of an auditory brainstem implant. Finally, in larger tumors there is increased risk of radiation necrosis of the adjacent brainstem and cerebellum.

Other Management Considerations

NF-2 is a heritable disease with significant morbidity; so, every patient must be fully educated and the family screened to identify other affected or at-risk individuals. Genetic counseling is important, and the geneticist should direct the family screening.

Auditory rehabilitation of all NF-2 patients should anticipate eventual hearing loss. Early training in speechreading, signing, and use of the telephone typewriter (TTY) will provide necessary skills when significant hearing loss occurs.

Other Tumors

Other intracranial and spinous tumors, as well as malignant tumors, occur in NF patients and must be evaluated. The surgical treatment of nonmalignant tumors is selectively introduced when clinically progressive disease is implicated. Ideally, intervention is accomplished without increasing the neurologic deficit.

DISCUSSION

In selected patients, careful observation of the tumors with serial audiometrics and serial MR scans may be most appropriate. This approach may be advisable in a patient with an apparently stable acoustic neuroma in one ear and no hearing in the opposite ear. The approach may be used in a patient with a family history of the Feiling and Gardner type in which the tumor occurs in the third or fourth decades of life and slow tumor progression has been documented in other family members.

The gamut of possibilities regarding hearing in surgical treatment of bilateral acoustic neuromas ranges from total removal with hearing preservation to removal with the application of sophisticated new technology incorporating electrical stimulation of the auditory system. It is hoped that if newly diagnosed bilateral tumors are treated more aggressively at the outset, hearing preservation surgery will be accomplished more frequently. When total removal and hearing preservation is not possible, cochlear implantation may be feasible if the cochlear nerve can be anatomically preserved. Cohen et al.[24] reported on such a patient, in whom total removal of bilateral acoustic neromas was accomplished but with loss of hearing. The cochlear nerve was preserved on one side, and a cochlear implant was performed in this ear. The patient was able to recognize various environmental sounds and had both closed- and open-set speech discrimination. When total removal of bilateral acoustic neuromas is performed and it is not possible to preserve the cochlear nerve, another treatment option is the auditory brainstem implant.[25] In this approach, an electrode is placed on the cochlear nucleus, and coded electrical signals are presented directly to the brainstem. Ongoing research is being conducted at the House Ear Institute to develop a multichannel brainstem stimulator to improve results over those obtained with the single-channel auditory brainstem implant, which has been under investigation since 1979.[26, 27] Yet another approach that has met with some success is the application of tactile devices that convert sound to tactile displays presented to the skin.[28]

References

1. National Institutes of Health Consensus Development Conference: Conference report—Neurofibromatosis Conference Statement. Arch Neurol 45: 575–578, 1988.
2. Hitselberger WE, Hughes RL: Bilateral acoustic tumors and neurofibromatosis. Arch Otolaryngol Head and Neck Surg 88 (Monograph II): 152–711, 1968.
3. Hughes GB, Sismanis A, Glasscock ME III, et al.: Management of bilateral acoustic tumors. Laryngoscope 92: 1351–1359, 1982.
4. Malis L: Neurofibromatosis. In Cummings CW, et al. (eds): Otolaryngology—Head and Neck Surgery. St. Louis, CV Mosby, 1986, pp 3449–3456.
5. Tator CH, Nedzelski JM: Preservation of hearing in patients undergoing excision of acoustic neuromas and other cerebellopontine angle tumors. J Neurosurg 63: 168–174, 1985.
6. Dutcher PO, House WF, Hitselberger WE: Early detection of small bilateral acoustic tumors. Am J Otol 8: 35–38, 1987.
7. Piffko P, Pasztor E: Operated bilateral acoustic neurinoma with preservation of hearing and facial nerve function. ORL Otorhinolaryngol Relat Spec 43: 255–261, 1981.
8. Miyamoto RT, Campbell RL, Fritsch M, Lochmueller G: Preservation of hearing in neurofibromatosis 2. Otolaryngol Head Neck Surg 103: 619–624, 1990.
9. Miyamoto RT, Roos KL, Cambell RL, Worth RM: Contemporary management of neurofibromatosis. Ann Otol Rhinol Laryngol 100: 38–43, 1991.
10. Miyamoto RT, Roos KL, Campbell RL: Hearing preservation in neurofibromatosis-2. In Tos M, Thomsen J (eds): Acoustic Neuroma. Amsterdam/New York, Kugler Publications, 1992, pp 843–847.
11. Miyamoto RT, Roos KL, Campbell RL: Hearing preservation in neurofibromatosis-2. In Samii M (ed): Proceedings of the First International Skull Base Congress. Hannover, Germany, June 14–20, 1992 [In press].
12. Eldridge R, Parry D: Neurofibromatosis 2: Evidence for clinical heterogeneity based on 54 affected individuals studied by MRI with gadolinium, 1987–1991. In Tos M, Thomsen J (eds): Acoustic Neuroma. Amsterdam/New York, Kugler Publications, 1992, pp 801–804.
13. Lubs MLE, Bauer MS, Formas ME, Djokic B: Lisch nodules in neurofibromatosis type I. N Engl J Med 324: 1264–1266, 1991.
14. Kaiser-Kupfer MI, Freidlin V, Datiles MB, et al.: The association of posterior capsular lens opacities with bilateral acoustic neuromas in patients with neurofibromatosis type 2. Arch Ophthalmol Head Neck Surg 107: 541–544, 1989.
15. Goldgar DE, Green P, Parry DM, Mulvihill JJ: Multipoint linkage analysis in neurofibromatosis type 1: An international collaboration. Am J Hum Genet 44: 6–12, 1989.
16. Ledbetter DH, Rich DC, O'Connell P, et al.: Precise localization of NF-1 to 17 q 11.2 by balanced translocation. Am J Hum Genet 44: 20–24, 1989.
17. Seizinger BR, Martuza RL, Gusella JF: Loss of genes on chromosome 22 in tumorigenesis of human acoustic neuroma. Nature 322: 644–647, 1986.
18. Seizinger BR, Rouleau G, Ozelius LJ, et al.: Common pathogenetic mechanism for three tumor types in bilateral acoustic neurofibromatosis. Science 236: 317–319, 1987.
19. Rouleau GA, Wetelecki W, Haines JL, et al.: Genetic linkage of bilateral acoustic neurofibromatosis to a DNA marker on chromosome 22. Nature 329: 246–248, 1987.
20. Wertelecki W, Rouleau GA, Supernau DW, et al.: Neurofibromatosis 2: Clinical and DNA linkage studies of a large kindred. N Engl J Med 319: 278–283, 1988.
21. Roos KL, Dunn DW: Neurofibromatosis. CA Cancer J Clin [In press].
22. Linthicum FH Jr, Brackmann DE: Bilateral acoustic tumors. A diagnostic and surgical challenge. Arch Otolaryngol Head Neck Surg 106: 729–733, 1980.
22a. House WF, Gardner G, Hughes RL: Middle cranial fossa approach to acoustic tumor surgery. Arch Otolaryngol 88: 631, 1968.
23. Gadre AK, Kwartler JA, Brackmann DE, et al.: Middle fossa decompression of the internal auditory canal in acoustic neuroma surgery: A therapeutic alternative. Laryngoscope 100: 948–951, 1990.
23a. Kemink JL, Langman AW, Niparko JK, Graham MD: Operative management of acoustic neuromas: The priority of neurologic function over complete resection. Otolaryngol Head Neck Surg 104:96–99, 1991.
24. Cohen NL, Ransohoff J, Kohan D, Hoffman R: Cochlear implants in the treatment of acoustic neuromas: A treatment algorithm for bilateral acoustic neuromas (BAN). In Tos M, Thomsen J (eds): Acoustic Neuroma. Amsterdam/New York, Kugler Publications, 1992, pp 857–862.
25. Nelson RA: Auditory brainstem implant. In Tos M, Thomsen J (eds): Acoustic Neuroma. Amsterdam/New York, Kugler Publications, 1992, pp 869–872.
26. Terr LI, Fayad J, Hitselberger WE, Rizkalla Z: Cochlear nucleus anatomy related to central electroauditory prosthesis implantation. Otolaryngol Head Neck Surg 102: 717–721, 1990.
27. Shannon RV, Otto SR: Psychophysical measures from electrical stimulation of the human cochlear nucleus. Hear Res 47: 159–168, 1990.
28. Miyamoto RT, Myres WA, Wagner M, Punch JL: Vibrotactile devices as sensory aid for the deaf. Otolaryngol Head Neck Surg 97: 57–63, 1987.
29. Leksell L: The stereotaxic method and radiosurgery of the brain. Acta Chir Scand 102: 316–319, 1951.
30. Larsson B, Leksell L, Rexed B, et al.: The high-energy proton beam as a neurosurgical tool. Nature 182: 1222–1223, 1968.
31. Thomsen J, Tos M, Borgesen S: Gamma knife: Hydrocephalus as a complication of the stereotactic radiosurgical treatment of acoustic neuroma. Am J Otol 11: 330–333, 1990.
32. Ferris NJ, Siu KH: Neurofibromatosis 2: Report of an affected kindred, with a discussion of imaging strategy. Australas Radiol 34(3): 229–233, 1990.

59

Auditory Brainstem Implant

WILLIAM E. HITSELBERGER, M.D.
FRED F. TELISCHI, M.D.

Patients who have lost integrity of the auditory nerves between the spiral ganglion of the cochlea and the cochlear nuclei in the brainstem were until recently confined to a world devoid of sound. Such patients cannot benefit from cochlear implants because they have no remaining eighth nerve to stimulate. Vibrotactile aids, lip reading, and sign language have been the only communication modes available to these patients. Technologic and surgical advances in neuro-otology now permit bypassing the sensory end organ and first-order neuron to stimulate the central auditory pathways. The auditory brainstem implant (ABI) is designed to bypass both the cochlea and the cochlear nerve and directly stimulate the cochlear nuclei, giving the sensation of sound to an otherwise deaf patient.

This chapter discusses the clinical and surgical aspects of implanting an electrode adjacent to the human cochlear nuclei. The techniques draw from the experience of implanting 28 patients with various devices since 1979 at the House Ear Clinic and Institute. Technical and theoretical considerations of central auditory implantation and stimulation have been reviewed elsewhere.[1,2]

PATIENT SELECTION

At this time, patients receive the ABI under a protocol monitored by the US Food and Drug Administration. The criteria for implantation are listed in Table 59–1. Only patients with neurofibromatosis type 2 (NF-2) manifesting bilateral acoustic neuromas may receive the device. At least 90 per cent of NF-2 patients exhibit bilateral eighth nerve neuromas.[3] An unpublished review of patients with NF-2 seen at the House Ear Clinic revealed that two thirds had bilateral internal auditory canal (IAC)–cerebellopontine angle (CPA) tumors alone or with one other tumor as the only central nervous system manifestation of their disease. The patients were young (average age, 28 years). With improvements in medical care and surgical techniques, the life span of many of these patients has been significantly prolonged. Restoration of even rudimentary auditory function can enhance their quality of life and ability to function in a hearing world.

The current protocol allows implantation only at the time of first or second tumor removal. Implantation during removal of the first tumor allows experience with the device and may enhance performance when the patient loses all hearing. Also, implantation in the first side gives the patient two chances at obtaining an optimally functioning system should the first side not be successful.

The management of bilateral acoustic neuromas

TABLE 59–1. Criteria for Implantation

Evidence of bilateral 7/8 nerve tumors involving the internal auditory canal or cerebellopontine angle
Competency in the English language
Age 15 years or older
Psychological suitability
Willingness to comply with the research follow-up protocol
Realistic expectations

should be highly individualized (see Chapter 58). Hearing preservation remains an ideal but elusive goal in the management of these tumors in patients with NF-2. No artificial means of restoring hearing can match an intact auditory system. Therefore, preserving any amount of the patient's own hearing is paramount. Patients meeting the criteria listed in Table 59–2 may be considered and observed accordingly. The availability of the ABI provides an alternative to a desperate attempt to preserve nonserviceable hearing when large tumors are removed and hearing conservation is unlikely.

Future applications of the ABI and similar devices include bilateral temporal bone fractures and demyelinating diseases affecting the eighth nerve but sparing at least one cochlear nucleus.

PREOPERATIVE EVALUATION AND COUNSELING

The goal of implantation is to place a safe and stable device that provides the patient with environmental sounds and improves lip reading without side effects. Prospective patients are apprised of the goals, limitations, and risks of the ABI through a series of three evaluation-counseling sessions similar to those of cochlear implantation. The implant candidate's expectations are evaluated as well, and informed consent is obtained. The role of an experienced multidisciplinary implant team—neuro-otologist, neurosurgeon, neuro/auditory physiologist, anatomist, radiologist, and others—cannot be overemphasized.

TABLE 59–2. Criteria for Auditory Brainstem Implant in NF-2 Patients*

Second tumor in an only-hearing ear
Any tumor in a hearing ear that measures greater than 1.5cm in the largest diameter
Short life expectancy due to other tumors, medical problems, or advanced age
Serviceable hearing with a tumor that shows no significant growth by sequential magnetic resonance scans and stable hearing by serial audiograms

*Situations in which to observe a tumor in a hearing ear that is not threatening life or neurologic function in an NF-2 patient with bilateral acoustic neuromas.

WILLIAM E. HITSELBERGER & FRED F. TELISCHI

DEVICE

The hardware of the ABI has undergone a number of modifications since the original ball electrode was inserted by Drs. William House and William Hitselberger in 1979.[1, 4] The electrode used at present employs eight disks in a silicone carrier connected to an implantable coil magnet receiver (Cochlear Corporation) (Fig. 59–1). The external device consists of a transcutaneous magnetic connector and sound processor similar to those of a cochlear implant. Signal processing strategies continuously evolve in an effort to improve patient performance.[2]

ANATOMIC CONSIDERATIONS

The target of the ABI electrodes is the cochlear nuclear complex—dorsal and ventral cochlear nuclei. In humans, the cerebellar peduncle that forms the base of the pons covers the auditory nuclei. This means that the nuclei are not visible to the surgeon and must be located from surface landmarks. Figure 59–2 illustrates the major structures of the pontomedullary junction region with the translabyrinthine approach surgical field of view within the dashed lines. The terminus of the sleevelike lateral recess forms the foramen of Luschka. Just inferior to the foramen is the root of the glossopharyngeal ninth nerve. Superior to the foramen lies the root entry and exit zones of the vestibulocochlear and facial nerves. This area is frequently distorted by the tumor, although a computer-assisted three-dimensional reconstruction of the cochlear nuclei in an acoustic neuroma patient showed the overall shape of the complex unchanged.

The cochlear nuclei come closest to the surface of the brainstem within the superior aspect of the lateral recess.[5, 6] The main target for stimulation is the ventral cochlear nucleus, which forms the main relay for eighth nerve input and the greater part of the ascending auditory pathway.[9] Placement of the electrodes completely within the recess gives the fewest side effects and preserves auditory stimulation even though in this position, some part of the electrode array lies adjacent to the dorsal cochlear nucleus.[2] Also, the disadvantage of lack of exposure is partially offset by positional stability provided to the electrode carrier by the limited space in the lateral recess.

SURGICAL CONSIDERATIONS

The surgical approach for tumor removal in ABI cases has been exclusively via translabyrinthine craniotomy (see Chapter 51). The translabyrinthine route has been

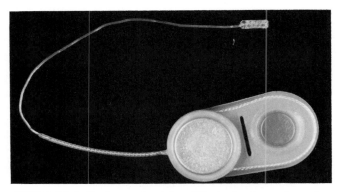

FIGURE 59–1. Photograph of the ABI electrode and receiver coil.

found to provide the most direct access to the lateral recess and surface of the cochlear nuclei.[8] Until the actual placement of the device, the surgery proceeds as in any other translabyrinthine acoustic neuroma excision with the following exceptions. The scalp hair shave is extended posteriorly to accommodate the percutaneous plug. Electrodes are placed for recording electrically evoked auditory brainstem responses and for monitoring cranial nerves V (motor), VII, and IX. A large C-shaped postauricular incision is made to cover the receiver coil so that no part of the device crosses the skin wound (Fig. 59–3).

Electrophysiologic monitoring is performed during implantation to ensure that the electrode activates the auditory system and to assess activation of nonauditory brainstem structures. To aid in placing the electrode array, electrically evoked auditory brainstem responses (EABRs) are recorded.[9] There may be considerable uncertainty about the correct position for the electrode array when a large tumor has distorted the anatomic landmarks at the brainstem. A repeatable EABR indicates that stimulation of the auditory system is occurring. Intraoperative EABRs obtained after tumor removal vary considerably from brainstem responses routinely recorded with acoustic stimulation (ABRs) in awake individuals. An experienced physiologist interprets these waveforms at the time of implantation based on data collected from previous implants (Fig. 59–4).

For recording EABRs, subdermal needle electrodes are inserted at the vertex of the head, over the seventh cervical vertebra in the neck, and at the hairline of the occiput prior to the draping of the sterile field. After the coil of the implant has been fastened to the skull and the electrode assembly has been placed on the brainstem, stimulating leads are connected from a current generator to the coil. Biphasic current pulses provide the stimuli to evoke responses. Scalp-recorded evoked signals are sampled and averaged by computer following suitable amplification and filtering.

FIGURE 59-2

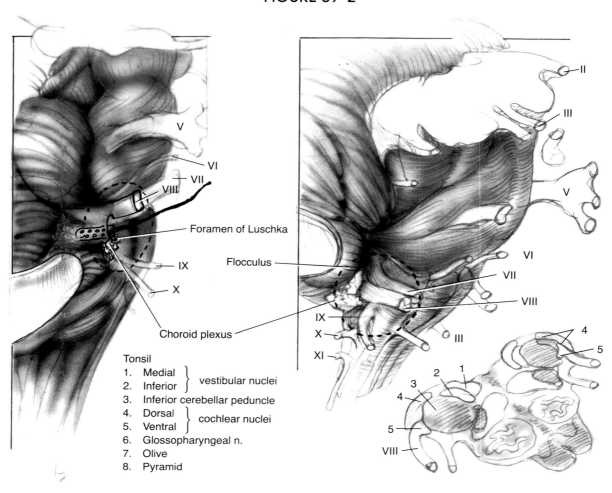

Foramen of Luschka

Flocculus

Choroid plexus

Tonsil
1. Medial ⎫
2. Inferior ⎬ vestibular nuclei
3. Inferior cerebellar peduncle
4. Dorsal ⎫
5. Ventral ⎬ cochlear nuclei
6. Glossopharyngeal n.
7. Olive
8. Pyramid

FIGURE 59-2. Schematic of cochlear nuclei region demonstrating relative location of various landmarks. Dashed area represents approximate surgical view. Electrode is fully inserted into proper position.

FIGURE 59-3. Location of incision with respect to planned site of receiver coil.

FIGURE 59-3

FIGURE 59-4

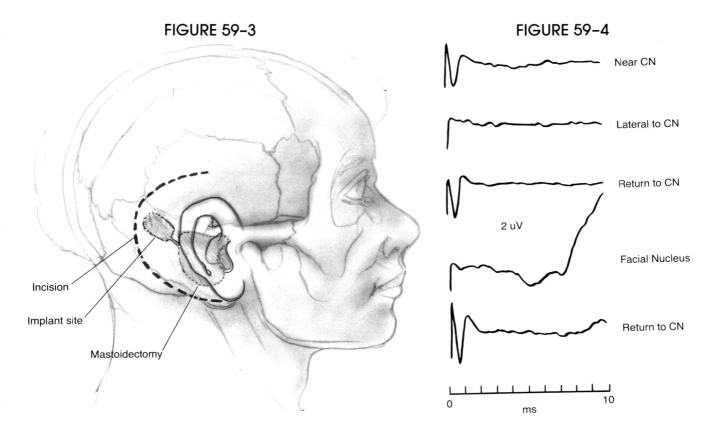

Incision

Implant site

Mastoidectomy

Near CN

Lateral to CN

Return to CN

2 uV

Facial Nucleus

Return to CN

0   ms   10

FIGURE 59-4. EABR tracings demonstrate intraoperative monitoring sequence. In the upper trace the electrode was positioned near the cochlear nuclei (CN), producing an auditory evoked response in the first 2 msec. In successive traces, the electrode was moved away from the CN, and no auditory response was observed. The electrode was returned to the CN region, and an auditory response was again observed. Moving the electrode in the direction of the facial nerve replaced the auditory response with a large muscle response after 5 msec. Finally, return of the electrode to the CN region produced an auditory response and no EMG response. (From Brackmann DE, et al.: Auditory brainstem implant: I. Issues in surgical implantation. Otolaryngol Head Neck Surg 108:624–633, 1993.)

Electrophysiologic monitoring also helps determine the electrode position that minimizes nonauditory side effects. In addition to monitoring the facial nerve in standard fashion,[10] bipolar electrodes are inserted in the ipsilateral masseter and pharyngeal muscles to monitor activation of cranial nerves V and IX, respectively. If the electromyographic recordings reveal activation of nonauditory centers during stimulation through the implant or if a muscle response is visually observed, the ABI is repositioned.

Electrode impedance is monitored when the electrode is placed and during and after wound closing. A high impedance value indicates a broken or cut wire, whereas a low impedance indicates a short circuit. In either case, the electrode can be repositioned or a new electrode–coil system implanted prior to final closing.

IMPLANTATION TECHNIQUE

Tumor dissection proceeds in the normal fashion via a translabyrinthine craniotomy. After tumor removal and hemostasis, an area of cortical bone posterior to the mastoid is flattened, and a trough to accept the wires from the electrodes to the coil is created in a fashion similar to that of cochlear implantation. Creation of the pedestal site begins with retraction of the posterior skin flap and periosteum. Using a replica of the coil as a guide, a circular area of bony cortex posterosuperior to the mastoid defect is drilled with cutting burrs (Fig. 59–5). A specially designed butterfly bit or other cylindrical bits associated with newer high-speed drills may be employed. Using a replica of the coil as a guide, the surgeon drills three or four screw holes into the bone to accept the tiedown suture. The coil is fixed with nylon suture prior to electrode positioning so that the manipulation of the leads does not alter the electrode placement. The receiver slides in medial to the temporalis muscle (Fig. 59–6). Because only bipolar cautery may be used after the electrode array is inserted to minimize the risk of current shunting through the device into the brainstem, meticulous hemostasis of the entire wound and cerebellopontine angle is ensured prior to implantation.

Anatomic landmarks lead the way to the surface of the cochlear nuclei. Normally intact choroid plexus marks the entrance to the lateral recess (foramen of Luschka) and the taenia obliquely traverses the roof of the lateral recess, marking the surface of the ventral cochlear nucleus. These structures may not be clearly visible, however, when a large tumor has significantly distorted the lateral aspect of the pons and medulla. Following the stump of the eighth nerve usually leads to the opening of the lateral recess in these cases. The ninth cranial nerve can also be used as a reference point for the lateral recess. A concavity sometimes visualized between the eight and ninth nerves should not be confused with the introitus of the recess. The location of lateral recess may be confirmed by noting the egress of cerebrospinal fluid as the anesthesiologist induces a Valsalva maneuver in the patient. This technique should be reserved as a final check after the opening to the recess has been located by standard landmarks because cerebrospinal fluid will be drained quickly and the advantage of this technique lost with multiple Valsalva maneuvers.

After identifying the opening to the foramen of Luschka, the electrode array is picked up atraumatically with a fine forceps. The carrier is passed into the lateral recess with the electrodes facing superiorly (Fig. 59–7). With experience, we have found that the system functions better, with fewer side effects, when the electrodes are placed fully within the lateral recess.[2] After placement, all the electrode plates are stimulated to confirm their position over the nucleus. They are tested for the presence of EABRs, stimulation of adjacent cranial nerves (V, VII, and IX), and vital sign changes. The position of the carrier usually needs some adjustment to maximize the EABRs and minimize electromyographic responses from the other nerves.

The carrier is secured by a small piece of fat packed into the meatus of the lateral recess. Fibrous tissue eventually stabilizes the implant in position. The reference electrode is embedded into the temporalis muscle, and the wires are positioned in the mastoid cavity and the bony trough previously drilled (Fig. 59–8). Abdominal fat obliterates the mastoid defect. The incision is closed in three layers, and care is taken not to disturb the wires. The wound is not drained routinely. A large mastoid-type dressing is left in place for 4 days.

FIGURE 59–5. Surgical view of completed translabyrinthine craniotomy, trough for wires and coil site being drilled.

FIGURE 59–6. Device secured in place with suture.

FIGURE 59-5

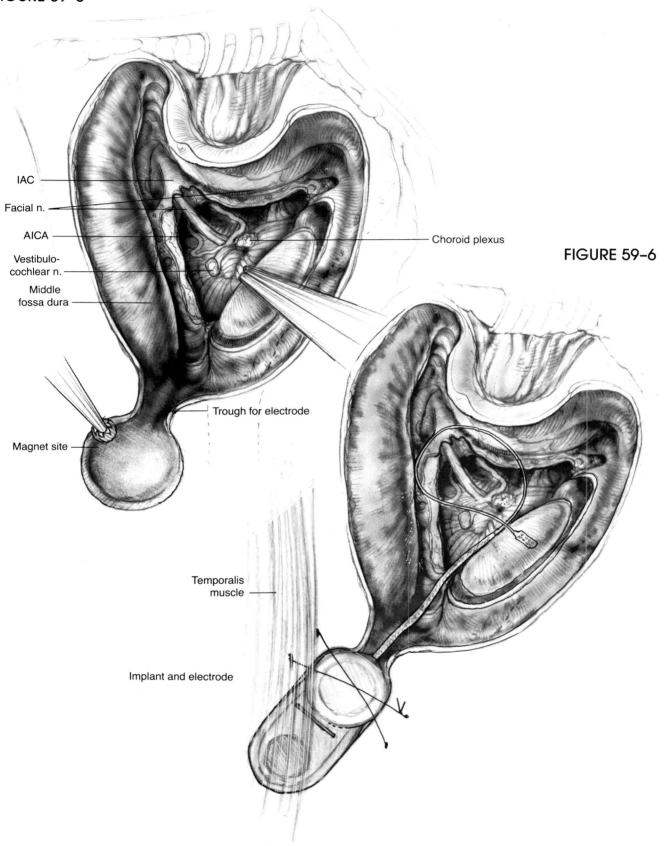

IAC

Facial n.

AICA

Vestibulo-
cochlear n.

Middle
fossa dura

Choroid plexus

FIGURE 59-6

Trough for electrode

Magnet site

Temporalis
muscle

Implant and electrode

POSTOPERATIVE CARE

The postoperative care after implantation shares many of the features with that for routine translabyrinthine tumor resections (see Chapter 51). A similar schedule for advancing patient activity and decreasing the level of intensity of nursing care is maintained. A mastoid dressing should remain in place for at least 4 days. Careful attention to any moisture on the bandages allows prompt identification of cerebrospinal fluid leak through the postauricular wound. Intravenous antibiotics are administered prophylactically 1 day preoperatively and continued through the fifth day postoperatively.

Initial testing of the appliance begins on the second postoperative day while the patient remains in the intensive care unit. Vital signs and oxygen saturation are closely monitored with an implant physician present. Electrode impedances are measured using a current level that is inaudible to the patient.

If the patient's condition permits, a pulsing stimulus is presented and slowly raised in amplitude. Stimulation with a 300Hz sinusoid has been shown to produce the lowest auditory thresholds and the fewest nonauditory side effects with the ABI.[11] Simulation charge densities should be maintained within safe limits for electrical stimulation of brain tissue.[12, 13] Behavioral measurements are obtained by instructing the patient to raise a hand when he or she hears the stimulus tone. The patient also reports nonauditory side effects, including facial movement (cranial nerve VII), vertigo (cranial nerve VIIIvest), sensations in the throat (cranial nerve IX), tingling in the shoulder and arm (long tracts of the brainstem), and vibratory sensation in the eye (cerebellar flocculus). Thresholds are recorded for auditory and nonauditory sensations for each electrode.

POSTOPERATIVE COMPLICATIONS

The most significant complication in the immediate postoperative period is cerebrospinal fluid leak around the percutaneous coil when this type of device is used. Unlike routine translabyrinthine surgery, in which the fluid usually takes the nasal route via the eustachian tube, the ABI electrode and wires provide a path along which cerebrospinal fluid can travel and extrude through the wound. Now that a fully implantable coil receiver has replaced the percutaneous coil, the rate of leak has decreased. Prevention of a leak begins with meticulous dural approximation and packing of the eustachian tube and mastoid cavity with various materials. Although the dural opening cannot be closed in a watertight manner, it should be approximated as closely as possible to minimize the opening. A dumbbell-shaped graft of fat will plug the residual space. Muscle, oxidized cellulose (Surgicel), and bone wax commonly are employed for eustachian tube closure, and autologous fat works well in the mastoid. Multilayered closure for the wound decreases pathways for cerebrospinal fluid egress.

Despite these precautions, patients with the ABI appear more prone to cerebrospinal fluid leak than those undergoing translabyrinthine procedures without implantation. Leaks from the nose and wound usually respond to reapplication of mastoid pressure dressing and bed rest. A lumbar-subarachnoid cerebrospinal fluid drain is added for persistent leaks. Finally, surgical exploration and repacking of the wound can be employed for leakage unresponsive to more conservative measures.

Meningitis can occur either spontaneously or as a result of postoperative cerebrospinal fluid leak. This unusual complication, when identified promptly, responds to antibiotics and cessation of the leak.

Normal healing to a stable implant situation usually takes 6 weeks. Avoidance of trauma and observance of careful local hygiene provide years of trouble-free use of the device.

RESULTS

Twenty-eight patients with NF-2 have been implanted between 1979 and 1993. The current fully implantable receiver coil device was placed in the four most recent cases. The tumor sizes for these patients averaged 3.8cm. Early on, device problems and failures limited the successful use of the implant in some cases. Technical refinements and experience have resulted in useful implantation in the more recent cases.

Nineteen patients have obtained auditory benefit without significant side effects in the testing labora-

FIGURE 59–7. Surgical view of the electrodes being passed into the lateral recess (magnified view of the dashed area in Figure 59–5).

FIGURE 59–8. Implant, wires, and fat in place prior to skin closure.

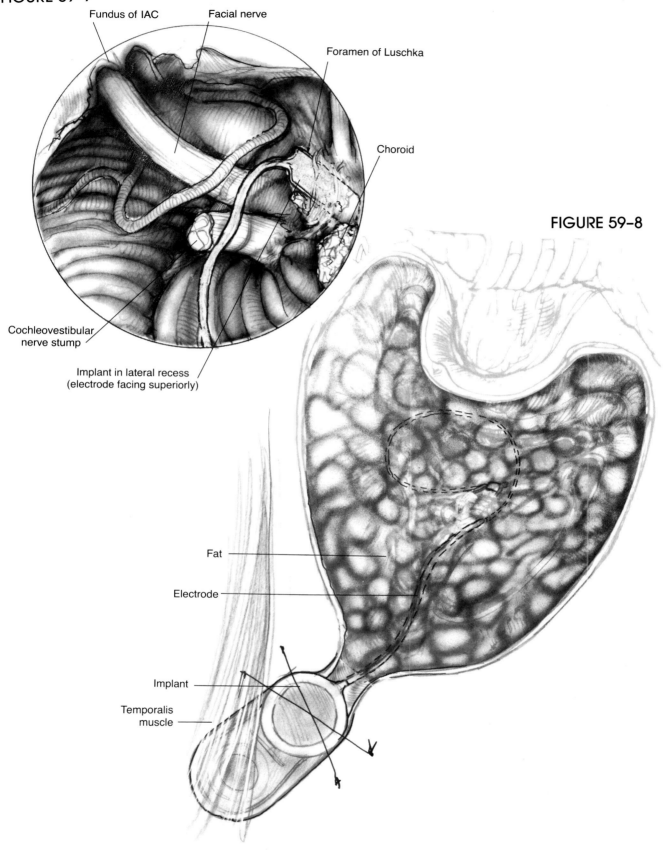

FIGURE 59-7

Fundus of IAC

Facial nerve

Foramen of Luschka

Choroid

Cochleovestibular
nerve stump

Implant in lateral recess
(electrode facing superiorly)

FIGURE 59-8

Fat

Electrode

Implant

Temporalis
muscle

tory, including 13 of the past 14 patients. Seventeen patients use the device at home; the other two have useful hearing contralaterally. All users have awareness of environmental sounds and improved lip-reading scores with the implant, with the exception of one patient, who has decreased vision. At this point, however, only a few ABI patients receive limited open-set speech recognition using their implant.

OTHER RESEARCH

Niparko et al.[14] demonstrated the feasibility of implanting and stimulating within the substance of the cochlear nucleus in guinea pigs. In a related study, el-Kashlan et al.[15] compared the effectiveness of surface electrodes with those placed into the nucleus. They found lower thresholds and a wider dynamic range in animals with penetrating electrodes than in those with surface placement. This more invasive technique may provide a future direction for cochlear nucleus implantation.

Luetje et al.[16] reported on one case in which they implanted a Nucleus mini–22-channel device during removal of a second-side tumor. The electrode array was placed along the root entry zone of the eighth nerve with the tip at the foramen of Luschka. Stimulation of the last five electrodes (#18–22) resulted in auditory sensation at the sixth postoperative day. Auditory stimulation ceased by 1 month after implantation. Workable multichannel configurations with new processing strategies may improve patient performance in the future.

SUMMARY

An electrode array for electrical stimulation can be safely and reliably placed on the brainstem of patients and chronically stimulated to produce auditory sensations by selective activation of the cochlear nucleus. Few side effects and minimal morbidity characterize the clinical course of patients with these implants.

Further research and improvements not only in the hardware but especially in the sound processing should give patients improved speech understanding in the future.

References

1. Brackmann DE, Hitselberger WE, Nelson RA, et al.: Auditory Brainstem Implant: I. Issues in Surgical Implantation. Otolaryngol Head Neck Surg 108:624–633, 1993.
2. Shannon RV, Fayad J, Moore JK, et al.: Auditory Brainstem Implant: II. Postsurgical issues and performance. Otolaryngol Head Neck Surg 108:634–642, 1993.
3. Ricardi VM: Neurofibromatosis. Neurol Clin 5(3): 337–349, 1987.
4. Hitselberger N, House WF, Edgerton BS, Whitaker S. Cochlear nucleus implant. Otolaryngol Head Neck Surg 92:52–54, 1984.
5. Terr LI, Edgerton BJ: Surface topography of the cochlear nuclei in humans: Two and three-dimensional. Hear Res 17: 51–59, 1985.
6. Sinha VK, Terr LI, Galey FR, Linthicum FH: Computer aided three-dimensional reconstruction of the cochlear nerve root. Otolaryngol Head Neck Surg 113: 651–655, 1987.
7. Morest DK, Ostapoff EM, Potashner SJ, et al.: The cellular basis for signal processing in the mammalian cochlear nuclei. In Merchan MA (ed): The Mammalian Cochlear Nuclei: Organization and Function. Europa Arts Graficas Salamanca, 1991.
8. Monsell EM, McElveen JT, Hitselberger WE, House WF: Surgical approaches to the human cochlear nucleus complex. Am J Otol 8(5): 450–455, 1987.
9. Waring M: Electrically evoked auditory brainstem response monitoring of auditory brainstem implant integrity during facial nerve tumor surgery. Laryngoscope 102(11): 1293–1295, 1992.
10. Niparko JK, Kileny PR, Kemink JL, et al.: Neurophysiologic intraoperative monitoring: II. Facial nerve function. Am J Otol 10: 55–61, 1989.
11. Shannon RV, Otto SR: Psychophysical measures from electrical stimulation of the human cochlear nucleus. Hear Res 47: 159–168, 1990.
12. McCreery DB, Agnew WF, Yven TGM, Bullara I: Charge density and charge per phase as cofactors in neural injury induced by electrical stimulation. IEEE Trans Biomed Eng 37: 996–1001, 1990.
13. Shannon RV: A model of safe levels for electrical stimulation. IEEE Trans Biomed Eng 39: 424–426, 1992.
14. Niparko JK, Altschuler RA, Xue XL, et al.: Surgical implantation and biocompatibility of central nervous system auditory prostheses. Ann Otol Rhin Laryngol 98: 965–970, 1989.
15. El-Kashlan HK, Niparko JK, Altschuler RA, Miller JM. Direct electrical stimulation of the cochlear nucleus: surface vs. penetrating stimulation. Otolaryngol Head Neck Surg 105:533–543, 1991.
16. Luetje CM, Whittaker CK, Geier L, et al.: Feasibility of multichannel human cochlear nucleus stimulation. Laryngoscope 102(1): 23–25, 1992.

60

Management of Postoperative Cerebrospinal Fluid Leaks

DERALD E. BRACKMANN, M.D.
GRAYSON K. RODGERS, M.D.

Egress of cerebrospinal fluid (CSF) from the subarachnoid space into surgical wounds often results in leakage of CSF from the wound, the ear canal (if the tympanic membrane is not intact), or the nose (via the eustachian tube). The spinal fluid follows the path of least resistance. Any procedure that encounters the subarachnoid space can be complicated by a postoperative CSF leak. These leaks result from failure to obtain watertight dural closure or from an inadequate seal of dural defects. CSF leaks are a concern because the defect provides a potential portal of entry for infection to seed the leptomeninges. Meningitis in this setting is met with significant morbidity and even mortality. CSF leaks, therefore, should be corrected promptly to avoid more serious complications. This chapter is dedicated to detailing the various techniques for treating postoperative CSF leaks.

PRESSURE DRESSING

For cases in which an abdominal fat graft has been used during closure to plug dural defects, a pressure dressing can be applied to control CSF leaks. The pressure dressing works by pushing the fat back into the dural defect, sealing off the subarachnoid space. In cases in which fat has been used, most leaks stop with a pressure dressing.

Technique

The dressing is applied in similar fashion to the initial postoperative dressing. First, a verticle gathering tie is placed in the temporal fossa. Four-by-four dressing sponges are folded in half and placed directly over the fat graft and in the postauricular sulcus to support the auricle (Fig. 60–1A). Next, fluffed Kerlix is placed over the 4 × 4 sponges and the auricle (Fig. 60–1B). A tight wrap of roller gauze is then applied (Fig. 60–1C). The direction of the wrap should be from the ear toward the occiput, which ensures that the auricle is not damaged by anterior folding. Also, the verticle tie must be as lateral as possible in the temporal fossa to avoid a pressure point on the forehead. Pressure necrosis of forehead skin can develop easily if attention is not given to this point.

The last layer of this dressing is a three-inch Ace bandage, which provides the final compression (Fig. 60–1D). The Ace bandage should be wrapped firmly, but patient comfort must be accommodated. Usually, the last several turns can be altered to adjust the exact amount of compression.

Ideally, a pressure dressing should be left in place for 4 or 5 days, which allows time for healing of the CSF leak site to occur. A minimum of 48 hours without leakage must pass before the dressing is removed.

Adjuncts:

In addition to the pressure dressing, other conservative actions should be undertaken. These measures all are directed at decreasing CSF pressure. Straining (Valsalva maneuver) is strictly avoided, and the patient is kept at bed rest with the head elevated 45 degrees. Limited activity, such as bathroom privileges or brief periods of sitting up in a chair, are at the surgeon's discretion. Stool softeners and cough suppressants can be used. Acetazolamide (Diamox) may be given to decrease CSF production.

LUMBAR DRAIN

The next step in CSF leak treatment is a lumbar subarachnoid spinal fluid drain. By removing CSF from the system at a site away from the dural defect, CSF pressure is decreased, and healing can occur. Some surgeons routinely place a lumbar drain at the time of surgery to assist with intraoperative CSF removal and decompression in the postoperative period.

Technique

To place the catheter, a lumbar puncture is performed at the L4-L5 level. The patient is placed in either a sitting or a lateral decubitus position. The spinous processes are palpated, and L4-L5 is identified at the level of the iliac crest. The patient is asked to flex the back and bring the knees and chin to the chest. A preprepared catheter kit contains all the necessary supplies for preparing, draping, and anesthetizing the sight. An 18-gauge Touey needle is introduced in the midline with a slight superior angle between the spinous processes (Fig. 60–2). The obturator is removed at intervals so the surgeon can look for a flow of CSF. Once a good flow of CSF is established, the epidural *site:* catheter is introduced through the needle and threaded into the epidural space. The opened side of the bevel of the needle faces the patient's left or right side on penetrating the spinous ligaments and arachnoid. Before the catheter is threaded, the bevel is turned to open superiorly, thereby facilitating directing the catheter cephalad. With a flow of CSF established, the needle is withdrawn, and the connector is placed on the end of the catheter so that a connection to intravenous tubing can be made. An empty intravenous fluid bag is attached to the tubing, and all connections are secured with tape.

rate: Several methods of regulating CSF output exist. This regulation is very important because if CSF is removed too rapidly, tension pneumocephalus and even brain herniation can occur.[1–3] Alternatively, if an inadequate amount of CSF is removed, the purpose of the drain is defeated. Humans produce approximately 18ml of CSF per hour. The natural mechanisms of CSF

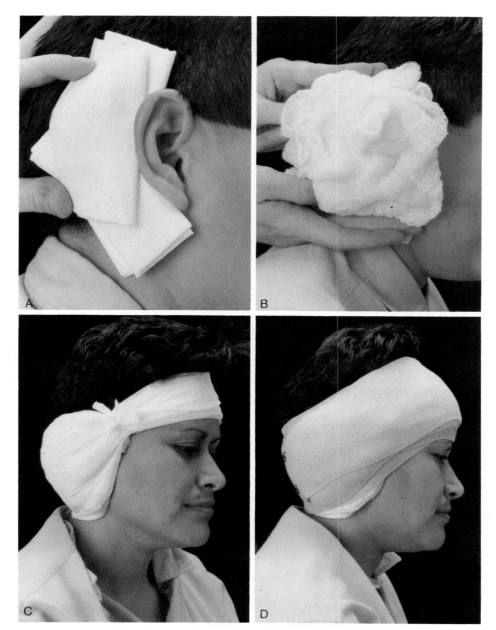

FIGURE 60-1. *A*, Folded 4 × 4 dressing sponges placed over the fat graft site after translabyrinthine acoustic tumor removal. The sponges are also placed in the postauricular crease to support the auricle. *B*, Fluffed Kerlix in place over the 4 × 4 sponges. *C*, Appearance of dressing after the roller gauze wrap. Tape can be applied to secure the position of the dressing. This is especially helpful on the forehead, where the dressing may slide inferiorly onto the brow. Note the laterally placed vertical gathering tie. *D*, Ace wrap in place. Again, tape can be helpful to stabilize the elastic dressing.

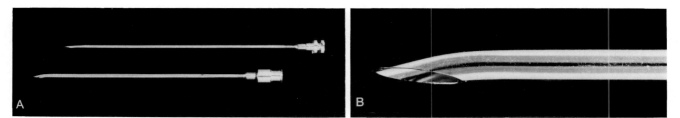

FIGURE 60-2. *A*, Touey needle used for lumbar puncture. *B*, Close-up of end of Touey needle.

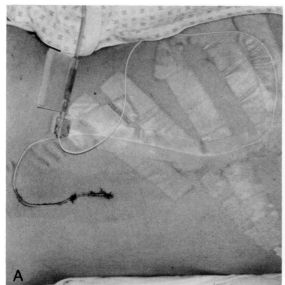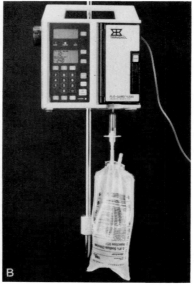

absorption reduce some CSF; therefore, the lumbar drain should remove less than 18ml of CSF per hour. Common neurosurgical practice is to order 50ml of CSF removed every 8 hours. Gravity is the standard method of effecting CSF drainage. The collection bag is placed at the level of the patient's heart or below to create increasing output of CSF as needed. This method requires extremely attentive nursing care to ensure the proper amount of drainage. Drains placed to respond to gravity have highly variable output, and a change in patient position may significantly increase or decrease flow. Establishing an even flow of spinal fluid is very difficult, and usually a bolus of fluid is removed, after which the drain is clamped. The system is at risk of occluding during these clamped periods. If flow becomes impaired, then removing the amount of CSF ordered becomes impossible.

To avoid some of these problems, we place the intravenous tubing in reverse direction through an intravenous infusion pump. The pump is set at 10ml per hour, and a slow, controlled, continuous flow of CSF is withdrawn from the patient (Fig. 60-3). Because this system is not gravity dependent, patients may move about without fear of a rapid discharge of CSF. Better patency of the catheter system is maintained because the flow is never stopped. Any occlusion of the system or air in the line is sensed, and an alarm is sounded as the pump stops. Other physicians have employed flow-regulated systems,[4,5] but the system described here is a definite improvement over those described. We have employed this system in a small series of patients and have found it vastly superior to gravity drainage.

While the lumbar drain is in place, the patient must be closely observed for signs of infection. The temper-

FIGURE 60-4. *A*, Postauricular approach and transection of the ear canal skin and dissection of cartilage from the canal skin. *B*, Everting stitches placed in the superior and inferior canal skin. These sutures are grasped with a hemostat placed through the canal and then pulled through, thus everting the canal skin. *C*, The everted canal skin is oversewn.

FIGURE 60-5. *A*, A mastoid periosteal flap is developed for a second layer of closure and is pedicled just posterior to the meatus. *B*, This flap is then rotated anteriorly and secured with absorbable sutures.

FIGURE 60-6. Middle fossa exposure with removal of the tegmen tympani and bony eustachian tube roof. The cochlea, vestibular labyrinth, facial nerve, and internal auditory canal are shown as well.

FIGURE 60-7. Obliteration of the bony eustachian tube with bone wax, bone paté, and muscle. Insert is a cross-section of the eustachian tube showing the relationship of the internal carotid artery (ICA), tensor tympani muscle, and greater superficial petrosal nerve.

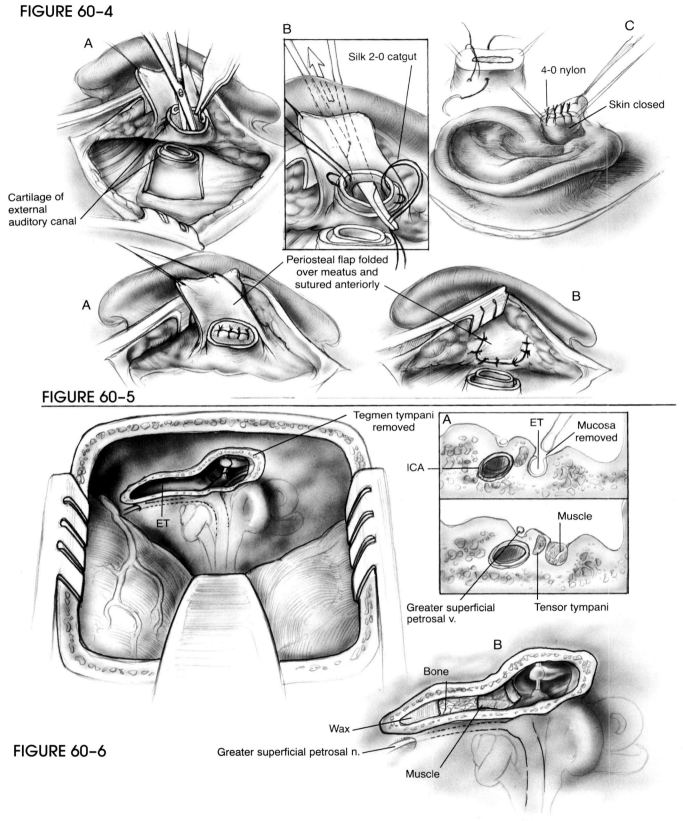

FIGURE 60-4

A

Cartilage of external auditory canal

A

B

Silk 2-0 catgut

Periosteal flap folded over meatus and sutured anteriorly

C

4-0 nylon

Skin closed

FIGURE 60-5

B

FIGURE 60-6

Tegmen tympani removed

ET

A

ET

ICA

Mucosa removed

Muscle

Greater superficial petrosal v.

Tensor tympani

B

Bone

Wax

Greater superficial petrosal n.

Muscle

FIGURE 60-7

ature, surgical wound, lumbar drain site, and white blood cell count must be monitored. Samples of CSF may be examined at any time. Headache during CSF drainage is common, but meningismus should not be present.

As with a pressure dressing, the lumbar drain should be left in place for 4 or 5 days. We often shut the pump off for the last 24 hours so that if the leak recurs, the drainage can be resumed.

WOUND EXPLORATION AND RECLOSURE

techniques:

When leaks do not resolve within 48 hours with a pressure dressing or lumbar drain, wound exploration with repacking of the abdominal fat and reclosure is indicated. In wounds in which a dural defect was packed with fat, dislodging of the fat from the defect may cause a CSF leak. When the wound is explored, the fat is removed and repacked (with additional fat as required) into the defect, as described in Chapter 51.[6] Some surgeons employ autologous fibrin glue as an adjunct to their closures.[7, 8] This material adds an additional seal to supplement the fat graft or, in other cases, a muscle or pericranial flap. A search should be made for opened mastoid air cells that can serve as pathways for spinal fluid. These air cell tracts can be occluded with bone wax. In cases of severe hearing loss, the eustachian tube should be packed off with Surgicel and temporalis muscle after removal of the incus and cutting of the tensor tympani tendon. *surgicel → bone patc → ME muscle*

Although a return to the operating room seems aggressive and is accompanied by the small risks brought by further surgery and anesthesia, this course of action has provided the most expedient control of CSF leaks that fail conservative therapy. The expeditious closure of a leak plays a very important part in the prevention of infection. The longer a leak remains open, the greater the chance for meningitis to develop. In a review of CSF leaks after translabyrinthine acoustic tumor removal at the House Ear Clinic, no statistically significant association between postoperative CSF leaks and the development of meningitis was found.[9] One explanation for this is that leaks are aggressively treated and stopped quickly, thus limiting the time available for contamination to occur.

REFRACTORY CEREBROSPINAL FLUID LEAKS

The techniques discussed earlier used separately or in combination stop the vast majority of CSF leaks.

Rarely, a leak is refractory to these measures. These leaks involve CSF that tracks through temporal bone cell tracts, finds its way to the middle ear, and subsequently discharges from the nose (eustachian tube) or the ear canal (tympanic membrane not intact). With an intact tympanic membrane, the eustachian tube is the final common pathway of most leaks. Although many methods involving repair of the source of the leakage are described, perhaps an easier and less risky approach is to block the final pathway.

Our management of these difficult leaks depends on the status of the patient's hearing and the tympanic membrane.① If no serviceable hearing exists or if the tympanic membrane is not intact, blind sac closure of the ear canal and obliteration of the middle ear and eustachian tube is performed.② If the tympanic membrane is intact and the patient has serviceable hearing, middle fossa closure of the eustachian tube is the procedure of choice.

Technique

Ear Canal Closure with Eustachian Tube and Middle Ear Obliteration

indx: poor hearing / TM not intact

Blind sac closure of the ear canal is accomplished through a postauricular incision with transection of the ear canal. The canal skin is separated from the cartilage of the lateral canal and then everted through the external auditory meatus. This everted canal skin is then oversewn with a nonabsorbable suture that is left in place for 10 days postoperatively (Fig. 60–4). A flap of mastoid periosteum is developed on a pedicle just posterior to the external auditory canal. This flap is then rotated anteriorly and secured as a second layer of closure for the meatus (Fig. 60–5). Next, all canal skin, the tympanic membrane, the malleus, and the incus are removed. To ensure complete removal of squamous epithelium and to enlarge the canal, a canalplasty is performed with a cutting burr. The eustachian tube is curetted and then packed with Surgicel and temporalis muscle. Before wound closure, the middle ear and remaining canal are packed with additional muscle. A pressure dressing is placed for 4 postoperative days, and a lumbar spinal fluid drain can also be used in the initial postoperative period.

Middle Fossa Obliteration of the Eustachian Tube

indx:

In cases in which the patient has good hearing and the tympanic membrane is intact, closure of the eustachian tube can be accomplished via the middle fossa. This procedure is approached as a middle fossa craniotomy, as outlined in Chapter 50. The bone flap is removed, and the dura is elevated from posterior to anterior. The arcuate eminence, greater superficial petrosal nerve, and middle meningeal artery are identified, and the middle fossa retractor is placed. A diamond burr is used to remove bone from the tegmen tympani and to expose the head of the malleus and the body of the incus (Fig. 60–6). Identification of the tensor tympani tendon and the cochleariform process allows identification of the eustachian tube, which is directly anterior. Also, the eustachian tube is just lateral to the greater superficial petrosal nerve. The bony eustachian tube is unroofed, and the mucosa is carefully curetted from the tube. The surgeon must be aware that the internal carotid artery can be dehiscent in the medial or inferior eustachian tube. The tube is packed first with bone wax, then bone paté, and finally, temporalis muscle (Fig. 60–7). A split-thickness piece of bone from the bone flap is placed over the tegmen defect to avoid fixation of the ossicles against the dura. The wound is closed in the usual manner. In this setting, a pressure dressing is not likely to be helpful, but a lumbar drain could be placed for several postoperative days.

SUMMARY

Postoperative CSF leak is a potential complication of any cranial base surgical procedure that violates the meninges. Although a CSF leak by itself is not a problem, it provides a portal of entry for bacteria to seed the meninges. Because postoperative meningitis is a serious complication, CSF leaks should be treated aggressively. This chapter discussed the methods for closing CSF leaks in a sequential manner from conservative to aggressive. Using this approach, the skull base surgeon should be able to seal all spinal fluid leaks.

References

1. Snow RB, Kuhel W, Martin SB: Prolonged spinal drainage after the resection of tumors of the skull base: A cautionary note. Neurosurgery 28: 880–883, 1991.
2. Effron MZ, Black FO, Burns D: Tension pneumocephalus complicating the treatment of postoperative CSF otorrhea. Arch Otolaryngol Head Neck Surg 107: 579–580, 1981.
3. Graf CJ, Gross CE, Beck DW: Complication of spinal drainage in the management of cerebrospinal fluid fistula: Report of three cases. J Neurosurg 54: 392–395, 1981.
4. Swanson SE, Kocan MJ, Chandler WF: Flow-regulated continuous spinal drainage: Technical note with case report. Neurosurgery 9: 163–165, 1981.
5. Swanson SE, Chandler WF, Kocan MJ: Flow-regulated continuous spinal drainage in the management of cerebrospinal fluid fistulas. Laryngoscope 95: 104–106, 1985.
6. House JL, Hitselberger WE, House WF: Wound closure and cerebrospinal fluid leak after translabyrinthine surgery. Am J Otol 4: 126–128, 1982.
7. Epstein GH, Weisman RA, Zwillenberg S, Schreiber A: A new autologous fibrinogen-based adhesive for otologic surgery. Ann Otol Rhinol Laryngol 95: 40–45, 1986.
8. Sierra DH, Nissen AJ, Welch J: The use of fibrin glue in intracranial procedures: Preliminary results. Laryngoscope 100: 360–363, 1990.
9. Rodgers GK, Luxford WM: Factors affecting the development of cerebrospinal fluid leak after translabyrinthine acoustic tumor surgery. Laryngoscope 103: 959–962, 1993.

61

Care of the Eye in Facial Paralysis

ROBERT E. LEVINE, M.D.

Rehabilitation of the facial paralysis patient depends on restoration of optimum lid position and function.[1-3] This chapter summarizes techniques that I have found to be most helpful in achieving that goal, based on more than 1000 patients with facial paralysis on whom I have operated during the past 2 decades.

For convenience, the chapter is divided into sections for lid reanimation procedures, lower lid reapposition procedures, and ancillary procedures. In practice, a combination of these techniques may be performed during the same operation. When the procedures are combined, the reanimation procedure is performed first because it is most influenced by the lid swelling that occurs during the course of the surgery. The lower lid reapposition procedure is performed next. Upper lid entropion correction is performed just before the upper lid incision is closed, and brow elevation is performed last. The final section of the chapter explains two very useful temporizing procedures.

CRITERIA FOR SURGERY

Three groups of patients with facial paralysis require lid surgery for functional reasons:

1. Those who are either symptomatic or who show signs of conjunctival or corneal injury, or both, despite maximum tolerated medical therapy.
2. Those who require rapid ocular rehabilitation to resume their usual occupation and responsibilities. For example, keeping the eye full of ointment might protect the cornea adequately but would not be a realistic option for a monocular patient or one who earns his or her livelihood flying an airplane.
3. Those whose ocular status is currently stable, but who are at high risk of corneal complications. Patients with hypoesthetic or anesthetic corneas secondary to associated fifth nerve involvement are the prime candidates in this group. If both fifth and seventh nerve deficits are present, even minimal lagophthalmos is a risk factor for corneal breakdown. Poor Bell's phenomenon or the absence of tears may further complicate the picture.

Patients with short-term problems (3 months or less to anticipated recovery of orbicularis oculi function) can usually be treated by conservative means. Patients with significant paralytic deficits who will require 6 months or more to recover, or who are not expected to recover, are generally best served by early surgical intervention.

The group of patients whose prognosis is unclear, for example, those who might improve in 3 months but could conceivably require 6 months or more to recover, poses the greatest challenges in surgical selection. In such patients, criteria such as the reliability of follow-up, the accessibility of medical care, the ability of the patient or family to care for the eye, and the patient's own needs, desires, and lifestyle all play a role in decision making. Where it is safe and feasible to do so, a prolonged trial of conservative management may allow the patient and the physician to decide if they are on the correct course.

PREPARATION OF THE PATIENT

The surgery is preferably done on an eye (or head and neck) gurney. Two advantages of this approach are ease of access to the eye area by the surgeon and the assistant and ability to crank up the bed so that the patient is brought to the seated position, thereby enabling the brow and lids to be checked with gravity operative. A doughnut is used to stabilize the head, and a nasal cannula with air is added to provide adequate circulation under the drapes. Some anesthesiologists prefer a carbon dioxide exhaust line as well. Air is used routinely instead of oxygen to eliminate the possibility of an accident resulting from the unhappy mixture of oxygen and cautery. If oxygen is required at any time, cautery is withheld until after the oxygen has been turned off.

ANESTHESIA AND SURGICAL PREPARATION

In lid reanimation procedures, in which the patient's cooperation is required, any medication that might make the patient drowsy and unable to cooperate fully throughout the operation is not used. Rather, short-acting intravenous medication, such as propofol (Diprivan), methohexital (Brevital), or a similar agent is given at the beginning of the surgery in amounts just adequate to cover the discomfort of the local injection. Lidocaine (Xylocaine), 2 per cent, with epinephrine (unless contraindicated by hypertension or cardiac problems) to which sodium bicarbonate, 7.5 per cent, (Neutracain) has been added (one part sodium bicarbonate to nine parts lidocaine with epinephrine) is used at the beginning of the surgery. Bupivacaine (Marcaine), 0.5 per cent, is used at the end of the surgery to reduce pain during the immediate postoperative period.

Local infiltration is placed in the areas to be operated, such as along the upper lid fold and along the lateral orbital rim for spring implantations, and at the canthi and brow areas, if surgery is to be performed there. Excessive infiltration should be avoided because it paralyzes the levator, impairs extraocular motility (making it harder to judge lid position), and distorts lid anatomy. The eyelids, both sides of the face above the mouth, and the forehead are prepared with green soap and then with povidone-iodine (Betadine), which is washed off.

DRAPING

The hair is covered with a small drape formed into a turban and secured with a clamp. A second small sheet is incorporated with that drape to cover the superior end of the table. A body sheet is also placed. The eyelids and brow are isolated by means of two No. 1000 Steri-Drapes cut in half (Fig. 61–1). Each of the four drapes forms a border of the surgical field, which includes both eyes and the forehead area. Before the Steri-Drape is placed over the nose, a thin cloth towel is placed over the nose to avoid the suffocating feeling resulting from plastic over the nose. In addition, the plastic drape over the towel inferior to the adhesive area is excised to prevent moisture accumulation. Care is taken to avoid distorting the lower lid anatomy or brow areas by undue traction from the drapes.

The body drape is fastened to the head drape on both sides with a towel clip so it does not slip down when the patient is brought to the seated position. The patient is secured on the table with a safety belt, and the belt is positioned so as to provide access for loosening it as needed when the patient is brought to the seated position.

The Mayo stand is brought over the drapes for easy access to the instruments. Although the tent effect obtainable by draping the Mayo stand would be desirable, it does not lend itself readily to moving the stand away when the patient needs to be brought to the seated position.

GENERAL CONSIDERATIONS

Procedures are generally performed on an outpatient basis, unless the patient is already hospitalized because of the neuro-otologic or head and neck surgery. Bipolar cautery is used for hemostasis during the lid surgery. At the end of the procedure, antibiotic ophthalmic ointment is applied to the wounds. Ophthalmic ointment is used because it is not irritating if any gets into the eye. The lids are not bandaged. An ice pack is applied to the closed lids and kept in place for 24 hours, after which time warm tap water compresses are used for at least 20 minutes four times a day until the swelling subsides. The antibiotic ointment is applied to the wounds twice a day until they are healed, and appropriate lubricating drops are prescribed for the eye.

UPPER LID REANIMATION PROCEDURES

The four procedures that I believe are the most useful in reanimating paralyzed lids are, in order of preference:

1. Enhanced palpebral spring implantation
2. Palpebral spring implantation
3. Gold weight implantation
4. Silicone rod prosthesis implantation

In all of these procedures, the principle is to create an external force that opposes the levator palpebrae superioris, the opening muscle of the lid. The respective forces are spring tension, gravity acting on the gold weight, and elasticity of the silicone band.

The relative merits and limitations of the various procedures are related to how they develop external closing forces and the consequences of increasing those forces. For example, the greater the force required by any device, the greater the pseudoptosis (lid droop in the primary position of gaze that results from the implant). If the palpebral spring, the gold weight, and the silicone rod prosthesis are all adjusted to provide the same closing force in a given patient, the pseudoptosis should be the same with each device. In the enhanced palpebral spring implantation procedure, the levator muscle is strengthened to balance the spring force, and therefore less pseudoptosis is possible with the same closing force, when compared with any of the other three procedures. Similarly, by tightening the levator and therefore using a stronger spring force, the surgeon makes increased blink speed possible.

Because the gold weight is gravity dependent, very large, unsightly gold weights may be required in lids that need a strong closing force. Also, because the gold weight is gravity dependent, lid closure may not be assured when the patient is supine, as in sleep. Further, blink speed is limited with the gold weight. However, the surgeon who does these procedures only infrequently can more easily master the techniques of the gold weight implant and silicone rod prosthesis than the technique of the palpebral spring implant or the enhanced palpebral spring implant.

The silicone rod prosthesis has the advantage of providing support for the lower lid as well. Its major disadvantage is its inevitable loss of elasticity over time, be it months or years. If facial nerve function does not recover before the prosthesis runs out of elasticity, it will need to be replaced. By contrast, a gold weight or palpebral spring can function over many years. A small percentage of springs may fail over time because of fatigue and breakage, thereby necessitating replacement.

An additional advantage of the palpebral spring is

that the tension on the wire can be adjusted postoperatively, either externally or through a small incision. This technique allows loosening of the spring when the patient recovers partial function but is not yet well enough to have the spring removed.

All prosthetic devices are subject to the potential hazards of extrusion or infection over the long term. However, with the techniques currently in use, these complications have been sufficiently infrequent as to not limit the usefulness of the devices.

In recent years, since I devised the enhanced palpebral spring procedure, I have used it with increasing frequency instead of nonenhanced spring implantation. The extra surgical effort is usually well rewarded by the diminished pseudoptosis and increased blink speed obtained by this procedure.

In summary, I prefer the enhanced palpebral spring implantation in most cases of significant upper lid closure deficits. When the patient has a strong levator or when the spring is being used only as a short-term remedy, the nonenhanced palpebral spring procedure may be used. Surgeons who are just beginning to undertake palpebral spring implantation should start off with the nonenhanced procedure and then move on to the enhanced procedure.

I find the gold weight of greatest benefit to those patients whose closure problem is relatively minimal, but nevertheless just exceeds the limits of conservative management. Patients who require definitive, reliable closure, such as those with coexistent poor Bell's phenomenon or fifth nerve involvement, are better protected with springs than with weights. Patients whose ocular management failed with weights in place have been successfully treated by removing the weight and replacing it with a spring. The silicone rod prosthesis is most useful in patients with an excellent prognosis for recovery in about 6 months, in whom significant lower lid lagophthalmos coexists.

Palpebral Spring Implantation [4-14]

Preparation of the Palpebral Spring

The palpebral spring is built preoperatively either in the office or at the bedside. Building the spring is time consuming, and both the surgeon and the patient should be comfortable during the procedure. Good light must be available, and if possible, the patient should be seated so that lid movement can be best evaluated.

Each spring is constructed from a plain piece of wire that is shaped to conform to the individual lid anatomy of the patient. Generally, a 0.010 inch wire provides suitable tension for most patients. Patients with very strong levators may require the use of 0.011 inch or even 0.012 inch wire. Patients with weak levators (when the levator is not going to be tightened)

may benefit from the use of 0.009 or even 0.008 inch wire.

The construction is begun by forming a 5mm loop at what is to become the fulcrum of the spring. The posterior aspect of that loop should be the superior arm of the spring. Because loosening the spring intraoperatively is easier than tightening it, the two arms should form an angle of about 120 degrees as they leave the fulcrum.

The fulcrum is then placed over the lateral orbital rim and held in position by the surgeon's fingers. Curves are then created in the lower arm to match the patient's lid anatomy. Curvature is also provided to accommodate the fact that the upper eyelid opens up and back, not straight up and down. Slight variations in spring position and curvatures may enhance its effect; therefore, these factors should be varied in the evaluation of the spring preoperatively. Sometimes, making more than one spring with slightly different curvatures is useful in determining which model will work best. Usually, the fulcrum should be placed as far laterally as possible without lengthening the spring so much that its design and placement are difficult. The completed spring is stored until the day of surgery, when it is placed on a gauze pad to prevent loss and is autoclaved with the instruments.

Surgical Technique

The eye is protected with a scleral shell. An incision is made along the lid fold at the junction of the medial one third and lateral two thirds of the palpebral aperture and is carried across the orbital rim (Fig. 61–2). Dissection is carried superolaterally, in the plane between the septum and orbicularis, to expose the orbital rim. Dissection is carried downward at the medial aspect of the incision to expose the tarsus.

A blunted 22 gauge spinal needle is then passed, beginning in the area of the exposed tarsus, 5mm superior to the lid margin. The needle passes in the plane between the orbicularis and the tarsus to a point 2mm above the lid margin at the lateral aspect of the lid. It then continues until it emerges at the anterior aspect of the lateral orbital rim. The stylette is then removed. The undersurface of the lid is inspected to ensure that the needle has not inadvertently perforated the tarsus.

The end of the lower arm of the previously prepared palpebral spring is then passed into the needle, and the needle and spring are withdrawn medially, thereby bringing the spring into the lid. The scleral shell is then removed, and the spring is positioned so that its previously determined curvature conforms to the lid anatomy. The upper arm of the spring is placed in position, and its length is determined. It usually needs to be about 3/4 of an inch long. A loop is

FIGURE 61-1

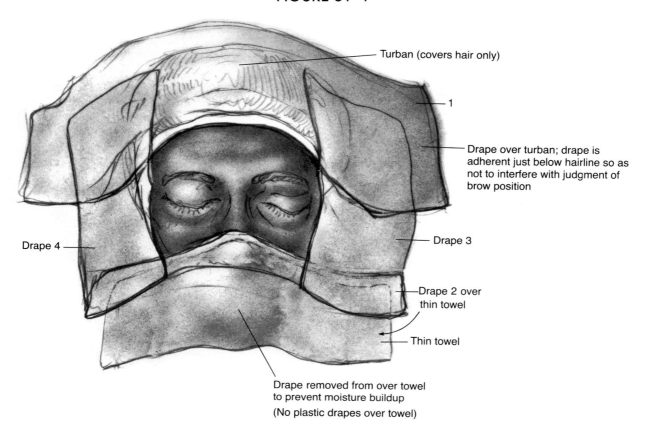

Turban (covers hair only)

1

Drape over turban; drape is adherent just below hairline so as not to interfere with judgment of brow position

Drape 3

Drape 4

Drape 2 over thin towel

Thin towel

Drape removed from over towel to prevent moisture buildup

(No plastic drapes over towel)

FIGURE 61-1. Draping the patient. After the hair has been covered with a turban, which is secured with a towel clip, two No. 1000 Steri-Drapes are cut in half. The first half-drape is placed with the edge as close to the hairline as possible so as not to interfere with judgment of brow position. A thin cloth towel is then placed over the nose, and a half-drape is placed to secure it into position, with the sticky end of the drape bridging the skin and the superior end of the towel. The nonsticky portion of the drape is then cut away and discarded, leaving only the towel over the nose. If the drape is not cut away, excess moisture builds up. A third half-drape is placed laterally, as far lateral to the lateral canthus as is practical, and a fourth half-drape is placed similarly on the contralateral side.

FIGURE 61-2. Palpebral spring implantation. *A,* With a protective scleral shell in place, an incision is made along the lateral two thirds of the lid crease and is carried across the orbital rim laterally. Dissection is carried downward at the medial end of the incision to expose the tarsal plate. Dissection is also carried upward and laterally to expose the orbital rim. *B,* A 22-gauge blunted spinal needle with the stilette in place is passed from the medial end of the dissection to emerge laterally in the plane between the orbicularis and the tarsus. The passage should be carried out overlying the midtarsus, and the needle is angulated slightly downward at its lateral extent. The exit of the needle tract should be close to its lateral orbital rim periosteum. The lid is everted to confirm that the needle has not inadvertently perforated the tarsus. The previously prepared wire spring (which has been autoclaved), is passed through the needle, and the needle is withdrawn. *C,* A cross-section of the lid illustrates placement of the needle over the midtarsus in the plane between the tarsus and orbicularis. The wire spring should be resting on the epitarsal surface. *D,* The scleral shell is removed, and the fulcrum of the spring is brought into the desired position along the orbital rim. The spring should be placed in a position in which its curves conform perfectly to the eyelid contour. (Inset: The fulcrum of the spring is secured to lateral orbital rim periosteum with three 4.0 Mersilene sutures, and an extra bite of the periosteum is taken with each stitch.) Loops are fashioned at each end, and the spring is cut to size. The loops should be flat and tightly closed to leave no sharp edges. The medial loop is enveloped in 0.2mm thick polyester (Dacron) patch material, to which it is secured by means of three 8.0 nylon sutures tied internally. The polyester patch is creased in an absorbable gelatin sponge (Gelfoam) press before surgery and is autoclaved with the other instruments. The folded polyester envelope is cut to size at surgery. The crease in the patch material should be directed downward so that the spring and patch together provide a smooth inferior surface. The loop at the end of the inferior arm is directed upward for the same reason. Suturing of the loop to the polyester is facilitated by resting the polyester on a retractor. *E,* The end of the spring with its polyester envelope is replaced into the lid between the tarsus and orbicularis. In time, the end of the spring will become fixed to the tarsus by granulation tissue integrating into the polyester patch. Securing the patch to the tarsus directly with an additional running 8.0 nylon suture helps to provide fixation until connective tissue grows into the polyester. The tension on the spring is checked, with the patient in both the upright and supine positions. The tension can be adjusted by grasping the upper end of the spring with forceps and changing its position. When the correct tension has been determined, the upper loop of the spring is secured to the orbital rim periosteum with a 4.0 Mersilene suture. An extra bite of the periosteum may be taken in the stitch before it is tied. When sutures are placed to secure either the fulcrum or the upper loop of the spring to the orbital rim periosteum, it is safer to sew in the direction away from the globe. Spring tension is again checked with the patient both seated and supine. Additional adjustments can be made by bending the wire or repositioning the loop. When the adjustments are completed, two additional 4.0 Mersilene sutures are placed through the upper loop in a manner similar to that of the initial suture. Deeper tissues overlying the spring are then closed with 5.0 plain gut suture to assure that the spring and Mersilene sutures are well covered. Skin and muscle are closed with running 6.0 plain gut fast-absorbing suture. *F,* The end of the spring should be between the pupillary axis and the medial limbus, with the eyes in the primary position of gaze. (*A–F,* From Tse D, Wright KW (eds): Oculoplastic Surgery. Philadelphia, JB Lippincott, 1992.)

FIGURE 61-2

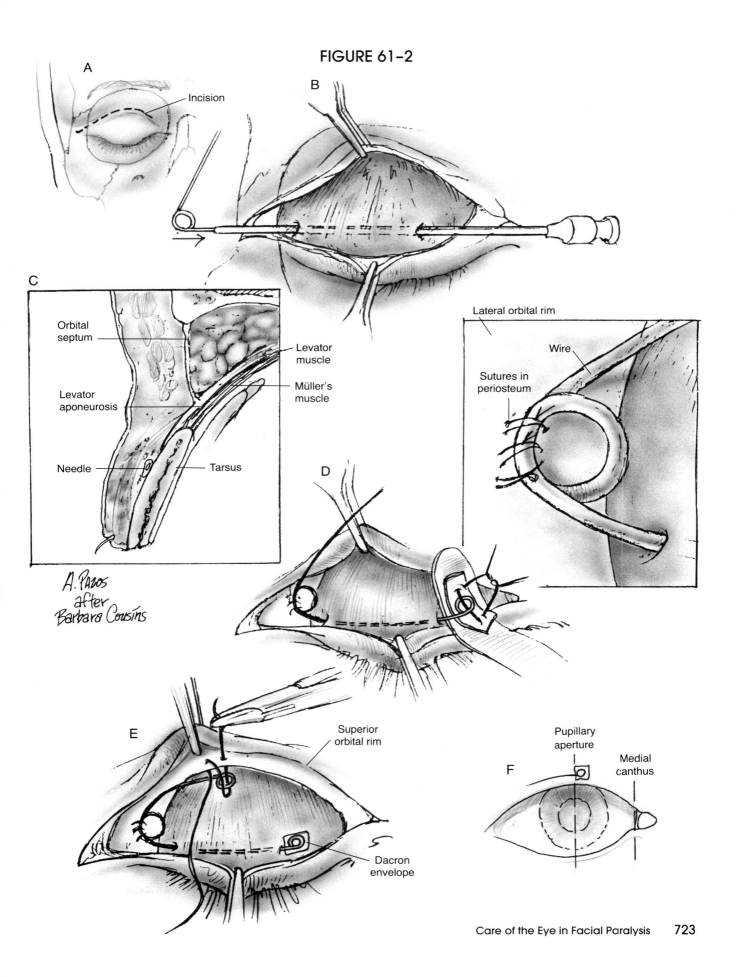

A — Incision

B

C

Orbital septum

Levator aponeurosis

Needle

Levator muscle

Müller's muscle

Tarsus

A. Pazos
after
Barbara Cousins

Lateral orbital rim

Wire

Sutures in periosteum

D

E

Superior orbital rim

Dacron envelope

F

Pupillary aperture

Medial canthus

Care of the Eye in Facial Paralysis   723

fashioned at the point that is to become the end of the upper arm, and the wire is cut to size. The loop is closed so as to leave no sharp ends. The loop at the fulcrum is then held in place with forceps, and the patient is asked to open and close the eye. The position at which the spring curvature best conforms to the lid anatomy is then found, with the eye both opened and closed, and the loop at the fulcrum is sutured in place. The suturing is accomplished with 4.0 Mersilene suture, and an extra bite of periosteum is taken with each stitch. Three such sutures are generally placed for the nonenhanced procedure, and five for the enhanced procedure because of the greater tensions involved.

The lower arm of the spring is cut to size, and a loop (which is also meticulously closed) is formed on its end. The loop should be formed upward to maintain a smooth inferior surface to the spring. The end of the spring should be between the pupillary axis and the medial limbus, with the eyes in the primary position of gaze. In very prominent eyes, terminating the spring slightly sooner, in the pupillary axis, may be preferable. Before the end of the spring is covered with polyester (Dacron) patch material, the angulation of the loop should be checked with the patient's eyes open and closed to ensure that the spring tracks well with lid movement and that the loop stays relatively parallel to the tarsus during opening and closing.

A piece of 0.2mm polyester patch material, which has been creased by its placement in a press that is used for compressing Gelfoam before it is autoclaved, is cut to size to fit over the inferior loop. This piece is converted into a pouch by closure of the sides with 8.0 nylon sutures tied internally. The creased side is directed downward. The open lateral side is then slipped over the spring, to which it is secured with an 8.0 nylon suture beginning within the pouch, is passed through the spring loop and the posterior end of the pouch, and is terminated by passing through the anterior side of the pouch. The knot is tied internally to prevent erosion. The polyester envelope is secured to the tarsus with one or more 8.0 nylon su-

tures, as needed, to prevent slippage of the polyester until granulation to the tarsus occurs.

Spring tension is then adjusted to just close the eye. This adjustment is accomplished by movement of the upper arm of the spring closer or farther from the orbital rim. A 4.0 Mersilene suture is used to secure the upper loop to the periosteum in this position, and an extra bite is taken with the stitch. Spring tension is checked with the patient both seated and supine. Additional adjustments can be made also by bending of the wire of the upper arm to loosen or tighten it.

Bending the wire of the lower arm near the fulcrum should be avoided at this time because such adjustments may be required during the postoperative period, and excess bending of the wire may increase its chance of breakage. Once the final position of the upper loop has been determined in the nonenhanced procedure, two additional 4.0 Mersilene sutures are placed, and an extra bite of periosteum is taken with each stitch. Four additional sutures are used in the enhanced procedure.

The deeper aspect of the wound overlying the orbital rim is closed with 5.0 plain gut suture, to cover the spring and Mersilene sutures at the upper loop and fulcrum. The lid fold incision is closed with running 6.0 plain gut suture. The eye is dressed with antibiotic ointment and an ice pack.

Enhanced Palpebral Spring Implantation

The enhancement of the palpebral spring operation consists of tightening of the levator during the same procedure (Fig. 61–3). The spring is prepared as described above, except that wire lighter than 0.10 inch is not used.

Surgical Technique

A scleral shell is placed. The initial skin fold incision is the same as that described earlier. Dissection is carried upward until preaponeurotic fat can be visual-

FIGURE 61–3. Enhanced palpebral spring implantation. *A,* The levator aponeurosis and the inferior aspect of the muscular portion of the levator are exposed. Centrally, the superior portion of the tarsus is also exposed. A double-armed 5.0 Mersilene suture is then placed through midtarsus. *B,* Each arm of the suture is brought superiorly through the levator to emerge just above the point at which the aponeurosis meets the levator muscle. Temporary knots are tied. If necessary, an additional lateral suture and possibly an additional medial suture are placed in a similar manner. Inset: The course of the suture is illustrated in cross-section. The surgeon should check to be sure that the suture has not perforated either the tarsus or the conjunctiva.

FIGURE 61-3

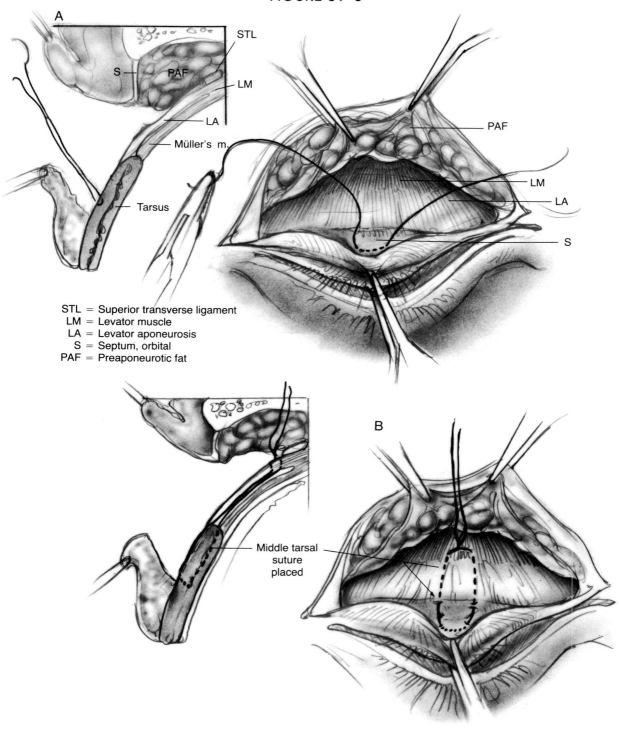

A

STL
PAF
S
LM
LA
Müller's m.
Tarsus

PAF
LM
LA
S

STL = Superior transverse ligament
LM = Levator muscle
LA = Levator aponeurosis
S = Septum, orbital
PAF = Preaponeurotic fat

Middle tarsal
suture
placed

B

ized through the septum. The septum is then opened, and dissection is carried down to expose the levator. Dissection is then carried inferiorly to expose the tarsus centrally. A 5.0 Mersilene suture is then placed through the midtarsus.

The undersurface of the lid is inspected to ensure that the suture has not perforated the tarsus. Both arms of the suture are then brought superiorly through the levator to emerge just above the point at which aponeurosis ends and levator muscle is visualized. A temporary knot is placed, and the patient is asked to open the eye.

The scleral shell is removed and the extent of levator tightening evaluated. If necessary, an additional lateral suture and possibly an additional medial suture are placed in a similar manner to achieve desired lid strengthening and maintenance of proper upper lid curvature. If the surgeon is not sure whether additional sutures are necessary, their placement can be deferred until after the spring has been placed and the overall effect of the spring and the initial suture can be evaluated.

Regardless of how many sutures are used, they are adjusted after the spring is in place, at the same time that the spring itself would otherwise be adjusted. The levator is tightened to a point at which maximum strengthening is achieved without inducing cicatricial lagophthalmos from an overly shortened levator.

The stronger the levator can be made, the greater the tension possible on the spring and, therefore, the more rapid the blink. The nuances of adjustment of both the levator and the spring can be appreciated only with experience. Nevertheless, once the general principles are understood, excellent results can be obtained (Fig. 61–4).

Gold Weight Implantation [15, 16]

The size of the weight is selected preoperatively. With the patient seated, a gold weight that is estimated to be suitable for the degree of lagophthalmos is selected and is secured to the patient's upper lid either with cyanoacrylate glue or with a temporary lid suture. The patient is then asked to open and close the eye, and the surgeon determines whether the weight of the gold is correct. The evaluation is repeated with the patient supine. Weights in the range of 1.2 to 1.5g are suitable for use in most patients.

Surgical Technique

The weight may be fixated either supratarsally (Fig. 61–5) or tarsally. Supratarsal fixation is preferable unless the weight is so large that is not practical. A scleral shell is placed. An incision is made in the lid fold, and dissection is carried upward to expose the orbital septum. The preaponeurotic fat can be seen through the septum, which is then opened and the weight secured to the levator with a single 5.0 polyester suture placed through the holes in the weight. The knot is buried. The function of the weight is then tested with the patient in the seated and supine positions. If the desired effect is not obtained, a different-sized weight may be tried. Overlying skin muscle is closed with running 6.0 plain gut suture.

Silicone Rod Prosthesis Implantation [17–19]

The prosthesis to be used is commercially available as a 1.0mm diameter rod.

Surgical Technique

While the eye is protected with a scleral shell, a curvilinear incision is made overlying the medial canthal tendon (Fig. 61–6). The incision should be just lateral to the angular vein to avoid the vein in the course of the dissection. Dissection is then carried posteriorly to expose the origin of the tendon. The prosthesis is

FIGURE 61–4. The patient is a 49-year-old woman with facial paralysis secondary to an acoustic neuroma. She had undergone two tarsorrhaphy procedures before she was first seen for evaluation. A, Eyes open, but eye function is largely blocked by tarsorrhaphy. Note also the brow droop. B, Attempted closure. Note that the tarsorrhaphy, although extensive, fails to protect the cornea well. C, Eyes open. The tarsorrhaphy has been opened and the lid margins reconstructed. The patient also has had enhanced palpebral spring implantation, medial and lateral canthoplasties, correction of upper lid entropion, and elevation of the brow. D, Attempted closure. Note excellent protection of the cornea by the spring.

FIGURE 61–5. Gold weight. The levator is exposed, and the gold weight is secured to it with a single 5.0 polyester suture placed through the holes in the weight. The knot is buried. Larger weights may be placed pretarsally in a similar manner.

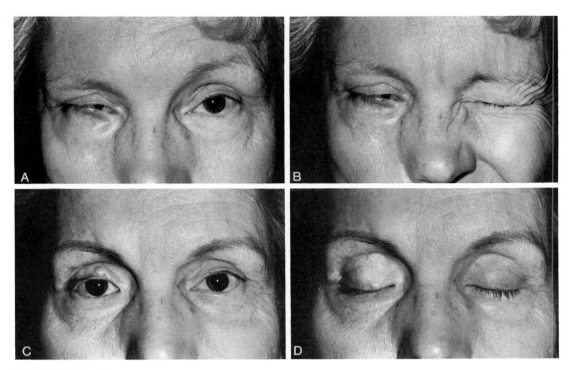

FIGURE 61-4

FIGURE 61-5

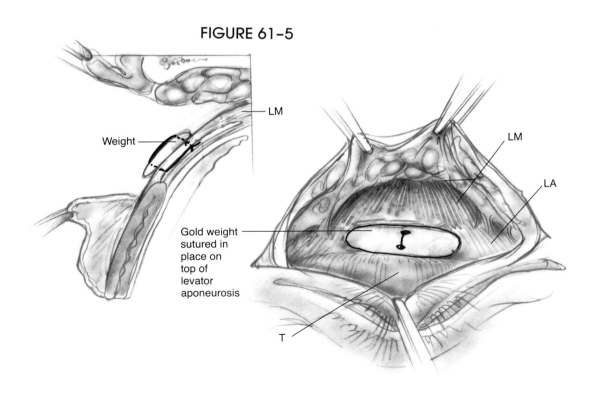

Weight

LM

Gold weight
sutured in
place on
top of
levator
aponeurosis

LM

LA

T

threaded on a large, noncutting needle and is sewn through the tendon twice. The lower arm should emerge from the posterior aspect of the tendon, which facilitates holding the lower lid against the globe.

A second incision is made at the lateral orbital rim, and dissection is carried to the periosteum. By use of sharp dissection, a tunnel is started in the plane between the orbicularis and the tarsus at the lateral aspect of the lower lid. A special introducer is then passed as close to the lid margin as possible across the lid to emerge medially close to where the silicone rod has been sewn through the tendon. The lower arm of the rod is then threaded onto the introducer, and the introducer is withdrawn laterally, thus bringing the rod through the lid. In a similar manner, the upper arm of the prosthesis is brought through the upper lid, except that passage is accomplished over the midtarsus.

The desired point of anchorage for the lower end of the prosthesis is determined, and a loop is formed at that point through periosteum by use of a 2.0 Prolene suture sewn through the periosteum twice at the orbital rim. The prosthesis must be secured at the inner aspect of the lateral orbital rim so as to pull the lid posteriorly. The point selected should be just above the horizontal raphe so as to draw the lid upward as well. In a similar manner, the upper arm of the prosthesis is secured just below the horizontal raphe, passing anterior to the lower arm.

With the patient in the seated position, suitable tension is placed on the lower arm to secure the lower lid in the desired position. (For additional discussion on how to best position the lid, see under *Assessing Lid Position*.) Similarly, the tension on the upper lid is adjusted to permit good opening and closing of the lid, and final knots are tied. Each arm of the prosthesis is further secured with additional bites through the lateral rim periosteum. A heavy suture, such as 2.0 Prolene, is selected to avoid cutting through the prosthesis. Deep tissues are closed with 5.0 plain gut suture medially and laterally, and the skin is closed with 6.0 plain gut suture.

LOWER LID REAPPOSITION PROCEDURES

Canthoplasty

Surgery may be performed at either the medial or lateral canthus to tighten and elevate the lower eyelid. Operating at the ends of the tarsus has the advantage of not creating an irregular lid margin or interfering with the visual field. Whereas tightening the lid only at the lateral canthus is usually the procedure of choice in patients with nonparalytic lid laxity, the paralyzed lid usually requires medial canthal tightening as well. Otherwise, tightening the lid only laterally may result in either marked displacement of the inferior punctum laterally or failure to elevate the lid. In some cases, tightening the lid only laterally can cause the lid to act as a shorter chord beneath the globe, thus actually lowering the lid rather than raising it. If only a limited amount of lid tightening and elevation is required, medial canthoplasty alone may be the procedure of choice.

Assessing Lid Position

Assuming that extraocular motility has not been impaired by excess local anesthesia infiltration, the position of the lid relative to the limbus (corneoscleral junction) can be used as a guideline in the adjustment of lid position. The gaze of the patient should be directed such that the limbus of the contralateral lid is placed just tangential to the inferior limbus. The lid being operated on can then be tightened to a position in which it, too, is tangential to the limbus, or it can

FIGURE 61–6. Silicone rod prosthesis. *A*, An incision is made medially just lateral to the angular vein; a second incision is made laterally over the orbital rim. *B*, Laterally, dissection is carried down to expose the orbital rim. Medially, the medial canthal tendon is exposed, and the prosthesis is sewn through it by use of a large noncutting needle. *C*, The prosthesis is further sewn through the tendon so that the lower arm emerges posterior to the tendon, thereby facilitating holding the lower lid against the globe. *D*, Each arm of the prosthesis is ready to be engaged on the introducer. *E*, With a special introducer, the upper arm of the prosthesis has been passed between the orbicularis and tarsus in the upper lid, at the level of midtarsus. The introducer is shown in the lower lid, in preparation for passing the lower lid of the prosthesis. The prosthesis must be as close to the lid margin as possible to prevent ectropion of the lid. *F*, The lower arm of the prosthesis is secured to orbital rim periosteum with 2.0 Prolene suture. *G*, Both arms of the prosthesis are further sutured to the periosteum with 2.0 Prolene. Note that the inferior arm is posterior to the superior arm because the lower lid must be pulled posteriorly.

FIGURE 61–6

Silicone
Elastic Prosthesis

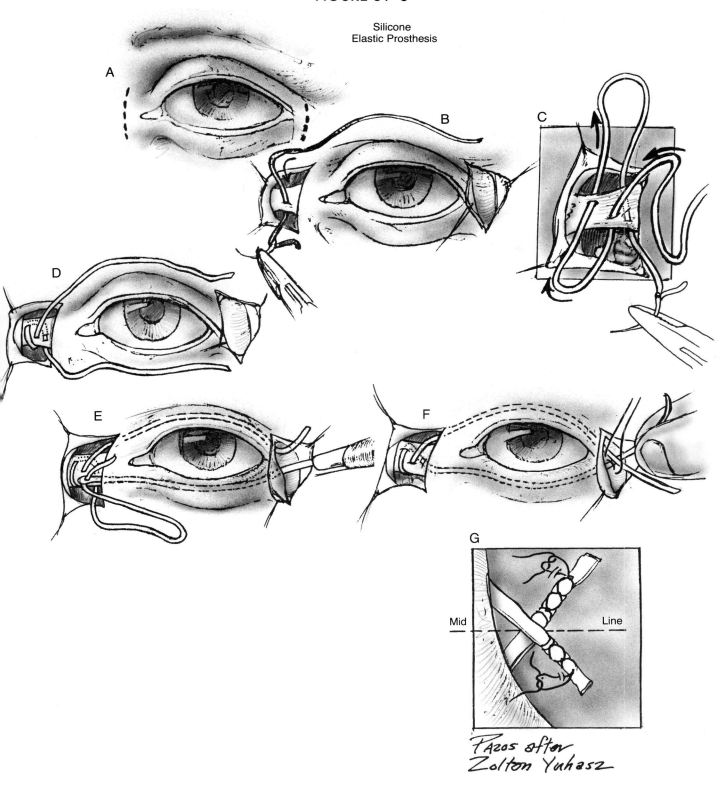

Pazos after
Zolton Yuhasz

be slightly overcorrected to allow for postoperative loosening. Matching this tangential position is more precise than judging the amount by which the lid crosses the cornea or comes inferior to it, compared with the other eye.

Medial Canthoplasty [20]

Medial canthoplasty consists of exposing the lower arm of the medial canthal tendon and the origin of the common tendon and tightening the lower arm. If additional effect is required, the upper arm of the tendon may also be exposed so that it, too, can be included in the surgical procedure.

Surgical Technique

To expose the medial canthal tendon, the globe is protected with a scleral shell, and the canaliculi are protected with probes. An incision is then made at the mucocutaneous junction, beginning 2mm medial to the lower punctum, along the mucocutaneous junction to the medial canthus, and for an additional 2mm beyond the canthus (Fig. 61–7). A skin-muscle flap is then elevated with scissors, and hemostasis is achieved with bipolar cautery. The insertion of the lower arm of the medial canthal tendon is then grasped with forceps and drawn superonasally, thereby permitting the placement of a 5.0 double-armed polyester suture through the insertion. Each arm of the suture is then woven through the tendon and sewn through the origin of the tendon. Temporary knots are tied.

The patient is then brought to the seated position, and the apposition of the lid and position of the punctum are evaluated. If a lateral canthoplasty is also being performed, sitting the patient up can be deferred, and tension on both sets of canthoplasty sutures can be adjusted simultaneously after completion of the lateral canthoplasty. If only a medial canthoplasty is being performed, the tension on the lid is adjusted, and final knots are tied. In the event that the punctum is not adequately inverted by the suture used to tighten the medial canthal tendon, the canthal tendon is exposed in the upper lid, and a second 5.0 polyester suture is placed. Each arm of that suture starts at the lower edge of the inferior canthal tendon and ends at the upper edge of the superior canthal tendon, further inverting the lower punctum.

The canthoplasty using a suture only in the lower lid is completed by re-forming the mucocutaneous junction with 8.0 Vicryl running or interrupted sutures. These may be allowed to dissolve or may be removed in 5 to 7 days. When a second canthal suture is required, the lid flaps are closed to each other with 6.0 plain gut sutures. Since a second canthal suture results in the blunting of the canthal angle and horizontal shortening of the palpebral fissure, such a suture should not be used unnecessarily.

Lateral Canthoplasty [21, 22]

The object of lateral canthoplasty is to pull the lid superoposteriorly against the globe. In lieu of the various lid shortening procedures that have been used in the past, the currently preferred method is to create a

FIGURE 61–7. Medial canthoplasty. *A*, While the globe is protected with a scleral shell and the canaliculi are protected with probes, an incision is made along the mucocutaneous junction and continued downward at a point 2mm medial to the punctum. *B*, An inferior flap is elevated, which exposes the inferior arm of the medial canthal tendon. The tendon is pulled medially to expose its junction with the lateral aspect of the tarsus (insertion of the tendon), and a 5.0 polyester double-armed suture is placed through the insertion. *C*, Each arm of the suture is woven through the tendon and brought through the origin of the tendon. The two sutures are then tied under appropriate tension, thereby tightening the lower lid. The mucocutaneous junction is then reconstructed with 8.0 Vicryl suture, thereby leaving the medial canthus with a normal appearance. *D*, If additional lower lid inversion is required, a second incision is made in the upper lid along the mucocutaneous junction, directed upward at a point 2mm medial to the punctum. *E*, A superior flap is elevated, which exposes the superior arm of the canthal tendon. *F*, A 5.0 polyester suture is placed as a horizontal mattress suture. The suture passes near the lower end of the lower tendon and near the upper end of the upper tendon, thus inverting the lids. *G*, The edges of the skin flaps are closed to each other with 6.0 plain gut suture. The steps shown in *D* through *G* may be performed independently when lid inversion is more important than lid tightening, or they may be combined with the steps shown in *A* through *C*. When the steps *D* through *G* are required, the result is a more blunted medial canthal angle, with some shortening of the horizontal fissure. Therefore, if the procedure shown in *A* through *C* suffices, it is preferable. Nevertheless, the additional steps may be required in patients with marked medial lid laxity or eversion.

FIGURE 61-7

MEDIAL CANTHOPLASTY

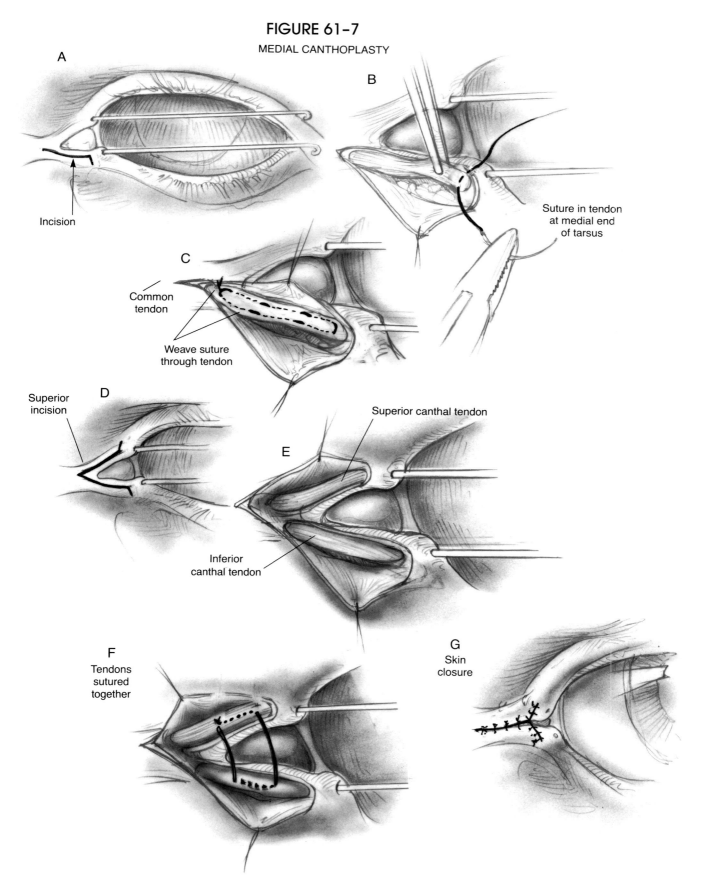

A

Incision

B

Suture in tendon
at medial end
of tarsus

C

Common
tendon

Weave suture
through tendon

D

Superior
incision

E

Superior canthal tendon

Inferior
canthal tendon

F

Tendons
sutured
together

G

Skin
closure

new lateral canthal tendon from the tarsus itself and to secure it to the orbital rim.

Surgical Technique

A hemostat is placed across the lateral canthal angle and removed (Fig. 61–8). The clamped area is then cut with scissors, accomplishing a canthotomy. The inferior crux of the lateral canthal tendon is then cut (inferior cantholysis) with scissors. At this point, the lateral aspect of the lower lid is freely movable. The lid is then pulled taut across the globe. If a medial canthoplasty has been performed, suitable tension should be placed on that canthoplasty suture before this maneuver.

The amount of excess lid is marked, and the skin-muscle lamina is separated from the tarsus lateral to this mark. The lid margin in this area is also removed. Some surgeons prefer to remove the conjunctiva at this point, thereby leaving a pure tarsal tongue. I have not found such removal necessary, and the tarsus may be damaged during such attempts. A double-armed 5.0 polyester suture is passed as a mattress suture beginning on the anterior surface of the tarsus, 3mm from the lateral end, with each needle emerging through the cut end. The lower arm of the suture is marked with a marking pen for future reference.

A tunnel is then made underneath the upper arm of the lateral canthal tendon, and a clamp is passed into the tunnel. The sutures are grasped within the clamp and brought through the tunnel. The desired location of the lid is determined, and the sutures are placed appropriately, with care taken to obtain a bite of orbital rim periosteum at the inside aspect of the rim, slightly superior to the desired lid position. In this manner, the lid is drawn up and posteriorly. The previously placed mark on the suture helps to avoid confusion about the location of the inferior arm of the suture. A temporary knot is tied, and the patient is brought to the seated position. Adjustments in lid position and tension can then be made, and final knots can be tied.

The surgeon completes the canthoplasty by trimming excess skin and muscle, re-establishing the canthal angle with a 5.0 plain gut suture, and closing the skin with 6.0 plain gut suture. In situations in which lateral canthoplasty is combined with palpebral spring implantation and the amount of lid tightening required is not too great, a variant of the technique may be used. In such circumstances, a separate canthal incision is not required. Rather, the upper arm of the lateral canthal tendon may be approached from the existent extended lid fold incision.

A tunnel is made under the upper arm of the tendon. With forceps placed into the tunnel, the lateral aspect of the tarsus of the lower lid is grasped and brought into the tunnel. A 5.0 polyester double-armed suture is then placed in the tarsus. This stitch is used to re-create the lateral canthal tendon in a manner similar to that described previously. However, if a great deal of lid tightening is required, it is not possible to omit the steps of canthotomy and inferior cantholysis and still adequately mobilize the lid to achieve the desired position.

FIGURE 61–8. Lateral canthoplasty. *A,* A hemostat is used to clamp the lateral canthal angle for hemostasis. *B,* The clamp is removed, and a lateral canthotomy is performed, *C,* The inferior canthal tendon is cut so that the lower lid is freely movable. *D,* The lower lid is approximated to the desired position with slight overcorrection. *E,* The excess skin-muscle and mucocutaneous junction tissue are excised, leaving a tarsal tongue. *F,* A double-armed 5.0 polyester suture is passed through the tarsal tongue, and one arm of the suture is marked with a marking pen for subsequent identification. A tunnel is then created under the superior arm of the lateral canthal tendon. A clamp is passed into the tunnel, and the sutures are grasped and withdrawn laterally. The tarsal tongue is brought into the tunnel and secured under the desired tension to the lateral orbital rim periosteum. By use of the identifying markings previously placed, the superior suture is kept superior, and the inferior suture is kept inferior, preventing twisting of the tarsus. The suture is tied under appropriate tension. The canthoplasty is completed with a 5.0 plain gut suture to re-establish the canthal angle and 6.0 plain gut suture to close skin muscle. *G,* When lateral canthoplasty is combined with spring implantation and only a moderate amount of lateral canthal tightening is required, the procedure can be accomplished through the prior lid fold incision. *H,* A tunnel is made under the superior arm of the lateral canthal tendon. A forceps is introduced into the tunnel, and the lateral aspect of the tarsus is grasped. *I,* The lateral end of the tarsus is drawn into the tunnel, and a doubled-armed 5.0 polyester suture is used to secure it. *J,* Each arm of the 5.0 polyester suture is secured through orbital rim periosteum under suitable tension.

FIGURE 61-8

LATERAL CANTHOPLASTY

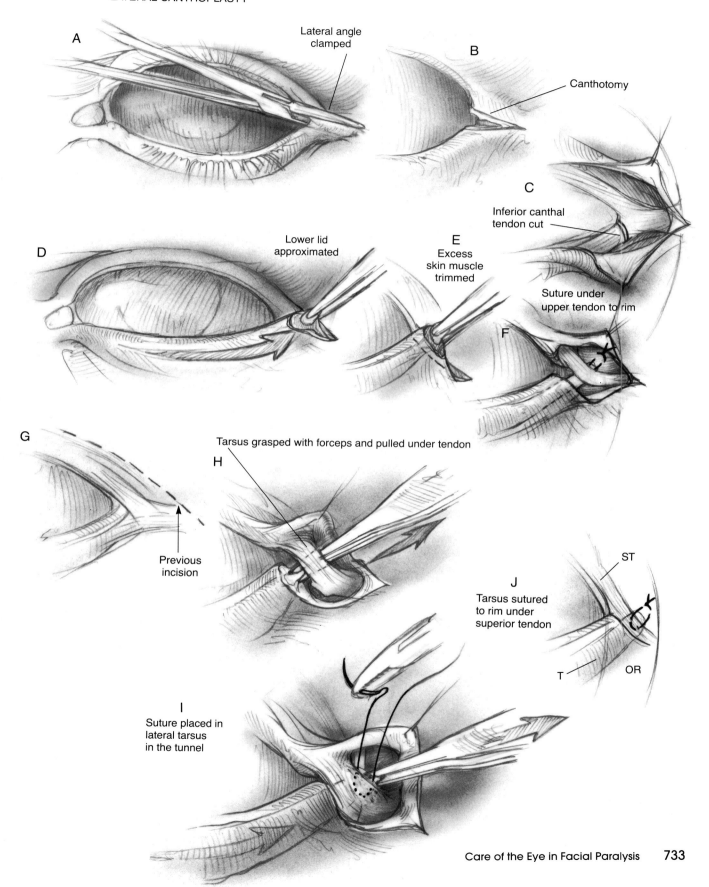

A

Lateral angle clamped

B

Canthotomy

C

Inferior canthal tendon cut

Suture under upper tendon to rim

D

Lower lid approximated

E

Excess skin muscle trimmed

F

G

Previous incision

H

Tarsus grasped with forceps and pulled under tendon

I

Suture placed in lateral tarsus in the tunnel

J

Tarsus sutured to rim under superior tendon

ST

T

OR

Fascia Lata Suspension of Lower Lid

In patients in whom medial and lateral canthoplasty together are inadequate to elevate the central portion of the lid, the lid may be supported by a fascia lata suspension. In this procedure, the fascia lata is anchored at each end of the lid and acts as a hammock to support the central lid.

Either autologous or banked fascia lata can be used. The preserved fascia lata is more subject to resorption over time; therefore, the autologous fascia lata is more likely to give a reliable long-term result. When autologous fascia lata is used, it is obtained from the leg by a general surgeon while the lid is being prepared for its placement.

Surgical Technique

A strip of fascia 3/16 of an inch wide and approximately 4 inches long is used. The technique for placing the fascia within the medial canthal tendon and in the lower lid is similar to that described in the section on the silicone rod prosthesis. The medial end of the fascia is anchored by means of a 5.0 polyester suture passed twice through the fascia and the medial canthal tendon (Fig. 61–9). The knot of the suture should be well buried to avoid later erosion.

The lateral end of the tendon is secured to the inner aspect of the lateral orbital rim with 5.0 polyester suture in a manner similar to that described for lateral canthoplasty and is adjusted in a similar way before final knots are tied. The suture, however, should encircle the fascia rather than go through it, to avoid tearing it. Once the fascia has been fixed in its position, additional bites through the periosteum and around the fascia are desirable to prevent slippage. Performing canthotomy and inferior cantholysis may be necessary to adequately mobilize the lid so that the fascial suspension holds it in the desired position.

ANCILLARY PROCEDURES

Patients with facial paralysis frequently manifest brow droop and entropion of the upper lid. These problems can be addressed surgically at the same time that upper lid reanimation surgery is undertaken. Elevation of the ptotic brow in a patient with facial paralysis should not be undertaken independent of a procedure to enhance lid closure. The droop of the brow tends to push the lid shut and thereby ameliorates the upper lid lagophthalmos. Therefore, correcting the brow position without concomitantly improving upper lid closure may significantly worsen the patient's lagophthalmos.

Brow Elevation[20]

An eyebrow can be elevated in three ways:

1. Excision of skin and muscle just above the brow
2. Suspension of the brow from the periosteum superior to it
3. Lifting of the forehead by a coronal approach

The coronal forehead lift requires extensive dissection, does not give as much effect as a direct lift, and may be difficult to control to elevate only one brow. A direct approach to brow elevation is generally preferable in facial paralysis patients. Skin and muscle excision alone is less effective in the paralyzed frontalis than in a normally innervated frontalis. I have found combining skin-muscle excision with brow suspension and simple brow suspension to be the two most useful brow-elevating procedures.

The choice of the procedure depends on several factors. First, will frontalis function return? If so, it is best not to excise tissue but only to suspend the brow. The second factor to consider is the effect of raising the brow without tissue excision. In some patients, this process induces a few brow wrinkles, which are actually welcome from an appearance standpoint in a previously abnormally smooth area. In others, only a bulge of tissue is created by elevation of the brow without tissue excision. In such patients skin muscle excision can be performed.

Elevating the entire brow is not always necessary. The point of maximum brow elevation should be noted on the contralateral side. A line drawn downward through this point usually passes at or near the lateral canthus. The exact position of such an imaginary line should be noted, and a comparable line should be marked on the side to be operated. Some patients have a different brow configuration and require more medial elevation.

Once the point of maximum brow elevation is determined and marked, the brow is raised. How much additional brow must be elevated to obtain a desirable contour can then be seen.

The extent of required brow elevation can also be judged by drawing a line tangential to the point of maximum brow elevation on the contralateral side. This line is drawn perpendicular to a vertical line bisecting the nose. Corresponding points on each brow are marked and measured relative to the horizontal reference line to determine the extent of brow elevation required at each point on the paralyzed side.

If it cannot be determined with certainty whether tissue excision will be required, the extent of the anticipated excision should be marked in advance of lid infiltration, so that the determination is not distorted by the swelling induced by the injection. The brow can then be suspended without tissue excision. If the result is not pleasing, skin-muscle excision can be carried out.

Be sure to assess the role of the ptotic brow in aiding lid closure. If a paretic brow that is assisting closure is raised without simultaneously performing a procedure such as spring implantation to enhance lid closure, the result may be worsened lagophthalmos.

Surgical Technique

The area in which brow elevation, tissue excision, or both, are required is marked as close to the superior extent of the brow as possible (Fig. 61–10), which will help to conceal the resultant scar. The skin is incised perpendicular to the skin surface with a scalpel blade until muscle is reached. Blunt dissection is then carried out at each site where a suspension suture is deemed necessary. The brow is elevated during the dissection so that the frontalis periosteum is encountered superior to the brow. A 4.0 Novafil suture on a very curved needle is passed through the periosteum and then through the dermis at the lower aspect of the wound as a horizontal mattress suture. Between one and four such sutures may be required, depending on the contour of the brow.

When all of the planned sutures have been placed and temporary knots have been tied, the patient is brought to the seated position, and the brow contour is adjusted to match that on the contralateral side in the primary position of gaze.

The normally innervated, nonfixated brow moves downward on lid closure—the suspended brow is not capable of doing this. Care must therefore be taken not to elevate the brow so much that a cicatricial lagophthalmos is induced. Especially in patients in whom lid skin is in short supply (e.g., in those who have undergone a previous blepharoplasty), fully elevating the paretic brow may not be possible without adversely affecting lid closure. In such cases, it is better to place the brow slightly lower than the contralateral side rather than induce lagophthalmos. Final knots are then tied. If skin muscle excision is required, it can then be carried out. The Novafil sutures are rotated to deeply bury the knots.

The brow should be closed in layers to minimize the scar. Depending on the thickness of the tissue, one or two rows of deep 5.0 or 6.0 Vicryl sutures are placed before skin closure with interrupted 6.0 plain gut sutures and a Steri-Strip.

Correction of Upper Lid Entropion

Correction of upper lid entropion is most easily carried out in combination with spring implantation, either enhanced or nonenhanced. This correction can be carried out as a separate procedure by opening the lid in the lid fold or, in combination with gold weight implantation, by extending the lid fold incision across the entire lid.

Surgical Technique

A series of 6.0 Vicryl sutures is placed across the lid (Fig. 61–11). Each of these sutures begins supratarsally, in the levator, and continues as a horizontal mattress suture through subcuticular tissue just inferior to the lower aspect of the skin incision. Tightening these sutures rotates the lid margin outward, thereby correcting the entropion resulting from the facial paralysis or from the downward pressure from an implanted prosthetic device. Tension on the sutures is adjusted at the time of surgery to give a slight overcorrection. The sutures also create a pleasing lid fold.

TEMPORIZING MEASURES

Two simple techniques are presented to protect the eye before a decision to undertake definitive surgery is made.

Lid Suture Taped to Cheek

A lid suture can easily be placed at the conclusion of a neuro-otologic or head and neck procedure in which the function of the fifth or seventh nerve is anticipated to be compromised postoperatively. The suture protects the eye during the immediate postoperative period without impairing the ability to check for pupillary or other neurologic signs involving the eye. If the patient subsequently requires temporary eye protection involving less than round-the-clock eye closure, the suture may be taped out of the way (to the forehead) during part of the day and used to close the eye at other times.

Surgical Technique

The eye is protected with a scleral shell. A 4.0 or 5.0 nonresorbable monofilament suture is passed through the skin and orbicularis, which have been pulled away from the tarsus with forceps (Fig. 61–12). The needle is passed parallel to the tarsus. The two arms of the suture are tied together with multiple knots to prevent slippage underneath the tape and are secured to the cheek with a strip of tape. The suture is then brought upward and locked with a second piece of tape. A third strip further locks the suture and keeps it out of the way. When it is necessary to inspect the eye or to check for pupillary signs, all three pieces of

FIGURE 61-9. Fascia lata suspension. This technique is analogous to that shown for placing the silicone rod prosthesis. The fascial strip is placed on a large needle and sewn through the medial canthal tendon, emerging behind the tendon. The end is locked with 5.0 polyester suture. With the special introducer, the fascia is brought laterally through the lid, where it is secured to orbital rim periosteum with 5.0 polyester suture in a manner similar to that described under lateral canthoplasty. Excess fascia lata is further secured to the periosteum by continuation of the same sutures after the initial knots are tied. These sutures encircle the fascia rather than perforate it, to avoid tearing it.

FIGURE 61-10. Brow elevation. *A,* If skin-muscle excision is not planned, an incision is made as close as possible to the brow over the area that needs to be suspended. Usually, this area consists of approximately the central two thirds of the brow. *B,* When skin-muscle excision is planned, the ellipse to be excised is marked, and skin incision is performed. *C,* Skin and muscle have been removed. *D,* Regardless of whether skin-muscle excision is required, suspension sutures are placed in a similar manner. Dissection is carried superiorly to expose periosteum. Sutures of 4.0 Novafil are placed through periosteum and then through subcuticular tissue at the lower end of the wound. After these have been tied under appropriate tension, the brow is closed in layers.

FIGURE 61-11. Correction of upper lid entropion. A series of 6.0 Vicryl horizontal mattress sutures are placed between the lower edge of levator aponeurosis and subcuticular tissue close to the inferior edge of the wound. Tightening these sutures under appropriate tension rotates the lashes outward and also creates a pleasing lid fold.

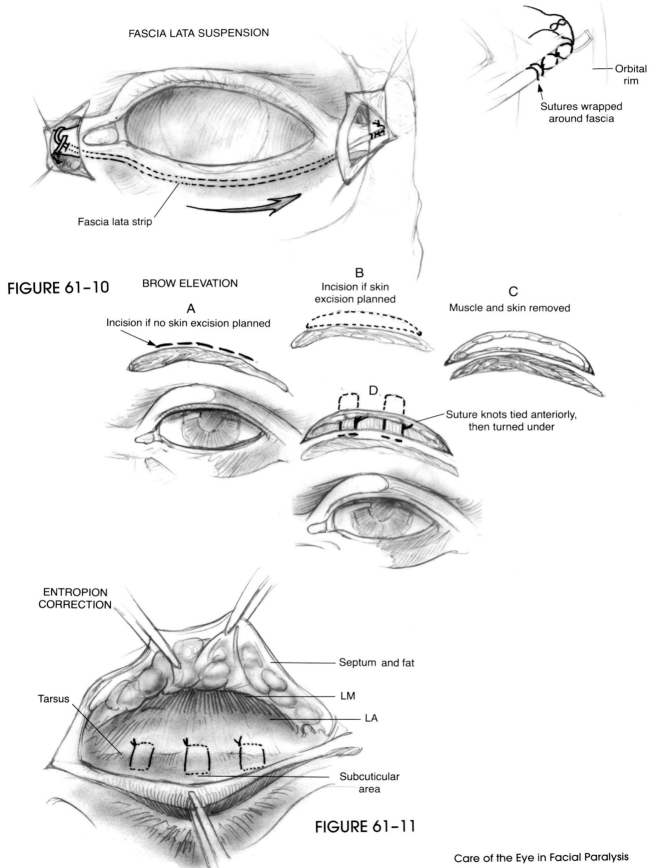

FIGURE 61-9

FASCIA LATA SUSPENSION

Orbital rim

Sutures wrapped around fascia

Fascia lata strip

FIGURE 61-10

BROW ELEVATION

B

Incision if skin excision planned

A

Incision if no skin excision planned

C

Muscle and skin removed

D

Suture knots tied anteriorly, then turned under

ENTROPION CORRECTION

Septum and fat

LM

LA

Tarsus

Subcuticular area

FIGURE 61-11

tape can be lifted together with the suture away from the cheek and then replaced. By placing antibiotic ointment at the suture sites in the lid, one can usually maintain a suture in the lid for 2 to 3 weeks without undue lid induration.

Temporary Tarsorrhaphy Suture

Temporary tarsorrhaphy suturing allows the lids to be kept securely closed over a several-week period without damage to the lid margins from the creation of a true tarsorrhaphy. It also permits one to inspect the eye at intervals by untying the suture, inspecting the eye, and retying the suture without having to replace it. It is particularly useful when there is a significant lower lid laxity component to the exposure problem.

Surgical Technique

The eye is protected with a scleral shell. Each arm of a double-armed, monofilament, nonresorbable suture is passed through the skin and orbicularis of the central third of the upper lid, beginning 5mm above the lid margin and exiting at the gray line of the lid margin (Fig. 61–13). The sutures continue into the gray line of the lower lid, exiting through the orbicularis and skin 5mm below the lid margin. The two arms of the suture are placed 1cm apart. Cotton bolsters are placed between the suture and skin before the suture is tied. The suture is tied like a shoelace, with a bow (leaving the ends of the suture long), to facilitate untying and retying in the future. The bow and ends of the suture are taped out of the way to the lid. Anti-

biotic ointment is applied to the suture sites twice daily, thus allowing the suture to be maintained for several weeks without undue induration of the lid.

CONCLUSIONS

By appropriate selection of the procedures presented, most patients with facial paralysis can be helped to obtain markedly improved lid position and function. Because eye problems frequently present major hurdles on the road to recovery, lid surgery greatly advances the patient's chances for successful overall rehabilitation.

The purpose of this chapter is to present procedures as I currently do them. Many of the modifications are my own, and tracing the historical evolution of procedures is not always possible. However, I would be remiss if I did not credit those who initially devised, pioneered, or popularized these procedures. This information is tabulated below.

Procedure	Author
Palpebral spring	Morel-Fatio and Lalardrie[4, 5]
	Levine and colleagues[6–14]
Enhanced palpebral spring	Levine
Gold weight	Jobe[15]
	May[16]
Silicone rod prosthesis	Arion[17]
	Marrone and Soll[18]
	Levine[7, 11, 13]
Medial canthoplasty and brow lift	Beard[20]
Lateral canthoplasty	Tenzel and colleagues[21, 22]

FIGURE 61–12. Lid suture. A 4.0 or 5.0 nonresorbable monofilament suture is passed through skin and orbicularis, which have been pulled away from the tarsus with forceps. The two arms of the suture are tied together with multiple knots to prevent slippage underneath the tape and are secured to the cheek with a strip of tape. The suture is then brought upward and locked with a second piece of tape.

FIGURE 61–13. Temporary tarsorrhaphy suture. A, Each arm of a double-armed nonresorbable monofilament suture is passed through the skin and orbicularis of the central third of the upper lid, beginning 5mm above the lid margin and exiting at the gray line of the lid margin. B, The sutures continue to the gray line of the lower lid, exiting through the orbicularis and skin 5mm below the lid margin. The two arms of the suture are placed 1cm apart. C, Cotton bolsters are placed between the suture and skin before the suture is tied. The suture is tied with a bow, and the ends are left long.

FIGURE 61-12

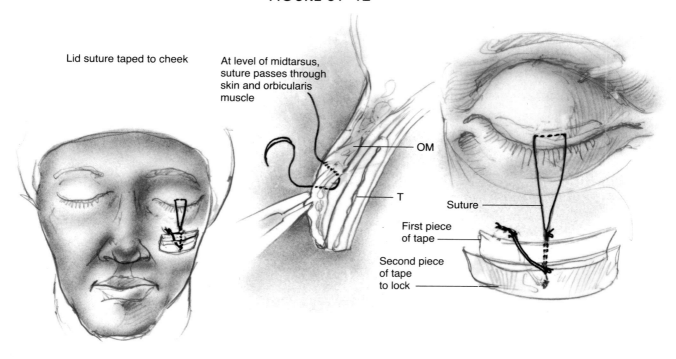

Lid suture taped to cheek

At level of midtarsus, suture passes through skin and orbicularis muscle

OM

T

Suture

First piece of tape

Second piece of tape to lock

FIGURE 61-13

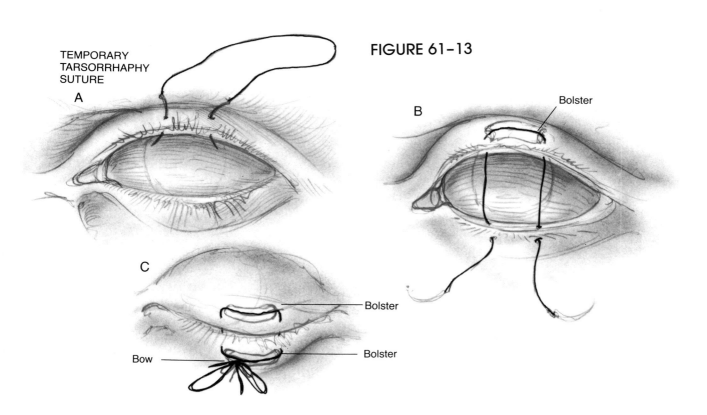

TEMPORARY TARSORRHAPHY SUTURE

A

B

Bolster

C

Bolster

Bolster

Bow

References

1. Jelks GW, Smith B, Bosniak S: The evaluation and management of the eye in facial palsy. Clin Plast Surg 6(3): 397–419, 1979.
2. Rosenstock TG, Hurwitz JJ, Nedzelski JM, Tator CH: Ocular complications following excision of cerebellopontine angle tumours. Can Opthalmol 21(4): 134–139, 1986.
3. Seiff SR, Chang J: Management of ophthalmic complications of facial nerve palsy. Otolaryngol Clin North Am 25(3): 669–690, 1992.
4. Morel-Fatio D, Lalardrie JP: Palliative surgical treatment of facial paralysis: The palpebral spring. Plast Reconstr Surg 33: 446, 1964.
5. Morel-Fatio D, Lalardrie JP: Le ressort palpebral: Contribution a l'etude de la chirurgie plastique de la paralysie faciale. Neurochirurgie 11: 303, 1965.
6. Levine RE, House WF, Hitselberger WE: Ocular complications of seventh nerve paralysis and management with the palpebral spring. Am J Ophthalmol 73: 219, 1972.
7. Levine RE: Management of the eye after acoustic tumor surgery. In House WF, Luetje CM (eds): Acoustic Tumors, Vol 2. Baltimore, University Park Press, 1979, pp 105–149.
8. Levine RE: Management of the ophthalmologic complications of facial paralysis. Trans Pac Coast Ophthalmol Otolaryngol Soc 61: 85–93, 1980.
9. Levine RE: Protection of the exposed eye. In Brackmann DE (ed): Neurological Surgery of the Ear and Skull Base. New York, Raven Press, 1982, pp 81–87.
10. Levine RE: Protection of the exposed eye in facial paralysis. In Graham MD, House WF (eds): Disorders of the Facial Nerve. New York, Raven Press, 1982, pp 336–375.
11. Levine RE: Eyelid reanimation surgery. In May M (ed): The Facial Nerve. New York, Thieme-Stratton, 1985, pp 681–694.
12. Levine RE: Palpebral spring for lagophthalmos due to facial nerve palsy. In Wesley RE (ed): Techniques in Ophthalmic Plastic Surgery. New York, John Wiley & Sons, 1986, pp 424–427.
13. Levine RE: Management of lagophthalmos with palpebral spring and silastic elastic prosthesis. In Hornblass A (ed): Ophthalmic and Orbital Plastic Reconstructive Surgery, Vol 1. Baltimore, Williams & Wilkins, 1989, pp 384–392.
14. Levine RE: Lid reanimation with the palpebral spring. In Wright K, Tse D (eds): Color Atlas of Ophthalmic Surgery. Philadelphia, JB Lippincott, 1992, pp 231–238.
15. Jobe RP: A technique for lid-loading in the management of lagophthalmos in facial paralysis. Plast Reconstr Surg 53: 29–31, 1974.
16. May M: Surgical rehabilitation of facial palsy. In May M (ed): The Facial Nerve. New York, Thieme-Stratton, 1985, pp 695–777.
17. Arion HG: Dynamic closure of the lids in paralysis of the orbicularis muscle. Int Surg 57: 48, 1972.
18. Marrone AC, Soll D: Modification of the Arion encircling silicone spring. Thesis for membership in the American Society of Ophthalmic Plastic and Reconstructive Surgery, 1977.
19. Wood-Smith D: Experience with the Arion prosthesis. In Tessier P (ed): Symposium on Plastic Surgery in the Orbital Region. St. Louis, CV Mosby, 1976.
20. Beard C: Canthoplasty and brow elevation for facial palsy. Arch Ophthalmol 71: 386–388, 1964.
21. Tenzel RR: Treatment of lagophthalmos of the lower lid. Arch Ophthalmol 81: 366–368, 1969.
22. Tenzel RR, Buffam FV, Miller GR: The use of the lateral canthal sling in ectropion repair. Can J Ophthalmol 12: 199–202, 1977.

62

Hypoglossal Facial Anastomosis

WILLIAM M. LUXFORD, M.D.

JAMES R. HOUSE, III, M.D.

Facial nerve injury is a debilitating problem both cosmetically and functionally. During the course of otologic and neurotologic surgery, sacrifice of the facial nerve is sometimes necessary and also may occur inadvertently, however meticulous the technique may be. In these cases, one must be prepared to rehabilitate and restore function as best as is possible. Direct repair of the injured nerve is currently the best option available to re-establish facial function. If a direct approximation of the nerve ends is not possible, then a graft connecting the two ends is the next best choice. Nevertheless, there are situations in which neither of these options is feasible. Perhaps the most common of these involves the extirpation of cerebellopontine angle tumors, in which the facial nerve is severed at the brainstem and there is no proximal stump in which to splice a graft. There are also cases in which a very attenuated but intact nerve regains no function. In these situations, an alternative to direct repair and nerve grafting is required.

Ideally, facial nerve restoration procedures should provide normal facial tone and symmetry, strong volitional and emotional facial movement, protection of the eye, facilitation of mastication, avoidance of dyskinesias, and no additional motor deficits. Unfortunately, even immediate direct anastomosis cannot attain these standards. Several methods to restore some facial function have been developed that require neither direct repair nor grafting. These include cross–facial nerve grafting, nerve muscle pedicle grafts, and nerve substitutions, such as the phrenic, accessory, hypoglossal, and ansa cervicalis.

Connection of a graft with the normal facial nerve and redirection of some of these fibers to the paralyzed side is known as cross-facial grafting. This method provides symmetry of movement, both volitionally and emotionally, while avoiding other motor deficits. However, this procedure partially compromises the normal nerve and provides a scant supply of neural elements to the recipient muscles, leading to inconsistent results.[1–4] As a consequence, this procedure has not met with widespread acceptance.[5–7]

Nerve muscle pedicle grafts have been used with some success but have also yielded inconsistent results.[8, 9] Because the results of nerve muscle pedicle grafts and faciofacial crossover grafts have been disappointing, modifications of these procedures have been developed that use combination cross-nerve grafting and microvascular free muscle flaps for facial reanimation.[8, 10] Efforts are also being made to use electrical stimulation of nerve pedicle grafts to overcome limitations seen with nerve muscle pedicle grafts.[11]

Nerve substitution procedures have the advantages of providing a large supply of axons to the recipient muscles and of being technically facile. The results are rather consistent and predictable. The major disadvantages include the loss of emotional facial function and the donor deficit. Because the loss of function of one side of the tongue proves not to be a major debility, and the relationship of tongue movement to facial movement is close, the hypoglossal-facial (XII–VII) anastomosis has proved to be a useful procedure in cases of facial paralysis in which a direct repair or graft is impossible. This chapter focuses on the hypoglossal-facial anastomosis.

PATIENT SELECTION

Patients with facial paralysis must receive a detailed evaluation to determine the etiology of the paralysis. In some cases, the cause is obvious, as in resection of the nerve in the course of removal of a neoplasm. The evaluation of facial palsy of unknown etiology is beyond the scope of this chapter. However, careful evaluation should precede any reanimation procedure to avoid missing treatable disease and to avoid destruction of a nerve that has potential for return of function.

In cases of known facial nerve discontinuity in which direct repair or grafting is impossible, the XII-VII anastomosis should be performed as soon as reasonably possible. Muscle atrophy and degeneration proceed rapidly after denervation.[12] Early repair provides axonal growth to the muscles and limits the amount of muscle degeneration.

The severed nerve also begins to experience fibrosis.[13, 14] In early anastomosis, new axons fill the nerve sheath prior to fibrosis and potentially allow a greater supply of axons to the muscles. Although earlier anastomosis gives a better functional result, the XII-VII anastomosis is also effective after a prolonged denervation and should be considered up to 2.5 years after injury.[6] Return of function can occur up to 4.5 years after injury.[15]

In other patients in whom the continuity of the nerve is in question, including those who suffer from trauma, idiopathic palsy, and nerves damaged in surgery, it is prudent to wait at least 1 year to make certain that no return is possible. Electrophysiologic testing is helpful in determining the innervation and viability of facial muscles. A positive response to electroneuronography or evoked electromyography indicates that at least some motor end plates are functional. These patients should be given the longest possible time to show improvement in function. However, some of these patients have so few remaining neural elements that they will never regain any useful function. In this situation, a XII–VII graft helps provide a sufficient amount of neurons to the muscles.

Electromyography helps detect polyphasic action potentials indicative of reinnervation, as well as fibrillation potentials indicative of denervation. In cases of long-standing paralysis (>2.5 years), a muscle biopsy in addition to electromyography may be useful to determine viability, atrophy, and fibrosis. In cases of severe muscle atrophy and neural fibrosis, the results of any reinnervation procedure will be poor, and muscle transfers and other augmentive procedures should be considered.

The clinician should also consider the status of the contralateral twelfth nerve when deciding on the XII–VII crossover. Contralateral hypoglossal paralysis is a contraindication to the XII–VII crossover, as are multiple lower cranial nerve deficits that already compromise swallowing and speech.

SURGICAL TECHNIQUE

In addition to standard head and neck surgical instrumentation, hypoglossal facial anastomosis requires jeweler's forceps to handle the nerve ends, a Castroviejo needle holder, and microforceps for knot tying. A sterile tongue blade is useful as a cutting surface to freshen the nerve ends. Colored plastic background material is also useful to improve visibility when the ends of the nerves are anastomosed under microscopic vision.

After satisfactory general endotracheal anesthesia has been obtained with the patient in the supine position, the neck is extended and the face turned toward the side opposite the paralysis. The ear, face, and neck are prepared and draped in sterile fashion. A standard lazy-S parotidectomy incision is made in the preauricular crease and extended behind the lobule and then anteriorly about 2cm below the angle of the mandible (Fig. 62–1). Skin flaps are raised anteriorly and posteriorly. The parotid is mobilized from the anterior border of the sternocleidomastoid muscle and from the external auditory canal. The angle formed by the cartilage of the anterior external canal, known as the tragal pointer, is then followed medially to the stylomastoid foramen, where the facial nerve exits the temporal bone. The nerve is dissected from the parotid gland to expose the pes anserinus and free the main trunk from the gland. The nerve is then transected at the stylomastoid foramen.

The hypoglossal nerve is identified by retracting the sternocleidomastoid muscle posteriorly and exposing the great vessels of the neck. The posterior belly of the digastric muscle is retracted superiorly, and the hypoglossal is found coursing inferiorly with the great vessels and then turning anteriorly as it supplies the ansa cervicalis, which descends in the carotid sheath (Fig. 62–2). The hypoglossal nerve is followed ante-

riorly and medially as it enters the tongue muscle. The nerve is freed from its fascial attachments in the neck. The network of veins and arteries entering the internal jugular vein and external carotid artery should be controlled during this maneuver. After the nerve is freed from its attachments, it is divided as far anteriorly as is possible to gain sufficient length. The free hypoglossal nerve is then rotated superiorly. Directing the nerve medial to the digastric in this rotation will give the most length but is not necessary for a satisfactory anastomosis.

There are many ways to anastomose the ends of the nerves, including collagen trays and fibrin glue, vein sheaths, laser welding, and various suture techniques. It is beyond the scope of this chapter to describe the various methods; however, several principles are almost universally agreed on. The two ends of the nerves should be free of all tension. This requirement is usually not a problem if the technique described earlier is followed. The ends should be cut sharply to provide a flush connection. The anastomosis should be as atraumatic as possible and yet provide strength to prevent disruption. It is also important to make sure, using frozen section histologic evaluation, that the distal facial nerve has not totally fibrosed in cases of long-standing paralysis. A conventional suture technique that yields reliable results is described as follows:

By use of the operating microscope, the distal end of the facial nerve and proximal end of the hypoglossal nerves are stripped of the epineurium 2mm to 3mm from the cut ends. The ends are freshened with a sharp, clean, perpendicular cut to provide a good flush connection. The perineurium is then approximated with two or three 9-0 nylon sutures (Fig. 62–3). The wound is closed in layers over a Penrose drain. A fluffed, snug parotidectomy dressing is applied, and the drain is removed the next day. Perioperative antibiotics are not necessary.

A modification of the standard XII-VII crossover graft uses a jump graft between the twelfth and seventh nerves. This procedure, as described by May et al., preserves tongue function as well as reinnervating the facial muscles.[16] The exposure of the twelfth and seventh nerves is identical to that described earlier (Fig. 66–2). In this incision, the great auricular nerve can be seen coursing across the sternocleidomastoid muscle. A 5cm length of this nerve is harvested (Fig. 62–4). The twelfth nerve is then cut through one half of its diameter in a bevelled fashion. The incision must be made in a portion of the nerve distal to the divergence of the ansa cervicalis to avoid tapping the fibers that constitute this nerve. Stimulation of the twelfth nerve with a nerve stimulator proximal to the partial transection should confirm preservation of tongue function. The great auricular graft and the distal segment of the facial nerve are then prepared for anastomosis in the manner described for the standard XII-VII crossover. The graft is sutured to the proximal segment of the partially severed twelfth nerve. The other end of the graft is sutured to the prepared distal end of the seventh nerve (Fig. 62–5). Two or three sutures are used for this connection. Enough length of graft must be used to avoid tension at the sites of anastomosis. The wound is then closed as in the standard procedure.

The patient is usually kept in the hospital overnight and discharged the following morning after removal of the drain. Although the patient may have some trouble with pooling of food in the ipsilateral oral vestibule, no special diet is necessary.

RESULTS

The patient with facial paralysis that is considered a candidate for the XII-VII crossover procedure should be counseled about the expected results from this procedure. The patient cannot expect normal facial function.[5, 6, 17–21] There are several reasons for this. As in a direct nerve repair, the axons directed to specific muscles find a random path. The muscles of the face include both agonists and antagonists for various expressions and movements. When agonist and antagonist muscles are simultaneously stimulated, the result is a canceling effect. This effect is similar to that occurring during stimulation of a flexor and extensor muscle at the same time. The hypoglossal nerve obviously controls different muscle groups, thereby allowing training of facial movement by attempting various tongue motions. The training is somewhat

successful but is not helpful in emotional facial response. This procedure will not reproduce the blink reflex, even though some investigators have demonstrated a trigeminal-hypoglossal reflex.[17] Therefore, problems with xerophthalmia and exposure keratitis may require adjunctive lid procedures, such as a palpebral spring or gold weight lid implant.

Within 4 to 6 months, the patient will begin to see tone in the muscles and a resting symmetry.[5, 6, 13, 21] With a rehabilitation program, volitional movement is possible, allowing the patient to smile with tongue movement. Electromyographic feedback–enhanced rehabilitation has shown some additional benefits.[1, 13, 22, 23] Because many facial movements are also coordinated with oral function, the XII–VII anastomosis improves the patient's ability to eat by providing tension to the buccal area and keeping the bolus in the oral vestibule. The natural interaction between the facial and hypoglossal nerves in eating, swallowing, and speaking facilitates the rehabilitation seen with this crossover graft as opposed to the accessory or phrenic nerve.

Because of the nonselective nature of reinnervation, movement of the face results in synkinesis and mass movement that varies from patient to patient. Synkinesis can be reduced by exercise and biofeedback early in the course of recovery.[23] Selective section of branches of the facial nerve is also useful in severe cases, as is the use of selective botulinum toxin injections.[24]

Because the function gained by reinnervation procedures cannot compare with normal facial function, a different method of grading facial function is used in evaluation of the results of the XII-VII crossover. A grading system used in a prior analysis of XII-VII

FIGURE 62–1. A lazy-S standard parotidectomy incision is used in this procedure. The scar is well hidden in the preauricular crease and in a natural skin crease in the submandibular area.

FIGURE 62–2. The parotid gland is mobilized anteriorly and superiorly as the sternocleidomastoid muscle is retracted posteriorly, thus exposing the facial and hypoglossal nerves.

FIGURE 62–3. The proximal end of the hypoglossal nerve is anastomosed to the distal end of the facial nerve. Care is taken to use the maximal length of each nerve to achieve a tension-free anastomosis.

FIGURE 62–4. In preparation for the XII-VII jump graft, the great auricular nerve is exposed and harvested as it courses superficially across the sternocleidomastoid muscle.

FIGURE 62–5. The great auricular nerve graft is spliced between the hypoglossal and the distal facial nerves at a point distal to the origin of the ansa cervicalis.

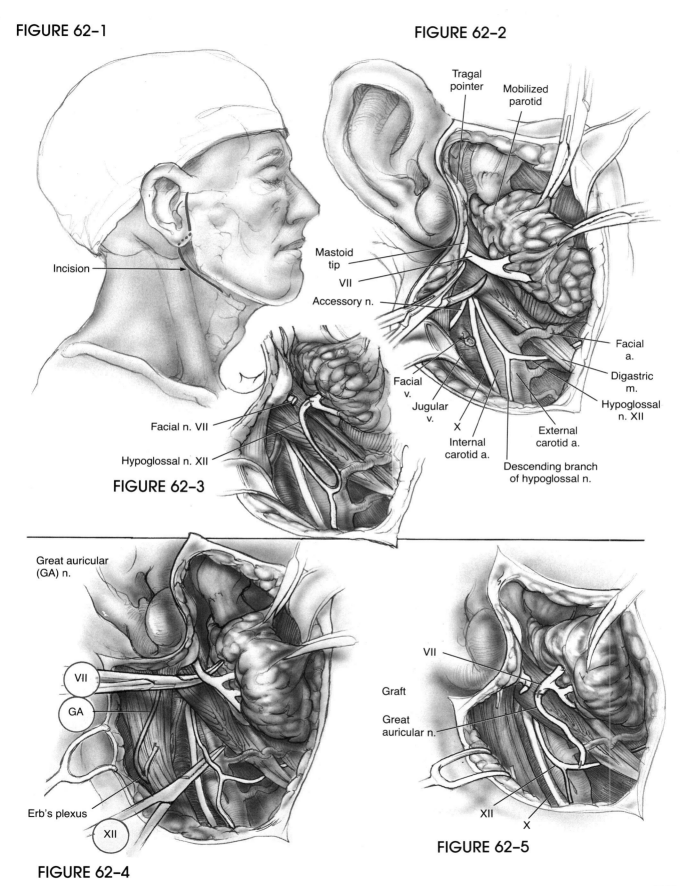

FIGURE 62-1

FIGURE 62-2

Tragal
pointer

Mobilized
parotid

Mastoid
tip

VII

Accessory n.

Facial
v.

Jugular
v.

X

Internal
carotid a.

Descending branch
of hypoglossal n.

External
carotid a.

Facial
a.

Digastric
m.

Hypoglossal
n. XII

Facial n. VII

Hypoglossal n. XII

FIGURE 62-3

Great auricular
(GA) n.

VII

GA

Erb's plexus

XII

FIGURE 62-4

VII

Graft

Great
auricular n.

XII

X

FIGURE 62-5

TABLE 62-1. Facial Nerve Function After XII–VII Anastomosis: Quality of Return Criteria

Poor	Tone without symmetry or movement
Fair	Tone, symmetry, limited movement
Good	Tone, symmetry, fair movement, moderate synkinesis
Excellent	Tone, symmetry, good movement, mild synkinesis

From Luxford WM, Brackmann DE: Facial nerve substitution: A review of 66 cases. Am J Otol (Suppl): 55–57, 1985.

crossover patients in our facility is presented in Table 62–1. Although the methods used to evaluate results vary from study to study, we have extrapolated the grading system in Table 62–1 to provide the results from several sizable studies (Table 62–2). This analysis should give the reader a good idea of reasonable expectations from this procedure.

The deficit incurred in sacrificing one hypoglossal nerve is easily overcome by most patients.[6, 13, 21] Initially, some pooling of food in the lingual sulcus is problematic. As the buccal musculature regains tone, and as the ipsilateral tongue atrophies, this problem lessens. In Conley and Baker's large series, about one quarter of the patients experienced severe or minimal atrophy, respectively, and the remaining half experienced moderate atrophy.[6] Very few patients have trouble with speech. The best results in regaining facial function and overcoming the twelfth nerve deficit are seen with early anastomosis compared with procedures performed on patients with long-standing paralysis.[6]

In patients with bilateral paralysis, May et al. proposed a partial graft of the twelfth nerve to retain function of the tongue.[16] In this procedure, the hypoglossal is partially severed, and a nerve graft is connected between the partially severed nerve and distal facial nerve. This procedure retains tongue function and provides tone and symmetry to the face. In this series, almost all of the patients had adjunctive procedures in addition to the XII-VII jump graft, making the results difficult to compare with those of the traditional XII-VII anastomosis.

Pitfalls to avoid in this surgery include use of the ansa cervicalis branch of the twelfth nerve instead of the twelfth nerve itself. This method has led to a much weaker result. The surgeon should also ensure that the distal facial nerve is not fibrosed and that the facial muscles are still viable.

SUMMARY

The XII–VII crossover graft is a relatively easy and reliable procedure in the rehabilitation of facial paralysis. A thorough preoperative evaluation is required, as is accurate timing. The patient can expect return of tone and symmetry as well as synkinesis and mass movement. The donor deficit is not significant when measured against the benefits gained from the procedure. Patients who are given realistic expectations are pleased with the improvement seen from this procedure.

References

1. O'Brien BM, Pederson WC, Khazanchi RK, et al.: Results of management of facial palsy with microvascular free-muscle transfer. Plast Reconstr Surg 86: 12–22, 1990.
2. Samii M: Rehabilitation of the face by facial nerve substitution: Panel discussion. In Fisch U (ed): Facial Nerve Surgery. Birmingham, AL, Aesculapius, 1977, pp 244–245.
3. May M: Management of cranial nerves I through VII following skull base surgery. Otolaryngol Head Neck Surg 88: 560–575, 1980.
4. Zini C, Sanna M, Gandolfi A: Hypoglosso-facial anastomosis in the rehabilitation of irreversible facial nerve palsies. In Portmann M (ed): Facial Nerve. New York, Masson, 1985, pp 519–522.
5. Chuang DCC, Wei FC, Noordhoff, MS: "Smile" reconstruction in facial paralysis. Ann Plast Surg 23: 56–65, 1989.
6. Conley J, Baker DC: Hypoglossal-facial nerve anastomosis for reinnervation of the paralyzed face. Plast Reconstr Surg 63: 63–72, 1979.
7. Tran Ba Huy P, Monteil JP, Rey A: Results of twenty cases of transfacio-facial anastomosis as compared with those of XII-VII

TABLE 62-2. Results of XII–VII Anastomosis From Selected Studies

STUDY	n	NO FOLLOW-UP	POOR (%)	FAIR (%)	GOOD (%)	EXCELLENT (%)
Sabin et al.[19]	134	13	9	48	43	*
Pensak et al.[18]	61	0	10	48	39	3
Luxford and Brackmann[21]	54	6	8	32	35	25
Gavron and Clemis[25]	36	6	7	20	33	40
Conley and Baker[6]						
Immediate	94	NA	5	18	77	*
Delayed	43	NA	30	29	41	*

*These studies did not use an "excellent" designation.
NA = not available.

anastomosis. *In* Portmann M (ed): Facial Nerve. New York, Masson, 1985, pp 85–87.

8. Tucker HM: Restoration of selective facial nerve function by the nerve-muscle pedicle technique. Clin Plast Surg 6: 293–300, 1979.

9. May M: Surgical rehabilitation of facial palsy. *In* May M (ed): The Facial Nerve. New York, Thieme, 1986, pp 695–777.

10. Harrison DH: The pectoralis minor vascularized muscle graft for the treatment of unilateral facial palsy. Plast Reconstr Surg 75: 206–216, 1985.

11. Broniatowski M, Grundfest-Broniatowski S, Davies CR, et al.: Dynamic rehabilitation of the paralyzed face: III. Balanced coupling of oral and ocular musculature from the intact side in the canine. Otolaryngol Head Neck Surg 105: 727–733, 1991.

12. Belal A Jr: Structure of human muscle in facial paralysis: Role of muscle biopsy. *In* May M (ed): The Facial Nerve. New York, Thieme, 1986, pp 99–106.

13. Pitty LF, Tator CH: Hypoglossal-facial nerve anastomosis for facial nerve palsy following surgery for cerebellopontine angle tumors. J Neurosurg 77: 724–731, 1992.

14. Ylikoski J, Hitselberger WE, House WF, et al.: Degenerative changes in the distal stump of the severed human facial nerve. Acta Otolaryngol (Stockh) 92: 239–248, 1981.

15. Hitselberger WE: Hypoglossal-facial anastomosis. *In* House WF, Luetje CM (eds): Acoustic Tumors, Vol 2: Management. Baltimore, University Park Press, 1979, pp 97–103.

16. May M, Sobol SM, Mester SJ: Hypoglossal-facial nerve interpositional-jump graft for facial reanimation without tongue atrophy. Otolaryngol Head Neck Surg 104: 818–825, 1991.

17. Stennert E: I. Hypoglossal facial anastomosis: Its significance for modern facial surgery. II. Combined approach in extratemporal facial nerve reconstruction. Clin Plast Surg 6: 471–486, 1979.

18. Pensak ML, Jackson CG, Glasscock ME III, Gulya AJ: Facial reanimation with the VII-XII anastomosis: Analysis of the functional and psychologic results. Otolaryngol Head Neck Surg 94: 305–310, 1986.

19. Sabin HI, Bordi LT, Symon L, Compton JS: Facio-hypoglossal anastomosis for the treatment of facial palsy after acoustic neuroma resection. Br J Neurosurg 4: 313–318, 1990.

20. Chang CGS, Shen AL: Hypoglossofacial anastomosis for facial palsy after resection of acoustic neuroma. Surg Neurol (21): 282–286, 1984.

21. Luxford WM, Brackmann DE: Facial nerve substitution: A review of sixty-six cases. Am J Otol (Suppl): 55–57, 1985.

22. Balliet R, Shinn JB, Gach-Y-Rita P: Facial paralysis rehabilitation: Retraining selective muscle control. Int Rehabil Med 4: 67–74, 1982.

23. Brudny J, Hammerschlag PE, Cohen NL, Ransohoff J: Electromyographic rehabilitation of facial function and introduction of a facial paralysis grading scale for hypoglossal-facial nerve anastomosis. Laryngoscope 98: 405–410, 1988.

24. Dressler D, Schonle PW: Hyperkinesias after hypoglossofacial nerve anastomosis-treatment with botulinum toxin. Eur Neurol 31: 44–46, 1991.

25. Gavron JP, Clemis JD: Hypoglossal-facial nerve anastomosis: A review of forty cases caused by facial nerve injuries in the posterior fossa. Laryngoscope 94: 1447–1450, 1984.

63

Facial Reanimation Techniques

DIETER F. HOFFMANN, M.D.
MARK MAY, M.D.

Numerous surgical techniques have been developed for rehabilitating the paralyzed face. The best procedure is usually one that re-establishes facial nerve continuity and can be performed within 30 days (and no longer than 1 year) after nerve injury. If the proximal facial nerve is unavailable for grafting, a hypoglossal-facial nerve anastomosis or hypoglossal-facial nerve jump graft procedure is preferred. This procedure gives optimal results when performed within 2 years after injury.

Static or other dynamic procedures provide significant improvement in the appearance and function of the paralyzed face, whether or not surgery is performed to re-establish facial nerve function. For example, procedures to reanimate the eye, including implantation of a gold weight or a palpebral spring in the upper lid, and tightening of the lower lid, with or without implantation of cartilage, are usually performed at the time of facial nerve reanimation surgery. Other procedures may also be used if facial nerve reinnervation procedures are inappropriate or have failed, or to provide immediate rehabilitation when reinnervation surgery is not expected to give results for 6 to 12 months. These other procedures are the focus of this chapter.

Dynamic procedures for facial reanimation, in addition to the eye procedures just mentioned, include regional muscle transposition with the temporalis or masseter muscle and reinnervated free muscle flaps. Temporalis muscle transposition is the technique most often used to reanimate the lower face and will be discussed at length in this chapter. Free muscle flaps are also reviewed.

Static procedures for facial reanimation include brow lift, adynamic slings, rhytidectomy, and lower lip procedures. These are discussed briefly, as are procedures such as neurolysis and myectomy that may be performed to manage hyperkinesis after facial reinnervation.

DYNAMIC PROCEDURES FOR FACIAL REANIMATION

Temporalis Muscle Transposition

Patient Selection

Patients who may be candidates for temporalis muscle transposition include those 1) who have absent or poor facial function, either with spontaneous recovery 2 years after the onset of paralysis or 2 years after nerve repair or nerve grafting; 2) who are not candidates for or refuse facial nerve repair or grafting or facial-hypoglossal nerve grafting; 3) who have neurofibromatosis, ipsilateral tenth cranial nerve paralysis, or another condition that is a contraindication to facial-hypoglossal nerve grafting; and 4) who have undeveloped facial nerves or facial musculature, such as may occur with Möbius's syndrome.[1, 2]

Temporalis muscle transposition has also been used recently in patients undergoing facial nerve repair or grafting. The transposition procedure provides two benefits in these cases: 1) immediate improvement in facial appearance during the 6 to 12 months before recovery can be expected after facial nerve repair or grafting, and 2) augmentation of the results of facial nerve repair or grafting.[3]

Temporalis muscle transposition may also be used in place of a classical facial-hypoglossal nerve anastomosis procedure to reanimate the lower face in combination with separate procedures to reanimate the eyelids and upper face. These multiple reanimation procedures result in separation of eyelid and mouth movement.

Patient Evaluation

When the cause of chronic facial paralysis is in question, a thorough evaluation is indicated before surgical rehabilitation of facial function is planned. The patient must be assessed for the presence of a tumor involving the facial nerve because if a tumor is present, it takes priority in planning management.

Systematic assessment of facial function in the patient who has elected to undergo temporalis muscle transposition includes evaluation of all areas of the face both at rest and with smiling. First, general facial tone and symmetry at rest are assessed. Next, the upper face is assessed, including brow position, degree of lagophthalmos, lower lid dropping, and ectropion.

The positions of the nasal alae, depths of nasolabial creases, and nasal airway structures are evaluated next. The appearance of nasolabial structures should be considered in the planning for temporal muscle transposition. Airway structures are evaluated because nasal valve collapse may have occurred, and if a nasal septal deformity is also present, nasal obstruction could result. Nasal obstruction may indicate the need for a nasoseptoplasty procedure to be performed at the time of temporalis muscle transposition.

The patient's smile on the unaffected side is classified, as described by Rubin, as 1) corner-of-the-mouth or "Mona Lisa" (67 per cent of the population), 2) canine or "Jimmy Carter" (31 per cent of the population), or 3) full-mouth or "Lena Horne" (2 per cent of the population).[4] The appropriate smile can be partly re-created on the affected side by temporalis muscle transposition with careful consideration of how the various muscles of the mouth contract to form each type of smile. Drooping, jowling, and draping of the cervical skin on the affected side of the face are also considered in planning surgery for facial reanimation.

Finally, to make an informed decision for surgery, the patient must understand what is realistically achievable in his or her case. Thus, the surgeon needs to discuss with the patient possible results of facial reanimation surgery. Spontaneous mimetic expression can be restored only with facial nerve reinnervation; however, temporalis muscle transposition can provide significant improvement in appearance and function of the paralyzed face.

Surgical Technique

Temporalis muscle transposition is performed with the patient under general anesthesia. Perioperatively, clindamycin is administered intravenously.

The patient is positioned supine for surgery with the head in a donut head holder and turned so that the affected side is exposed. The affected eyelid is protected during this procedure by a suture tarsorrhaphy, which is released at the end of the procedure. The hair is parted along the proposed scalp incision site, which begins superior to the preauricular crease and extends vertically to the temporoparietal region. Hair is trimmed with a scissors on either side of the part (extensive shaving of the scalp is unnecessary); then povidone-iodine solution is applied to the skin of the scalp, face, and neck and blotted dry.

Draping begins with clipping sterile towels along the scalp incision site and around the patient's face and neck. Then, a clear sticky drape is placed over the operative site so that it envelops the endotracheal tube. Ideally, the sticky drape can be used to anchor the tube to the patient's chin and neck without altering mobility of the lips.

The scalp and lip-cheek incision sites are infiltrated with a solution of 1 per cent lidocaine with 1:100,000 epinephrine to improve hemostasis. The initial incision is made in the scalp with a blade and continued through subcutaneous tissue and loose aponeurotic tissue with cutting, needle-tip cautery. After the temporalis muscle fascia has been identified, it is widely exposed from the zygomatic arch to just above the superior temporal line. Then a 4cm-wide segment (about two fingerbreadths) of the midportion of the muscle is outlined with the cautery (Fig. 63–1). If necessary, the scalp incision is extended superiorly above the fascial-pericranial border so that the edge of the muscle can be included in the flap.

A heavy periosteal elevator is used to elevate the muscle off the squamous portion of the temporal bone, beginning superiorly and moving inferiorly to the level of the zygomatic arch (Fig. 63–2). Care must be taken as the medial aspect of the muscle is elevated inferiorly to preserve its neurovascular supply from deep temporal nerves and vessels.

Next, a tunnel is made into which the temporalis muscle will be transposed. The tunnel is begun by developing a pocket off the scalp incision, superficial to the superficial musculoaponeurotic system (SMAS), in the direction of the corner of the mouth. Remaining superficial to the SMAS protects underlying facial nerve branches, which is particularly important in patients with some intact facial function or in whom a chance exists for spontaneous recovery or for whom a facial nerve reinnervation procedure is planned.

The lip-cheek incision is then made near the mouth with a razor-blade knife. In patients with a prominent lip-cheek crease, this incision is made in this crease. In patients with no lip-cheek crease, this incision is made in the vermilion-cutaneous border. The lower-face terminus of the tunnel to accept the transposed temporalis muscle is begun by making a pocket off the lip-cheek incision, in the direction of the scalp incision. Fine scissors are used to create this pocket, and, as with the scalp pocket, this pocket is made superficial to the SMAS and facial muscles.

The pockets off the scalp and lip-cheek incisions are connected to form a tunnel large enough to accommodate two of the surgeon's fingers. This tunnel is made with face-lift scissors, which have two cutting edges on each blade, and a long bayonet bipolar cautery for hemostasis. Injecting the subcutaneous tissues of the face with saline protects the facial nerve fibers and allows for rapid dissection with less bleeding and trauma.

After the tunnel has been made, the temporalis muscle flap is bisected longitudinally, creating two 2cm-wide pedicles. A 2-0 Prolene suture is placed through each pedicle in a figure 8, and the needle is left on the suture (Fig. 63–3). Then, large clamps are used to pull the needles with sutures and attached muscle pedicles through the subcutaneous tunnel (Fig. 63–4). The pedicles of the temporalis muscle are sutured to facial muscle, if present, and submucosal layers such that one slip is above the oral commissure and one slip below the commissure (Fig. 63–5). Additional sutures are used to secure the muscle such that the corner of the mouth is pulled toward the angle between the two pedicles to create a lateral smile that is overcorrected to show the first molar (Fig. 63–6).

An implant may be placed in the temporal deficit. A soft triangular silicone sheeting block made by Mentor Corporation had been found satisfactory but is no longer available. An alternative, presented at the Ohio State University Head and Neck Reconstruction Seminar (June 3, 1992) by Dr. Mack Cheney is to use a flap of superficial temporal fascia. This flap is pedicled on the temporalis artery and vein and elevated before elevation of the temporalis muscle flap. After

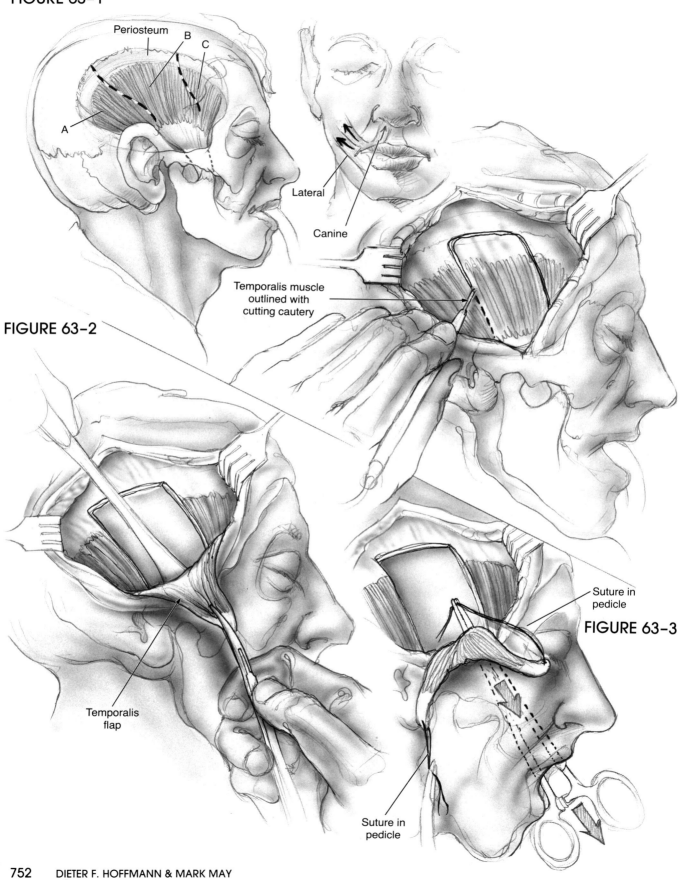

FIGURE 63–1

Periosteum

B   C

A

Lateral

Canine

Temporalis muscle
outlined with
cutting cautery

FIGURE 63–2

Temporalis
flap

Suture in
pedicle

FIGURE 63–3

Suture in
pedicle

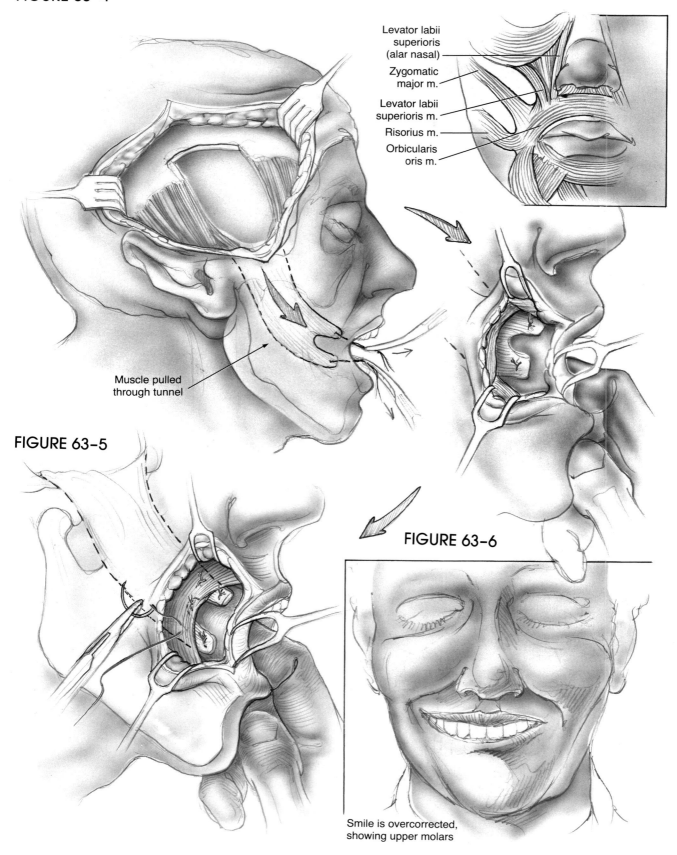

FIGURE 63-4

Levator labii
superioris
(alar nasal)

Zygomatic
major m.

Levator labii
superioris m.

Risorius m.

Orbicularis
oris m.

Muscle pulled
through tunnel

FIGURE 63-5

FIGURE 63-6

Smile is overcorrected,
showing upper molars

the temporalis muscle flap has been positioned, the fascia flap is rotated and sutured over the defect created by the transposed muscle.

At the completion of the procedure, a test tube drain is placed at the corner of the mouth and a Jackson-Pratt drain is positioned in the tunnel alongside the transposed muscle and brought out of the scalp behind the scalp incision. The lip-cheek incision is closed with 4-0 chromic sutures in the subcutaneous layer, a running subcuticular 5-0 Prolene suture, and a 6-0 fast-absorbing gut suture in the skin. The scalp incision is closed with 3-0 absorbable suture and skin staples. Antibiotic ointment is applied to the incisions, and each is covered with a Telfa pad; then a bulky pressure dressing is placed over the entire operative area.

Postoperatively, most patients have moderate facial edema and ecchymosis for about 10 days. The drains and dressings are removed and intravenous administration of antibiotics discontinued on the second postoperative day; most patients can be discharged on the third postoperative day. The patient is instructed to follow a soft diet and not to chew vigorously for the first 3 weeks after the operation. Lip sutures absorb, and skin staples are removed in 14 days.

Results

The results of temporalis muscle transposition begin to be evident 3 to 6 weeks postoperatively, with the appearance of facial symmetry and resolution of the overcorrected smile.

At 6 weeks postoperatively, patients are instructed to create a smile on the affected side by biting down. They learn to balance this voluntary smile with the smile on the unaffected side by practicing in front of a mirror. In some cases, these efforts can be enhanced by motor sensory re-education, a biofeedback technique in which a therapist uses electromyography to help the patient identify which muscles are being activated by voluntary effort. With time, the amount of conscious effort involved in creating a balanced smile decreases.

The results of temporalis muscle transposition continue to improve for about a year after the procedure. Results are judged to be 1) excellent, if voluntary smiling results in the ability to show teeth, 2) good, if voluntary smiling moves the corner of the mouth, 3) fair, if the face is symmetrical at rest, and 4) poor, if no improvement is noted. Good-to-excellent results may be expected in about 85 per cent of patients; 10 per cent of patients actually have some spontaneous emotional movement of the face. In addition, myoneurotization of denervated facial muscles may occur via trigeminal nerve fiber extension. Fair (10 per cent of cases) or poor (5 per cent of cases) results of tem-

poralis muscle transposition may often be improved with revision surgery.

Complications

The complications that occur most frequently after temporal muscle transposition are formation of a hematoma or seroma (2 per cent of cases) and infection (2 per cent of cases). Inflammatory reactions to implant or suture materials may also occur.

A hematoma that forms early in the postoperative period usually must be drained in the operating room. A small seroma can be managed by needle aspiration and application of pressure dressings.

Postoperative infections are rare when prophylactic antibiotic therapy is given perioperatively and two drains are used in the wound. If a wound infection occurs, any abscess present must be incised and drained. A specimen of infectious material should be sent for laboratory culture and sensitivity testing; even before laboratory results are received, however, antibiotic therapy should be instituted with an agent effective against oral pathogens, including anaerobes, and *Staphylococcus aureus.* The antibiotic agent can be adjusted if necessary, based on the results of culture and sensitivity testing.

Extrusion of a silicone sheeting temporal implant has occurred after three of 250 procedures in the senior author's (MM) series, and some patients have experienced granuloma formation around Prolene sutures. Suture granulomas are treated by removal of the offending suture. Violation of the parotid duct also occurred in one patient, probably during creation of the cheek tunnel to accept the temporalis muscle. A sialocele formed in this patient and subsequently required parotidectomy. This last problem can be avoided by creating the cheek tunnel lateral or superficial to the SMAS.

Other complications of temporalis muscle transposition include separation or slipping of the sutures at the corner of the mouth, resulting in increased drooping of the mouth and loss of ability to create a smile. Surgery can be performed in such cases, through the lip-cheek or vermilion incision, to reattach the temporalis muscle pedicles. Another complication is bulging of the temporalis muscle over the zygomatic arch. Usually due to retraction of the muscle, this problem can be corrected by revision of the transposed muscle's attachment at the lip-cheek crease; occasionally, interposition of fascia lata may be needed to extend and relieve tension on the retracted temporalis muscle. Very rarely, the smile may remain overcorrected on the operated side. This condition is relieved by reopening the lip-cheek incision and adjusting the sutures at the corner of the mouth.

Evolution of the Technique

The technique reported here for temporalis muscle transposition was first described by Rubin and modified by Conley (Conley lengthens the muscle by leaving a portion of pericranium attached rather than by using fascial strips, as Rubin described). Temporalis muscle transposition has been used in the past to reanimate the affected eye as well as mouth, but using the technique for mouth reanimation alone, in combination with other techniques to reanimate the eye area, permits separation of eyelid closure and efforts to smile, which is preferred.

The type of temporalis muscle flap raised, and its placement, affect the results of surgery. Using the midportion of the temporalis muscle is all that is necessary to achieve the desired result, in contrast to the procedure described by Rubin, in which the entire temporalis muscle is used. In addition, using only the middle third of the temporalis muscle and a cheek tunnel two fingerbreadths wide have resulted in minimal bulging over the zygomatic arch and in the cheek. The temporal depression left by elevation of the temporal muscle flap is also less prominent when less temporalis muscle is transposed.

Another difference in our technique from that of Rubin and Conley is use of a vermilion-cutaneous incision rather than a nasolabial-crease incision in patients with little or no nasolabial skin crease. The vermilion incision reduces scarring in these patients.

Rubin has described attaching *muscle-fascia* strips at specific sites along the vermilion border to recreate a lateral or canine smile. Alternatively, Conley brings *muscle-pericranial* slips through small puncture wounds and sutures them to underlying dermis. Our method of placing multiple sutures for direct *muscle-submucosal layer* attachment provides secure attachment and consistently good results. If a nasolabial crease is to be created or exaggerated, this procedure can be performed by placing additional sutures in the dermis underlying the crease.

Use of the masseter muscle for regional facial reanimation, either alone or in combination with temporal muscle transposition, was described by both Rubin and Conley. We have found, however, that in most cases, the use of the temporalis muscle alone gives the best results: this muscle provides the upward pull desirable for lifting the corner of the mouth in a smile, and using the masseter muscle is unnecessary and adds more bulk in the cheek. This extra bulk may be desirable, however, if radical parotid or temporal bone surgery has left a large defect in the cheek. In such cases, the masseter muscle may be used to augment facial reanimation by temporal muscle transposition. The masseter muscle is elevated completely from the mandible and attached to the mouth in a manner similar to that used to attach the temporalis muscle.

Free Muscle Flaps

Twenty years ago, Thompson first described the use of free (non-neurovascularized) autogenous muscle transplants to reanimate the paralyzed face; denervated muscle was placed in direct contact with muscle on the nonparalyzed side of the face. Subsequently, Frielinger introduced the use of free nonvascularized muscle grafts innervated by cross-facial nerve grafting.[5] The techniques described by Thompson and Frielinger had limited success but spurred interest in use of revascularized and innervated free muscle flaps.

Harii et al. reported using a free gracilis muscle graft to reanimate the chronically paralyzed face.[6] The vascular supply to the graft was provided by microvascular anastomosis to the superficial temporal vessels. At first, innervation was supplied by anastomosis of the graft nerve to the deep temporal nerve, but later, cross-face grafting was performed instead to provide the possibility of symmetric, mimetic facial function.[7]

Numerous donor muscles have been proposed for free muscle graft rehabilitation of the paralyzed face, including the gracilis, rectus abdominus, serratus anterior, latissimus dorsi, and pectoralis minor.[8] Ideally, the donor muscle will have 1) a long neurovascular pedicle, 2) cross-sectional area adequate to provide a flap of the width needed, 3) fiber length suitable to reproduce muscle action on the unaffected side, and 4) anatomy and physiology that permit harvesting with minimal morbidity at the donor site.[9]

Currently, the primary candidate for a free muscle graft procedure is a young person with chronic facial paralysis who is not a candidate for facial nerve repair, nerve grafting, or a muscle transposition procedure. Candidates include those with developmental facial paralysis and those with atrophy or fibrosis of the distal facial nerve or musculature such that standard reinnervation procedures are unlikely to succeed.

The reported results of free muscle grafting to restore facial movement are encouraging. In particular, some patients who have undergone the procedure have achieved a symmetric, mimetic smile.

Free muscle grafting has the disadvantage over muscle transposition of requiring several procedures, which also lengthens the time to final results. Further, the results of free muscle grafting are as yet unpredictable because of limited experience with each of the various donor muscles and techniques. When techniques for this procedure have become standardized so that results are predictable, free muscle grafting may replace regional muscle transposition as the preferred surgical therapy for most patients with facial paralysis.

STATIC PROCEDURE FOR FACIAL REHABILITATION

Brow Lift

Ptosis of a paralyzed eyebrow is a cosmetic and functional problem that is a frequent residuum of Bell's palsy or herpes zoster oticus, persisting even after spontaneous recovery or surgical correction of other facial function deficits. Patients with brow ptosis complain of a heavy feeling in the upper eyelid and visual field obstruction.

This condition is evaluated by noting the position of the brow on the affected side in relation to the ipsilateral supraorbital rim and contralateral brow, both at rest and with the patient elevating the unaffected brow (if both brows are ptotic, bilateral brow-lift procedures may be indicated). Blepharoplasty may also be planned if manual elevation of the affected brow shows significant dermatochalasis or persistent lateral hooding. If orbicularis oculi muscle function is also decreased, an eyelid reanimation procedure, such as implantation of a gold weight or spring may be indicated. In such patients, the brow lift procedure or blepharoplasty must be planned so as not to worsen lagophthalmos or detract from the success of the reanimation procedure.

The procedure to lift the brow is performed with the patient under local anesthesia so that the surgeon can assess the adequacy of eyelid closure throughout the operation. The choice of technique used depends on whether the patient has prominent forehead wrinkling and whether one or both brows will be operated on. If both brows need to be raised, a midforehead lift can be performed.

When one brow is operated on, the incision is made horizontally along the top of the brow hair line. Skin and subcutaneous tissue are excised, and the lower flap is undermined to the level of the orbicularis oculi muscle. The brow is suspended to the frontal periosteum with one or two 4-0 permanent sutures (Fig. 63–7) such that the arch of the brow on the operative side corresponds to that on the normal side. The incision is closed meticulously to minimize postoperative scarring.

Static Slings

A static sling (muscle plication procedure) may be performed to elevate paralyzed lower face tissues. Although it does not affect facial function, plication of the angular elevator muscles of the mouth may improve facial symmetry at rest. Patients who may be candidates for such a procedure are those in whom a facial reinnervation or other facial reanimation procedure has failed and those who are not candidates for a dynamic procedure.

A lower face muscle plication procedure is performed through a nasolabial or vermilion-cutaneous incision. Fascia lata grafts or palmaris longus muscle tendon are used to suspend the corner of the mouth and collapsed nasal ala from the zygomatic arch in a procedure similar to that for temporalis muscle transposition. (Note: Allografts such as Gore-Tex are no longer used because of the high incidence (15 of 50 patients) of patients who experienced delayed [1 to 2 years] infection or extrusion.) The grafts are first fixed to the muscle and submucosal tissue around the mouth, and the mouth or ala is elevated and slightly overcorrected by pulling the grafts toward the malar bone. The tendon or fascia grafts are then fixed to the zygomatic arch with a miniplate and screws. In addition to this technique to suspend deeper muscles, a standard rhytidectomy procedure is usually performed to suspend sagging skin.

Lower Lip Rehabilitation

Many procedures have been developed to depress the lower lip during smiling to create a "full-mouth" smile. Patients who have complete facial paralysis are not candidates for such a procedure, because depression of the lower lip would decrease oral competence, particularly if a procedure was also performed to elevate the corner of the mouth. Rehabilitation of the paralyzed lower lip is appropriate, however, when this is an isolated problem.

One method for rehabilitating the lower lip is to transpose the tendon of the anterior belly of the digastric muscle to the paralyzed orbicularis oris muscle.[10] A tunnel is created between the tendon of the anterior belly of the digastric muscle and the lower lip depressor muscles. Then, the anterior belly of the digastric muscle is left attached to the mandible, and the tendon is brought through the tunnel and attached to the lip depressor muscles. This procedure provides a symmetric smile in the patient with isolated lower lip paralysis because downward pull of the digastric muscle tendon counteracts upward pull of muscles elevating the lips.

In patients with oral incompetence, a procedure to reduce the size of the oral sphincter and transpose innervated muscle from the normal side to the denervated side can improve oral sphincter function. One such cheiloplasty procedure is V-wedge excision of a portion of the paralyzed lower lip; another is commissure Z-plasty. Others have been described.

FIGURE 63-7

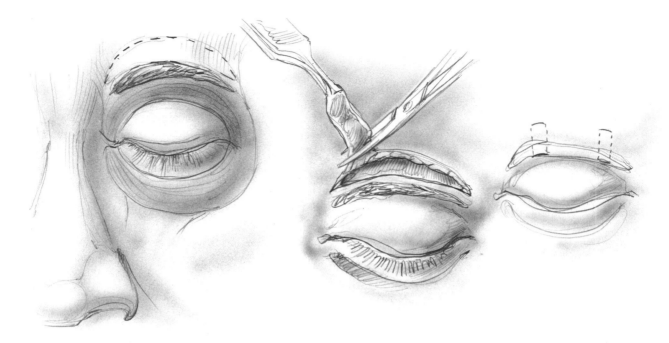

Surgical Management of Hyperkinesis

Some degree of synkinesis, hypokinesis, and hyperkinesis accompanies reinnervation of the face, whether nerve regeneration occurs with nerve grafting or nerve substitution techniques or with spontaneous recovery from a denervating injury. Synkinesis can be improved by sensorimotor re-education in which the patient practices in front of a mirror, with the help of electromyography, to separate facial muscle activities. Hyperkinesis may be treated medically or surgically.[11]

Botulinum toxin injected into muscles involved in hyperkinesis causes temporary paralysis and thus temporary relief from hyperkinesis. When the effects of the toxin dissipate (3 to 6 months after injection), botulinum toxin injection can be repeated. Surgery—selective neurolysis or regional myectomy—provides longer-lasting treatment for hyperkinesis. Selective neurolysis involves weakening or paralyzing innervation to the hyperkinetic muscle. The results of neurolysis are difficult to predict, however, and hyperkinesis may return, even after excision of a segment of nerve. For these reasons, regional myectomy is the currently preferred surgical technique for management of hyperkinesis.

Hyperkinesis of muscles around the eye, which results in squinting and diminished vision, can be treated by excision of a portion of the orbicularis oculi muscle. A large part of this muscle can be excised, through standard upper and lower blepharoplasty incisions, without compromising eyelid closure as long as a strip of pretarsal muscle is left intact. Additional plastic surgery procedures, such as a brow-lift procedure, blepharoplasty, and lower lid tightening procedure, may be performed simultaneously with myectomy to treat orbital muscle hyperkinesis. Excision of a portion of the orbicularis oculi muscle may also be performed to treat blepharospasm and hemifacial spasm.

Hyperkinesis of the oral levator muscles, which results in pulling of the mouth to the affected side, can be improved by selective resection of the zygomaticus and levator labii superioris muscles. Chin spasm may be improved by mentalis myectomy, which is performed through a submental incision. Platysma hyperkinesis, which results in unsightly cords being evident in the neck, can usually be treated satisfactorily by excision of a portion of this muscle through a horizontal cervical incision.

SUMMARY

Surgical rehabilitation of the paralyzed face is a challenging, yet rewarding, area of specialization. When the patient is not a candidate for a standard facial reinnervation procedure or when such a procedure has failed, a combination of static and dynamic procedures may successfully improve the appearance and function of the face. Facial symmetry, eyelid closure, and a balanced smile can usually be restored by standard techniques, and recent innovations as well as future developments in this field promise the possibility of re-establishing spontaneous mimetic motion of the face.

References

1. May M (ed): The Facial Nerve. New York, Thieme Medical Publishers, 1986.
2. May M: Muscle transposition for facial reanimation. Arch Otolaryngol Head Neck Surg 110: 184–189, 1984.
3. Sobol SM, May M, Mester S: Early facial reanimation following radical parotid and temporal bone tumor resections. Am J Surg 160: 382–386, 1990.
4. Rubin L: Reanimation of the paralyzed face. St. Louis, CV Mosby, 1977.
5. Frielinger G: A new technique to correct facial paralysis. Plast Reconstr Surg 56: 44–48, 1975.
6. Harii K, Ohmori K, Torii S: Free gracilis muscle transplantation with microneurovascular anastomoses for the treatment of facial paralysis. Plast Reconstr Surg 57: 133–143, 1976.
7. Harii K: Microneurovascular free muscle transplantation for reanimation of facial paralysis. Clin Plast Surg 6: 361–375, 1979.
8. O'Brien BM, Pederson WC, Khazanchi RK, et al.: Results of management of facial palsy with microvascular free-muscle transfer. Plast Reconstr Surg 86: 12–22, 1990.
9. Wells MD, Manktelow RT: Surgical management of facial palsy. Clin Plast Surg 17: 645–653, 1990.
10. Conley J, Baker DC, Selfe TW: Paralysis of the mandibular branch of the facial nerve. Plast Reconstr Surg 70: 569–576, 1982.
11. May M, Croxson GR, Klein SR: Bell's palsy: Management of sequelae using EMG rehabilitation, botulinum toxin, and surgery. Am J Otol 10: 220–229, 1981.

64

Intraoperative Neurophysiologic Monitoring

AAGE R. MØLLER, Ph.D.

During the past decade, it has become evident that the application of relatively standard electrophysiologic techniques can help reduce neurologic deficits of both motor and sensory systems.

The use of such intraoperative neurophysiologic monitoring techniques is based on the assumption that injury caused by surgical manipulation to a specific neural structure results in detectable changes in the recorded potentials before the injury has reached a level that causes a permanent neurologic deficit. Another assumption is that reversal of the specific surgical manipulation that caused the injury can reverse or at least halt the progression of the injury.[1]

When small acoustic tumors are removed in patients who still have hearing, the remaining hearing must be preserved. Preservation of hearing is particularly important in patients who have bilateral tumors from neurofibromatosis type II or in patients in whom tumors may develop later on the side opposite to that being operated on.

Although no method for monitoring vestibular function exists, two ways exist for monitoring hearing intraoperatively: 1) by recording the brainstem auditory evoked potentials (BAEPs), which are the far-field evoked potentials from the auditory system, or 2) by recording evoked potentials directly from the eighth nerve.

Monitoring auditory function also helps reduce the risk of hearing loss in microvascular decompression operations to relieve hemifacial spasm, trigeminal neuralgia, or disabling positional vertigo. Intraoperative recording of BAEPs helps determine when surgical manipulations have caused changes in the function of the ear and the auditory nerve before these changes have reached a level that causes permanent hearing loss.[1-7]

In situations in which the eighth cranial nerve is exposed during surgery, monitoring of the compound actions potentials (CAPs) recorded directly from the eighth nerve is better suited than BAEPs to detect injuries to the auditory nerve because the amplitude of the CAPs allows these potentials to be viewed directly on an oscilloscope or after only a few responses have been added.[5, 8] In addition, the amplitude of the BAEP is so low that 1000 to 2000 responses must be added before an interpretable recording can be obtained. This method of recording CAP from the eighth nerve was developed for use in microvascular decompression operations to relieve hemifacial spasm, trigeminal neuralgia, and disabling positional vertigo, and it is also useful in operations on acoustic tumors in patients who still have useful hearing and in whom attempts are made to save the hearing postoperatively.[9, 10, 11]

Monitoring auditory evoked potentials can also be of value in operations on the ear; in such operations, recording auditory evoked potentials directly from the ear by electrocochleography (ECoG) can be useful,[12-15] as can recording of BAEP.

When operations to remove acoustic tumors were first introduced, the main goal was to save the life of the patient. As progress continued in surgical and anesthesiologic techniques, the risk of death was reduced to very small numbers, and the focus is now to maintain the quality of life postoperatively. Avoiding loss of facial function following operations on acoustic tumors, which was almost inevitable earlier, became the operating team's goal; it is now possible to do so in most such operations. Intraoperative neurophysiologic monitoring has contributed to the accomplishment of this goal.[5, 11, 16-26]

Intraoperative neurophysiologic monitoring of the facial nerve can also be useful in preserving the peripheral portion of the facial nerve, for example, in operations to remove parotid tumors[27] and in operations on the face, for example, in trauma cases. For this purpose, the facial nerve is stimulated electrically, and the elicited contractions of the facial muscles are detected. Numerous techniques have been described for detecting facial muscle contractions. Some of these techniques make use of mechanical sensors for detecting muscle movements,[9, 23, 28, 29] but recording electromyographic (EMG) potentials is now the most common way to detect facial muscle contractions.[11, 17, 18, 21, 23-26] When used with electrical stimulation of the facial nerve using a hand-held stimulating electrode,[5, 11, 18] this method is an efficient aid in identifying the facial nerve in the surgical field as well as in detecting muscle activity elicited by surgical manipulation of the facial nerve. This method is also valuable for identifying in which portions of a tumor no facial nerve is present so that such portions of a tumor can be removed without risk of injury to the facial nerve.

More recently, intraoperative monitoring of cranial motor nerves has been found useful in operations on skull base tumors.[5, 20, 30-32] In such operations, not only the seventh and eighth cranial nerves may be involved but also other cranial motor nerves. Intraoperative monitoring of EMG potentials recorded from the extraocular muscles is useful in cases in which the nerves that innervate the extraocular muscles are at risk of being injured during surgical manipulations.[5, 20, 30] Monitoring of the motor portion of the fifth cranial nerve, which may also be involved in skull base tumors, can also be done by recording EMG potentials from the masseter or temporal muscles.[5] In cases in which tumors involve the caudal brainstem, intraoperative monitoring of the eleventh and twelfth cranial nerves can be very useful in preserving the function of these nerves.[5, 31, 33]

In this chapter, I describe the technique for intraoperative neurophysiologic monitoring and discuss interpretations of the obtained results. I first discuss the principles of intraoperative monitoring and then the use of specific techniques for monitoring auditory evoked potentials and the EMG potentials for monitoring cranial motor nerves.

GENERAL PRINCIPLES OF INTRAOPERATIVE MONITORING

Although the electrophysiologic techniques of recording evoked potentials and EMG potentials intraoperatively are similar to techniques that have been used clinically for many years, important differences exist in the practical application of these methods in the operating room. The importance of time during intraoperative monitoring is one of the major differences. Although test results in the clinic do not need to be interpreted while they are being collected, interpretation of recordings obtained in the operating room is necessary immediately. This requirement has implications regarding the technique and the equipment used as well as the specific qualifications of the personnel who perform the intraoperative monitoring.

Quality control of the recorded potentials in the operating room is essential. Repeating each recording is optimal in the operating room, because this method essentially doubles the time it takes to obtain an interpretable record; thus, other methods that are more suitable than repeating the recorded potentials must be applied.

In clinical testing, malfunctions in equipment or other technical problems usually do not have a major impact on the test results, except for maybe causing some inconvenience to the patient; also, it is almost always possible to repeat a test in the clinic if the results are unsatisfactory. This repetition is not possible in the operating room. Intraoperative monitoring may be worthless if a technical problem in the operating room cannot be corrected immediately.

Personnel who perform intraoperative monitoring must be present in the operating room well before electrodes are placed on the patient so that he or she can be certain that all equipment is available and has been prepared for use. The recording equipment must be checked well before the beginning of the operation. Psychologically, and indeed practically, other activities in the operating room must not be detained because of preparations for intraoperative neurophysiologic monitoring.

The equipment selected for intraoperative monitoring must be of a good quality to assure reliability and must be easy to operate. Therefore, one should not select more complex equipment than is necessary to conduct the specific tasks. Most intraoperative neurophysiologic monitoring consists of relatively simple tasks, such as recording and displaying neuroelectric potentials. This monitoring can usually be done with standard basic equipment. There is a trend to make equipment universally applicable and to design it so that it offers many options, but in the operating room it is usually better to use simple equipment, even if it can perform only one or two different tasks. Complex equipment is not only costly but in many cases the operation of such equipment is also complex and results in more frequent mistakes than if simple equipment had been used. The setup of more complex equipment may also require more time.

The operating room environment is different from that of the clinic—in the operating room, a high degree of both acoustic and electrical noise is usually present and may interfere with the recordings. This electrical interference can be reduced by an appropriate arrangement of the equipment. Recording electrodes should be routed away from equipment that causes electrical interference. The sources of electrical interference should be identified before the operation, most conveniently, on the afternoon or evening before the operation when no other activity is occurring in the operating room, so that any equipment that may cause interference can be switched on and off freely to identify the source of interference (for more details see reference 5).

The most practical type of electrode both for recording far-field evoked potentials (BAEP) and EMG potentials is the subdermal needle electrode (e.g., Type E2, Grass Instrument Co., Quincy, MA). When held in place with a good-quality adhesive tape that will not be affected by the moistening of the skin that sometimes occurs during an operation (e.g., Blenderm, 3M Company, St. Paul, MN), such electrodes provide a stable recording condition for many hours. Surface electrodes take a longer time to place and tend to provide less stable recordings than do needle electrodes during operations that last many hours. It is important that earphones, electrodes, and other such equipment be placed on the patient when this activity will not interrupt the normal operating room routine. This can usually be done when the patient is being shaved or during other such activities.

We have found that creating and following a checklist that notes everything to be taken to the operating room; specifies how to set amplification, filters, and stimulus parameters; and describes computer start-up routines and the necessary parameters to be entered considerably reduces the number of mistakes and enables personnel to concentrate on important issues rather than on trivial matters.

Because the purpose of intraoperative monitoring of sensory evoked potentials is to detect changes in the recorded potentials, they should be compared with a baseline recording obtained in the same patient before the beginning of the operation. It is not, as it is in the clinic, important to determine whether the recorded potentials deviate from normal. If auditory evoked potentials are to be monitored intraoperatively, a preoperative BAEP should be obtained. If obtaining a satisfactory BAEP is not possible before the operation, there is little chance that obtaining one in the operating room will be possible. Similarly, if a reproducible BAEP is obtained from the patient preoperatively and it is not possible to obtain a satisfactory BAEP intraoperatively, then most likely technical problems exist in the operating room that need to be corrected immediately.

Patients in whom injury to the ear or the auditory nerve may occur intraoperatively should have a complete hearing test in the clinic before the operation. If no preoperative record of the patient's hearing threshold and speech discrimination was obtained before the operation, then it is not possible to determine quantitatively if the patient's preoperative hearing status was preserved. Relying on the patient's own assessment of changes in hearing is not satisfactory. Likewise, if, for example, facial nerve monitoring is to be done, the status of the patient's facial function should be checked before the operation.

ANESTHESIA RESTRICTIONS DURING INTRAOPERATIVE MONITORING

Although anesthesia does not noticeably affect BAEP or other short-latency auditory evoked potentials,[34–36] muscle relaxants must not be used during monitoring of motor nerves when recordings of muscle contractions are being used to detect stimulation of the motor nerve, regardless of what method is used to detect muscle movements. Paralysis from the use of muscle end-plate–blocking agents prevents the recording of muscle movements as well as the recording of EMG potentials. This means that the muscle relaxants that are commonly used for "balanced anesthesia" (nitrous oxide, a strong narcotic, and a muscle relaxant) cannot be used when muscle movement recordings or EMG recordings are to be made. In our institution, patients in whom EMG recordings are to be made intraoperatively are intubated with a short-acting muscle relaxant of the end-plate depolarizer type (succinylcholine) in addition to a small amount of D-tubocurarine (3mg). Anesthesia is maintained with inhalation agents, such as isoflurane, or with intravenously administered drugs, such as barbiturates and propofol, often together with other drugs, such as midazolam. Such restrictions in the anesthesia regimen have been in general use in our institution with no known adverse effects for more than 10 years during operations in which monitoring of EMG potentials is done.

If it is known that testing of motor nerves will be done early in the operation, intubation can be performed with a short-acting muscle end-plate–blocking agent, such as vecuronium or atracurium; however, when the motor nerves are to be tested, it must be ascertained that no muscle relaxing effects remain so that a strong contraction can be achieved. Partial muscle relaxation causes rapid fatigue of a muscle, and although the response to the first stimulus may be of normal amplitude, the following stimuli will evoke responses of much smaller amplitudes. Continuous muscle activity, such as that elicited from surgical manipulation of a motor nerve, may not be detectable if the muscle is still being affected by the muscle end-plate–blocking agent.

Recently, investigators suggested that it may be possible to maintain a constant level of partial muscle relaxation such that it would be possible to obtain EMG responses while still providing some protection against patient movement. If this method is used during intraoperative monitoring, the paralyzing agent must be administered through servocontrolled infusion (Bloom and Stiller, personal communication, 1992).[37]

AUDITORY EVOKED POTENTIALS

Several forms of auditory evoked potentials are important in monitoring auditory function during otologic and neuro-otologic operations. The most common is BAEPs, which are recorded from electrodes placed on the scalp and which represent the electrical activity of the auditory nerve and nuclei and fiber tracts of the ascending auditory pathway. ECoG is the recording of the different sound-evoked electrical potentials that are generated in the ear, such as the cochlear microphonics, summating potential, and action potential of the auditory nerve. ECoG potentials are traditionally recorded from an electrode that is passed through the tympanic membrane to rest on the promontorium,[12] but they can also be recorded noninvasively by placing an electrode in the ear canal near the tympanic membrane.[38] ECoG potentials are useful in monitoring the function of the ear, but these potentials do not detect changes beyond the ear and thus cannot be used to detect changes in the neural conduction of the intracranial portion of the auditory nerve.

CAPs recorded directly from the exposed eighth nerve intracranially are useful when the eighth nerve is exposed, as it is in operations to remove acoustic tumors and in microvascular decompression[9] of cranial nerves.[8] The CAPs recorded from the intracranial portion of the eighth nerve reflect neural activity in the portion of the auditory nerve that is distal to the recording electrode. Recordings of such potentials can therefore be used to detect changes in ear function as well as in the intracranial portion of the auditory nerve peripheral to the location of the recording electrode.

Monitoring auditory evoked potentials such as BAEPs, ECoG changes, and CAPs recorded from the exposed eighth nerve in the operating room is done primarily to preserve hearing in patients undergoing operations in which the eighth nerve is being manipulated, but BAEPs are also of value for monitoring brainstem function, and they can be used to detect the effect of surgical manipulations on the brainstem and on brainstem ischemia.

Brainstem Auditory Evoked Potentials

BAEPs consist of five to seven vertex-positive peaks. These potentials are sometimes shown with the vertex-positive peaks as upward deflections and sometimes as downward deflections, and different types of filtering will affect the waveform of these potentials (Fig. 64–1). The first five peaks are constant in most

individuals who have normal hearing and no neurologic pathologies affecting the ascending auditory nervous system.

Recording Technique

Recording electrodes are placed on the vertex and the ipsilateral earlobe. Because the amplitude of the BAEP is so small compared with the background electrical activity (electroencephalographic activity and electrical interference), 1000 to 2000 responses must be added to get an interpretable record. Because this process is time consuming, every possibility to improve the signal-to-noise ratio should be implemented. The most important means to attain this goal are 1) selecting the optimal (high) repetition rate of the stimulation, 2) using adequate stimulus intensity, 3) reducing electrical noise in the recordings as much as possible, and 4) using optimal spectral filtering.

The operating room should be checked carefully, and the sources of electrical interference should be

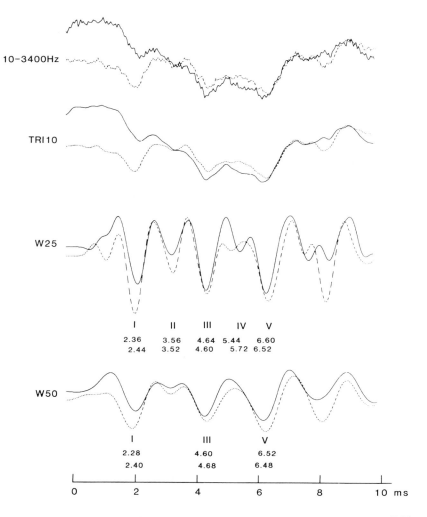

FIGURE 64–1. Brainstem auditory evoked potentials (BAEPs) recorded in the traditional way (differentially between vertex and mastoid) obtained from a person with normal hearing while the background noise was low to show the effects of different types of digital filtering. Note that the vertex-positive peaks (indicated by Roman numerals I through VI) are shown as downward deflections, in accordance with common practice for displaying neuroelectric potentials. Some investigators, however, prefer to display the BAEP with the vertex-positive peaks as upward deflections. The upper tracings were averaged responses to 2048 stimulus presentations (rarefaction clicks, *solid lines;* condensation clicks, *dashed lines)* and filtered only by traditional electronic filters (10Hz to 3400Hz). The other tracings represent the same data as the upper tracings, but after different kinds of zero-phase digital filtering and after removal of the stimulus artifact. The TRI10 filter is a lowpass filter, whereas the W25 and W50 filters are bandpass filters. The data were obtained in a patient with normal hearing who was undergoing a microvascular decompression operation.

identified.[5] Because the latencies of the peaks in the BAEPs are important, they should be enhanced as much as possible by appropriate filtering to facilitate their identification and to obtain their accurate measurements. Digital (filtering) techniques are suitable for such filtering (Fig. 64–1).[39] Digital filters can be designed so that they do not shift the peaks in time (zero-phase digital filters).[5, 39–41] Digital filtering is usually implemented on the averaged waveform, which has the same effect as implementing filtering before signal averaging is performed. Spectral filtering using conventional electronic filters can be performed, but it will shift the peaks of the BAEPs in time to a degree that depends on the waveform of the peaks. If digital filtering is available, the electronic filters that are integral parts of physiologic amplifiers should be set at 10Hz to 3000Hz, but if digital filtering is not available, settings such as 150Hz to 1500Hz are more suitable. The aggressive filtering that zero-phase digital filtering provides also makes the records so clean that automatic computer programs can be used to identify the individual peaks and to measure the latencies without human intervention.[5, 39]

Sound Stimulation

BAEPs can be elicited by different kinds of transient sounds, but the most suitable stimuli for use in the operating room are clicks. The stimulus repetition rate should be at least 30 pps, and probably 40 pps is even closer to the optimal stimulus rate.[11, 42] A stimulus intensity of about 105dB PeSPL (65dB to 70dB above normal threshold) is appropriate. Although standard audiometric earphones are commonly used in the clinic when BAEPs are obtained, such earphones are not suitable for intraoperative monitoring of BAEPs. We use miniature stereo earphones (Realistic, Radio Shack, Ft. Worth, TX) that are normally used with the "Walkman" type of sound equipment,[5] but many other types of earphones are suitable for use in the operating room, such as the Tubephone, Etymotic Research, Elk Grove Village, IL. Using light earphones eliminates the need for contralateral masking. Such masking is necessary only when old-fashioned earphones (such as the Telephonic TDH-39) are used; such earphones are heavy and therefore a considerable amount of their energy is expended as bone-conducted sound.

Interpretation of Results

Because only the changes in the recorded auditory potentials (BAEPs) that occur during the operation are of interest, the interpretation of the recorded potentials consists of detecting deviations in the BAEPs from a baseline recording obtained in the same patient. The best time to obtain the baseline recording is just after the patient has been anesthetized but before the operation begins, using the same equipment and electrode placements that are to be used during the operation. Changes in the latencies of any of the peaks (except peak I) of the BAEPs presumably reflect changes in neural conduction of the auditory nerve as a result of surgical manipulations of the auditory nerve. Usually, peak V is selected for scrutiny, because this peak has the largest amplitude of the different peaks of the BAEPs. However, events other than a change in the conduction time of the auditory nerve may cause the latency of peak V to change during an operation. Therefore, if peak III can be clearly identified, it may be better to use this peak as an indicator of changes in conduction velocity of the auditory nerve.

Studies of the changes that occur in the CAPs recorded from the exposed eighth nerve during microvascular decompression operations have revealed that impairment of neural transmission does not necessarily result in a change of the conduction velocity in the auditory nerve, but that it may result in a conduction block in parts of the auditory nerve fibers.[5] Such partial conduction blocks do not necessarily result in an increased latency of BAEPs but rather a decrease in the amplitudes of the peaks of the BAEPs. We regard a decrease of 50 per cent or more in the amplitudes of the peaks of the BAEPs to be a strong indication of injury, and we consider changes in both amplitude and latency during an operation to be even more serious.

Neural Generators of the BAEPs

The BAEPs are generated by the auditory nerve and the nuclei and fiber tracts of the ascending auditory pathway. On the basis of results from intracranial recordings from different structures of the ascending auditory pathway, it became evident that the auditory nerve in humans is the generator of both peaks I and II,[43–45] whereas in animals (even monkeys), only peak I is generated by the auditory nerve.[46, 47] The reason for this difference is that the auditory nerve in man is 2.5cm long,[48] and the conduction time in human auditory nerve fibers is relatively low (20 to 40m per sec).[49, 50] Peak III of the human BAEP is mainly generated by the cochlear nucleus, peak V by the termination of the lateral lemniscus in the inferior colliculus, and the slow potential that sometimes can be seen to follow peak V (SN_{10})[51] is probably generated by the inferior colliculus.[52] Peak IV is rather variable, even in patients with normal hearing, and the neural generator of this peak is generally unknown. Although it is almost certain that peaks I and II are exclusively generated by the auditory nerve, peaks III, IV, and V most likely have multiple generators, and the same nucleus or fiber tract may contribute to more than one peak. Not all of the nuclei of the ascending auditory pathway are represented in the BAEP, however, because some nuclei have an internal organization that makes the electrical field decrease rapidly with distance.[5, 45–47, 53] A schematic illustration of the neural generators of the BAEP is seen in Figure 64–2.

On the basis of our present knowledge of the neural generators of the BAEP, it can thus be assumed that a similar prolongation of the latencies of both peak III and peak V is a result of increased conduction time in the auditory nerve. An increase of the latency of only peak V (increased interpeak latency III to V) or a decrease in the amplitude of peak V with no change

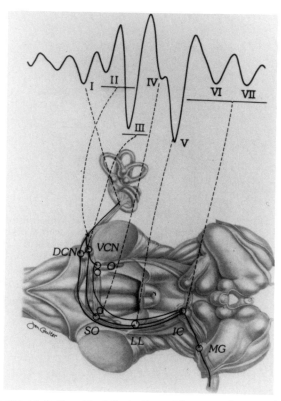

FIGURE 64–2. Simplified illustration of the neural generators of the brainstem auditory evoked potentials based on the results of intracranial recordings in patients undergoing neurosurgical operations. (From Møller AR, Jannetta PJ: Neural generators of the auditory brainstem response. *In* Jacobson JT (ed): The Auditory Brainstem Response. San Diego, College-Hill Press, 1984, pp 13–31.)

in the amplitude of peak III is a clear indication that the brainstem has been manipulated. Such changes can also be a result of ischemia possibly caused by low blood pressure (Fig. 64–3).

Electrocochleography

ECoG potentials are generated in the ear by the cochlea and consist of cochlear microphonics, the summating potential, and auditory nerve action potentials, which are generated in the most distal portion of the auditory nerve.

Recording Technique and Sound Stimulation

ECoG potentials are recorded in the clinic as well as in the operating room from the surface of the promontorium by penetrating the tympanic membrane with the recording electrode.[12] However, ECoG may be recorded noninvasively by placing a suitable electrode close to the tympanic membrane.[38, 54] Such an electrode will record potentials whose waveshape is similar to that of the potentials recorded from the promontorium, but the amplitudes of the potentials recorded noninvasively are somewhat smaller. Intraoperative monitoring of ECoG potentials has an advantage over that of BAEPs because the ECoG potentials have much larger amplitudes; therefore, only a few responses need to be collected and added to obtain an interpretable record.[11, 15, 55, 56] When insert earphones are used, the same sound delivery system as was described for use for recording of BAEPs can be used to generate stimuli for recording ECoG responses.

Interpretation of ECoG Potentials

ECoG has been used during operations on acoustic tumors to monitor hearing.[15, 55, 56] However, the ECoG potentials include only potentials that are generated in the ear; therefore, ECoG cannot be used to detect changes beyond the ear, such as in the intracranial portion of the auditory nerve. However, the neural component of the ECoG will be affected by a compromise in cochlear blood flow, which is only one of several causes of hearing impairment that may occur during removal of acoustic tumors; injury to the intracranial portion of the auditory nerve is another and more important cause of postoperative hearing loss. Also, if the cochlear blood supply is compromised during removal of an acoustic tumor, there is little chance that intervention will restore it. Therefore, in-

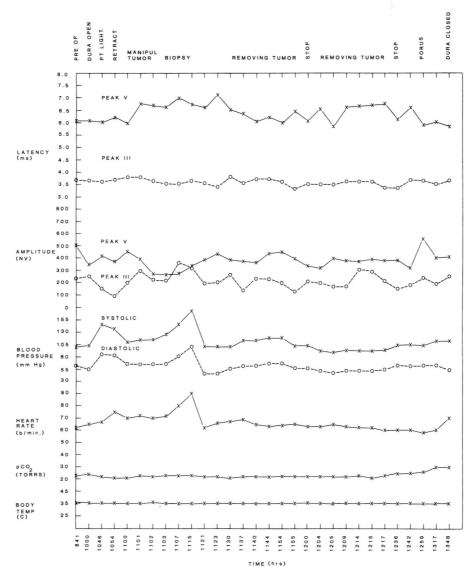

FIGURE 64-3. Changes in the latencies and amplitudes of peaks III and V of the brainstem auditory evoked potential (BAEP) as a function of time, displayed together with cardiovascular changes, during an operation to remove a large acoustic tumor. The BAEPs were elicited by stimulating the ear opposite the side of the tumor. (From an unpublished thesis by Richard Angelo, 1992.)

traoperative monitoring of ECoG potentials is of limited value in operations on acoustic tumors.

Recording of ECoG potentials is of value during operations on patients with Ménière's disease because the summating potential.[57, 58] Because this abnormal summating potential seems to be a result of abnormal pressure in the cochlea that is typical in patients with Ménière's disease, and because it seems to normalize rather rapidly when the pressure is normalized, monitoring this potential during operations for Ménière's disease is valuable when endolymphatic sac shunts are being inserted.[13, 57]

Recording Directly From the Intracranial Portion of the Eighth Nerve

CAPs that can be recorded from an electrode placed directly on the intracranial portion of the exposed eighth nerve[5, 8] have much larger amplitudes than the BAEPs; therefore, fewer responses need to be averaged to obtain an interpretable record. This type of recording was developed to detect injuries to the auditory nerve resulting from surgical manipulations during microvascular decompression operations,[8] but

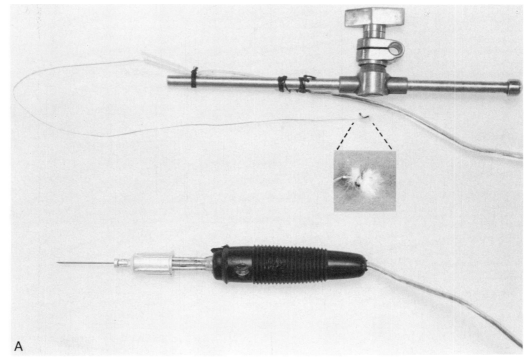

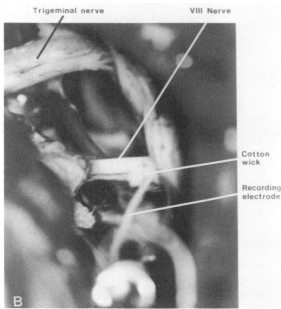

Trigeminal nerve   VIII Nerve

Cotton
wick

Recording
electrode

FIGURE 64-4. *A,* Electrode used to record compound action potentials from the eighth nerve. *B,* Electrode in place on the exposed eighth nerve. (From Møller AR: Evoked Potentials in Intraoperative Monitoring. Baltimore, Williams & Wilkins, 1988.)

it is also useful during operations on acoustic tumors. When the recording electrode is placed central to the tumor, a transpiring injury to the cochlear nerve where the nerve passes through the tumor can be detected nearly instantly.[9] This technique is especially useful during operations on relatively small tumors that have not reached the brainstem, thus allowing the recording electrode to be placed directly on the eighth nerve.

Recording CAPs from the exposed eighth nerve can also be helpful in the identification of the demarcation line between the vestibular nerve and the auditory nerve. This is important in operations in which the vestibular portion of the eighth nerve must be severed to treat vestibular disorders.

Recording Technique and Sound Stimulation

For the purpose of monitoring the integrity of the auditory nerve, the CAPs from the intracranial portion of the auditory nerve are recorded by placing a monopolar recording electrode in contact with the exposed nerve (Fig. 64–4). A fine, malleable, multi-

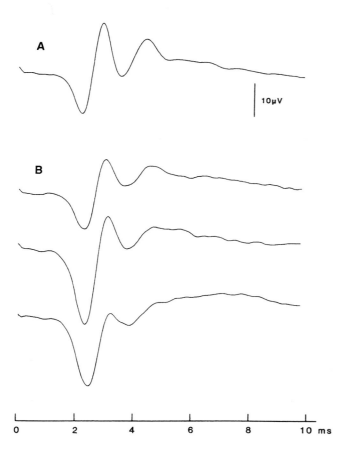

10μV

0   2   4   6   8   10 ms

FIGURE 64–5. Recordings from the eighth nerve before *(A)* and after *(B)* the eighth nerve was subjected to heat from electrocoagulation. The results were obtained in a patient with normal hearing who was undergoing a microvascular decompression operation to relieve disabling positional vertigo. (From Møller AR: Evoked Potentials in Intraoperative Monitoring. Baltimore, Williams & Wilkins, 1988.)

strand, polytetrafluoroethylene (Teflon)–coated silver wire with a cotton wick sutured to its uninsulated tip is a suitable electrode for such recordings.[5, 8] The reference electrode should be placed on the opposite earlobe. It is practical to record BAEPs simultaneously with CAPs from the auditory nerve on a second channel, so that BAEPs are available if the direct eighth nerve recording electrode becomes dislocated during the operation.

A monopolar electrode is not sufficiently selective to make it suitable for determining the extent of the auditory portion of the eighth nerve so that the vestibular nerve can be cut without injuring the auditory portion of the eighth nerve. A bipolar electrode is more suitable for this work: such an electrode can be made with two wires of the same type used for the monopolar electrode but without cotton wicks and with both wires cut so that their tips are equal in length and about 1mm apart. Such an electrode must be placed so that a line through the tips is parallel to the longitudinal axis of the eighth nerve. Such a bipolar electrode should be used with caution because its metal tips are not protected by a cotton wick, as is the tip of a monopolar electrode.

The same sound stimulation that was used to record BAEPs can be used.

Interpretation of Results

CAPs provide more detailed information about injuries to the auditory nerve because these potentials are recorded from the exposed eighth nerve and therefore reflect the discharge pattern of the auditory nerve fibers more directly than do the different peaks in BAEPs. To use CAPs for more detailed interpretations, it is necessary to understand how such potentials are generated.

CAP recordings from the exposed eighth nerve using the technique described earlier may be regarded as monopolar recordings from a long nerve in which a distinct volley of neural activity is propagated. Such potentials have a triphasic waveshape when recorded from an individual with normal hearing (Fig. 64–5*A*), and they can be interpreted by using the theories developed and described by Lorente de No.[59]

The initial positivity seen in the CAPs is a sign that a volley of neural excitation is approaching the location of the recording electrode, and the following (large) negative deflection is generated when this volley passes under the site of the recording electrode. The following small positive deflection is generated when the volley of neural excitation is leaving the site of the electrode. This description refers to a situation in which the auditory stimulus generates a single short volley of neural activity that occurs at nearly the same time in all activated nerve fibers, as is the case in patients with normal hearing when the neural activity is elicited by a click sound. If a total conduction block is located distal to the location of the recording electrode, the volley of neural activity approaches the recording electrode but never passes under it, and a single positive deflection is recorded. A partial conduction block results in a CAP in which the amplitude of the initial positive deflection is larger than normal and the amplitude of the negative deflection is smaller (Fig. 64–5B). If the eighth nerve is stretched, for example, because of retraction of the cerebellum, the neural conduction time increases and the negative peak may become broader.

This rather simplistic description applies to individuals with normal hearing. Hearing loss of the cochlear type results in a more complex waveform of the CAP.[60, 61] Consequently, the interpretation becomes more complex, but in general the rules mentioned earlier apply in these instances also.

When a bipolar electrode is used to determine the exact location of the auditory nerve so that the vestibular nerve can be cut without injury to the auditory nerve, the amplitude of the recorded potentials drop considerably when the electrode is moved from a location on the auditory nerve to a location on the vestibular nerve. This drop makes it possible to identify the border between these two nerves accurately.

Changes in Evoked Potentials From Nonsurgical Factors

Several factors that are not directly related to surgical manipulations may affect the recorded evoked potentials. A fall in the patient's body temperature may produce prolongations of the latencies of BAEPs similar to that caused by surgical manipulations of the eighth nerve.[62, 63] Irrigation around the eighth nerve with a solution that has a temperature lower than normal body temperature will also result in changes in auditory evoked potentials.[64] Anesthesia, on the other hand, does not seem to affect the recordings of short-latency auditory evoked potentials as noticeably as it does BAEPs.[34–36]

MONITORING CRANIAL MOTOR NERVES

One of the earliest attempts to improve the preservation of cranial motor nerves through intraoperative monitoring was applied to the facial nerve in operations to remove acoustic tumors.[65] However, not until the early 1980s did intraoperative monitoring of facial function during neurosurgical operations become routine practice.[5, 11, 18, 21, 23–25, 28, 66]

Intraoperative monitoring of other cranial motor nerves, such as those that innervate the extraocular muscles and the muscles of the shoulder and tongue, are important if these nerves are involved in a tumor and if surgical manipulation involves manipulation of these nerves.[20, 30] These methods are now routinely used in many institutions where operations on skull base tumors are performed.[5, 26, 31–33, 67]

Preserving the Facial Nerve in Operations on Acoustic Tumors

Intracranial electrical stimulation in conjunction with direct observation of facial movements was one of the first techniques designed specifically to aid in preserving facial function following removal of acoustic tumors.[65] At that time, when the facial nerve and the surrounding tissue were rather coarsely stimulated electrically to find the facial nerve, the stimulus parameters were mostly uncontrolled, and in many instances, the stimulus current (or its duration) exceeded what today is regarded as innocuous to the facial nerve.

More recently, electronic methods to detect facial movements have been devised, and more adequate ways to electrically stimulate the facial nerve have been introduced. This development has made it possible to identify the facial nerve where it may not be visible, and it has made it possible to identify areas of a tumor in which facial nerve is not present so that portions of a tumor can be removed without risking injury to the facial nerve.[18] This reduces not only the risk of injury to facial function but also the operating time. The most common methods make use of recording EMG potentials from electrodes placed in facial muscles.[11, 17, 18, 24, 25, 31, 32] Other methods to detect the movement of facial muscles make use of accelerometers[28] or movement detectors placed on the face.[29]

Recording EMG Potentials

Subdermal needle electrodes are suitable for recording EMG potentials. One of these can be placed in the upper face and one in the lower face so that all facial muscles on one side will be contained in the response recorded on one channel. We have found this to be a convenient and practical way to monitor facial muscle activity,[5, 18] whereas others prefer to have two channels, one recording from the upper face and one from the lower face. In the latter method, two electrodes are placed in, for example, the orbicularis oculi muscles for one channel and two in the orbicularis oris muscles for the second channel. When the facial nerve is monitored, it has been found that in addition to having an oscillographic display of the recorded potentials, it is advantageous to make the EMG potentials audible so that the surgeon can hear the EMG.[11, 18, 24, 25]

Stimulation

A monopolar, hand-held, stimulating electrode provides electrical stimulation that is suitable for probing the surgical field in operations on acoustic tumors to find the facial nerve as well as areas of a tumor where no nerve is present. It is equally well suited for testing the integrity of the facial nerve during an operation in which the nerve's location is known (Fig. 64–6A). The use of a semiconstant voltage in the delivery of the stimuli prevents the efficiency of the stimulation from being affected by shunting, which is caused by alternating changes in the surgical field from a relatively dry condition to a wet one from cerebrospinal fluid that sometimes flows onto the area.[5, 11, 18] The conventional way to electrically stimulate peripheral nerves makes use of a constant current to reduce the influence of changes in skin resistance when surface electrodes are used. If constant-current stimulation is used intracranially, the effectiveness of the stimulation of a nerve changes when the shunting of the current varies due to the condition of the surgical field becoming more or less wet. Some authors[68] prefer to use constant current when stimulating with electrodes that are insulated completely to the tip (flush tip). Some investigators advocate the use of bipolar stimulating electrodes because a bipolar electrode stimulates a smaller area of tissue than a monopolar electrode and is thus more selective.[69] Unfortunately, a bipolar electrode is also more difficult to use because its ability to stimulate nervous tissue depends on its orientation. Although high selectivity is valuable for distinguishing between two nerves that are located close to each other, it is a disadvantage when used to identify sections of a tumor in which no motor nerve is present. We therefore prefer to use a monopolar stimulating electrode that is connected to a stimulator that has a low impedance (semiconstant voltage) because we are convinced that such stimulation provides less variation in the effectiveness of stimulation on the facial nerve (or for that matter, any motor nerve) when the nerve is buried in tumor tissue or when we are attempting to identify regions of a tumor where no facial nerve is present.[5, 18]

Interpretation of Results

When combined with adequate ways to electrically stimulate the facial nerve, either of the methods described earlier to record facial muscle activity represents a very useful tool for the surgeon to easily and safely identify the facial nerve long before it becomes visible surgically. Both methods for recording facial muscle contractions also make it possible to continuously monitor facial EMG activity for the purpose of detecting when surgical manipulations imply a risk of permanent injury to the facial nerve. When using a single EMG channel, contraction of the mastication muscle will be included in the recording, and thus, electrical stimulation of the motor portion of the fifth nerve will give rise to EMG potentials from the mastication muscles. Although the sound of these potentials is indistinguishable from those of the facial muscles, their latency will be much shorter (1.5 milliseconds to 2.0 milliseconds versus 5 milliseconds to 6 milliseconds).[5] The EMG response to stimulation of the motor portion of the fifth nerve and that to stimulation of the facial nerve can therefore be distinguished on the basis of the oscillographic display of these potentials (Fig. 64–6B).

It is not only EMG activity elicited by electrical stimulation of the facial nerve that is important, however. Various kinds of non–stimulus evoked EMG activity may occur during removal of acoustic tumors and may take the form of short bursts of activity or more continuous repetitive or nonrepetitive activity.[25] Such activity may indicate heat being transferred to the facial nerve from electrocoagulation, or more likely, it may indicate surgical manipulation of the facial nerve. Such activity may indicate that a postoperative deficit will result, and the operation should be halted until this activity disappears. Similar EMG activity can be elicited by events that are probably harmless, such as irrigation with fluid, the temperature of which is below normal body temperature.

Monitoring Other Cranial Motor Nerves

The third, fourth, and sixth cranial nerves, which control the extraocular muscles, can be conveniently monitored by methods similar to those used for monitoring the facial nerve. Loss of function of the extraocular muscles, particularly of those innervated by the third cranial nerve, has severe consequences for patients who suffer such a loss, the result being a useless eye. Every possible effort must therefore be applied to avoid this unfortunate complication. Also, the motor portion of the fifth cranial nerve may be involved in skull base tumors. The ninth, tenth, eleventh, and twelfth cranial nerves may be involved in skull base tumors that extend far caudally.

The quality of life of a patient in whom the twelfth cranial nerve is injured on both sides so that the tongue cannot move is severely degraded. The probability of this loss from operations on tumors that affect the medulla and upper spinal cord in the area

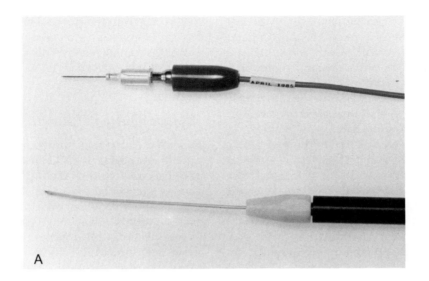

A

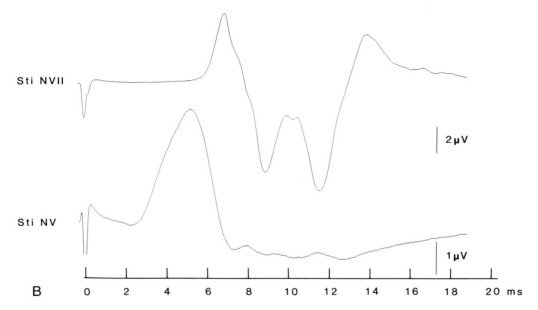

Sti NVII

Sti NV

2 μV

1 μV

B   0   2   4   6   8   10   12   14   16   18   20 ms

FIGURE 64–6. *A,* Hand-held stimulating electrode for intracranial nerve stimulation (Grass Instrument Co.). The all-metal hypodermic needle is placed in the wound near the opening in the bone and is used as a return electrode. (From Møller AR: Evoked Potentials in Intraoperative Monitoring. Baltimore, Williams & Wilkins, 1988.) *B,* Recordings of electromyographic activity typical of those obtained from a set of electrodes, one placed in the upper face and one in the lower face, when the intracranial portion of the facial nerve is being stimulated electrically with rectangular impulses of 100-microsecond duration set at about 0.8V using the electrode shown in *A* (Sti NVII), and recordings obtained when the intracranial portion of the trigeminal nerve (portio minor) is being stimulated with the hand-held stimulating electrode (Sti NV).

of the foramen magnum can be reduced by proper intraoperative monitoring of evoked EMG potentials.

The third, fourth, sixth, ninth, tenth, eleventh, and twelfth cranial nerves are often difficult to identify visually when tumors have altered the anatomy. However, localizing these cranial nerves is rather easy with a technique similar to that described for monitoring the facial nerve during operations on acoustic tumors, in which electrical stimulation of the area where these nerves are assumed to be located is done in combination with recording of EMG potentials from muscles that are innervated by these cranial nerves. Continuous monitoring of activity in the muscles that are innervated by these nerves provides important information about surgical manipulations that may place the respective nerve at risk for permanent injury.

Recording Technique

Recording EMG potentials from the extraocular muscles can be done with needle electrodes (such as type E2 subdermal, Grass Instrument Co.) placed subcutaneously in the extraocular muscles that are innervated by a respective cranial motor nerve (Fig. 64–7). Naturally, great care should be exercised when such needles are inserted so that they do not injure the globe. Reaching the lateral rectus muscle for monitoring of the sixth cranial nerve or the medial rectus muscle for monitoring of the third cranial nerve is usually not difficult, but reaching the superior oblique muscle or its close vicinity may take some practice for satisfactory monitoring of the fourth cranial nerve. It is important to secure the electrodes with a good-quality adhesive tape so that the location of the electrodes is not altered when the patient is moved. For this reason, the electrodes should always be secured to the patient's face by the adhesive tape at a distance from the electrodes.

Because for practical reasons only one electrode can be placed in each muscle, one reference electrode for each of the recording electrodes must be placed in a different location. We have used the forehead area on the opposite side to avoid contamination of the recorded potentials from EMG potentials from the facial muscles.

Others have recorded from the extraocular muscles after surgically exposing the muscles and placing recording electrodes directly on these muscles.[70] Recently, a noninvasive method was described for recording EMG potentials from the extraocular muscles. This method makes use of electrodes in the form of wire loops that are placed under the eyelids.[71]

Recording of the EMG potentials from the soft palate and from the tongue represents a convenient way to monitor the ninth and twelfth cranial nerves. Recording from electrodes placed in the false vocal cords can be used to monitor the tenth cranial nerve.[5, 33]

Recording from the sternocleidomastoid muscle or the trapezoid muscle is a suitable way to monitor the eleventh cranial nerve. This can be done by placing two needle electrodes in each location about 1cm apart.[72]

Interpretation of Results

Recorded in the way shown in Figure 64–7, the EMG potentials are large and can be easily viewed on an oscilloscope without averaging (Fig. 64–8). The response elicited by electrical stimulation of respective motor nerves provides information about the location and identity of a respective nerve. As was mentioned in the section concerning monitoring of the facial nerve, continuous EMG activity may be an indication of injury or mechanical irritation to the nerve. It is therefore important to continuously monitor the EMG potentials from the muscles and not simply observe the responses elicited by electrical stimulation.

Recording of EMG potentials from muscles that are innervated by these cranial motor nerves should be done on separate channels so that the responses from different muscles can be viewed separately. However, although several channels on an oscilloscope can easily be watched simultaneously, listening to the sound of more than one channel at a time is not easy. The loudspeaker in the operating room must therefore be switched to the channel that is at any given time most important to listen to while all channels are watched on an oscilloscope.

When to Inform the Surgeon About Changes in Evoked Potentials

Few would disagree that it is important to reverse an injury that may cause a permanent neurologic deficit as quickly as possible. It has, however, been disputed at what magnitude the changes in the recorded potentials must reach when the surgeon should be informed. We have taken a different approach: namely, to routinely inform the surgeon about any change in evoked potentials as soon as these changes reach a magnitude that is larger than normal spontaneous variations and about *any* abnormalities in EMG potentials. Although we do not believe that all small changes can cause a noticeable postoperative deficit, informing the surgeon immediately when these changes occur makes it possible for him or her to precisely identify what caused a certain change in the recorded potentials. It also leaves him or her the option of intervening immediately or waiting to see if the changes increase to values that might indicate a noticeable risk of permanent postoperative deficit. If a surgeon is informed that changes that began several minutes ago have now reached a level at which there

FIGURE 64-7. A, Schematic illustration of the placement of electrodes for recording electromyographic activity from the extraocular muscles as well as from the facial muscles, the masseter muscle, and the tongue. (From Møller AR: Intraoperative monitoring of evoked potentials: An update. In Wilkins RH, Rengachary SS (eds): Neurosurgery Update I. Diagnosis, Operative Technique, and Neuro-oncology. New York, McGraw-Hill, 1990, pp 169–176.) B, The placement of the electrodes shown in A in a patient undergoing an operation to remove a skull base tumor. (From Møller AR: Evoked Potentials in Intraoperative Monitoring. Baltimore, Williams & Wilkins, 1988.)

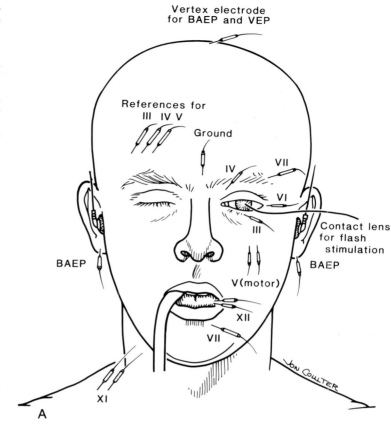

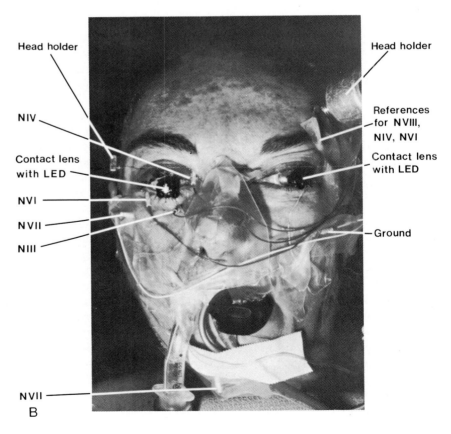

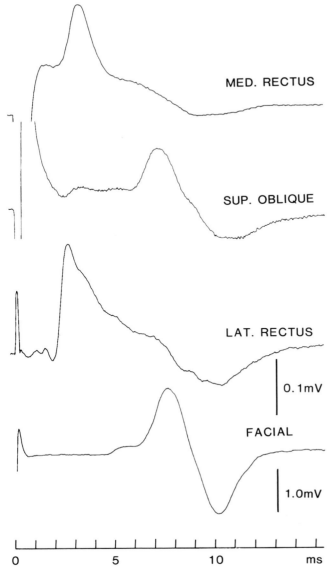

MED. RECTUS

SUP. OBLIQUE

LAT. RECTUS

0.1mV

FACIAL

1.0mV

0   5   10   ms

FIGURE 64-8. Recordings typical of those obtained from the extraocular muscles and facial muscles in response to electrical stimulation of the respective motor nerves intracranially. The stimuli were rectangular impulses of 150-microsecond duration set at 0.8V to 1.5V. Stimulation of the respective cranial nerves intracranially was performed with the hand-held electrode shown in Fig. 64-6. (From Møller AR: Evoked Potentials in Intraoperative Monitoring. Baltimore, Williams & Wilkins, 1988.)

may be a risk of permanent neurologic deficit, then he or she will not be able to identify specifically which manipulation caused the change. Consequently, it would be difficult to reverse the manipulation. If the surgeon is immediately informed when a change occurs, and if that change progresses to a level at which there is a certain risk of a permanent postoperative neurologic deficit, then the surgeon can reverse the manipulation because he or she would then know what specific manipulation caused the injury. We do, however, find it much more satisfactory to reverse the

manipulation as soon it is detected instead of taking the "wait and see" stance, because the levels of change in evoked potentials that indicate a risk of neurologic deficit are poorly defined and because the surgeon then does not need to be concerned with how the injury will develop.

The results of intraoperative monitoring of evoked potentials should therefore not be used as warnings of imminent disasters but rather as a support system that informs the surgeon that he or she has manipulated a specific neural tissue, and that reversal of the manipulation may reverse the injury so that it does not result in a permanent postoperative neurologic deficit.

Because the surgeon must make the decision of how to respond to a change in the recorded potentials, the information must be given when the change occurs in a form that the surgeon understands. It is usually not satisfactory to just convey raw data, for example, that a change in the latencies of peaks of the BAEP have occurred, because not all surgeons have sufficient knowledge in the field of neurophysiology to interpret and understand the implications of such information.

DOCUMENTATION OF THE BENEFITS OF INTRAOPERATIVE NEUROPHYSIOLOGIC MONITORING

Although most surgeons who have been introduced to the use of intraoperative neurophysiologic monitoring agree that these techniques are valuable in reducing neurologic deficits and, in some cases, help achieve the therapeutic goals of an operation, it has been difficult to prove that these methods reduce the number of postoperative neurologic deficits in a strictly statistical sense. One of the reasons is that it has not been possible to apply traditional methods, such as the double-blind method, for testing of the efficacy of intraoperative neurophysiologic monitoring. In only a few cases has it been possible to determine the efficacy of intraoperative neurophysiologic monitoring of BAEP using statistical methods.[6] A few published studies, some of which have been based on historical data, have shown a clear reduction in postoperative permanent hearing loss following microvascular decompression operations for hemifacial spasm, trigeminal neuralgia, disabling positional vertigo, and glossopharyngeal neuralgia.[7] However, it can be argued that improvements in techniques during the same time period may also have been responsible for this improvement in results, or may at least have contributed to it. With regard to the benefits of facial nerve monitoring during acoustic tumor operations as well as during operations on skull base tumors, recent studies have shown a clear improvement in outcome as a result of intraoperative monitoring of facial function.[21–23, 73] However, different ways to evaluate results hamper comparison of facial nerve preservation in different hospitals, but the increased use of common classification methods, such as the House-Brackmann classification,[74] has improved the possibilities of comparing results from different institutions.

It is also generally recognized that the introduction of neurophysiologic methods for intraoperative monitoring in the operating room has fostered better operating methods, and that intraoperative neurophysiologic monitoring has played an important role in teaching residents.

References

1. Grundy BL: Evoked potentials monitoring. *In* Blitt CD (ed): Monitoring in Anesthesia and Critical Care Medicine. New York, Churchill-Livingstone, 1985, pp 345–411.
2. Grundy BL: Intraoperative monitoring of sensory evoked potentials. Anesthesiology 58: 72–87, 1983.
3. Hardy RW Jr, Kinney SE, Lueders H, Lesser RP: Preservation of cochlear nerve function with aid of brain stem auditory evoked potentials. Neurosurgery 11: 16–18, 1982.
4. Raudzens PA: Intraoperative monitoring of evoked potentials. Ann N Y Acad Sci 388: 308–326, 1982.
5. Møller AR: Evoked Potentials in Intraoperative Monitoring. Baltimore, Williams & Wilkins, 1988*a*.
6. Radtke RA, Erwin W, Wilkins RH: Intraoperative brainstem auditory evoked potentials: Significant decrease in post-operative morbidity. Neurology 39: 187–191, 1989.
7. Møller AR, Møller MB: Does intraoperative monitoring of auditory evoked potentials reduce incidence of hearing loss as a complication of microvascular decompression of cranial nerves? Neurosurgery 24: 257–263, 1989.
8. Møller AR, Jannetta PJ: Monitoring auditory functions during cranial nerve microvascular decompression operations by direct recording from the eighth nerve. J Neurosurg 59: 493–499, 1983.
9. Silverstein H, Norrell H, Hyman S: Simultaneous use of CO_2 laser with continuous monitoring of eighth cranial nerve action potential during acoustic neuroma surgery. Otolaryngol Head Neck Surg 92: 80–84, 1984.
10. Jannetta PJ, Møller AR, Møller MB: Technique of hearing preservation of small acoustic neuromas. Ann Surg 200: 513–523, 1984.
11. Linden RD, Tator CH, Benedict C, et al.: Electro-physiological monitoring during acoustic neuroma and other posterior fossa surgery. J Sci Neurol 15: 73–81, 1988.
12. Eggermont JJ: Electrocochleography. *In* Keidel WD, Neff WD (eds): Handbook of Sensory Physiology, Vol 3, New York, Springer-Verlag, 1976, pp 625–705.
13. Ferraro JA, Best LG, Arenberg IK: The use of electrocochleography in the diagnosis, assessment, and monitoring of endolymphatic hydrops. Otolaryngol Clin North Am 16: 69–82, 1983.
14. Lambert PR, Ruth RA: Simultaneous recording of noninvasive ECoG and ABR for use in intraoperative monitoring. Otolaryngol Head Neck Surg 98: 575–580, 1988.
15. Levine RA, Ojemann RG, Montgomery WW, McGaffigan PM: Monitoring auditory evoked potentials during acoustic neuroma surgery. Insights into the mechanism of the hearing loss. Ann Otol Rhinol Laryngol 93: 116–123, 1984.
16. Kartush JM, Bouchard KR: Intraoperative facial monitoring. Otology, neurotology, and skull base surgery. *In* Kartush JM, Bouchard KR (eds): Neuromonitoring in Otology and Head and Neck Surgery. New York, Raven Press, 1992, pp 99–120.
17. Delgado TE, Buchheit WA, Rosenholtz HR, Chrissian S: Intraoperative monitoring of facial muscle evoked responses obtained by intracranial stimulation of the facial nerve: A more accurate technique for facial nerve dissection. J Neurosurg 4: 418–421, 1979.
18. Møller AR, Jannetta PJ: Preservation of facial function during removal of acoustic neuromas: Use of monopolar constant-voltage stimulation and EMG. J Neurosurg 61: 757–760, 1984*a*.
19. Møller AR, Jannetta PJ: Neural generators of the auditory brainstem response. *In* Jacobson JT (ed): The Auditory Brainstem Response. San Diego, College-Hill Press, 1984*b*, pp 13–31.
20. Møller AR: Electrophysiological monitoring of cranial nerves in operations in the skull base. *In* Sekhar LN, Schramm V (eds): Tumors of the Cranial Base: Diagnosis and Treatment. Mt. Kisco, NY, Futura Publishers, 1987, pp 123–132.
21. Harner SG, Daube JR, Ebersold MJ, Beatty CW: Improved preservation of facial nerve functions with use of electrical monitoring during removal of acoustic neuromas. Mayo Clin Proc 62: 92–102, 1987.
22. Harner SG, Daube JR, Beatty CW, Ebersold MJ: Intraoperative monitoring of the facial nerve. Laryngoscope 98: 209–212, 1988.
23. Dickins JRE, Graham SS: A comparison of facial nerve monitoring systems in cerebellopontine angle surgery. Am J Otol 12: 1–6, 1991.
24. Prass R, Lueders H: Acoustic (loudspeaker) facial electromyographic monitoring. Part I. Neurosurgery 19: 392–400, 1986.
25. Prass RL, Kinney SE, Hardy RW, et al.: Acoustic (loudspeaker) facial electromyographic monitoring: Part II. Use of evoked EMG activity during acoustic neuroma resection. Otolaryngol Head Neck Surg 97: 541–551, 1987.
26. Benecke JE, Calder HB, Chadwick G: Facial nerve monitoring during acoustic neuroma removal. Laryngoscope 97: 697–700, 1987.
27. Schwartz DM, Rosenberg SI: Facial nerve monitoring during parotidectomy. *In* Kartush J, Bouchard K (eds): Intraoperative Monitoring in Otology and Head and Neck Surgery, New York, Raven Press, 1992, pp 121–130.
28. Sugita K, Kobayashi S: Technical and instrumental improvements in the surgical treatment of acoustic neurinomas. J Neurosurg 57: 747–752, 1982.
29. Silverstein H, Smouha E, Jones R: Routine identification of facial nerve using electrical stimulation during otological and neurotological surgery. Laryngoscope 98: 726–730, 1988.
30. Sekhar LN, Møller AR: Operative management of tumors involving the cavernous sinus. J Neurosurg 64: 879–889, 1986.
31. Daube JR: Intraoperative monitoring of cranial motor nerves. *In* Schramm J, Møller AR (eds): Intraoperative Neurophysiologic Monitoring in Neurosurgery. Heidelberg, Springer-Verlag, 1991, pp 246–267.
32. Daube JR, Harper CM: Surgical monitoring of cranial and peripheral nerves. *In* Desmedt JE (ed): Neuromonitoring in Surgery. Amsterdam, Elsevier Science Publishers, 1989, pp 115–138.
33. Lanser MJ, Jackler RK, Yingling CD: Regional monitoring of the lower (ninth through twelfth) cranial nerves. *In* Kartush J, Bouchard K (eds): Intraoperative Monitoring in Otology and Head and Neck Surgery. New York, Raven Press, 1992, pp 131–150.
34. Smith DI, Mills JH: Anesthesia effects: Auditory brain stem response. Electroencephalogr Clin Neurophysiol 72: 422–428, 1989.
35. Duncan PG, Sanders RA, McCullough DW: Preservation of auditory brainstem responses in anesthetized children. Can J Anaesth 26: 492–495, 1979.
36. Sanders RA, Duncan PG, McCullough DW: Clinical experience with brain stem audiometry performed under general anesthesia. J Otolaryngol 8: 24–32, 1979.
37. O'Hara DA, Derbyshire GJ, Overdyk FJ, et al.: Closed look infusion of atracurium with four different anesthetic techniques. Anesthesiology 74: 258–263, 1991.
38. Coats AC: Human auditory nerve action potentials and brainstem evoked responses-latency-intensity functions in detection of cochlear and retrocochlear pathology. Arch Otolaryngol Head Neck Surg 104: 709–717, 1978.
39. Møller AR: Use of zero-phase digital filters to enhance brainstem auditory evoked potentials (BAEPs). Electroencephalogr Clin Neurophysiol 71: 226–232, 1988*b*.

40. Doyle DJ, Hyde ML: Analogue and digital filtering of auditory brainstem responses. Scand Audiol 10: 81–89, 1981.
41. Møller AR: A digital filter for brain stem evoked responses. Am J Otolaryngol 1: 372–377, 1980.
42. Campbell KCM, Abbas PJ: The effect of stimulus repetition rate on auditory brainstem response in tumor and nontumor patients. J Speech Hear Res 30: 494–502, 1987.
43. Møller AR, Jannetta PJ, Møller MB: Neural generators of brainstem evoked potentials. Results from human intracranial recordings. Ann Otol Rhinol Laryngol 90: 591–596, 1981.
44. Møller AR, Jannetta PJ: Auditory evoked potentials recorded intracranially from the brainstem in man. Exp Neurol 78: 144–157, 1982a.
45. Hashimoto I, Ishiyama Y, Yoshimoto T, Nemoto S: Brainstem auditory evoked potentials recorded directly from human brain-stem and thalamus. Brain 104: 841–859, 1981.
46. Møller AR, Burgess JE: Neural generators of the brain-stem auditory evoked potentials (BAEPs) in the rhesus monkey. Electroencephalogr Clin Neurophysiol 65: 361–372, 1986.
47. Legatt AD, Arezzo JC, Vaughn HG: Short-latency auditory evoked potentials in the monkey. II. Intracranial generators. Electroencephalogr Clin Neurophysiol 64: 53–73, 1986.
48. Lang J: Clinical Anatomy of the Head, Neurocranium, Orbit, and Cranio-cervical Region. New York, Springer-Verlag, 1983.
49. Lazorthes G, Lacomme Y, Gaubert J, Planel H: La constitution du nerf auditif. Presse Med 69: 1067–1068, 1961.
50. Spoendlin H, Schrott A: Analysis of the human auditory nerve. Hear Res 43: 25–38, 1989.
51. Davis H, Hirsh SK: A slow brain stem response for low-frequency audiometry. Audiology 18: 445–461, 1979.
52. Møller AR, Jannetta PJ: Evoked potentials from the inferior colliculus in man. Electroencephalogr Clin Neurophysiol 53: 612–620, 1982b.
53. Møller AR: Neural generators of auditory evoked potentials (BAEP). In Jacobson JT (ed): Principles and Applications in Auditory Evoked Potentials. San Diego, Allyn & Bacon, 1994, pp 23–46.
54. Ferraro JA, Murphy GB, Ruth RA: A comparative study of primary electrodes used in extratympanic electrocochleography. Semin Hear 7: 279–287, 1986.
55. Sabin HI, Bentivoglio P, Symon L, et al.: Intra-operative electrocochleography to monitor cochlear potentials during acoustic neuroma excision. Acta Neurochir (Wien) 85: 110–116, 1987.
56. Ojemann RG, Levine RA, Montgomery WM, McGaffigan PM: Use of intraoperative auditory evoked potentials to preserve hearing in unilateral acoustic neuroma removal. J Neurosurg 61: 938–948, 1984.
57. Kanzaki J, Ouchi T, Yokobbori H, Ino T: Electrocochleographic study of summating potentials in Ménière's disease. Audiology 21: 409–424, 1982.
58. Coats AC: The summating potential and Ménière's disease. I. Summating potential amplitude in Ménière and non-Ménière ears. Arch Otolaryngol Head Neck Surg 107: 199–208, 1981.
59. Lorento de No R: Analysis of the distribution of action currents of nerve in volume conductors. Stud Rockefeller Inst Med Res 132: 384–482, 1947.
60. Møller AR, Møller MB, Jannetta PJ, Jho HD: Auditory nerve compound action potentials and brain stem auditory evoked potentials in patients with various degrees of hearing loss. Ann Otol Rhinol Laryngol 100: 488–495, 1991a.
61. Møller AR, Møller MB, Jannetta PJ, Jho HD: Compound action potentials recorded from the exposed eighth nerve in patients with intractable tinnitus. Laryngoscope 102: 187–197, 1991b.
62. Markand ON, Lee BI, Warren C, et al.: Effects of hypothermia on brainstem auditory evoked potentials in humans. Ann Neurol 22: 507–513, 1987.
63. Sohmer H, Gold S, Cahani M, Attias J: Effects of hypothermia on auditory brain-stem and somatosensory evoked response. A model of a synaptic and axonal lesion. Electroencephalogr Clin Neurophysiol 74: 50–57, 1989.
64. Sekiya T, Hatayama T, Iwabuchi T, Takiguchi M: Thermal effect of irrigation in the cerebellopontine angle on brainstem auditory evoked potentials: Experimental and clinical study. Clin Thermometry 12: 72–79, 1992. [Abstract]
65. Rand RW, Kurze TL: Facial nerve preservation by posterior fossa transmeatal microdissection in total removal of acoustic tumours. J Neurol Neurosurg Psychiatry 28: 311–316, 1965.
66. Møller AR, Jannetta PJ: Monitoring of facial function during removal of acoustic tumor. Am J Otol (Suppl): 27–29, 1985.
67. Møller AR: Neuromonitoring in operations in the skull base. Keio J Med 40: 151–159, 1991.
68. Prass RL, Lueders H: Constant-current versus constant-voltage stimulation. J Neurosurg 62: 622–623, 1985.
69. Babin RM, Jai HR, McCabe BF: Bipolar localization of the facial nerve in the internal auditory canal. In Graham MD, House WF (eds): Disorders of the Facial Nerve: Anatomy, Diagnosis, and Management. New York, Raven Press, 1982, pp 3–5.
70. Sekiya T, Iwabuchi T, Suzuki S, et al.: Recordings of evoked electromyographic response from the extraocular muscle to monitor the oculomotor, trochlear, and abducens nerve function during skull base and orbital surgery. No Shinkei Geka 18: 447–451, 1990.
71. Sekiya T, Hatayama T, Iwabuchi T, Maeda SH: A ring electrode to record extraocular muscle activities during skull base surgery. Acta Neurochir (Wien) 117: 66–69, 1992.
72. Møller AR: Intraoperative monitoring of evoked potentials: An update. In Wilkins RH, Rengachary SS (eds): Neurosurgery Update I. Diagnosis, Operative Technique, and Neuro-oncology. New York, McGraw-Hill, 1990, pp 169–176.
73. Leonetti JP, Brackmann DE, Prass RL: Improved preservation of facial nerve function in the infratemporal approach to the skull base. Otolaryngol Head Neck Surg 101: 74–78, 1989.
74. House JW, Brackmann DE: Facial nerve grading system. Otolaryngol Head Neck Surg 93: 146–167, 1985.

Index

Note: Pages in *italics* indicate illustrations; those followed by t refer to tables.

A

Abdomen, trauma to, perilymphatic fistula from, 374
Abducens nerve, aneurysm and, petrosal approach to, *682–683*
Abscess, brain, dural herniation in, 278, 279
ear canal wall reconstruction in, contraindications to, 243
epidural, *205*
extradural, 202, 204, *205*
granulation tissue, 206, *208*
intraluminal, 206
retrograde thrombophlebitis and, 204
stages of, 204
subdural, 202, 210
suppurative otitis media and, 202, 204, *205*, 206, *208*, 210
Acoustic neuroma, bilateral, brain tumor with, 695–696
clinical approaches to, 695–696
clinical manifestations of, 694
cochlear implant in, 696
cochlear nerve in, 694, 695
magnetic resonance imaging of, 694
neurofibromatosis type 2 and, 692
observation of, 695–696
spinal tumor with, 695–696
stereotactic surgery for, 696
surgery for, hearing preservation in, 694, 695, 696
surgical approaches to, 694, 695
treatment of, 691–697
chronic otitis media with, surgical approach in, 623
computed tomography of, *606–607*
incomplete removal of, 633
magnetic resonance imaging of, *606–607*
middle fossa approach to, 647
neurofibromatosis type 2 and, 694
of cerebellopontine angle, 623
extradural retraction in, 618
retrosigmoid approach to, 619–636, 620, *620–621*
results of, 633
stages of, 625
technique for, 625–632
suboccipital approach to, 647
surgery for. See also surgical approaches under *Cerebellopontine angle.*
approach selection in, 647

Acoustic neuroma *(Continued)*
cranial nerve preservation in, 622
facial nerve preservation in, 633
goals of, 622
hearing preservation in, 622–623, 633, 760
intraoperative monitoring in, 760
transcochlear approach to, 620–626
translabyrinthine approach to, 606, *606–607*, 617–618, 647
transotic approach to, 637–647
translabyrinthine approach vs., 647
Acoustic tumor(s). See also *Acoustic neuroma.*
facial nerve hemangioma as, 414
intracanalicular, hearing preservation in, 597
middle fossa approach to, 595–603
arcuate eminence in, 598, *598–599*
auditory brain stem responses before, 596
Bill's bar in, 598, *600–601*
complications of, 602
counseling in, 597
craniotomy in, 598, *598–599*
electronystagmography in, 596–597
facial nerve function after, 602, 603t
facial nerve manipulation in, 596
facial paralysis from, 597
facial-cochlear nerve dissection in, *600–601*, 602
geniculate ganglion in, 598, *600–601*
greater superficial petrosal nerve in, 598, *600–601*
healing in, 602
hearing preservation in, 602, 603t
tumor location and, 596–597
House-Urban retractor in, 598, *600*
incision in, 598, *598–599*
indications for, 596
internal auditory canal dura division in, *600–601*, 602
internal auditory canal skeletonization in, 598, *600–601*
labyrinthectomy with, 596
labyrinthine facial nerve in, 598
middle meningeal artery in, 598, *598–599*
patient selection in, 602–603
petrous ridge in, 598, *598–599*

Acoustic tumor(s) *(Continued)*
posterior fossa bleeding in, 596
preoperative evaluation in, 596–597
preoperative preparation in, 597
results of, 602–603
success of, 602, 603t
technique for, 598, *598–602*, 602
temporal bone anatomy in, 597–598, *598–599*
tinnitus after, 597
tumor size and, 602–603
vestibular nerve dissection in, *600–601*, 602
of vestibular nerve, hearing preservation in, 596–597
surgery for, brain stem auditory evoked potentials during, *766*
electrocochleographic monitoring during, 765–766
facial nerve preservation in, intraoperative monitoring in, 769–770, *770–771*
translabyrinthine approach to, 595–608
air embolism and, 606
anesthesia in, 608
bleeding in, 614
cerebellopontine angle exposure in, 606, *606–607*
cerebellopontine angle hematoma in, 614
cerebrospinal fluid leakage in, 614–615
closure in, 612
cochlear aqueduct in, 610, *610–611*
complications of, 614–615
facial nerve exposure in, 606, *606–607*
facial nerve in, 610, 612, *612–613*, 614
hearing status and, 596, 608
House-Urban dissector in, 610, *612–613*
internal auditory canal exposure in, 606, *606–609*, 610, *610–613*
labyrinthectomy in, 608, *610–611*
mastoidectomy in, 608, *610–611*
neurosurgical technique in, 617–618
patient positioning in, 606, *608–609*
patient selection in, 606, 608
posterior fossa exposure in, 610, *610–613*
postoperative care in, 614
postoperative hematoma in, 614
preoperative preparation in, 608